OXFORD MEDICAL PUBLICATIONS

Oxford Desk Reference
Nephrology

Oxford Desk Reference
Nephrology

Jonathan Barratt

Senior Lecturer and Honorary Consultant Nephrologist,
John Walls Renal Unit,
Leicester General Hospital,
Leicester

Kevin Harris

Reader and Honorary Consultant Nephrologist,
John Walls Renal Unit,
Leicester General Hospital,
Leicester

and

Peter Topham

Reader and Honorary Consultant Nephrologist,
John Walls Renal Unit,
Leicester General Hospital,
Leicester

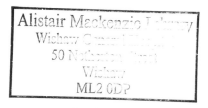
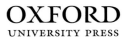
OXFORD
UNIVERSITY PRESS

OXFORD
UNIVERSITY PRESS

Great Clarendon Street, Oxford OX2 6DP

Oxford University Press is a department of the University of Oxford.
It furthers the University's objective of excellence in research, scholarship,
and education by publishing worldwide in

Oxford New York

Auckland Cape Town Dar es Salaam Hong Kong Karachi
Kuala Lumpur Madrid Melbourne Mexico City Nairobi
New Delhi Shanghai Taipei Toronto

With offices in

Argentina Austria Brazil Chile Czech Republic France Greece
Guatemala Hungary Italy Japan Poland Portugal Singapore
South Korea Switzerland Thailand Turkey Ukraine Vietnam

Oxford is a registered trade mark of Oxford University Press
in the UK and in certain other countries

Published in the United States
by Oxford University Press Inc., New York

© Oxford University Press 2009

The moral rights of the author have been asserted
Database right Oxford University Press (maker)

First published 2009

British Library Cataloguing in Publication Data
Data available

Library of Congress Cataloguing in Publication Data
Data available

Typeset by Cepha Imaging Private Ltd., Bangalore, India
Printed in CPI Antony Rowe,
Chippenham, Wiltshire

ISBN 978–0–19–922956–7

10 9 8 7 6 5 4 3 2 1

Preface

In this era of evidence-based medicine, one of the biggest challenges confronting clinicians is keeping abreast with often rapidly changing recommendations that guide clinical practice. While it is clearly helpful to have research-based guidelines and protocols to draw upon it is not always easy to access this information, particularly at the time when it is needed most, such as on a ward round or in a busy outpatient clinic. These evidence-based guidelines, produced by national organizations (The Renal Association, British Hypertension Society, National Institute for Health and Clinical Excellence) and international organizations (International Society of Nephrology, National Kidney Federation – KDOQI) are often found in a variety of locations and published media and therefore timely access is not always possible.

To overcome this problem we have aimed to produce a comprehensive textbook of nephrology which focuses on aspects of renal disease that are important to the clinician. The book brings together the key recommendations found in current evidence-based guidelines and presents them in a uniform and accessible format. It has been designed and written so that locating information is both quick and simple, and the layout of the chapters allows the reader to identify and assimilate information rapidly.

The book is aimed at clinicians with a specialist interest in Nephrology (including consultants and specialist trainees in Nephrology) but it should also prove to be a valuable resource for any generalists who encounter a nephrological problem in their day-to-day practice.

We hope that this book will become an integral part of your working day.

Dr Jonathan Barratt
Dr Kevin Harris
Dr Peter Topham

vi

Acknowledgements

Many people are involved in the production of a book like this and it is impossible to recognize every contribution. We would, however, like to thank specifically the chapter authors who without exception have produced work of the highest quality. In addition we thank Chris Reid, Helen Liepman, and Marionne Cronin from Oxford University Press who have been instrumental in driving the production of the book. Finally we owe particular thanks to our wives and children who have provided endless support, encouragement and patience during the writing and editing process.

Brief contents

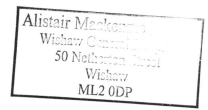

Detailed contents

Abbreviations

ACEI	angiotensin-converting enzyme inhibitor
ACR	albumin:creatinine ratio
ADH	antidiuretic hormone
ADMA	asymmetric dimethyl arginine
ADPKD	autosomal dominant polycystic kidney disease
ADQI	Acute Dialysis Quality Initiative
AG	anion gap
AGE	advanced glycation end-products
AIDS	acquired immune deficiency syndrome
AIN	acute interstitial nephritis
AKI	acute kidney injury
AKIN	Acute Kidney Injury Network
ANA	antinuclear antibodies
ANCA	antineutrophil cytoplasmic antibodies
APD	automated peritoneal dialysis
ARAS	atheromatous renal artery stenosis
ARB	angiotensin-receptor blocker
ARPKD	autosomal recessive polycystic kidney disease
ARVD	atherosclerotic renovascular disease
ASOT	antistreptolysin O titre
ATN	acute tubular necrosis
AVF	arteriovenous fistula
AXR	abdominal X-ray
bd	twice daily
BCG	bacillus Calmette–Guérin
BNF	British National Formulary
BP	blood pressure
CAKUT	congenital abnormalities of the kidneys and urinary tract
CAPD	continuous ambulatory peritoneal dialysis
CAVH	continuous arteriovenous hemofiltration
CCPD	continuous cycling peritoneal dialysis
cfu	colony-forming units
CH_{50}	dose of complement required to hemolyse 50% of erythrocytes
CKD	chronic kidney disease
CMV	cytomegalovirus
CNI	calcineurin inhibitor
CNS	central nervous system
COX	cyclo-oxygenase
CRP	C-reactive protein
CRRT	continuous renal replacement therapy
CsA	ciclosporin
CT	computed tomography
CVP	central venous pressure

CVVHF	continuous venovenous hemofiltration
CVVHD	continuous venovenous hemodialysis
CVVHDF	continuous venovenous hemodiafiltration
CXR	chest X-ray
DBP	diastolic blood pressure
DEXA	dual energy X-ray absorptiometry
DI	diabetes insipidus
DIC	disseminated intravascular coagulation
DM	diabetes mellitus
DMSA	dimercaptosuccinic acid
DOPPS	Dialysis Outcomes & Practice Patterns Study
dsDNA	double-stranded DNA
DTPA	diethylenetriamine penta-acetic acid
ECF	extracellular fluid
ECG	electrocardiograph
EDD	extended daily dialysis
EDTA	ethylenediamine tetra-acetic acid
ENaC	epithelial sodium channel
eGFR	estimated glomerular filtration rate
eKt/V	equilibrated Kt/V
ELISA	enzyme-linked immunosorbent assay
EM	electon micrograph
ENA	extractable nuclear antigen
EPO	erythropoietin
ERF	established renal failure
ESA	erythropoiesis-stimulating agent
ESR	erythrocyte sedimentation rate
ESRD	end-stage renal disease
FSGS	focal and segmental glomerulosclerosis
FE_{Na}	fractional excretion of sodium
FMD	fibromuscular disease
FSGS	focal segmental glomerulosclerosis
GBM	glomerular basement membrane
GDP	glucose degradation products
GFR	glomerular filtration rate
GI	gastrointestinal
H&E	hemotoxylin and eosin
HAART	highly active antiretroviral therapy
HbSS	homozygous sickle cell anemia
HD	hemodialysis
HDF	hemodiafiltration
HELLP	Hemolytic anemia, Elevated Liver enzymes and Low Platelet count
HF	hemofiltration
HIT	heparin-induced thrombocytopenia
HIV	human immunodeficiency virus

HMG CoA	3-hydroxy-3-methylglutaryl coenzyme A	OCPD	optimized cycling peritoneal dialysis
HP	hemoperfusion	PCR	protein:creatinine ratio
HPF	high power field	PD	peritoneal dialysis
HRS	hepatorenal syndrome	PE	plasma exchange
HTN	hypertension	PET	peritoneal equilibration test
HUS	hemolytic uremic syndrome	PeT	per-eclampsia
IF	immunofluorescence	pmp	per million population
IHD	intermittent hemodialysis	PNA	protein equivalent of total nitrogen appearance
IHF	intermittent hemofiltration	PO	per oral
IL	interleukin	PRA	panel reactive antibodies
iPTH	intact parathyroid hormone	PRCA	pure red cell aplasia
ISPD	International Society of Peritoneal Dialysis	PSA	prostate-specific antigen
ITU	intensive therapy unit	PTFE	polytetrafluoroethylene
IV	intravenous	PTH	parathyroid hormone
IVU	intravenous urogram	PTLD	post-transplant lymphoproliferative disease
K/DIGO	Kidney Disease Improving Global Outcomes	PUJ	pelviureteric junction
K/DOQI	Kidney Disease Outcomes Quality Iniative	qds	four times daily
		RAS	renin–angiotensin–aldosterone system
KUB	kidneys, ureters and bladder	RBF	renal blood flow
LDH	lactate dehydrogenase	RCC	renal cell carcinoma
LDL	low density lipoprotein	RCIN	radio contrast-induced nephropathy
LFTs	liver function tests	RI	resistive index
LMWH	low molecular weight heparin	RIFLE	risk, injury, failure, loss, end-stage disease
LV	left ventricle	RTA	renal tubular acidosis
MAG3	mercaptoacetylglycine	RR	relative risk
MARS	molecular adsorbent recirculating system	RRT	renal replacement therapy
MCUG	micturating cystourethrogram	SBP	systolic blood pressure
MDRD	Modification of Diet in Renal Disease study	SC	subcutaneous
		SEP	sclerosing encapsulating peritonitis
MMF	mycophenolate mofetil	SGA	subjective global assessment
MRI	magnetic resonance imaging	SHPT	secondary hyperparathyroidism
MW	molecular weight	SIRS	systemic inflammatory response syndrome
NIPD	nocturnal intermittent peritoneal dialysis	SLEDD	slow low-efficiency daily dialysis
nPCR	normalized protein catabolic rate	SNS	sympathetic nervous system
NHANES	National Health and Nutrition Examination Surveys	SPA	standardized permeability analysis
		SPEP	serum protein electrophoresis
NICE	National Institute for Health and Clinical Excellence (renamed in 2005)	spKt/V	single-pool Kt/V
		stdKt/V	standardized Kt/V
NIDDKD	National Institute of Diabetes and Digestive and Kidney Diseases	SVR	systemic vascular resistance
		TCC	transitional cell carcinoma
NKF	National Kidney Foundation	tds	three times daily
NODAT	new-onset diabetes after transplantation	TIPS	transjugular intrahepatic portosystemic shunt
NPHP	nephronophthisis		
nPNA	normalized protein equivalent of total nitrogen appearance	TMP	transmembrane pressure
		TNF-α	tumor necrosis factor-α
NSAID	nonsteroidal anti-inflammatory drug	TNM	tumor, node, metastases
NSF	nephrogenic systemic fibrosis	TPN	total parenteral nutrition
OAT-1	organic anion transporter-1	TRUS	transrectal ultrasound
od	once daily	TTP	thrombotic thrombocytopenic purpura

TURBT	transurethral resection of bladder tumor	URR	urea reduction ratio
		USRDS	US Renal Data System
TURP	transurethral resection of prostate	USS	ultrasound scan
U&Es	urea, creatinine and electrolytes	UTI	urinary tract infection
UF	ultrafiltration	VHL	von Hippel–Lindau
UFH	unfractionated heparin	VUJ	vesicoureteric junction
UKM	urea kinetic modeling	VUR	vesicoureteric reflux
UPEP	urine protein electrophoresis		

Contributors

Dr Samuel Ajayi
Consultant Nephrologist
Department of Medicine
University of Abuja Teaching Hospital
Abuja, FCT
Nigeria

Dr Reem Al Jayyousi
Consultant Nephrologist and Honorary
Senior Lecturer
John Walls Renal Unit
Leicester General Hospital
Leicester

Dr Karen Anderson
Consultant Nephrologist
The Richard Bright Renal Unit
Southmead Hospital
Bristol

Professor Mustafa Arici
Professor of Medicine
Hacettepe University Faculty of Medicine
Department of Nephrology
Ankara
Turkey

Dr Richard Baines
Clinical Lecturer in Nephrology
John Walls Renal Unit
Leicester General Hospital
Leicester

Mr Ali Bakran
Consultant Transplant & Vascular Surgeon
Royal Liverpool University Hospital
Liverpool

Mr Adam Barlow
Clinical Research Fellow
Department of Transplant Surgery
Leicester General Hospital
Leicester

Dr Jonathan Barratt
Senior Lecturer and Honorary Consultant
Nephrologist
John Walls Renal Unit
Leicester General Hospital
Leicester

Professor Rashad Barsoum
Professor of Medicine
Kasr El-Aini Medical School
Cairo University
The Cairo Kidney Center
Cairo
Egypt

Dr Anne Barton
Reader and Honorary Consultant
Rheumatologist
ARC Epidemiology Unit
Division of Epidemiology
and Health Sciences
Stopford Building
Oxford Road
Manchester

Dr Linda M Barton
Consultant Haematologist
Department of Haematology
Leicester Royal Infirmary
Leicester

Dr Sunita Bavanandan
Consultant Nephrologist
Department of Nephrology
Institute of Urology and Nephrology
Hospital Kuala Lumpur
Kuala Lumpur
Malaysia

Professor Daniel Bichet
Professor of Medicine and Physiology
Renal Genetics
Montreal Sacré-Coeur Hospital
University of Montreal
Quebec
Canada

Dr Anne Blanchard
Centres d'Investigations Cliniques
Hopital Europeen Georges Pompidou
Paris
France

Dr Detlef Böckenhauer
Consultant Paediatric Nephrologist
Department of Nephrology
Great Ormond Street Hospital for
Children NHS Trust
London

Professor Nigel Brunskill
Professor of Renal Medicine
John Walls Renal Unit
Leicester General Hospital
Leicester

Dr Katharine Buck
Consultant Nephrologist
Queen Margaret Hospital
Dunfermline

Mr Paul Butterworth
Consultant Urological Surgeon
Department of Urology
Leicester General Hospital
Leicester

Professor J Stewart Cameron
Emeritus Professor of Renal Medicine
Elm Bank
Melmerby
Penrith
Cumbria

Professor Giovambattista Capasso
Professor of Nephrology
Department of Internal Medicine
Second University of Naples
Naples
Italy

Dr S J Carr
Consultant Nephrologist and Honorary Senior Lecturer
John Walls Renal Unit
Leicester General Hospital
Leicester

Dr Claire S Chapman
Consultant Haematologist
Department of Haematology
Leicester Royal Infirmary
Leicester

Dr Chern Li Chow
Specialist Registar in Nephrology
Kidney Genetics Group
Academic Nephrology Unit
The Henry Wellcome Laboratories for Medical Research
School of Medicine and Biomedical Sciences
University of Sheffield
Sheffield

Miss Alexandra J Colquhoun
Specialist Registrar in Urology
Department of Urology
Leicester General Hospital
Leicester

Professor Christian Combe
Professor of Nephrology
Centre Hospitalier Universitaire de Bordeaux
Service de Néphrologie
Université de Bordeaux,
Unité INSERM U889
Bordeaux
France

Dr Andrew Davenport
Consultant Nephrologist and Honorary Senior Lecturer
UCL Centre for Nephrology
Royal Free & University College Medical School
Hampstead Campus
London

Dr Frédéric Debelle
Consultant Nephrologist
Department of Nephrology
Hôpital Erasme
Université Libre de Bruxelles
Brussels
Belgium

Professor Chris Denton
Professor of Experimental Rheumatology
Department of Medicine
Royal Free Campus
University College
London

Dr Stephen J Dickinson
Specialist Registrar in Nephrology
John Walls Renal Unit
Leicester General Hospital
Leicester

Dr Haresh Dodeja
Consultant Nephrologist and Transplant Physician
Wockhadt Hospitals Ltd
Mulund-Mumbai
India

Dr Christopher Dudley
Consultant Nephrologist
The Richard Bright Renal Unit
Southmead Hospital
Bristol

Dr Tony Elliott
Consultant Clinical Oncologist
The Christie Hospital
Withington
Manchester

Dr Hossam El Shazly
Consultant Nephrologist
Department of Renal Medicine
Cairns Base Hospital
Cairns 4870
Australia

Dr Sally Feather
Consultant Paediatric Nephrologist
Department of Paediatric Nephrology
St James's University Hospital
Leeds

Professor John Feehally
Professor of Renal Medicine
John Walls Renal Unit
Leicester General Hospital
Leicester

Professor Jürgen Floege
Professor of Nephrology
Division of Nephrology
University Hospital
Aachen
Germany

Dr John Frew
Registrar in Clinical Oncology
Northern Centre for Cancer Treatment
Newcastle General Hospital
Westgate Road
Newcastle-upon-Tyne

Dr Trevor Friedman
Consultant Liaison Psychiatrist
Brandon Unit
Leicester General Hospital
Leicester

Dr Julian Gillmore
Senior Lecturer and Honorary Consultant Nephrologist
National Amyloidosis Centre
Royal Free and University College Medical School
Royal Free Hospital
London

Mr Leyshon Griffiths
Senior Lecturer and Honorary Consultant Urological Surgeon
Urology Section
Department of Cancer Studies & Molecular Medicine
University of Leicester Clinical Sciences Unit
Leicester General Hospital
Leicester

Prof Krishan Lal Gupta
Professor of Nephrology
Postgraduate Institute of Medical Education and Research
Chandigarh
India

Dr Pankaj Gupta
Specialist Registrar in Chemical Pathology
Leicester Royal Infirmary
Leicester

Dr Shikha Gupta
Specialist Registrar in Dermatology
Leicester Royal Infirmary
Leicester

Dr Jenny Hainsworth
Clinical Psychologist
Leicestershire Partnership NHS Trust and
Leicester General Hospital
Leicester

Dr Andrew Hall
Clinical Research Fellow
Centre for Nephrology
Royal Free and University College Medical School
London

Dr Matt Hall
Specialist Registrar in Nephrology
John Walls Renal Unit
Leicester General Hospital
Leicester

Dr Lorraine Harper
Senior Lecturer and Honorary Consultant Nephrologist
Division of Immunity and Infection
The Medical School
University of Birmingham
Edgbaston
Birmingham

Dr Steve Harper
Consultant Nephrologist
The Richard Bright Renal Unit
Southmead Hospital
Bristol

Dr Kevin Harris
Reader and Honorary Consultant Nephrologist
John Walls Renal Unit
Leicester General Hospital
Leicester

Professor Philip N Hawkins
Professor of Medicine
National Amyloidosis Centre
Department of Medicine
Royal Free and University College Medical School
Royal Free Hospital
London

Professor Friedhelm Hildebrandt
Professor of Pediatrics and of Human Genetics
Frederick G.L. Huetwell Professor for the Cure and Prevention of Birth Defects
Doris Duke Distinguished Clinical Scientist
University of Michigan
Department of Pediatrics
Ann Arbor
Michigan
USA

Dr Richard Holt
Consultant Paediatric Nephrologist
Royal Liverpool Children's Hospital
Alder Hey
Liverpool

Prof Pascal Houillier
Professor of Physiology
Departement de Physiologie
Hopital Europeen Georges Pompidou
Paris
France

Dr Peter Houtman
Consultant Paediatrician
Leicester Royal Infirmary
Leicester

Dr Alastair Hutchison
Consultant Nephrologist
Department of Renal Medicine
Manchester Royal Infirmary
Manchester

Dr David Jayne
Consultant Nephrologist
Renal Unit
Addenbrookes Hospital
Cambridge

Dr Graham Johnston
Consultant Dermatologist
Leicester Royal Infirmary
Leicester

Dr Caroline Jones
Consultant Paediatric Nephrologist
Royal Liverpool Children's Hospital
Alder Hey
Liverpool

Dr Philip A Kalra
Consultant Nephrologist and Honorary Senior Lecturer
Dept of Renal Medicine
Hope Hospital
Salford

Dr Jens Kannmacher
Renal Fellow
Division of Nephrology
University Hospital
Aachen
Germany

Professor Robert Kleta
Professor of Nephrology
Centre for Nephrology
Royal Free and University College Medical School
London

Mr Roger Kockelbergh
Consultant Urological Surgeon
Leicester General Hospital
Leicester

Dr George Kosmadakis
Nephrologist and Clinical Research Fellow
John Walls Renal Unit
Leicester General Hospital
Leicester

Dr Andrew J P Lewington
Consultant Nephrologist and Honorary Senior Lecturer
Department of Renal Medicine
St James's University Hospital
Leeds

Dr Robert Mactier
Consultant Nephrologist
Renal Unit
Glasgow Royal Infirmary
Glasgow

Dr Webster Madira
Consultant Chemical Pathologist
Leicester Royal Infirmary
Leicester

Dr Stephen D Marks
Consultant Paediatric Nephrologist
Department of Nephrology
Great Ormond Street Hospital for Children NHS Trust
London

Dr Nick Mayer
Consultant Histopathologist
Department of Pathology
Leicester General Hospital
Leicester

Dr Simon Maxwell
Senior Lecturer in Clinical Pharmacology
Queens Medical Research Institute
Edinburgh

Dr Catherine McBain
Consultant Clinical Oncologist
The Christie Hospital
Withington
Manchester

Professor John K Mellon
Professor of Urology
Urology Section
Department of Cancer Studies & Molecular Medicine
University of Leicester Clinical Sciences Unit
Leicester General Hospital
Leicester

Dr Christopher Mitchell
Consultant Paediatric Oncologist
John Radcliffe Hospital
Headington
Oxford

Dr Henry Morgan
Consultant Paediatric Nephrologist
Royal Liverpool Children's Hospital
Alder Hey
Liverpool

Dr Francis J Mussai
Fellow in Paediatric Haematology and Oncology
John Hopkins University Hospital
Baltimore
Maryland
USA

Dr Chas Newstead
Consultant Nephrologist
Department of Renal Medicine
St James's University Hospital
Leeds

Professor Michael Nicholson
Professor of Transplant Surgery
Department of Transplant Surgery
Leicester General Hospital
Leicester

Dr Joëlle Nortier
Head of the Department of Nephrology
Hôpital Erasme
Université Libre de Bruxelles
Brussels
Belgium

Dr Albert CM Ong
Reader and Honorary Consultant Nephrologist
Kidney Genetics Group, Academic Nephrology Unit
The Henry Wellcome Laboratories for Medical Research
School of Medicine and Biomedical Sciences
University of Sheffield
Sheffield

Dr Rakesh S Patel
Specialist Registrar in Nephrology and General Medicine
John Walls Renal Unit
Leicester General Hospital
Leicester

Dr Sue Pavord
Consultant Haematologist
Leicester Royal Infirmary
Leicester

Dr Henry Penn
Clinical Research Fellow
Centre for Rheumatology
Royal Free Hospital
London

Dr Liam Plant
Consultant Nephrologist
Department of Renal Medicine
Cork University Hospital
Cork
Ireland

Dr Pradeep Rao
Specialist Registrar in Psychiatry
Brandon Unit
Leicester General Hospital
Leicester

Dr Yvonne Rees
Consultant Radiologist
Department of Radiology
Leicester General Hospital
Leicester

Professor Vincent Rigalleau
Professor of Nutrition
Centre Hospitalier Universitaire de Bordeaux
Service de Diabétologie Nutrition
Université de Bordeaux
Bordeaux
France

Dr Alan D Salama
Senior Lecturer and Honorary Consultant Nephrologist
Renal Section
Division of Medicine
Hammersmith Hospital
London

Dr Moin A Saleem
Reader and Consultant Paediatric Nephrologist
University of Bristol
Children's Renal Unit
Bristol Royal Hospital for Children
Bristol

Dr Andy Salmon
Clinical Lecturer in Nephrology
The Richard Bright Renal Unit
Southmead Hospital
Bristol

Mr Richard FJ Stanford
Clinical Research Fellow
Department of Cancer Studies & Molecular Medicine
University of Leicester

Dr John Schollum
Consultant Nephrologist
Department of Nephrology
Dunedin Hospital
Dunedin
New Zealand

Dr John E Scoble
Consultant Nephrologist
New Guys House
London

Dr Adrian Stanley
Consultant Physician and Clinical Pharmacologist
Leicester Royal Infirmary
Leicester

Professor Vladisav Stefanovic
Professor of Medicine
Institute of Nephrology
Faculty of Medicine
University of Nis
Nis
Serbia

Dr Daniel Teta
Consultant Nephrologist
Privat-Docent & MER
Service de Néphrologie
CHUV, 1011 Lausanne
Switzerland

Mr James F Thorpe
Clinical Research Fellow
Department of Cancer Studies & Molecular Medicine
University of Leicester

Dr Charles Tomson
Consultant Nephrologist
The Richard Bright Renal Unit
Southmead Hospital
Bristol

Dr Peter Topham
Senior Lecturer and Honorary Consultant Nephrologist
John Walls Renal Unit
Leicester General Hospital
Leicester

Dr Kjell Tullus
Consultant Paediatric Nephrologist
Department of Nephrology
Great Ormond Street Hospital for Children NHS Trust
London

Professor Robert Unwin
St Peter's Professor of Nephrology
Centre for Nephrology
Royal Free and University College Medical School
London

Professor Jean-Louis Vanherweghem
Emeritus Professor of Nephrology
Department of Nephrology
Hôpital Erasme
Université Libre de Bruxelles (ULB)
Brussels
Belgium

Dr William Van't Hoff
Consultant Paediatric Nephrologist
Department of Nephrology
Great Ormond Street Hospital
London

Dr Stephen Walsh
Clinical Research Fellow
Centre for Nephrology,
Royal Free and University College Medical School,
London

Dr Graham Warwick
Consultant Nephrologist
John Walls Renal Unit
Leicester General Hospital
Leicester

Professor Alan Watson
Professor of Paediatric Nephrology
Children's Renal and Urology Unit
Nottingham University Hospitals
Nottingham

Dr Rachel Westacott
Specialist Registrar in Nephrology
John Walls Renal Unit
Leicester General Hospital
Leicester

Dr Stanley White
Senior Lecturer
Institute of Membrane and Systems Biology
University of Leeds
Leeds

Dr Christopher Winearls
Consultant Nephrologist
Oxford Radcliffe Hospitals
Oxford

Dr Matthias TF Wolf
Senior Research Fellow
Department of Pediatrics
University of Michigan
Ann Arbor
Michigan
USA

Dr Graham Woodrow
Consultant Renal Physician
Department of Renal Medicine
St James's University Hospital
Leeds

Dr Rosnawati Yahya
Consultant Nephrologist
Department of Nephrology
Hospital Kuala Lumpur
Jalan Pahang
Kuala Lumpur
Malaysia

Dr Janak R de Zoysa
Consultant Nephrologist
Department of Renal Medicine
Auckland City Hospital
Auckland
New Zealand

Chapter 1

Assessment of renal disease

Chapter contents

History and clinical examination of patients with renal disease

A patient with renal disease can present in different ways:
- The patient complains of a symptom or shows physical signs typically associated with renal disease.
- The patient is asymptomatic and comes to attention through pathological results of clinical or laboratory examination.
- A systemic disease is diagnosed that can lead to renal involvement.
- The patient is examined because he has been exposed to nephrotoxic agents.
- The family history of the patient reveals inherited renal disorders.

Investigation methods which often lead to the detection of asymptomatic renal patients are biochemical analysis, urine analysis and blood pressure measurement.

Cardinal symptoms suggesting underlying renal disease are disorders of micturition, disorders of urine volume, alteration in urinary composition, edema, loin pain and hypertension. Furthermore there is a large variety of symptoms or medical problems associated with advanced renal failure and uremia respectively (Table 1.1.1).

Disorders of micturition

Frequency
Frequent emptying of the bladder can be associated with normal or increased urine volume (polyuria). The former may be due to inflammation, stone or tumor of the bladder or a reduced bladder capacity. Frequency is often accompanied with nocturia.

Poor urinary stream
The most common cause is prostatic enlargement in men past middle age. Urethral obstruction leads to retention and back pressure.

Dysuria
Pain or discomfort during micturition is usually a result of bladder, prostatic or urethral inflammation. Cystitis also causes frequency and urgency of micturition. Perineal or rectal pain in men indicates prostatitis.

Disorders of urine volume

Polyuria
Urine output of >3 L per day is defined as polyuria. It is often difficult for patients to differentiate between polyuria and frequency. Thus the measurement of daily urine excretion is necessary to elucidate the symptom. In many cases patients complain of thirst instead of increased urine volume. The possible causes for polyuria are listed in Table 1.1.2.

Oliguria
A reduction in urine volume to <500 mL per day indicates AKI leading to a situation in which homeostasis cannot be maintained.

Anuria
The sudden development of urine output of <100 mL per day is most commonly due to obstruction of the urinary tract. Other possible causes are renal infarction or cortical necrosis.

Table 1.1.1 Typical symptoms and complications in patients with advanced renal failure

General nonspecific symptoms	Malaise, weakness, diminished appetite, sleep disorders, headache
Water–electrolyte, acid–base imbalance	Water overload, dehydration, hyperkalemia, metabolic acidosis
Gastroenterological problems	Anorexia, nausea and regurgitation, peptic ulcer, gastrointestinal bleeding, diverticulosis
Cardiovascular and pulmonary problems	Hypertension, pulmonary edema, pleurisy, pericarditis, cardiomyopathy, cardiac arrhythmia
Endocrinological and metabolic problems	Secondary hyperparathyroidism, osteomalacia, infertility, disturbance of growth in children
Neuromuscular problems	Peripheral polyneuropathy, restless legs syndrome, cramps, seizures, tremor, coma
Dermatological disorders	Many different skin alterations, such as palor, hyperpigmentation, pruritus, scratch marks
Hematological and immunological disorders	Renal anemia, bleeding tendency, immunodeficiency

Table 1.1.2 Conditions which may cause polyuria

Increased renal water loss	
Endocrinologic disorders	Central (cranial) diabetes insipidus
	Addison's disease
	Hyporeninemic hypoaldosteronism
Renal tubular disorders	Nephrogenic diabetes insipidus
	Acquired tubular defects, e.g. salt-losing nephropathy
	- Pyelonephritis
	- Analgesic nephropathy
	- Multiple myeloma
	- Obstructive uropathy
	- Sarcoidosis
	- Hypercalcaemia, chronic potassium depletion
	Toxic agents (e.g. aminoglycosides, lithium, cisplatinum)
	Diuretic therapy
	Bartter's syndrome
	Polyuric phase of acute or acute-on-chronic renal failure
Osmotic diuresis	Glycosuria in diabetes mellitus
	Administration of mannitol
	Administration of large volume of contrast agents
Increased water intake	
Psychogenic	
Medication	Drugs causing xerostomia or thirst (e.g. anticholinergics or clonidine)

Alteration in urinary composition

Hematuria

Hematuria may originate from any part of the renal tract and there are many possible underlying conditions, such as glomerulonephritis, infection, calculi, tumors, thrombocytopenia or disordered coagulation.

- The most common cause is urinary tract infection.
- Recurrent macroscopic hematuria is often seen in IgA nephropathy, but may also be due to intermittent bleeding from a structural lesion.
- Blood from the urethra only appears in the initial urinary stream.
- Blood from the bladder or prostate appears usually at the end of micturition.
- Intense exercise can cause transient hematuria.
- Alteration in urine colour does not always indicate the presence of blood (see Chapter 1.2).

Proteinuria

A urinary protein loss of up to 150 mg/24 h is normal. Patients with higher concentrations sometimes report frothy urine, but mostly proteinuria is only determined chemically. Usually a dipstick test is used, but this method does not detect immunoglobulin light chains or microalbuminuria.

- Proteinuria arising from interstitial disease is generally mild (up to 2 g/24 h).
- Proteinuria caused by glomerular disorders is variable (up to 10 g/24 h and more).
- Orthostatic proteinuria (proteinuria noted after being upright and absent in the first urine passed in the morning after lying down) is usually harmless.
- The type of proteinuria can help in establishing a diagnosis (see page 9).

Bacteriuria

Bacteria in the urine do not always cause symptoms. Usually it is only considered significant if there are >10^5 organisms per mL.

Leukocyturia

There are different conditions that lead to the presence of leukocytes in the urine such as nephrocalcinosis, analgesic nephropathy and papillary necrosis. In immunologically mediated tubulointerstitial nephritis, eosinophils may be present in the urine.

Pyuria

Pyuria always indicates a significant infection. Sterile pyuria may be due to chlamydial infection or tuberculosis.

Pneumaturia

This suggests a vesicocolonic fistula, which may arise as a consequence of Crohn's disease, diverticular disease or carcinoma of the colon.

Edema

An increase of fluid in the interstitium in patients with renal disease may be caused by hypoproteinemia. If this is the consequence of proteinuria (typically >3.5 g/24 h) it is part of the nephrotic syndrome. Initially this kind of edema is typically most visible around the eyes in the morning and in the feet and ankles in the evening.

Edema may also be caused by salt and water retention as a result of CKD, congestive cardiac failure and chronic hepatic disease, or increased capillary permeability due to allergy, inflammation or ischemia.

As a consequence of long-term renal failure or nephrotic syndrome, up to 20 additional liters of fluid can accumulate in the body, leading to generalized swelling called anasarca. In advanced fluid overload, interstitial pulmonary edema is common.

Administration of drugs such as calcium-channel antagonists and steroids or diuretic abuse may also lead to edema.

Pain

If pain occurs as a symptom of renal disease, it mostly indicates inflammation or obstruction. Pain arising from pyelonephritis usually develops gradually and has a constant intensity, whereas an acute obstruction typically causes a sudden severe and colicky pain radiating to the scrotum or groin.

Clinical syndromes and other modes of presentation

Nephrotic syndrome

This is a consequence of severe proteinuria (usually defined as >3.5 g/24 h) and is characterized by hypoalbuminemic edema and hyperlipoproteinemia. The underlying diseases are diverse, and include different types of glomerulonephritis, diabetic nephropathy, myeloma or amyloidosis.

Acute nephritic syndrome

This is characterized by hematuria with red blood cell casts in the urine, proteinuria, oliguria and hypertension. Common causes are post-streptococcal glomerulonephritis and the acute exacerbation of a chronic glomerular disorder such as IgA nephropathy.

Acute kidney injury (AKI)

AKI is a rapid reduction of the glomerular filtration rate, resulting in the retention of waste products such as urea, creatinine and other uremic toxins. It may cause metabolic disturbances and disorders of the fluid balance. AKI may be oliguric (urine volume reduced to <500 mL/day) or nonoliguric. The underlying conditions are varied and can be subdivided into pre-renal, renal and post-renal causes.

Chronic kidney disease (CKD)

CKD irrespective of aetiology is classified into five stages based on the GFR. Chronicity is defined as an abnormality for >3 months:

1 GFR normal or increased, but findings indicating kidney damage (e.g. proteinuria or hematuria)
2 GFR of 89–60 mL/min/1.73 m^2 (with abnormal urinalysis or structural renal lesion)
3 GFR of 59–30 mL/min/1.73 m^2
4 GFR of 29–15 mL/min/1.73 m^2
5 GFR of <15 mL/min/1.73 m^2 or necessity for renal replacement therapy (dialysis or transplantation)

The early forms of CKD are asymptomatic.

Macroscopic (visible) hematuria

The underlying conditions of patients presenting with grossly visible hematuria are diverse and vary with age. The most common causes are inflammation of the bladder or prostate, stones and, particularly in older patients, benign prostatic hyperplasia and malignancy. In most young patients it is transient and of no consequence. Nevertheless a urologic evaluation is essential in all cases of macroscopic hematuria.

Microscopic (nonvisible) hematuria

Isolated microscopic hematuria is defined as the presence of >2 red blood cells per high-power field in a urine sediment. It is very common and mostly a chance finding. At first benign causes should be excluded, e.g. menstruation, physical exercise or infection. If the hematuria persists and the etiology remains unclear, or if the history points towards a specific cause, further investigation is necessary (e.g. laboratory analysis, radiologic imaging, urologic evaluation). If microscopic hematuria is accompanied by proteinuria >1 g/day a 'urologic' cause is unlikely and an intra-renal origin should be sought.

Asymptomatic proteinuria

While proteinuria >1–2 g/day usually indicates glomerular disease, proteinuria <1 g/day usually should be closely followed but does not usually warrant invasive procedures such as renal biopsy, at least as long as it is not accompanied by a decreased GFR or an otherwise active urine sediment.

Clinical history of the patient with renal disease

History of the current complaint

The chronological order of the patient's presenting symptoms should be established. This should include a full description of the course of their intensity and quality. It is important to encourage the patient to describe his complaints in his own words, as otherwise essential information might be lost.

Details of associated symptoms should be obtained. For example, upper respiratory tract symptoms at the time of visible hematuria may suggest a diagnosis of IgA nephropathy.

Hypertension is often related to renal disease and therefore should always be investigated in detail.

Patients suffering from pain should be asked about its localization and character, the mode of onset and aggravating or relieving factors.

Any factors accompanying the presenting illness should be determined carefully.

Past history

Previous major illnesses and hospitalizations should be determined, including those in childhood and adolescence. Special attention must be paid to systemic diseases that are known to be associated with renal disease, e.g. systemic lupus erythematosus or Wegener's granulomatosis. Some metabolic diseases are closely related to renal disease, such as diabetes mellitus, oxalosis or Fabry's disease. Examples of pre-existing conditions that may be associated with renal disease are listed in Table 1.1.3. To complete the past history, previous medical records should be obtained with particular emphasis on prior renal function tests.

Gynecologic and obstetric history

In females information about menstruation, contraception and pregnancy should be obtained.
- Impaired renal function can be associated with delayed menarche and amenorrhea.
- In women taking combined estrogen–progesterone contraceptives, renal disease significantly increases the risk of hypertension.
- Initiation or exacerbation of renal disease may be associated with pregnancy. The increase of pre-existing proteinuria during pregnancy can lead to the development of nephrotic syndrome.
- Repeated fetal loss may suggest underlying systemic lupus erythematosus and antiphospholipid antibody syndrome.

Table 1.1.3 Conditions associated with renal disease

Condition	Associated renal disease
Hypertension	Hypertensive nephrosclerosis
	Secondary hypertension due to renal disease
Diabetes mellitus	Diabetic nephropathy
Gout	Urate calculi
Recurrent cystitis and pyelitis	Reflux nephropathy
Chronic headache	Analgesic nephropathy due to analgesic abuse
Raynaud's syndrome	Systemic sclerosis
	Systemic lupus erythematosus
	Cryoglobulinemia with renal involvement
Recurrent sinusitis or ENT problems	Wegener's granulomatosis
Pleurisy, pericarditis	Rheumatoid arthritis
	Systemic lupus erythematosus
Haemoptysis	Wegener's granulomatosis
	Goodpasture's syndrome
Recurrent thrombosis and fetal loss	Antiphospholipid antibody syndrome
Impaired hearing	Alport syndrome
Tonsillitis, scarlet fever	Post-streptococcal glomerulonephritis
Liver cirrhosis	Hepatorenal syndrome
Hepatitis B or C	Membranous or membranoproliferative glomerulonephritis
Diarrhea	Hemolytic uremic syndrome
Tuberculosis	Urogenital tuberculosis
	Amyloidosis
	Sterile leukocyturia
HIV infection	HIV nephropathy
Malignancy	Membranous glomerulonephritis

Drug history

Complete details about recent drug intake should be obtained, including onset, duration and dosage of ingestion. The use of nonprescription drugs, especially nonsteroidal anti-inflammatory drugs, should also be noted.

Social and occupational history

Social status may have considerable influence on the development of renal disease. For example bacteriuria is more common in pregnant women of low socio-economic class, whereas calcium stones occur more often in men of higher social standing. During therapy poor compliance may be a serious problem, which is more frequent among patients of lower socio-economic status.

It is important to ask patients about tobacco consumption. Smoking may contribute to the development and progression of renal failure and is a risk factor for renovascular hypertension. Drug addiction is associated with several renal complications, e.g. acute renal failure due to rhabdomyolysis, virus-related renal disease, or infections.

Development of renal disease may be associated with certain occupational factors.

- It has been shown that there is an increased incidence of urothelial tumors in aniline dye workers.
- Miners, sewage workers and farm labourers are at higher risk of leptospirosis leading to AKI.
- Hantavirus infection originating from bank voles (*Myodes glareolus*) is more common in people working outdoors or engaging in outdoor activities in endemic areas.
- Exposure to lead may cause CKD due to lead nephropathy.

Family history
Medical information on relatives may help in elucidating cases of inherited kidney diseases. Furthermore familial predispositions to systemic lupus erythematosus, IgA nephropathy or the development of diabetic nephropathy are known. The classification of inherited renal diseases is listed in Table 1.1.4.

Ethnic and geographic factors
The ethnic background of a patient is an important factor associated with different incidences of kidney disease.

- Renal failure associated with hypertension or diabetes mellitus is more common in black patients.
- In the UK the incidence of end-stage renal disease in South Asians and African Caribbeans is at least three times higher than in Caucasians.
- IgA nephropathy is more common in white populations and in certain parts of Asia than in black populations.
- The incidence and aggressiveness of systemic lupus erythematosus is higher in oriental, hispanic and black populations than in Caucasians.
- Amyloidosis as a complication of familial Mediterranean fever occurs more often in Arabs, Turks and Sephardic Jews from the Mediterranean area compared to Sephardic Jews from other regions, Ashkenazi Jews and Armenians.
- The risk of developing tuberculosis during immunosuppressive therapy, e.g. after transplantation, is higher in patients originating from high prevalence regions such as India or Russia.

Clinical examination
Direct examination of the kidneys is usually not possible so a careful general examination is necessary to identify any abnormalities suggesting underlying renal disease.

Examination of the kidneys and the urinary tract
Inspection
In some patients an enlarged kidney may be visible, e.g. in cases of advanced polycystic kidney disease. Rarely in patients with bladder outflow obstruction an extreme distension may be visible.

Palpation
Palpation of the kidneys is possible but practicable only in thin patients. If the patient lies with both arms beside the body, the kidneys are palpated by placing the left hand posteriorly in the loin and the right hand on the abdomen lateral to the umbilicus. With the patient taking a deep breath the lower kidney pole may be palpable by pushing the right hand inwards and upwards. The right kidney is more accessible to palpation than the left one, due to its lower abdominal position. Size and shape of the kidneys should be estimated. The surface normally feels smooth and relatively hard. Irregularities may suggest cystic disease or malignancy.

Percussion
In patients suffering from pyelonephritis or acute glomerulonephritis slight percussion of the renal region may be sufficient to cause severe pain, also referred to as costovertebral tenderness. Pyelonephritis is rather accompanied by fever and dysuria, whereas hematuria, hypertension and oliguria suggest glomerulonephritis.

Auscultation
Abdominal auscultation is essential in patients with hypertension, as the presence of a bruit may suggest renal artery stenosis.

General examination
Every patient with renal disease has to be examined completely to detect any abnormality that might be of diagnostic value.

Table 1.1.4 Classification of the most important inherited kidney diseases

---

1. **Polycystic kidney disease**
2. **Alport's syndrome and variants** (e.g. 'benign' familial hematuria)
3. **Inherited metabolic diseases with renal involvement**
   - *without glomerular involvement*   Cystinosis, hyperoxaluria, inherited urate nephropathy
   - *with glomerular involvement*   Fabry's disease, lecithin-cholesterol acyltransferase deficiency
4. **Other inherited diseases with glomerular or nonglomerular involvement**
   - *with glomerular involvement*   congenital nephrotic syndrome
   - *with nonglomerular involvement*   nephronophthisis
   - *with cystic kidney disease*   renal angiomyolipoma in tuberous sclerosis
     renal cell carcinoma in von Hippel–Lindau's disease
5. **Familial IgA nephropathy or focal segmental glomerulosclerosis**
6. **Inherited tubular disorders**
   - cystinuria
   - various other inherited tubular defects
7. **Renal diseases with variable polygenetic influence**
   - diabetic nephropathy
   - reflux nephropathy
   - calcium nephrolithiasis
8. **Unclassified cases**

Facial appearance

An abnormal facial appearance may suggest underlying disease. In patients with systemic sclerosis a typical facies with thickening and rigidity of the skin is visible. A loss of the buccal pad accompanied by fat loss from the upper part of the body (partial lipodystrophy) is associated with mesangiocapillary glomerulonephritis (MCGN) type 2. In Wegener's granulomatosis a characteristic facies may appear due to loss of the nasal cartilaginous septum. Patients receiving steroids frequently develop typical mooning of the face.

Skin

The skin should always be examined thoroughly, as there is a wide variety of cutaneous alterations associated with renal disease.

- Skin turgor is an important sign to detect fluid imbalances.
- Patients with uremia frequently have a dry and flaky skin of yellowish-brown colour. Depigmented scratch marks or reddish-brown papules may indicate pruritus. Pallor is common in patients with chronic renal failure as a consequence of renal anemia, but there may also be diffuse hyperpigmentation of sun-exposed areas. Due to impaired coagulation and fragile small vessels there may be a tendency to hematoma formation (Figure 1.1.1).
- Subcutaneous nodules may appear due to the deposition of calcium salts within the skin (calcinosis cutis) in patients with secondary hyperparathyroidism.
- Palpable purpura, particularly on the lower limbs and the buttocks, is a common sign of Henoch–Schönlein purpura.

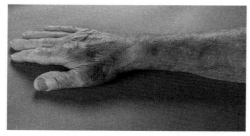

Fig. 1.1.1 Typical skin alterations in a patient with chronic renal failure.

Note the diffuse hyperpigmentation, the local deposition of hematin and the depigmented scratch marks.

- Allergic exanthema accompanied by renal failure may suggest interstitial nephritis (Figure 1.1.2).
- The appearance of vasculitis may be variable (Figure 1.1.3).
- Patients receiving long-term immunosuppression may develop hyperkeratotic lesions, which can transform into malignant lesions.
- In patients with Fabry's disease small reddish-purple papules (angiokeratoma) appear on the skin with predominance on the lower abdomen and the groin area.
- Uremic frost is a manifestation of terminal renal failure which is now rarely seen. It is due to the crystallization of urea and other nitrogenous waste products in sweat presenting as a white crystalline material on the skin, particularly on the face.

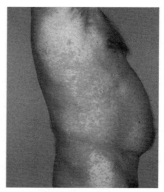

Fig. 1.1.2 Allergic rash in a patient.

Nails

Patients with CKD may have variable nail abnormalities. The most common anomalies are absence of the lunula and half-and-half nails characterized by a proximal white band and a distal red brown band. Transverse ridges (Beau's lines) may be a result of serious preceding illness. Patients with vasculitis or endocarditis may have splinter hemorrhages. Dystrophic nail alterations accompanied by absent or hypoplastic patella are seen in patients with the nail–patella syndrome, which is associated with renal failure.

Eyes

Examination of the eyes may show peri-limbal calcification following longstanding uremia, subconjunctival hemorrhages in patients with vasculitis, or lenticonus in Alport's syndrome. Fundoscopy may reveal typical alterations in patients with diabetes mellitus, hypertension, vasculitis, or MCGN type 2.

Heart

During cardiac auscultation particular attention should be paid to murmurs, which may be due to renal anemia, and a pericardial rub which indicates pericarditis in terminal uremia.

Chest

When examining the chest of patients with renal disease one should consider the possibility of pleural effusions and listen for crepitations and pleural rubs. Increased breathing with an open mouth may indicate compensation of metabolic acidosis (Kussmaul's respiration).

Abdomen

Important findings on abdominal examination include organomegaly or hernias, especially in patients who might subsequently require continuous ambulatory peritoneal dialysis.

Limbs

Attention should be paid to edema, which is mostly obvious in the lower limbs, but may also appear in the face and the arms or even occur as anasarca. In bedridden patients edema usually occurs in the calves, the sacrum and the loins. In children, edema is predominantly visible in the face.

The vascular tree should be examined by taking the pulse on all limbs and looking for trophic disorders. In longstanding

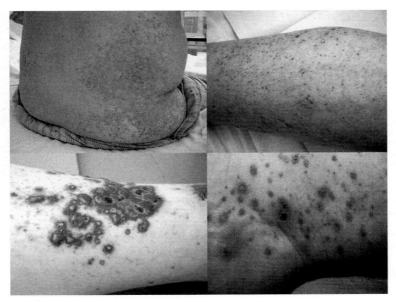

Fig. 1.1.3 Different manifestations of vasculitis.

Note the wide range of appearances from an allergic-like exanthema to the presence of necrosis and hemorrhages.

renal failure atherosclerosis is very common and may cause problems for subsequent dialysis access.

A neurological examination is essential to exclude polyneuropathy, which may be secondary to uremia or diabetes mellitus. Polyneuropathy due to renal disease is symmetric with predominance of the lower limbs. It may cause sensory loss, paresthesias, dysesthesias, itch and muscular cramps.

Measurement of blood pressure

Taking the blood pressure in both arms is an essential part of the clinical examination of renal patients. The measurement conditions should be as standardized. Overestimation of systolic blood pressure may occur due to hard, calcified vessels. This can be detected by a positive Osler's sign, in which the radial artery is palpable in spite of the cuff inflated above systolic blood pressure.

Further reading

Dyachenko P, Monselise A, Shustak A, Ziv M, Rozenman DJ. Nail disorders in patients with chronic renal failure and undergoing haemodialysis treatment: a case–control study. Eur Acad Dermatol Venereol 2007;21:340–344.

Feehally J. Ethnicity and renal disease: questions and challenges.. Clin Med 2003;3:578–582.

Nuyts GD, Van Vlem E, Thys J, De Leernijder D, D'Haese PC, Elseviers MM, De Broe ME. New occupational risk factors for chronic renal failure. Lancet 1995;346:7–11.

Picó MR, Lugo-Somolinos A, Sànchez JL, Burgos-Calderón R. Cutaneous alterations in patients with chronic renal failure. Int J Dermatol 1992;31:860–863.

See also

Urinalysis and microscopy p. 8

Clinical assessment of renal function p. 12

Urinalysis and microscopy

Urine examination is one of the basic diagnostic evaluations in patients with disease of the kidneys or the urinary tract.

Collection of urine samples

The method of obtaining and handling urine specimens has a great effect on the result. It is therefore essential to standardize these procedures as far as possible.

- The patient should not perform arduous physical exercise for 72 h before collecting the urine, otherwise proteinuria, hematuria or cylindruria might be induced.
- Urinalysis should not be performed in females during menstruation because of possible blood contamination.
- The first or second morning urine is preferred for analysis.
- To prevent contamination, females should spread the labia, males withdraw the foreskin and the genitalia should have been washed. The first few milliliters of urine are discarded.
- Urine collection through bladder catheters may be associated with hematuria, bacteriuria or leukocyturia.
- In small children urine bags are commonly used, but they increase the probability of contamination.
- Written instructions for the patient contribute to the optimization of urine collection.

Physical characteristics of urine

Color and turbidity

Depending on the urochrome concentration, the normal color of urine ranges from pale yellow to amber. An abnormal coloration may be caused by several pathologic conditions and the intake of certain drugs or foods (Table 1.2.1). It is important to remember that red urine is not always due to hematuria.

Table 1.2.1 Causes of abnormal color changes in urine

Underlying condition	Possible urine coloration
Hematuria, hemoglobinuria, myoglobinuria	Pink, red, brown or black
Jaundice	Dark yellow to brown
Chyluria	White and milky
Massive uric acid crystalluria	Pink
Porphyrinuria	Red (possibly darkening upon standing or fluorescence in UV light)
Alkaptonuria	Brown to black
Drugs	
Rifampicin	Orange to red
Phenytoin	Red
Chloroquine	Brown
Triamterene	Green
Methylene blue	Blue
Metronidazole, imipenem/ cilastatin, methyldopa	Darkening upon standing
Foods	
Beetroot	Red
Rhubarb, senna	Yellowish-brown or red
Carotene	Brown

Normally urine is transparent. An increased concentration of particles may cause turbidity. The underlying conditions are diverse, but the most common causes are urinary tract infections, hematuria and contamination from genital secretions.

Odor

In urinary tract infections with bacteria producing ammonia a pungent smell can often be noted. A sweet, fruity odor may be due to ketonuria. In some rare metabolic diseases characteristic odours of urine are described:

- phenylketonuria (distinctive musty or 'mousy' odor);
- maple syrup urine disease (maple syrup odor);
- isovaleric acidemia (sweaty feet odor);
- hypermethioninaemia (fishy or rancid butter odor).

Relative density

Relative density provides a measure of the urine concentration and can provide information about the fluid balance of a patient. It can also suggest whether the patient has a normal ability to adjust the urine concentration in states of dehydration or fluid overload. There are different methods to measure relative density:

- Specific gravity (SG) depends on the number and weight of the solute particles. It is determined with a weighted float called a urinometer and normal SG ranges from 1003 to 1035 g/L.
- Osmolality is defined as the number of particles per kg. Urine osmolality is determined by measuring the freezing point and physiologically it ranges from 50 to 1200 mosmol/kg.
- Refractometry is a method based on the measurement of the refractive index which correlates with osmolality.
- The most common means to determine relative density is dipstick testing based on dry chemistry with cations in the urine causing the colour change of an indicator substance. This method is not very accurate but is adequate for everyday use. As dipstick use is widespread, it is important to pay attention to conditions that may confound the results (Table 1.2.2).

Chemical characteristics of urine

pH

Urine pH is useful in evaluating acid–base disorders and for the interpretation of certain dipstick tests and microscopic findings. The commonly used dipsticks can measure pH values from 5.0 to 9.0.

- Urine pH normally ranges from 4.8 to 7.6.
- Acidic urine may be due to high meat intake or acidosis.
- Alkaline urine may be due to vegetarianism, infections of the urinary tract with ammonia-producing bacteria (e.g. *Proteus* spp.), prolonged storage of the specimen or alkalosis.

Hemoglobin

The detection of hemoglobin by dipsticks utilizes the pseudoperoxidase activity of the heme moiety to produce a colored product. In the presence of intact erythrocytes green spots become visible, whereas a homogeneous color change may occur following hemolysis due to longer storage of the specimen, alkaline urine or low relative urine density. With a high erythrocyte concentration there may also be a diffuse colour change.

Table 1.2.2 Main causes for false dipstick results

Measurement	False-negative results	False-positive results
Specific gravity	Underestimation in glucosuria, pH >6.5	Overestimation in proteinuria >7 g/L, ketoaciduria
pH	Reduced values in presence of formaldehyde	
Hemoglobin	Ascorbic acid, standing before examination, high relative density, formaldehyde	Myoglobinuria, bacterial peroxidases, intravascular hemolysis, hydrochloric acid
Glucose	Ascorbic acid, bacteria	Hydrochloric acid, oxidizing agents
Albumin	Light chains, tubular proteins, hydrochloric acid	pH >9, quaternary ammonium detergents
Leukocyte esterase	High relative density, vitamin C, proteinuria >5 g/L, glucosuria >20 g/L, cephalosporins	Oxidizing detergents
Nitrites	No vegetable intake, vitamin C, bacteria that do not reduce nitrates	
Ketones		Drugs containing free sulfhydryl groups

This dipstick method has low sensitivity but high specificity. False-positive results may be seen in patients with intravascular hemolysis, myoglobinuria or infection with bacteria showing pseudoperoxidase activity (Enterobacteriaceae, staphylococci and streptococci). Therefore phase-contrast microscopy of a fresh specimen of urine may be useful to confirm positive cases or those where the result is unclear.

Glucose

Dipstick testing is also commonly used for the detection of glucosuria. By using this method glucose concentrations of 0.5–20 g/L can be measured. Usually glucosuria is a consequence of hyperglycemia due to diabetes mellitus, but renal glucosuria may occur as a result of certain tubular disorders. See Table 1.2.2 for causes of false-positive or -negative results.

Protein

Normally, daily urinary protein excretion does not exceed 150 mg (140 mg/m^2 for children), as most of the filtered protein is reabsorbed in the proximal tubules.

A dipstick can provide a rough quantification of proteinuria. This method has a high sensitivity to albumin, but only low sensitivity to other proteins, e.g. immunoglobulin light chains. For more detailed assessment other laboratory techniques are necessary. The most reliable results are obtained by 24 h urine collection. The results should be denoted as g/L or g/24 h.

Alternatively spot or better timed urine collections can be assessed for albumin or protein concentration and this is then normalized for urinary dilution by dividing it by the urinary creatinine concentration (albumin:creatinine ratio (ACR) or protein:creatinine ratio (PCR)). There is a good correlation between carefully performed 24 h urine collection for protein estimation and ACR/PCR on spot urine

and therefore the latter a used routinely in everyday clinical practice to quantify proteinuria.

To analyze proteinuria qualitatively, electrophoretic protein separation can be done on the basis of molecular weight. Thus information can be obtained about the origin of the excreted proteins and help to inform possible underlying disorders. Alternatively, specific marker proteins can indicate tubular damage (see below).

Prerenal (overload) proteinuria. An increased serum concentration of a protein results in urinary excretion without a glomerular or tubular defect. Examples are Bence–Jones proteinuria in monoclonal gammopathy, myoglobinuria following rhabdomyolysis or hemoglobinuria due to hemolytic crisis. In the case of Bence–Jones proteinuria, immunofixation of serum should be performed.

Glomerular proteinuria. Increased permeability of the glomerular filtration membrane causes pathologic proteinuria. Further differentiation is made based on the pattern of protein excretion.

- Selective glomerular proteinuria means that predominantly albumin and transferrin are detected, which suggests the presence of a moderate glomerular disorder (e.g. minimal change nephritis).
- Nonselective glomerular proteinuria implies that higher molecular weight proteins (e.g. IgG) appear in the urine, which indicates severe glomerular damage.
- The selectivity can be assessed by determining the ratio of IgG clearance to transferrin clearance. Values <0.1 reflect selective proteinuria, whereas values >0.2 indicate nonselective proteinuria.

Microalbuminuria implies an albumin excretion of 30–300 mg/day or 20–200 mg/L (ACR of 2.5–30 mg/mmol in men, or 3.5–30 mg/mmol in women). It is a typical early albeit nonspecific feature of diabetic or hypertensive nephropathy.

Tubular proteinuria. This is characterized by the presence of low molecular weight proteins, which are normally filtered in the glomeruli and reabsorbed in the tubules, such as α_1-microglobulin or β2-microglobulin. Their increased concentration in the urine indicates tubular damage.

Leukocyte esterase

Dipstick testing for leukocyturia as a marker for urinary tract infection is based on the activity of leukocyte esterase released from lysed macrophages and neutrophil granulocytes. High glucose or protein concentrations may cause false-negative results (see Table 1.2.2).

Nitrites

Most Gram-negative uropathogenic bacteria are capable of reducing nitrates to nitrites. *Pseudomonas* spp., *Staphylococcus albus* and *Enterococcus* spp. lack this ability. Thus dipstick testing for nitrite can help to characterize the causative agent of urinary tract infection. The test is dependent on an adequate nitrate intake (e.g. from vegetables).

Ketones

Acetoacetate and acetone are detected using dipsticks. They may occur in the urine due to diabetic ketoacidosis, fasting, vomiting or arduous exercise.

Urine microscopy

Urine microscopy can complement the physicochemical results and add critical information when properly performed. The interpretation is subjective and requires an experienced investigator.

General procedure

- After collecting the urine as described above it should be examined as soon as possible – any cellular elements within the urine will lyse with prolonged storage.
- An aliquot of 10 mL is centrifuged for 5 min at 2000–3000 rpm.
- The supernatant is discarded almost completely and the sediment is resuspended in ~0.5 mL of the residual urine.
- An aliquot of the suspension is transferred to a slide and covered with a coverslip.
- The use of a phase-contrast microscope is recommended. For the proper differentiation of lipids and crystals, polarized light should be used.
- Several microscopic fields should be examined with both low and high magnification.

Cells

Cells may originate from the blood circulation or from the epithelia of the urinary tract. A cell count is performed at ×400 magnification. Note that alkaline pH and a low relative density may cause lysis of erythrocytes and leukocytes.

Erythrocytes

Erythrocytes may appear as round cells with a regular contour and without a nucleus (Fig. 1.2.1). In these cases they are referred to as isomorphic and most probably originate from the lower urinary tract. Erythrocytes with irregular shapes are called dysmorphic. Normally the number of erythrocytes does not exceed two per high power microscopic field.

Acanthocytes show a characteristic contour with vesicle-like protrusions poking out of a ring-shaped body. Although they are very specific for glomerular damage, the sensitivity is low. Furthermore many different types of dysmorphic erythrocytes can be differentiated (e.g. anulocytes, echinocytes or stomatocytes), but these are rather nonspecific for glomerular bleeding.

Leukocytes

Under normal conditions there should not be more than five leukocytes per high power microscopic field.

- Neutrophils constitute the majority of leukocytes and can be recognized by a granulated cytoplasm and lobulated nucleus. They are indicators of urinary tract infection and may also be seen in patients with interstitial nephritis or proliferative forms of glomerulonephritis. Urine contamination also frequently results in their appearance in urine (Fig. 1.2.2).
- Eosinophils are nonspecific and may be seen in cases of acute interstitial nephritis, glomerulonephritis, chronic pyelonephritis or prostatitis.
- The proper identification of lymphocytes requires specific staining, which is not widely practised. Their occurrence in urine is considered an indicator of acute cellular rejection after renal transplantation.
- Macrophages appear as cells of variable size. They may be granular, phagocytic or vacuolar, and in patients with nephrotic syndrome they may contain lipid droplets ('oval fat bodies'). In clinical practice they are of low significance.

Epithelial cells

Renal tubular epithelial cells are of variable size and shape, but mostly they have a large nucleus, which is often positioned eccentrically. Their appearance is nonspecific and may be due to acute tubular necrosis, interstitial nephritis, acute renal transplant rejection, or intake of acetylsalicylic acid.

Uroepithelial cells have their origin in the urinary tract from the renal calyces to the bladder (or proximal urethra in men). Typically a large, round nucleus is visible in the centre of the cells. Uroepithelium is a multilayered epithelium, which contains small cells in the deep layers and larger cells in the superficial layers. Whereas superficial cells are visible in many patients, cells of the deep layers may suggest significant urological disease, such as neoplasia or calculi.

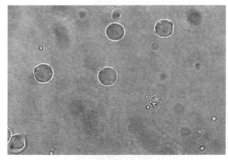

Fig. 1.2.1 Erythrocyturia. Some isomorphic erythrocytes with a regular smooth surface.

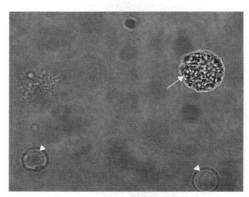

Fig. 1.2.2 Granulocyte in urine sediment. Note the size and shape of the granulated cell (arrow) compared to the smaller erythrocytes (arrowheads).

Squamous cells are the largest cells in urinary sediment and contain a round, central nucleus and smooth or granular cytoplasm. They derive from the urethra or external genitalia. Large numbers may be seen due to contamination from genital secretions.

Casts

Casts are cylindrically shaped elements, which form in the lumen of distal renal tubules and collecting ducts and subsequently are eliminated in the urine. Their matrix consists mainly of Tamm–Horsfall glycoprotein, which is secreted into the tubules and precipitates in an acidic environment. An alkaline pH prevents the formation of casts. Different types of cast may form due to embedding of different particles. Useful information for establishing a diagnosis may be obtained by regarding the different visible casts together with other abnormal microscopic findings.

- Hyaline casts are homogeneous, translucent, colorless elements with a smooth surface. They are common and do not necessarily indicate disease.

- Granular casts contain small granules originating from degenerated cells (Fig. 1.2.3). They may be found in a variety of renal diseases. Thus they are of low diagnostic value.
- Waxy casts have an opaque wax-like matrix and square ends. These casts suggest chronic renal disease, such as glomerulonephritis, diabetic nephropathy or amyloidosis.
- Fatty casts contain lipid droplets in variable forms and typically are visible in patients with marked proteinuria or nephrotic syndrome. Under polarized light cholesterol drops appear as 'Maltese crosses'.
- Erythrocyte casts contain various amounts of intact or dysmorphic erythrocytes (Fig. 1.2.4). Brownish hemoglobin casts may develop due to degradation of the erythrocytes. These casts reflect glomerular hematuria, e.g. in glomerulonephritis. A so-called nephritic sediment as a marker for active glomerulonephritis is characterized by erythrocyte casts, dysmorphic erythrocytes, leukocytes and renal tubular epithelial cells.

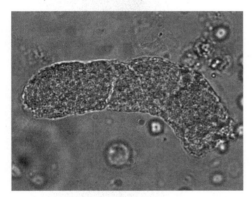

Fig. 1.2.3 Granular cast. The cast contains small granules and no included cells can be seen.

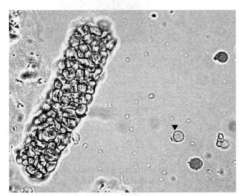

Fig. 1.2.4 Red cell cast. This cast contains many erythrocytes, which are of similar size as the single erythrocyte on the right (arrowhead).

- Leukocyte casts contain leukocytes with polymorphic nuclei, sometimes together with epithelial cells or erythrocytes. Their presence suggests pyelonephritis or acute interstitial nephritis.
- Epithelial casts contain exfoliated tubular epithelial cells recognizable by their prominent nucleus. These casts

may indicate acute interstitial nephritis or acute tubular necrosis and may also be seen in glomerular disorders.

Lipids

Lipids may be visible as spherical, translucent or yellow drops of variable size, which may appear free in the urine, within casts, as cholesterol crystals, and intracellular in epithelial cells or macrophages. Urinary lipids suggest glomerular disorders with marked proteinuria, but they may also be detected in sphingolipidoses, such as Fabry disease.

Crystals

Several different types of crystal can be differentiated by morphology and appearance under polarized light. The majority of crystals have hardly any clinical significance. Their formation depends on urine pH, urine temperature and food intake. The most frequently found crystals consist of uric acid, calcium oxalate, phosphates and urates.

- Uric acid crystals have an amber color and appear in a large variety of shapes. They are detected only in acidic urine (pH ≤5.8).
- Calcium oxalate crystals can be found at pH 5.4–6.7. Monohydrated crystals appear in various shapes, bihydrated crystals mostly appear bipyramidal. Only the latter polarize light.
- Amorphous urates and phosphates are small granules of irregular appearance that are morphologically indistinguishable. Urates, however, form in acid urine and are birefringent, whereas phosphates precipitate in alkaline urine (pH ≥7.0) and do not polarize light.

Some crystals always indicate underlying disease, such as cystine crystals (hexagonal plates with irregular sides, precipitation in acidic urine) as indicators of cystinuria or cholesterol crystals (transparent thin plates with sharp edges) in patients with marked proteinuria.

Bacteria and other organisms

Bacteria are identified frequently, as urine specimens are usually not obtained under sterile conditions. The detection of 10^5 bacteria per mL in an appropriately collected specimen strongly indicates urinary tract infection. In patients with dysuria or leukocyturia, lower bacteria concentrations are regarded as pathologic. *Candida* and *Trichomonas* are frequently found due to contamination from genital secretions. The microscopic detection of eggs of *Schistosoma hematobium* is an essential diagnostic tool in areas endemic for schistosomiasis.

Further reading

Aspevall O, Hallander H, Gant V, Kouri T. European guidelines for urinalysis: a collaborative document produced by European clinical microbiologists and clinical chemists under ECLM in collaboration with ESCMID. *Clin Microbiol Infect* 2001; **7**: 173–178.

D'Amico G, Bazzi C. Urinary protein and enzyme excretion as markers of tubular damage. *Curr Opin Nephrol Hypertens* 2003; **12**: 639–643.

Fogazzi GB, Ponticelli C, Ritz E. *The urinary sediment. An integrated view*, 2nd edn. Oxford: Oxford University Press; 1999.

Fogazzi GB, Saglimbeni L, Banfi G, Cantu M, Moroni G, Garigali G, Cesana BM. Urinary sediment features in proliferative and non-proliferative glomerular diseases. *J Nephrol* 2005; **18**: 703–710.

Köhler H, Wandel E, Brunck B. Acanthocyturia – a characteristic marker for glomerular bleeding. *Kidney Int* 1991; **40**: 115–120.

See also

Clinical assessment of renal function, p. 12

Clinical assessment of renal function

Glomerular filtration rate (GFR)

Measurement of the GFR is considered the 'gold standard' measure of excretory renal function. It is difficult to measure in routine clinical practice and the most commonly used marker of kidney function is an estimated GFR (see below) which is reported automatically alongside the serum creatinine concentration (this is universal in UK laboratories).

GFR is the multiplication product of the average filtration rate of single nephrons and the total number of nephrons in both kidneys. The normal GFR level ranges from ~80 to 120 mL/min/1.73 m^2, with significant interindividual variation depending on many different factors, such as age, body size, physical activity and diet.

GFR also changes during pregnancy, increasing by ~50% in the first trimester and normalizing soon after delivery. After the fourth decade of life, GFR declines by ~0.75 mL/min/1.73 m^2 per year.

In an individual patient GFR is a relatively constant parameter. A reduction in GFR may result from a decline in the number of nephrons or from a decline in the GFR of single nephrons (SNGFR). As a reduction in the number of nephrons may be compensated by an increased SNGFR due to glomerular hypertrophy or elevated glomerular capillary pressure, early substantial kidney damage is not always associated with a decline in the GFR.

In patients who are at increased risk for chronic kidney disease (CKD), investigations should be made to detect albuminuria or a decrease in GFR. The GFR is also used as a parameter to stage the severity of CKD.

GFR measurement

Urinary clearance

Direct measurement of the GFR is not a routine clinical test and remains a research tool only. GFR can be determined from the urinary clearance of certain suitable marker substances.

In general, clearance of a substance is defined as the virtual volume of plasma cleared of this substance by excretion per unit of time. For a substance 'x' it is defined as:

$$C_x = A_x/P_x$$

where A_x is the amount of x eliminated from the plasma and P_x is the plasma concentration. The value reflects the efficacy of the elimination of a certain substance and is expressed in units of volume per time. It comprises both urinary and extrarenal excretion.

For the assessment of renal excretion, urinary clearance is determined. For a substance x it can be calculated as follows:

$$C_{U(x)} = (U_x \times V)/P_x$$

where U_x is the urinary concentration of x, V is the urinary flow rate and P_x is the plasma concentration of x.

It depends on glomerular filtration, tubular secretion and tubular reabsorption.

- The urinary clearance of a substance that is filtered, but neither secreted nor reabsorbed, equals GFR. Thus substances that fulfill these criteria constitute ideal markers for the measurement of GFR.
- Urinary clearance is larger than GFR for substances, which are both filtered and secreted.
- Urinary clearance is smaller than GFR for substances, which are filtered and reabsorbed.

Exogenous filtration markers

For the measurement of urinary clearance these substances have to be administered to the patient by infusion or injection.

Inulin (5.2 kDa) is a polymer of fructose, which meets the aforementioned criteria for ideal GFR markers, is nontoxic, and is not metabolized. It is therefore regarded as the gold standard marker, which can be used for the evaluation of other markers.

Since the protocol for the measurement of inulin clearance is labour intensive (requiring continuous infusion of the substance to generate a constant serum concentration and accurate assessment of urine flow with multiple urine collections) it cannot be used in clinical practice.

There are several other suitable exogenous marker substances, such as iohexol, [^{51}Cr]EDTA, [^{99m}Tc]DTPA and [^{125}I]iothalamate, but due to the complex measurement protocols GFR is commonly estimated using endogenous filtration markers.

Endogenous filtration markers

For the calculation of the urinary clearance of a substance according to the aforementioned equation, the determination of serum concentration and a timed urine collection are required. The results depend on a complete timed urine collection. In patients in whom the serum levels of the marker are not constant, the precision of the investigation can be increased by taking multiple blood samples to calculate the average serum concentration.

Creatinine

Creatinine is the most commonly used marker for the assessment of renal function.

- It derives from muscle catabolism, and meat or creatine intake, and hence varies according to body muscle mass and food intake.
- With a molecular weight of 113 Da it is freely filtered by the glomerulus. As it is additionally secreted by the tubules, creatinine clearance systemically overestimates the GFR, particularly in patients with impaired renal function.
- The serum creatinine concentration varies inversely with the GFR, but this relationship is not linear. Renal function may be significantly impaired before increased creatinine levels are measured. In patients with early renal dysfunction small changes in serum creatinine may reflect considerable diminutions of GFR. However, in advanced renal failure great changes in creatinine level reflect only small changes in GFR. Furthermore there is a great variability of GFR for a given serum creatinine concentration due to individual variation in muscle mass.
- To a negligible degree, creatinine is secreted by the intestine and can be degraded by bacteria. This extrarenal excretion is increased when the GFR is reduced. Antibiotics may inhibit this pathway due to elimination of the intestinal flora, and thereby increase serum creatinine levels.
- Several factors have been identified, which are associated with an increase or decrease in production and excretion of creatinine, and hence may affect the serum concentration (see Table 1.3.1).

Table 1.3.1 Extrarenal factors which may influence serum creatinine levels

Increase of serum creatinine	Decrease of serum creatinine
Increased production	**Reduced production**
Higher muscle mass due to physical exercise	Reduced muscle mass due to malnutrition or following amputation
Higher average muscle mass in African-Americans	Decline in muscle mass with age
Meat-rich diet	Lower muscle mass in females
	Vegetarian diet
Impaired tubular secretion	
Drugs, such as trimethoprim, cimetidine or certain fibrates	
Impaired intestinal elimination	
Destruction of the intestinal flora due to antibiotics	

Table 1.3.2 Interpretation of the fluid deprivation test

	Plasma osmolality	Urine osmolality	Urine osmolality after DDAVP
Primary polydipsia	<296 mOsmol/kg	>900 mOsmol/kg	no increase
Central diabetes insipidus	>296 mOsmol/kg	increase of <10 mOsmol/kg/h	increase of >10%
Nephrogenic diabetes insipidus	>296 mOsmol/kg	increase of <10 mOsmol/kg/h	no increase

- Creatinine measurement by the Jaffe reaction may produce falsely elevated values in the presence of acetoacetate due to diabetic ketoacidosis.

For the calculation of creatinine clearance (CrCl) the above-mentioned equation can be modified as follows:

$$C_{U(crea)} = (U_{crea} \times V)/(P_{crea} \times t)$$

where U_{crea} is the urinary creatinine concentration [mg/dL], V is the volume of collected urine [mL], P_{crea} is the plasma creatinine concentration [mg/dL] and t is the collection time [min].

Assuming a steady state with equal production and excretion of creatinine, GFR can also be estimated from serum levels using equations that incorporate additional demographic and clinical variables, such as age, sex, race and body size.

- The *Cockcroft–Gault formula* (see below) incorporates age, sex and body weight. In patients who are overweight and edematous this equation overestimates GFR, whereas it is probably underestimated in patients of African origin. As the formula estimates creatinine clearance there is a systematic overestimation of GFR.

$$CrCl \ [mL/min] = \frac{(140 - age) \times lean\ body\ weight\ [kg]}{(Creat\ [\mu mol/L]/88.4) \times 72}$$

For women multiply the result by 0.85.

- The *MDRD (Modification of Diet in Renal Disease) Study formula* incorporates a correction for race. The equation underestimates GFR in patients with high levels of GFR, e.g. people evaluated as kidney transplant donors. There are several population groups, for which the equation has not yet been validated, e.g. children, patients older than 70 years or pregnant women. The four-variable MDRD formula is:

GFR [mL/min/1.73 m^2] = 186 × (Creat [μmol/L]/88.4)$^{-1.154}$ × (age)$^{-0.203}$ × (0.742 if female) × (1.21 if Black).

- In some studies it has been shown that GFR estimation by using the MDRD Study formula is more precise than the Cockroft–Gault formula or measurement of creatinine clearance.
- As both equations assume a steady state, quick changes in GFR may cause incorrect results, thus overestimating a rapidly declining GFR and underestimating a rapidly rising one.
- It should be kept in mind that both formulae are not reliable for GFR values >60 mL/min/1.73 m^2.
- In patients with very high or low creatinine generation (see Table 1.3.1) both equations are of limited accuracy.
- There is considerable variability in measured serum creatinine levels between different laboratories. Therefore GFR estimations based on serum creatinine are not necessarily directly comparable, if they are obtained from different laboratories, unless a correction has been applied to allow for this variation (in the UK all laboratories report the four-variable MDRD eGFR appropriately corrected to allow for the different creatinine assays in use).

Urea

Urea is a 60 Da product that is derived from hepatic protein catabolism. It is freely filtered in the glomerulus and reabsorbed to a variable extent in the proximal and distal tubules. Its generation is increased in states of hyperalimentation, after the absorption of blood due to gastrointestinal hemorrhage or in catabolic situations due to infection or chemotherapy. Malnutrition or liver disease may result in decreased urea generation. A reduction in kidney perfusion may cause increased tubular reabsorption.

The variability in generation and reabsorption of urea mean that it is not of value for estimating GFR.

Cystatin C

Cystatin C is a 1300 Da protein produced by all nucleated human cells. It appears to be generated at a constant rate. It is freely filtered by the glomerulus and subsequently reabsorbed and degraded in the tubular epithelial cells. Therefore urinary excretion is minimal. Thus it is not possible to measure a urinary clearance for cystatin C.

Normal serum levels range from 0.54 to 1.55 mg/L with a constant concentration from the age of ~1–50 years. Furthermore the levels are not influenced by muscle mass, gender or body height. After the seventh decade cystatin C levels increase, possibly due to the decline in GFR in older people.

It has been shown that in patients with acute renal failure increased cystatin C levels can be detected prior to an increase in serum creatinine. Compared to serum creatinine, cystatin C seems to be a better marker for GFR, but in comparison to estimations based on creatinine no significant superiority of cystatin C has been shown and its measurement is considerably more costly. As further research and standardization of the laboratory assay is required, the measurement of cystatin C in everyday clinical practice is not currently recommended.

Markers of tubular damage
The urinary excretion of certain proteins is associated with tubular disorders. A variety of such substances have been identified, but only some of them have so far made their way into clinical practice.

Low molecular weight proteins
These proteins are freely filtered by the glomerulus. In healthy individuals they are reabsorbed by the proximal tubule. The urinary excretion of these substances increases in cases of impaired proximal tubular reabsorption.

- α1-Microglobulin (33 kDa) is a glycosylated protein originating from the liver, which is stable in urine and therefore suitable for measurement in clinical practice. In patients with chronic glomerulonephritis the measurement may allow prediction about the outcome of the disease, as in these cases the level of urinary loss is proportional to the severity of tubulointerstitial damage.
- β2-Microglobulin (11.8 kDa) constitutes the light chain of class I major histocompatibility antigens. It is unstable in acidic urine (pH <6.0) and hence bicarbonate needs to be administered to the patient for it to be measured.
- Retinol-binding protein (21 kDa) binds retinol circulating in the plasma and also appears to be a suitable marker for proximal tubular damage, since it is stable in urine.

N-Acetyl-β-glucosaminidase (NAG)
NAG is a hydrolytic enzyme with activity in the whole nephron, particularly in the proximal tubule. With a molecular weight of ~130 kDa it is not filtered by the glomerulus, so NAG measured in the urine mainly derives from the tubules.

Tubular damage, e.g. in tubulointerstitial nephritis or renal transplant rejection, results in an increase in urinary NAG excretion. The substance is commonly regarded as a marker for early drug nephrotoxicity. In patients with glomerular proteinuria, NAG may partially originate from the plasma.

Urine osmolality
The measurement of urine osmolality reveals information about the ability of the kidneys to adjust the urine concentration in response to water balance.

In patients with an osmolality of ≥800 mOsmol/kg in an early morning urine, a defect of renal concentrating ability is very unlikely.

For the further investigation of patients with unexplained polyuria a fluid deprivation test can be administered, after having excluded glucosuria or hypercalcemia as causes for increased diuresis.

After a period of thirst for ~12 h, urine osmolality normally rises to >1000 mosmol/kg and plasma osmolality is <295 mOsmol/kg. To prevent severe dehydration, regular measurements of urine excretion, urine osmolality and body weight are required during the test. At the end of the test period, plasma osmolality and sodium are also determined. Desmopressin (DDAVP) is then administered to the patient. The interpretation of the test is summarized in Table 1.3.2.

Further reading
D'Amico G, Bazzi C. Urinary protein and enzyme excretion as markers of tubular damage. *Curr Opin Nephrol Hypertens* 2003; **12**: 639–643.

Filler G, Bokenkamp A, Hofmann W, Le Bricon T, Martinez-Bru C, Grubb A. Cystatin C as a marker of GFR – history, indications, and future research. *Clin Biochem* 2005; **38**: 1–8.

K/DOQI clinical practice guidelines for chronic kidney disease: evaluation, classification, and stratification. *Am J Kidney Dis* 2002; **39**: 1–266.

Perrone RD, Madias NE, Levey AS. Serum creatinine as an index of renal function: new insights into old concepts. *Clin Chem* 1992; **38**: 1933–1953.

Rule AD, Larson TS, Bergstralh EJ, Slezak JM, Jacobsen SJ, Cosio FG. Using serum creatinine to estimate glomerular filtration rate: accuracy in good health and in chronic kidney disease. *Ann Intern Med* 2004; **141**: 929–937.

Stevens LA, Levey AS. Measurement of kidney function. *Med Clin North Am* 2005; **89**: 457–473.

See also
The aging kidney, p. 18

Urinalysis and microscopy, p. 8

Nephrogenic diabetes insipidus, p. 220

Renal function in the newborn infant

The neonatal kidney can adapt to the usual physiological processes occurring after birth. It is less able to adapt to endogenous and exogenous stress such as hypotension, hypoxia and fluid overload and this is more pronounced in the more immature infants. The understanding of renal function in the neonate will aid the clinician in the appropriate management of fluid, electrolytes, nutrition and acid–base in either the sick or preterm neonate. It helps in the interpretation of biochemical investigations and drug handling in the neonate. Normative biochemical data for newborn infants are listed in Table 1.4.1.

Table 1.4.1 Normative biochemical data for newborn infants

	Age	Reference range
Serum		
Bicarbonate	<1 month	17–26 mmol/L
Base excess	Newborn	−10 to −2 mmol/L
Calcium (total)	Premature	1.5–2.5 mmol/L
	≤2 weeks	1.9–2.8 mmol/L
Phosphate	1 month	1.4–2.8 mmol/L
Potassium	1 month	3.5–6.0 mmol/L
Sodium	<1 month	130–145 mmol/L
Creatinine	1 week	40–125 µmol/L
	2 weeks	35–105 µmol/L
	3 weeks	25–90 µmol/L
	4 weeks	20–80 µmol/L
GFR	1 week	26–60 mL/min/1.73 m^2
	1 month	28–68 mL/min/1.73 m^2
Urine		
Maximal osmolality	1–14 days	210–650 mosm/kg
	2–4 weeks	780–1100 mosm/kg

Water homeostasis

In early postnatal life there is a reduction in total body water, extracellular water, and extracellular sodium (Na^+) and chloride (Cl^-). There is an increase in intracellular water and its main components protein, magnesium and potassium (K^+).

Total body water as a percentage of body weight is ~75% and the extracellular fluid (ECF) is 35–40% of total body water.

The reduction in total body water is reflected in the weight loss observed in early postnatal life. This is greater in low birth weight premature infants where a weight loss of up to 10% can occur.

Fluid prescriptions need to be adjusted for increased insensible water loss because of:
• increased relative body surface area;
• increased metabolic rate;
• increased transepidermal water loss, particularly in the premature infant exposed to phototherapy and overhead heaters.

Sodium homeostasis

Neonates have a limited capacity to excrete a Na^+ load or to conserve Na^+ if there is Na^+ restriction. In the first week of life fractional Na^+ excretion is high and this is greater in the more immature neonates.

Early hyponatremia (occurring shortly after birth) can be caused by:
• excessive fluid given to the mother;
• release of antidiuretic hormone secondary to neonatal pathology such as asphyxia;
• inadequate Na^+ content of feed/fluid.

Late hyponatremia can be caused by:
• inadequate Na^+ content of feed/fluid;
• deranged renal tubular function;
• Na^+ losses from the gastrointestinal tract.

Prolonged hyponatremia is associated with a reduction in brain function and growth.

Hypernatremia can be caused by:
• sodium bicarbonate infusions for acidosis;
• insufficient free water administration when insensible water losses are high.

Hypernatremia induces a fluid shift from the intracellular compartment causing cell shrinkage and tearing of the cerebral capillaries. This mechanism reduces the physiologic contraction of the ECF, increasing the risk of patent ductus arteriosus, cardiac failure, bronchopulmonary dysplasia and intracranial hemorrhage.

Potassium homeostasis

In the neonate the rate of K^+ excretion is low. This reduction in K^+ excretion is partly explained by the low activity of the Na^+K^+-ATPase in the K^+ secreting epithelium, and a reduction in the number of K^+ channels.

Plasma K^+ in term infants falls in the first week of life. In preterm infants plasma K^+ reaches its maximum in the 3rd or 4th week of life as a result of metabolic acidosis, oliguric renal failure and catabolic activity.

Acid–base balance

Following birth, neonates have a mixed respiratory/metabolic acidosis as a result of changes in the cardiopulmonary circulation and the effects of the birthing process. Later they develop a self-limited metabolic acidosis which is influenced by the protein load, weight gain, ability of the renal tubules to excrete an acid load, and the renal threshold for bicarbonate reabsorption. This has usually resolved by the end of the fourth week.

Glomerular filtration rate

The glomerular filtration rate is low after birth and is closely correlated to gestational age. It is ~5 mL/m^2 in neonates of 28 weeks gestation and 12 mL/m^2 in term infants. Postnatally there is a rapid increase in GFR with a two-fold increase in GFR occurring in the first 2 weeks of life. Adult values are achieved between 1 and 2 years of age. Factors involved in the maturation of GFR include:
• increase in renal blood flow as a consequence of an increase in BP and a fall in intravascular resistance;

- increase in the number of superficial nephrons involved in filtration;
- increase in the surface area of the glomerular basement membrane.

Creatinine is usually used as a measure of renal function as [^{51}Cr]EDTA GFR measurements are invasive and expensive. This may underestimate GFR if the patient has a high bilirubin level and the analyzer does not correct for noncreatinine cromogens.

Creatinine in the first few days after birth is a measurement of maternal plasma creatinine.

Plasma creatinine is usually higher in more immature infants and does not fall steadily from birth, but rises in the first few days of life, reaching a peak and then falling to reach an equilibrium level. In more immature infants the rise in creatinine is higher and the decrease is much slower. This trend is the result of slower maturation of glomerular function and increased tubular reabsorption and may not indicate renal insufficiency.

The Schwartz formula (eGFR = $\kappa \times$ height/creatinine) can be used to estimate GFR once the plasma creatinine has stabilised with the constant $k = 33$ for full term infants and 24 for low birth weight infants.

Tubular function

Neonates have a lower urinary concentrating capacity but an obligatory water loss even when water-depleted. Normal urinary volume is 1–3 mL/kg/h and it is usually dilute.

Urinary concentrating ability matures rapidly after birth and by 8 weeks of age maximal urine osmolality is 1000–1200 mosm/kg H$_2$O.

Glycosuria is common in neonates and is greatest in preterm infants.

Urinary amino acid loss is higher in the neonate as a result of reduced tubular reabsorption. The maturity of renal reabsorption varies between different amino acids and these factors need to be considered when intrepreting urinary amino acid profiles for metabolic conditions.

Urinalysis may be positive for protein and does not always indicate renal disease. This decreases with increasing maturity and by 2 weeks of life is usually <50 mg/L.

Fractional reabsorption of phosphate is greater in the neonate to allow bone accretion of phosphate. Neonates have a lower ability to secrete anions and this is more pronounced in the preterm infant. Drugs used in the neonate that are organic anions include folic acid, benzylpenicillin, methotrexate and phenobarbitone.

Timed urines to measure tubular function require urethral catheterization and are not practical for routine use.

Spot urines to look at tubular function expressed as a ratio of creatinine are also unreliable because of the variation in urinary creatinine and the unreliable normative data.

Renin–angiotensin system

Renal renin activity is higher in the neonate than in the adult and falls after birth reaching adult levels between ages 6 and 9 years. Neonates have a highly activated renin–angiotensin–aldosterone system but the decline in plasma Na$^+$ and rise in plasma K$^+$ reflect a relative unresponsiveness to aldosterone.

The location of angiotensin receptors within the kidney changes during development and the observation that the use of angiotensin-II receptor blockers and angiotensin-converting enzyme inhibitors in the mother cause renal dysplasia in the neonate indicates that the renin–angiotensin system has a role in nephrogenesis.

Neonatal renal handling of drugs

Listed below are a few pharmacologic agents commonly used in the neonate.

Furosemide

Furosemide is excreted by both glomerular filtration and secretion in the tubules by an organic acid tubular transport mechanism. These mechanisms are both immature and reduced in the neonatal kidney. The half-life of furosemide may be >24 h in the neonate and therefore if given more frequently it will accumulate in the plasma and exceed the threshold for ototoxicity.

Indomethacin

Indomethacin is typically used in preterm infants to close the ductus arteriosus. Indomethacin inhibits prostaglandin synthesis and consequently reduces renal perfusion and induces acute renal failure in approximately a quarter of neonates <30 weeks gestation. These effects are usually transient and reverse after the drug has been stopped. This effect is also observed with ibuprofen.

Severe and irreversible renal insufficiency has been reported in neonates after prenatal exposure to NSAIDs.

Contrast agents

Hypertonic radiographic contrast material is associated with renal artery thrombosis, medullary necrosis and ischemia. These high osmolar agents increase plasma osmolality and may also cause intravascular hemorrhage. The risk of nephrogenic systemic fibrosis (nephrogenic fibrosing dermopathy) following the use of gadolinium-containing contrast agents in neonates with borderline renal function has not been quantified.

Aminoglycosides

Aminoglycosides are eliminated by glomerular filtration and therefore the dose needs to be adjusted with increasing conceptional age. Changes in tubular and glomerular function as a result of aminoglycoside nephrotoxicity are usually reversible.

Further reading

Arant BS. Developmental patterns of renal functional maturation compared in the human neonate. *J Pediatr* 1978; **92**: 705–712.

Brion LP, Fleischman AR, McCarron C, Schwartz GJ. A simple estimate of glomerular filtration rate in low birth weight infants during the first year of life: non-invasive assessments of body composition and growth. *J Pediatr* 1986; **109**: 698–707.

Guignard JP, Drukker A. Why do newborn infants have a high plasma creatinine? *Pediatrics* 1999;**103**:e49–52.

Guignard JP, Torrado A, Cunha OD, Gautier E. Glomerular filtration rate in the first three weeks of life. *J Pediatr* 1975; **87**: 268–272.

Karlsson FA, Hardell LI, Hellsing K. A prospective study of urinary proteins in early infancy. *Acta Paediatr Scand* 1979; **68**: 663–667.

Schwartz GJ, Feld LG, Langdorf DJ. A simple estimate of glomerular filtration rate in full-term infants during the first year of life. *J Pediatr* 1984; **104**: 849–854

Simmons MA, Adock EW, Bard H. Hypernatraemia and intracranial haemorrhage in neonates. *N Engl J Med* 1974; **291**: 6–10.

The aging kidney

Aging is a physiological process which incorporates degenerative changes in many organs. The involvement of the kidney is accompanied by a decrease in renal function associated with certain structural and functional alterations. A wide variety of mechanisms promoting renal change with age have been proposed, such as elevated angiotensin II levels, reduced nitric oxide production by endothelial cells or chronic hyperuricemia (see Table 1.5.1).

Structural changes

The maximum size of the kidneys is reached at the age of ~40 years, followed by a decrease of ~10% per decade. In males this trend seems to be greater than in females. The renal cortex becomes thinner and the number of nephrons declines.

Some anatomical alterations that affect the glomeruli can be identified.

- The preserved glomeruli often hypertrophy.
- There is a thickening of the glomerular basement membrane.
- Focal and segmental glomerulosclerosis can be found affecting an increasing number of glomeruli. This is associated with the expansion of the mesangial matrix and a loss of capillary loops.

Both tubules and interstitium also undergo structural changes.

- Tubular dilatation and atrophy particularly appear in the outer medulla.
- Interstitial fibrosis occurs due to collagen deposition and is accompanied by interstitial infiltration of macrophages and myofibroblasts.
- Small tubular diverticuli may be detectable, which possibly promote the development of recurrent pyelonephritis by constituting reservoirs for bacteria.

Furthermore several vascular changes occur with aging.

- In patients with hypertension thickening of the arterioles can frequently be seen. Arteriolar hyalinosis is typical for elderly people.
- The development of vascular shunts from afferent to efferent arterioles may result in bypassing of glomeruli.

Functional changes

Glomerular filtration rate (GFR)

In elderly patients serum creatinine is of limited use as a marker of renal function, because of a reduction in muscle mass with aging. Whereas normal daily creatinine excretion is 20–25 mg/kg body weight for males and 15–20 mg/kg body weight for females, this value progressively declines after the 6th decade of life. In spite of a decrease in creatinine clearance the serum level of creatinine may remain stable due to reduced muscle mass. Both the MDRD equation and Cockcroft–Gault formula underestimate GFR in patients aged >65 years.

With advancing age there may be a reduction in the so-called renal reserve, which describes the ability of the kidneys to increase GFR following a protein load or food intake.

Renal plasma flow (RPF)

There is a decrease in RPF with age, measured by para-aminohippurate clearance, from ~650 mL/min in the 4th decade to ~300 mL/min in the 9th decade. This decrease is greater for the renal cortex than for the medulla.

Capillary permeability

In elderly people a higher prevalence of microalbuminuria and albuminuria has been detected. Microalbuminuria is regarded as an independent risk factor for cardiovascular events.

Electrolyte problems

Sodium. In aging there is impaired sodium excretion following a salt load, and the ability to conserve salt during sodium restriction is also reduced. In developed countries very sodium-rich diets are common, leading to the risk of sodium excess in elderly people.

The trend to increased total body sodium may promote the development of hypertension with aging, in addition to other factors, such as endothelial dysfunction. This might explain why, in most elderly patients, sodium restriction results in a significant fall in blood pressure.

Potassium. As a result of impaired potassium excretion and reduced aldosterone levels elderly people are more likely develop hyperkalemia than younger subjects.

Impaired distal tubular acidification in elderly patients contributes to the tendency to develop acid–base disturbances.

Water balance

In older patients urine-concentrating and -diluting abilities are impaired. There may be a predisposition to develop dehydration, due to production of urine with an inappropriately reduced urine osmolality and a weaker thirst response to an increasing plasma osmolality. As excretion following a water load also is impaired, there may be a tendency to hyponatremia.

Clinical implications

The treatment of elderly patients requires some general considerations.

- The fluid, electrolyte and acid–base balances of elderly patients are more likely to become abnormal in response to disease. In particular this must be taken into consideration in, for example, patients with diarrhea, those receiving intravenous fluids or those suffering from hypoxemia.
- Due to comorbidity, renal disease in elderly patients is often the result of more than one pathology. For example diabetic or hypertensive nephropathy often coexists with other lesions such as glomerulonephritis.
- The prevalence of many diseases differs between young and old people. This must be considered when establishing a diagnosis. Table 1.5.2 provides examples for diseases, which exhibit significant differences in prevalence with aging.
- The clinical manifestations of certain diseases may be atypical compared to younger patients. For example a considerable number of elderly patients with IgA nephropathy present with acute renal failure, whereas this is less common in younger patients.
- Older persons are more prone to the nephrotoxic effects of many drugs, such as NSAIDs, aminoglycosides, COX-2 inhibitors and chemotherapy.
- The incidence and prevalence of end-stage renal disease is higher for elderly people.

Table 1.5.1 Possible mechanisms causing renal affects of aging

Free oxygen-derived radicals	Cumulative injury to all kinds of tissue over time
Telomere shortening of chromosomal DNA	General senescence due to impaired replication capacity
Decrease in the number of glomeruli	Hypertrophy of remaining glomeruli due to hyperfiltration, subsequent scarring
Intrarenal activation of the renin–angiotensin system	Glomerular hypertension, nonhemodynamic effects (podocyte injury)
Endothelial dysfunction	Impaired renal autoregulation and ischemia due to reduced nitric oxide production
Renal overexpression of transforming growth factor-β	Mediation of renal fibrosis
Chronic hyperuricemia	Inhibition of nitric oxide availability, activation of the renin–angiotensin system

Table 1.5.2 Diseases more/less frequent with aging

Increase in incidence with aging
  Membranous glomerulonephritis
  Malignancy-associated glomerular disease
  Acute renal failure (e.g. following cardiovascular surgery)
  Acute-on-chronic renal failure
  Renovascular disease
  Urinary calculi
  Malignancies of the urinary tract
  Obstructive uropathy
  Urinary incontinence

Decrease in incidence with aging
  Systemic lupus erythematosus
  Wegener's granulomatosis

Further reading

Epstein M. Aging and the kidney. *J Am Soc Nephrol* 1996; **7**: 1106–1122.

Fliser D, Franek E, Joest M, Block S, Mutschler E, Ritz E. Renal function in the elderly: impact of hypertension and cardiac function. *Kidney Int* 1997; **51**: 1196–1204.

Lindeman, RD, Goldman R. Anatomic and physiologic age changes in the kidney. *Exp Gerontol* 1986; **21**: 379–406.

See also

Clinical assessment of renal function, p. 12

Imaging in renal disease

Imaging of the renal tract has changed dramatically over recent years with advances in the technology of all imaging modalities.

The basic underlying principle of renal imaging remains obtaining the diagnosis by the quickest and safest route possible.

Plain X-ray KUB (kidney, ureters, bladder)

This is a plain radiograph of the abdomen, centered on the umbilicus, that includes the upper poles of the kidneys and the pubic symphysis (Fig. 1.6.1).

It provides only limited information.

The main value of plain radiography is:

● Identification of calcification and its relationship to the renal tract. Approximately 85% of renal calculi are radio-opaque.
● Assessment of the renal outlines which can be identified due to the contrasting density of the kidneys with the perirenal fat. This may be difficult due to overlying bowel gas obscuring the outlines.
● Identification of bone abnormalities that may be associated with renal tract disease, e.g. renal osteodystrophy, and sclerotic bone metastases in prostate cancer.

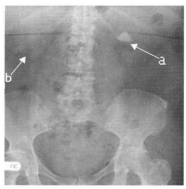

Fig. 1.6.1 Plain X-ray in renal tract disease. Plain X-ray showing (a) a triangular calculus overlying the pelvis of the left kidney, and (b) renal outline.

Ultrasound scanning (USS)

Ultrasound is the first-line investigation for most renal diseases (Fig. 1.6.2).

It is relatively quick to perform, requires minimal patient preparation, and does not involve the use of ionizing radiation or contrast agents.

However, it is operator dependent, gives no functional information, and offers little in the assessment of pelviureteric abnormalities.

Indications for USS in native kidneys

To assess the size and position of the kidneys.

● The normal renal size range is 9.0–12 cm and cortical thickness is normally >1.5 cm.
● USS gives very good anatomical detail. The demonstration of small shrunken kidneys implies advanced CKD.

The causes of abnormally sized kidneys are listed in Table 1.6.1.

To look for renal cortical scarring.

To demonstrate interstitial renal disease.

● As the severity of intrinsic renal disease increases, the echogenicity of the kidneys tends also to increase.

To demonstrate and characterize renal masses.

● Cystic lesions: simple cysts are anechoic; complex cysts may contain multiple internal septae and abnormal soft tissue.
● Solid lesions: renal tumors cannot be characterized further except for angiomyolipomas which are increased in echogenicity due to the fat content. CT or MRI is required for further evaluation.
● Although CT is used for the staging of renal tumors, USS may be used to demonstrate metastases in the liver, enlarged retroperitoneal lymph nodes and tumor thrombus in the renal veins.

Table 1.6.1 Causes of abnormally sized kidneys

Large kidneys	
Bilateral	*Unilateral*
Polycystic kidney disease	Compensatory hypertrophy
Infiltration (lymphoma, oedema)	Hydronephrosis
HIV-associated nephropathy	Renal vein thrombosis
Renal vein thrombosis	Tumor
	Cysts
Small kidneys	
Bilateral	*Unilateral*
Congenital hypoplasia/dysplasia	Congenital hypoplasia/dysplasia
Renal artery stenosis	Renal artery stenosis
Chronic intrinsic renal disease (glomerulonephritis, interstitial nephritis)	Chronic intrinsic renal disease (glomerulonephritis, interstitial nephritis)
Reflux nephropathy	Reflux nephropathy
Renal tuberculosis	Renal tuberculosis

Ultrasound is poor at demonstrating transitional cell carcinomas of the kidney as they merge into the fat of the renal sinus. These may, however, be identified because of secondary effects of the tumor, e.g. obstruction, especially in high risk patients.

● To demonstrate bladder abnormalities.
  Bladder tumors may be diagnosed on USS but cystoscopy remains the gold standard for diagnosis. USS is also useful for the assessment of bladder emptying.
● To provide evidence of renal tract obstruction. Obstruction rarely occurs without dilatation of the collecting system but dilatation may occur without obstruction. The level and cause of the obstruction may also be identified on USS.
● To demonstrate renal calcification.
  Calcification including calculi can be demonstrated but the sensitivity is dependent on the size of the stone. Other techniques (e.g. CT scanning) are more sensitive.

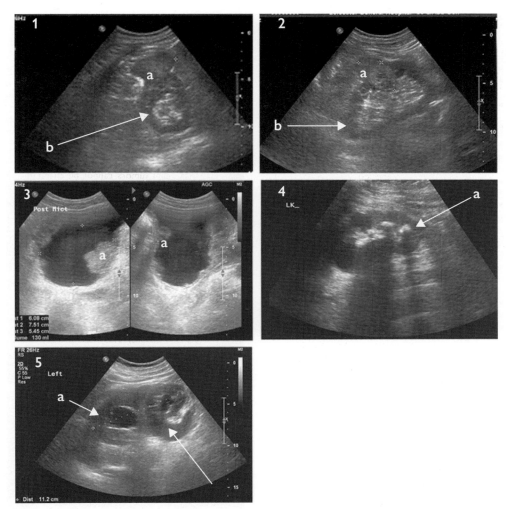

Fig. 1.6.2 Ultrasound in renal tract disease. 1. Transverse image of kidney showing (a) a renal tumor, and (b) the kidney. 2. Longitudinal image of kidney showing (a) a renal tumor, and (b) the kidney. 3. Longitudinal and transverse images of bladder showing (a) bladder tumors. 4. Longitudinal image of kidney showing (a) a collection of calculi. 5. Longitudinal image of kidney showing hydronephrosis. (a) Renal parenchyma and (b) dilated pelvis.

Indications for USS in renal transplants

Renal transplants are very amenable to ultrasound scanning because:

- there is little respiratory movement;
- the renal artery is well positioned for accurate assessment of flow velocities to investigate renal artery stenosis.

Doppler ultrasound is valuable in the assessment of the patency of the renal vessels and overall flow velocity.

Measurement of the resistive index (RI), which is an indication of the resistance to arterial flow in the renal vascular bed, is useful in the assessment of graft dysfunction.

$$RI = \frac{(\text{peak systolic velocity} - \text{end diastolic velocity})}{\text{peak systolic velocity}}$$

RI of up to 0.8 is normal. A value above this indicates graft dysfunction, but this is a nonspecific finding and does not differentiate between the different causes of graft dysfunction.

Minimal dilatation of the collecting system in renal transplants is normal. Care must therefore be taken to differentiate dilatation due to reflux from that due to obstruction.

Ultrasound is also useful in identifying perinephric collections that may subsequently be drained percutaneously.

Intravenous urography (IVU)

The role of IVU in renal imaging is declining as other modalities take its place.

Indications
- Can provide good anatomical detail of the urinary tract.
- Useful particularly for the diagnosis of conditions involving the urothelium.
- Effective in the evaluation of patients with ureteral colic but this role has been superseded by CT (Fig. 1.6.3).

Disadvantages
- Involves the use of iodinated contrast media.
- Involves a radiation dose.
- May fail to identify some calculi.
- Masses, especially those lying anteriorly or posteriorly, may be missed.
- Unable to differentiate solid from cystic masses.

Procedure

After a plain KUB radiograph is performed, iodinated contrast medium is injected IV. As the contrast is excreted, a series of images of the abdomen are taken:

5 min post injection: an X-ray of the renal area is obtained to visualize the renal parenchyma (nephrogram). Delayed nephrograms may be seen with:
- obstruction;
- ATN;
- reduced renal perfusion;
- renal vein thrombosis.

Renal scars may also be identified.

Abdominal compression is then applied to impede the passage of contrast into the bladder.

15 min post injection: an X-ray of the renal area is obtained to visualize the calyces, pelves, and proximal ureters (pyelograms).

Immediately after abdominal compression is released, a radiograph is obtained to visualize the ureters and the bladder.

The study is completed by obtaining a post-void radiograph.

Other contrast radiography

Retrograde pyelography

This is the visualization of the ureter and pelvicalyceal system using a direct retrograde injection of contrast medium introduced via a catheter placed in the ureter during cystoscopy.

Indications
- To investigate possible transitional cell carcinoma in the ureters or renal pelvis, when other imaging modalities either have failed to identify a lesion, or are contraindicated.
- To further evaluate defects seen on other investigations.

Advantages
- Provides excellent anatomical detail of the ureters and collecting system.

Disadvantages
- Invasive, requiring a catheter to be placed up the ureter and into the collecting system.
- Requires iodinated contrast. However, the contrast is extravascular unless extravasation occurs.
- Requires radiation.

- May cause ureteric trauma with perforation and/or stricture formation.
- Infection may be introduced into the upper urinary tract.

Antegrade pyelography

This is the visualization of the upper urinary tract by direct injection of contrast media into the renal pelvis. This is rarely done apart from as a prelude to an interventional procedure.

The renal pelvis or preferably a calyx is percutaneously punctured using a narrow gauge needle under USS or fluoroscopic (after an IV injection of contrast media) guidance.

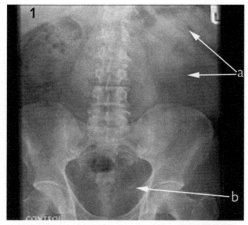
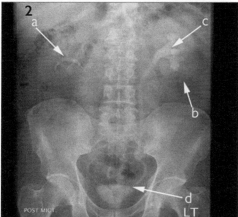

Fig. 1.6.3 Intravenous urography. 1. Control image showing (a) outline of left kidney and (b) a small opacity in the left side of the pelvis. 2. Postmicturition image showing (a) a normal right collecting system, (b) a dense nephrogram on the left, (c) a dilated pelvicalyceal system on the left, and (d) a dilated ureter down to the level of the opacity demonstrated in image 1.

Indications
- To identify the cause of upper tract obstruction when IV urography/CT urography or retrograde pyelography is unsatisfactory or cannot be undertaken.

- To determine in a renal transplant whether a dilated collecting system represents obstruction in the face of deteriorating function.
- It is part of upper tract urodynamic testing (Whitaker test).

Disadvantages
- Relative contra-indications are an uncorrected bleeding diathesis, cutaneous infection, or anatomy that precludes safe renal puncture.
- Can be complicated by puncture of adjacent structures (renal vein, liver, spleen, colon) although these are rarely significant given the small needle size.
- In an obstructed system some contrast extravasation may occur post procedure.
- It is time-consuming and may be unsuccessful if the collecting system is nondilated.

Cystography
Contrast is introduced via a bladder catheter to fill up the bladder and X-ray images are then taken of the bladder (Fig. 1.6.4).

The patient can then be asked to micturate to obtain further information (micturating cystography).

Indications
Cystography is used to demonstrate:
- bladder anatomy;
- urinary leaks (which are usually iatrogenic);
- vesico-enteric fistulae;
- ureteric reflux;
- urethral anatomy.

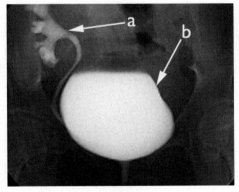

Fig. 1.6.4 Cystogram. (a) Bladder, and (b) urinary reflux into the collecting system of a transplant kidney.

Ascending urethrography
Contrast is introduced into the urethra through a narrow-bore catheter and X-ray images are obtained (Fig. 1.6.5).

It provides good anatomical detail of the urethra and can be performed by ultrasound or fluoroscopy.

Indications
- Following trauma it is used to demonstrate continuity of the urethra and urethral leaks.
- To evaluate penile strictures prior to intervention.

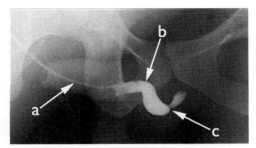

Fig. 1.6.5 Urethrogram. (a) Catheter, (b) penile urethra, and (c) a stricture in the membranous urethra.

Computed tomography
CT without contrast enhancement
This is now the gold standard for the diagnosis of renal calculi especially in the setting of acute ureteral colic (Fig. 1.6.6).

Noncontrasted CT has a sensitivity and specificity of >95% for the detection of stone disease.

Contrast is not usually required since almost all calculi, even those traditionally considered radiolucent on plain imaging, are seen as high density structures (the only exception is stones caused by indinavir sulphate). Contrast may be required to differentiate phleboliths from calculi in the pelvis.

It involves a significant radiation dose especially in those patients requiring repeated examinations.

In up to 30% of cases another cause for flank or abdominal pain may be demonstrated.

The site of renal tract obstruction can be determined.

Primary signs of stone disease
- Calculus within the ureteric lumen.

Secondary signs of stone disease
- Hydronephrosis.
- Perinephric or periureteric stranding.
- Ureteric dilatation.
- Blurring of the sinus fat.
- Enlarged kidney.

CT with intravenous contrast enhancement
Scanning is performed after the intravenous injection of contrast media (Fig. 1.6.6). The acquisition of images at different times after injection provides additional information:

Arterial: This is used to image renal arteries primarily for evidence of renal artery stenosis. To optimize the visualization of the arteries, bolus tracking is done first so that the scan can be performed at the time of peak enhancement of the aorta.

Corticomedullary phase: 25–80 s post injection. During this phase the cortex is enhanced while the (hypovascular) medulla remains relatively unenhanced. It is useful for evaluating the vascularity of tumors and inflammatory lesions. Hypovascular medullary tumors or hypervascular cortical tumors may, however, be missed during this phase.

Nephrographic phase: 85–100 s post injection. The renal parenchyma should appear homogeneous during this phase. This is the best phase for detecting and evaluating renal lesions.

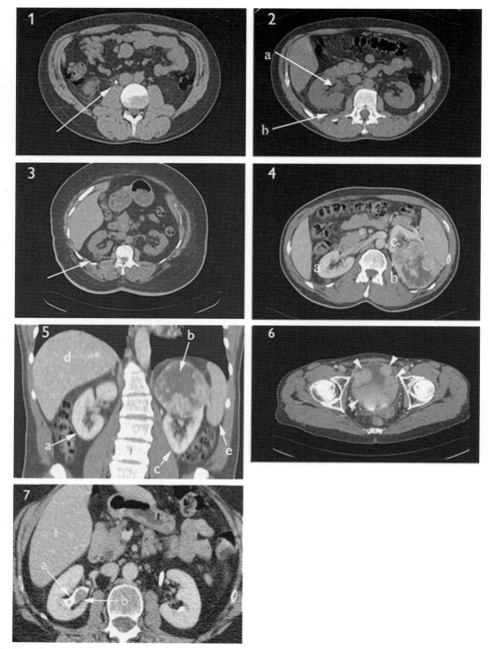

Fig. 1.6.6 CT scanning in renal disease. 1. Abdominal CT scan without contrast showing a calculus in the mid-ureter with stranding around it (arrow). 2. CT scan without contrast showing (a) a dilated pelvis and (b) peri-renal stranding. 3. CT scan without contrast demonstrating a small solid lesion (arrow) containing fat (low attenuation), therefore most likely to be an angiomyolipoma. 4. CT scan with contrast demonstrating (a) a normal right kidney, (b) a left renal tumor, and (c) remaining normal renal parenchyma on the left. 5. Reconstructed CT scan with contrast demonstrating (a) a normal right kidney, (b) a renal tumor in the left upper pole, (c) normal lower pole of the left kidney, (d) normal liver, and (e) spleen. 6. CT scan demonstrating multiple bladder tumors (arrowheads). 7. CT urogram demonstrating (a) contrast in the right collecting system, and (b) a filling defect in the collecting system consistent with a transitional cell carcinoma.

Excretory phase: 3–5 min post injection. The collecting system is enhanced and this is primarily useful in detecting urothelial lesions (see 'CT urography' below).

Indications

- To stage urogenital cancers: may be used in conjunction with MRI.
- To demonstrate obstruction, the level of obstruction, and its cause. If contrast is given, calculi may be more difficult to identify.
- To demonstrate collections associated with the renal tract, e.g. perinephric collections.
- To demonstrate soft tissue abnormalities related to the renal tract, e.g. retroperitoneal fibrosis.
- To demonstrate mass lesions in the renal tract.
- To differentiate cystic from solid tumors.
- To characterize the vast majority of angiomyolipomas so that they do not require tissue confirmation.
- To aid in the diagnosis of infection, including tuberculosis.
- To evaluate the renal tract after trauma to demonstrate:
  - the anatomy of the renal tract and any pre-existing anomalies;
  - the type and severity of parenchymal injury;
  - the extent of perinephric hemorrhage;
  - urinary extravasation/leaks;
  - injuries to the vascular pedicle.

CT urography

The patient first undergoes a noncontrast enhanced scan to exclude calcification.

This is followed by an arterial phase scan to demonstrate enhancing tumors including transitional cell carcinomas.

A final scan is undertaken 5–7 min after the IV injection of contrast media, by which time contrast has accumulated in the collecting system (Fig. 1.6.6).

It is undertaken mainly to diagnose congenital abnormalities of the urinary tract, and to detect and evaluate urothelial lesions (e.g. transitional cell carcinomas).

Magnetic resonance imaging

Indications

- To characterize renal mass lesions (Fig. 1.6.7). Noncontrasted and gadolinium-enhanced T1-weighted scans are undertaken during the phases described under contrasted CT.
- To stage bladder and prostate carcinomas.
- To assess tumor thrombus in renal tumors.

MRI does not require iodinated contrast media but the risk of nephrogenic systemic fibrosis if gadolinium-based MR contrast agents are used in patients with reduced GFR must be considered.

There is no cross-sensitivity between iodinated contrast agents and MR contrast agents. The risk of anaphylaxis with MR contrast agents is ~0.04%.

MRI may be used in early pregnancy.

MR angiography

This is an effective and noninvasive method to evaluate renovascular disease in native kidneys (Fig. 1.6.7).

For the diagnosis of renal artery stenosis the sensitivity is >93% and the specificity >83%.

No radiation is required.

Nephrotoxic contrast agents are avoided. The risk of nephrogenic systemic fibrosis needs to be considered in those with impaired renal function.

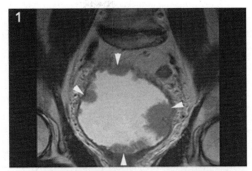

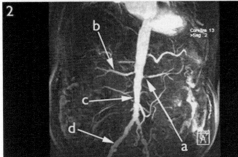

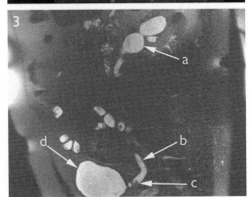

Fig. 1.6.7 MRI of the renal tract. 1. MRI demonstrating multiple bladder tumors (arrowheads). 2. MR angiography demonstrating (a) left ostial renal artery stenosis, (b) normal right renal artery, (c) aorta, and (d) iliac artery. 3. MR urogram demonstrating (a) left hydronephrosis, (b) dilated left ureter, (c) a ureteric filling defect, and (d) the bladder.

MR urography

This can be an effective method for imaging the urinary tract (Fig. 1.6.7). It provides good anatomical detail but the resolution is not as good as CT.

It can be undertaken in two ways:

- Heavily T2-weighted image acquisition provides good detail of static fluid in the collecting system, particularly when it is obstructed and dilated. IV contrast is not required, therefore this method is useful even in the absence of urine production.

- T1-weighted images can be obtained during the excretory phase following IV gadolinium injection. This is analogous to CT urography.

Nuclear medicine

Nuclear medicine techniques can provide both functional and structural information in the investigation of renal disease.

There are broadly three types of nuclear medicine study:

- GFR estimation (this is discussed in Chapter 1.3).
- Dynamic: serial scans are obtained to determine uptake, transit and excretion of the tracer.
- Static: tracer is taken up and retained in the kidney. Scanning is performed in multiple projections to identify structural abnormalities.

The four most widely used radiopharmaceuticals are:

- [51Cr]Ethylenediamine tetra-acetic acid ([51Cr]EDTA). It is excreted exclusively by glomerular filtration and is used for the accurate estimation of GFR. It is not used for imaging.
- [99mTc]Diethylenetriamine penta-acetic acid ([99mTc]DTPA). Again this is excreted by glomerular filtration. It is used in dynamic imaging studies. This has fallen out of favor and is being replaced by [99mTc]MAG3.
- [99mTc]Mercaptoacetyltriglycine ([99mTc]MAG3). This is excreted by tubular secretion. It is used in dynamic studies and produces better scintigraphic images than [99mTc]DTPA, particularly when the GFR is reduced.
- [99mTc]Dimercaptosuccinic acid ([99mTc]DMSA). This compound becomes retained and concentrated in the renal cortex and is therefore used in static studies to provide high resolution anatomic images.

Dynamic renography

[99mTc]MAG3 (or [99mTc]DTPA) is usually used in these studies.

Indications

- To determine the percentage of renal function contributed by each kidney.
- To diagnose obstruction. IV furosemide is often given as part of this study (diuresis renography) (Fig. 1.6.8).
- To differentiate obstruction from a dilated, but nonobstructed, collecting system.
- To assess renal perfusion.
- To assess perfusion and urine drainage in a renal transplant.
- To evaluate potential renal artery stenosis (RAS). Captopril is often used as part of this study since in the presence of significant renal artery stenosis, renal perfusion is dependent on angiotensin II. A captopril-induced fall in GFR (determined by reduced and delayed uptake of tracer) is suggestive of RAS.

Static renography

[99mTc]DMSA is used in these studies (Fig. 1.6.8).

Indications

- To accurately assess the percentage of function contributed by each kidney.
- To demonstrate renal scarring or other anatomical abnormalities of the parenchyma.
- To localize ectopic renal tissue.

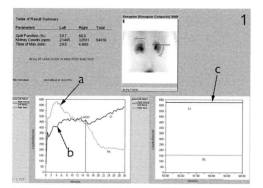

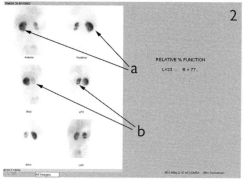

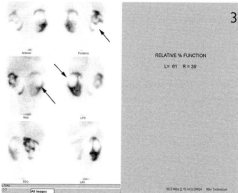

Fig. 1.6.8 Radioisotope studies. 1. Renogram showing left-sided obstruction. (a) Normal right kidney trace. (b) Accumulation of tracer isotopes after furosemide. (c) Persistence of tracer in the left kidney on delayed imaging. 2. DMSA renogram: (a) a normal right kidney and (b) a scarred left kidney. 3. DMSA renogram demonstrating multiple photopenic areas due to cysts in polycystic kidney disease.

Other nuclear medicine studies used in renal medicine

Isotope bone scintigraphy

[99mTc]Diphosphonate or polyphosphonate becomes fixed to hydroxyapatite in bone. Therefore uptake of tracer is increased in areas of high bone turnover.

It is useful in identifying metastatic lesions in bone, particularly from prostate carcinoma. However, it is unhelpful in myeloma since bone deposits to not incorporate the tracer.

Cystic brown tumors (of hyperparathyroidism) may also not take up the tracer.

Percutaneous nephrostomy

This involves the percutaneous insertion of a catheter into the renal pelvis (Figures 1.6.9 and 1.6.10).

Indications

Emergency indications:
- Drainage of a pyonephrosis.
- Drainage of a kidney in a patient with acute kidney injury caused by obstruction.

Other indications:
- Drainage of an obstructed kidney.
- Diversion of urine from the collecting system to allow leaks or fistulae (iatrogenic or otherwise) to heal.
- To provide access for other endourological procedures, e.g. antegrade stenting, percutaneous nephrolithotomy, pyeloplasty.
- To provide access for the administration of drugs/treatments, e.g. chemotherapy, solutions for stone dissolution.
- Nephrostogram: after the procedure, contrast can be injected via the nephrostomy catheter and the site of obstruction can be determined.

Preassessment

Full blood count and coagulation studies. Although abnormal coagulation is not an absolute contraindication, all efforts should be made to reverse the abnormalities before the procedure is undertaken.

If coagulation abnormalities are severe and/or not correctable, alternative approaches should be considered, e.g. retrograde ureteric stenting.

Obtain informed consent.

Administer prophylactic antibiotics (even if the patient is not overtly septic prior to the procedure).

Procedure

It is usually performed under ultrasound guidance but fluoroscopic or CT guidance may also be used (Fig. 1.6.10).

The patient is placed in the prone oblique position.

If possible, the skin puncture is made under the 12th rib to prevent pneumothorax, and lateral to the paraspinous muscles.

Local anaesthetic is applied.

The kidney puncture is made at the tip of a calyx, usually in the lower pole, to avoid the arcuate arteries. The track through the kidney should be posterolateral through the renal parenchyma. This ensures that the relatively avascular zone (Broedel's line) is traversed and avoids direct entry to the pelvis which is associated with more complications (laceration of renal pelvis, bleeding from large hilar vessels).

A wire is placed through the puncture needle and is manipulated into renal pelvis.

The tract is dilated over the wire.

The nephrostomy catheter is inserted and secured.

Complications

Immediate

Pain. This is common and should be anticipated.

Bleeding:
- Minor bleeding is common, and requires no treatment.
- In <4% of cases bleeding is heavy and may require transfusion. Less commonly bleeding continues, and embolisation of the bleeding point, or (even more rarely) nephrectomy may be needed.

Catheter blockage as a result of clots.

Infection: <4% risk of bacteremia.

Pneumothorax.

Perforation of other abdominal organs.

Failed access <5%.

Death. This is rare.

Long-term

Infection.

Catheter blockage. Therefore long-term nephrostomies require regular changing.

Catheter displacement.

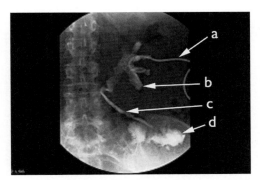

Fig. 1.6.9 Nephrostogram showing urinary leak. (a) Nephrostomy catheter, (b) pelvicalyceal system, (c) ureter, and (d) contrast extravasation.

Arteriography

Inspite of the advent of newer imaging techniques, arteriography remains the 'gold standard' investigation for renovascular disease.

It is an invasive investigation, therefore renal arteriography should only be performed as a prelude to a therapeutic procedure. It should not be used as a screening test.

Indications

- Renovascular disease. It may confirm the presence of RAS. Renal artery angioplasty and/or stenting can be undertaken at the same time.
- Acute renal ischemia. Renal artery thrombosis or embolization may be diagnosed which may be amenable to thrombolysis.
- Unexplained macroscopic hematuria (after full urological evaluation). It may identify arteriovenous malformations or angiomata that may be amenable to embolization.
- Polyarteritis nodosa. Arteriography may identify intrarenal microaneurysms.

- Bleeding post renal biopsy. To identify site of bleeding and possibly allow embolization.
- Renal trauma. Embolization to control bleeding may be possible (Fig. 1.6.11).

Venography/fistulography

These investigations are used in the preparation for, and the management after, arteriovenous fistula (AVF) formation.

Indications

- To assess the vessels for anatomical mapping prior to AVF formation.
- To assess vascular problems in a fistula, e.g. poor flow, recirculation, high venous pressure. Ultrasound with or without Doppler ultrasound may be used in conjunction with fistulography.
- In some cases fistuloplasty can be undertaken to treat fistula strictures (Fig. 1.6.12).

Contrast-induced nephrotoxicity

Risk factors

- Pre-existing renal disease: the risk of nephrotoxity is proportional to the severity of the underlying renal disease.

- Diabetes mellitus: particularly when associated with impaired renal function.
- Volume depletion.
- Concurrent use of nephrotoxic drugs, e.g. NSAIDs.
- Heart failure.
- Gout.
- Age >70 years.

Preventative measures

- If possible, use alternative imaging tests which do not require iodinated contrast agents.
- Stop nephrotoxic drugs before the study.
- Ensure patients are volume replete. Start IV volume expansion to induce a diuresis before the study (unless this is contraindicated by heart failure or advanced CKD with volume overload).
- Use nonionic contrast agents.
- Use the smallest dose of contrast required to obtain the diagnostic result.
- Currently there is insufficient evidence that other strategies (e.g. N-acetylcysteine or sodium bicarbonate infusion) can protect against contrast-induced nephrotoxicity.

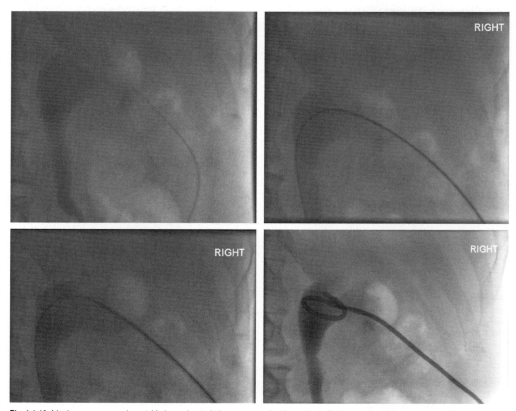

Fig. 1.6.10 Nephrostomy procedure. 1. Hydronephrotic kidney punctured with needle. 2. Guidewire placed through needle. 3. Tract dilated. 4. Pigtail catheter inserted.

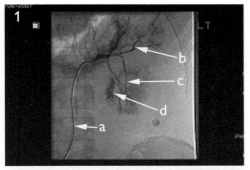

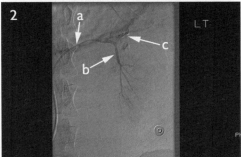

Fig. 1.6.11 Renal arteriography for renal bleeding. 1. Arteriogram. (a) Catheter, (b) upper pole arteries, (c) lower pole arteries, (d) extravasation of contrast. 2. Arteriogram post-coil embolization. (a) Catheter, (b) lower pole renal artery, (c) coils with no further contrast extravasation.

Nephrogenic systemic fibrosis (NSF)

This is a rare scleroderma-like skin condition that affects patients with renal insufficiency. It was first described in 1997.

It was previously called nephrogenic fibrosing dermopathy, although with the realization that the sclerosis was not skin-limited, the term NSF has been adopted.

Recent evidence has suggested that gadolinium-containing contrast agents (particularly gadodiamide (Omniscan), and gadopentetic acid (Magnevist)) may play a role in causing this disorder (>95% of patients with NSF have been exposed to gadolinium).

It occurs exclusively in patients with moderate-to-severe renal failure (there are no reports in patients with GFR >60 mL/min).

It has been seen mainly in hemodialysis patients, but can also occur in patients: on peritoneal dialysis; with failing renal transplants; and with severe renal impairment not requiring dialysis (GFR <30 mL/min/1.73 m^2).

It has been associated with liver failure and liver transplantation, although always in association with renal failure.

An association with the use of erythropoietin-simulating agents has been suggested but not established.

Male:female involvement is equal. The majority of cases are in patients aged 45–50 years, although children can also be affected. Cases have been reported in Europe, USA and Asia.

It is a progressive, sometimes fatal disease affecting the skin, muscle and internal organs, including striated muscle, myocardium and lungs.

It manifests with erythema, plaques, a peu d'orange appearance, and induration initially on the legs.

A typical distribution of lesions is from the ankles to below the knees, the mid-thighs, and between the wrists and upper arms.

It progresses to involve other parts of the body and ultimately involves tendons and peri-articular tissues causing contractures and immobility. The trunk is less commonly affected and the head is spared.

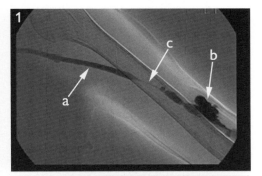

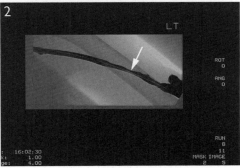

Fig. 1.6.12 Fistulogram and fistuloplasty. 1. Fistulogram of a brachio-cephalic AVF demonstrating (a) the cephalic vein, (b) the fistula, and (c) a tight stenosis in the vein. 2. Post-fistuloplasty the cephalic vein is widely patent (arrow).

Histologically the appearances are different from systemic sclerosis. Early changes include dermal fibrocyte proliferation, with progression to extensive dermal thickening and fibrocyte proliferation in advanced disease. Gadolinium can usually be identified in the skin if appropriate investigations are undertaken.

There is currently no effective treatment. Restoration of renal function with renal transplantation offers the best hope for improvement in symptoms.

Prevention

If possible, avoid gadolinium in high risk patients (i.e. those with GFR <30 mL/min, and those with concurrent liver disease) through the use of alternative imaging modalities.

Gadodiamide (Omniscan) is contraindicated in patients with impaired renal function (GFR <30 mL/min).

Other gadolinium-based contrast agents should be used with caution in patients with severe renal impairment (GFR <30 mL/min/1.7 m^2).

The minimum dose of contrast agent that gives the desired diagnostic information should be used. It is suggested that the dose of any gadolinium-based contrast agent should not exceed 0.3 mmol/kg.

In patients on hemodialysis it is sensible to dialyse the patient as soon as possible after the procedure, and then again 24 h later. There is no evidence, however, that this will prevent the development of NSF.

Patients with CKD 5 who are not currently on dialysis should not be commenced on hemodialysis purely to enhance gadolinium removal. The risks of establishing access for hemodialysis and the procedure itself outweigh the risks of developing NSF.

Further reading

Federle M, Brooke JR, Venkat Sridhar A. *Diagnostic Imaging: Abdomen (Diagnostic Imaging)*. AMIRSYS; 2004.

Grainger & Allison's Diagnostic Radiology: A Textbook of Medical Imaging, 5th edn. Edinburgh: Churchill Livingstone; 2007.

Royal College of Radiologists. *Making the best use of clinical radiology services*, 6th edn. London: RCR; 2007.

Sutton D, Reznek R, Murfitt J. *Textbook of radiology and imaging*, 5th edn. Edinburgh: Churchill Livingstone; 2002.

Internet resources

Guidelines on the use of gadolinium-based contrast agents:

http://www.esur.org/Nephrogenic_Fibrosis.30.0.html

Information about gadolinium-based contrast agents and risk of NSF:

http://www.mhra.gov.uk

Information about gadolinium-based contrast agents and risk of NSF:

http://www.fda.gov

Gadolinium-bases Contrast Media and Nephrogenic Systemic Fibrosis:

http://www.rcr.ac.uk/docs/radiology/pdf/BFCR0714_Gadolinium_NSF_guidanceNov07.pdf

ESUR Guidelines on contrast media version 6.0:

http://www.esur.org/fileadmin/Guidelines/ESUR_2007_Guideline_6_Kern_Ubersicht.pdf

See also

Drug-induced nephropathies, p. 698

Dermatologic disorders in CKD, p. 450

Renal biopsy

Percutaneous renal biopsy was first described in the early 1950s. Since then the procedure has been refined and now provides a tissue diagnosis in >95% of cases with a life-threatening complication rate of <0.1%.

Indications

The biopsy should be able to provide a specific diagnosis, reflect the level of disease activity, and guide the use of appropriate treatment. Common indications for renal biopsy are listed in Table 1.7.1.

Table 1.7.1 Indications for renal biopsy

Nephrotic syndrome
Acute renal failure
Systemic disease with renal dysfunction
Renal transplant dysfunction
Nonnephrotic proteinuria
Isolated microscopic hematuria
Unexplained chronic renal failure
Familial renal disease

Nephrotic syndrome

The cause of nephrotic syndrome cannot be reliably predicted noninvasively in adults and older children after puberty; a renal biopsy is therefore indicated.

In children between 1 year and puberty, a presumptive diagnosis of minimal change disease can be made. Renal biopsy is reserved for those with atypical features (microscopic hematuria, reduced complement levels, persistent renal impairment, nonresponse to steroids).

Acute kidney injury

In most cases of acute kidney injury the cause (pre-renal, obstruction, acute tubular necrosis) can be confidently diagnosed without a renal biopsy. However, if a confident diagnosis cannot be made a renal biopsy should be undertaken urgently, particularly if there is an active urine sediment (microscopic hematuria, proteinuria, and cellular casts).

Renal dysfunction with systemic disease

Diabetes mellitus

If the clinical setting is compatible with diabetic nephropathy (isolated proteinuria, diabetes of long duration, evidence of other microvascular complications) a biopsy is not necessary.

However, the presence of atypical features (microscopic hematuria with or without proteinuria, absence of retinopathy or neuropathy (type 1 diabetes only), proteinuria within 5 years of onset of diabetes, atypical changes in renal function or the presence of immunologic abnormalities) should prompt consideration of a renal biopsy.

Systemic vasculitis and Goodpasture's disease

Even though the availability of serologic testing for MPO- and PR3-specific ANCA and antiglomerular basement membrane antibodies allows a confident diagnosis of renal vasculitis or Goodpasture's disease to be made in many cases, a renal biopsy should still be performed in order to confirm the diagnosis and to clarify the degree of active inflammation and chronic scarring. This will help guide the type and intensity of immunosuppressive treatment.

Lupus nephritis

This can usually be diagnosed using noninvasive criteria. However a renal biopsy will clarify the type of pathological lesion, and will indicate the level of acute activity and the degree of chronic damage. This provides a robust basis for evidence-based treatment.

Other diseases

Amyloidosis, sarcoidosis, allergic drug reactions, and myeloma can all be diagnosed on renal biopsy. Renal biopsy is reserved for those cases where the diagnosis cannot be made by noninvasive means.

Renal transplant dysfunction

In the absence of ureteric obstruction, urinary sepsis, renal artery stenosis, or toxic levels of calcineurin inhibitors, a renal biopsy is required to determine the cause of renal allograft dysfunction.

Non-nephrotic proteinuria

The value of renal biopsy in this situation is unclear. If proteinuria is >1 g per day a renal biopsy can be justified since it will provide prognostic information, may identify a disease for which a different therapeutic approach is needed, and may provide clinically important information about the future risk of disease recurrence following renal transplantation.

Isolated microscopic hematuria

If a structural cause for microscopic hematuria has been ruled out, a glomerular source for the hematuria needs to be considered.

50–75% of such patients will have a glomerular lesion with IgA nephropathy being the commonest abnormality.

However, in the absence of hypertension or proteinuria the renal prognosis is excellent. In such cases a renal biopsy will only provide diagnostic information and is unlikely to alter therapy and therefore is often not considered necessary.

Renal biopsy should be performed only if the result would provide reassurance to the patient, avoid repeated urological investigations, provide specific information (e.g. in the evaluation of potential living kidney donors), or for life insurance and employment purposes.

Unexplained chronic renal failure

A renal biopsy in patients with chronic renal failure and normal-sized kidneys can be informative. It may identify unexpected pathology in almost 50% of cases. If the kidneys are small (<9 cm) the risks of the biopsy are increased and the utility may be compromised by extensive glomerular and tubulo-interstitial fibrosis which is not amenable to any specific therapy.

Familial renal disease

A biopsy performed on one family member may secure the diagnosis for the whole family and avoid the need for repeated investigation. Conversely a renal biopsy may unexpectedly identify a lesion that has a hereditary basis and prompt investigation of other family members.

Pre-biopsy evaluation

Before undertaking a renal biopsy it is important to identify issues that may compromise the safety of the procedure. The pre-biopsy evaluation is shown in Table 1.7.2.

Evaluation should determine whether the patient has: two normal-sized unobstructed kidneys; sterile urine;

controlled blood pressure; and no abnormality of coagulation.

The value of the bleeding time in this setting has never been prospectively tested.

Retrospective studies have shown a three- to five-fold increase in bleeding complications after renal biopsy in patients with prolonged bleeding times.

Prospective studies in liver biopsy patients have shown a five-fold increase in bleeding complications in those with uncorrected bleeding times.

There is a consensus view that the bleeding time is a poor predictor of post-surgical bleeding, but that it does correlate with bleeding episodes in uremic patients.

For this reason many centres include the bleeding time in their pre-biopsy evaluation and if prolonged beyond 10 min administer 1-desamino-8-D-arginine (DDAVP).

An alternative but equally acceptable approach is to administer DDAVP to all patients with significant uremia (urea >20 mmol/L or serum creatinine >250 μmol/L) without performing a bleeding time.

Table 1.7.2 Renal biopsy work-up

	Pre-biopsy requirement
Renal imaging	2 normal-sized, unscarred, unobstructed kidneys
Blood pressure	Systolic BP <160 mmHg, diastolic <95 mmHg
Urine culture	Sterile
Coagulation status	• No aspirin, clopidogrel, NSAID, warfarin for 1–2 weeks pre-biopsy • Platelet count >100 × 10⁹/L • Prothrombin time <1.2 times control • Activated partial thromboplastin time <1.2× control (if prolonged consider presence of lupus anticoagulant) • Bleeding time <10 min (measure if urea >20 mmol/L) (see text). If prolonged (or if urea >20 mmol/L, high risk biopsy, and bleeding time unavailable (see text)) give DDAVP 0.4 μg/kg 3–4 h before the biopsy.

Contraindications to renal biopsy

These are listed in Table 1.7.3.

Absolute

An uncorrectable bleeding diathesis is the only absolute contraindication to percutaneous biopsy. If the biopsy is indispensable alternative approaches can be used (open biopsy, laparoscopic biopsy, or transvenous (usually transjugular) biopsy).

Relative

Hypertension (>160/95), hypotension, perinephric abscess, pyelonephritis, hydronephrosis, severe anemia, large renal tumours, and renal cysts are all relative contraindications to renal biopsy. Where possible they should be corrected before undertaking the biopsy.

The presence of a solitary functioning kidney is considered to be a relative contraindication to percutaneous biopsy. It has been argued that performing the biopsy with direct visualization is required in this circumstance. However, the postbiopsy nephrectomy rate of 1:2000 to 1:5000 is similar to the mortality associated with a general anesthetic. Therefore percutaneous biopsy of a solitary kidney can be justified in the absence of risk factors for bleeding.

Table 1.7.3 Contraindications to renal biopsy

Kidney status
Multiple cysts (R)
Solitary kidney (R)
Acute pyelonephritis/perinephric abcess (R)
Renal neoplasm (R)

Patient status
Uncontrolled bleeding diathesis (A)
Uncontrolled blood pressure (R)
Uremia (R)
Obesity (R)
Uncooperative patient (R)

A, absolute contraindication; R, relative contraindication.

Renal biopsy technique

Percutaneous renal biopsy

Native renal biopsy

Typically a renal biopsy is performed by nephrologists using continuous (real-time) ultrasound guidance and disposable automated biopsy needles. 16 gauge needles may be used as a compromise between the greater tissue yield of larger needles and the trend to fewer bleeding complications of smaller needles.

- Sedation is only rarely required.
- The patient lies prone with a pillow under the abdomen to straighten the spine and splint the kidneys.
- Ultrasonography is used to localize the lower pole of the kidney to be biopsied and the skin is marked with an indelible pen at the point of entry of the biopsy needle.
- The skin is then prepped and anesthetized with 1–2% lidocaine.
- Under ultrasound guidance a narrow gauge spinal needle is advanced to the renal capsule and further local anesthetic is infiltrated along the needle track.
- A stab incision is made through the dermis to ease passage of the biopsy needle.
- The biopsy needle is directed under ultrasound guidance towards the kidney capsule.
- The biopsy is taken after patients are instructed to hold their breath. The biopsy needle is withdrawn immediately and the patient resumes breathing.
- Usually a second core of tissue is required for immunofluorescence and electron microscopy.
- If insufficient material is obtained, further passes of the needle can be made. There is a modest increase in the postbiopsy complication rate if the needle is passed more than four times.
- Once sufficient renal tissue has been obtained the skin incision is dressed and the patient is rolled directly into bed for observation.

Since no single fixative allows good quality immunofluorescence, light or electron microscopy to be performed on the same sample, the biopsy cores are divided into three and placed in:

- Formalin for conventional light microscopy.
- Normal saline for subsequent snap-freezing in liquid nitrogen for immunofluorescence microscopy.
- Glutaraldehyde for electron microscopy.

There are a number of variations of the percutaneous renal biopsy technique. For example, some operators use ultrasound to localize the kidney and to determine its depth and the angle of approach of the needle. The biopsy is then performed without further ultrasound guidance. The success and complication rates of this technique appear to be no different from that seen with continuous ultrasound guidance.

Computed tomography guidance has been advocated for patients in whom the biopsy can be technically challenging.

Renal transplant biopsy

The general technique for renal transplant biopsy is similar to that of the native kidney. The proximity of the allograft to the anterior abdominal wall and the lack of movement on respiration facilitate its biopsy.

If the biopsy is being performed to identify the cause of acute allograft dysfunction a formalin-fixed sample for conventional light microscopy is usually sufficient. A snap-frozen sample for C4d immunostaining should be obtained if antibody-mediated rejection is suspected. If recurrent or de-novo glomerulonephritis is suspected, additional samples for electron microscopy and immunofluorescence microscopy should be collected.

Post-biopsy monitoring

Following the biopsy the patient is placed supine and is put on strict bed rest for 6–8 h.

The blood pressure is monitored frequently, the urine is examined for macroscopic hematuria, and the skin puncture site is examined for excessive bleeding.

If after 6–8 h there is no evidence of bleeding the patient is sat up in bed and subsequently allowed to mobilize.

If macroscopic hematuria develops, bed rest is continued until the bleeding settles.

Historically patients were observed in hospital overnight following the renal biopsy.

Day case renal biopsy

Day case renal biopsy with same-day discharge after 6–8 h of observation has become increasingly popular.

This has been largely driven by the financial and resource implications of overnight hospital admission and has been justified by the perception that any significant complications of renal biopsy will develop within 6–8 h post-biopsy.

However, a recent study has suggested that only 67% of the major complications observed after renal biopsy in 750 patients became apparent within 8 h after biopsy.

Up to half of our renal biopsies are performed as day cases. Patients with the highest risk of complications – significantly impaired renal function (serum creatinine >250 µmol/L; small kidneys; and uncontrolled hypertension – should not be considered for a day case renal biopsy.

In properly selected cases up to 5% of patients can develop a self-limiting postbiopsy complication within 8 h that requires a short hospital admission for observation, and 0.75% of patients return 1–4 days after same-day discharge with either macroscopic hematuria or loin pain due to perirenal hematoma. Typically such complications settle with conservative management.

Therefore, day case biopsy is acceptably safe when a low-risk patient population is selected.

Alternatives to the percutaneous approach

When a percutaneous approach is contraindicated, alternative approaches to renal biopsy have been described. The choice of technique in any situation depends on the safety, morbidity, recovery period, and adequacy of the technique, but above all on the local expertise that is available.

Transvenous (transjugular or transfemoral) renal biopsy

Transvenous sampling of the kidney is theoretically safer than the percutaneous approach because:

- the needle passes from the venous system into the renal parenchyma and is directed away from large blood vessels;
- it is suggested that any bleeding that occurs should be directed back into the venous system;
- if capsular perforation occurs, significant bleeding points can be immediately identified and controlled by coil embolization.

The transjugular renal biopsy cannot be regarded as routine because it requires specialist skill, and involves additional time and expense.

Indications for this approach are:

- an uncontrollable bleeding diathesis;
- the need to obtain tissue from more than one organ including the kidney, liver, or heart;
- large volume ascites (precludes the prone position);
- uncontrolled hypertension;
- morbid obesity;
- severe respiratory insufficiency;
- solitary right kidney;
- failed percutaneous approach;
- coma.

Studies report diagnostic yields for transjugular biopsy of between 73 and 98%. Despite these being high risk patients, the complication rate appears to be similar to that seen in percutaneous renal biopsy

Open renal biopsy

This is a safe alternative to percutaneous biopsy when uncorrectable contraindications exist. Published studies report tissue adequacy of 100% with no major complications. However, the risk of general anesthesia and the delayed recovery time have prevented its widespread adoption.

It is most useful when a renal biopsy is required in patients who are undergoing an abdominal procedure for other reasons.

Laparoscopic renal biopsy

This procedure requires general anesthesia and two laparoscopic ports in the posterior and anterior axillary lines to gain access to the retroperitoneal space. Laparoscopic biopsy forceps are used to obtain cortical samples, and the biopsy sites are coagulated with laser and packed to prevent hemorrhage.

The largest published study reported that adequate tissue was obtained in 96% of 74 patients. Significant bleeding occurred in three patients, the colon was injured in one, and a biopsy was performed inadvertently on the spleen and liver in two others.

Complications of renal biopsy

The complication rates compiled from large series of renal biopsies are shown in Table 1.7.4. Hemorrhagic complications still occur but other serious complications are now rare.

Table 1.7.4 Complications of renal biopsy (1990 to present)

No. of biopsies	3884
Hematoma	3%
Macroscopic hematuria	3%
Arteriovenous fistula formation	0.2%
Surgery	1 case
Death	1 case

Pain

A dull ache around the needle entry site is almost invariable when the local anesthetic wears off. Patients should be warned about this in advance.

This can be managed with simple analgesia such as paracetamol or paracetamol/codeine combinations.

More significant pain may indicate significant perirenal hemorrhage. Opiate analgesia may be necessary and appropriate investigations should be undertaken to clarify the severity of the bleed.

Macroscopic hematuria may be associated with ureteral colic (clot colic).

Hemorrhage

Some perirenal bleeding postbiopsy is inevitable. On average hemoglobin may fall by 1 g/dL post biopsy.

Significant perirenal hematomas are almost invariably associated with severe loin pain.

Both macroscopic hematuria and painful hematoma are seen in 3% of patients after biopsy.

The initial management involves strict bed rest and maintenance of normal coagulation indices.

If the bleeding is either associated with hypotension or prolonged and fails to settle with bed rest, renal arteriography should be performed to identify the source of bleeding. Coil embolization can be performed during the procedure and this has largely eliminated the need for open surgical intervention and nephrectomy.

Arteriovenous fistula

When specifically sought by duplex USS or contrast-enhanced CT they can be found in as many as 18% of patients.

Since most are clinically silent and >95% resolve spontaneously within two years, routine screening is not recommended.

Unusually arteriovenous fistulae can lead to macroscopic hematuria, hypertension, and renal impairment, in which case embolization is appropriate.

Other complications

Other rare complications have been reported, including:

- biopsy of other organs (liver, spleen, pancreas, bowel, and gallbladder);
- pneumothorax;
- hemothorax;
- calyceal–peritoneal fistula;
- dispersion of carcinoma;
- Page kidney (compression of the kidney by a perirenal hematoma leading to renin-mediated hypertension).

Death

Death resulting directly from the renal biopsy has become much less common according to recent biopsy series when compared with earlier reports. The vast majority of deaths are the result of uncontrolled hemorrhage in high risk patients, particularly those with acute kidney injury.

Further reading

Appel GB. Renal biopsy: how effective, what technique, and how safe. *J Nephrol* 1993; **6**: 4.

Hergesell O, Felten H, Andrassy K, *et al.* Safety of ultrasound-guided percutaneous renal biopsy-retrospective analysis of 1090 consecutive cases. *Nephrol Dial Transplant* 1998; **13**: 975.

Madaio MP. Renal biopsy. *Kidney Int* 1990; **38**: 529.

Manno C, Strippoli GF, Arnesano L, *et al.* Predictors of bleeding complications in percutaneous ultrasound-guided renal biopsy. *Kidney Int* 2004; **66**: 1570.

Sam R, Ing TS. Transjugular renal biopsy: when to do it and when not to? *Int J Artif Organs* 2001; **24**: 595.

Schwarz A, Gwinner W, Hiss M, *et al.* Safety and adequacy of renal transplant protocol biopsies. *Am J Transplant* 2005; **5**: 992.

Stiles KP, Yuan CM, Chung EM, *et al.* Renal biopsy in high-risk patients with medical diseases of the kidney. *Am J Kidney Dis* 2000; **36**: 419.

Internet resources

National Kidney Federation biopsy information:

http://www.kidney.org.uk/Medical-Info/kidney-disease/biopsy.html

Renal biopsy information for patients:

http://patients.uptodate.com/topic.asp?file=kidn_dis/6752

Immunological investigation of renal disease

Immunological tests on blood and urine are never diagnostic of kidney disease.

Results must always be interpreted in the light of clinical evaluation.

Commonly useful tests include:
- serum immunoglobulins (Igs);
- serum and urine protein electropheresis;
- complement: C3, C4, CH_{50};
- antineutrophil cytoplasm antibodies (ANCA);
- anti-GBM (glomerular basement membrane) antibodies;
- anti-DNA antibodies;
- anti-ENA antibodies;
- anti-C1q antibodies;
- antiphospholipid (APL) antibodies.

Clinical context

Immunological testing is useful in the following contexts:
- urgent evaluation of unexplained renal failure – usually as an inpatient;
- evaluation before renal biopsy;
- to obtain additional diagnostic information in the light of renal biopsy findings;
- follow-up when the diagnosis is known to assess progress, including the response to treatment.

Tables 1.8.1–1.8.3 show the use of tests in these contexts

Serum immunoglobulins

Reduced serum immunoglobulins

Serum IgG, IgA, IgM are reported in g/L.

Serum IgG and IgA are typically low in nephrotic syndrome because of urinary loss; serum IgM is not reduced, since the larger pentameric IgM is not lost in urine.

A monoclonal increase in Ig in myeloma may be accompanied by reductions in other serum Igs (immune paresis).

Raised serum immunoglobulins

Serum IgA is raised in about one-third of people with IgA nephropathy.

Raised levels of serum Igs must be interpreted in the context of the results from serum and urine protein electrophoresis (SPEP and UPEP respectively):
- polyclonal increases in Igs accompany a number of inflammatory states, including systemic lupus erythematosis and vasculitis;
- a monoclonal increase in Ig is characteristic of myeloma.

Serum and urine protein electrophoresis

Serum protein electrophoresis (SPEP)

SPEP showing a monoclonal Ig band with reduction in other Igs (immune paresis) strongly suggests myeloma.

However, this does not prove that the renal disease is myeloma cast nephropathy. Amyloid and monoclonal immunoglobulin deposition disease (MIDD) cannot be excluded.

SPEP showing a monoclonal band without immune paresis often means MGUS (monoclonal gammopathy of uncertain significance), but this does not exclude a diagnosis of amyloid or MIDD.

Urine protein electrophoresis (UPEP)

This detects urine free immunoglobulin light chains.

It has replaced Bence–Jones proteinuria as the routine test for light chains.

The presence of free light chains in the urine strongly suggests myeloma kidney, amyloid, or MIDD.

Cryoglobulins

Cryoglobulins are measured as g/L or as a 'cryocrit' – the percent precipitate as a function of the total serum volume tested.

They must be measured in serum kept at 37°C from the time of venesection until the serum has been separated.

Cryoglobulins may be monoclonal or polyclonal.

Clinical features of cryoglobulin-related disease include livedo reticularis, liver dysfunction, neuropathy ± suspicion of lymphoproliferative disease.

If there is a clinical suspicion of cryoglobulinemia but the cryoglobulin test is negative, repeat twice since specimen collection requirements can make testing unreliable.

Complement

C3 and C4 components are reported in g/L or mg/dL.

C3 and C4 measure the circulating amount, but do not assess complement activation, which requires measurement of CH_{50} (50% hemolyzing dose of complement); or C3d (or other breakdown products of C3).

A low C3 usually implies tissue injury with activation of complement (classical or alternative pathway).

A low C4 implies activation of classical pathway or the presence of a hereditary null allele.

In most clinical situations C3 and C4 are sufficient when interpreted with clinical and other laboratory information.

Nephritic factor

C3 nephritic factor (C3Nef) is a circulating IgG auto-antibody against C3 convertase; it stabilizes C3 convertase producing gain-of-function and C3 consumption.

C3Nef is associated with mesangiocapillary GN type II (dense deposit disease).

C3Nef should be measured in glomerulonephritis if the serum C3 is persistently reduced.

C4 Nef and Nef against the alternative pathway convertase occur rarely.

Factor H

Genetic deficiency in factor H, an alternative pathway regulatory protein, is associated with familial hemolytic–uremic syndrome, and predisposes to mesangiocapillary GN type II.

The variations in complement associated with renal disease are shown in Table 1.8.4.

Table 1.8.1 Immunological testing for urgent evaluation of renal disease

Clinical setting	Tests
Rapidly progressive renal failure with active urine sediment	ANCA Anti-GBM Anti-DNA C3, C4
If also suspicion of lymphoproliferative disease or cryoglobulinemia	SPEP UPEP Cryoglobulins
Nephrotic syndrome, especially in women with clinical evidence of multisystem extrarenal disease	Serum Igs Anti-DNA C3, C4
Nephrotic syndrome age >40 years	Serum Igs Anti-DNA C3, C4 SPEP UPEP
Unexplained renal failure age >40 years with clinical suspicion of myeloma (anemia, hypercalcemia, bone pain)	Serum Igs SPEP UPEP
Unexplained renal failure age >70 years with bland urine	Serum Igs SPEP UPEP
Thrombotic microangiopathy without infective prodrome	Anti-ADAMTS13

Table 1.8.3 Immunological testing during follow-up of renal disease

Diagnosis	Test	Comments
ANCA-associated vasculitis	ANCA	Rising titer usually precedes relapse
		Occasionally persistently positive in remission
Anti-GBM disease	Anti-GBM	Early testing to follow disappearance of antibody with or without treatment
		Once antibody negative, test only if clinical suspicion of relapse
Lupus nephritis	Anti-DNA C3, C4 Anti-C1q	Anti-PL, anti-ENA for specific clinical indications

Immunological testing should not be unnecessarily frequent; it is rarely required more often than monthly unless there are rapid changes in the clinical state.

Table 1.8.2 Immunological testing before nonurgent renal biopsy

Clinical setting	Extra-renal disease	Tests	Comment
Microscopic hematuria	None	(Anti-GBM)	Rare presentation of anti-GBM disease
Proteinuria Proteinuria and hematuria Nephrotic syndrome	None	Serum Igs Anti-DNA C3, C4 Age >50 years, add SPEP UPEP	
Nephrotic syndrome	Including those with multisystem extra-renal disease	Serum Igs Anti-DNA C3, C4 ANCA	
Nephrotic syndrome age >40 years		Serum Igs Anti-DNA C3, C4 ANCA SPEP UPEP	

Table 1.8.4 Altered complement levels in renal disease

Pathway affected	Complement changes	Glomerular diseases	Nonglomerular diseases
Classical pathway activation	$C3 \downarrow$, $C4 \downarrow$, $CH_{50} \downarrow$	Lupus nephritis (especially class IV) Mixed essential cryoglobulinemia	
	$C3 \downarrow$, $C4 \downarrow$, $CH_{50} \downarrow$ [± C4 nephritic factor]	Mesangiocapillary GN type I	
Alternative pathway activation	$C3 \downarrow$, C4 normal, $CH_{50} \downarrow$	Post-streptococcal GN GN associated with other infection: • endocarditis • shunt nephritis • hepatitis B Hemolytic uremic syndrome	Atheroembolic renal disease
	$C3 \downarrow$, C4 normal, $CH_{50} \downarrow$ + C3 nephritic factor Factor H deficiency	Mesangiocapillary GN type II (dense deposit disease)	
Reduced complement synthesis	Acquired		Hepatic disease Malnutrition
	Hereditary C4 null allele Hereditary C2 deficiency Factor H deficiency	Systemic lupus erythematosis Familial hemolytic uremic syndrome	

In GN associated with visceral abscesses, complement usually normal or raised (elevations because complement components are acute phase reactants).

Table 1.8.5 Autoantibodies in systemic lupus and allied conditions

	Class III and IV lupus nephritis		Comments
	Sensitivity	Specificity	
ANA	>98%	Low: 30% healthy women positive	Also positive in CREST syndrome, scleroderma Sjögren's syndrome, Mixed connective tissue disease (MCTD)
Anti-dsDNA	95%	95%	
Sm (a small nuclear riboprotein)	20–30%	90%	Associated with lupus AND with nephritis
Anti-C1q antibodies	95%		35% in inactive nephritis 25% in lupus without nephritis
Anti-Ro (SSA) and anti-La (SSB)	Very low	Very low	MCTD: 90% positive Sjögren's syndrome: 70–80% positive Increased congenital heart block
Antiphospholipid (IgG or IgM) antibodies	–	–	Anti-PL syndrome: 95% positive Prolong APTT and KCT *in vitro*, but associated with thrombosis *in vivo*
Anti-Scl 70 (topoisomerase 1)	–	–	Scleroderma: 60% positive; associated with lung involvement and extent of cutaneous change
Anticentromere Ab	–	–	CREST syndrome: 95% positive

CREST: Calcinosis, Raynaud's syndrome, Esophageal dysmotility, Sclerodactyly, Telangiectasia.

Antineutrophil cytoplasmic antibodies (ANCAs)

IgG ANCAs may be detected by a fluorescence binding test.

ANCA are categorized according to the neutrophil antigen specificity of the antibodies (either PR3 (proteinase 3) or MPO (myeloperoxidase)) and reported in arbitrary units (AU).

ANCAs are strongly associated with small vessel vasculitis with renal involvement, although ~10% are ANCA negative at presentation.

PR3 antibodies are most commonly seen in Wegener's granulomatosis; MPO antibodies are most commonly seen in microscopic polyangiitis. However, these associations are not absolute.

ANCAs with other antigen specificities occur, but not usually in association with renal disease.

ANCA titers fall in response to treatment, and in many become negative.

There can be persistent ANCA positivity during remission.

Anti-glomerular basement antibodies

These are reported in AU of antibody against purified GBM.

They are strongly associated with anti-GBM disease.

They are diagnostic in the context of pulmonary hemorrhage and rapidly progressive GN, and therefore renal biopsy may not be necessary.

The anti-GBM titer follows disease activity.

The titer is useful in following treatment response (falls with plasma exchange and immunosuppression).

Antibodies are absent in remission, and reappear with relapse.

Anti-DNA antibodies

Anti-ds (double-stranded) DNA antibodies are characteristic of systemic lupus (Table 1.8.5).

Active lupus nephritis (ISN/RPS Class III/IV) is almost always associated with high titer anti-DNA antibodies.

Less active lupus nephritis (ISN/RPS Class I, II, V) is typically associated with low titer anti-dsDNA antibodies.

The antibody titer parallels renal disease activity in some patients only.

Always interpret the antibody titer in the context of complement levels (C3, C4 low in active nephritis) and the clinical features.

Antiphospholipid antibodies

These can be found with or without systemic lupus and are associated with recurrent venous thrombosis (antiphospholipid syndrome), and intrarenal small vessel thrombosis.

Anti-C1q antibodies

Anti-C1q antibodies are highly specific for active lupus nephritis (ISN/RPS II, III, IV).

Autoantibodies against ADAMTS13

ADAMTS13 is a metalloprotease which normally prevents accumulation in the circulation of large multimers of von Willebrand factor. Low ADAMTS13 activity, either due to genetic deficiency, or to an acquired autoantibody to ADAMTS13, is associated with atypical, often recurrent, thrombotic microangiopathy.

Other autoantibodies

A number of other autoantibodies are associated with lupus and associated immune disorders, but because of low specificity they have a limited role in investigation of renal disease (Table 1.8.5).

Further reading

Berden JHM, Wetzels JFM. Immunological investigation of the patient with renal disease. In: Davison AM *et al.* (eds), *Oxford Textbook of clinical nephrology*, 3rd edn. Oxford: Oxford University Press; 2004. pp.183–193.

See also

Mesangiocapillary glomerulonephritis, p. 112

Mixed cryoglobulinemia and hepatitis C infection, p. 176

Systemic lupus erythematosus, p. 180

Infection related glomerulonephritis, p. 128

Antiglomerular basement membrane disease, p. 124

Crescentic glomerulonephritis, p. 120

Systemic vasculitis, p. 168

Amyloid or immunotactoid glomerulopathy, p. 150

Rheumatoid arthritis, connective tissue diseases and Sjögrens syndrome, p. 188

Scleroderma – systemic sclerosis, p. 186

Hemolytic uremic syndrome and thrombotic thrombocytopenic purpura, p. 348

Fluid and electrolyte disorders

Chapter contents

Hypo-/hypernatremia: disorders of water balance

Sodium (Na^+) is the major cation in the extracellular fluid (ECF). It is also the major determinant of serum osmolality.

The serum sodium concentration ($[Na^+]$) reflects the relative amount of sodium to water. Serum $[Na^+]$ disorders therefore result from changes in water balance.

Water balance is controlled by osmoreceptors in the hypothalamus that regulate water intake (thirst mechanism) and renal water excretion (antidiuretic hormone (ADH) or vasopressin).

ADH decreases renal free water excretion through engagement of V2 receptors in the collecting duct.

Serum $[Na^+]$ disorders usually occur as a result of altered thirst (excess or inadequate water intake) and aberrant ADH action.

Serum $[Na^+]$ disorders usually result in alterations in serum osmolality. Changes in serum osmolality cause significant free water shifts in and out of the intracellular compartment to maintain osmotic equilibrium.

The rapid transcellular shift of water can lead to cellular damage, particularly in the central nervous system (CNS). Most cases are mild, but in acute or inappropriately managed cases of hypo- or hypernatremia, substantial morbidity and mortality may develop due to CNS damage.

Hyponatremia
Serum $[Na^+]$ <135 mmol/L.

Epidemiology
Hyponatremia is the most frequent electrolyte abnormality with an incidence of 1% and a prevalence of 15–22% in hospitalized patients.

Its prevalence is ~7% in ambulatory patients.

It is more frequent in the elderly, with reported incidences as high as 30–50%.

Hyponatremic encephalopathy risk is highest in children, menstruating females, hypoxic patients and patients with brain injury.

Pathophysiology
Hypo-osmolal hyponatremia occurs when the ingestion of water exceeds excretion.

The most common pathophysiological mechanism is the persistent secretion of antidiuretic hormone (ADH, vasopressin) that prevents maximal urinary dilution.

Persistent ADH release is most commonly due to: decreased effective circulating volume, cortisol deficiency or hypothyroidism, and the syndrome of inappropriate ADH secretion (SIADH).

Etiology
Hyponatremia can be associated with low, normal or high osmolality:

Hyponatremia with hyperosmolality (translocational hyponatremia)
This results from the shift of water out of cells in response to the presence of a nonsodium solute in plasma.

The most common cause is hyperglycemia. Each 5.6 mmol/L increase in the serum glucose concentration decreases the serum $[Na^+]$ by ~1.6 mmol/L.

Mannitol, glycine and radiocontrast infusions may also cause translocational hyponatremia

Hyponatremia with iso-osmolality (pseudohyponatremia)
This is the result of a laboratory artifact caused by hyperlipidemia and hyperproteinemia when the $[Na^+]$ is measured by flame photometry.

This is not a problem when direct ion-selective electrode measurement is utilized, which is currently the standard method for measuring $[Na^+]$. Pseudohyponatremia is therefore currently rarely a clinical issue.

Hyponatremia with hypo-osmolality (true hyponatremia)
This is due to a relative excess of water and can occur with hypo-, eu- or hypervolemia

Clinical evaluation of the underlying causes of hypo-osmolar hyponatremia is facilitated by clinical assessment of the ECF volume status (Fig. 2.1.1).

Decreased ECF volume indicates renal and extra-renal salt and water losses. Loss of Na^+ exceeds loss of water. Thiazide diuretic use is a common cause. Water excretion is prevented by baroreceptor-mediated ADH secretion.

The most common cause of euvolemic hyponatremia is SIADH. SIADH is also the most common cause of hyponatremia among hospitalized patients. The causes of SIADH are malignant disease, pulmonary disease, disorders of the CNS, and drugs.

The presence of edema indicates an increase in total body Na^+. Hyponatremia occurs as the increase in total body water exceeds that of Na^+. Congestive heart failure, cirrhosis, nephrotic syndrome and renal failure are common causes. Water excretion is prevented by baroreceptor-mediated ADH secretion.

Signs and symptoms
A low $[Na^+]$ concentration is usually associated with hypo-osmolality. Low serum osmolality results in water movement into cells, and thus causes cellular swelling, which is clinically most important in brain cells. This osmolar shift of water is primarily responsible for the neurologic symptoms and potentially life-threatening complications. Brain cells compensate for hypo-osmolality by excreting electrolytes and osmolytes, but this process can take up to 48 h.

Symptoms depend on the absolute level of serum $[Na^+]$ and the rapidity of onset of hypo-osmolality.

At any $[Na^+]$ level, patients with 'acute' hyponatremia (duration <48 h) will have more severe symptoms. In chronic cases, symptoms are fewer, milder and less specific.

Most patients with a serum $[Na^+]$ >125 mmol/L are asymptomatic. Patients with a serum $[Na^+]$ ≤125 mmol/L may have anorexia, malaise, nausea and vomiting. Headache, lethargy, disorientation, confusion and depressed reflexes may occur with serum $[Na^+]$ <120 mmol/L. With severe (serum $[Na^+]$ usually <110 mmol/L) and rapidly evolving hyponatremia, seizures, coma, brain stem herniation, respiratory arrest and death may occur.

Diagnosis
Hyponatremia is rarely suspected from the clinical presentation; the diagnosis is made by measurement of the serum $[Na^+]$.

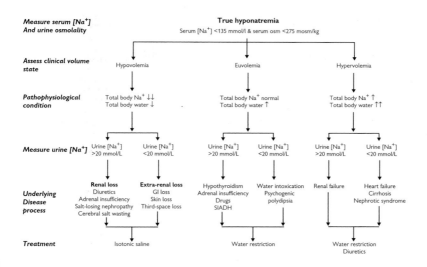

Fig. 2.1.1

Take a careful history (for water intake and loss, medications, underlying disease).

Clinically assess the ECF volume status and perform a neurologic evaluation including fundoscopy.

Laboratory studies:

- Serum electrolytes and osmolality.
- Glucose, urea, creatinine, uric acid, triglycerides and albumin.
- Urine [Na⁺] concentration and osmolality.
- Adrenal and thyroid function tests (in selected cases).

SIADH is a diagnosis of exclusion. Essential diagnostic features are:

- Low plasma osmolality (<275 mOsmol/kg H$_2$O).
- Elevated urine osmolality (>100 mOsmol/kg H$_2$O in the face of a low plasma osmolality).
- Presence of clinical euvolemia.
- Urine [Na⁺] >40 mmol/L with normal dietary salt intake.
- Normal thyroid, adrenal, and kidney function.
- No recent diuretic use.
- Hypouricemia (<238 µmol/L) and low [urea] (<3.5 mmol/L) are supplementary features of SIADH.

A diagnostic algorithm for hypo-osmolal hyponatremia is shown in Fig. 2.1.1.

In a euvolemic patient with hyponatremia, a urine osmolality <100 mosm/L indicates the presence of primary polydipsia, reset osmostat or beer potomania.

Treatment

Treating the underlying cause and restricting fluid intake is sufficient in most cases.

Morbidity and mortality are related to neurologic complications of either acute cerebral edema in severe, acute cases or central pontine myelinolysis (CPM) due to improper management (too rapid correction or overcorrection).

Treatment choices are dependent on the rapidity of onset of hyponatremia, the severity of symptoms and the ECF volume state.

Acute and symptomatic hyponatremia

The [Na⁺] is usually <120 mmol/L and needs to be promptly treated. Failure to treat promptly risks further brain edema, tentorial herniation and death.

Administer hypertonic saline (3% NaCl, 1–2 ml/kg/h) with IV furosemide (20–40 mg) with a maximal rate of correction of serum [Na⁺] in the range of 1–2 mmol/L/h until symptoms resolve.

The total magnitude of correction should not exceed 8–10 mmol/day. The target is to raise the serum [Na⁺] to safe levels (120–125 mmol/L).

During treatment close monitoring of the patient, serum [Na⁺], fluid intake, urine output and neurologic symptoms are necessary and should preferably be undertaken in an intensive care setting.

Several formulae can be used to calculate the Na⁺ requirement (Formula 1), water excess (Formula 2) or to estimate the effect on serum [Na⁺] concentration of any infused solution (Formula 3) (Table 2.1.1). These formulae can be used to determine the initial rate of hypertonic saline infusion, but the rate of infusion should be adjusted according to the [Na⁺] that is measured every 2–3 h.

Chronic, symptomatic hyponatremia

Patients with hyponatremia of over 48 h duration with mild to moderate symptoms need to be treated with caution as overaggressive correction risks CPM. The maximal rate of correction of serum [Na⁺] should not exceed 0.5–1.0 mmol/L/h.

Asymptomatic hyponatremia

Treatment should focus on underlying causes.

- In the hypovolemic patient, prevent further fluid loss and replace the ECF volume deficit with normal saline. Once euvolemia is established, ADH production will be suppressed and excess water will be excreted.
- For hypervolemic patients, treat the underlying disorder. Restrict salt and water intake and administer diuretics if necessary. Ultrafiltration and dialysis may be required in those with resistant heart failure or renal failure.

- In euvolemic patients, fluid restriction (<800–1000 mL/day) is the treatment of choice. Some patients may need pharmacologic antagonism of ADH with demeclocycline or lithium. Supplementation of the diet with additional solute in the form of protein, salt or urea may also be helpful.

A new class of drugs known as vasopressin receptor antagonists induces free water diuresis without natriuresis or kaliuresis (aquaretics) by antagonizing V2 receptors in the collecting duct. Conivaptan (V1a and V2 antagonist) has been approved by the Food and Drug Administration for IV treatment of euvolemic and hypervolemic hyponatremia. Several orally active drugs that are specific to V2 receptors are still being investigated.

Prevention
Avoid hypotonic fluid use in high risk hospitalized patients, especially in the postoperative period.

Be cautious with thiazide use in the elderly.

Hypernatremia
Serum $[Na^+]$ >145 mmol/L.

Epidemiology
In hospitalized patients the prevalence of hypernatremia is 0.5–3.5%.

The highest risk is in patients with altered mental status, the elderly, intubated patients and infants.

Pathophysiology
Hypernatremia is generated by net water loss or hypertonic Na^+ gain, but maintained by a failure to sense thirst and/or an inability to access water. Normally the development of thirst prevents the maintenance of hypernatremia.

A defect in urine concentration with an inadequate water intake will cause hypernatremia. A decrease in the level or activity of ADH prevents maximal urinary concentration.

Hypernatremia is most often due to net water loss in excess of sodium. This may be due to renal or extrarenal water loss.

Etiology
Hypernatremia is always associated with hyperosmolality. Hypernatremic conditions are classified according to the ECF volume status (Fig. 2.1.2)

Hypernatremia with decreased ECF volume indicates renal or extrarenal salt and water losses in which the loss of water exceeds that of sodium.

Euvolemic hypernatremia is usually caused by diabetes insipidus (DI). In DI, there is either an abnormality in ADH secretion (central DI) or resistance to ADH action in the kidney (nephrogenic DI).

Hypervolemic hypernatremia indicates net sodium gain. Most cases are iatrogenic.

Signs and symptoms
High serum osmolality results in water movement out of cells, leading to cellular dehydration and cell shrinkage, particularly in brain cells. This osmolar shift of water is primarily responsible for the neurologic symptoms and potentially life-threatening complications.

Brain cells compensate for hyperosmolality by increasing intracellular electrolyte and osmolyte concentrations over a 24–48 h period.

Symptoms of hypernatremia depend on the absolute level of serum $[Na^+]$ and the rapidity of onset of hyperosmolality.

In severe, acute hypernatremia (duration <48 h) brain shrinkage may be substantial, resulting in cerebral and subarachnoid hemorrhage.

In less severe chronic hypernatremia, manifestations are nonspecific (nausea, muscle weakness, and alterations in mental status ranging from lethargy to coma).

Elderly patients have generally few symptoms unless serum $[Na^+]$ is >160 mmol/L.

Diagnosis
Hypernatremia is rarely suspected from the clinical presentation; the diagnosis is made by measurement of the serum $[Na^+]$.

Take a careful history (for water intake and loss, polyuria, medications, underlying diseases).

Clinically assess the ECF volume status and perform a neurologic evaluation.

Laboratory studies:
- serum electrolytes and osmolality;
- glucose, urea, creatinine, calcium;
- urine sodium concentration and osmolality.

Most patients have signs and symptoms of hypovolemia.

Euvolemic patients are usually mildly hypernatremic, but complain of polyuria.

Polyuria is defined as a urine output of >3 L/day. The water deprivation test followed by administration of ADH helps to differentiate central from nephrogenic DI (Chapter 5.5 for details).

A diagnostic algorithm for hypernatremia is shown in Fig. 2.1.2.

In a hypo- or euvolemic patient with hypernatremia, a urine osmolality >700 mOsm/L indicates the presence of an extrarenal source for water loss.

Table 2.1.1 Formulae used in calculating initial therapeutic targets of hypo- and hypernatremia

Formula 1:
  Sodium requirement = TBW × (Desired serum $[Na^+]$ − Actual serum $[Na^+]$)

Formula 2:
  Water excess (in L) = TBW × {1 − (Actual serum $[Na^+]$/Desired serum $[Na^+]$)}

Formula 3:
  Serum $[Na^+]$ change (after 1 L of IV fluid) = ($[Na^+]$ concentration in IV fluid − Actual serum $[Na^+]$)/(TBW + 1)

Formula 4:
  Water deficit (in L) = TBW × {(Actual serum $[Na^+]$/Desired serum $[Na^+]$) − 1}

TBW: total body water (in L) is estimated as body weight × 0.6 in men and × 0.5 in women.

Treatment

Treating the underlying cause and giving water is sufficient in most cases.

Acute symptomatic hypernatremia

In this situation rapid correction of the water deficit is required. Water should be administered (usually as IV 5% dextrose solution) at a rate that reduces the serum [Na^+] by 1 mmol/L/h until symptoms have resolved. The total magnitude of correction should not exceed 8–10 mmol/day. During treatment close monitoring of the patient, the serum [Na^+], fluid intake, urine output and neurologic symptoms are necessary and should preferably be done in an intensive care unit.

Several formulae can be used to calculate the water deficit (Formula 4) or to estimate the effect on serum [Na^+] concentration of any infused solution (Formula 3) (Table 2.1.1).

Chronic asymptomatic hypernatremia

Rapid correction of chronic hypernatremia can cause cerebral edema. The rate of correction should not exceed 0.5 mmol/L/h. Water may be administered orally, by nasogastric tube or IV (as 5% dextrose in water).

In hypovolemic patients with circulatory compromise, normal saline should be given until euvolemia is restored.

In euvolemic patients, oral tap water, 5% dextrose in water or hypotonic saline (0.45% sodium chloride) may be given to correct hypernatremia.

In hypervolemic patients, diuretics plus 5% dextrose in water are administered to remove the excess sodium. In massive volume overload or renal failure, dialysis may be needed.

For chronic treatment of central DI, desmopressin is the drug of choice. In nephrogenic DI, treatment involves: reducing solute intake to reduce the obligate urinary solute excretion; administering thiazide diuretics to induce mild volume contraction; and administering nonsteroidal anti-inflammatory drugs to suppress prostaglandin-mediated antagonism of ADH.

Prevention

Administering adequate fluid avoids hypernatremia in high risk settings.

Be cautious with hypertonic solution (such as sodium bicarbonate) administration.

Further reading

Adrogue HJ, Madias NE. Hypernatremia. *N Engl J Med* 2000; **342**: 1493–1499.

Adrogue HJ, Madias NE. Hyponatremia. *N Engl J Med* 2000; **342**: 1581–1589.

Cawley MJ. Hyponatremia: current treatment strategies and the role of vasopressin antagonists. *Ann Pharmacother* 2007; **41**: 840–850.

Ellison DH, Berl T. The syndrome of inappropriate antidiuresis. *N Engl J Med* 2007; **356**: 064–2072.

Kumar S, Berl T. Sodium. *Lancet* 1998;**352**:220–228.

Reynolds RM, Padfield PL, Seckl JR. Disorders of sodium balance. *Br Med J* 2006; **332**: 702–705.

Smellie WSA, Heald A. Hyponatremia and hypernatremia: pitfalls in testing. *Br Med J* 2007; **334**: 473–476.

Verbalis JG, Goldsmith SR, Greenberg A, Schrier RW, Sterns RH. Hyponatremia treatment guidelines 2007: expert panel recommendations. *Am J Med* 2007; **120**(11 Suppl 1): S1–21.

Internet resources

Overview of fluid physiology:

`http://www.anaesthesiamcq.com/FluidBook/index.php`

Review of diseases of water metabolism:

`http://www.kidneyatlas.org/book1/ADK1_01.pdf`

Review of diseases of sodium balance:

`http://www.kidneyatlas.org/book1/ADK1_02.pdf`

See also

Nephrogenic diabetes insipidus, p. 220

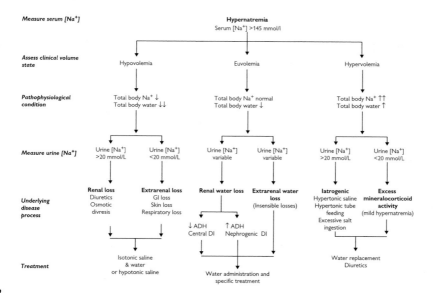

Fig. 2.1.2

Hypo-/hyperkalemia

Potassium (K^+) is the major intracellular cation. 98% of total body K^+ is in the cells. The intracellular/extracellular K^+ ratio is the major determinant of the resting membrane potential, and is therefore critical for the proper function of excitable tissues, such as heart and neuromuscular cells.

Potassium balance and serum K^+ concentration ($[K^+]$) is controlled:
- in the short term by transcellular shift of potassium:
  - this is controlled by insulin, epinephrine (via β_2 adrenergic receptors( ), acid–base status and serum $[K^+]$;
- in the longer term by renal K^+ handling:
  - this is mainly regulated by distal K^+ secretion;
  - distal K^+ secretion is augmented by aldosterone, high distal sodium delivery, high urine flow rate, and high intracellular $[K^+]$ in the tubule cells.

Serum $[K^+]$ disorders can alter membrane excitability, thus causing serious complications, including fatal cardiac arrhythmias, paralysis and respiratory failure.

Hypokalemia
Serum $[K^+]$ <3.5 mmol/L.

This increases the morbidity and mortality risk in patients with cardiovascular disease.

Epidemiology
Hypokalemia is found in >20% of hospitalized patients. The frequency increases with age.

It is found in 10–40% of patients treated with non-K^+-sparing diuretics.

Pathophysiology
Hypokalemia may develop because of either:
- increased shift of K^+ into the cells (redistribution hypokalemia; total body K^+ is usually normal); or
- total body K^+ depletion due to either decreased intake or increased renal or extrarenal losses.

Increased K^+ loss is the major cause of hypokalemia.

Etiology
Pseudohypokalemia (spurious hypokalemia)

This is seen in patients with leukocyte counts >50–100×10^9/L, particularly if the sample is stored at room temperature.

This can be avoided by prompt centrifugation of the specimen.

Redistribution hypokalemia

This is a relatively uncommon cause but when it coexists with mild K^+ depletion it can lead to severe hypokalemia.

Most common causes are:
- Alkalosis (serum $[K^+]$ decreases 0.2–0.3 mmol/L per 0.1 unit increase in pH).
- Excess insulin (acute glucose load, exogenous insulin or insulinoma).
- Increased β-adrenergic activity (e.g. acute myocardial infarction, head trauma) or exogenous administration of β-adrenergic agonists (adrenaline, salbutamol, terbutaline, fenoterol).

Rare causes are hypokalemic periodic paralysis, hypothermia, chloroquine intoxication, and rapid cell synthesis during B12 therapy.

Total potassium depletion

Poor dietary intake is an uncommon cause. Alcoholics, the elderly and poor, and patients with eating disorders are prone to inadequate dietary intake.

Increased K^+ loss may be due to renal or extrarenal losses. Urinary indices of K^+ (Table 2.2.1), acid–base status, blood pressure, urinary chloride (Cl^-) and plasma renin and aldosterone levels are helpful in determining the source of potassium loss (Figure 2.2.1).

This is commonly seen in patients who either are on diuretics (thiazide or loop diuretics) or have gastrointestinal diseases (most commonly with diarrhea).

Vomiting and nasogastric suctioning are also common causes. These result in volume depletion, metabolic alkalosis, and increased urinary K^+ loss.

Endogenous or exogenous mineralocorticoid excess (primary or secondary) is also a frequent cause

Hypomagnesemia often accompanies hypokalemia. Hypokalemia cannot be reversed until the magnesium deficit is corrected.

Rare causes of renal K^+ loss are renal tubular acidosis and the hypokalemic tubulopathies (Gitelman's, Bartter's, and Liddle's syndromes).

Signs and symptoms
Mild hypokalemia (3.0–3.5 mmol/L) is often asymptomatic. Symptoms are more common in patients with moderate (2.5–3.0 mmol/L) or severe (<2.5 mmol/L) hypokalemia.

Most signs and symptoms involve the cardiovascular, neuromuscular, renal and endocrine systems (Table 2.2.2).

Cardiac arrhythmias are common in patients with underlying heart disease (acute myocardial infarction, left ventricular hypertrophy, heart failure) and may be fatal.

In digoxin-treated patients, hypokalemia of any degree can precipitate arrhythmias.

Diagnosis
Measure serum $[K^+]$; exclude spurious or redistribution hypokalemia.

Undertake a detailed history (for dietary intake, medication history, severe diarrhea) and physical examination particularly for blood pressure and neuromuscular signs.

Perform an ECG to determine the effects on cardiac conduction (Figure 2.2.2) and to detect evidence of digoxin toxicity.

Laboratory studies:
- Measure serum electrolytes, glucose, urea and creatinine.
- Assess urine K^+ indices (Table 2.2.1).
- Assess acid–base status.
- Measure magnesium, renin, aldosterone and cortisol in selected cases.

Treatment
Treat the underlying cause; stop ongoing K^+ losses.

Replete K^+ according to:
1. Underlying pathophysiology (redistribution vs K^+ loss).
2. Severity of hypokalemia (actual level of $[K^+]$ ± neuromuscular symptoms ± ECG alterations ± presence of cardiac disease).

Table 2.2.1 Urinary indices of potassium excretion

Index	Equation	Hypokalemia		Hyperkalemia		Caution
		Extrarenal loss	Renal loss	↑ Load	↓ Renal excretion	
Spot urinary [K^+] (mmol/L)	–	<15–20	>15–20	>100	<200	Convenient, but less accurate
Spot urine K^+/Creat (mmol/mmol)	–	<1	>2	>15	<15	Convenient, but with a large 'grey' area
24 h urinary K^+ (mmol/day)	–	<15–20	>15–20	>100	<200	Accurate but inconvenient, needs 24 h urine collection
Fractional excretion of potassium (FEK)	$\dfrac{U_K^+/S_K^+ \times 100\%}{U_{Cre}/S_{Cre}}$	<5%	>5%	>20%	<20%	–
Transtubular potassium gradient (TTKG)	$\dfrac{U_K^+/S_K^+}{U_{osm}/S_{osm}}$	<3	>7	>10	<5–7	Not useful when $U_{osm} < S_{osm}$

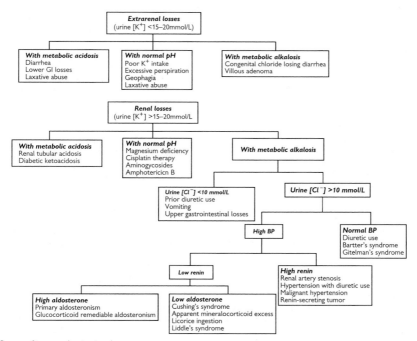

Fig. 2.2.1 Causes of increased potassium loss.

In redistribution hypokalemia, treating the underlying cause is sufficient. Potassium supplementation is not indicated and can even be dangerous.

Serum $[K^+]$ decreases by 0.25–0.30 mmol/L for every 100 mmol reduction in total body K^+.

In acute, life-threatening conditions (paralysis, malignant ventricular arrhythmias and digoxin intoxication), potassium chloride (KCl) should be given IV in a nondextrose-containing solution (10–20 mmol/h into a peripheral vein or 20–40 mmol/h (never >40 mmol/h) into a central vein) with continuous ECG monitoring. Serum $[K^+]$ should be checked every 2–3 h.

Asymptomatic and mild hypokalemia (3.0–3.5 mmol/L) can simply be treated with a K^+-rich diet. The only exception is following myocardial infarction when K^+ supplementation is recommended to keep the serum $[K^+]$ >4.5 mmol/L.

In all other cases of hypokalemia (moderate hypokalemia with no indications for urgent treatment), K^+ supplementation should be undertaken orally. Potassium chloride (KCl) should be used in most circumstances (in divided doses of 20–160 mmol/day). KCl can be administered IV (<10 mmol/h) if the oral route is not possible.

Replete magnesium if it is low.

Patients with hyperaldosteronism may require K^+-sparing diuretics (spironolactone 25–400 mg/day, amiloride 5-40 mg/day, or triamterene 100–400 mg/day) until the underlying disorder can be corrected.

Overtreatment of hypokalemia leading to hyperkalemia is a life-threatening complication. A conservative approach is recommended in most situations and where active treatment is instituted, close monitoring of the response to treatment is mandatory.

Prevention

Check serum $[K^+]$ regularly in patients treated with thiazide diuretics and in those with ongoing sources of K^+ loss.

Hyperkalemia

Serum $[K^+]$ >5.0 mmol/L.

This is the most common electrolyte disorder associated with life-threatening cardiac arrhythmias and sudden death.

Epidemiology

Reported incidence is between 1 and 10% of hospitalized patients.

Most cases are related to drugs interfering with K^+ excretion (renin–angiotensin–aldosterone inhibitors) in combination with pre-existing or acute renal failure.

Advanced age, presence of diabetes, renal failure, congestive heart failure and polypharmacy are the main risk factors.

Pathophysiology

Hyperkalemia may develop because of:

- decreased shift of K^+ into the cells (redistribution hyperkalemia, the total body K^+ is usually normal);
- increased total body K^+ due to either excessive potassium ingestion or, more commonly, decreased renal excretion.

In most situations, persistent hyperkalemia is associated with impairment of urinary K^+ excretion.

Etiology

Pseudohyperkalemia (spurious hyperkalemia)

Prolonged tourniquet application, difficult venepuncture, hemolysis, marked leukocytosis (>50–100 × 10^9/L) and thrombocytosis (>1000 × 10^9/L) may cause pseudohyperkalemia.

In marked leukocytosis or thrombocytosis, parallel measurements of serum and plasma (sample with heparin) $[K^+]$ will identify spurious hyperkalemia.

Redistribution hyperkalemia

This is rarely an important cause of hyperkalemia unless it is accompanied by impaired K^+ excretion.

Most common causes are:

- metabolic acidosis (serum $[K^+]$ rises 0.7 mmol/L per 0.1 unit decrease in pH during a mineral acidosis, i.e. hyperchloremic acidosis);
- insulin deficiency or resistance;
- hyperosmolality (e.g. hyperglycemia, mannitol infusion);
- β-adrenergic antagonist treatment (e.g. propranolol, labetolol, carvedilol, etc.).

Rare causes are hyperkalemic periodic paralysis, digoxin toxicity and succinylcholine administration.

Increased total body potassium

Since the excretory capacity of the kidneys for potassium is so great, excessive K^+ ingestion causes hyperkalemia only rarely. A massive potassium load in a short time (e.g. 300 mmol as a single dose orally or >40 mmol/h IV; or massive cell lysis, such as in tumor lysis or rhabdomyolysis) may overwhelm the renal excretory capacity and cause hyperkalemia.

Impairment of renal K^+ excretion is the cause of hyperkalemia in >80–90% of cases (Table 2.2.3).

Patients with a GFR of <5–10 ml/min have an intrinsic risk of developing hyperkalemia.

If hyperkalemia develops in a patient with less severe renal failure (i.e. GFR >20 mL/min), there is usually an associated condition which further impairs K^+ excretion. These are:

1. Effective circulating volume depletion (congestive heart failure).
2. Diminished aldosterone activity (primary adrenal insufficiency, hyporeninemic hypoaldosteronism, drug-induced hypoaldosteronism).
3. Decreased tubular secretion (tubulointerstitial diseases, pseudohypoaldosteronism, potassium sparing diuretics).

Signs and symptoms

Hyperkalemia may be classified as mild (5.5–6.0 mmol/L), moderate (6.0–6.5 mmol/L) and severe (>6.5 mmol/L or any $[K^+]$ associated with muscle symptoms or ECG changes).

Table 2.2.2 Major clinical manifestations of hypo- or hyperkalemia

System	Hypokalemia	Hyperkalemia
Cardiovascular	ECG alterations (Fig. 2.2.2)	ECG alterations (Fig. 2.2.2)
	Ventricular tachycardia/fibrillation, long QT syndrome, torsade de pointes, hypertension	Life-threatening ventricular arrythmias including sudden death, hypotension
Neuromuscular	Muscular weakness, cramps, rhabdomyolysis, ileus, constipation, bladder dysfunction, ascending symmetric paralysis, respiratory impairment	Muscular weakness, paresthesias, ascending paralysis, respiratory impairment
Renal	Nephrogenic diabetes insipidus, increased ammonia production, metabolic alkalosis, hypokalemic nephropathy (vacuolization in proximal tubules, medullary cyst formation and interstitial fibrosis)	Reduced ammoniagenesis, type IV renal tubular acidosis, natriuresis
Endocrine/metabolic	Increased renin, decreased aldosterone, decreased insulin secretion, growth retardation	Decreased renin, increased aldosterone, increased insulin secretion

Table 2.2.3 Causes of impaired potassium excretion

Glomerular filtration rate <5–10 mL/min	Glomerular filtration rate >20 mL/min
Oliguria of any cause	Low aldosterone
Endogenous potassium load	Low renin
Gastrointestinal bleeding	Hyporeninemic hypoaldosteronism
Hemolysis	Diabetes mellitus
Rhabdomyolysis	NSAIDs
Catabolic state	High renin
Exogenous potassium load	Addison's disease
Dietary intake	Heparin
Salt substitutes	ACEIs
Stored blood	ARBs
Drugs	Normal–high aldosterone
Aldosterone antagonists	Aldosterone antagonists
K^+-sparing diuretics	K^+-sparing diuretics
ACEIs	Trimethoprim
ARBs	Tubulointerstitial nephritis
Beta-blockers	Systemic lupus erythematosus
NSAIDs	Amyloidosis
Trimethoprim	Sickle cell disease
Heparin	Pseudohypoaldosteronism types I and II (Gordon's syndrome)

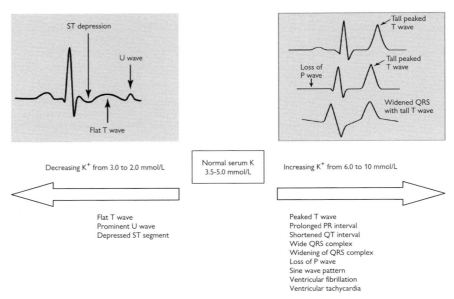

Fig. 2.2.2 Typical electrocardiographic changes in a spectrum of potassium disorders from hypo- to hyperkalemia. (ECG tracings from Slovis C, Jenkins R. ABC of clinical electrocardiography: conditions not primarily affecting the heart. *BMJ* 2002;324:1320-1323, with permission.)

Most signs and symptoms involve the cardiovascular, neuromuscular, renal and endocrine systems (Table 2.2.2).

Cardiac toxicity is enhanced by hypocalcemia, hyponatremia, acidosis and a rapid rise in [K+].

Cardiac toxicity usually precedes neuromuscular manifestations. Muscle weakness usually only becomes apparent when [K+] >8.0 mmol/L.

Patients with hypoaldosteronism may also complain of weight loss and symptoms related to salt wasting.

Diagnosis

Measure serum [K+], exclude pseudohyperkalemia and look for potential causes of redistribution hyperkalemia.

A thorough history (for dietary intake, history of kidney disease, medication history including K+ supplements, K+-sparing diuretics, renin–angiotensin–aldosterone system inhibitors) and physical examination (for blood pressure and muscle weakness) should be undertaken.

Perform an ECG to determine the effects on cardiac conduction and the need for urgent treatment (Figure 2.2.2).

Laboratory studies:
- Measure serum electrolytes, glucose, urea and creatinine.
- Calculate the estimated GFR.
- Assess urine K+ indices (Table 2.2.1).
- Assess acid–base status.
- Measure renin, aldosterone and cortisol levels in selected cases.

Treatment

Treat urgently if:
- there are ECG abnormalities and signs of neuromuscular dysfunction, or
- the serum [K+] is >6.5 mmol/L without any ECG abnormalities.

If urgent treatment is required, continuous cardiac monitoring should be instituted.

The aims of treatment are to:
1. Antagonize the cell membrane actions of hyperkalemia to protect the heart and respiratory muscles.
   - Infuse 10 mL of 10% calcium gluconate or chloride over 2–3 min; action starts in 1–3 min, but the effect is transient.
   - Repeat the dose after 5–10 min if ECG changes persist.
   - Use calcium cautiously in patients taking digoxin as it may precipitate toxicity.
2. Increase K+ entry into the cells.
   - Administer 10 U of soluble insulin with 50 mL of 50% dextrose in water (DW) as an intravenous bolus, followed by an insulin infusion (1–4 U/h) with 5% DW. The effect is apparent in ~15–30 min and lasts ~2–4 h. Blood glucose must be monitored because of the risk of hypoglycemia.
   - Administer high-dose β2-adrenergic agonist (salbutamol (albuterol) 0.5 mg IV in 5% DW for 10–15 min or 10–20 mg by nebulized inhaler for 10 min). Action of IV and nebulized salbutamol begins in ~20–30 min and lasts ~2–4 h. Patients treated with this will also become very tremulous.
   - Combining insulin–dextrose with salbutamol probably leads to greater reductions in potassium than either alone.
   - Administer sodium bicarbonate (50–100 mmol IV for 5 min) only if there is a metabolic acidosis. Onset of action may be delayed by hours, so the efficacy is questionable. In addition caution should be used in patients with renal failure since the sodium load may precipitate pulmonary edema.

3. Eliminate excess potassium from the body.

- Volume expand with saline followed by furosemide (20–40 mg IV) administration once volume replete. This may be helpful if there is prerenal acute renal failure or residual renal function. Onset of action is within 1 h; however, it is unlikely to work in patients with advanced renal failure.

- Resin exchanger sodium or calcium polystyrene sulfonate (kayexalate or calcium resonium respectively) mixed with sorbitol can be given orally (30 g) or as a retention enema (50 g). Each gram of resin removes 0.5–1.0 mmol of potassium. The onset of action is within 1–2 h. The dose may be repeated every 3–4 h (oral) or 2–4 h (rectal).

- Dialysis is indicated if all of the above measures fail to correct hyperkalemia.

Most patients with mild hyperkalemia (5.5–6.0 mmol/L) can be treated by eliminating the underlying cause (such as discontinuing K^+ supplements or aldosterone antagonists) and restricting dietary potassium.

In patients with moderate hyperkalemia (6.0–6.5 mmol/L) consider additional maneuvres such as loop diuretics (provided that renal function is relatively maintained), resin exchanger or synthetic mineralocorticoids (in cases of mineralocorticoid deficiency).

Prevention

Check $[K^+]$ regularly in susceptible patients, especially those taking drugs that impair K^+ excretion.

An increasing incidence of hyperkalemia is observed with combined use of aldosterone antagonists with renin–angiotensin system (RAS) inhibitors in heart failure patients.

In chronic kidney disease patients, if hyperkalemia develops during RAS inhibitor treatment, other measures (dietary K^+ restriction, stopping contributory drugs, adding a diuretic or reducing the dose of RAS inhibitors) should be tried before discontinuing the RAS inhibitors.

Further reading

Alfonzo AVM, Isles C, Geddes C, *et al*. Potassium disorders – clinical spectrum and emergency management. *Resuscitation* 2006; 70: 10–25.

Gennari FJ. Hypokalemia. *N Engl J Med*1998; **339**: 451–458.

Halperin ML, Kamel KS. Potassium. *Lancet* 1998; **352**: 135–140.

Mahoney BA, Smith WAD, Lo DS, *et al.* Emergency interventions for hyperkalemia. *Cochrane Database Syst Rev* 2005; CD003235.

Rastergar A, Soleimani M. Hypokalaemia and hyperkalaemia. *Postgrad Med J* 2001; **77**: 759–764.

Smelli WSA, Shaw, Bowlees R, *et al.* Best practice in primary care pathology: Review 9. *J Clin Pathol* 2007; **60**: 966–974.

Internet resources

Review of disorders of potassium metabolism:

http://www.kidneyatlas.org/book1/adk1_03.pdf

See also

Hypo-/hypercalcemia

Calcium is the most abundant mineral in the body.

98% of the total body calcium is stored in bone and the rest is in the soft tissues and extracellular fluid.

Calcium circulates in the plasma in the bound and free form. The normal range for total calcium is 2.25–2.65 mmol/L.

Approximately 40% of plasma calcium is bound to proteins (mainly albumin), and 10% is complexed to anions such as bicarbonate, citrate, sulphate, phosphate and lactate.

The remaining 50% of plasma calcium is in the ionized form and is physiologically active.

Functions of calcium

The functions of calcium in the body include:
- maintenance of skeletal and dental structure;
- muscle contraction and relaxation;
- stimulation of blood clotting;
- maintenance of cell membrane integrity;
- nerve transmission;
- regulation of intracellular signalling;
- stimulation of hormone secretion;
- augmentation of enzyme activity (enzyme cofactor).

Calcium homeostasis

The serum calcium concentration is maintained in a very narrow range with <2% variability.

The three key organs involved in calcium homeostasis are the gut, bone, and kidney.

The main calcium regulators are parathyroid hormone (PTH) and $1,25\text{-}(OH)_2$ vitamin D.

A critical level of serum magnesium concentration is required for PTH secretion, thus severe hypomagnesemia may impair PTH release even in the presence of significant hypocalcemia.

Gut

Gastrointestinal absorption of calcium can be passive or active.

About 40% of the daily dietary calcium intake (~25 mmol) is absorbed in the gut (10 mmol). The absorption can be greatly increased if the body is in negative calcium balance.

Passive absorption is by the paracellular junctions driven by the concentration gradients between the gut lumen and the serosal surfaces.

Active transport is mediated by entry of luminal calcium through apical calcium channels, binding to the calcium binding protein, calbindin, and extrusion by an active Na/Ca-ATPase and Na/Ca exchanger. This is a saturable process which is tightly regulated by $1,25\text{-}(OH)_2$ vitamin D.

Calcium absorption can be inhibited by citrates, phytates, and drugs such as colchicine and theophylline.

Bone

Both PTH and $1,25\text{-}(OH)_2$ vitamin D play a key in bone metabolism through regulation of both bone formation and resorption.

Under normal circumstances in adults, bone formation and resorption are in balance and there is no net movement of calcium from bone.

With $1,25\text{-}(OH)_2$ vitamin D deficiency and/or hyperparathyroidism, osteoclastic activity may be enhanced resulting in increased bone resorption.

There is a steep inverse relationship between the serum ionised calcium concentration and PTH release that is mediated by the calcium-sensing receptor (CaSR) on the chief cells of the parathyroid gland.

Kidney

Sixty-five percent of filtered calcium is reabsorbed in the proximal tubule. This is not under hormonal regulation but is closely associated with sodium and water balance.

Approximately 25% of the filtered calcium is reabsorbed in the loop of Henle and ~10% in the distal convoluted tubule under the influence of PTH.

PTH also stimulates 1α-hydroxylase activity in the kidney, leading to increased formation of $1,25\text{-}(OH)_2$ vitamin D and thus indirectly regulates intestinal calcium and phosphate absorption.

There is also evidence that vitamin D may independently increase renal calcium reabsorption.

Hypocalcemia

Hypocalcemia is regarded as mild when the serum calcium concentration (adjusted for albumin) is 1.75–2.10 mmol/L, and severe when it is <1.75 mmol/L.

Causes of hypocalcemia

- 25-(OH) vitamin D deficiency
  Nutritional deficiency in Asians, the elderly in nursing homes or those who are home-bound and vegetarian.
  Malabsorption of fat soluble vitamins, e.g. Crohn's disease, chronic pancreatitis, hepatobiliary disorders.
  In renal diseases such as nephrotic syndrome, vitamin D binding proteins may be lost leading to vitamin D deficiency.
  Antiepileptic drugs such as phenytoin and phenobarbital.
- $1,25\text{-}(OH)_2$ vitamin D deficiency
  Chronic renal failure with GFR <30 mL/min.
  Inherited disorders, e.g. vitamin D-dependent rickets type I due to 1-α-hydroxylase deficiency; and vitamin D dependent rickets type II due to end-organ unresponsiveness to $1,25\text{-}(OH)_2$ vitamin D.
- Hypoparathyroidism
  Postoperative.
  Autoimmune.
  Congenital (e.g. activating mutations of the CaSR, parathyroid aplasia).
  Infiltrative disorders.
  Pseudohyperparathyroidism.
- Hyperphosphatemia (resulting in increased calcium × phosphate (Ca × P) product causing ectopic calcification)
  Renal failure.
  Tumor lysis syndrome.
  Rhabdomyolysis.
  Intravenous phosphate administration.
- Severe magnesium deficiency/depletion.
- Acute pancreatitis.
- Hungry bone syndrome.
- Sepsis, burns or severe illness.

- Drugs, e.g. bisphosphonates, cinacalcet.
- Artefactual, e.g. chelation with EDTA.

Clinical manifestations of hypocalcemia

Both the rate of fall and the severity of hypocalcemia determine the severity of the signs and symptoms.

Patients may be asymptomatic or have subtle symptoms and signs but they may also present acutely with life-threatening manifestations.

Hypomagnesemia, hypokalemia and alkalosis may coexist and worsen the clinical picture.

Neuromuscular
- Tetany and seizures.
- Trousseau's and Chvostek's sign.
- Muscle cramps/tenderness/myopathy.
- Laryngeal stridor, bronchospasm and respiratory arrest.
- Perioral numbness and paresthesias.
- Calcifications of the basal ganglia, cerebrum and cerebellum.
- Depression and irritability.
- Dementia and movement disorders.
- Papilloedema.

Cardiovascular
- Syncope, rarely congestive heart failure and angina.
- Prolongation of QT interval, ventricular fibrillation and heart block.

Other manifestations
- Biliary and intestinal cramps.
- Resistance to digoxin therapy.
- Cataracts.
- Poor dentition (age of ≤5 years).
- Dry, coarse skin, brittle nails, alopecia.
- Bone changes (rickets) and osteodystrophy.

Investigation of hypocalcemia

Measure:
- Serum urea, creatinine and electrolytes, calcium, phosphate, albumin, alkaline phosphatase and magnesium.
- PTH and 25-(OH) vitamin D.
- Serum bicarbonate and arterial blood gases if acidosis is suspected.
- 24 h urine calcium excretion (reference range: 2.5–7.5 mmol/24 h). This is useful for monitoring patients on treatment for hypoparathyroidsm.

Treatment of hypocalcemia

The decision to treat hypocalcemia will depend on the presenting symptoms, their severity and rapidity of onset.

Acute symptomatic hypocalcemia (particularly if calcium <1.75 mmol/L)

Treat the underlying cause
- 10 ml of 10% calcium gluconate is given IV over 10 min. This may be followed by slow IV infusion of up to 20 mL of 10% calcium gluconate over >6 h with ECG monitoring. This may be repeated once within a 24 h period.
- Hypomagnesemia and hypokalemia may coexist and should be treated as appropriate. If correction of hypomagnesemia is undertaken it should be done cautiously in patients with CKD as they have impaired renal excretion of magnesium.

- If hyperphosphatemia is present (e.g. in renal failure), saline infusions should be administered cautiously since this may worsen the hypocalcemia. Dialysis may be necessary in severe hyperphosphatemia.
- Oral calcium and vitamin D supplements may be given concurrently with IV infusions. Once the patient can tolerate adequate oral supplements, the infusions may be stopped.

Chronic hypocalcemia
- In patients with CKD the goal is to prevent metabolic bone disease and vascular mineralization. Serum calcium should be maintained within the target range and Ca × P kept at <4.8 mmol^2/L^2 and ideally <4.2 mmol^2/L^2.
- In dialysis patients, serum calcium should ideally be kept at <2.5 mmol/L.
- PTH measurement is not routinely required in the absence of suspected disorder of bone and mineral metabolism in CKD stages 1 and 2 or in nonprogressive stage 3, although PTH levels should be maintained within normal reference ranges.
- PTH needs to be routinely measured 3-monthly in patients with CKD 5. Measurement of PTH should also be considered in earlier stages of CKD (CKD 4 and possibly CKD 3) although opinion varies about the required frequency and utility of this. In stage 4, the PTH should be between the upper limit and two times the upper limit of the normal range, and in stage 5 patients not on dialysis it should be between two and four times the upper limit of the normal range. If necessary, surgical treatment for hyperparathyroidism may be considered.
- In patients with hypocalcemia and CKD stages 3–5, therapy with active oral vitamin D sterols (calcitriol, alfacalcidol) is indicated with close monitoring of serum calcium and phosphate, and to maintain plasma PTH within the defined limits.
- Patients with hypoparathyroidism are treated with 1,25-(OH)$_2$ vitamin D and the 24 h urine calcium excretion is monitored in order to avoid hypercalciuria.

Hypercalcemia

A serum total calcium concentration (adjusted for albumin) of >2.60 and <3.0 mmol/L is considered mild, >3.0 and <3.5 mmol/L is moderate and >3.5 mmol/L severe hypercalcemia.

Causes of hypercalcemia
- Primary hyperparathyroidism (adenoma 80–85%, multiglandular or associated with MEN1 and MEN2 A 15–20%, and rarely due to carcinoma 1%) accounts for >50% of all cases of hypercalcemia.
- Malignancy (30% of all cancers: 35% of lung cancers, 25% of breast and 14% of hematological malignancies particularly myeloma). This is mediated mainly by parathyroid-hormone-related peptides (PTHrP) whose N-terminal is similar to that of PTH or by cytokines (IL-1, IL-6, TGF, TNF etc.). Lymphoma cells may activate conversion of 25-(OH) vitamin D to 1,25-(OH)$_2$ vitamin D.
- Drugs, e.g. thiazides, lithium.
- Vitamin D toxicity.
- Vitamin A toxicity.
- Tertiary hyperparathyroidism.
- During recovery from acute renal failure.
- Granulomatous diseases, e.g. sarcoidosis, tuberculosis.

- Immobilization.
- Familial hypocalciuric hypercalcemia.
- Endocrine e.g. thyrotoxicosis, Addison's disease, pheochromocytoma, acromegaly.
- Milk alkali syndrome.
- Aluminium toxicity.
- Parenteral nutrition.

Clinical manifestations of hypercalcemia

About 80% of cases of hypercalcemia are asymptomatic.

The occurrence of symptoms depends on the severity of hypercalcemia and rapidity of onset.

Neurological

- Lethargy, drowsiness and coma.
- Apathy and cognitive impairment.
- Confusion.
- Depression.
- Hypotonia and decreased deep tendon reflexes.

Gastrointestinal

- Dyspepsia with or without peptic ulcer disease.
- Acute pancreatitis.
- Constipation.
- Abdominal pain.
- Anorexia, nausea and vomiting.

Renal

- Polyuria and polydipsia.
- Hypercalciuria, nephrolithiasis and nephrocalcinosis.

Cardiovascular

- Arrhythmias.
- Hypertension.
- Increased sensitivity to digoxin.

Other manifestations

- Osteopenia and osteoporosis.
- Soft tissue calcification with chondrocalcinosis and band keratopathy.

Investigation of hypercalcemia

Measure:

- Serum urea, creatinine, electrolytes, total calcium, inorganic phosphate, albumin, alkaline phosphatase.
- PTH (and 25-(OH) vitamin D where indicated).
- ECG.

Treatment of hypercalcemia

The treatment of hypercalcemia depends on its severity, chronicity and the underlying cause.

Symptoms of hypercalcemia are more common at calcium concentrations >3.0 mmol/L.

Calcium concentrations >3.5 mmol/L are considered severe and require emergency treatment.

Acute symptomatic hypercalcemia

- Initial treatment in patients with preserved renal function is volume expansion with normal saline (2–6 L for a period of 24 h).
- Loop diuretics may be given cautiously with close monitoring of the volume status. These measures may reduce serum calcium by ~0.5 mmol/L.

- The main treatment for hypercalcemia is IV bisphosphonates, e.g. pamidronate 30–90 mg over 2–4 h depending on the degree of the hypercalcemia. It may take up to 4 days to achieve normocalcemia. Persistent or recurrent hypercalcemia may require repeated infusions at 3–4 week intervals but paradoxical hypocalcemia may occur with repeated infusions. Bisphosphonates should be used with caution in patients with renal impairment.
- Calcitonin (200–400 U per day in divided doses) may be given and acts within minutes, but due to tachyphylaxis it is effective for only up to 48 h.
- Glucocortocoids are particularly effective in hypercalcemia due to granulomatous disorders, multiple myeloma and other hematological malignancies, and may be tried in these cases for a period of 10 days.

Chronic hypercalcemia

- The general measures in the treatment of chronic hypercalcemia are adequate oral hydration and avoidance of thiazide diuretics.
- In CKD patients with hypercalcemia who are taking calcium-based phosphate binders, dose reduction or use of noncalcium containing binders is appropriate. Again, for the CKD patients on vitamin D sterols, the therapy can be stopped or dose reduced when the target serum calcium levels have been reached. In patients on dialysis, low calcium dialyzate can be used for a short period of ~3–4 weeks.
- During the course of renal failure, parathyroid hyperplasia and associated hyperparathyroidism often develops and may persist following renal transplantation when hypercalcemia may result. Hypercalcemia due to tertiary hyperparathyroidism may require parathyroidectomy. Cinacalcet, a calcium mimetic drug, may offer an alternative to surgery. Cinacalcet directly decreases PTH levels and thus calcium concentrations by directly activating the CaSR in the parathyroid gland.

Further reading

Baker SB, Worthley LIG. The essentials of calcium, magnesium and phosphate metabolism: Part 1 and 2. *Crit Care Resusc* 2002; **4**: 301–315.

Body J, Bouillon R. Emergencies in calcium homeostasis. *Rev Endocr Metab Dis* 2003; **4**: 167–175.

Bushinsky DA, Monk RD. Calcium. *Lancet* 1998; **352**: 306–311.

Clines GA, Guise TA. Hypocalcaemia of malignancy and basic research on mechanisms responsible for osteolytic and osteoblastic metastasis to bone. *Endocr-Rltd Cancer* 2005; **12**: 549–583.

Davison AM, Cameron JS, Grunfield J-P, Ponticelli C, Ritz E, Winearls CG, Ypersele CV. Hypo- hypercalcaemia. *Oxford textbook of clinical nephrology*, vol. 1. Oxford: OUP; 2005. pp. 269–286.

Dusso AS, Brown AJ, Slatopolsky E. Vitamin D. *Am J Physiol – Renal Physiol* 2005; **289**: F8–F28.

Gunn IR, Gaffney D. Clinical and laboratory features of calcium-sensing receptor disorders: a systemic review. *Ann Clin Biochem* 2004; **41**: 441–458.

Leca N, et al. Early and severe hyperparathyroidism associated with hypercalcaemia after renal transplant treated with Cinacalcet. *Am J Transpl* 2006; **6**: 2391–2395.

Moe SM, Drüeke TB. Management of secondary hyperparathyroidism: the importance and the challenge of controlling parathyroid hormone levels without elevating the calcium, phosphorus and calcium-phosphorus product. *Am J Nephrol* 2003; **23**: 368–379.

Silverberg SJ, Bilezikian JP. The diagnosis and management of asymptomatic primary hyperparathyroidism. *Nat Clin Pract Endocrinol Metab* 2006; **2**: 94–503.

Singh J, Moghal N, Pearce SHS, Cheetham T. The investigations of hypocalcaemia and rickets. *Archs Dis Childh* 2003; **88**: 403–407.

Tfelt-Hansen J, Brown EM. The calcium-sensing receptor in normal physiology and pathophysiology: a review. *Crit Rev Clin Lab Sci* 2005; **42**: 35–70.

Internet resources

National Kidney Foundation: K/DOQI clinical practice guidelines for bone metabolism and disease in chronic kidney disease. http://www.kidney.org/professionals/kdoqi/guidelines_bone/index.htm

Porter RS, Kaplan JL, Beer MH (eds), *The Merck manual*, 18th edn; 2006–2007:

http://www.merck.com/mmpe/index.html

Skugor M, Milas M (2004). Hypocalcaemia. The Cleveland Clinic: http://www.clevelandclinicmeded.com/medicalpubs/diseasemanagement/endocrinology/hcalcemia/hcalcemia.htm

The Renal Association. *Clinical Practice Guidelines* (2007): http://www.renal.org/guidelines/index.html

See also

Skeletal disorders in CKD, p. 432

Hypo-/hyperphosphatemia, p. 56

Hypo-/hypermagnesemia, p. 60

Nephrocalcinosis, p. 278

Medical management of stone disease, p. 270

Sarcoidosis , p. 164

Hypo-/hyperphosphatemia

Phosphate is the most abundant intracellular anion.

It is stored predominantly in the bones and teeth, 80% of which is in the form of hydroxyapatite.

Approximately 9% of phosphate is in skeletal muscles and 10.9% in the viscera.

Only 0.1% of the total body phosphate is in the extracellular compartment.

The normal serum phosphate concentration ranges from 0.80 to 1.40 mmol/L and is slightly higher in children.

Functions of phosphate

- Phosphate is a component of lipid membranes, phospholipids, nucleic acids and nucleoproteins.
- It is essential for adenosine triphosphate (ATP) synthesis and is required for the function of most metabolic pathways.
- It is important for signalling pathways that involve protein phosphorlyation.
- It is an important buffer.
- It also upregulates osteopontin gene activity, thereby playing a role in bone mineralization.

Phosphate homeostasis

Phosphate regulation is closely linked to calcium homeostasis.

The plasma phosphate concentration is dependent on dietary inorganic phosphate intake, intestinal absorption, renal filtration and reabsorption, and exchange between the intracellular and bone reservoirs.

Gastrointestinal absorption of phosphate

Phosphorus is ubiquitous in food and there is usually an excess of phosphate in the diet.

Up to 80% of the ingested phosphate (~40 mmol/day) is absorbed, mainly in the duodenum and upper jejunum.

Phosphate absorption occurs by an active, saturable process in the duodenum and jejunum (mediated by the sodium phosphate cotransporter: NaPi IIb), and by passive paracellular diffusion along a concentration gradient in the rest of the small intestine.

$1,25\text{-}(OH)_2$ vitamin D increases intestinal absorption by increasing the transcription of the NaPi cotransporter.

Raised parathyroid hormone (PTH) levels and low serum phosphate indirectly increase absorption via $1,25\text{-}(OH)_2$ vitamin D.

3–4 mmol/day of phosphate is secreted into the intestinal lumen.

Renal excretion of phosphate

The kidney is the key organ in maintaining phosphate homeostasis.

Approximately 180 mmol of phosphate is filtered daily, of which 80% is reabsorbed in the proximal tubules along with sodium through the NaPi IIa cotransporter. This can be increased to >95% in deficiency states.

There is a renal threshold for reabsorption of phosphate (Tm) that varies with GFR. The Tm/GFR ratio can be used as a surrogate marker of proximal tubular function.

A decrease in GFR to <30 mL/min (CKD 4) will impair phosphate excretion.

PTH and PTH-related peptides (PTHrP) decrease phosphate reabsorption by activating intracellular signaling pathways which increase internalization of NaPi IIa.

Glucocorticoids, hypokalemia, chronic hypocalcemia, and volume expansion will also cause hypophosphatemia.

Phosphatonins such as fibroblast growth factor 23 (FGF-23) and frizzled-related protein-4 are also important phosphaturic agents.

Important factors that increase phosphate reabsorption are:
- $1,25\text{-}(OH)_2$ vitamin D.
- other hormones including thyroid hormones, growth hormone, and insulin;
- high calcium intake increases phosphate reabsorption probably as a result of suppression of PTH secretion;
- low dietary phosphate intake stimulates 1α-hydroxylase activity which increases $1,25\text{-}(OH)_2$ vitamin D levels and thereby enhances phosphate resorption.

Bone remodeling

The release and uptake of phosphate from and into bone depends on bone resorption and formation respectively.

The serum phosphate concentration is critical for bone mineralization and resorption.

The vast majority of phosphate in the bone is in the form of hydroxyapatite.

The factors affecting bone remodelling are listed in Table 2.4.1.

Hypophosphatemia

The plasma phosphate concentration refers to the concentration of the inorganic moiety. This varies with age, gender and dietary intake.

In adults hypophosphatemia is considered mild when the serum phosphate concentration is 0.5–0.75 mmol/L, moderate 0.3–0.5 mmol/L and severe when <0.3 mmol/L.

Patients susceptible to severe hypophosphatemia include those with:
- sepsis;
- severe trauma;
- malnutrition (especially with a BMI <18 kg/m², and/or lack of nutrition for >5–10 days);
- diabetic ketoacidosis;
- alcoholism;
- chronic obstructive pulmonary disease.

Causes of hypophosphatemia

Gastrointestinal causes
- Malabsorption.
- Vitamin D deficiency/resistance.
- Prolonged vomiting.
- Prolonged intake of high doses of phosphate-binding antacids (containing magnesium or aluminium).

Low intake alone rarely causes hypophosphatemia, since phosphate is ubiquitously present in food.

Renal causes
- Hyperparathyroidism or secretion of PTHrP.
- Vitamin D deficiency or resistance.
- Renal tubular dysfunction (e.g. Fanconi syndrome).

Table 2.4.1 Hormonal factors regulating bone formation and resorption: direct/indirect effects

	Formation	Resorption
Calcium-regulating hormones		
Parathyroid hormone	Increase	Increase
1,25-(OH)$_2$ vitamin D	Increase/decrease	Increase
Calcitonin	–	Decrease
Systemic hormones		
Glucocorticoids	Decrease	Increase
Insulin	Increase	–
Growth hormone	Increase	–
Insulin-like growth factor-1	Increase	–
Thyroxine	Increase	Increase (in excess)
Sex hormone deficiency	Decrease	Increase
Leptin/neuropeptide Y	Decrease	–
Other circulating and local factors		
Postaglandin E2	–	Increase
Interleukin-1	Increase	Increase
Interleukin-6	–	Increase
Transforming growth factor	Increase	Increase/decrease
RANK ligand/RANK receptor	–	Increase
Osteoprotegerin	–	Decrease
Lipoprotein receptor-related protein 5	Increase	–
PTHrP	Increase	Increase
Interferon-γ	Decrease	Decrease

RANK, receptor activator of NF-κβ; PTHrP, PTH-related peptides.

- Postrenal transplantation.
- Post dialysis.
- Osmotic diuresis (e.g. with glycosuria).
- Volume expansion.
- Diuretics.
- Glucocorticoid excess.
- Tumor-induced osteomalacia (oversecretion of FGF-23 by mesenchymal tumors).
- Genetic defects:
  - X-linked dominant hypophosphatemic rickets: mutations have been identified in the phosphate-regulating (PHEX) gene.
  - Autosomal dominant hypophosphatemic rickets and oncogenic osteomalacia: FGF-23 gain-of-function gene mutations have been identified as causing autosomal dominant hypophosphatemic rickets, and overproduction of FGF-23 arises from some oncogenic tumors.

Internal redistribution
- Refeeding syndrome. This usually occurs within 3–4 days after starting feeds in malnourished patients.
  - Malnourished patients may have depletion of phosphate even though the serum levels appear normal due to redistribution from the intracellular compartment.
  - In these circumstances administration of glucose with increased insulin secretion may lead to a rapid uptake of glucose, magnesium and phosphate into cells resulting in potentially life-threatening hypophosphatemia.
- Recovery from diabetic ketoacidosis.
- Respiratory alkalosis.

- Increased cell turnover or formation (hungry bone syndrome or acute leukemia).
- Increased steroid production resulting in metabolic alkalosis.

Clinical manifestations of hypophosphatemia
There is a four-fold increase in mortality in patients with severe hypophosphatemia.

Low serum phosphate levels do not necessarily imply depletion since hypophosphatemia may be due to shifts from the extracellular to the intracellular compartments.

The symptoms of hypophosphatemia and phosphate depletion are generally associated with decreased availability of intracellular ATP and impaired oxygenation.

Musculoskeletal effects
- Muscle weakness.
- Proximal myopathy.
- Rhabdomyolysis, especially in alcoholic and severely malnourished patients with acute hypophosphatemia.
- Bone pain and fractures.
- Osteomalacia.
- Respiratory failure (from poor diaphragmatic function).

Cardiac effects
- Reduced myocardial contractility.

Central nervous system effects
- Altered mental state.
- Polyneuropathy similar to Guillain–Barré syndrome.
- Paresthesias.
- Metabolic encephalopathy.
- Convulsions and coma.

Hematological effects
- Impaired leukocyte chemotaxis and phagocytosis.
- Impaired platelet function.
- Increased affinity of red blood cells for oxygen.

Renal effects
- Decreased buffering capacity.
- Hyperchloremic metabolic acidosis.
- Glycosuria and bicarbonaturia.
- Increased 1,25-(OH)$_2$ vitamin D synthesis.
- Hypercalciuria due to increased bone turnover and hypercalcemia.
- Increased magnesium excretion.

Investigation of hypophosphatemia
Measure the serum urea, creatinine, electrolytes, bicarbonate, chloride calcium, phosphate, albumin, alkaline phosphatase, and magnesium.

Liver function tests.

Arterial blood gases (especially if respiratory alkalosis is suspected).

PTH and 25-(OH) vitamin D levels

24 hour urine phosphate excretion:
- Reference range is 15–20 mmol/24 h.
- <10 mmol/24 h suggests the presence of a gastrointestinal cause such as malabsorption, antacid use, or chronic alcohol abuse.
- If excretion is >20 mmol/24 h, estimate the maximal rate of tubular reabsorption of phosphate (TRP) from

nomograms or calculate the phosphate/creatinine clearance ratio (Cp/Ccr):

$$Cp/Ccr = \frac{urine\ PO_4 \times serum\ creatinine}{serum\ PO_4 \times urine\ creatinine}$$

- TRP = $(1 - Cp/Ccr) \times 100$ (reference range: 78–98%).
- A low TRP indicates an inappropriate renal loss of phosphate.

Skeletal X-rays and bone densitometry if osteopenia and/or osteomalacia suspected.

Treatment of hypophosphatemia

The treatment of hypophosphatemia depends on the underlying cause and its severity.

Mild hypophosphatemia

Mild hypophosphatemia, particularly when it is due to redistribution with increased uptake into the cells, may not necessarily require specific treatment.

Severe or symptomatic hypophosphatemia

Phosphate concentrations <0.3 mmol/L are likely to require IV treatment.

Phosphate infusion should be given at a rate of 9 mmol every 12 h and in critically ill patients the dose can be increased up to a maximum of 50–60 mmol over 24 h.

It is recommended that plasma phosphate should be monitored 6-hourly and where possible oral supplementation should be commenced when the serum concentration is >0.6 mmol/L.

Administration of IV phosphate can be associated with potentially serious adverse effects due to precipitation with calcium. This can lead to hypocalcemia, renal failure and potentially fatal arrhythmias. It is therefore essential to closely monitor serum calcium, potassium and magnesium concentrations during the infusion.

Treatment with oral phosphate (~30 mmol per day) should be considered in patients with mild to moderate hypophosphatemia.

In the refeeding syndrome, patients may become symptomatic with phosphate levels of <0.5 mmol/L and therefore may require IV phosphate replacement.

Patients at high risk of refeeding syndrome include those with a BMI <16 kg/m^2, an unintentional weight loss of >15% in the preceding 3–6 months, or no food intake for ≥10 days. In such patients oral or IV nutrition should be given at a maximum of 5–10 kcal/kg per day and increased slowly over the following 4–7 days.

Hyperphosphatemia

The normal serum phosphate concentration is 0.8–1.4 mmol. The Renal Association clinical practice guidelines recommend that in patients with CKD stages 3 and 4:

- serum phosphate should be maintained at 0.9–1.5 mmol/L, and in patients on dialysis 1.1–1.8 mmol/L.
- serum calcium × phosphate (Ca × P) product should be kept to <4.8 mmol^2/L^2 and ideally <4.2 mmol^2/L^2.

Causes of hyperphosphatemia

Renal causes

- Acute kidney injury or chronic kidney disease (almost universal in those with GFR <30 mL/min)
- Hypoparathyroidism.
- Pseudohypoparathyroidism.

Increased release from the intracellular compartment

- Rhabdomyolysis.
- Tumor lysis syndrome (common).
- *In vivo* hemolysis.

Redistribution

- Metabolic or respiratory acidosis.

Increased intake

- Can occur due to vitamin D intoxication, although this is rare.
- Absorption of very large amounts of phosphate (can be caused by phosphate enemas).

Endocrine causes

- Acromegaly.
- Thyrotoxicosis.
- Glucocorticoid deficiency.

Miscellaneous causes

- Tumor calcinosis.

Artifactual causes

- *In vitro* hemolysis.
- Raised immunoglobulins.

Clinical manifestations of hyperphosphatemia

There are no specific symptoms and signs related to hyperphosphatemia, but patients may present with features of hypocalcemia.

The calcium × phosphate (Ca × P) product needs to be maintained at <4.2 mmol^2/L^2.

A raised Ca × P product may lead to ectopic calcification and/or deposits in acral tissue, skin or subcutaneous tissue causing painful necrosis. Asymptomatic corneal calcification, conjunctivitis and large deposits around joints may also develop.

Ectopic calcification in the medial wall of blood vessels may result in hypertension and left ventricular hypertrophy. Calcification may also involve the myocardium and heart valves.

Persistent hyperphosphatemia plays an important role in the pathogenesis of secondary hyperparathyroidism and contributes to the development of osteitis fibrosa cystica.

Investigation of hyperphosphatemia

Investigations for hyperphosphatemia are similar to those for hypophosphatemia.

In addition, serum creatine kinase and urine myoglobin (for rhabdomyolysis), and potassium, urate, and lactate dehydrogenase (for tumor lysis syndrome) should be measured as appropriate.

Treatment of hyperphosphatemia

Acute and severe hyperphosphatemia

This may be life-threatening, particularly when associated with symptomatic hypocalcemia.

When kidney function is intact, resolution of hyperphosphatemia can be achieved by enhancing renal phosphate excretion with saline infusion. Care must be taken to avoid the development of hypocalcemia.

Hemodialysis is often required in patients with concurrent renal impairment and symptomatic hypocalcemia.

Chronic hyperphosphatemia

Depending on the stage of CKD, renal patients may require ongoing therapy to control chronic hyperphosphatemia.

- The dietary phosphate intake should be restricted to 800–1000 mg/day. Renal dietetic input is required for this to be achieved.
- Phosphate binders may be required for CKD stages 4 and 5 as dietary phosphate restriction alone may be insufficient in controlling hyperphosphatemia. The choice of binder depends on calcium requirements for individual patients and local practice guidelines.
- The calcium intake should be restricted to <2 g daily.
- PTH is usually measured every 3 months in patients with stage 5 CKD.
- Measurement of PTH should also be considered in earlier stages of CKD (CKD 4 and possibly CKD 3) although opinion varies about the required frequency and utility of this.
- There is no indication to measure PTH in CKD 1 and 2 in the absence of a suspected disorder of bone and mineral metabolism.
- In stage 4, the PTH should be between the upper limit and two times the upper limit of the normal range, and between two and four times the upper limit of the normal range in CKD stage 5 patients not on dialysis. These PTH targets may be achieved by the use of 1,25-$(OH)_2$ vitamin D and/or calcimimetics, and if necessary parathyroidectomy.

Further reading

Amanzadeh J, Reilly Jr, RF. Hypophosphataemia: an evidence-based approach to its clinical consequences and management. *Nat Clin Pract Nephrol* 2006; **2**: 136–148.

Baeksgaard L, Sorensen JB. Acute tumor lysis syndrome in solid tumors: a case report and review of the literature. *Cancer Chemother Pharmacol* 2003; **51**: 187–192.

Baker SB, Worthley LIG. The essentials of calcium, magnesium and phosphate metabolism: Part 1 and 2. *Crit Care Resusc* 2002; **4**: 301–315.

Berndt TJ, Schiavi S, Kumar R. Phosphatonins and the regulation of phosphorus homeostasis. *Am J Physiol, Renal Physiol* 2005; **289**: F1170–F1182.

Bessmertny O, Robitaille LM, Cairo SM. Rasburicase: a new approach for preventing and/or treating tumor lysis. *Curr Pharm Design* 2005; **11**: 4177–4185.

Block GA. Control of serum phosphorus: implications for coronary artery calcification and calcific uraemic ateriolopathy (calciphylaxis). *Curr Opin Nephrol Hypertens* 2001; **10**: 741–747.

Brunelli SM, Goldfarb S. Hypophosphataemia: clinical consequences and management. *J Am Soc Nephrol* 2007; **18**: 1999–2003.

Davison AM, Cameron JS, Grunfield J-P, Ponticelli C, Ritz E, Winearls CG, Ypersele C V. Hypo- hyperphosphataemia. *Oxford Textbook of Clinical Nephrology*, vol. 1; 2005. pp. 287–308.

Gaasbeek A, Meinders E. Hypophosphataemia: an update on its aetiology and treatment. *Am J Med* 2005; **118**: 1094–1101.

Giachelli CM, Speer MY, Li X, Rajachar RM, Yang H. Regulation of vascular calcification: roles of phosphate and osteopontin. *Circuln Res* 2005; **96**: 717–722.

Jan de Beur SM. Tumoral calcinosis: a look into the metabolic mirror of phosphate homeostasis. *J Clin Endocrinol Metab* 2005; **90**: 2469–2471.

Ketteler, M. Phosphorus control in chronic kidney disease. *Eur Renal Dis* Issue 1 2007; 24–26.

Moe S, Drüke TB. Management of secondary hyperparathyroidism: the importance and the challenge of controlling parathyroid hormone levels without elevating the calcium, phosphorus and calcium-phosphorus product. *Am J Nephrol* 2003; **23**: 368–379.

Murer H, Hernando N, Forster I, Biber J. Proximal tubular phosphate: a molecular perspective. *Kidney Int* 2006; **70**: 1548–1559.

Nordin BEC, Fraser R. Assessment of urinary phosphate excretion. *Lancet* 1960; **60**: 947–951.

Quinbi WY. Consequences of hyperphosphataemia in patients with end-stage renal disease (ESRD). *Kidney Int* 2004; **66**: S8–S12.

Sinclair D, Smith H, Woodhead P. Spurious hyperphosphataemia caused by IgA paraprotein: a topic revisited. *Ann Clin Biochem* 2004; **14**: 119–124.

Internet resources

National Collaborating Centre for Acute Care (2006) Nutrition Support in Adults: Oral nutrition support, enteral tube feeding and parenteral nutrition. London (UK): National Institute for Health and Clinical Excellence: http://www.guideline.gov/summary/summary.aspx?doc_id=8739

National Kidney Foundation. K/DOQI clinical practice guidelines for bone metabolism and disease in chronic kidney disease: http://www.kidney.org/professionals/kdoqi/guidelines_bone/index.htm

The Renal Association (2007) Clinical Practice Guidelines: http://www.renal.org/guidelines/index.html

See also

Hypo-/hypermagnesemia

Magnesium is the second most abundant intracellular cation. It is stored predominantly in bone, muscle and soft tissue.

Less than 1% of the total body magnesium stores are in the extracellular fluid of which ~55–70% is ionized (physiologically active), 20–30% is protein-bound (mainly to albumin) and 10–15% is complexed to serum anions (e.g. phosphate, citrate, bicarbonate).

The normal serum magnesium concentration is 0.7–1.0 mmol/L.

Functions of magnesium

Magnesium is an essential part of many metalloenzymes and acts as a cofactor of many enzyme systems, especially those associated with the metabolism of ATP, proteins, carbohydrates, and DNA.

Magnesium acts as a calcium channel antagonist and modulates activities that are dependent on intracellular calcium fluxes, e.g. muscle contraction and insulin release.

Along with potassium and calcium ions, magnesium also regulates neuromuscular function and the clotting mechanism.

Magnesium, calcium and potassium are closely linked functionally and metabolically, including in their handling by the kidney.

Magnesium homeostasis

Magnesium balance is normally regulated by intestinal absorption and renal excretion.

Gastrointestinal absorption of magnesium

About 30–40% of dietary magnesium intake (10–15 mmol/day) is absorbed in the small intestine with smaller amounts being absorbed in the colon. The TRPM6 protein, which is a transient receptor potential cation channel, is crucial for the epithelial absorption of magnesium in both the intestine and the distal convoluted tubule. Mutations in TRPM6 lead to severe hypomagnesemia and hypocalcemia.

Absorption can vary from 25 to 80% depending on the intracellular magnesium stores.

Absorption is by both saturable active transcellular transport and by nonsaturable paracellular passive transport.

Approximately 1 mmol/day of magnesium is secreted into the intestinal lumen. This may increase during diarrheal episodes and lead to significant losses.

Renal excretion of magnesium

About 100 mmol of magnesium is filtered daily, of which >95% is reabsorbed by the renal tubule:

- 15–20% in the proximal convoluted tubule (PCT).
- 60–70% in the thick ascending limb (TAL) of the loop of Henle. This occurs by passive and paracellular transport that is to some extent stimulated by parathyroid hormone, glucagon and antidiuretic hormone. Passive diffusion depends on the electrochemical gradient created by the Na-K-2Cl transporter and the potassium-rectifying channel, ROMK. The gradient is abolished by factors that reduce the positive luminal charge (e.g. loop diuretics, hypercalcemia). Magnesium reabsorption is also decreased by increased tubular flow (e.g. osmotic diuresis, saline infusion). Paracellular transit of magnesium

and calcium in the TAL is facilitated by the tight junction protein, claudin 16. Mutations in this protein result in hypomagnesemia with associated hypercalciuria and nephrocalcinosis.

- 5–15% in the distal convoluted tubule (DCT). This involves an active transcellular transport process (stimulated by aldosterone, antidiuretic hormone and glucagon) and is the site where fine adjustments of magnesium excretion are made. The understanding of the hormonal regulation of magnesium homeostasis remains incomplete.

Approximately 3–5% of the filtered magnesium is excreted in the urine (~4 mmol/day) but this may vary considerably in order to maintain magnesium homeostasis.

The fractional reabsorption of magnesium can decline from 95% to nearly zero in hypermagnesemic states or when the GFR is severely reduced (<5–10 mL/min), or increase to 99.5% in severe hypomagnesemic states (i.e. magnesium excretion <0.5 mmol/day).

There are several inherited disorders of magnesium handling, many of which are directly or indirectly associated with disturbed calcium metabolism and homeostasis. These are listed in Table 2.5.1.

Hypomagnesemia

Hypomagnesemia is defined as a serum magnesium concentration <0.7 mmol/L, and is considered severe when <0.5 mmol/L.

A magnesium deficit may exist even when the serum magnesium concentration is normal (serum magnesium levels may remain normal even when total body stores are depleted by 20%).

Since ~30% of serum magnesium is bound to protein, 75% of which is albumin, the routinely measured total magnesium concentration is affected by the serum albumin concentration.

Epidemiology

The prevalence of severe hypomagnesemia (serum magnesium <0.5 mmol/L) in hospital populations is high (10–20%) but may be as high as 65% among critically ill patients.

Patients at particular risk of hypomagnesemia include:

- the elderly (up to one-third of elderly subjects living in residential homes are hypomagnesemic);
- alcoholics (30% are hypomagnesemic and nearly all are magnesium deplete);
- the chronically ill;
- those receiving parenteral nutrition (high incidence of hypomagnesemia with or without refeeding syndrome);
- those with refractory hypokalemia and/or hypocalcemia;
- those with ventricular arrhythmias (particularly following an ischemic event), and rarely atrial arrhythmias;
- postoperative patients in the first 24 h after major surgery.

Serum magnesium is not routinely requested and measured, therefore hypomagnesemia may be undiagnosed. Magnesium deficiency is also often associated with an imbalance of other electrolytes such as hypokalemia and hypocalcemia.

Table 2.5.1 Inherited diseases of magnesium handling

Thick ascending limb (TAL)

Mutations in TAL transporters
- Bartter's syndrome

Calcium sensor receptor disorders
- Mutation activating Mg^{2+}/Ca^{2+} sensing (autosomal dominant hypoparathyroidism)
- Mutation inactivating Mg^{2+}/Ca^{2+} sensing (familial hypocalciuric hypercalcemia)

Claudin 16 (paracellin-1) (protein involved in controlling the magnesium and calcium permeability of the cortical TAL)
- Familial hypomagnesemia associated with hypercalciuria and nephrocalcinosis

Distal convoluted tubule (DCT)

Gitelman's syndrome
- Hypomagnesemia associated with abnormal renal NaCl transport (mutations in thiazide-sensitive co-transporter)

Isolated dominant hypomagnesemia with hypocalciuria (mutation in δ-subunit of ATPase)

Hypomagnesemia with secondary hypocalcemia (mutation in $TRPM6-Mg^{2+}$ channel)

Causes of hypomagnesemia

Gastrointestinal causes:

- Inflammatory bowel disease.
- Short bowel syndrome.
- Biliary or intestinal fistulae.
- Small intestinal bypass surgery.
- Celiac disease.
- Congenital malabsorption.
- General malabsorption syndromes.
- Acute or chronic pancreatitis.
- Acute or chronic diarrhea.
- Prolonged vomiting or nasogastric suction.
- Alcoholism.
- Laxative abuse.
- Malnutrition.
- Prolonged IV administration of magnesium-free fluids.

Renal causes:

- Drugs
  - Loop or thiazide diuretics.
  - Cisplatin (hypomagnesemia very common and routine monitoring in all patients on cisplatin therapy is recommended).
  - Amphotericin B.
  - Ciclosporin.
  - Aminoglycosides (hypokalemia, hypocalcemia and magnesium wasting may persist for months after cessation of treatment).
  - Pentamidine toxicity.
  - Foscarnet.
- Tubulointerstial nephropathies.
- Postrenal transplantation.
- Postobstructive diuresis.
- Diuretic phase of acute tubular necrosis.
- Hypercalcemia and hyperparathyroidism.

- Renal tubular acidosis.
- Osmotic diuresis.
- Chronic alcoholism.
- Diabetes type I and II.
- Diabetic ketoacidosis.
- Hyperaldosteronism.
- Hyperthyroidism.
- Hypoparathyroidism.
- Congenital magnesium renal wasting.
- Bartter's syndrome (one-third of cases).
- Gitelman's syndrome (universal).

Miscellaneous causes

- Major burns.
- Hungry bone syndrome postparathyroidectomy.
- Syndrome of inappropriate ADH secretion.
- Insulin infusion.
- Excessive lactation and sweating.

Clinical manifestations of hypomagnesemia

Although hypomagnesemia is usually asymptomatic, the clinical spectrum of its manifestations include dysfunction of the cardiac, neuromuscular and CNS systems.

Seizures, tetany and cardiac arrhythmias are commoner at serum magnesium levels <0.5 mmol/L whereas neuromuscular irritability, hypokalemia and hypocalcemia may be seen even with levels of 0.5–0.70 mmol/L.

However, the severity of the symptoms may not be directly related to the serum magnesium concentration.

Clinical consequences of hypomagnesemia

Hypokalemia occurs in 30–60% of patients with hypomagnesemia and conversely 60% of patients with hypokalemia are hypomagnesemic. This may be due to common etiologies.

Hypocalcemia is found in ~12–50% of patients with hypomagnesemia.

Cardiovascular:

- Cardiac arrhythmias (some ventricular arrhythmias may only respond to magnesium infusion):
  - Premature ventricular contractions.
  - Ventricular fibrillation.
  - Torsade de Pointes.
  - Increased susceptibility to digoxin induced arrhythmias.
  - Atrial fibrillation and tachycardia.
- Hypertension.
- Coronary artery spasm.
- Symptomatic mitral valve prolapse.
- Sudden death.
- ECG changes (similar to those seen in hypokalemia):
  - ST segment depression.
  - T wave changes which may be progressive.
  - Prolongation of the PR interval.
  - Widening of the QRS complex.
- Magnesium has membrane stabilizing properties and some of the cardiac complications may reflect abnormal cardiac repolarization resulting mainly from the effects of low magnesium concentration on the Na/K-ATPase pump.

Neuromuscular:
- Tetany.
- Tremors, muscle twitching with positive Trousseau's and Chvostek's signs.
- Seizures (tonic, clonic or multifocal).
- Respiratory muscle weakness or paralysis.

Central nervous system:
- Confusion.
- Apathy, depression, psychosis.
- Anxiety, delirium.
- Weakness, fatigue.
- Vertigo, vertical nystagmus.
- Wernicke's encephalopathy.
- Coma.

Investigation of hypomagnesemia

Measure serum magnesium, electrolytes, urea, creatinine, albumin, calcium, and inorganic phosphate.

The serum magnesium concentration may be an unreliable indicator of total body stores as serum levels may be normal in the presence of significant magnesium depletion.

When serum levels are significantly low, however, this does indicate depletion of magnesium stores.

Total body stores may be assessed by a magnesium loading test but this is not a routine investigation.

Since about 30% of serum magnesium is protein-bound, the magnesium concentration should be corrected for the albumin concentration. There is no general agreement about how this may be achieved but the following formula has been proposed:

$$Mgc = MgT + 0.005 (40 - Alb)$$

where Mgc is the corrected magnesium concentration (mmol/L), MgT is the measured total serum magnesium concentration (mmol/L), and Alb is the concentration of albumin in g/L. The adjustment may not be reliable for serum albumin concentrations of 39–45 g/L.

The cause of hypomagnesemia may be determined (in patients without significant renal impairment) by measuring the fractional excretion of magnesium (FeMg). This requires a blood and spot urine sample:

$$FeMg = \frac{(sCr \times uMg)}{(0.7 \times sMg \times uCr)} \times 100$$

where sCr is serum creatinine (mmol/L), sMg is serum magnesium (mmol/L), uMg is urine magnesium (mmol/L) and uCr is urine creatinine (mmol/L). The serum magnesium is multiplied by 0.7 to correct for the 30% of magnesium that is protein bound and therefore not filtered.

In the presence of hypomagnesemia, a FeMg >2% indicates inappropriate renal wasting whereas a FeMg <2% is compatible with appropriate renal magnesium conservation (indicating extrarenal loss).

The normal 24 h urine magnesium excretion is 1.0–7.0 mmol. In the presence of hypomagnesemia a 24 h magnesium excretion of <0.5 mmol indicates appropriate renal magnesium conservation.

Treatment of hypomagnesemia

The type of treatment and the speed of correction of hypomagnesemia are determined by the underlying cause and the severity of the clinical signs and symptoms.

Asymptomatic hypomagnesemia

Patients should be given oral magnesium in divided doses, 15–30 mmol daily for severe depletion or 5–15 mmol daily for mild deficiency.

Symptomatic hypomagnesemia

In patients with hypomagnesemic tetany, seizures or ventricular arrhythmias, rapid intravenous administration of 4–8 mmol magnesium over 10–60 min with close cardiac monitoring is indicated. This is followed by magnesium infusion: 12–90 mmol over a period of 24 h depending on the severity of the symptoms, signs, and magnesium depletion. Up to 160 mmol of magnesium may be required over 5–6 days to replenish the deficit and maintain serum magnesium at >0.5 mmol/L.

Hypocalcemia and hypokalemia may coexist with hypermagnesemia and should be treated as appropriate.

In patients with significant renal impairment, the magnesium infusion rate should be reduced by 25–50% and serum levels monitored more frequently.

Amiloride or triamterene may be helpful in reversing diuretic-induced renal magnesium wasting, and in treating the renal loss due to Gitelman's or Bartter's syndromes, or cisplatin nephrotoxicity.

Hypermagnesemia

Hypermagnesemia (serum magnesium >1.0 mmol/L) is relatively rare and has a prevalence of 4–5% in the hospital population.

Normally the kidney excretes ~3–5% daily of the filtered magnesium but is capable of increasing FeMg to nearly 100% in the presence of hypermagnesemia in patients with normal GFR.

When the GFR falls to <30 mL/min and magnesium intake is maintained or increased, hypermagnesemia may occur.

Causes of hypermagnesemia

Acute or chronic renal failure (GFR <30 mL/min), often in association with excess magnesium intake (e.g. magnesium infusions, antacids, laxative abuse, Epsom salts, cathartics and enemas).

Causes of mild to moderate hypermagnesemia include:
- Hypothyroidism.
- Lithium therapy.
- Addison's disease.
- Familial hypocalciuric hypercalcemia.
- Cell necrosis, rhabdomyolysis, especially with renal failure.

Clinical manifestations of hypermagnesemia

Serum magnesium concentrations <2.0 mmol/L are not usually associated with any symptoms.

Neuromuscular toxicity

With serum magnesium levels of 2.1–2.9 mmol/L, lethargy, flushing, drowsiness, nausea and vomiting, and suppression of deep tendon reflexes may occur.

With concentrations of 2.9–5.0 mmol/L, loss of deep tendon reflexes becomes more evident and with levels >5.0 mmol/L paralysis, coma and apnea may ensue.

Other neuromuscular toxic effects include ileus, urinary retention, and parasympathetic nervous system inhibition with fixed dilated pupils.

Cardiovascular toxicity

These usually become evident with serum magnesium concentrations >2.9 mmol/L and include bradycardia, hypotension, ECG changes (prolongation of PR and QT intervals, and widening of the QRS complex).

With higher levels, complete heart block, ventricular fibrillation and cardiac arrest may develop.

Metabolic disturbance

Mild hypocalcemia and variable degrees of hyperkalemia have been observed.

Investigation of hypermagnesemia

The investigation of hypermagnesemia is very similar to that for hypomagnesemia.

In the presence of hypermagnesemia, FeMg <2% indicates inappropriate renal conservation of magnesium, whereas FeMg of >2% is compatible with an appropriate renal response.

Treatment of hypermagnesemia

Mild magnesium toxicity requires no treatment except to stop further administration of magnesium.

For symptomatic patients with cardiovascular toxicity and respiratory depression, 10 mL of 10% calcium gluconate is given IV and slowly over 10 min, and can be repeated as necessary. Calcium gluconate will antagonise the effects of the high magnesium concentration.

Volume expansion with normal saline followed by IV furosemide will greatly increase FeMg. Serum potassium should be monitored.

Hemodialysis or peritoneal dialysis with a low or zero magnesium dialyzate may be necessary and will reduce serum magnesium by 30–50% within 3–4 h. Repeated dialysis treatment may be necessary.

Further reading

Agus ZS. Hypomagnesaemia. *J Am Soc Nephrol* 1999;**10**:1616–1622.

American Heart Association Guidelines for: Cardiopulmonary resuscitation and emergency cardiovascular care. Life-threatening electrolyte abnormalities: *Circulation* 2005; **112**(Suppl): IV-121–IV-125.

Cole DEC, Quamme GA. Inherited disorders of renal magnesium handling. *J Am Soc Nephrol* 2000; **11**: 1937–1947.

Davison AM, Cameron JS, Grunfield J-P, *et al.* Hypo- hypermagnesaemia. *Oxford Textbook of Clinical Nephrology*, vol. 1; 2005. pp. 309–319.

Dubé L, Granry J-C. The therapeutic use of magnesium in anaesthiology, intensive care and emergency medicine: a review. *Can J Anaesth* 2003; **50**: 732–736.

Innerarity S. Hypomagnesaemia in acute and chronic illness. *Crit Care Nurs Quart* 2000; **23**: 1–19.

Konrad M, Schlingmann KP, Gudermann T. Insights into the molecular nature of magnesium homeostasis. *Am J Physiol, Renal Physiol* 2004; **286**: F599–F605.

Kroll MH, Elin RJ. Relationships between magnesium and protein concentrations in serum. *Clin Chem* 1985; **31** 244–246.

Long-Jun D, *et al.* Magnesium transport in the renal distal convoluted tubule. *Physiol Rev* 2001; **81**: 51–84.

Topf JM, Murray PT. Hypomagnesaemia and hypermagnesaemia. *Rev Endocr Metabol Dis* 2003; **4**: 195–206.

Internet resources

Review of hypomagnesemia:

http://www.emedicine.com/emerg/topic274.htm

Review of hypermagnesemia:

http://www.intox.org/databank/documents/treat/treate/trt23_e.htm

See also

Hypo-/hypercalcemia, p. 52

Hypo-/hyperkalemia, p. 46

Hypokalemic tubular disorders, p. 200

Clinical acid–base disorders

A normal daily diet generates nonvolatile acids such as sulfuric acid and phosphoric acid from protein metabolism, and lactate from anerobic breakdown of glucose.

In addition, volatile acid (CO_2) is produced primarily from carbohydrate metabolism.

Acid–base homeostasis maintains systemic pH within a narrow range (7.35–7.45) by the integration of a number of physiological processes including intracellular and extracellular buffering, and compensatory processes in the kidneys and lungs.

The kidney both excretes the acid load generated from dietary protein and reclaims filtered bicarbonate.

The lungs mediate the excretion of CO_2.

Bicarbonate is the most important buffer at physiological pH.

The primary changes in bicarbonate concentration are metabolic whereas those in CO_2 concentration are respiratory.

Respiratory causes of acid–base disturbance are compensated for by the kidneys and metabolic causes are compensated for by the lungs.

Acid–base homeostasis

Intracellular and extracellular physiological buffers serve to attenuate the changes in pH that would occur with retention of either acids or bases.

The regulation of CO_2 tension by the respiratory system and the control of the bicarbonate concentration by the kidney constitute the regulatory processes that act together with physiological buffers to stabilize the arterial pH.

The major buffer systems are comprised of:
- a base (H^+ acceptor) which is predominantly bicarbonate;
- an acid (H^+ donor) which is predominately carbonic acid.

The addition of acid leads to the conversion of bicarbonate to CO_2.

For the pH to be maintained, CO_2 is eliminated by the lungs.

$$H^+ + HCO_3^- \leftrightarrow H_2CO_3 \leftrightarrow H_2O + CO_2$$

In order for acid–base homeostasis to be maintained the correct ratio of HCO_3^- to CO_2 (~5:1) is required.

$$pH = 6.1 + \log \frac{[HCO_3^-]}{0.03 \times PCO_2}$$

$$[H^+] \propto \frac{PCO_2}{HCO_3^-}$$

Therefore, any condition which alters the concentration of either HCO_3^- or PCO_2 will change the pH.

In addition to the HCO_3^-/PCO_2 buffer system, other buffer systems are physiologically important and these include:
- hemoglobin and other proteins;
- organophosphate complexes;
- bone apatite.

The role of the respiratory system in acid–base metabolism

Following the addition or generation of an acid or an alkali, buffers attenuate the change in pH, but do not remove acid/alkali from the body.

The respiratory system contributes to acid–base homeostasis by regulating the elimination of CO_2 by the lungs.

CO_2 generated in the tissues passes into red blood cells down a concentration gradient and combines with water to form carbonic acid (catalyzed by carbonic anhydrase).

Carbonic acid then dissociates into HCO_3^- and hydrogen ions, and the hydrogen ions bind to reduced hemoglobin to form HHb.

Through an exchange process with chloride, the generated HCO_3^- passes back into plasma.

This process is reversed in the lungs and the H^+ ions bound to hemoglobin recombine with HCO_3^- to form CO_2 which diffuses into the alveoli.

An increase in nonvolatile acid production lowers pH and HCO_3^- concentrations and leads to increased alveolar ventilation which lowers PCO_2.

Thus even small changes in ventilation can profoundly change the hydrogen ion concentration and pH.

Mixed respiratory–metabolic acid–base disorders should be considered when the PCO_2 is too high or too low for a given abnormal serum HCO_3^- concentration.

In general, respiratory compensation does not entirely normalize blood pH.

In any case, the buffer system would become depleted if there were no other mechanism(s) for elimination of nonvolatile acids from the body.

The kidneys provide the ultimate route of excretion of nonvolatile acids.

The role of the kidneys in acid–base metabolism

The kidney's role in acid–base homeostasis includes:
- Reclamation of filtered HCO_3^-.
- Regeneration of HCO_3^- consumed in the buffering of nonvolatile acids.
- Excretion of hydrogen ions buffered by phosphate or ammonia (to form of ammonium).

Reclamation of filtered bicarbonate

The kidneys reclaim all of the 4000 mmol of HCO_3^- that is filtered daily. Of this amount, 70–80% occurs in the proximal convoluted tubule (PCT) and the rest is reabsorbed by the thick ascending loop (TAL) of Henle (10–25%) with a minor contribution by the distal nephron (5–10%).

This reclamation process prevents bicarbonaturia but does not result in the elimination of acid from the body.

Excretion of hydrogen ions

In addition to reclamation of HCO_3^-, the kidney must excrete the hydrogen ions produced from the dissociation of H_2CO_3.

The excreted hydrogen ions are trapped in the lumen by urinary buffers (principally phosphate and ammonia) and then excreted.

Phosphate buffers contribute to the excretion of ~20–30 mmol of H^+ per day. The capacity of this system is limited by the fixed quantity of phosphate that is filtered into the tubular fluid.

The remaining 20–40 mmol per day of H^+ are buffered by ammonia that is generated in the renal tubule from glutamine and other amino acids. The capacity of the system can be increased ten-fold in conditions where enhanced H^+ excretion is required.

Urine pH can vary from 4.5–8 depending on the acid–base load that needs to be excreted.

The PCT and the distal convoluted tubule (DCT) are able to maintain pH gradients of 1 and 3 units respectively. Therefore, the minimum pH of the final urine is ~4.5. This acidification process is impaired in distal renal tubular acidosis.

There are many factors which regulate renal acidification.

Reabsorption of HCO_3^- in the PCT is mediated by Na^+/H^+ exchange.

The peritubular HCO_3^- concentration, pH and the prevailing PCO_2 influence HCO_3^- reabsorption.

A decrease in extracellular volume enhances HCO_3^- reabsorption and vice versa.

Reabsorption of HCO_3^- is also stimulated by increased arterial PCO_2 and potassium depletion, and it is inhibited by hypocapnia, PTH and phosphate depletion.

Net hydrogen excretion in the DCT is influenced by the electrical gradient in the tubule cells and lumen with sodium reabsorption favoring H^+ secretion. This process can be enhanced by aldosterone and the availability of buffers (NH_3 and HPO_4^-).

Disorders of acid–base homeostasis

Disturbances in acid–base homeostasis are due to processes that lead to either:
- production or retention of an excess of hydrogen ions (acidosis); or
- retention of bicarbonate ions (alkalosis).

If these processes are severe enough then there may be:
- increase in arterial hydrogen ion concentration (acidemia: blood pH <7.35);
- reduction in arterial hydrogen ion concentration (alkalemia: blood pH >7.45).

Respiratory (i.e. changes in ventilation leading to altered PCO_2) or nonrespiratory (metabolic) causes are responsible for these disturbances.

Metabolic acidosis

Metabolic acidosis is characterized by:
- low arterial blood pH (acidemia);
- reduced serum HCO_3^- concentration;
- decreased PCO_2 (from respiratory compensation).

Etiology of metabolic acidosis

Metabolic acidosis may result from:
- inability of the kidneys to excrete the obligate dietary hydrogen load;
- inappropriate loss of bicarbonate in the kidneys or the gastrointestinal tract;
- increase in the generation of the hydrogen ions (such as in lactic acidosis or ketoacidosis).

Impaired excretion of the dietary acid load
- Uremic acidosis (usually GFR <15–20 mL/min).
- Type 1 (distal) renal tubular acidosis (RTA).
- Type 4 RTA.

Excessive loss of renal bicarbonate
- Type 2 (proximal) RTA.
- Carbonic anhydrase inhibitors, e.g. acetazolamide.

Excessive loss of gastrointestinal bicarbonate
- Diarrhea.
- External loss of pancreatic or biliary secretions.
- Urinary–gastrointestinal connections.

Increased acid production
- Ketoacidosis (diabetes mellitus or alcohol excess).
- Lactic acidosis.
- Inborn errors of metabolism (methylmalonic aciduria, propionic aciduria, isovaleric aciduria).
- Poisoning (ethylene glycol, methanol, salicylate, iron, paraldehyde).

Systemic effects of metabolic acidosis

Metabolic acidosis may lead to a variety of changes in tissues and organs.

The associated symptoms and signs will depend on the rate and magnitude of fall of the pH and the underlying pathology.

Cardiovascular
- Tachycardia or bradycardia.
- Reduced cardiac contractility.
- Chest pain.
- Fatal cardiac arrhythmia.
- Vascular changes resulting in hypotension and congestive cardiac failure.
- Life-threatening hyperkalemia.

Pulmonary
- Hyperpnea.
- Kussmaul respiratory pattern.

Gastrointestinal
- Nausea and vomiting.
- Abdominal pain.
- Gastric distension.
- Diarrhea.

Neurological
- Confusion.
- CNS depression progressing to coma.

Nutritional
- Systemic inflammation.
- Increased protein catabolism and hypoalbuminemia.
- Insulin resistance.
- Decreased leptin.

Bone
- Decreased function of osteoblasts.
- Increased function of osteoclasts.
- Increased parathyroid hormone secretion and action.
- Hypercalciuria.
- Reduced activity of 1α-hydroxylase.

Others
- Natriuresis.
- Hypertriglyceridemia.
- Leukocytosis.

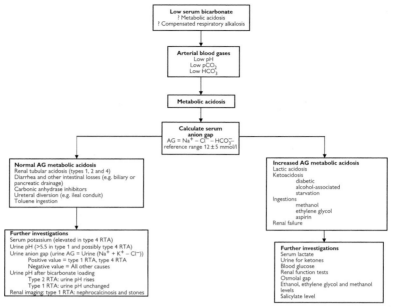

Fig. 2.6.1 Algorithm for the investigaation of metabolic acidosis.

Table 2.6.1 Etiology of renal tubular acidosis (RTA)

Type 1 (distal RTA)	Type 2 (proximal RTA)	Type 4 (distal RTA)
Primary or idiopathic • familial • sporadic	**Primary or idiopathic** • familial • sporadic	**Hyper-reninemic hypoaldosteronism** • Addison's disease • congenital adrenal hyperplasia (21-hydroxylase deficiency) • drugs (ACEIs, ARBs, heparin, ketoconazole)
Genetic • Ehlers–Danlos syndrome • Marfan's syndrome	**Inherited systemic diseases** (Fanconi-like syndromes): • cystinosis • galactosemia • Wilson's disease • glycogen storage disease (type 1) • inherited fructose tolerance • tyrosinemia	**Hypo-reninemic hypoaldosteronism** • diabetes mellitus • drugs (NSAIDs, cyclosporin, tacrolimus) • interstitial nephritis • urinary tract obstruction • sickle cell disease • gout
Immunological diseases • Sjögren's syndrome • systemic lupus erythematosus • primary biliary cirrhosis • chronic renal transplant rejection • hypergammaglobulinemia	**Disorders associated with hyperparathyroidism** • primary hyperparathyroidism • vitamin D deficiency • vitamin D resistance	**Distal tubule dysfunction** • chronic tubulointerstitial disease
Diseases associated with nephrocalcinosis • vitamin D toxication • idiopathic hypercalcuria • primary hyperparathyroidism	**Drugs/toxins** • lead poisoning • cadmium poisoning • mercury poisoning • acetazolamide • gentamicin and • topiramate and zonisamide	**Drugs/toxins** • spironolactone • amiloride • triamterene • trimethoprim
Drugs/toxins • amphotericin • toluene • lithium	**Miscellaneous renal diseases** • multiple myeloma • amyloidosis • nephrotic syndrome • medullary cystic disease • renal transplantation (early)	
Significant volume depletion		

Evaluation of metabolic acidosis

The following investigations are required to evaluate patients with suspected metabolic acidosis (reduced serum bicarbonate).

An algorithm for the evaluation of such patients is described in Fig. 2.6.1.

Initial investigations

Step 1

Measure the blood pH on an arterial blood sample (arterial blood gases (ABGs)) to:
- confirm the presence of acidemia
- exclude respiratory alkalosis as cause of low HCO_3^-

Step 2

Calculate the serum anion gap:
- Serum AG = $Na^+ - (HCO_3^- + Cl^-)$
- (reference range 12 ± 5 mmol/L)

or
- Serum AG = $(Na^+ + K^+) - (HCO_3^- + Cl^-)$
- (reference range 16 ± 5 mmol/L).

In the critically ill patient, a correction for the albumin concentration (AGc) may be necessary:

AGc = AG + 0.25[40 − albumin]

The anion gap will be either:
- normal: due to the presence of an acid in which the anion is Cl^- (hyperchloremic metabolic acidosis); or
- high: due to the presence of an acid in which the anion (unmeasured) is not Cl^-

The causes of 'normal' and 'high' AG metabolic acidosis are listed in Fig. 2.6.1.

Investigations to determine the etiology of the acidosis
- Serum electrolytes, urea, creatinine (uremic acidosis).
- Blood glucose (ketoacidosis).
- Liver function tests (lactic acidosis).
- Full blood count (sepsis and profound anemia).
- Plasma lactate (lactic acidosis).
- Serum osmolality.
- Serum osmolal gap (methanol/ethylene glycol).
- Urine pH (see Fig. 2.6.1).
- Urine anion gap = Urine $(Na^+ + K^+ - Cl^-)$ (see Fig. 2.6.1).
- Toxin assays as appropriate, e.g. methanol, ethylene glycol, paraldehyde, salicylates, lead, mercury.
- Bacteriological culture(s) as appropriate.

Serum osmolal gap (OG)

This is the measured − calculated serum osmolality.

Calculated osmolality = 2(Na⁺ + glucose + urea).

Normal OG is <10 mOsm/kg.

An OG >10 mOsm/kg when accompanied by a high AG metabolic acidosis should raise the possibility of methanol or ethylene glycol intoxication. However, late presentation after intoxication may show a normal OG and a raised AG.

Ketoacidosis and lactic acidosis can also increase the OG (usually by only a modest amount, i.e. <25 mOsm/kg), but these can usually be readily identified (clinically and with urgent investigations).

Ethanol will also increase the OG, making interpretation difficult. The measured ethanol concentration can be included in the calculated osmolality to correct for this.

An increased OG (particularly if >25 mOsm/kg) in the presence of a high AG metabolic acidosis, without evidence of lactic or ketoacidosis, should prompt treatment for methanol/ethylene glycol intoxication (i.e. ethanol infusion) pending results of methanol and ethylene glycol assays.

Renal tubular acidosis (RTA)

Hyperchloremic, normal AG metabolic acidosis is the hallmark of renal tubular acidosis.

RTA results from a defect in tubular function which causes a decrease in either net tubular hydrogen secretion or HCO_3^- reabsorption.

There are three main types of RTA:
- type 1 (distal);
- type 2 (proximal);
- type 4.

The causes of these forms of RTA and the clinical differences between them are indicated in Tables 2.6.1 and 2.6.2 respectively.

Renal tubular acidosis is discussed in more detail in Chapter 5.3.

Uremic acidosis

Metabolic acidosis occurs in renal failure due to a decreased ability to excrete H^+ or due to an inability to produce ammonia.

In the early stages of chronic kidney disease (CKD) (GFR <40 mL/min), metabolic acidosis with a normal anion gap (AG) (see below) may become evident. As CKD progresses (GFR <20 mL/min) a high AG metabolic acidosis may result.

In ~80% of patients with CKD and GFR <20–30 mL/min, there is mild to moderate metabolic acidemia with the pH usually remaining >7.2 and bicarbonate levels of 12–22 mmol/L.

In advanced CKD an increased AG is typical due to the presence of retained acids such as sulphates, phosphates, urate and hippurate. The presence of normal AG acidosis in this setting would imply a second pathology such as HCO_3^- wasting.

A serum HCO_3^- concentration <10 mmol/L and an AG >20 mmol/L are infrequent in renal failure and may be indicative of coexistent disorders, e.g. lactic acidosis or ketoacidosis.

Serum levels of HCO_3^- and pH in dialysis patients are determined by the dialysis process, exogenous alkali ingestion and endogenous acid production.

In hemodialysis patients, a predialysis $[HCO_3^-]$ of 17.5–20 mmol/L has been shown to be associated with the lowest risk of death.

Postdialysis metabolic alkalosis which may result from complete correction of predialysis metabolic acidosis may lead to hypoventilation, phosphate transfer into cells and vascular calcification.

Although there is no general agreed guidance on the optimal pre-dialysis bicarbonate concentration, a value of 20–26 mmol/L has been recommended as good practice.

Lactic acidosis

Lactic acidosis is classically defined as a plasma lactate level >5 mmol/L associated with a high AG metabolic acidosis (lactate is the unmeasured anion).

Table 2.6.2 Clinical manifestations of renal tubular acidosis (RTA)

	Type 1 (distal RTA)	**Type 2** (proximal RTA)	**Type 4** (distal RTA)
Plasma potassium	Low	Low or normal	High
Plasma bicarbonate	Low	Low (↑ urine bicarbonate)	Low
Plasma chloride	Increased	Increased	Increased
Urine pH with acidosis	>5.5	<5.5	<5.5 or >5.5
Fractional bicarbonate excretion	<5%	>10–15%	<5–10%
Bone and calcium metabolism	Nephrocalcinosis, rickets, osteomalacia and nephrolithiasis	Rickets and osteomalacia (hypercalciuria and nephrolithiasis rare)	Hypercalciuria and nephrolithiasis does not occur
Response to treatment	Good	Fair	Poor

Table 2.6.3 Causes of lactic acidosis

Type A lactic acidosis (tissue hypoxia)
  Left ventricular failure
  Septic shock
  Cardiogenic shock
  Hemorrhagic shock
  Respiratory failure
  Carbon monoxide poisoning
  Acute anemia
  Methemoglobinemia

Type B lactic acidosis (No tissue hypoxia)
  Renal failure
  Sepsis
  Hepatic failure
  Inborn errors of metabolism
  Leukemia, lymphoma, large tumors
  Grand mal seizures
  Strenuous muscular exercise
  Drugs or toxins
    Ethanol, methanol, ethylene glycol
    Biguanides
    Salicylates
    Isoniazid
    Iron
    Nitroprusside
    Cyanide
    Nalidixic acid
    Paracetamol
    Cocaine, amphetamines
    Paraldehyde
    Theophylline
    Lactulose
    Parenteral nutrition
    Antiretroviral drugs

Glucose metabolism generates pyruvate during anaerobic glycolysis.

Pyruvate is converted to lactate by reduction under anaerobic conditions.

The entry of pyruvate into the tricarboxylic acid (TCA) cycle depends on aerobic oxidation.

Glucose $\rightarrow$ pyruvate $\leftrightarrow$ lactate

Pyruvate + NADH + H^+ $\leftrightarrow$ lactate + NAD^+

Lactate itself cannot be broken down for energy production.

Reduction of pyruvate to lactate is reversible and excessive production of lactate will lead to depletion of NADH.

Approximately 1400 mmol of lactate are produced per day and under normal conditions the plasma lactate level is maintained at ~1–2 mmOl/L.

This is achieved by the buffering capacity of bicarbonate and the metabolism of lactate by the liver (60%), kidneys (30%) and perhaps muscle.

Approximately 50% of lactate is converted to glucose by gluconeugenesis and the rest is metabolised to pyruvate and then CO_2 and H_2O.

From the above it can be seen that an increased lactate concentration can result from three processes:

1 Increased pyruvate synthesis with a normal lactate/pyruvate ratio (glucose infusion, epinephrine administration, respiratory alkalosis). Lactate usually <5 mmol/L.

2 Increase in the NADH/NAD^+ ratio resulting in an increased lactate/pyruvate ratio.

3 Combination of 1 and 2. This results in severe metabolic acidosis.

Lactic acidosis is classified into two types (A and B), and the causes are outlined in Table 2.6.3.

D-Lactic acidosis

Lactic acid exists in two forms: L-lactate and D-lactate. D-Lactate cannot be metabolized, and is produced by gut bacteria in patients with short bowel syndrome and other malabsorptive disorders.

D-Lactate is not measured by the routine laboratory methods but can cause an increased AG metabolic acidosis.

Ketoacidosis

Diabetic ketoacidosis (DKA)

DKA is characterized by hyperglycemia, usually with a high AG metabolic acidosis due to the accumulation of ketone bodies (acetoacetate, β-hydroxybutyrate).

A normal AG metabolic acidosis may also be seen in DKA particularly when the extracellular volume is near normal.

Acetoacetate and β-hydroxybutyrate are metabolically interchangeable and the primary determinant of the balance is the NADH/NAD^+ ratio. A high ratio favours the formation of β-hydroxybutyrate and lactate.

A relative or absolute insulin deficiency and a compensatory rise in counter-regulatory hormones such as glucagon, cortisol, growth hormone and catecholamines occur in all cases of DKA.

The usual precipitant of DKA is infection or inadequate/missed insulin therapy.

The severity of DKA is graded as:
- moderate (when pH is 7.0–7.24);
- severe (when pH is <7.0).

A pH <6.7 is thought to be incompatible with life.

In DKA peripheral glucose utilization is impaired and gluconeogenesis is stimulated. This results in an osmotic diuresis leading to volume depletion and loss of electrolytes (sodium, potassium, magnesium, phosphate).

Alcoholic ketoacidosis
Alcoholic ketoacidosis is a recognized complication of ethanol abuse.

The ketoacidosis occurs after binge drinking in chronic alcohol abusers who have decreased food intake. It is often accompanied with gastritis, nausea, vomiting and abdominal pain, and occasionally with acute pancreatitis.

The symptoms may render the patients incapable of further ethanol consumption, and at presentation ethanol may not be detectable in blood.

The acidosis is thought to be due to an exaggerated normal response to fasting, i.e. low insulin levels and increased counter-regulatory hormones leading to lipolysis.

Lactic acidosis often coexists with ketoacidosis in alcohol abusers, in particular if hypoxia, hypoperfusion, hypothermia and convulsions are present.

Starvation ketoacidosis
Mild ketoacidosis may appear after an overnight fast but typically severe acidosis requires 3–14 days of starvation. This is accentuated by exercise and pregnancy.

Similar to the ketosis of alcohol abuse, starvation ketoacidosis is also thought to be due to an exaggerated normal response to fasting, with low insulin levels and increased lipolysis.

More fulminant ketoacidosis is unlikely as the islet cells respond to synthesis of ketone bodies by increasing insulin release which inhibits further lipolysis. This compensatory process does not take place in patients with type 1 diabetes mellitus.

Ethylene glycol
The ingestion of ethylene glycol (motor vehicle antifreeze), typically by alcoholics, leads to a high AG gap metabolic acidosis.

The high AG is caused by the generation of ethylene glycol metabolites, particularly oxalate, glycolate and glyoxylate.

These metabolites are more toxic than the parent compound and lead to an increase in the $NADH/NAD^+$ ratio, favoring the production of lactate from pyruvate.

Ingestion of ~50–100 mL of ethylene glycol may be enough to cause severe toxicity. A fatal dose is ~100 mL.

The early toxic effects of ethylene glycol are cardiovascular collapse and noncardiogenic pulmonary edema. Later flank pain and renal failure ensue due to extensive intratubular calcium oxalate crystal deposition.

Methanol
Toxic exposure to methanol is usually through ingestion but may also occur by inhalation or absorption through the skin.

Methanol is metabolized in the liver and converted to formaldehyde and formic acid which accounts for most of the toxic features.

Methanol has few toxic effects before it is metabolized.

In addition, lactic acid, keto acids, and other unidentified organic acids may contribute to the metabolic acidosis.

The toxic effects of methanol metabolites are pancreatitis, blindness, seizures and coma. A delayed onset parkinsonian syndrome may also develop due to hemorrhage in the putamen.

Salicylate
Adult patients with salicylate overdose usually present with respiratory alkalosis as a direct effect of salicylate poisoning or have a mixed respiratory alkalosis–metabolic acidosis.

Salicylate also uncouples oxidative phosphorylation, leading to overproduction of lactic and other organic acids.

In children, ketoacid production may also be increased.

Treatment principles in metabolic acidosis
Patients with metabolic acidosis are often very ill and their condition tends to deteriorate rapidly.

The cause of the acidosis should be established quickly and accurately as treatment needs to be directed towards the underlying cause.

Below are a few examples of specific treatments for underlying disorders.

Fluid, insulin and electrolyte replacement should be administered for diabetic ketoacidosis.

Severe lactic acidosis may be associated with a high mortality and if there is evidence of hypovolemia, fluid resuscitation with colloid should be commenced promptly while the diagnosis is being established.

Certain toxins may require specific antidotal therapies (e.g. ethanol or fomepizole for methanol or ethylene glycol, pyridoxine for isoniazid) and/or hemodialysis (e.g. lithium, salicylate, methanol, ethylene glycol).

Hemodialysis is often required for toxin-induced metabolic acidosis complicated by renal failure.

The routine administration of sodium bicarbonate in metabolic acidosis is controversial.

The potential complications of sodium bicarbonate administration include volume overload, especially in patients with renal or cardiac function impairment, hypernatremia, hypokalemia, hypocalcemia and alkalosis.

A rapid elevation of plasma sodium concentration may also occur which can induce demyelination of subcortical brain structures.

However, in cases of methanol or ethylene glycol poisoning, sodium bicarbonate should be given in order to maintain an arterial pH of up to 7.2 (plasma bicarbonate of ~10 mmol/L) whilst avoiding the adverse hemodynamic effects.

If ethanol or fomepizole are not administered in methanol or ethylene glycol poisoning, organic acids may continue to be produced. This may lead to the so-called bicarbonate-resistant acidosis where the administration of larger amounts of bicarbonate may be required with the potential hemodynamic complications.

In salicylate poisoning, bicarbonate should be given to maintain blood pH >7.4 to promote renal salicylate elimination and reduce salicylate penetration into the tissues.

The amount of bicarbonate required (in mmol) can be estimated as follows:

(target plasma HCO_3^- (mmol/L) − current plasma HCO_3^- (mmol/L)) × 40% of body weight (kg)

The management of patients with severe metabolic acidosis should be carried out on the critical care unit and liaison with the toxicology/poison services is essential.

Metabolic alkalosis

Metabolic alkalosis is characterized by:
- high arterial blood pH (alkalemia);
- increased serum HCO_3^- concentration;
- increased PCO_2 (from respiratory compensation).

The clinical effects of metabolic alkalosis are in part due to coexisting problems such as hypovolemia, hypokalemia, hypophosphatemia, reduced ionized calcium concentration and chloride depletion.

Etiology of metabolic alkalosis

Metabolic alkalosis may result from:
- alkali administration;
- accumulation of HCO_3^- due to acid loss;
- HCO_3^- retention or intracellular shift of H^+ as occurs in hypokalemia.

Exogenous alkali
- Antacids, milk alkali syndrome.
- Sodium bicarbonate, sodium citrate, gluconate, acetate administration.
- Massive blood transfusion.

Loss of hydrogen
- Gastrointestinal loss:
  - vomiting;
  - nasogastric suction;
  - chloride losing diarrhea;
  - villous adenoma;
  - antacid therapy;
  - laxative abuse.
- Renal loss:
  - loop and thiazide diuretics;
  - mineralcorticoid excess (renovascular hypertension, primary aldoesteronism, Cushing's, liquorice);
  - hypercalcemia;
  - magnesium deficiency;
  - Bartter's syndrome;
  - Gitelman's syndrome;
  - Liddle's syndrome.

H^+ redistribution into cells
- Hypokalemia.

Systemic effects of metabolic alkalosis

Pulmonary
- Hypoventilation.
- Impaired unloading of oxygen peripherally (oxygen dissociation curve shifted to the left).

Cardiovascular
- Arrhythmias, especially in patients with hypoxemia.
- Decreased myocardial contractility.
- Nitric oxide-mediated vasodilatation.

Nervous system
- Decreased cerebral blood flow.
- Neuromuscular excitability.
- Confusion, lethargy and seizures.

Renal
- Increased tubular reabsorption of calcium.

Investigation of metabolic alkalosis

Symptoms of metabolic alkalosis may be evident but the diagnosis is made following routine biochemical investigations.

The diagnosis of metabolic alkalosis is often suspected from the clinical and drug history, physical examination and the presence of hypertension.

Routine biochemical investigations
- Arterial blood gas analysis:
  - confirm the presence of alkalemia;
  - exclude respiratory acidosis as cause of high HCO_3^-.
- Serum urea, creatinine, electrolytes, chloride and bicarbonate.
- Spot urine sodium, potassium, chloride and pH.
- ECG.

Specialized investigations
- Plasma renin activity and aldosterone concentration.
- Serum cortisol and ACTH concentration.
- Urine laxative and diuretic assay.

An algorithm for the evaluation of patients with suspected metabolic alkalosis is described in Fig. 2.6.2.

In addition, the following points can help to clarify the underlying cause of the metabolic alkalosis.

Chloride-responsive alkalosis
A urine chloride <10 mmol/L.

In the presence of normotension the causes include:
- vomiting;
- nasogastric aspiration;
- diuretics;
- potassium deficiency;
- bicarbonate therapy;
- diarrhea;
- ingestion of nonabsorbable antacids.

Chloride-resistant alkalosis
A urine chloride >20 mmol/L.

In the presence of normotension or hypotension causes include:
- severe magnesium deficiency;
- severe potassium deficiency;

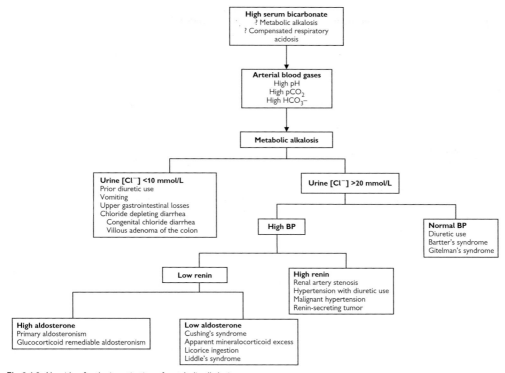

Fig. 2.6.2 Algorithm for the investigation of metabolic alkalosis.

- Bartter's syndrome;
- Gitelman's syndrome;
- diuretics.

In the presence of hypertension causes include:
- primary hyperaldosteronism;
- Cushing's syndrome;
- renal artery stenosis;
- congenital adrenal hyperplasia (11β-hydroxylase or 17α-hydroxylase deficiencies);
- apparent mineralcorticoid excess;
- renin producing tumor;
- Liddle's syndrome.

Treatment of metabolic alkalosis
The underlying cause must be identified and treated, with particular attention to the correction of hypovolemia and hypochloremia.

Chloride-responsive alkalosis
Urinary chloride <10 mmol/L indicates significant renal chloride reabsorption and hence a chloride-responsive cause; therefore these patients should be treated with normal saline until the urinary chloride rises to >25 mmol/L and the urine pH normalizes.

If chloride-responsive alkalosis occurs with volume depletion, it should be treated with normal saline; if there is associated hypokalemia, this should be treated with potassium replacement.

However, if the patient is edematous, normal saline should be avoided. Potassium-sparing diuretics (e.g. spironolactone, amiloride, triamterene) or a carbonic anhydrase inhibitor (acetazolamide) may be used to correct the alkalosis.

Chloride-resistant alkalosis
A urinary chloride >20 mmol/L suggests a chloride-unresponsive form of alkalosis and these patients rarely benefit from volume expansion. Treatment of chloride-resistant metabolic alkalosis will depend on the underlying etiology, e.g. primary hyperaldosteronism may be treated with aldosterone antagonists, adrenal adenoma or carcinoma with surgery, and glucocorticoid remediable hyperaldosteronism with dexamethasone.

In severe metabolic alkalemia (e.g. pH >7.6), particularly if associated with fluid overload, hemodialysis/hemofiltration may be required.

Respiratory acidosis

Respiratory acidosis is characterized by:
- low arterial blood pH (acidemia);
- increased PCO_2;
- normal or increased serum HCO_3^- concentration (due to renal compensation).

Respiratory acidosis and elevated PCO_2 (hypercapnia) is due to alveolar hypoventilation which results in a lower HCO_3^-/PCO_2 ratio and a decreased blood pH.

Thus, hypercapnia and respiratory acidosis occur when there is an imbalance between the production of CO_2 by the tissues and its elimination by the lungs.

Respiratory acidosis can be acute such as when there is abrupt failure of ventilation, or chronic such as in chronic obstructive pulmonary disease (COPD).

Respiratory acidosis results from:
- severe pulmonary disease;
- respiratory muscle fatigue;
- depression of the ventilatory drive.

Etiology of respiratory acidosis
Lung/chest disorders
- Emphysema, COPD, asthma.
- Laryngospasm.
- Restrictive lung disease.
- Aspiration.
- Pneumoconiosis.
- Bronchitis, infections.
- Pulmonary edema.
- Respiratory distress syndrome.
- Inadequate mechanical ventilation.
- Chest trauma: flail chest, contusion, hemothorax.

Neuromuscular disease
- Diaphragm paralysis.
- Severe kyphoscoliosis.
- Guillan–Barré syndrome.
- Muscle relaxant drugs.
- Multiple sclerosis.
- Poliomyelitis.
- Tetanus.
- Myasthenia gravis.
- Various myopathies.
- Toxins, e.g. organophosphates, snake venom.

Central nervous system disease (with a direct effect on the respiratory centre)
- Drugs: narcotics, sedatives, anesthetics, alcohol intoxication.
- Cerebrovascular disorders.
- CNS infections/encephalitis.
- CNS trauma, infarct, hemorrhage or tumor.
- Primary alveolar hypoventilation.

Miscellaneous causes
- Obesity.
- Cervical cord trauma/lesions.
- Cardiac arrest with cerebral hypoxia.

Systemic effects of respiratory acidosis
The systemic and clinical effects of respiratory acidosis will vary depending on its severity and duration, the underlying cause, and the severity of accompanying hypoxemia.

In acute respiratory acidosis, the initial response is cellular buffering which occurs over minutes or hours and slightly elevates plasma HCO_3^-. This is followed by renal compensation in the next 3–5 days when carbonic acid excretion and HCO_3^- reabsorption are both increased.

The acidosis tends to increase the concentration of plasma ionized calcium and causes the extracellular shift of potassium. These changes are rarely significant, however.

Depending on the degree of hypercapnia, the clinical effects of a rapid increase in PCO_2 may result in:
- increased intracranial pressure;
- anxiety;
- confusion;
- psychosis;
- hallucinations;
- depressed tendon reflexes.

If severe and prolonged this may progress to:
- stupor;
- seizures;
- coma;
- death.

In chronic hypercapnia, the clinical effects may be less severe and include:
- headaches (due to the vasodilator effects of CO_2);
- personality changes;
- daytime somnolence;
- sleep;
- memory and motor disturbances e.g. tremor, myoclonic jerks.

The effects of hypercapnia on the respiratory system include breathlessness, central and peripheral cyanosis (especially when breathing room air) and pulmonary hypertension.

The effects on the cardiovascular system are varied and will also depend on the severity of the hypercapnia. These include warm/flushed skin, bounding pulse, diaphoresis, cor pulmonale, decreased cardiac output with systemic hypotension, cardiac arrhythmias, renal impairment and peripheral edema.

When there is concomitant renal impairment, mixed acid–base disturbances should be suspected.

Investigation of respiratory acidosis
The clues to the diagnosis of respiratory acidosis can be obtained from a detailed history, physical examination and ultimately measurement of arterial blood gases.

Investigations include
Arterial blood gas analysis:
- confirm the presence of acidemia;
- exclude metabolic alkalosis as cause of high HCO_3^-.

If chronic respiratory acidosis then the pH may be normal.

Serum/plasma urea, creatinine, electrolytes, bicarbonate (usually a compensatory rise in HCO_3^-).

Full blood count: in chronic hypercapnia, patients may have secondary polycythemia.

Drug screens as appropriate.

Chest X-ray.

CT and MRI scans of the chest and brain as appropriate when chest radiography inconclusive.

Pulmonary function tests, e.g. spirometry.

Treatment of respiratory acidosis
The treatment of respiratory acidosis will depend on its severity, rate of onset, and etiology.

The underlying cause must be identified and treated, and adequate alveolar ventilation must be restored; mechanical ventilation may even be required.

Oxygen should be used with care in patients with severe COPD who are breathing spontaneously. In this situation, aggressive use of oxygen may worsen respiratory acidosis (through loss of hypoxic respiratory drive).

Furthermore, rapid correction of hypercapnia may provoke complications such as cardiac arrhythmias and reduced cerebral perfusion which may lead to seizures.

In chronic respiratory acidosis, general measures such as cessation of cigarette smoking, use of oxygen, bronchodilators, corticosteroids and diuretics should be carefully considered.

Respiratory alkalosis

Respiratory alkalosis is characterized by:
- high arterial blood pH (alkalemia);
- reduced PCO_2;
- normal or reduced serum HCO_3^- concentration (due to renal compensation).

Respiratory alkalosis and decreased PCO_2 (hypocapnia) is due to increased alveolar ventilation which increases the HCO_3^-/PCO_2 ratio as well as the blood pH.

Thus hypocapnia develops when ventilation is increased and the elimination of PCO_2 from the lungs is increased relative to its production in the tissues.

The most commonly observed acid–base disturbance in critically ill patients is respiratory alkalosis and when severe it is associated with a poor prognosis.

It may be associated with mechanical ventilation and many cardiopulmonary disorders.

Increased bicarbonate excretion occurs in acute respiratory alkalosis and within hours is followed by reduced net acid excretion.

In chronic hypocapnia, the serum bicarbonate concentration is reduced but rarely falls to <12 mmol/L in uncomplicated respiratory alkalosis.

Etiology of respiratory alkalosis

Central nervous system disease (with a direct effect on the respiratory centre)
- Head injury.
- Pain.
- Anxiety, psychogenic.
- Fever.
- Meningitis/encephalitis.
- Cerebrovascular accident.
- Tumor.
- Trauma.
- Various endogenous toxins, e.g. toxins in patients with chronic liver disease, progesterone in pregnancy, cytokines during sepsis.

Drugs
- Salicylates.
- Analeptics (respiratory stimulants).
- Methylxanthines.
- Nicotine.

Hypoxemia
- High altitude.
- Severe anemia.
- Pneumonia.
- Pulmonary edema

- Aspiration.
- Right-to-left shunts.

Stimulation of chest receptors
- Pneumothorax/hemothorax.
- Pneumonia.
- Pulmonary edema, pulmonary embolism.
- Aspiration.
- Flail chest.
- Cardiac failure.
- Interstitial lung disease.

Miscellaneous
- Septicemia.
- Mechanical ventilation.
- Heat exhaustion.
- Recovery phase of metabolic acidosis.
- Thyrotoxicosis.

Systemic effects of respiratory alkalosis

The systemic and clinical effects of respiratory alkalosis will depend primarily on the duration, severity and underlying cause.

The cardiovascular effects of acute hypocapnia are generally minimal in the awake individual but may be significant in anesthetized or mechanically ventilated patients. This may be due to a concomitant fall in cardiac output and systemic blood pressure resulting from the effects of sedation and positive pressure ventilation on venous return, systemic vascular resistance and heart rate.

Cardiac contractility may also be reduced in patients with hypocapnia.

Patients with ischemic heart disease and respiratory alkalosis are more susceptible to cardiac arrhythmias as a result of the left shift in the hemoglobin–oxygen dissociation curve, thus impairing oxygen unloading.

Acute hypocapnia may cause cerebral vasoconstriction, leading to reduced blood flow, resulting in a variety of neurological symptoms.

These include:
- paresthesias (circumoral tingling, numbness);
- tetany and carpopedal spasm;
- dizziness;
- mental confusion;
- syncope;
- seizures.

Acute respiratory alkalosis may also result in reduced ionized calcium, intracellular shifts of potassium and phosphate but these effects are rarely significant.

Investigation of respiratory alkalosis

The diagnosis and evaluation of respiratory alkalosis requires measurement of arterial pH and PCO_2 as well as a detailed clinical history and physical examination.

Investigations include

Arterial blood gas analysis:
- confirm the presence of alkalemia;
- exclude metabolic acidosis as cause of low HCO_3^-.

Serum/plasma urea, creatinine, electrolytes, bicarbonate and chloride.

Drug screen as appropriate.

Chest X-ray.

In the evaluation of a patient suspected of hyperventilation syndrome, the organic and metabolic disorders such as pulmonary embolism, cardiac ischemia and hyperthyroidism should be considered and excluded.

Treatment of respiratory alkalosis

As respiratory alkalosis is rarely life-threatening, treatment should focus on identifying and alleviating the underlying cause.

Rebreathing from a paper bag during symptomatic attacks, reassurance, and awareness of the underlying psychological stress are useful in the management of patients with the hyperventilation syndrome.

Further reading

Chairat SA, Seth LA. Inherited renal tubular acidosis. *Curr Opin Nephrol Hypertens* 2000; **9**: 541–546.

Dubin A, *et al.* Comparison of three different methods of evaluation of metabolic acid–base disorders. *Crit Care Med* 2007; **35**: 1264–1270.

Dubose Jr, TD. Acid–base disorders. In: Brenner BM (ed.), *Brenner and Rector's "The Kidney"*. Philadelphia: WB Saunders; 2004. pp. 921–996.

English P, Williams G. Hyperglycaemic crises and lactic acidosis in diabetes mellitus. *Postgrad Med J* 2004; **80**: 253–261

Fall PJ, Szerlip HM. Lactic acidosis: from sour milk to septic shock. *J Intens Care Med* 2005; **20**: 255–271.

Figge J, *et al.* Anion gap and hypoalbuminaemia. *Crit Care Med* 1998; **26**: 1807–1810.

Gluck SL. Acid–base. *Lancet* 1998; **352**: 9126.

Heusel JW, Siggaard-Andersen O, Scott MG. Physiology and disorders of water, electrolyte, and acid–base metabolism. In: Burtis CA, Ashwood ER (eds), *Tietz Textbook of Clinical Chemistry*. Philadelphia: Saunders; 1999. pp. 1095–124.

Hood VL, Tannen RL. Mechanisms of disease: protection of acid–base balance by pH regulation of acid production. *N Engl J Med* 1998; **339**: 819–826.

Kellum JA, *et al.* The first international consensus conference on continuous renal replacement therapy. *Kidney Int* 2002; **62**: 1855–1863.

Kopple JD, Kalantar-Zadeh K, Mehrotra R. Risks of chronic metabolic acidosis in patients with chronic kidney disease. *Kidney Int* 2005; **67**: S21–S27.

Kraut JA, Krutz I. Metabolic acidosis of CKD: diagnosis, clinical characteristics and treatment. *Am J Kidney Dis* 2005; **45**: 978–993

Kraut JA, Krutz I. Use of base in the treatment of severe acidaemic states. *Am J Kidney Dis* 2001; **38**: 703–727.

Morgan TJ. What exactly is the strong ion gap and does anybody care? *Crit Care Resusc* 2004; **6**: 155–159.

Penney MD, Oleesky DA. Renal tubular acidosis. *Ann Clin Biochem* 1999; **36**: 408–422.

Schwartz GJ. Plasticity of intercalated cell polarity: effect of metabolic acidosis. *Nephron* 2001; **87**: 304–313.

Wagner CA, *et al.* Renal acid–base transport: old and new players. *Nephron Physiol* 2006; **103**: 1–6.

Internet resources

The Renal Association (2007) Clinical Practice Guidelines:

`http://www.renal.org/guidelines/index.html`

Review of the management of metabolic acidosis:

`http://www.intox.org/databank/documents/treat/treate/trt34_e.htm`

Review of the management of metabolic alkalosis:

`http://www.intox.org/databank/documents/treat/treate/trt35_e.htm`

Review of renal physiology:

`http://www.brucegilbertmd.com/publications/chapters/BRGcambells.htmL`

Review of acid–base disorders:

`http://www.kidneyatlas.org/book1/adk1_06.pdf`

Overview of acid–base physiology:

`http://www.anaesthesiamcq.com/AcidBaseBook/ABindex.php`

See also

Hypo-/hyperkalemia, p. 46

Renal tubular acidosis, p. 208

Hypokalemic tubular disorders, p. 214

Dialysis and hemoperfusion treatment of acute poisoning, p. 336

Chapter 3

Glomerular disease

Chapter contents

Proteinuria and/or hematuria

General principles

Proteinuria and hematuria are two cardinal features of kidney disease.

Urine dipstick testing to detect them is simple and widely available.

Persistent proteinuria or hematuria is much more likely to indicate significant renal disease.

The combination of proteinuria and hematuria is more likely to indicate significant and potentially progressive kidney disease than either alone.

Urine testing is mostly opportunist.

Symptomless individuals often have a urine test if they require medical approval for some key life event, e.g. life insurance, employment, entry into armed forces.

Screening is only for high risk populations, e.g. those patients with diabetes, hypertension, cardiovascular disease, family history of renal disease.

Not all people with kidney disease have proteinuria or hematuria.

Proteinuria is most characteristic of glomerular disease. In tubulointerstitial and vascular renal parenchymal disease, proteinuria often develops later or not at all.

Not all people with proteinuria or hematuria have kidney disease. Hematuria has many other possible causes in the renal tract.

Initial evaluation

Repeat the urine dipstick 2–3 times to confirm it is persistent.

Ignore trace hematuria or proteinuria (the sticks are very sensitive).

Urine culture.

If the dipstick is persistently positive in the absence of infection:

History
Enquire about:
- lower urinary tract symptoms;
- visible hematuria;
- frothy urine;
- swelling;
- symptoms suggestive of multisystem immune disease (skin, eyes, joints, etc.);
- history of hypertension;
- history of deafness;
- Family history of kidney disease or hypertension.

Examination
Look for:
- edema;
- hypertension;
- renal masses;
- abnormalities on urine microscopy (if a skilled observer is available).

Investigations
Quantify proteinuria: either urine albumin:creatinine ratio (ACR) or protein:creatinine ratio (PCR) on a random (preferably early morning) urine specimen. In glomerular disease albumin is the major protein excreted in the urine.

24 h urine collections are tedious for patients and therefore inaccurate. Urine ACR or PCR on a random sample is sufficient in routine clinical practice.

Measure the excretory renal function: serum creatinine and calculation of estimated GFR.

Immediate microscopy of the urine may be helpful (only if a skilled observer is available – see below).

Renal imaging: ultrasound and plain abdominal radiograph (radiograph is more sensitive for ureteric stones).

If there is persistent proteinuria and/or hematuria with normal renal imaging:
- immunological tests (see Chapter 1.8);
- consider renal biopsy (see below for specific criteria and Chapter 1.7).

Tests of coagulation are only indicated for hematuria if there is clinical suspicion of a bleeding disorder or as preparation for a renal biopsy.

Interpreting proteinuria values

Normal
Urine protein:creatinine ratio (uPCR) <15 mg protein/mmmol creatinine (approximately equivalent to <150 mg/24 h).

Nephrotic-range proteinuria
uPCR >350 mg/mmol.

Absolutely characteristic of glomerular disease.

Non-nephrotic proteinuria
uPCR 15–350 mg/mmol.

This is much less specific. It occurs with a wide range of nonglomerular parenchymal renal diseases as well as with urinary tract conditions beyond the kidney.

Microalbuminuria
30–300 mg albumin/day (it is usually measured as urine ACR: microalbuminuric range is 2.5–30 mg/mmol in men, and 3.5–30 mg/mmol in women).

This is below the sensitivity of the urine dipstick.

It is used to identify early diabetic nephropathy.

It may also be used to assess cardiovascular risk, for example in patients with hypertension (controversial).

Interpreting evidence of hematuria

Hematuria is usually detected by dipstick testing.

The dipstick is very sensitive, therefore ignore 'trace' readings.

The dipstick does not differentiate between hematuria and hemoglobinuria so should be interpreted in the clinical context.

Microscopic hematuria has a quantitative definition based on the number of red cells seen on urine microscopy.

This is not helpful in clinical practice; there is no value in confirming the presence of red cells by routine microscopy in the laboratory (they are often absent because of cell lysis in hypotonic urine before it reaches the laboratory).

Glomerular disease is no less likely if the dipstick is positive and routine urine microscopy is negative.

Immediate microscopy of urine by a skilled observer is useful (but often unavailable):

- casts indicate parenchymal renal disease;
- dysmorphic red cells under phase contrast microscopy indicate glomerular hematuria.

Asymptomatic proteinuria (Fig. 3.1.1)

'Functional' proteinuria

This is transient non-nephrotic proteinuria that can occur with fever, exercise, or heart failure. It is benign and assumed to have a hemodynamic cause.

Overflow proteinuria

This is caused by increased filtration of proteins through a normal glomerular barrier.

It is typical of urinary light chain excretion in myeloma.

Suspect if the urine dipstick is negative for albumin despite large amounts of proteinuria by other tests.

Tubular proteinuria

In addition to the loss of tubular proteins (such as α1- or β2-microglobulin), tubular injury will also lead to some albuminuria owing to impaired tubular reabsorption of filtered albumin. Tubular proteinuria accompanying glomerular (nonselective) proteinuria is an adverse prognostic sign in various glomerular diseases as it usually indicates advanced tubulointerstitial damage.

Orthostatic proteinuria

In this benign condition, proteinuria does not occur in the recumbent position, so there is no protein in the early morning urine.

Proteinuria appears later in the day (uPCR usually <100) and is isolated proteinuria (i.e. no hematuria, normal BP, normal GFR). The prognosis is uniformly good and renal biopsy is therefore not indicated.

Persistent non-nephrotic proteinuria

Persistent non-nephrotic proteinuria is usually caused by glomerular disease.

If the GFR is preserved and the uPCR <100, renal biopsy is not required.

Prolonged follow-up is necessary while proteinuria persists, since there is a small risk of progressive renal disease.

Role of renal biopsy

Although controversial, many nephrologists will perform a renal biopsy in patients with a normal GFR and no hematuria if there is persistent non-nephrotic proteinuria (PCR >100), especially if it persists following ACEI or ARB treatment.

Tubulointerstitial disease can also cause low-grade proteinuria (usually uPCR <200) and typically indicates a poor long-term renal prognosis.

Asymptomatic proteinuria with hematuria

The risk of significant glomerular injury, hypertension, and progressive renal dysfunction is much higher compared with proteinuria or hematuria alone.

In general the prognosis is worse, whatever histological pattern is identified by renal biopsy.

Renal biopsy is indicated if hematuria is accompanied by uPCR >50.

Proteinuria with hematuria and with multisystem disease

Thresholds for renal biopsy are lower when proteinuria and/or hematuria accompany clinical and laboratory

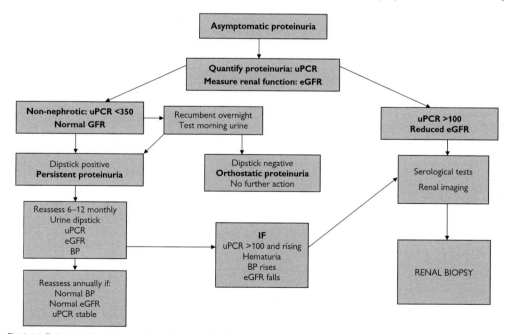

Fig. 3.1.1 Evaluation of asymptomatic isolated proteinuria without hematuria.

evidence of multisystem immune disease, most commonly systemic lupus erythematosus or systemic vasculitis; active glomerular disease requiring therapeutic intervention is more likely.

Isolated microscopic (nonvisible) hematuria (Fig. 3.1.2)

Microscopic hematuria (without proteinuria) is common in many glomerular diseases, especially IgA nephropathy (IgAN), thin basement membrane nephropathy (typically an autosomal dominant condition), and Alport syndrome (usually X-linked and occurs with deafness).

There are, however, many other causes of hematuria in the genitourinary tract beyond the kidneys.

The prevalence of isolated microscopic hematuria is high, increases with age, and is more common in women than men. A single positive test for blood is found in up to 20% of older women. Persistent microsopic hematuria requires further evaluation.

Any detectable proteinuria coinciding with microscopic hematuria virtually excludes 'urological' bleeding and strongly suggests a glomerular origin.

If urine microscopy is available, suspect glomerular hematuria if:
- >5% of the red cells are 'acanthocytes';
- red cell casts are present (usually only seen with proteinuria).

Urine cytology (looking for malignant cells) is not useful.

Renal imaging will identify macroscopic structural kidney disease (e.g. polycystic kidneys), stones, tumors, or (rarely) arteriovenous malformations.

Urological evaluation

Persistent isolated microscopic hematuria in patients aged >40 years (without evidence of a glomerular cause): cystoscopy is mandatory to exclude uroepithelial malignancy.

Persistent isolated microscopic hematuria in patients aged <40 years: uroepithelial malignancy is so rare that cystoscopy is not recommended.

If age is >40 years and there is hematuria with proteinuria, the possibility of two coincidental diagnoses should not be forgotten. If in doubt and particularly if risk factors for urothelial malignancy are present, undertake cystoscopy to exclude malignancy.

Role of renal biopsy

If all these evaluations are negative, consider a glomerular cause for isolated microscopic hematuria. Renal biopsy is usually not indicated since the prognosis is excellent if there is normal renal function, normal blood pressure, and low grade proteinuria (uPCR <50).

Renal biopsy will identify the cause of familial hematuria (where no affected family member has previously had a biopsy) and therefore may avoid other family members undergoing extensive evaluation.

Renal biopsy may be needed to facilitate medical certification, e.g. for immigration requirements, for life or health insurance, or for recruitment to public or military service.

Whether or not the cause of hematuria is defined by renal biopsy, repeated clinical evaluation (urinalysis, eGFR, blood pressure) is mandatory while hematuria persists, since a good long-term renal prognosis cannot be absolutely guaranteed.

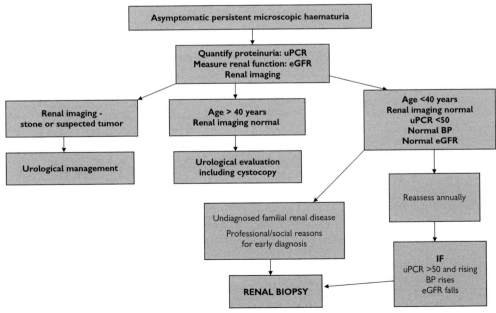

Fig. 3.1.2 Evaluation of asymptomatic microscopic hematuria without proteinuria.

Macroscopic (visible) hematuria

Macroscopic hematuria associated with glomerular disease is usually episodic and is brown or 'smoky' rather than red, and clots are unusual. It is usually painless although the kidneys may ache.

It must be distinguished from other causes of red or brown urine:

- hemoglobinuria;
- myoglobinuria;
- porphyrias;
- consumption of food dyes, particularly beetroot;
- drugs, particularly rifampicin.

Macroscopic hematuria caused by glomerular disease is usually seen in children and young adults and becomes rare beyond the age of 40 years.

The commonest cause is IgAN, but it may occur with other glomerular diseases.

In IgAN, the frank hematuria is usually episodic, occurring within a day of an upper respiratory infection. This is a clear distinction from the 2–3 week latency between an upper respiratory tract infection and hematuria that is highly suggestive of postinfectious (usually post-streptococcal) GN, when there may also be other features of nephritic syndrome.

Macroscopic hematuria requires urological evaluation including renal imaging and cystoscopy at any age unless it occurs in a young person and the history is characteristic of glomerular hematuria.

Further reading

Cameron JS. The patient with proteinuria and/or haematuria. In: Davison AM, *et al.* (eds), *Oxford Textbook of Clinical Nephrology*, 3rd edn. Oxford: Oxford University Press; 2004. pp. 389–414.

Floege J, Feehally J. Introduction to glomerular disease: clinical presentations. In: Feehally J, Floege J, Johnson R (eds), *Comprehensive Clinical Nephrology*. St Louis, MO: Mosby; 2007. pp. 193–207.

See also

Nephrotic syndrome

Nephrotic syndrome is the term given to the constellation of:

- heavy proteinuria (>40 mg/m^2/h or >50 mg/kg/day (i.e. >3.5 g/day in a 70 kg adult));
- hypoalbuminemia (<25 g/L);
- edema;
- hyperlipidemia;
- lipiduria.

It is associated with a variety of other complications including, hypercoagulability, negative nitrogen balance, and infection.

Etiology

Common causes of nephrotic syndrome are listed in Table 3.2.1.

Substantial proteinuria may also be seen in the absence of edema or the other complications of the nephrotic syndrome. This usually results from glomerular disease with the same etiologies as the nephrotic syndrome, but is not associated with the same clinical and management complications. Heavy proteinuria in this setting is often due to secondary FSGS.

Clinical features, complications, and pathogenesis

Presenting features

Patients with the nephrotic syndrome characteristically present with edema.

This is often first noticed in a periorbital distribution first thing in the morning.

This is characteristic of nephrotic syndrome: facial edema is rare in heart failure or cirrhosis because in those conditions patients are unable to lie flat due to the development of pulmonary edema or pressure on the diaphragm from massive ascites in heart failure and cirrhosis respectively.

As the degree of edema increases, fluid will accumulate around the ankles, sacrum and elbows in a gravity-dependent manner, and then become more generalized. Genital edema may ensue and cause significant distress.

Severe edema may be associated with striae, even in the absence of steroid therapy.

Pleural effusions and ascites may develop.

In children, the edema is less gravity dependent and ankle edema may be absent even in the presence of ascites and pleural effusions.

Hypoalbuminemia is also associated with loss of normal pink coloration of the nail. This results in white nails or, if the nephrotic syndrome is transient, white bands (Muerhrcke's bands).

Xanthelasma may also develop as a result of the associated hyperlipidemia.

Proteinuria

Nephrotic range proteinuria is almost always due to glomerular disease.

Under normal circumstances the passage of most plasma proteins (particularly albumin) into the urine is prevented by the glomerular capillary wall (GCW).

The GCW is a trilaminar structure comprised of fenestrated glomerular endothelial cells, the glomerular basement membrane (GBM), and podocytes.

It is richly decorated throughout with an anionic glycocalyx which electrostatically repels negatively charged proteins.

In addition, the structure of the GBM and the podocyte intercellular junctions (slit-diaphragms) restricts the passage of proteins according to molecular size.

Proteinuric disease is almost invariably associated with structural or functional changes in the GCW. In particular, it is now recognized that most nephrotic diseases are associated with podocyte injury and dysfunction (manifest on electron microscopy as foot process effacement), and the loss of anionic charge in the GCW.

Thus proteinuria usually results from a loss of both charge and size selectivity in the GCW.

The precise mechanism underlying these changes is unknown for most diseases, but in inflammatory conditions, a variety of cytokines, eicosanoids, and complement components (e.g. C5b-9, TNF-α, interleukin-1β) may be implicated.

Hemodynamic changes in the glomeruli may also promote proteinuria. Experimentally, an increase in intraglomerular pressure results in proteinuria, and the corollary of this is that currently available therapies which reduce intraglomerular pressure are antiproteinuric.

Hypoalbuminemia

This largely results from urinary losses of protein.

A contribution from protein catabolism by tubular epithelial cells may also be relevant.

In response, hepatic albumin synthesis is increased but this is insufficient to prevent a fall in serum albumin concentration.

Hepatic synthesis of other proteins is also enhanced and if these proteins are too large to be lost in the urine, their plasma concentration may actually increase. This underlies some of the other complications of the nephrotic syndrome, e.g. hypercoagulability and hyperlipidemia.

Edema

Edema is thought to result from two distinct mechanisms:

Underfill model

This is thought to be more common in children.

The reduced plasma oncotic pressure promotes the translocation of fluid from the vascular compartment into the extracellular fluid compartment.

The reduction in plasma volume stimulates both activation of the renin–angiotensin–aldosterone system, and release of vasopressin, which results in sodium and water reabsorption in the distal nephron.

Capillary hydrostatic pressure is increased and this promotes further fluid movement into the extravascular compartment.

Overfill model

This results primarily from a defect of sodium excretion in the distal nephron. The cause of the natriuretic defect is unclear but may relate to tubulointerstitial inflammation that often accompanies proteinuria.

Table 3.2.1. Common causes of nephrotic syndrome

	Prevalence (%)		
	Children	Young adults	Middle and old age
Minimal change disease	77	23	18
Focal segmental glomerulosclerosis	8	18	15
Mesangiocapillary glomerulonephritis	7	13	5
Membranous nephropathy	2	10	34
Other proliferative glomerulonephritis	6	30	15
Amyloid	0	2	16

Sodium retention results in an increased blood volume associated with suppressed vasopressin and angiotensin/aldosterone levels.

The increased intracapillary hydrostatic pressure and the low oncotic pressure favors movement of fluid into the extravascular compartment.

Hyperlipidemia

This is very common in nephrotic patients (>90% of patients with >3 g proteinuria per day will have serum cholesterol >5.2 mmol/L). Therefore hyperlipidemia is usually included in the definition of nephrotic syndrome.

Serum cholesterol concentrations may be extremely elevated, as much as >10 mmol/L in 25% of patients. Triglyceride concentrations are more variable.

The degree of hyperlipidemia correlates inversely with the serum albumin concentration. The enhanced hepatic lipoprotein synthesis is stimulated primarily by reduced plasma oncotic pressure.

The nephrotic lipid profile is regarded as atherogenic (increased LDL (particularly the more atherogenic LDL III), IDL and VLDL; increased lipoprotein (a); reduced HDL-2 and -3) and nephrotic patients (with the exception of those with minimal change disease) have five-fold increased risk of cardiac death.

Hyperlipidemia may also independently promote progressive renal dysfunction.

Hyperlipidemia results from:
- Increased hepatic synthesis of very low density lipoprotein (VLDL). This leads to a downstream increase in both intermediate density lipoprotein (IDL), and low density lipoprotein (LDL).
- Reduced catabolism of lipoproteins due to inhibition of endothelial lipoprotein lipase activity. This further increases VLDL levels.
- Urinary loss of high density lipoprotein (HDL)-3 and reduced activity of lecithin cholesterol acyltransferase (LCAT) leads to reduced levels of the cardioprotective HDL-2.

Hypercoagulability and thrombosis

10% of nephrotic adults and 2–3% of children will have a clinically apparent thrombotic complication.

Subclinical thrombosis can be identified in up to 50% of adults and 28% of children when sought.

Thrombotic episodes are typically venous, but arterial involvement can rarely occur.

The risk of thrombosis is inversely proportional to the serum albumin concentration, and is increased markedly at levels <20 g/L.

Membranous nephropathy is more frequently complicated by thrombotic events than other causes of nephrotic syndrome. The reason for this is unknown.

The pathogenesis of the increased thrombotic risk is multifactorial (Table 3.2.2).

Table 3.2.2. Coagulation abnormalities that promote thromboembolism in patients with the nephrotic syndrome

Physical factors	Immobility
	Hemoconcentration
	Increased viscosity (increased fibrinogen levels)
Clotting factor abnormalities	*Increased concentration (increased hepatic synthesis)*
	Fibrinogen
	Factors V and VII
	Von Willebrand factor
	Protein C
	α1-Macroglobulin
	Unchanged/reduced concentration (increased hepatic synthesis offset by increased urinary loss)
	Factors IX, X, XI, XII
	Antithrombin III
Enhanced platelet function	Altered prostaglandin metabolism
	Altered membrane lipids
	Increased von Willebrand factor
Abnormal endothelial function	Possibly resulting from lipid abnormalities

Infection

Historically infection was a common cause of death in childhood nephrotic syndrome. With the advent of effective treatment with steroids, infection is now less of a problem but remains a significant concern in developing countries.

The characteristic infections are primary peritonitis (usually pneumococcal) and cellulitis (β-hemolytic streptococci).

The pathogenesis of the increased infection risk is multifactorial:
- Edema results in fragile skin that can break down easily, and dilution of local humoral defences. In addition it provides fluid collections in which bacteria can grow easily.
- Urinary loss of IgG and complement components (particularly factor B).
- Urinary loss of zinc and transferrin (required for lymphocyte function).
- Neutrophil and T-lymphocyte dysfunction.

Metabolic abnormalities

A variety of metabolic complications can arise:

Urinary loss of vitamin-D-binding protein. Plasma 25-(OH) vitamin D levels are reduced but free vitamin D levels are usually normal. Osteomalacia and hyperparathyroidism are therefore rare.

Urinary loss of thyroid-binding globulin. Total thyroxine is usually low but free T4 and thyroid-stimulating hormone levels are usually normal.

Rarely copper, zinc, and iron deficiency can result from urinary loss of binding proteins.

Hypoalbuminemia affects the free drug levels of drugs that are protein-bound. This usually does not require dose alteration but warfarin activity may be enhanced, and it may have an impact on the response to furosemide (see later).

Protein wasting/negative nitrogen balance

Many nephrotic patients become seriously wasted during the course of their illness.

Loss of 10–20% of lean body mass is not uncommon.

This is often masked by the edema.

It results from a combination of urinary protein loss and enhanced tubular catabolism of protein.

Increasing protein intake (>1.5 g protein/kg/day) can be counterproductive since it increases intraglomerular hydrostatic pressure and increases proteinuria, without any effect on serum albumin.

Protein restriction (≤0.8 g/kg/day), may reduce proteinuria, but tends to worsen the negative nitrogen balance.

Renal dysfunction

Acute kidney injury

Patients with nephrotic syndrome are at risk of developing acute renal insufficiency.

This is most common in adults with minimal change/FSGS.

It is usually present at the time of the initial presentation with the nephrotic syndrome and only unusually develops after diagnosis.

The potential causes of this are listed in Table 3.2.3.

Table 3.2.3. Causes of acute kidney injury in nephrotic syndrome

- Pre-renal failure due to volume depletion/sepsis (potentially compounded by the use of ACEIs, ARBs, and NSAIDs).
- Acute tubular necrosis due to volume depletion/sepsis.
- Acute interstitial nephritis. Usually due to drugs including diuretics.
- Intrarenal edema causing tubular (and vascular) compression.
- Transformation of underlying glomerulopathy, e.g. crescentic glomerulonephritis in patient with membranous nephropathy.
- Renal vein thrombosis.

Chronic kidney disease (CKD)

With the exception of minimal change disease, nephrotic range proteinuria is associated with an increased risk of progressive renal dysfunction and CKD.

The risk is proportional to the degree of proteinuria and is largely independent of the underlying cause.

While the link between proteinuria and progressive renal disease may be due to the severity of the underlying glomerular disorder, there is increasing evidence that proteinuria is a mediator of tubulointerstitial inflammation and fibrosis.

In support of this, strategies that reduce proteinuria also limit the development of tubulointerstitial fibrosis and renal impairment.

Tubular dysfunction

Fanconi syndrome has been described rarely in patients with nephrotic syndrome.

This may result from proteinuria-induced tubular injury, or from tubular injury mediated by the underlying disease process.

In children, evidence of tubular dysfunction favours a diagnosis of FSGS rather than minimal change disease.

Management

The first stage of management is to determine the underlying cause of nephrotic syndrome using serological investigations and renal biopsy in order to determine whether specific therapy is indicated.

Treatment of the specific causes of nephrotic syndrome is dealt with in their respective chapters.

However, in addition, the clinical consequences of nephrotic syndrome need to be addressed for as long as nephrosis persists.

Edema

Nephrotic edema is managed using a combination of sodium restriction (50–80 mmol/day (this also potentiates the antiproteinuric effect of RAS inhibition)), and loop diuretics.

Nephrotic patients are relatively diuretic resistant because:

- Diuretics are protein-bound. Hypoalbuminemia increases the proportion of unbound drug which increases its volume of distribution. Plasma concentrations are therefore reduced.
- Diuretic that enters into the renal tubules becomes bound to the urinary proteins, limiting its effectiveness.
- The loop of Henle is relatively resistant to loop diuretics.
- Absorption of oral diuretic may be delayed in severely nephrotic patients due to intestinal edema.

Diuretics should be administered in a stepwise fashion until an appropriate response is achieved (e.g. Fig. 3.2.1).

If high-dose loop diuretic fails to induce a diuresis, the addition of a thiazide may be effective. Spironolactone is rarely effective in this setting and should not be used.

If there is concern about drug absorption, IV administration (either as bolus or infusion) should be considered.

Infusion of salt-poor albumin prior to IV loop diuretic can induce a diuresis in some resistant cases. Caution needs to be exhibited since pulmonary edema can be precipitated if a diuresis is not induced.

Finally, patients resistant to these measures may require mechanical ultrafiltration although this may precipitate acute kidney injury as a result of intravascular volume depletion.

In any patient and with any treatment the rate of fluid loss should be limited to <2 kg per day, to avoid severe volume depletion and the risk of precipitating acute kidney injury.

Close monitoring of electrolytes is required. If hypokalemia develops, potassium supplements or a potassium-sparing diuretic should be added.

Proteinuria

Given the evidence that persistent heavy proteinuria predicts progressive renal dysfunction, reduction of proteinuria is an important therapeutic goal.

In the absence of disease-specific therapy, a number of approaches are available.

Antiproteinuria therapy works mainly by altering glomerular hemodynamics to reduce intraglomerular hydrostatic pressure.

RAS inhibition
The most commonly used drugs are inhibitors of the renin–angiotensin system. These result in efferent arteriolar dilatation.

There is accumulating evidence that a combination of ACEIs and ARBs provides an additional antiproteinuric effect, and further slows renal function decline when compared with either agent alone.

Therefore both an ACEI and an ARB at the maximum dose tolerated may be used in nephrotic patients.

The serum potassium concentration needs to be carefully monitored. Hyperkalemia can usually be managed with dietary measures.

Excessive sodium intake can eliminate the benefit of RAS blockade. Therefore, the dietary sodium intake should be limited to 50–70 mmol/day.

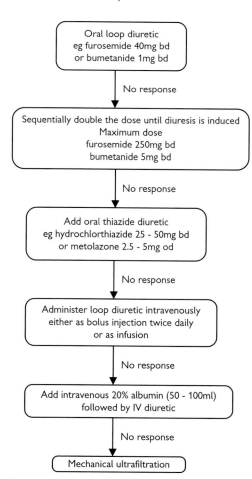

Fig. 3.2.1 An approach to the management of edema in the nephrotic syndrome.

Low protein diet
Dietary protein restriction reduces intraglomerular pressure (via constriction of afferent arterioles).

However, in nephrotic patients dietary protein restriction risks making the negative nitrogen balance worse.

It is therefore recommended that dietary protein intake should be 0.8 g/kg/day plus 1 g of protein per gram of proteinuria.

Other pharmacological approaches
NSAIDs and ciclosporin both cause afferent arteriolar constriction, and dipyridamole causes efferent arteriolar dilatation.

They have all been used in nephrotic patients but the clear benefit (and safety) of RAS inhibition has led to other agents being used less commonly.

In morbidly nephrotic patients with an inadequate response to RAS inhibition, NSAIDs can be very effective.

They may, however, precipitate AKI, particularly in volume-depleted patients, and therefore need to be used very cautiously.

Nephrectomy
Rarely, the nephrotic syndrome can be very severe and resistant to treatment. In such patients the complications of nephrotic syndrome can become potentially life-threatening; nephrectomy, dialysis and intensive nutrition may be the preferred treatment.

Nephrectomy can be achieved surgically, radiologically by renal artery embolization, or medically using high dose diuretics, RAS inhibitors, and NSAIDs.

Hyperlipidemia
The severity of hyperlipidemia is proportional to the degree of proteinuria. Therefore successful disease-specific treatment or antiproteinuria treatment usually leads to an improvement in the lipid profile.

Dietary fat restriction has only a modest effect on hyperlipidemia in nephrotic patients.

Statins (HMG CoA reductase inhibitors) are the most commonly used agents for the treatment for nephrotic hyperlipidemia.

LDL cholesterol can be reduced by 35–40% and triglycerides by 15–30%.

Lipoprotein (a) concentrations are not affected.

Statins are generally safe and indeed there is some evidence to suggest that statins may reduce proteinuria and slow renal function decline.

Reversible myopathy can complicate statin use. Rarely this can lead to rhabdomyolysis and AKI. Serum creatine kinase levels should be monitored after initiation of a statin.

Fibrates have a less potent effect on LDL-cholesterol than statins, and since lowering LDL is the main aim in nephrotic patients, fibrates are uncommonly used.

Fibrate-induced muscle injury is also more common in patients with renal impairment.

Hypercoagulability
Prophylactic anticoagulation
The role of anticoagulation in nephrotic patients without evidence of thrombosis is unclear.

Relatively immobile patients, e.g. during hospitalization, with a serum albumin <25 g/L should be given low-dose anticoagulation (e.g. heparin 5000 U bd SC) until normal mobility has returned.

Many clinicians would also administer full-dose anticoagulation to those at particularly high risk of thromboembolic events, i.e. serum albumin <20 g/L, underlying membranous nephropathy, substantial proteinuria (>10 g/day), particularly when additional risk factors are present, e.g. reduced mobility, massive edema, heart failure, substantial diuresis. However, the evidence base to support this approach is weak.

The response to heparin may be blunted due to reduced levels of antithrombin III, therefore higher doses may be necessary.

In contrast, the response to warfarin is enhanced because of reduced protein binding. This is of particular relevance during remission of proteinuria, when the anticoagulant effect of a stable dose of warfarin decreases.

An alternative approach is treatment with aspirin and dipyridamole, which may also be beneficial given the associated cardiovascular risk.

Therapeutic anticoagulation

Patients with clinically apparent thromboembolic disease should be anticoagulated with heparin followed by warfarin.

Treatment should be continued for the duration of the nephrotic syndrome (or at least until serum albumin rises to >25 g/L) unless the risks of anticoagulation become excessive.

The optimal treatment of clinically silent thromboembolism is less clear-cut.

Asymptomatic pulmonary emboli should prompt full anticoagulation, and most clinicians would fully anticoagulate those with silent deep venous thrombosis.

Further reading
Charlesworth JA, Gracey DM, Pussell BA. Adult nephrotic syndrome: Non-specific strategies for treatment. *Nephrology (Carlton)* 2008; **13**: 45–50.

Crew RJ, Radhakrishnan J, Appel G. Complications of the nephrotic syndrome and their treatment. *Clin Nephrol* 2004; **62**: 245–259.

Glassock RJ. Prophylactic anticoagulation in nephrotic syndrome: a clinical conundrum. *J Am Soc Nephrol* 2007; **18**: 2221–2225.

Koomans HA. Pathophysiology of oedema in idiopathic nephrotic syndrome. *Nephrol Dial Transpl* 2003; **18**(Suppl 6): vi30–32.

Internet resources

Nephrotic syndrome information:

http://www.kidney.org.uk/Medical-Info/kidney-disease/nephsyn_adult.html

Patient information about childhood nephrotic syndrome:

http://www.ich.ucl.ac.uk/factsheets/families/F040225/

Overview of nephrotic syndrome – suitable for patient information:

http://www.merck.com/mmhe/sec11/ch144/ch144c.html

See also

History and clinical examination of patients with renal disease, p. 2

Urinalysis and microscopy, p. 8

Renal biopsy, p. 32

Immunological investigation of renal disease, p. 36

Proteinuria and/or hematuria, p. 76

Minimal change disease, p. 86

Focal segmental glomerulosclerosis, p. 92

Membranous nephropathy, p. 106

Diabetes mellitus, p. 144

Minimal change disease

Minimal change disease (MCD) is the cause of nephrotic syndrome in 90% of children, 50% of postpubertal children, and 10–15% of adults.

Epidemiology
MCD is most common in children but can be seen in adults of all ages.

There is geographical variation in incidence:
- 1 pmp in the UK;
- 27 pmp in USA.

It is more common in South Asians and Native Americans and less common in Africans.

Before puberty, the male:female ratio is 2:1; the gender difference disappears after puberty.

Etiology
This is unknown but a disorder of T-lymphocytes has been proposed. This is supported by:
- the association with lymphoma (particularly Hodgkin's disease);
- the association with HLA-DR7;
- the association with atopy (up to 30% of children in some series);
- MCD relapse following allergen exposure in sensitive individuals;
- remission of nephrotic syndrome with intercurrent measles infection.

In addition, a circulating factor of T-cell origin has also been postulated:
- supernatants from patient-derived T-cell hybridomas induce proteinuria and podocyte foot process effacement in rats;
- a single report of proteinuria resolution after a renal transplant from a donor with MCD.

Although most cases of MCD are idiopathic, infrequent cases have an identifiable cause. These are listed in Table 3.3.1.

Clinical presentation
The typical presentation is with edema of rapid onset.

Up to two-thirds present after an infective episode (typically infection of the upper respiratory tract).

Symptoms and signs are the same as for any cause of the nephrotic syndrome (see Chapter 3.2).

Microscopic hematuria is rare in MCD: its presence is more typical of focal segmental glomerulosclerosis (FSGS).

Hypertension occurs in 30–89% of adults and 14–21% of children.

Complications of nephrotic syndrome
These occur uncommonly in patients with MCD:

Acute kidney injury
This usually occurs following aggressive diuresis but other causes include:
- renal vein thrombosis;
- drug-induced interstitial nephritis;
- interstitial edema leading to tubular compression.

Thromboembolism
This can involve conventional sites; however, in children cerebral venous thrombosis and arterial thrombosis are rare but devastating consequences of nephrosis.

Peritonitis
This remains a significant problem, particularly in the developing world. It occurs mainly in children and is caused by encapsulated organisms.

Table 3.3.1 Causes of minimal change disease

Drugs
- NSAIDs
- Interferon-α
- Lithium (rare)
- Gold (rare, usually causes membranous nephropathy)
- Pamidronate (rare, usually causes FSGS)

Allergy
- Pollens
- House dust
- Insect stings
- Immunizations

Malignancy
- Hodgkin's disease
- Mycosis fungoides
- Chronic lymphocytic leukemia (uncommon)

Others
- Associations with lupus nephritis and IgA nephropathy (uncommon)
- Chronic graft-versus-host disease

Laboratory investigations
Urinalysis
Nephrotic range proteinuria is invariably found in MCD:
- >50 mg/kg/day or >40 mg/h/m^2 in children;
- >3.5 g/day in adults.

The proteinuria in MCD is highly selective (i.e. mainly involves loss of albumin and low molecular weight proteins).

Protein selectivity can be determined from the ratio of IgG to albumin or transferrin clearance.

A ratio of <0.1 indicates highly selective proteinuria.

Values >0.15–0.2 imply loss of higher molecular weight proteins and raise doubt about a diagnosis of MCD.

Glycosuria can result from transient proteinuria-induced tubular dysfunction.

Blood chemistry
The albumin concentration is reduced often to <20 g/L.

Serum IgG is also considerably reduced. By contrast, IgM is increased and IgA tends to be unchanged.

Electrolytes are usually normal.

Hyponatremia may result from volume-depletion-induced ADH release.

Ionized calcium may be reduced in prolonged nephrosis due to 25-(OH) vitamin D3 loss in the urine.

Hypokalemia can result from transient proteinuria-induced tubular dysfunction.

Increased urea and creatinine may be seen as the result of AKI.

Hematology

Hemoglobin concentrations can be increased acutely due to intravascular volume contraction.

Chronic nephrosis can be associated with microcytic anemia due to urinary transferrin loss.

Pathology

By definition MCD is associated with completely normal light microscopic and immunohistological appearances (Fig. 3.3.1).

By electron microscopy the abnormalities are limited to podocyte effacement. This appearance is not specific and can be seen in nonsclerosed glomeruli in primary FSGS.

It is accepted that small numbers of patients with clinical courses compatible with MCD may have:
- mild mesangial hypercellularity (3–5%);
- small amounts of mesangial IgG, complement C3, and occasionally IgA deposition.

Mesangial IgM deposition (often with mild mesangial hypercellularity) can be seen but many regard this as a separate entity (IgM nephropathy).

IgM deposition is associated with reduced steroid responsiveness (50% vs 90%).

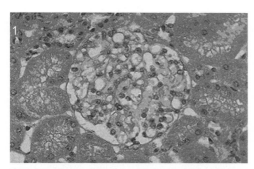

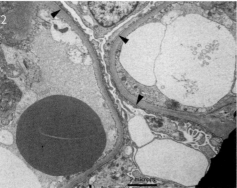

Fig. 3.3.1 (1) Light micrograph of H&E-stained renal biopsy section showing normal glomerular morphology. (2) Electron micrograph demonstrates extensive effacement of podocyte foot processes (arrowheads) but otherwise normal glomerular ultrastructure. (Courtesy of Dr Nick Mayer, Consultant Histopathologist, University Hospitals of Leicester, UK.)

Diagnosis

In children aged between 1 year and puberty, nephrotic syndrome is assumed to be due to MCD.

Renal biopsy is reserved for those children with an atypical presentation:
- microscopic hematuria;
- reduced complement levels;
- impaired renal function;
- marked hypertension;
- absence of steroid response.

In addition, if ciclosporin treatment is being contemplated, a baseline renal biopsy should be performed so that an assessment of nephrotoxicity can be made on later biopsies.

In adults and older children without systemic disease there is no reliable way to predict the glomerular pathology with confidence by noninvasive criteria alone, therefore a renal biopsy should be performed.

The biopsy is not always able to discriminate between MCD and FSGS.

The latter diagnosis relies upon the identification of segmental sclerosing lesions. Since these are focal, they may be missed through sampling error.

Sampling the corticomedullary junction improves the chances of identifying FSGS if it is present.

Natural history

In adults 5–10% of patients will have a spontaneous remission within a few months.

By 18 and 36 months the spontaneous remission rate increases to 50% and 70% respectively. This has to be balanced against the significant morbidity and mortality that accompanies untreated nephrosis.

MCD tends to run a relapsing–remitting course.

The length of the disease course is determined by the age at onset: onset at a young age predicts a longer course before long-term remission is achieved:
- two-thirds of children have at least one relapse;
- 50% of children have more than four relapses.

Long-term remission occurs in 75% of responders who remain in remission for >6 months.

Relapsers tend to achieve long-term remission after an average of 3 years.

Fewer than 5% of children have further relapses after entering adulthood.

MCD does not progress to renal failure.

If renal failure develops, a repeat biopsy will usually demonstrate FSGS. Whether this represents evolution of MCD into FSGS, or a missed diagnosis of FSGS on the initial biopsy, is unknown.

Treatment

Corticosteroids are the treatment of choice in MCD and are effective in most patients.

Complete remission occurs in >90% of patients.

Children tend to respond rapidly with >80% remission within 4 weeks and almost all within 8 weeks.

Adults respond more slowly with >25% taking as long as 16 weeks to remit.

Initial approach

General measures to deal with consequences of nephrotic syndrome are described the Chapter 3.2.

Children

1. Treatment of the first episode

Prednisolone 60 mg/m^2 (maximum 60 mg) per day:

- 75% respond within 2 weeks;
- 80–85% respond within 4 weeks;
- >90% respond within 8 weeks.

Continue steroids at the initial dose for 4 weeks after the urine becomes protein-free.

Switch to alternate day dosing for 8 weeks, then taper every 2 weeks by 15 mg/m^2 on alternate days until stopped.

The relapse rate is lower if steroids are maintained for 3–4 months rather than for 2 months.

Treatment failure may be due to poor compliance or poor absorption from an edematous gut.

If proteinuria persists at 4 weeks consider increasing the dose of oral steroids or giving three pulses of methylprednisolone (1 g/1.73 m^2) on alternate days. Failure to respond to this is defined as steroid resistance.

Potential outcomes:

- 30% of children have only one episode and no relapses.
- 10–20% relapse several months after treatment is discontinued. Most have three or four steroid-responsive episodes before prolonged remission is achieved.
- 40–50% relapse rapidly after stopping steroids and relapse frequently (four or more relapses per year), or relapse while still on steroids (frequent relapsing and steroid-dependent disease respectively).

2. Treatment of first relapse

Following remission, patients should monitor their weight frequently and test their urine daily. A finding of 3+ protein for 3 consecutive days indicates relapse and should be treated promptly to avoid nephrotic complications.

The first relapse is treated with a second course of prednisolone as indicated above although a shorter course may be appropriate (dose reduction 3–5 days after proteinuria has resolved).

3. Treatment of frequently relapsing or steroid-dependent disease

A number of treatment options are available:

(1) Prednisolone 60 mg/m^2 per day until the urine has been protein-free for 3 days, then 40 mg/m^2 on alternate days for 4 weeks.

(2) Prednisolone 40–60 mg/m^2 per day until the urine has been protein-free for 4–5 days. Alternate day therapy is then begun and the dose tapered to 15–20 mg/m^2 on alternate days (depending on the steroid dose at which relapse has occurred). This dose is continued for 6–12 months.

Option (2) may be better since the duration of high dose steroid therapy is shorter, therefore steroid side-effects may be minimized.

Repeated or prolonged courses of steroids may be complicated by significant steroid side-effects:

- growth impairment;
- weight gain;
- cataracts;
- osteoporosis;
- Suppression of the hypothalamic–pituitary–adrenal axis.

To avoid serious side-effects of steroids with prolonged or repeated use, 'second-line agents' are often used in this circumstance.

(1) Cyclophosphamide (2–2.5 mg/kg/day orally) for 8–12 weeks or chlorambucil (0.2 mg/kg orally) for 8 weeks.

These induce sustained remission at 2 years in 67% treated for 12 weeks versus 30% treated for 8 weeks (others have not shown this difference).

Frequent relapsers are more likely to respond than steroid-dependent children (70% versus 30%).

Cyclophosphamide has potentially serious side-effects including:

- infection;
- alopecia;
- gonadal toxicity;
- hemorrhagic cystitis;
- longer-term risks of hematological malignancy.

The risks are probably minor given the doses used in an 8 or 12 week regimen but nonetheless need to be weighed against the fact that MCD is usually self-limiting.

(2) Levamisole (2.5 mg/kg on alternate days for 3 months) can induce remission in just under 50% of patients but most relapse within 3 months of stopping the drug. However, it is a relatively safe steroid-sparing alternative that may be used until spontaneous remission occurs. The most serious side-effect is reversible neutropenia.

(3) Ciclosporin 150 mg/m^2 per day in two doses (aiming for trough levels of 100–200 ng/ml) leads to remission in 85% of frequently relapsing or steroid-dependent patients. However, relapse usually occurs within several months of stopping treatment. Prolonged treatment may therefore be necessary which runs the risk of nephrotoxicity. Some advocate renal biopsy after 18 months of treatment to identify evidence of subclinical nephrotoxicity. The optimal length of treatment is unclear but many advocate 1 year of treatment followed by slow withdrawal.

(4) Mycophenolate mofetil. There are only limited data for its use in children. A small number of retrospective series have been described which suggest benefit in preventing relapse once remission is achieved; however, well-designed trials need to be performed before it can be recommended for use in childhood MCD.

4. Steroid-resistant nephrotic syndrome in children

10% of children will not respond to steroid treatment. In this setting a renal biopsy should be performed and genetic screening should be undertaken to guide further treatment.

10–30% of patients with sporadic steroid-resistant nephrotic syndrome will have mutations of *NPHS2*, the gene encoding the podocyte protein, podocin. Such patients tend to have early onset of disease and a high risk of progressive renal dysfunction. Treatment with steroids or 'second-line' agents is ineffective.

A further 10% of patients with sporadic steroid-resistant nephrotic syndrome will have mutations of WT1 (the Wilms' tumor suppressor gene). Such patients are also resistant to treatment.

In the absence of an identifiable genetic cause, further treatment options need to be considered:

- *Alkylating agents.* There is no evidence to support the use of cyclophosphamide or chlorambucil in this setting.
- *Ciclosporin.* Remission rates of 40–50% can be achieved with 150–200 mg/m^2/day of cyclosporin A. Remission is seen within 1 month in 50% of these patients. Subsequent relapses can also become steroid-sensitive and the risk of developing progressive renal impairment is also reduced.
- *Mycophenolate.* There is insufficient evidence about its effectiveness in this setting.
- *Methylprednisolone.* Aggressive regimens using pulse methylprednisolone (30 mg/kg given IV every other day for 2 weeks, weekly for 8 weeks, every other week for 8 weeks, monthly for 9 months, and then every other month for 6 months), oral prednisone (2 mg/kg every other day), and cyclophosphamide (2–2.5 mg/kg/day) if no response is observed after 2 weeks of pulse therapy, have been shown to induce remission in 60% of patients. The presence of segmental sclerosis on the renal biopsy reduces the efficacy of this regimen.
- *Renin–angiotensin system blockade.* There are few data about the use of ACEIs and ARBs in children. Nonetheless by extrapolation from adult data, they should be used in children with persistent nephrotic-level proteinuria. Obviously they should be discontinued if refractory hyperkalemia or progressive renal dysfunction ensues.

Adults

1. Treatment of the first episode
There is no consensus about the optimal steroid regimen to be used in the treatment of adult MCD.

However, a typical treatment regimen is:

Oral prednisolone 1 mg/kg/day (maximum dose 80 mg/day) for 8 weeks even if remission is induced before this. If remission is not achieved by 8 weeks, prednisolone is continued until 1 week after remission has been induced, to a maximum of 16 weeks. Alternatively IV methylprednisolone can be considered in those without remission at 8 weeks.

Gastric protection with an H2 blocker or proton pump inhibitor should be commenced. Bone protection with calcium/vitamin D or bisphosphonates should also be considered.

On remission reduce to half dose for 4–6 weeks, then gradually reduce the dose over next 4–6 weeks, then stop.

Several outcomes can be observed:
- 80–95% of patients will remit.
- <50% remit within 4 weeks; 10–25% will only remit after 3–4 months of treatment.
- Older patients in general take longer to remit.
- 50–75% will relapse after remission is achieved. This usually occurs within 1 year of steroid cessation although occasionally relapses can develop after years of remission. Relapses can be triggered by infection or allergy.
- 10–25% of patients will have frequent relapses.
- 25–30% will relapse while still taking steroids ('steroid-dependent').

- 0–20% will have persistent heavy proteinuria after 16 weeks of steroid treatment and are classified as steroid-resistant.

2. Treatment of the first relapse
The first relapse is treated with a further course of prednisolone identical to that described above.

3. Treatment of frequently relapsing and steroid-dependent disease
Oral cyclophosphamide 2 mg/kg/day for 8 weeks.

75% and 66% of frequent relapsers will be relapse-free at 2 and 5 years respectively with this regimen.

The success rate is lower in steroid-dependent disease but the success rate may be enhanced by increasing the duration of therapy to 12 weeks although the benefit of this approach has not been universally noted.

Ciclosporin. Further relapses or steroid-dependent disease after cyclophosphamide treatment can be treated with ciclosporin 4–6 mg/kg/day.

70–90% of patients will completely or partially remit.

However, 60–90% will relapse after therapy is withdrawn (usually within 6 months).

There is some evidence that if ciclosporin is continued for 1 year and then gradually withdrawn, prolonged remission can be achieved.

Evidence suggests that ciclosporin doses of <5.5 mg/kg/day do not produce nephrotoxicity even after 20 months of treatment.

Other treatment options:
- Mycophenolate mofetil (MMF). There is limited published experience with MMF suggesting potential benefit in patients with steroid-dependent and -resistant disease. Further studies are required before the role of MMF in MCD can be determined.
- Azathioprine, levamisole and rituximab have been shown to be effective in very small studies. However, the data are so limited that their use cannot be recommended.

4. Treatment of steroid-resistant disease
Steroid-resistant MCD is uncommon and often represents:
- a missed diagnosis of FSGS;
- the presence of another MCD variant such as mesangial hypercellularity;
- inadequate treatment (<8 weeks treatment, <1 mg/kg/day of prednisolone, or alternate day treatment).

For truly steroid-resistant MCD the options are:
- *Cyclophosphamide* (2 mg/kg/day for 8–12 weeks), usually started while the patient is taking steroids, induces remission in many patients. Relapses can occur but these are often steroid responsive.
- *Ciclosporin* (4–6 mg/kg/day). This regimen will induce partial or complete remission in ~50% of patients. Since early withdrawal will often lead to early relapse, continuation of full-dose treatment for 12 months followed by slow tapering of the dose is recommended and will often maintain prolonged remission.

Follow-up
Once remission is achieved patients should monitor their weight and dipstick test the urine regularly.

Weight gain, edema, and 3+ proteinuria on dipstick on at least 3 consecutive days should be treated as a relapse and medical attention should be sought immediately.

Regular nephrology follow-up is not essential for those who stay in remission for at least 1 year.

Frequent relapsers or steroid-dependent or -resistant patients should continue with regular nephrology follow-up.

Internet resources

Nephrotic syndrome in children support group:

http://www.nephrotic.co.uk/

National Kidney Federation:

http://www.kidney.org.uk/

Further reading

Brodehl J. The treatment of minimal change nephrotic syndrome: lessons learned from multicentre co-operative studies. *Eur J Pediatr* 1991; **150**: 380–387.

Korbet SM. Management of idiopathic nephrosis in adults, including steroid-resistant nephrosis. *Curr Opin Nephrol Hypertens* 1995; **4**: 169–176.

Niaudet P. Nephrotic syndrome in children. *Curr Opin Pediatr* 1993; **5**: 174–179.

Waldman M, Crew RJ, Valeri A, *et al.* Adult minimal-change disease: clinical characteristics, treatment, and outcomes. *Clin J Am Soc Nephrol* 2007; **2**: 445–453.

See also

Urinalysis and microscopy, p. 8

Renal biopsy, p. 32

Nephrotic syndrome, p. 80

Focal segmental glomerulosclerosis, p. 92

Focal segmental glomerulosclerosis

Focal segmental glomerulosclerosis (FSGS) is not a single disease entity but rather a group of clinicopathological syndromes that present with similar histological appearances on renal biopsy.

Usually FSGS presents with proteinuria or nephrotic syndrome. It accounts for up to 35% of nephrotic syndrome in adults but is uncommon in children.

It is associated with progressive renal dysfunction with a risk that is proportional to the level of proteinuria.

FSGS can be classified as primary (idiopathic) or secondary (to a wide variety of disease processes).

Epidemiology

The prevalence of FSGS is increasing in both adults and children.

Primary FSGS is marginally more common in males. The risk of progressing to ESRD is two times higher in males than in females.

It is two to three times more common in Blacks than in Caucasians (it accounts for up to 50% of nephrotic syndrome in adult Blacks in the USA). Progression to ESRD is also four times more likely in Blacks than in Caucasians.

There is geographic variation in prevalence. For example:
- in the USA, FSGS is the commonest cause of nephrotic syndrome in adults (35–50%) and is the commonest primary glomerular cause of ESRD (2.3% of all ESRD patients);
- by contrast, in Spain FSGS accounts for 12% of adult nephrotic syndrome.

Etiology

The causes of FSGS are listed in Table 3.4.1.

Primary FSGS

By definition the etiology of primary FSGS is unknown. The focus of injury is the podocyte although the mediators of this injury are unknown.

Some argue that primary FSGS and minimal change disease (MCD) may be part of the same disease spectrum and therefore share a common etiology. This is supported by:
- the morphological similarity of MCD glomeruli with nonsclerosed glomeruli in FSGS;
- the observation in a small number of cases of MCD of apparent evolution with time into FSGS;
- the presence of a circulating factor in some patients with FSGS. This factor is thought to be responsible for the early recurrence of proteinuria after transplantation in some patients. This factor has not yet been characterized.

This view is not universally held, however. The differential expression of cyclin-dependent kinase inhibitors, dystroglycans, TGF-β, and cytotoxic T-lymphocyte effectors in MCD and FSGS argue that MCD and FSGS have divergent etiologies.

Table 3.4.1 Causes of FSGS

Primary (idiopathic) FSGS
Secondary FSGS

Familial FSGS due to mutations in:
- α-Actinin 4 (autosomal dominant)
- Podocin (autosomal recessive)
- TRPC6 (autosomal dominant)

Virus-associated:
- HIV (HIV-associated nephropathy)
- Parvovirus B19

Drugs:
- Pamidronate
- Lithium
- Interferon-α
- Heroin

Secondary FSGS due to adaptive responses:
Reduced renal mass
- Oligomeganephronia
- Unilateral renal agenesis
- Renal dysplasia
- Reflux nephropathy
- Chronic allograft nephropathy
Normal renal mass
- Hypertension
- Obesity
- Sickle cell anemia
- Cyanotic congenital heart disease

Secondary FSGS

Genetic disease
α-Actinin 4
- This is inherited in an autosomal dominant pattern.
- α-Actinin 4 is an actin cross-linking protein the mutant form of which binds to actin with higher affinity. It is postulated that this causes alterations to the podocyte cytoskeleton and dysfunction.
- It characteristically causes subnephrotic proteinuria.

Podocin
- This is inherited in an autosomal recessive pattern.
- It characteristically causes steroid-resistant disease in childhood.
- Sporadic cases have also been described in both children and adults. This is more common in children and 20–30% of sporadic FSGS in children have podocin (*NPHS2* gene) mutations.
- Podocin is an integral membrane protein that interacts with nephrin and CD2-associated protein (CD2-AP) and therefore has a critical role in maintaining glomerular permselectivity.

TRPC6
- Mutations of the transient receptor potential cation 6 channel cause autosomal dominant FSGS.
- TRPC6 localizes to the slit-diaphragm in association with podocin and nephrin.
- Alterations in calcium fluxes caused by the TRPC6 mutations probably underlie the development of FSGS through alteration of podocyte cytoskeletal structure.

CD2-AP
- CD2-AP interacts with nephrin and podocin and is probably important for the maintenance of slit-diaphragm integrity. CD2-AP mutations have been identified in a small number of cases of FSGS, although causality has not been established.

Viral-mediated FSGS
Parvovirus B19
- This has been detected in 80% of biopsies and >85% of serum samples from patients with collapsing FSGS.
- It is highly prevalent in the general population, and therefore causality has not yet been established.

Human immunodeficiency virus (HIV)
- There is robust evidence that HIV causes collapsing FSGS.
- HIV can directly infect podocytes.
- A number of HIV gene products have been shown to disrupt podocytes: Nef induces dedifferentiation and proliferation of podocytes and also disrupts the cytoskeleton; Tat suppresses nephrin expression; vpr synergizes with nef and enhances podocyte injury.

Drug-induced FSGS
- Heroin, pamidronate, lithium, and α-interferon have been associated with FSGS.
- The mechanism of injury is unclear but direct podocyte toxicity is likely.
- FSGS can remit following drug withdrawal.

Structural maladaptive FSGS
- Common forms of secondary FSGS are caused by adaptive glomerular responses. These usually relate to:
- congenital renal mass reduction (renal dysplasia, oligomeganephronia, unilateral renal agenesis);
- acquired renal mass reduction (reflux nephropathy, surgical resection, chronic allograft nephropathy);
- hemodynamic stress (obesity, hypertension, sickle cell disease).

In these conditions the unifying process is an increase in intraglomerular hydrostatic pressure that causes glomerular hyperfiltration (either to maintain GFR in the face of a reduced nephron number, or as a direct consequence of the underlying pathological process).

Whilst initially adaptive, these changes eventually become maladaptive with glomerular hypertension and hyperfiltration leading to glomerular scarring.

Clinical presentation
FSGS presents with nephrotic syndrome or asymptomatic proteinuria.

In children with FSGS 70–90% will have nephrotic syndrome. In adults 50–70% will have nephrotic syndrome.

Secondary FSGS due to hyperfiltration injury tends to present with subnephrotic proteinuria and CKD.

In adults and children with FSGS:
- hypertension is present in 30–50% at presentation;
- invisible hematuria is present in 25–75%;
- reduced GFR is present in 20–30%.

Proteinuria can vary from <1 g/day to >30 g/day, and is typically nonselective.

Complement levels and other soluble immunological investigations are normal.

Tubular dysfunction (aminoaciduria, phosphaturia, glycosuria) may develop as a consequence of proteinuria-induced injury.

Pathology
FSGS is classified into a number of histological variants based on their light microscopic appearances.

This classification is used for both primary and secondary forms but first requires exclusion of other glomerulopathies that may result in an FSGS pattern of injury (e.g. hereditary nephritis, healed inflammatory GN) by immunofluorescence and electron microscopy, and clinical correlation.

In this classification five variants have been described (Table 3.4.2). In addition, other variants have been proposed to fall within the FSGS spectrum (e.g. C1q nephropathy, FSGS with diffuse mesangial hypercellularity).

It should be understood that these variants are simply pathological descriptions and their clinical implications have not yet been tested prospectively.

Table 3.4.2 Morphologic variants of FSGS

FSGS, not otherwise specified (NOS) (classic FSGS)
FSGS, perihilar variant
FSGS, cellular variant
FSGS, collapsing variant (collapsing glomerulopathy)
FSGS, tip variant

FSGS not otherwise specified (NOS) (classic FSGS)
This is the common form of FSGS.

It is defined by segmental sclerosis involving any portion of the tuft, in some, but not all, glomeruli.

The other FSGS variants must be excluded first.

Glomerular capillaries are occluded by hyaline deposits (insudation of plasma proteins into the permeable capillary wall) and foam cells (Fig. 3.4.1A)

Juxtamedullary glomeruli are affected first, therefore the sclerotic lesions may be missed in early disease if the corticomedullary junction is not sampled in the renal biopsy.

Immunofluorescence microscopy reveals no immune deposits although granular deposition of IgM, C3 and C1 may be seen in sclerotic lesions (thought to be due to passive trapping).

Electron microscopy demonstrates podocyte foot process effacement both in sclerosed areas, and also in nonsclerosed glomeruli. This indicates that although at the light microscopic level this is a focal disease, it is in fact a diffuse podocyte disease.

FSGS, perihilar variant
This is defined as perihilar hyalinosis and sclerosis in >50% of the glomeruli with sclerotic lesions (Fig. 3.4.1B).

The cellular, tip, and collapsing variants must be excluded first.

This variant is often seen in the secondary forms of FSGS mediated by hyperfiltration (although it can also be indicative of primary FSGS).

If caused by secondary FSGS, glomerular hypertrophy is often apparent.

Immunofluorescence microscopy reveals IgM and C3 in sclerosed areas only.

Electron microscopy demonstrates variable foot process effacement.

FSGS, cellular variant

This is defined by the presence of at least one glomerulus with segmental endocapillary hypercellularity that occludes the capillary lumen (Fig. 3.4.1C).

Capillary occlusion is caused by foam cells, infiltrating leukocytes, karyorrhectic debris, and hyaline.

Podocytes may be hyperplastic, and occasionally they form a pseudocrescent.

The tip and collapsing variants must be excluded.

Immunofluorescence microscopy demonstrates C3 and IgM in the sclerosed areas.

Electron microscopy demonstrates widespread and severe podocyte foot process effacement.

FSGS, collapsing variant (collapsing glomerulopathy)

This is defined by the presence of at least one glomerulus with segmental or global tuft collapse and overlying hypertrophy/hyperplasia of podocytes (Fig. 3.4.1D).

The lesion is usually global rather than segmental.

The hyperplastic/hypertrophied podocytes often contain protein resorption droplets and fill Bowman's space forming pseudocrescents.

There is no endocapillary proliferation which differentiates it from the cellular variant.

Collapsing variant changes may be seen with FSGS NOS in the same biopsy.

Tubulointerstitial disease with tubular atrophy and interstitial fibrosis is prominent.

Immunofluorescence microscopy demonstrates IgM and C3 in sclerosed areas.

Electron microscopy demonstrates severe and widespread foot process effacement.

Endothelial tubuloreticular inclusions are characteristic of HIV-associated collapsing FSGS.

FSGS, tip variant

This is defined by the presence of at least one segmental lesion involving the tip domain (the outer 25% of the tuft next to the origin of the proximal tubule) (Fig. 3.4.1E).

The affected segment may herniate into the tubular lumen.

The lesions may be cellular or sclerosing. Foam cells and hyalinosis are common.

The presence of perihilar sclerosis or collapsing sclerosis rules out the tip variant.

Tip lesions occur in isolation in approximately one-quarter of cases, and in association with other peripheral FSGS lesions in the remainder.

Immunofluorescence microscopy changes are the same as seen with other lesions.

Foot process effacement is severe and widespread.

Other variants of FSGS

C1q nephropathy

This is an idiopathic glomerulopathy characterized by FSGS or MCD morphology (with variable mesangial hypercellularity) and predominant deposition of C1q (with IgG, IgA, IgM and other complement components).

Exclusion of immune-complex-mediated disease (e.g. lupus nephritis, MCGN) is necessary to make the diagnosis.

Electron-dense deposits are found in a paramesangial distribution.

There is variable foot process effacement.

Although the morphology resembles FSGS, there is debate whether C1q nephropathy represents an FSGS variant or whether it should be regarded as a separate entity.

FSGS with diffuse mesangial hypercellularity

This is defined by the identification of FSGS lesions on a background of diffuse mesangial hypercellularity.

Immunofluorescence microscopy demonstrates diffuse mesangial deposition of IgM, with variable amounts of C3.

Electron microscopy demonstrates extensive foot process effacement without electron-dense deposits.

This variant is seen almost exclusively in children.

Secondary FSGS

Generally the appearances of secondary FSGS are the same as those of primary FSGS.

A few additional pathological features may be identified that help to determine the etiology:

HIV-associated disease

This causes the collapsing variant of FSGS but in addition tubular microcysts and glomerular endothelial cell tubuloreticular inclusions are characteristically seen.

Structural maladaptive FSGS

These usually have glomerulomegaly and perihilar sclerosing lesions.

Podocyte hyperplasia and hypertrophy are unusual.

Podocyte foot process effacement is less severe than in other forms of FSGS and usually affects <50% of the glomerular capillary surface.

Diagnosis

The diagnosis of FSGS requires a renal biopsy, and for the biopsy sample to contain glomeruli with sclerosed lesions.

In addition, the identification of sclerosed lesions within a biopsy depends on the affected glomeruli being sectioned at the appropriate level.

The chances of identifying the lesions of FSGS are increased by:

• sampling the corticomedullary junction;
• obtaining a biopsy with a substantial number (>20) of glomeruli;
• sectioning the biopsy sample at multiple levels.

In those with no sclerosing lesions on biopsy, a repeat biopsy may be prompted by failure to respond to steroid therapy. The additional sampling in itself increases the likelihood of identifying sclerosing lesions.

If FSGS lesions are identified, primary and secondary forms need to be differentiated, since this will determine the subsequent management.

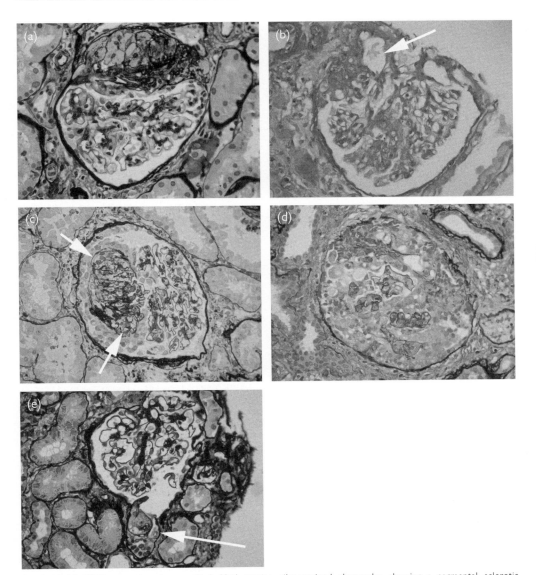

Fig. 3.4.1 (a) FSGS not otherwise specified. Methanamine silver-stained glomerulus showing a segmental sclerotic lesion with hyalinosis and extracellular matrix accumulation. The nonsclerosed capillary loops are otherwise normal. (b) FSGS perihilar variant. A segmental sclerosing lesion is located at the vascular pole (arrow). (c) FSGS cellular variant. The indicated segment (arrows) demonstrates endocapillary occlusion with foam cells, inflammatory cells, and pyknotic debris. The overlying podocytes are hypertrophied and hyperplastic. (d) FSGS collapsing variant. There is global collapse of the glomerular tuft with hypertrophy and hyperplasia of the overlying podocytes. (e) FSGS tip lesion variant. The arrow indicates an area of hyalinosis and adhesion to the tubular pole. This area has become detached from the remaining glomerular tuft. (Courtesy of Dr Nick Mayer, Consultant Histopathologist, University Hospitals of Leicester, UK.)

Secondary FSGS due to structural maladaptive changes is usually associated with less proteinuria, higher serum albumin levels, and less foot process effacement on the biopsy.

A family history of proteinuria and young age at onset is suggestive of genetic forms of FSGS.

A thorough drug history should be obtained and appropriate viral studies undertaken.

Natural history

This is very variable.

However, most untreated patients (or treated patients with no response) with primary FSGS will have a progressive rise in proteinuria and progression to ESRD.

Only 5–25% of patients will have a spontaneous remission. ESRD develops after 5–20 years of proteinuria (by 5 years in 50%).

The risk of renal failure is increased by:
• nephrotic range proteinuria;
• elevated serum creatinine;
• Black race;
• collapsing variant;
• tubulointerstitial fibrosis;
• failure to respond to treatment.

The histological variant also determines outcome.
• The NOS, cellular, and tip variants have a 50% to almost 80% chance of complete or partial remission with treatment.
• The collapsing variant is the least responsive to therapy and progresses most rapidly to ESRD.
• Raised serum creatinine and tubulointerstitial fibrosis at presentation heralds a particularly poor prognosis.

In those that develop ESRD due to primary FSGS, recurrence can occur following renal transplantation (see below).

Treatment

General treatment

General measures to deal with consequences of nephrotic syndrome are described in Chapter 3.2.

For patients with FSGS and CKD 3, 4 and 5 close attention should be paid to cardiovascular risk management. Patients should be encouraged to:
• stop smoking;
• eat a healthy and balanced diet;
• take regular exercise.

Hypertension should be treated to national guidelines using:
• dietary sodium restriction;
• diuretics;
• renin–angiotensin system blockade.

Secondary hyperlipidemia should be managed using:
• dietary measures;
• HMG CoA reductase inhibitors (aim LDL-cholesterol <3 mmol/l, total cholesterol <5 mmol/l, or a 30% reduction from baseline for either parameter; extrapolated from national targets).

Proteinuria should be minimized using renin–angiotensin system (RAS) blockade with ACEIs and/or ARB titrated to a maximal dose (alone or in combination) as long as there are no adverse effects on systemic BP, GFR or serum potassium.

Anticoagulation should be considered in those with severe nephrotic states (serum albumin <20–25 g/l, proteinuria >10 g/day).

Disease-specific treatment

Until recently primary FSGS was regarded as a steroid-resistant disease.

However, longer courses of steroids at higher doses have been shown to induce remission (complete or partial) in 50–70% of patients.

There are no large-scale randomized trials that help to guide the optimal therapy of FSGS. However, the available studies have highlighted some general principles:
• Given the poor prognosis of untreated nephrotic FSGS, such patients should be offered corticosteroid treatment.
• When corticosteroids are used, they should be administered at an appropriately high dose (1 mg/kg/day of prednisolone).
• Corticosteroids should be given for an appropriate length of time. Four months of treatment may be necessary before remission is induced.

Who to treat

There is no way to predict in advance who will respond to steroids.

Steroids should be offered to those with primary FSGS and nephrotic range proteinuria.

Significant renal function impairment (GFR <35 mL/min) predicts a poorer response to steroids unless it is due to AKI, and the renal biopsy demonstrates little tubulointerstitial fibrosis.

The risk of steroid side-effects in individual cases needs to be considered and weighed against the potential benefit given the necessity for high dose and prolonged steroid treatment.

Steroid treatment is usually not given to those with:
• subnephrotic proteinuria and preserved renal function since the prognosis in this setting is usually good;
• subnephrotic proteinuria and impaired renal function since the response to therapy is poor (may indicate secondary FSGS or primary FSGS of long duration).

These patients should be managed primarily with general treatment measures, particularly RAS blockade.

Initial treatment approach

There is no consensus about the optimal steroid regimen to be used in the treatment of FSGS.

A typical regimen is:

Prednisolone 1 mg/kg/day (or 2 mg/kg on alternate days) for up to 12–16 weeks.

Several outcomes may be observed:
• Complete remission (<300 mg proteinuria/day) within 12 weeks. Continue prednisolone at full dose for 2 weeks after remission, then gradually taper to stop over 2–3 months.
• Partial remission (>50% fall in proteinuria to <3.5 g/day) within 12 weeks. Taper the prednisolone dose over 6–9 months. An alternate-day steroid regimen can be used in this situation. If proteinuria increases during the taper (defined as steroid dependence) second-line treatments can be used (see below).

- Reduction in proteinuria at 12–16 weeks but fall <50% and proteinuria still >3.5 g/day. If proteinuria is still falling and if steroid side-effects are minimal, high-dose prednisolone may be continued (or an alternate-day regimen used). If proteinuria has plateaued or if steroid side-effects are significant, second-line agents can be considered.
- No significant improvement in proteinuria by 12–16 weeks. These patients are defined as steroid resistant. A trial of second-line therapy can be used with brisk withdrawal of steroids (over 4–6 weeks).

Relapsing disease
If after a complete or partial remission is induced, a relapse occurs after 1 year, the steroid course is repeated.

If relapse occurs either within 1 year of remission, or while on a steroid taper, or after a previous relapse, second-line agents should be considered.

Second-line treatment
Second-line agents should be considered in those patients with:
- unacceptable steroid side-effects (or likelihood of poor tolerance of steroids e.g. morbid obesity, diabetes mellitus);
- incomplete remission (i.e. <50% reduction in proteinuria, or >3.5 g/day proteinuria after treatment);
- steroid-dependent FSGS;
- relapsing disease (i.e. more than one relapse);
- steroid-resistant FSGS.

Ciclosporin
This is the most commonly used second-line agent.

It is able to induce remission in 20–70% of patients with steroid-resistant FSGS, although the longer-term efficacy is unknown.

Ciclosporin should be given at a dose of 3–4 mg/kg/day in 2 doses, with low dose prednisolone (0.15 mg/kg/day). Target ciclosporin trough levels are 100–200 ng/mL.

Remission usually occurs within 3 months.

Relapse is common after early withdrawal therefore many clinicians continue for ≥6 months (perhaps ideally >1 year) after remission is achieved followed by a slow taper.

The prednisolone dose can be halved after 6 months and then continued for the duration of the ciclosporin treatment (or withdrawn if steroid side-effects are significant).

Because of the potential nephrotoxic effects of ciclosporin, alternative agents (e.g. mycophenolate or cyclophosphamide) should be considered in those with GFR <40 mL/min.

Cytotoxic agents
The use of cyclophosphamide and chlorambucil in the treatment of FSGS has only been reported in retrospective, uncontrolled studies.

In children with steroid-dependent or relapsing idiopathic nephrotic syndrome, cyclophosphamide induces remission in 75%, but in only 25% of those with steroid-resistant disease.

In the treatment of FSGS, cyclophosphamide should be reserved for those with an incomplete response to steroids in whom ciclosporin is contraindicated (e.g. extensive tubulointerstitial fibrosis, GFR <40 mL/min). In this setting, however, many would prefer to use mycophenolate mofetil because of its better side-effect profile.

Cyclophosphamide (2 mg/kg/day) should be given for 8–12 weeks, while the patient is still taking steroids.

Mycophenolate mofetil
In uncontrolled studies mycophenolate has induced complete or partial remission in ~40% of patients with steroid-resistant or steroid-dependent FSGS.

An National Institutes of Health/NIDDK-sponsored prospective randomized trial comparing ciclosporin and mycophenolate in steroid-resistant patients is currently underway.

It can be considered in those with no response to prednisolone and/or ciclosporin, contraindications to ciclosporin use, or evidence of ciclosporin nephrotoxicity.

A dose of 750–1000 mg/bd should be given for 4–6 months.

Tacrolimus
There is some evidence, albeit from uncontrolled studies, that tacrolimus may be of benefit in patients with FSGS.

Although it has not been directly compared with ciclosporin, case reports have described response to tacrolimus in patients who have had no response to ciclosporin.

It should be primarily reserved for patients in whom side-effects (excluding nephrotoxicity) preclude the use of ciclosporin.

Sirolimus
A small number of reports have described a variable outcome with sirolimus.

Two studies have described episodes of AKI, deteriorating renal function, and no remissions.

A further study has described a 50% remission rate.

A further concern is that the use of sirolimus in proteinuric renal transplant recipients is associated with worsening of proteinuria and the development of focal sclerosing lesions on biopsy.

For these reasons there is currently insufficient evidence to support the use of sirolimus in the treatment of FSGS.

Rituximab
The use of rituximab (monoclonal anti-CD20 antibody) in the treatment of childhood and adult FSGS in native and transplant kidneys has been described in a few case reports.

The outcome has been variable and its use in the treatment of FSGS cannot be recommended.

Plasmapheresis
The role of plasmapheresis in the treatment of primary FSGS has only been evaluated in a small number of uncontrolled studies in patients with steroid- and cytotoxic-resistant disease. Its use is based upon the benefit seen in patients with early recurrence of FSGS post-transplantation, and the identification of a circulating permeability factor in some patients with primary FSGS.

The reported remission rate has varied from 25 to 75%.

It is currently not possible to identify patients who may benefit from plasmapheresis. An assay for the permeability factor is not widely available, and the relationship between the presence of permeability factor and proteinuria is not strong.

Based on this evidence plasmapheresis should only be considered in those with severe FSGS-related nephrosis that is resistant to all other treatment modalities.

Follow-up

Routine blood chemistries, including eGFR, and the urine PCR should be measured at 2–4 week intervals during the first 2–3 months of treatment.

Before reducing immunosuppression, the level of proteinuria should be confirmed with two urine PCR measurements.

Once drug therapy is stabilized and/or is being tapered, monitoring at 1–2 month intervals is appropriate.

Recurrent FSGS post-transplantation

Primary FSGS can recur in a renal allograft.

It is thought to be due to the presence of a circulating permeability factor (or possibly to the loss of a normal serum component).

The overall risk of recurrence is 20%; however, an increased risk of recurrence can be seen in those:
- aged <20 years;
- with a rapid course from diagnosis to ESRD (<3 years);
- with previous recurrence in a transplant;
- with mesangial proliferation on native renal biopsy.

The onset of recurrence may be very rapid (within hours of the transplant), the nephrosis may be severe, and allograft dysfunction is common. Most cases present within 1 month post-transplant (median 14 days in children) although late recurrence can also occur.

The diagnosis is made by detecting increasing proteinuria (a baseline measurement of protein excretion form the native kidneys is helpful in this regard), and from a renal biopsy. The renal biopsy in the early stages may just demonstrate foot process effacement. Given the association of FSGS with viral infection, polymerase chain reaction for Parvovirus B19, CMV, EBV, BK virus, and hepatitis C virus should be performed.

Treatment

Although never subjected to randomized prospective study, plasmapheresis is the treatment of choice for recurrent FSGS.

Retrospective studies have shown that most people who commence plasmapheresis within 2 weeks of disease onset will remit.

A typical treatment regimen would be:
- Nine plasmapheresis treatments (removal of 1.5 plasma volumes with 4.5% albumin as replacement fluid): daily for 3 days then three times a week for 2 weeks.

- Standard immunosuppression regimen (steroid, calcineurin inhibitor, mycophenolate). Avoid mTOR (mammalian target of rapamycin) inhibitors.
- RAS blockade.

If remission is induced (urine PCR <100), monitor proteinuria monthly.

If remission is not induced:
- continue plasmapheresis (weekly for 6 weeks);
- consider switching the immunosuppression regimen to cyclophosphamide (1–2 mg/kg/day) and prednisolone 0.5–1 mg/kg/day for up to 3 months, then revert to standard transplant regimen.

Although recurrent FSGS can cause graft loss, the incidence of allograft loss at 10 years due to recurrent FSGS is only ~12%.

Further reading

Burgess E. Management of focal segmental glomerulosclerosis: evidence-based recommendations. *Kidney Int* 1999; **70**(Suppl): S26.

D'Agati V. The many masks of focal segmental glomerulosclerosis. *Kidney Int* 1994; **46**: 1223.

D'Agati V. Pathologic classification of focal segmental glomerulosclerosis. *Semin Nephrol* 2003; **23**: 117–134.

Matalon A, Valeri A, Appel GB. Treatment of focal segmental glomerulosclerosis. *Semin Nephrol* 2000; **20**: 309.

Meyrier A. Nephrotic focal segmental glomerulosclerosis in 2004: an update. *Nephrol Dial Transplant* 2004; **19**: 2437.

Rydel JJ, Korbet SM, Borok RZ, Schwartz MM. Focal segmental glomerular sclerosis in adults: presentation, course, and response to treatment. *Am J Kidney Dis* 1995; **25**: 534.

Internet resources

NIH/NIDDK cyclosporin/mycophenolate trial information:
`http://www.fsgstrial.org/welcome.htmL`

See also

Urinalysis and microscopy, p. 8

Renal biopsy, p. 32

Nephrotic syndrome, p. 80

Minimal change disease, p. 86

Infection-related glomerulonephritis, p. 128

Recurrent disease and *de novo* disease postrenal transplantation, p. 572

Immunoglobulin A nephropathy and Henoch–Schönlein purpura

Immunoglobulin A nephropathy (IgAN) is the commonest pattern of glomerulonephritis seen in the Western world.

It is an important cause of progressive kidney disease with 25–30% of patients developing ESRD within 25 years of diagnosis. The diagnosis of IgAN always requires a renal biopsy.

Closely associated with IgAN is Henoch–Schönlein purpura (HSP), a small vessel systemic vasculitis characterized by small blood vessel deposition of IgA predominantly within the skin, joints, gut and kidney. The nephritis of HSP is also characterized by mesangial IgA deposition and may be histologically indistinguishable from IgAN.

IgA nephropathy

IgAN is defined by the predominant deposition of polymeric IgA1 in the glomerular mesangium.

Epidemiology

There is a male predominance.

Peak incidence is in the 2nd and 3rd decades.

There is wide geographic variation in the incidence, the highest being reported in the Pacific rim (this may reflect differing approaches to renal biopsy for minor urine abnormalities).

Prevalence of subclinical (asymptomatic and undiagnosed) IgAN may be as high as 16% of the general population.

Etiology

<10% of cases have familial IgA nephropathy.

- Genome-wide linkage analysis has demonstrated linkage of IgAN to 6q22–23 and the putative gene locus IGAN1.
- There are no obvious candidate genes within the linked interval.
- It is not certain that genetic findings from these families will have direct bearing on more typical sporadic cases of IgAN.

>90% of cases are sporadic and the etiology is unknown.

- No evidence for involvement of a specific infectious agent despite association of macroscopic hematuria with mucosal inflammation.
- No evidence for hypersensitivity to food antigens in the majority of cases with exception of a small group of patients with celiac disease.
- Abnormal O-glycosylation of IgA1 hinge region thought to promote formation of circulating IgA immune complexes with propensity for mesangial deposition and mesangial cell activation.

Natural history

The perceived overall cohort risk is heavily influenced by different diagnostic approaches.

Centres with a low threshold for renal biopsy for patients with mild urine abnormality, particularly those working in countries where urine screening programs are established, will likely diagnose IgAN in a larger number of patients with mild disease and good prognosis, thus favorably influencing the overall outcome of the cohort.

It is generally accepted that:

- <10% have complete resolution of urinary abnormalities;
- episodes of macroscopic hematuria become less frequent with time after diagnosis although the majority of patients will have persistent microscopic hematuria;
- 1.5% will reach ESRD per year;
- 25–30% will require renal replacement therapy within 20–25 years;

Recurrence after renal transplantation:

- This is assuming increasing importance as a cause of graft failure as control of rejection improves.
- It is typically slowly progressive although occasional patients will have a rapidly progressive course.
- At 5 years a 5% risk of graft failure due to recurrence, a 13% risk of significant graft dysfunction, and a risk of IgA deposition of ≥50%.
- The risk of graft loss increases to 25% if first graft was lost to recurrence.
- There is no consistent evidence that these risks differ between living and cadaveric donors.
- There is no evidence that the immunosuppressive regimen alters the incidence of IgAN recurrence or the prognosis of recurrence in the short term.

Clinical features

Symptoms

30–40% of patients present with macroscopic hematuria 12–72 h after the development of a mucosal infection (most commonly upper respiratory tract).

30–40% of patients are asymptomatic and are identified following incidental urine testing with microscopic hematuria and/or proteinuria.

5% of patients develop nephrotic syndrome.

<5% of patients present with AKI.

<5% of patients present with malignant hypertension.

Remaining patients are identified following investigation of hypertension, usually associated with microscopic hematuria and or proteinuria.

Signs

There are no specific physical signs diagnostic of IgAN.

Occasionally patients may exhibit loin pain (unilateral or bilateral). The relationship of loin pain to active glomerulonephritis is ill-understood.

Differential diagnosis

The diagnosis of IgAN requires a renal biopsy.

Primary IgAN must be distinguished from other secondary forms of IgAN associated with:

- Chronic liver disease, particularly alcoholic cirrhosis (thought to be due to impaired IgA immune complex clearance by the liver).
- HIV and AIDS (associated with high serum IgA level).
- Celiac disease (in a small proportion of patients adherence to a gluten-free diet can lead to reduced proteinuria and improvement of renal function).
- Henoch–Schönlein purpura (a small vessel vasculitis with renal biopsy appearances indistinguishable from IgA nephropathy).

Mesangial deposition of IgA, along with other immunoglobulin classes and complement may also be a feature of lupus nephritis but the clinical and serologic features usually present no diagnostic difficulty.

There have also been a number of reports of an IgA-dominant post-infectious glomerulonephritis associated with methicillin-sensitive and -resistant *Staphylococcus aureus* infection. This disease is marked by severe glomerular changes on renal biopsy, nephrotic range proteinuria and rapid decline in renal function with many patients developing irreversible ESRD.

Investigations

General investigations
Assessment of renal function, urinary protein leak and renal size are mandatory for the investigation of suspected glomerulonephritis.

Raised serum IgA1 levels are found in 30–50% of all patients, but are less common in children and do not correlate with disease activity or severity.

A high proportion of λ light chain, rather than the normal predominance of the κ isotype, is also a distinctive feature of serum IgA in IgAN although the significance of this is unknown.

Complement components C3 and C4, and CH_{50} in the serum are usually normal but there is some evidence of systemic complement activation with more specific testing.

Circulating autoantibodies, IgA-rheumatoid factors and IgA-containing immune complexes have been reported in IgAN but none appear to be disease specific.

Laboratory checks for liver function and hepatitis B status are sufficient to exclude the common causes of secondary IgAN.

Special investigations
The diagnosis of IgAN requires a renal biopsy.

No accumulation of clinical and laboratory evidence has sufficient specificity and sensitivity to avoid the need for diagnostic biopsy.

There has been a single report suggesting measurement of IgA1 O-glycosylation may in the future be used to diagnose IgAN but this remains speculative at present.

Renal biopsy features
Mesangial IgA deposits are the defining hallmark of IgAN and can be identified by immunofluorescence or immunoperoxidase techniques.

IgA deposits are diffuse and global even if light microscopic changes are focal and segmental.

Heavy mesangial IgA deposition may be seen with no light microscopic change.

- Light microscopy

  Light microscopic abnormalities may be minimal, but the commonest appearance is mesangial hypercellularity which is usually diffuse and global (Fig. 3.5.1).

  Progressive disease is associated with relentless accumulation of mesangial matrix.

  Crescentic change may be superimposed on diffuse mesangial proliferative glomerulonephritis with or without associated segmental necrosis.

Crescents are common in biopsies performed during episodes of macroscopic hematuria with renal impairment.

Tubulointerstitial changes do not differ from those seen in other forms of progressive glomerulonephritis.

- Immunohistology

  IgA is the sole immunoglobulin in 15% of biopsies (Fig. 3.5.2).

  IgG is present in 50–70% and IgM in 31–66% of biopsies although staining is usually less intense than IgA.

  Codeposition of IgG and IgM is unrelated to the extent of glomerular injury or clinical outcome.

  C3 deposition is usual and has the same distribution as IgA. The pathological significance is uncertain.

  IgA deposits may extend beyond the mesangium to the periphery of the glomerular capillaries and this has been associated with a worse prognosis.

- Electron microscopy

  Mesangial and paramesangial electron-dense deposits are the ultrastructural manifestation of mesangial IgA deposition (Fig. 3.5.3).

  Capillary loop deposits are usually subendothelial but can be intramembranous or subepithelial and are associated with a worse clinical outcome in adults.

  The quantity, size, shape and density of deposits vary from glomerulus to glomerulus and from one mesangial zone to another.

  The glomerular basement membrane (GBM) shows localized abnormalities in 15–40% cases. GBM abnormalities are associated with heavy proteinuria, more severe glomerular changes and crescent formation.

  A proportion of patients have diffuse uniform global thinning of the GBM indistinguishable from thin membrane nephropathy. It is not clear whether this group of patients has any defining clinical or prognostic characteristics compared with most IgAN.

A number of classifications of IgAN based on light microscopic findings are in use (for example those of Lee and Haas), but there is little agreement about their relative utility. The International IgA Nephropathy Network with the Renal Pathology Society are presently developing an international consensus on a pathological classification for IgAN which is expected to be published in 2009.

Risk stratification

Many studies have identified features at presentation which mark a poor prognosis (Table 3.5.1).

Although prognostic formulae using simple clinical and laboratory data have been proposed there is not yet sufficient consensus to recommend them in clinical practice for the prediction of individual progression risk.

Treatment

General measures
As with all causes of CKD, patients with IgAN and CKD 3, 4 and 5 must pay close attention to cardiovascular risk and:

- stop smoking;
- eat a healthy and balanced diet;
- take regular exercise.

Table 3.5.1 Prognostic markers at presentation in IgA nephropathy

Clinical	Histopathologic	
Poor prognosis	**Poor prognosis**	
Increasing age	*Light microscopy*	Capsular adhesions and crescents
Duration of preceding symptoms		Glomerular sclerosis
Severity of proteinuria		Tubule atrophy
Hypertension		Interstitial fibrosis
Renal impairment		Vascular wall thickening
Increased body mass index		
	Immunofluorescence	Capillary-loop IgA deposits
	Ultrastructure	Capillary wall electron-dense deposits
		Mesangiolysis
		GBM abnormalities
Good prognosis	**Good prognosis**	
Recurrent macroscopic hematuria	Minimal light microscopic abnormalities	
No impact on prognosis	**No impact on prognosis**	
Gender	Intensity of IgA deposits	
Ethnicity	Codeposition of mesangial IgG, IgM or C3	
Serum IgA level		

Recurrent macroscopic hematuria
No specific treatment required.

No role for prophylactic antibiotics.

No role for tonsillectomy.

Microscopic hematuria and <1 g/24 h proteinuria
No specific treatment required.

Consider ACEI and/or ARB.

Nephrotic syndrome
Consider corticosteroids if the histological features are consistent with superimposed minimal change disease.

Generic management of nephrotic syndrome.

Acute kidney injury
A renal biopsy is almost always required.
- Acute tubular necrosis: provide supportive care.
- Crescentic IgAN: if there is active glomerular inflammation, deteriorating renal function and no significant chronic damage then treat with cyclophosphamide and corticosteroids (as for small vessel vasculitis); otherwise provide supportive management.

Slowly progressive IgAN
Blood pressure control: aim for <125/75 mmHg; greatest benefit is with maximal renin–angiotensin system blockade.

Proteinuria >1 g/24 h: aim for maximal renin angiotensin system blockade.

There is no conclusive evidence for:
- corticosteroids;
- mycophenolate mofetil;
- cyclophosphamide;
- fish oil;
- anticoagulation or antiplatelet agents.

Follow-up
Patients with CKD 1–3 can be followed up in primary care (see algorithm in Appendix). Patients with progressive renal decline and CKD 4 and 5 require continued nephrological review on a 2–6-monthly basis dependent upon their eGFR.

Pregnancy
As with other chronic glomerulonephritides, pregnancy-related complications in IgAN are increased when there is:
- renal impairment (Cr >150 μmol/l);
- proteinuria (>1 g/24 h);
- hypertension (either on treatment or >140/90).

Patients with high-risk clinical profiles should be offered preconception counselling and when pregnant careful monitoring in a combined renal–obstetric clinic.

Prognosis
25–30% of patients will require renal replacement therapy within 20–25 years.

Those at greatest risk of progressive renal failure are patients with significant proteinuria, hypertension and impaired renal function at the time of renal biopsy (Table 3.5.1).

Future prospects
The International IgAN Network is shortly to report on an international consensus on a pathological classification for IgAN. This will hopefully help with stratification of patients according to the risk of progressive renal failure and help in the development of new clinical trials where recruitment is based on renal biopsy features of disease activity (as in lupus nephritis) rather than on blunt clinical parameters such as proteinuria which may reflect both active disease and chronic irreversible parenchymal damage.

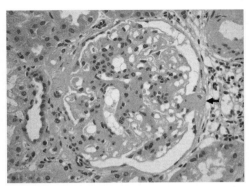

Fig. 3.5.1. Light microscopic changes in IgA nephropathy. An H&E-stained section demonstrating mesangial expansion with mesangial cell proliferation. A capsular adhesion can also be seen (arrowed).

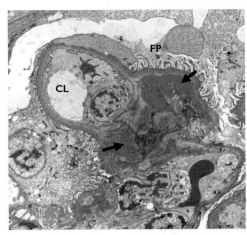

Fig. 3.5.3. An electron micrograph demonstrating IgA immune complex deposition within the mesangium and paramesangium. Electron-dense IgA immune complexes (arrowed). Normal podocyte foot processes (FP) and capillary loops (CL) can be seen. (All images courtesy of Dr Nick Mayer, Consultant Histopathologist, University Hospitals of Leicester, UK.)

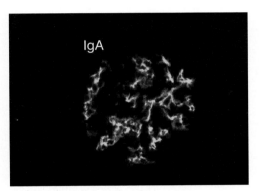

Fig. 3.5.2. Immunofluorescence micrograph demonstrating mesangial IgA staining.

Two ongoing trials will hopefully resolve the issue of whether immunosuppression is appropriate in progressive IgAN: the STOP-IgAN trial comparing maximal supportive therapy with immunosuppression; and an Italian-based study which is comparing ACEI and prednisolone versus ACEI alone.

Henoch–Schönlein purpura

Henoch–Schönlein purpura (HSP) is a small-vessel systemic vasculitis characterized by IgA deposition in affected blood vessels. The purpuric rash is a cutaneous vasculitis and the renal lesion (HSP nephritis) is a mesangial proliferative GN usually indistinguishable from IgAN.

Epidemiology

HSP can occur at any age but is commonest in the first decade of life.

There is a slight male predominance.

Etiology

There is much indirect evidence to suggest a close relationship between IgAN and HSP:

- Monozygotic twins have been described: one who developed IgAN and the other HSP at the same time.
- HSP developing on a background of proven IgAN has been described in both adults and children.
- Many abnormalities of the IgA immune system, including abnormal IgA1 glycosylation, have been described in both IgAN and HSP.

Why some individuals suffer renal-limited disease (IgAN) and others a systemic disease (HSP) is not known.

Natural history

Much of the renal disease in HSP is transient.

Asymptomatic hematuria or proteinuria usually disappears within a few weeks of presentation.

Of those with persistent evidence of renal disease the most common feature is persistent asymptomatic hematuria and proteinuria.

~20% will develop the nephrotic syndrome.

~25% patients will develop CKD.

AKI due to crescentic HSP nephritis usually occurs early and is more common than crescentic IgAN.

HSP nephritis can recur after renal transplantation.

Overall transplant success and graft longevity do not differ between HSP and other forms of primary renal disease.

Changes in immunosuppressive regimens over the last two decades have not altered the recurrence rate or its prognosis.

Clinical features

Symptoms

The presenting feature is a palpable purpuric rash caused by cutaneous vasculitis.

The rash has a characteristic extensor surface distribution with sparing of the trunk and face.

Crops of rash, often provoked by intercurrent infection, may continue for some time but rarely beyond one year from first presentation.

Polyarthralgia is common.

Abdominal pain, due to gut vasculitis, is usually mild and transient but severe pain and bloody diarrhea may develop due to intussusception.

Signs

Apart from the rash there are no other distinctive physical signs.

Differential diagnosis

In children HSP is the commonest form of vasculitis.

A clinical diagnosis is often made from the characteristic rash and abdominal pain.

A definitive diagnosis requires identification of tissue IgA deposition which can be found in the vessels of affected skin as well as the kidney.

In adults the differential diagnosis is wider including many other forms of small vessel vasculitis which must be distinguished on the basis of clinical, serological and histopathological findings.

Investigations

General investigations

Assessment of renal function, urinary protein leak and renal size are mandatory for the investigation of suspected glomerulonephritis.

Serum IgA is raised in 50%, but complement C3 and C4 are normal.

Special investigations

The diagnosis of HSP nephritis requires a renal biopsy.

No accumulation of clinical and laboratory evidence has sufficient specificity and sensitivity to avoid the need for a diagnostic biopsy.

Renal biopsy features

HSP nephritis is defined by the presence of mesangial IgA detected by immunofluorescence or immunoperoxidase.

Renal biopsy features are the same as those for IgAN.

Risk stratification

There is limited information but case series suggest that, as with IgAN hypertension, the degree of proteinuria and impaired renal function at biopsy predict a poorer prognosis.

Treatment

General measures

As with all causes of CKD, patients with HSP and CKD3, 4 and 5 must pay close attention to cardiovascular risk and:

- stop smoking;
- eat a healthy and balanced diet;
- take regular exercise.

Specific treatment

There is very little information to guide treatment of HSP nephritis.

There are no published randomized controlled trials and most studies in IgAN exclude those with HSP so it is unclear whether their conclusions can be extrapolated to HSP.

Transient early nephritis requires no specific treatment.

There is no evidence that corticosteroids or other immunosuppressive regimens alter the natural history of nephrotic syndrome or slowly progressive glomerular damage in HSP.

Crescentic HSP nephritis is more common than crescentic IgAN. Regimens used for renal vasculitis have also been applied to crescentic HSP nephritis with apparent benefit, although there are no controlled trials.

Follow-up

Follow-up should be the same as for patients with IgAN.

Evidence from cohort studies of children with HSP suggests that all women with a history of HSP should be carefully monitored during pregnancy, even if they had no evidence of renal disease at the time of diagnosis.

Prognosis

The long-term outcome of patients with HSP is generally considered to be very good unless they develop HSP nephritis.

The risk of ESRD in children and adults with HSP nephritis is unclear but appears low (<10%).

Future prospects

There is a clear need for randomized controlled trials of immunosuppressive regimens in HSP nephritis in both adults and children.

In all likelihood, however, it will be advances in the understanding of the pathogenesis and treatment of IgAN that will make the most impact on the management of HSP nephritis.

Further reading

Barratt J, Feehally J. IgA nephropathy. *J Am Soc Nephrol* 2005; **16**: 2088–2097.

Barratt J, Feehally J. Treatment of IgA nephropathy. *Kidney Int* 2006; **69**: 1934–1938.

Barratt J, Feehally J. IgA nephropathy. *Semin Nephrol* 2008; **28**: 1–3.

Barratt J, Smith AC, Molyneux KM, Feehally J. Immunopathogenesis of IgA nephropathy. Semin Immunopathol 2007; **29**: 427–443.

Davin JC, Ten Berge IJ, Weening JJ. What is the difference between IgA nephropathy and Henoch–Schönlein purpura nephritis? *Kidney Int* 2001; **59**: 823–834.

Feehally J, Barratt J, Coppo R, Cook T, Roberts I. International IgA nephropathy network clinico-pathological classification of IgA nephropathy. *Contrib Nephrol* 2007; **157**: 13–18.

Floege J Recurrent IgA nephropathy after renal transplantation. *Semin Nephrol* 2004; **24**: 287–291.

Ronkainen J, Nuutinen M, Koskimies O. The adult kidney 24 years after childhood Henoch Schönlein purpura: a retrospective cohort study. *Lancet* 2002; **360**: 666–670.

Sano H, Izumida M, Shimizu H, et al. Risk factors of renal involvement and significant proteinuria in Henoch Schönlein purpura. *Eur J Pediatr* 2002; **161**: 196–201.

Internet resources

The International IgA nephropathy network:

http://www.igan-world.org

IgA nephropathy factsheets for children and adults:

http://www.gosh.nhs.uk/factsheets/families/F060415/index.html

http://www.emrn.org.uk/documents/IgANephropathy.pdf

Henoch–Schönlein purpura factsheet for children and families:

http://www.ich.ucl.ac.uk/factsheets/families/F050244

See also

Proteinuria and/or hematuria, p. 76

Nephrotic syndrome, p. 80

Minimal change disease, p. 86

Membranous nephropathy

Membranous nephropathy (MN) is the commonest cause of nephrotic syndrome in Caucasian adults. Approximately one-quarter of patients have an underlying systemic disease ('secondary MN'). The routine use of immunosuppressive therapies remains controversial.

Definition

MN is a histological diagnosis, usually made in the context of nephrotic range, or persistent nonnephrotic, proteinuria. Fine granular immune deposits of IgG and complement components are present in a diffuse pattern in the subepithelial space, resulting in thickening of the glomerular basement membrane (GBM). The absence of associated hypercellularity or glomerular inflammation confirms the diagnosis.

Epidemiology

The UK incidence is ~11 cases pmp per year.

It is most commonly diagnosed in the 5th–6th decades of life, and is uncommon in children.

Male:female ratio is 2:1.

It is a more common cause of unexplained nephrotic syndrome in Caucasian than Black individuals.

There is little variation in the incidence of idiopathic MN across geographical regions; variations in the incidence of secondary causes in different parts of the world reflect variations in the incidence of the underlying (particularly infectious) causes.

HLA-DR3 confers a three-fold increased risk.

Progressive renal dysfunction is more common in individuals with HLA-DR3 and HLA-DR5.

Etiology

Primary ('idiopathic') MN

Classification of MN as idiopathic indicates, by definition, an unknown etiology.

Primary MN accounts for ~75% of cases in adults, but only 25% of cases in children.

Secondary MN

MN can occur with a wide variety of underlying diseases and treatments. It is most commonly associated with the following.

Malignancy

Malignancy accompanies MN in 7–8% of cases, although the incidence is reported to be as high as 22% in patients aged >60 years.

Tumors of lung, breast and gastrointestinal tract are most common.

MN may precede evidence of malignancy in 40% of patients, and by up to 12–18 months.

Systemic lupus erythematosis (SLE)

MN accounts for ~20% of nephrotic syndrome in patients with SLE.

Anti-DNA and antinuclear antibodies are typically of low titer and low avidity, whereas complement levels are frequently normal.

Infection

Hepatitis B virus (HBV) infection is the most common infectious disease associated with MN.

MN is the most common renal manifestation of HBV infection.

MN typically develops in the chronic carrier state.

HBV accounts for up to 40% of MN cases in endemic regions, and is particularly common in young males.

Hepatitis C virus infection and a number of tropical diseases (including malaria) have been reported in association with MN.

Drugs

Penicillamine, gold and NSAIDs are the agents most commonly associated with MN.

MN usually appears in the first 6–12 months of treatment.

Renal transplantation

MN may recur in the renal transplant, typically in patients whose initial disease demonstrated rapid deterioration to end-stage renal failure (ESRF). Recurrence usually occurs in the first year after transplantation.

De novo MN accounts for 30% of cases of nephrotic syndrome in renal transplant recipients.

Pathogenesis

A number of lines of evidence indicate an autoimmune pathogenesis of idiopathic MN:

- the association with autoimmune diseases such as SLE and diabetes;
- case series in which transplacental transfer of maternal antibodies directed against a podocyte cell membrane antigen (neutral endopeptidase: NEP) caused membranous nephropathy in the fetus;
- the observation of comparable histology in animal models, following induction of synthesis of antibodies directed against the rat podocyte surface antigen megalin by injection of brush border proteins ('Heymann nephritis').

Studies of Heymann nephritis suggest that:

- immune deposits form in situ;
- antipodocyte antibodies induce complement activation, leading to podocyte cell activation and secretion of oxidants, proteases and other molecules that impair the function of the glomerular filtration barrier;
- alterations in podocytes and the composition of the GBM lead to loss of size- and charge-molecular selectivity, and to decreased hydraulic conductance;
- ongoing proteinuria initiates interstitial fibrosis, which further impairs excretory renal function.

Immune complexes in secondary MN are specific to the underlying disease (e.g. HBeAg and HBeAb in HBV infection).

Natural history

Traditionally known as the 'disease of thirds'; epidemiological studies indicate likely outcomes for patients with MN:

- One-third exhibit spontaneous remission of disease, usually in the first 2 years after diagnosis, although remission can occur at any time.
- One-third exhibit chronic persistent proteinuria with preservation of renal function.

- One-third progress slowly to ESRF.

Outcome variability contributes to the different conclusions reached by therapeutic trials and meta-analyses, particularly when small numbers and short follow-up are employed.

Symptoms and signs

There are no specific clinical features of MN.

80% of patients present with nephrotic syndrome; asymptomatic non-nephrotic proteinuria is detected in the remaining 20%.

50% of adult patients have microscopic hematuria at presentation.

Additional clinical features of underlying associated diseases (see 'Secondary MN'), or complications of MN (see 'Special investigations'), should be sought.

Differential diagnosis

Prior to renal biopsy, the differential diagnoses are the causes of unexplained nephrotic syndrome, including:
- minimal change disease;
- FSGS;
- mesangiocapillary glomerulonephritis (types I and II);
- amyloidosis;
- light chain deposition disease.

Following renal biopsy, the differential diagnosis lies between idiopathic and secondary MN.

General investigations

Assessment of renal function, blood pressure, urinary protein excretion and serum albumin, urinalysis and renal size are mandatory for the investigation of suspected glomerulonephritis.

Special investigations

The diagnosis of MN requires a renal biopsy.

A number of additional investigations directed at the most frequent underlying causes of secondary MN should include:
- anti-dsDNA and antinuclear antibodies;
- complement levels;
- hepatitis B serology;
- fasting glucose;
- thyroid function tests;
- CXR.

For patients aged >50 years, recommended investigations for malignancy include:
- CXR.
- mammography (in women).
- stool for fecal occult blood.
- colonoscopy.
- measurement of tumor markers, such as prostate-specific antigen (PSA).

For patients with acutely deteriorating renal function and an active urinary sediment, anti-GBM antibodies should be sought. Development of these antibodies is a rare but well-recognized complication of MN.

For patients with suspected thromboembolic events, including those with flank pain and hematuria, renal venography should be considered to look for renal vein thrombosis.

For patients with nephrotic syndrome in the presence of solid-organ malignancy:
- MN is the histological diagnosis in 60–80% of cases;
- the need for renal biopsy under these circumstances should be carefully balanced against tumor prognosis, and the possibility of alternative glomerular diagnosis (more common in hematological malignancies).

Renal biopsy findings

IgG-positive deposits limited to the subepithelial space are characteristic of MN. Fig. 3.6.1 shows the characteristic histological appearances of MN.

Light microscopy

This can be normal in early disease.

Later changes are characterised by:
- glomerular capillary wall thickening;
- GBM projections evident on silver-methanamine staining ('silver spikes');
- absence of glomerular hypertrophy.

Mesangial hypercellularity may indicate underlying SLE.

Renal function is best predicted by the magnitude of interstitial (rather than glomerular) changes. These are:
- diffuse infiltrate (mononuclear cells);
- tubular atrophy;
- interstitial fibrosis.

Immunohistology

Immune deposits consist of IgG (predominantly IgG4) and complement components (C3 and the C5b-9 'membrane attack complex').

Fine, granular, diffuse staining is present in all capillary loops.

Positive staining for IgA or IgM, or staining in mesangial areas, suggests underlying SLE.

Electron microscopy

Electron-dense deposits (responsible for IgG-positive staining) are observed in the subepithelial space.

Foot process effacement overlies the deposits.

GBM projects between electron-dense deposits (responsible for silver spikes).

GBM becomes thickened and engulfs the electron-dense deposits.

Staging

Electron microscopy findings are used to categorize MN into four stages:
- stage I: subepithelial deposits with podocyte foot process effacement and normal GBM thickness;
- stage II: GBM projection between deposits;
- stage III: new GBM surrounds deposits;
- stage IV: highly thickened GBM, with loss of clear 'spike' pattern of GBM projections and with increasing deposit lucency.

These biopsy stages do not correlate with clinical disease severity, treatment response, or outcome.

Important histological variants

Focal sclerosis

This finding predicts rapid progression to ESRF.

Glomerular crescents

The presence of anti-GBM antibodies is associated with the development of crescentic glomerulonephritis on a background of MN.

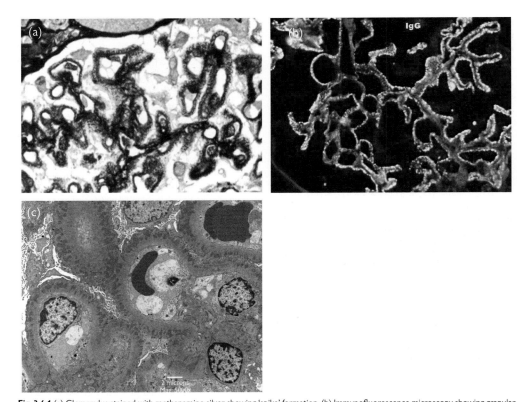

Fig. 3.6.1 (a) Glomerulus stained with methanamine silver showing 'spike' formation. (b) Immunofluorescence microscopy showing granular deposition of IgG around capillary loops. (c) Electron micrograph showing numerous subepithelial electron-dense deposits and foot process effacement. (Courtesy of Dr Nick Mayer, Consultant Histopathologist, University Hospitals of Leicester, UK.)

Atypical deposits

IgA- or C1q-positive immunofluorescence, mesangial cell proliferation and mesangial or subendothelial deposits indicate an increased likelihood of underlying malignancy.

Panimmunoreactivity

Positive immunofluorescence for IgM and/or IgA, alongside IgG, particularly in mesangial areas, indicates underlying SLE.

Risk stratification

Older age and male gender adversely affects prognosis.

Persistent proteinuria (>8 g/day for >6 months, >6 g/day for >9 months, or >4 g/day for >1 year) has a high (>65%) positive predictive value for progression to ESRF.

Impaired renal function is a useful index (positive predictive value >60%) of progression to ESRF.

The rate of change of creatinine clearance over time is a better index of disease severity than creatinine at presentation.

Published algorithms augment the specificity and positive predictive value of prognostically important clinical factors.

The use of published methods of risk stratification is variable, both in practice and in therapeutic trials.

Patient advice

General

As with all causes of chronic kidney disease, patients with MN and CKD 3, 4 and 5 must pay close attention to cardiovascular risk and:

- stop smoking;
- eat a healthy and balanced diet;
- take regular exercise.

Pregnancy

ACEIs or A2R blockers should be avoided in women considering pregnancy

When pregnant, patients should be monitored in a renal–obstetric clinic.

90% of pregnancies in patients with MN result in live births. Repeated pregnancies do not alter the outcome of MN.

Pharmacological treatment

Nonspecific measures

Blood pressure: treat to National Guidelines.

- Dietary sodium restriction.
- Diuretics.
- Renin–angiotensin system blockade.

Secondary hyperlipidemia
- Dietary measures.
- HMG CoA reductase inhibitors (aim LDL-cholesterol <3 mmol/L, total cholesterol <5 mmol/L, or a 30% reduction from baseline for either parameter; extrapolated from national targets).

Anticoagulation
- Decision analysis models predict benefit from prophylactic warfarin therapy. Recommendations are for treatment in severe nephrotic states (serum albumin <20 g/l).

Decrease urinary protein excretion
- Renin–angiotensin system blockade with ACEIs or A2R blockers should be titrated to a maximal dose (alone or in combination) as long as there are no adverse effects on systemic BP, GFR or serum potassium.

In individuals with well-maintained serum albumin the above measures may be all that is required. For those who are overtly nephrotic corticosteroids alone are often sufficient to induce clinical remission, although the use and enthusiasm for such treatment varies between centers and countries.

Disease-specific measures
Routine use of cytotoxic therapies is still controversial and these are often reserved for those at the highest risk of progression to ESRF (usually those with severe and/or resistant nephrosis and those with deteriorating renal function). There is often considerable delay between the start of therapy and a reduction in urinary protein excretion. Several treatment regimens have been described:

Corticosteroids plus chlorambucil
Methylprednisolone 1 g IV for 3 days, then 0.5 mg/kg prednisolone orally for 1 month, alternating with 1 month of chlorambucil 0.1–0.2 mg/kg/day for 6 months.

Outcome: Decreased proteinuria, slower rate of decline of renal function, and decreased progression to ESRF.

Corticosteroids + cyclophosphamide
Methylprednisolone 1 g IV for 3 days, then 0.5 mg/kg prednisolone orally for 1 month, alternating with 1 month of cyclophosphamide 2.5 mg/kg/day for a total of 6 months.

Comparable efficacy to the corticosteroid + chlorambucil regimen, with a better adverse effect profile.

Ciclosporin
3.5–5 mg/kg/day

Higher rates of complete or partial remission of nephrotic syndrome, and short-term preservation of renal function, when compared with placebo.

Short (<12–24 month) courses are associated with a higher relapse rate.

Alternative third-line strategies
Some preliminary evidence supports the consideration of mycophenolate mofetil, IV immunoglobulin, pentoxyfylline, rituximab, and eculizumab.

Further clinical trials are necessary to evaluate the utility of these agents.

Underlying disease
Malignancy
Primary treatment should be directed at the underlying malignancy.

The use of immunosuppression should be balanced against the risk of worsening the malignant disease.

Systemic lupus erythematosis
Evidence-based recommendations for therapy specific to SLE-related MN are lacking.

The natural history and therapeutic approaches are similar to idiopathic MN.

HBV
In the minority of children in whom MN does not spontaneously remit, interferon-α therapy is effective and well-tolerated.

Successful therapy with interferon-α and lamivudine has been reported in adult patients with HBV-associated MN.

Drugs
Withdraw any drug therapy considered to be causative.

De novo MN in renal allografts
No formal evidence supports changes to immunosuppressive therapy although, if accompanied by deteriorating graft function, use of calcineurin inhibitors can be minimized.

Prognosis and follow-up
Idiopathic MN
Patients with partial remissions or normal renal function after 3 years have an excellent prognosis.

Of the one-third of patients who progress to ESRF, the proportion who are dead or dialysis dependent is 30% at 5 years, 70% at 10 years and 80% at 15 years.

Secondary MN
Malignancy
Nephrotic syndrome frequently, though not invariably, resolves with treatment of the malignant disease given time (6–18 months).

Tumor prognosis determines outcome, but is often poor (75% mortality 3 months after the diagnosis of malignancy).

Systemic lupus erythematosis
Monitoring for transformation into the more aggressive forms of lupus nephritis (e.g. proliferative nephritis) is important.

HBV
The course is more benign than idiopathic MN.

Most children exhibit spontaneous remission within 5 years.

50–75% of patients treated with anti-HBV therapy experience sustained remission.

Drugs
Drug discontinuation leads to resolution of nephrotic syndrome within 12–36 months.

Progressive renal failure is very uncommon in this setting.

Renal transplantation
De novo MN in renal transplant recipients does not adversely affect graft survival and is not considered a contraindication to retransplantation.

Further reading
Burstein DM, Korbet SM, Schwartz MM. Membranous glomerulonephritis and malignancy. *Am J Kidney Dis* 1993; 22: 5–10.

Cattran DC. Mycophenolate mofetil and cyclosporine therapy in membranous nephropathy. *Semin Nephrol* 2003; **23**: 272–277.

Cattran DC, Pei Y, Greenwood CM, Ponticelli C, Passerini P, Honkanen E. Validation of a predictive model of idiopathic membranous nephropathy: its clinical and research implications. *Kidney Int* 1997; **51**: 901–907.

Cattran DC, Appel GB, Hebert LA, *et al.* Cyclosporine in patients with steroid-resistant membranous nephropathy: a randomized trial. *Kidney Int* 2001; **59**: 1484–1490.

Glassock RJ. Diagnosis and natural course of membranous nephropathy. *Semin Nephrol* 2003; **23**: 324–332.

Haas M, Meehan SM, Karrison TG, Spargo BH. Changing etiologies of unexplained adult nephrotic syndrome: a comparison of renal biopsy findings from 1976–1979 and 1995–1997. *Am J Kidney Dis* 1997; **30**: 621–631.

Hariharan S, Peddi VR, Savin VJ, *et al.* Recurrent and de novo renal diseases after renal transplantation: a report from the renal allograft disease registry. *Am J Kidney Dis* 1998; **31**: 928–931.

Jefferson JA, Couser WG. Therapy of membranous nephropathy associated with malignancy and secondary causes. *Semin Nephrol* 2003; **23**: 400–405.

Malik GH, Al-Harbi AS, Al-Mohaya S, *et al.* Repeated pregnancies in patients with primary membranous glomerulonephritis. *Nephron* 2002; **91**: 21–24.

Ponticelli C, Zucchelli P, Passerini P, *et al.* A 10-year follow-up of a randomized study with methylprednisolone and chlorambucil in membranous nephropathy. *Kidney Int* 1995; **48**: 1600–1604.

Ponticelli C, Altieri P, Scolari F, *et al.* A randomized study comparing methylprednisolone plus chlorambucil versus methylprednisolone plus cyclophosphamide in idiopathic membranous nephropathy. *J Am Soc Nephrol* 1998; **9**: 444–450.

Reichert LJ, Koene RA, Wetzels JF. Prognostic factors in idiopathic membranous nephropathy. *Am J Kidney Dis* 1998; **31**: 1–11.

Internet resources

MGN Support Group:

http://www.mgninfo.co.uk/

National Kidney Foundation:

http://www.kidney.org.uk/

See also

Nephrotic syndrome, p. 80

Renal biopsy, p. 32

Systemic lupus erythematosis, p. 180

Malignancy-associated glomerular disease, p. 134

Mesangiocapillary glomerulonephritis

Mesangiocapillary, or membranoproliferative, glomerulonephritis (MCGN) is an uncommon cause of glomerulonephritis.

MCGN is typically related to complement-mediated glomerular damage, either through immune complex (or cryoglobulin) deposition and complement activation *in situ*, or through chronic activation of complement pathways.

Idiopathic disease is most common in children, whereas hepatitis C virus (HCV)-related disease is most common in adults.

There is no clear consensus about the optimal treatment of MCGN.

Definition

MCGN is a histological diagnosis, characterized by profuse glomerular hypercellularity (proliferation of mesangial cells and matrix), thickening of capillary walls with dense deposits, and splitting of the basement membrane ('double contouring') due to mesangial interposition.

It is classified into types I, II and III, primarily according to the distribution and morphology of electron-dense deposits on electron microscopy.

Epidemiology

The European incidence is ~0.9 cases pmp per year, where it accounts for ~10% of cases of nephrotic syndrome.

MCGN is more common in South America, Asia and Africa, where it accounts for 30–40% of cases of nephrotic syndrome, predominantly because of associations with chronic infection.

Peaks of incidence are between the ages of 6 and 30 years (commonly associated with nephritic factors) and in older adults (commonly associated with HCV).

MCGN type I is more common in females than in males; MCGN type II occurs with approximately equal frequency in males and females.

It is more common in Caucasian than in Black individuals.

Familial forms of all three types of MCGN are reported, albeit infrequently.

Etiology

Etiology of MCGN varies according to the histological subtype.

MCGN type I is associated with:

Mixed cryoglobulinemia (type II or III).

Viral infection (particularly HCV, but also hepatitis B virus (HBV) and HIV).

Bacterial infection (particularly bacterial endocarditis and abscesses).

Parasitic infection (Malaria (*Plasmodium malariae*) and schistosomiasis).

Complement deficiency (hereditary or acquired).

Systemic lupus erythematosis (SLE) and Sjögren's syndrome.

Sickle cell disease.

Chronic liver disease (cirrhosis and α1-antitrypsin deficiency).

Malignancy (chronic lymphocytic leukemia, lymphoma).

MCGN type II is associated with:

The presence of C3 nephritic factor (often in association with partial lipodystrophy).

Impaired factor H function (deficiency, defect or autoantibodies).

MCGN type III

Two lines of evidence support the hypothesis that MCGN types I and III are different histological phenotypes of the same disease.
- Reports of MCGN types I and III in siblings.
- Similar etiological agents are associated with both MCGN types I and III.

Pathogenesis

MCGN types I and III

A number of steps contribute to the pathogenesis of MCGN type I.

The persistence of either:
- circulating immune complexes, either through continued formation (e.g. chronic infection) or impaired elimination (hepatic and splenic disease); or
- cryoglobulins.

Glomerular deposition of immune complexes (or cryoglobulins).

Complement activation, via the classical pathway, within the glomerular capillary wall (with the involvement of the 'nephritic factor of the terminal pathway' (NFt) in some cases of MCGN type III).

Leukocyte recruitment.

Subsequent capillary wall damage, mediated by growth factors, cytokines and proteases.

MCGN type II

This results from persistent activation of the alternative pathway of complement at the level of C3. This usually occurs because of:
- the presence of an autoantibody (C3 nephritic factor: (C3Nef)) that binds to and activates the alternative pathway C3 convertase (C3bBb).

Less commonly it occurs because of:
- impaired function of an inhibitor of the alternative pathway (factor H).

MCGN type II may occur in association with partial lipodystrophy, because adipocytes display surface expression of complement components, the inappropriate activation of which by C3Nef results in adipocyte cell loss.

Natural history

Idiopathic MCGN has a relatively unfavorable prognosis.

Adverse prognostic markers include:
- abnormal renal function.
- nephrotic-range proteinuria.
- hypertension.
- interstitial fibrosis.

MCGN may recur in a renal allograft:
- types II and III 85% risk of recurrence;
- type I 25% risk of recurrence.

Recurrent disease has a negative impact on graft survival.

The addition of cyclophosphamide to standard immunosuppressive therapy may be considered in these circumstances.

Symptoms and signs

There are five major clinical patterns of presentation, which are usually associated with significant hypertension:

- asymptomatic microscopic hematuria and non-nephrotic proteinuria (~20%).
- nephrotic syndrome and minor renal function impairment (~50%).
- acute nephritic syndrome (~15%).
- recurrent macroscopic hematuria (~10%).
- end-stage renal failure (either acute or chronic) (~5%).

MCGN type II, although relatively uncommon, may be associated with:

- absent SC tissue in the face and upper limbs (partial lipodystrophy).
- visual field defects and mottled retinal pigmentation (Drusen bodies).

Cryoglobulin-associated MCGN (usually in adults) may present with:

- arthralgia, weakness and purpuric rash;
- ulcerative skin lesions;
- peripheral neuropathy;
- Raynaud's phenomenon.

Additional clinical features of underlying associated diseases (see 'Etiology') should be sought.

Differential diagnosis

Following renal biopsy, careful consideration should be given to the presence of:

- post-streptococcal glomerulonephritis;
- paraproteinemias;
- thrombotic microangiopathy;
- transplant glomerulopathy (in renal allografts);

particularly because many of these diseases also cause complement consumption.

General investigations

Assessment of renal function, blood pressure, urinary protein excretion and serum albumin, urinalysis and renal size are mandatory for the investigation of suspected glomerulonephritis.

Special investigations

The diagnosis of MCGN requires a renal biopsy.

Once confirmed on renal biopsy, investigations directed towards underlying diseases associated with MCGN should be instituted.

Complement levels/factors help to distinguish between the different types of MCGN.

MCGN type I

- Low C3 in ~50% of patients.
- Low classical pathway components (C2, C4, C1q).
- Low or normal terminal components (C5, C8, C9).
- NFt may be present.

MCGN type II

- Low C3 in ~75% of patients.
- Normal levels of classical pathway (C2, C4, C1q) and terminal (C5, C8, C9) components.

- C3NeF present in ~75% of patients.

MCGN type III

- As for MCGN type I, except that classical pathway components (C4, C1q) are usually normal

Serological markers provide no information about disease severity or activity.

Renal biopsy findings

Light microscopy

Glomeruli are hypercellular and enlarged, due to:

- mesangial cell proliferation and matrix expansion;
- leukocyte (neutrophil and monocyte) infiltration.

Glomerular hypertrophy is absent.

Glomerular capillary walls are thickened, due to expansion of mesangial cells and/or matrix into the capillary wall. This gives rise to the 'double contour' appearance of the glomerular capillary wall that is best appreciated with silver-methanamine staining.

In MCGN type II, basement membranes in many locations (e.g. Bowman's capsule, tubules, peritubular capillaries) are thickened.

Crescents are present in <10% of biopsies.

Impaired renal function is accompanied by interstitial inflammation, tubular atrophy, and interstitial fibrosis.

MCGN type II is considered by some to be a different disease from MCGN types I and III, and the diseases are classified together merely because of similar histological appearances on light microscopy.

Immunohistology

The classic pattern is granular C3 positivity in the capillary wall and mesangial areas. This may be accompanied by:

- other early complement components (e.g. C1q), IgG and occasionally IgM in MCGN type I;
- little or no immunoglobulin positivity in MCGN type II;
- C5, properdin, IgG and IgM detected in the capillary walls in MCGN type III.

Electron microscopy

Different appearances on electron microscopy define the different types of MCGN.

MCGN type I is characterized by the presence of subendothelial electron-dense deposits. These are occasionally accompanied by mesangial and subepithelial deposits.

MCGN type II is characterized by the deposition of amorphous electron-dense deposits (hence the alternative name of this disease: 'dense deposit disease') in the lamina densa of the GBM, leading to basement membrane thickening.

MCGN type III is characterized by dense deposits in:

- subendothelial regions;
- mesangial areas;
- subepithelial regions.

These deposits result in a laminated appearance of the basement membrane in MCGN type III.

Risk stratification

Adverse prognostic clinical features include:

- older age;
- renal impairment;
- nephrotic syndrome;
- hypertension at presentation.

Adverse prognostic histological features include:
- interstitial fibrosis;
- tubular atrophy;
- glomerular crescents;
- a high proportion of sclerotic glomeruli.

Patient advice

General

As with all causes of chronic kidney disease patients with MCGN and CKD 3, 4 and 5 must pay close attention to cardiovascular risk and:
- stop smoking;
- eat a healthy and balanced diet;
- take regular exercise.

Pregnancy

Patients with high risk clinical profiles (particularly those receiving ACE inhibitors or A2R blockers) should be offered preconception counselling and, when pregnant, undergo careful monitoring in a combined renal–obstetric clinic.

Adverse fetal outcome is more likely in offspring of women with MCGN type I as compared with those with MCGN type II.

Patients with MCGN are more likely to experience deteriorating renal function, proteinuria and hypertension during pregnancy, as compared with many other glomerular diseases.

Pharmacological treatment

Nonspecific measures

Blood pressure: treat to National Guidelines.
- Dietary sodium restriction.
- Renin–angiotensin system blockade.
- Diuretics.
- Additional agents where necessary.

Secondary hyperlipidemia:
- Dietary measures.
- HMG CoA reductase inhibitors (aim LDL-cholesterol <3 mmol/l, total cholesterol <5 mmol/l, or a 30% reduction from baseline for either parameter; extrapolated from current national targets).
- Reduce urinary protein excretion.

Decrease urinary protein excretion:

Renin–angiotensin system blockade with ACEIs or A2R blockers should be titrated to a maximal dose (alone or in combination) as long as there are no adverse effects on systemic BP, GFR or serum potassium.

Anticoagulation:

Preliminary reports document improvements in renal function and proteinuria with the combined use of anticoagulation and antiplatelet therapy in MCGN.

Renal vein thrombosis is reported in patients with nephrotic syndrome due to MCGN. Anticoagulation should be considered, as in other glomerulonephritides, in severe nephrotic states (serum albumin <20 g/L).

Disease-specific measures

MCGN type I

Disease-modifying treatment is recommended for those with nephrotic-range proteinuria or deteriorating renal function.

Benefit has been demonstrated for:
- children with idiopathic MCGN type I treated with corticosteroids;
- adults treated with antiplatelet agents (small studies also demonstrate benefit in children).

Evidence is lacking for the use of steroids in adults.

Corticosteroids (in children)

Alternate-day prednisolone (40 mg/m^2) (for ≥3–6 months and for up to 10 years), when compared with control, has been shown to improve:
- creatinine clearance;
- renal survival;
- biopsy findings.

Antiplatelet agents

Aspirin (375–925 mg/day) + dipyridamole (150–300 mg/day) improves:
- renal survival at 5 (but not 10) years (when administered for 1 year);
- proteinuria.

Purported mechanisms include altered glomerular hemodynamics, decreased mesangial proliferation and antiplatelet effects.

Alkylating agents

In patients with rapidly deteriorating renal function and crescentic disease on biopsy, methylprednisolone followed by oral prednisolone and cyclophosphamide should be considered.

Alternative strategies

Preliminary evidence supports the use of mycophenolate mofetil, particularly in steroid-resistant cases. Ciclosporin in combination with prednisolone may also be of benefit.

Further randomized controlled trials are necessary to evaluate the utility of mycophenolate mofetil and ciclosporin.

MCGN type II

Steroids and calcineurin inhibitors are ineffective.

Plasma exchange has been effective when disease is due to inactivating mutations of factor H, but less effective when the cause is C3Nef.

The utility of mycophenolate mofetil is not yet established.

Rituximab has been suggested for use in patients with C3Nef, but again its role needs to be more clearly defined.

Underlying disease

HCV

Interferon-α has been shown to improve renal function, cryoglobulin levels, and HCV RNA load.

Relapse commonly occurs on drug withdrawal, although this is usually reversible with reinstitution of therapy.

Promising anecdotes report successful therapy with interferon-α and ribavarin in combination, although ribavarin is contraindicated once creatinine clearance is <50 mL/min.

Aggressive therapy with:
- steroids + cyclophosphamide;
- plasmapheresis;
- rituximab.

has been reported in severe cases.

SLE and rheumatological diseases
Standard treatment of the underlying disease should be instituted.

HBV
Spontaneous remission is common, and therefore immunosuppression is rarely required.

Prognosis and follow-up

MCGN type I
Prognosis is heavily dependent on the presence or absence of nephrotic syndrome at presentation.

Nephrotic syndrome
• 50% ESRF at 10 years;
• 90% ESRF at 20 years.

Absence of nephrotic syndrome
• 15% ESRF at 10 years.

MCGN type II
Prognosis is less favorable than MCGN type I (median renal survival 5–10 years).

MCGN type III
There is no concordance in the literature about the outcome of MCGN type III.

Recurrent disease post-transplantation
Recurrence is both common (20–30%) and likely to lead to graft failure (≤40%) in MCGN type I.

Recurrence occurs in 50–100% of cases of MCGN type II, although recurrences tend to be mild and <20% of grafts are lost as a result.

Recurrent MCGN must be differentiated from transplant glomerulopathy, which has similar appearances on light microscopy, but without the presence of immune deposits.

References

Appel GB, Cook HT, Hageman G, *et al.* Membranoproliferative glomerulonephritis type II (dense deposit disease): an update. *J Am Soc Nephrol* 2005; **16**: 1392–1403.

D'Amico G, Ferrario F. Mesangiocapillary glomerulonephritis. *J Am Soc Nephrol* 1992; **2**(10 Suppl): S159–166.

Hariharan S, Adams MB, Brennan DC, *et al.* Recurrent and de novo glomerular disease after renal transplantation: a report from Renal Allograft Disease Registry (RADR). *Transplantation* 1999; **68**: 635–641.

Miller G, Zimmerman R, Radhakrishnan J, Appel G. Use of mycophenolate mofetil in resistant membranous nephropathy. *Am J Kidney Dis* 2000; **36**: 250–256.

Zimmerman SW, Moorthy AV, Dreher WH, Friedman A, Varanasi U. Prospective trial of warfarin and dipyridamole in patients with membranoproliferative glomerulonephritis. *Am J Med* 1983; **75**: 920–927.

Internet resources
The British Kidney Patient Association:
`http://www.britishkidney-pa.co.uk/`
National Kidney Federation:
`http://www.kidney.org.uk/`
National Kidney Foundation:
`http://www.kidney.org/`

See also
Immunological investigation of renal disease, p. 36
Mixed cryoglobulinemia and hepatitis C infection, p. 176
Systemic lupus erythematosis, p. 180

Acute endocapillary glomerulonephritis

Acute endocapillary glomerulonephritis (AEGN) is the most common form of glomerular lesion worldwide and results from an infection-stimulated immunological response that initiates inflammation and cellular proliferation within the glomerulus.

When appropriate clinical support is available the prognosis is generally good, especially in children.

The primary treatment is directed at eradicating the underlying infection.

Definition

AEGN is a histological diagnosis, usually made in the context of the 'nephritic' syndrome.

Characteristically light microscopy reveals neutrophil infiltration and immunohistochemistry demonstrates immunoglobulin and complement deposition.

Epidemiology

The UK incidence is now very low although many subclinical cases are likely to go unnoticed.

It is most commonly seen in the developing world but the incidence is falling with the slowly improving healthcare infrastructure and socioeconomic conditions.

The male:female ratio is 2:1.

Most cases occur in infancy, childhood and adolescence. Only 5–10% of cases occur in patients aged >40 years.

Seasonal variations have been reported but these often differ between geographic regions.

Etiology

Glomerular lesions in AEGN are believed to result from glomerular antigen deposition and in situ formation of immune complexes with subsequent immune-mediated glomerular injury.

The nature of the antigen deposition is speculative except in the case of post-streptococcal glomerulonephritis (PSGN).

Pathogenesis

PSGN

Antigenic moieties derived from streptococcal proteins are thought to be deposited or 'planted' in glomeruli.

Host antibodies directed against the infecting organism result in in situ immune complex formation.

The immune complexes (and possibly streptococcal derivatives) activate complement and induce an inflammatory response.

Two prominent serotypes of β-hemolytic streptococci (Lancefield Grp A) have been highlighted as causative agents in PSGN: serotypes 12 and 49, that cause respiratory and skin infections respectively. Other serotypes that have been implicated are: 1, 2, 4 (respiratory), 47, 55, 57 (skin).

Nonstreptococcal infection-associated glomerulonephritis

AEGN has been associated with a wide variety of clinical infections including endocarditis, infected CSF shunts, infected grafts, and tissue abscesses associated with IV drug abuse. A large number of causative organisms have also been reported including:

- *bacteria*: staphylococci (occasionally MRSA), mycobacteria, meningococci, salmonella;
- *viruses*: Hepatitis B virus, Epstein–Barr virus, cytomegalovirus, rubella, mumps;
- *fungi*: candida, coccidioides, histoplasma;
- *parasites*: malaria, schistosomiasis, toxoplasmosis, filiariasis.

Natural history

The outcome of AEGN is generally good with 100% recovery reported in some pediatric series.

Complement levels return to normal within a few months.

Proteinuria and microscopic hematuria generally resolve after 3–4 years.

Even in adults the prognosis is favorable, although cases where recovery is absent or incomplete are well-recognized and this outcome becomes more common with increasing age.

Symptoms and signs

In addition to nonspecific symptoms of weakness, nausea and malaise, individuals usually present with features of the 'nephritic' syndrome and impaired renal function 1–4 weeks after onset of the infection.

Common presenting features:

- Loin pain (thought to be due to capsular stretching).
- Hypertension (sometimes severe).
- Oliguria.
- Hematuria. This is said to be universal, is often associated with red cell casts, and is sometimes macroscopic. The time interval from infection to hematuria contrasts with IgA nephropathy in which macroscopic hematuria appears hours or days post infection.
- Edema (often facial).

Differential diagnosis

The differential diagnoses are the causes of unexplained rapidly declining renal function in the context of an active urinary sediment:

- Renal vasculitis.
- Systemic lupus erythematosis.
- Anti-GBM disease.
- Cryoglobulinemia.
- Henoch–Schönlein purpura.
- Hemolytic uremic syndrome.

General investigations

Assessment of renal function, blood pressure, urinary protein excretion and serum albumin, urinalysis and renal size are mandatory for the investigation of suspected glomerulonephritis.

Special investigations

The diagnosis requires a renal biopsy.

Investigations relating to the underlying infection:

- Infection screen of blood, urine, stool, sputum as appropriate.
- Echocardiography and CXR as appropriate.
- Antistreptolysin antibody titers.

- Other serology may be required to identify other causative organisms.

Investigations directed at excluding the differential diagnoses would include:
- Antinuclear and anti-dsDNA antibodies.
- Complement levels.
- ANCA.
- Anti-GBM antibodies.
- Cryoglobulins.
- Blood film.

Renal biopsy findings
The principal abnormality is glomerular hypercellularity.

Light microscopy
Two aspects contribute to the hypercellularity of the glomeruli:
- Resident glomerular cell (endothelial and mesangial) proliferation.
- Inflammatory cell infiltration (neutrophils initially, monocytes and lymphocytes later. A lymphocytic interstitial infiltrate is also typical).

The glomerular basement membrane is normal.

Crescent formation is described but is rare.

Immunofluorescence
Immune deposits are found in the GBM and mesangium.

The deposits usually contain C3, C5b–C9 and immunoglobulins (typically IgG and IgM).

The pattern and distribution of immunofluorescence staining is said to vary according to the time after onset of disease and with the degree of proteinuria.

Electron microscopy
Subepithelial deposits ('humps') are typical in post-streptococcal glomerular lesions.

Subendothelial and intramembranous electron-dense deposits also occur in post-streptococcal and nonstreptococcal AEGN.

Risk stratification
Older age, male gender, persistent proteinuria (beyond 4 years) and long-term impaired renal function are poor prognostic markers.

The presence of acute renal failure at presentation is not necessarily associated with a poor outcome.

Patient advice
General
Those in whom renal function returns to normal can be reassured, and long-term follow-up is not required. However, in individuals in whom AEGN leads to CKD, in line with the management of other glomerular lesions that may lead to progressive renal impairment, attention should be paid to cardiovascular risk:
- stop smoking;
- eat a healthy and balanced diet;
- exercise regularly.

Pharmacological treatment
Nonspecific measures
For the minority in whom long-term renal impairment develops, the general management should be as in any other GN lesion.

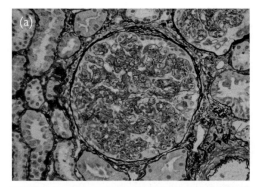

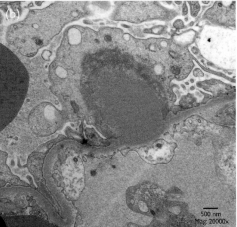

Fig. 3.8.1. (a) Methanamine-silver-stained glomerulus showing diffuse proliferative changes with endocapillary proliferation. (b) Electron micrograph demonstrating a well-demarcated subepithelial electron-dense deposit. (Courtesy of Dr Nick Mayer, Consultant Histopathologist, University Hospitals of Leicester, UK.)

Blood pressure: treat to levels suggested by National Guidelines.
- Dietary sodium restriction.
- Diuretics.
- Renin–angiotensin system blockade.
- Additional antihypertensive agents where necessary.

Secondary hyperlipidemia:
- Dietary measures.
- HMG CoA reductase inhibitors (aim for LDL-cholesterol <3 mmol/L, total cholesterol <5 mmol/L, or a 30% reduction from baseline for either parameter; extrapolated from current national targets).

Decrease urinary protein excretion:
Renin–angiotensin system blockade with ACEI or A2R blockers, titrated to a maximal dose (alone or in combination) as long as adverse effects on systemic blood pressure, GFR or serum potassium concentration (a greater risk if oliguric) are avoided.

Anticoagulation:

This is usually considered if the presentation is primarily with nephrotic syndrome and in those in whom there is significant hypoalbuminemia (<20 g/L) and low bleeding risk.

Supportive measures

Acute kidney injury: supportive renal replacement therapy as required.

Hypertensive encephalopathy is rare but requires aggressive therapy.

Primary infection should be appropriately treated avoiding nephrotoxic antimicrobials whenever possible.

Disease-specific measures

The primary aim is to treat the underlying infective lesion with the notional aim of removing the offending putative antigen.

There is no controlled trial data to suggest that the use of corticosteroids or other anti-inflammatory/ immunosuppressant agents are of any benefit and these are often relatively contraindicated by the underlying infective process.

However, in severe disease in which there is widespread crescent formation on biopsy, corticosteroids are sometimes considered although usually after definitive treatment for the primary infection is well underway.

References

Levy M. Infection-related proteinuric syndromes. In: Cameron JS, Glassock RG (eds), *The nephrotic syndrome*. New York: Dekker; 1988. pp. 745–804.

Moroni G, Pozzi C, Quaglini S, *et al.* Long-term prognosis of diffuse proliferative glomerulonephritis associated with infection in adults. *Nephrol Dial Transplant* 2002; **17**: 1204–1211.

Naicker S, Fabian J, Naidoo S, Wadee S, Paget G, Goetsch S. Infection and glomerulonephritis. *Semin Immunopathol* 2007; **29**: 397–414.

Simon P, Ramée MP, Autuly V, *et al.* Epidemiology of primary glomerular diseases in a French region. Variations according to period and age. *Kidney Int* 1994; **46**: 1192–1198.

Sotsiou F. Postinfectious glomerulonephritis. *Nephrol Dial Transplant* 2001; **16**(Suppl 6) :68–70.

Yoshizawa N. Acute glomerulonephritis. *Intern Med* 2000; **39**: 687–694.

See also

Infection-related glomerulonephritis, p. 128

Glomerular disease in the tropics, p. 138

Crescentic glomerulonephritis

Definitions

A crescent is an area of extracapillary cell accumulation within Bowman's space, associated with severely damaged glomerular tufts (Fig. 3.9.1). It is so-named because of its appearance on renal biopsy.

Crescents consist of:

- proliferating parietal and visceral epithelial cells (podocytes);
- leukocytes: predominantly monocytes, macrophages and lymphocytes;
- fibroblasts;
- fibrin;
- other serum components leaking from the ruptured glomerular tuft.

Crescents may enlarge rapidly and compress the glomerular tuft, preventing effective glomerular blood flow and filtration.

Crescentic glomerulonephritis (CGN) is a pathological definition, which may result from a number of different etiological processes.

Diffuse CGN (DCGN) is defined as crescent formation in >50% of glomeruli in a kidney biopsy.

DCGN is clinically associated with a rapid decline in renal function over weeks to months. This is known as rapidly progressive glomerulonephritis.

The diagnosis of CGN requires a renal biopsy to be performed.

Further assessment by immunohistochemistry, electron microscopy and serological analysis is required to identify the particular underlying condition.

A rapid assessment of the particular form of crescentic GN is essential for appropriate therapy to be instituted in order to avoid permanent renal failure.

CGN may heal by scarring and lead to glomerular sclerosis with permanent glomerular damage and some degree of chronic kidney disease.

Treatment may lead to complete resolution of the crescentic change or healing with scarring.

Based on the histological similarities in all forms of CGN, similar treatment protocols have initially been tried for the different underlying conditions.

More recently these have been refined based on our current understanding of the pathogenesis of individual diagnoses.

Classification

Pathologically, crescentic glomerulonephritis has been classified according to the pattern of IgG and complement deposition in the glomerulus, determined by immunofluorescence or immunoperoxidase staining.

Three patterns have been described:

- linear capillary loop deposition (anti-GBM disease);
- granular capillary and/or mesangial deposition, (associated with immune complex deposition (e.g. SLE or postinfectious GN));
- little or no deposition (pauci-immune) (mostly due to antineutrophil cytoplasm antibody (ANCA)-associated disease);

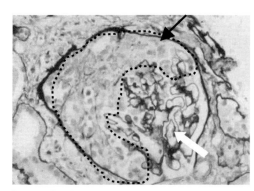

Fig. 3.9.1 The glomerular crescent is outlined by the dotted line and black arrow. The compressed glomerular tuft is shown by the solid white arrow.

Pathogenesis

Crescents form following severe damage to the glomerular tuft by activated leukocytes, resulting in rupture of the GBM or, when periglomerular inflammation occurs, of Bowman's capsule.

This releases cells and soluble mediators into Bowman's space where they stimulate proliferation of epithelial cells, as well as recruitment of further leukocytes from the circulation along chemotactic gradients.

Fibrin may be deposited and fibroblasts may be recruited and activated leading to the production of fibrocellular or fibrous crescents.

Differential diagnosis

Other conditions may present with a rapidly progressive decline in renal function that is not caused by a diffuse crescentic glomerulonephritis. Examples of these are:

- thrombotic microangiopathy (occasional crescents may be seen in association with intraglomerular thrombosis);
- acute tubulointerstitial nephritis;
- myeloma.

These have particular clinical features that may give clues to the cause of the rapid renal failure, but ultimately renal biopsy is required to confirm or exclude DCGN.

Etiology and epidemiology

The particular conditions giving rise to CGN, classified according to the pattern of IgG and complement staining, have been reported from large kidney biopsy series (Figure 3.9.2).

In the UK and USA, the largest proportion were pauci-immune CGN, now known to be mostly associated with ANCA, followed by immune complex-mediated CGN, and anti-GBM disease.

Causes of CGN:

- pauci-immune CGN.
- immune complex CGN including:
  - SLE;
  - cryoglobulinemia;
  - IgA disease;

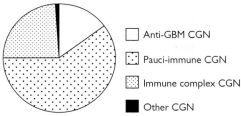

Fig. 3.9.2 Percentage of underlying disease causing CGN from >600 renal biopsies. Adapted from Jennette and Nickeleit (2006).

• Henoch–Schönlein purpura;
• postinfectious glomerulonephritis;
• mesangiocapillary glomerulonephritis;
• nonlupus membranous glomerulopathy;
• fibrillary glomerulonephritis.
• anti-GBM disease-associated CGN.

These proportions vary according to the geographical location and the age of the patients studied (Fig. 3.9.3):

In China, immune complex-mediated CGN predominates (half of these cases are due to SLE), whereas in Eastern Europe postinfectious CGN is most common, possibly due to the presence of certain common local infectious agents.

In children Henoch–Schönlein purpura and mesangiocapillary CGN were most common.

Since ANCA-associated vasculitis is more common in older patients, it is not surprising that pauci-immune CGN is the most frequent cause of CGN in adult patients.

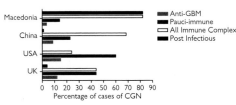

Fig. 3.9.3 Differences in reported percentages of each type of CGN (and the percentage of postinfectious CGN) in adults from various series.

Clinical presentation

Patients may present with loin pain due to nephromegaly and capsule distension, systemic malaise and symptoms relating to their underlying disorder.

They will have deteriorating renal function, an active urinary sediment, with microscopic hematuria, proteinuria, and red cell casts.

With more advanced renal impairment, patients may have uremic symptoms and, in some, symptoms relating to pulmonary hemorrhage may be present.

However, pulmonary hemorrhage may be subclinical, and radiological assessment, pulmonary function tests or bronchoscopy may be required in order to make the diagnosis.

Investigations in CGN

Renal biopsy

• Light microscopy of hematoxylin and eosin-, Periodic acid–Schiff (PAS)-, and methanamine-silver-stained tissue

sections to confirm the presence of CGN, to assess the degree of glomerular involvement, and determine the degree of renal scarring.
• Immunohistochemistry for IgG, IgA, IgM, C3 and C4, and C1q.

Serological investigations

• Anti-GBM antibodies.
• ANCA, antimyeloperoxidase (MPO) antibodies, antiproteinase 3 (PR-3) antibodies.
• Antinuclear antibodies (ANA), Anti-dsDNA antibodies, ENA.
• Complement components C3, C4, CH50.
• Antistreptolysin-O titre (ASOT).
• IgG, IgA and IgM.
• Serum protein electrophoresis or free light chain assay.
• Urine protein electrophoresis for Bence–Jones protein.
• Cryoglobulins.
• C-reactive protein (CRP).

Other investigations

• Blood cultures: for evidence of infection-related immune complex disease.
• FBC and blood film for evidence of thrombotic microangiopathy.
• Biochemistry profile.
• CXR, pulmonary function tests (with KCO), and/or bronchoscopy for evidence of pulmonary involvement (hemorrhage).

General management principles

Treat the underlying condition.

Not all forms of CGN require immunosuppression.

The degree of crescentic change and the rate of decline in renal function will influence the choice of therapeutic options.

In certain severe aggressive forms of CGN early immunosuppressive therapy prevents further renal function decline.

The outcome is mostly dependent on the renal function at presentation, although certain conditions fair better than others with similar degrees of renal dysfunction.

Generally, CGN associated with ANCA or anti-GBM antibodies requires treatment as it is likely to progress, while CGN associated with postinfectious GN is less severe and should resolve spontaneously (or following treatment of the causative infection).

CGN associated with IgA nephropathy has a poor prognosis even with treatment, while CGN associated with SLE responds to treatment of class IV lupus nephritis.

Individual management principles

Pauci-immune CGN

This is generally associated with ANCA.

The autoantigens are PR-3 and MPO, which are constituents of neutrophil granules and monocyte lysosomes.

Three clinical syndromes are recognized:
• Wegener's granulomatosis;
• Microscopic polyangiitis;
• Churg–Strauss syndrome.

(ANCA-associated renal-limited vasculitis causing CGN is considered a form of limited microscopic polyangiitis.)

These three conditions cannot be distinguished histologically, therefore classification is dependent on the associated clinical features.

Treatment protocols are dependent on disease severity.

Patients with mild–moderate renal impairment (<500 μmol/L) require induction treatment with steroids and cyclophosphamide, and maintenance therapy with steroids and azathioprine.

At least 18 months of therapy are required. Longer treatment is required for anti-PR3-associated disease which has a greater tendency for relapse.

More severe renal failure (serum creatinine >500 μmol/L or if dialysis dependent) or the presence of pulmonary hemorrhage requires the above treatment with additional plasmapheresis (shown to be more effective than methylprednisolone pulses).

Plasmapheresis regimen is 60 mL/kg exchange, maximum 4 L, using human albumin solution as replacement (with additional FFP if there is active bleeding or if a renal biopsy has been performed recently).

Prophylaxis against *Pneumocystis jiroveci* (previously known as *Pneumocystis carinii*) pneumonia with cotrimoxazole (or pentamidine or dapsone in those allergic to cotrimoxazole) should be provided while taking cyclophosphamide.

In addition, to prevent the adverse effects of corticosteroids, a proton pump inhibitor, oral nystatin, fluconazole, or amphotericin, and bone protection with calcium/ergocalciferol and bisphosphonates when appropriate should be provided.

Novel treatment strategies with alternative induction agents are currently being trialled.

The outcome is dependent on the severity of renal failure and the presence of alveolar hemorrhage at presentation.

Approximately 50% of patients presenting with dialysis-dependent renal failure will regain independent renal function if treated aggressively.

Relapses are common with a 30–40% relapse rate overall.

Anti-GBM disease

The autoantigen is the noncollagenous domain of the α3 chain of type IV collagen, which is located in glomerular and alveolar basement membranes.

Approximately 60% of patients present with associated pulmonary hemorrhage.

Treatment is with plasmapheresis, and oral cyclophosphamide and steroids for up to 3 and 6 months respectively.

Relapses are rare, unlike ANCA-associated disease.

Treatment should be offered for all patients with renal failure unless they are dialysis dependent with 100% crescents on renal biopsy, when they are unlikely to regain independent renal function.

Immune complex disease

This group encompasses a diverse number of disease processes.

Generally immune complex disease involves less severe crescentic GN than is seen in either anti-GBM antibody or ANCA-associated disease.

Treatment is variable and dependent on the underlying disease.

Severe immune complex-mediated crescentic glomerulonephritis has been treated with immunosuppression using steroids, cyclophosphamide and in some cases plasmapheresis or pulsed steroid therapy, in a way that is analagous to the treatment of anti-GBM disease.

The outcome of crescentic immune complex disease appears to be dependent on the underlying condition.

In crescentic IgA disease, cyclophosphamide and steroids with plasmapheresis have been used, but many series show continued decline to ESRF despite immunotherapy (over 12 months).

Lupus class III/IV nephritis has been successfully treated with steroids and cyclophosphamide (low or high dose) or mycophenolate mofetil (MMF) with equal success, and such regimens would be used in CGN, possibly with the addition of plasmapheresis.

Postinfectious crescentic GN requires immunosuppression only in the face of rapidly declining renal function and DCGN. Pulsed steroids, and combined steroids and cyclophosphamide have been used. Treatment of the underlying infection is a prerequisite.

CGN with membranous GN has been successfully treated with steroids and cyclophosphamide (or chlorambucil) ('Ponticelli regimen'). Small series suggest that MMF or tacrolimus may be as effective although these have not specifically addressed membranous with CGN changes.

In cryoglobulinemic CGN, steroids, cyclophosphamide, plasmapheresis and more recently rituximab have been used. Care needs to be taken with immunosuppression in hepatitis B or C virus-related disease because of the risk of enhancing viral replication.

Further reading

Angangco R, Thiru S, Esnault VL, et al. Does truly 'idiopathic' crescentic glomerulonephritis exist? *Nephrol Dial Transplant* 1994; **9**: 630–636.

Booth AD, Almond MK, Burns A, et al. Outcome of ANCA-associated renal vasculitis: a 5-year retrospective study. *Am J Kidney Dis* 2003; **41**: 776–784.

Dewan D, Gulati S, Sharma RK, et al. Clinical spectrum and outcome of crescentic glomerulonephritis in children in developing countries. *Pediatr Nephrol* 2008; **23**: 389–394.

Grcevska L, Polenakovic M. Crescentic glomerulonephritis as renal cause of acute renal failure. *Renal Fail* 1995; **17**: 595–604.

Jardim HM, Leake J, Risdon RA, et al. Crescentic glomerulonephritis in children. *Pediatr Nephrol* 1992; **6**: 231–235.

Jayne D, Rasmussen N, Andrassy, et al. A randomized trial of maintenance therapy for vasculitis associated with antineutrophil cytoplasmic autoantibodies. *N Engl J Med* 2003; **349**: 36–44.

Jayne DR, Gaskin G, Rasmussen N, et al. Randomized trial of plasma exchange or high-dosage methylprednisolone as adjunctive therapy for severe renal vasculitis. *J Am Soc Nephrol* 2007; **18**: 2180–2188.

Jennette JC. Rapidly progressive crescentic glomerulonephritis. *Kidney Int* 2003; **63**: 1164–1177.

Jennette JC, Nickeleit V. Antiglomerular basement membrane glomerulonephritis and Goodpasture's syndrome. In: Jennette JC, Olso, JL, Schwartz MM, Silva FG (eds), *Pathology of the kidney*. Philadelphia: Lippincott Williams & Wilkins 2006; 613–643.

Tang Z, Wu Y, Wang Q, et al. Clinical spectrum of diffuse crescentic glomerulonephritis in Chinese patients. *Chin Med J (Engl)* 2003; **116**: 1737–1740.

Internet resources

The EUVAS group website with all the details of current and previous trials, classifications, disease assessment tools and other ANCA-related resources: www.vasculitis.org

See also

Antiglomerular basement membrane (Goodpasture's) disease

Antiglomerular basement membrane (anti-GBM) disease, or Goodpasture's disease, is a rare pulmonary–renal syndrome characterized by crescentic glomerulonephritis which generally manifests as rapidly progressive renal failure and, in more than half of patients, concurrent pulmonary hemorrhage.

Epidemiology

Anti-GBM disease has an incidence of ~0.5–1 pmp per year with two age peaks in 20–30- and 60–70-year-olds.

It is marginally more common in men, and occurs almost uniquely in Caucasians.

Men tend to present at a younger age than women (median age 35 years compared with 45 years respectively).

Pulmonary hemorrhage occurs in ~60% of cases and is more common in younger patients.

Etiology

Anti-GBM disease is associated with:
- Exposure to hydrocarbons.
- Smoking (pulmonary hemorrhage).
- Direct renal insults, e.g. lithotripsy.
- Other forms of glomerulonephritis, e.g. membranous nephropathy.

One explanation linking these provoking factors with anti-GBM disease is that they all result in damage to the GBM (or alveolar basement membrane in the case of smoking and other inhaled agents), which exposes cryptic immunological epitopes, which in turn stimulates a novel autoimmune response.

Although originally described during the influenza pandemic, and despite clinical associations between disease activity and infectious episodes, there have been no firm associations with any particular infectious agents.

Pathogenesis

Anti-GBM disease remains one of the few human autoimmune diseases in which the autoantigen has been fully characterized, and this has led to considerable understanding of the immune perturbations that underlie the condition.

Both humoral and cellular arms of the immune response contribute to kidney injury.

Humoral immunity

The deposited and circulating anti-GBM antibodies react with the noncollagenous domain of the α3 chain of type IV collagen, termed the Goodpasture antigen.

This collagen chain is found only in specialized basement membranes in the kidney, lung, choroid plexus, retina and cochlea. The similar collagen composition of alveolar and glomerular basement membranes explains the clinical features of the pulmonary–renal syndrome.

The pathogenicity of the autoantibodies was established following transfer experiments using eluted human autoantibodies transferred into primates, and from the observation of rapid disease recurrence in transplanted kidneys if circulating anti-GBM antibodies were present in the recipient at the time of transplantation.

With the recognition of the pathogenicity of the antibody, plasmapheresis was introduced as a mainstay of treatment.

Subsequent clinical data demonstrated that anti-GBM antibody levels broadly correlate with disease activity, while rapid resolution of disease occurs following antibody depletion.

Cell-mediated immunity

Data from both animal models and patients demonstrate that disease is also critically dependent on autoreactive T-cells.

Crescentic glomerulonephritis, identical to that found in anti-GBM disease, can be induced by immunization of animals with the α3 chain of type IV collagen, even when animals are incapable of producing antibodies. By contrast, anti-GBM antibody transfer into T-cell-deficient mice does not result in disease, demonstrating that α3(IV)collagen-reactive cellular immune effectors are also required.

In patients, T-cells reactive against the Goodpasture antigen can be found at high frequencies in patients with acute disease, and at much lower frequencies following treatment and disease resolution.

Additional evidence for T-cell involvement includes the observations that:
- disease is strongly HLA-associated, with nearly all patients carrying the HLA-DRB1 1501 or 0401 alleles;
- T-cells are found in the affected glomeruli of patients with anti-GBM disease;
- anti-GBM autoantibody is a class-switched IgG implicating the involvement of T-cell help.

Following acute disease, regulatory T-cells (expressing CD4 and CD25), inhibiting α3(IV)collagen-reactive effector T-cells are generated which persist long term; this may explain the rarity of disease relapse.

Disease associations

A proportion of patients are positive for both anti-GBM antibodies and antineutrophil cytoplasm antibodies (ANCA) (generally pANCA with antimyeloperoxidase (MPO) specificity).

These double-positive patients behave more like patients with anti-GBM disease rather than patients with ANCA-associated vasculitis, in that they have a low likelihood of recovering renal function once they are established on dialysis.

Anti-GBM disease is also associated with membranous nephropathy (MN), which may precede or follow the episode of anti-GBM disease.

The diagnosis of MN may be suspected if heavy proteinuria develops in a patient with known anti-GBM disease. Alternatively, if a patient with MN develops a rapid decline in renal function, anti-GBM disease should be suspected.

The diagnosis is confirmed on renal biopsy with electron microscopy demonstrating the characteristic subepithelial deposits of membranous GN.

Clinical features

Patients may present early with macroscopic hematuria, loin pain, or pulmonary hemorrhage, which may be acute or subclinical, or late with rapidly progressive renal impairment and oliguanuria.

Other major systemic symptoms are often lacking, differentiating it to some extent from systemic vasculitis.

Lung hemorrhage occurs in over half the patients and is generally found in smokers. It may result in breathlessness, cough and hemoptysis. In some cases it may be subclinical and only found following investigation, with evidence of iron deficiency anemia, shadowing on chest radiography or an elevated carbon monoxide gas transfer coefficient (KCO).

Bronchoalveolar lavage may demonstrate frank blood or hemosiderin-laden macrophages.

Rarely, anti-GBM-mediated pulmonary hemorrhage may occur in the absence of glomerulonephritis.

Investigations

The diagnosis is suggested by the clinical features but is established on serology and renal biopsy.

Appropriate investigations for a patient presenting with the features of anti-GBM disease include:
- serum urea and electrolytes, creatinine.
- FBC and MCV.
- C-reactive protein.
- anti-GBM antibody.
- ANCA.
- anti-MPO, anti-PR3 antibodies.
- complement C3, C4.
- immunoglobulins, serum protein electrophoresis.
- hepatitis B sAg and HCV Ab, HIV Ab test.
- urinalysis.
- urine microscopy.
- urine protein/creatinine ratio.
- CXR.
- pulmonary function tests with KCO.
- renal biopsy.

Urinalysis demonstrates hematuria and proteinuria, though generally not in the nephrotic range (unless associated with membranous GN – see above).

Urine microscopy may demonstrate red cell casts.

Anti-GBM antibodies are found almost exclusively in patients with disease, and very rarely in healthy individuals, thus they have high specificity and sensitivity for Goodpasture's disease.

False-positive tests may occur in the context of viral infections such as hepatitis C virus or HIV. In such cases, renal biopsy should effectively exclude anti-GBM disease.

Rarely anti-GBM disease may occur in the absence of circulating anti-GBM antibodies (on conventional ELISA) and again these cases require biopsy to confirm the diagnosis.

Renal biopsy

Although positive anti-GBM antibody serology may be sufficient evidence to make the diagnosis and begin treatment, renal biopsy should be performed to confirm the diagnosis, provide an assessment of the extent and severity of glomerular involvement, and assess the severity of any accompanying acute tubular necrosis (ATN).

Anti-GBM disease is characterized by crescentic glomerulonephritis and segmental glomerular fibrinoid necrosis, with the glomeruli containing crescents of similar age (in contrast to ANCA-associated vasculitis in which crescents of different stages of evolution are typically seen ( )) (Figure 3.10.1).

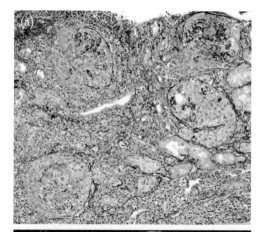

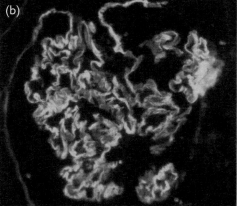

Fig. 3.10.1 (a) Renal biopsy showing crescentic glomerulonephritis with all glomeruli affected with crescents of a similar age. (b) Immunofluorescence microscopy demonstrating linear IgG staining around the capillary loops.

There is often associated ATN.

Immunohistochemistry demonstrates linear deposition of IgG and C3 (Figure 3.10.1), with IgA, IgM and other complement components being deposited less frequently.

Linear basement membrane IgG deposition may occur in other conditions, particularly diabetes, and in older patients with atherosclerosis. However, the associated glomerular pathology and additional immunohistochemical tests should easily permit exclusion of these conditions.

Treatment

Due to the relative rarity of anti-GBM disease, no randomised controlled clinical trials have been performed with regards to immunosuppressive regimens.

Standard therapy

This consists of:
- oral cyclophosphamide (starting at 2–3 mg/kg/day and adjusted for age);
- prednisolone (starting at 1 mg/kg/day with a maximum starting dose of 60 mg/day);

- plasmapheresis (60 mL/kg exchange, maximum 4 L, using human albumin solution as replacement with additional FFP if either there is active bleeding or a renal biopsy has been performed recently). This is continued for at least 14 treatments or until anti-GBM antibodies become undetectable. Anti-GBM antibody levels, platelets and fibrinogen levels need to be closely monitored;
- prophylaxis with cotrimoxazole (or pentamidine or dapsone in those allergic to cotrimoxazole) against *Pneumocystis jiroveci* (previously known as *Pneumocystis carinii*) pneumonia should be provided while on cyclophosphamide;
- additionally, to prevent the adverse effects of corticosteroids, a proton pump inhibitor, oral nystatin or fluconazole, and bone protection with calcium/ergocalciferol and biphosphonates when appropriate should be provided.

The optimal duration of immunosuppressant therapy is unknown; however, 3 months of cyclophosphamide and prednisolone, followed by a further 6 months of prednisolone alone (reducing dose) is a regimen that is widely adopted.

It is not usually necessary to combine prednisolone with alternative, less toxic immunosuppressants once cyclophosphamide is stopped, although azathioprine may be used if patients remain anti-GBM positive after 3 months of cyclophosphamide treatment.

Alternative therapy

Anecdotal case reports of successful treatment with other induction therapies, such as mycophenolate mofetil and rituximab have been published, but direct comparison with standard therapy has not been made.

Less aggressive treatment has been suggested for dialysis-dependent patients without pulmonary hemorrhage, since most series report renal recovery rates of only 0–18% if the presenting serum creatinine is >600 μmol/L.

However, a report on a large series of patients with serum creatinine >500 μmol/L, some of whom required dialysis, suggests that some (with less severe biopsy changes) do recover renal function. Therefore, use of immunosuppression with the treatment regimens described above should be instituted regardless of renal function at presentation, unless patients are dialysis dependent with 100% crescents on renal biopsy.

Who should be immunosuppressed?

Patients with pulmonary hemorrhage.

Patients with rapidly declining renal function.

Patients recently started on dialysis, unless biopsy demonstrates 100% glomerular crescents.

Adjunctive therapeutic strategies

Volume overload should be avoided in patients with alveolar hemorrhage since this can provoke further bleeding.

Severe hemorrhage may require ventilation in the prone position.

Disease relapses are infrequent but are generally found in patients who continue to smoke (therefore advice regarding smoking cessation is critically important) or in those with intercurrent infections (therefore infectious episodes should be treated promptly).

Disease outcome

Survival of patients with anti-GBM disease treated with immunosuppression and plasmapheresis is dependent on their presenting renal function, dialysis requirements and the presence of pulmonary hemorrhage.

Outcome is best in those with less severe renal failure or in those in whom dialysis is not immediately required.

Therefore, at 1 year, independent renal function was achieved in 95% of patients presenting with a creatinine <500 μmol/L, in 82% of those with a creatinine >500 μmol/L but not requiring immediate dialysis, but in only 8% of patients who presented dialysis dependent.

Pulmonary hemorrhage is associated with an increased early mortality.

Renal transplantation

In those patients who develop end-stage renal failure, transplantation is a safe option, with no risk of disease relapse unless circulating anti-GBM antibodies are present at the time of transplantation.

A period of 6 months of disease remission with undetectable anti-GBM antibodies is generally required prior to transplantation.

Standard transplantation immunosuppressive protocols are appropriate.

Alport's syndrome and post-transplantation anti-GBM disease

Patients with classical Alport's disease lack a normal α5 chain of type IV collagen, and cannot therefore synthesize a normal type IV collagen triple helix (consisting of α3, 4 and 5 chains) within their GBM.

Following transplantation with a kidney expressing normal GBM collagen α chains, these are recognized as neoantigens and an immune response directed towards these antigens is stimulated. As a result anti-GBM disease may develop that is indistinguishable on biopsy from classical anti-GBM disease, although the antibodies may be predominantly directed towards the α5 chain, and may thus be undetectable on standard anti-GBM ELISA.

Approximately 5% of transplanted Alport's disease patients will develop anti-GBM disease.

Treatment is with immunosuppression and plasmapheresis as for classical anti-GBM disease, although graft outcome is universally poor.

Further reading

Browne G, Brown PA, Tomson CR, *et al*. Retransplantation in Alport post-transplant anti-GBM disease. *Kidney Int* 2004; **65**: 675–681.

Burns AP, Fisher M, Li P, *et al*. Molecular analysis of HLA class II genes in Goodpasture's disease. *Q J Med* 1995; **88**: 93–100.

Kalluri R, Danoff TM, Okada H, Neilson EG. Susceptibility to anti-glomerular basement membrane disease and Goodpasture syndrome is linked to MHC class II genes and the emergence of T cell-mediated immunity in mice. *J Clin Invest* 1997; **100**: 2263–2275.

Levy JB, Turner AN, Rees AJ, Pusey CD. Long-term outcome of anti-glomerular basement membrane antibody disease treated with plasma exchange and immunosuppression. *Ann Intern Med* 2001; **134**: 1033–1042.

Levy JB, Hammad T, Coulthart A, Dougan T, Pusey CD. Clinical features and outcome of patients with both ANCA and anti-GBM antibodies. *Kidney Int* 2004; **66**: 1535–1540.

Rees AJ, Lockwood CM, Peters DK. Enhanced allergic tissue injury in Goodpasture's syndrome by intercurrent bacterial infection. *Br Med J* 1977; **2**: 723–726.

Salama AD, Chaudhry AN, Ryan JJ, *et al*. In Goodpasture's disease, CD4(+) T cells escape thymic deletion and are reactive with the autoantigen alpha3(IV)NC1. *J Am Soc Nephrol* 2001; **12**: 1908–1915.

Salama AD, Dougan T, Levy JB, *et al*. Goodpasture's disease in the absence of circulating anti-glomerular basement membrane antibodies as detected by standard techniques. *Am J Kidney Dis* 2002; **39**: 1162–1167.

Salama AD, Chaudhry AN, Holthaus KA, *et al*. Regulation by CD25+ lymphocytes of autoantigen-specific T-cell responses in Goodpasture's (anti-GBM) disease. *Kidney Int* 2003; **64**: 1685–1694.

Turner N, Mason PJ, Brown R, *et al*. Molecular cloning of the human Goodpasture antigen demonstrates it to be the alpha 3 chain of type IV collagen. *J Clin Invest* 1992; **89**: 592–601.

See also

Membranous nephropathy, p. 106

Crescentic glomerulonephritis, p. 120

Systemic vasculitis, p. 168

Alport's syndrome, p. 606

Infection-related glomerulonephritis

Glomerulonephritis (GN) may occur in association with a variety of infections caused by bacterial, viral, fungal and other pathogens.

Bacterial infections

Post-streptococcal GN (PSGN)

Epidemiology

Globally ~0.5 million cases of PSGN occur annually.

The incidence is decreasing in developing countries.

Sporadic cases occur worldwide.

The peak incidence is between 2 and 14 years of age.

Male: female 2:1.

Etiology/pathogenesis

PSGN is caused by nephritogenic strains of group A *Streptococcus pyogenes* (particularly strains 47, 49, 55 and 57 following skin infection and 1, 2, 4 and 12 following throat infection).

GN is immune-mediated but the precise nature of the antigen–antibody interaction is unclear. Planting of streptococcal antigen in glomeruli is thought to be an early event.

Deposition of immune complexes in the glomerulus results in activation of the complement cascade (predominantly the alternative pathway).

Clinical features

>90% of patients present with an acute nephritic syndrome (edema, hypertension, hematuria, proteinuria and impaired renal function).

Rapidly progressive glomerulonephritis (RPGN) is uncommon, but if present suggests extensive glomerular crescent formation.

Although most patients have a history of previous skin or throat infection, the infection may have resolved by the time the renal disease becomes apparent.

Diagnosis

Reduced CH_{50} and C3, with normal C4 reflect alternate complement pathway activation.

A renal biopsy is not always required.

If a biopsy is performed the pathological appearances are:

- diffuse, proliferative, endocapillary GN, with the inflammatory cell infiltrate comprising mainly neutrophils. Crescents may be present.
- C3, IgG and IgM deposition in the mesangium and/or around capillary walls.
- subepithelial electron-dense deposits ('humps') are seen on electron microscopy.

Treatment

In the absence of renal failure, treatment is mainly supportive with antihypertensive agents and diuretics.

Temporary dialysis may rarely be required.

If the renal failure is severe and prolonged (>2 weeks duration) and the renal biopsy shows extensive crescent formation, steroid therapy may be useful.

Prognosis

In children, the prognosis is excellent with >95% of patients recovering renal function within 3–4 weeks. No long-term sequelae are usually observed even when renal failure is severe enough to need dialysis.

In adults, up to 25% have been reported to be left with some degree of CKD.

Endocarditis-associated GN

Epidemiology

GN may occur in 20% of cases of bacterial endocarditis (acute and subacute).

Etiology/pathogenesis

The causative organisms are typically *Streptococcus viridans* (subacute) or *Staphylococcus aureus* (acute).

Deposition of immune complexes containing bacterial antigen (similar to PSGN) has been identified.

Type III cryoglobulins can be found in up to 50% of patients.

Clinical features

Fever, arthralgia, anemia, leukocytosis, raised ESR and purpura are typical.

Other characteristic findings of endocarditis such as Osler's nodes, Janeway lesions and splinter hemorrhages may occasionally be seen, but are often absent.

Typical renal manifestations are microscopic hematuria, and non-nephrotic proteinuria with or without renal failure. Crescentic GN may occur and may result in acute kidney injury.

Diagnosis

Reduced C3 and C4 reflect classical complement pathway activation.

High titers of rheumatoid factor, circulating immune complexes and type III cryoglobulins are commonly found.

cANCA (without myeloperoxidase (MPO) or proteinase-3 (PR3) specificity) may occasionally be identified.

Renal biopsy findings include:

- subacute disease – predominantly focal, segmental proliferative GN with more diffuse immune complex deposition on immunohistochemistry;
- acute disease – acute, diffuse, exudative, proliferative GN. Crescents can be observed in 50% of such cases.

Treatment

Treatment should be focused on eradication of the endocarditis with 4–6 weeks of appropriate antibiotics.

In crescentic GN, pulse steroid therapy has been used in addition to antibiotic but carries risk of exacerbating the underlying infection.

Prognosis

Mortality in patients with bacterial endocarditis is ~20% and increases to 36% in patients who have renal failure.

Shunt nephritis

Epidemiology

Approximately 30% of atrioventricular (AV) shunts become infected, and of those, 0.7–2% are associated with GN.

Ventriculoperitoneal (VP) shunts are rarely complicated by GN.

Etiology/pathogenesis

Causative organisms include *Staphylococcus epidemidis*, *S. aureus*, *Propionibacterium acne*, diphteroids, *Pseudomonas* and *Serratia* spp.

GN results from chronic low-level bacteremia, antibody production and immune complex formation. Deposition of bacterial immune complexes in the glomeruli is associated with activation of both the classical and alternative complement pathways.

Clinical features

Common features are low-grade fever, arthralgia, weight loss, anemia, skin rash, hepatosplenomegaly, hypertension and signs of raised intracranial pressure.

Renal manifestations are microscopic hematuria and proteinuria which may be heavy (25% of cases have nephrotic syndrome).

Diagnosis

Reduced C3, C4 and CH_{50}.

Rheumatoid factors and mixed cryoglobulins may be detected in some patients.

Blood cultures are positive for the causative organism.

Renal biopsy findings are most commonly mesangiocapillary GN (MCGN) type 1, although occasionally diffuse proliferative GN or mild mesangial proliferative GN can be seen.

IgM, IgG and C3 deposition is typical.

Electron-dense deposits are observed in the subendothelial region.

Treatment

Appropriate antibiotic therapy by itself is usually insufficient, and prompt removal of the infected AV shunt is necessary with subsequent placement of a VP shunt.

If dialysis is required, hemodialysis is the modality of choice since peritonitis complicating peritoneal dialysis may lead to meningitis in patients with VP shunts.

Prognosis

The renal outcome is good if early diagnosis and prompt treatment is provided.

Other bacterial infections causing GN are listed in Table 3.11.1.

Viral infections

Viral infections can result in various forms of renal disease (Table 3.11.2).

Hepatitis B virus (HBV)

Renal disease associated with hepatitis B infection may manifest in several ways:

Serum sickness

This occurs during acute infection.

It is characterized by fever, arthralgias/arthritis, hepatitis, rash (urticaria/maculopapular) and renal involvement (microscopic hematuria, sterile pyuria, and proteinuria).

Renal biopsy, if performed, shows mesangial proliferative GN.

The kidney involvement resolves when the hepatitis recovers.

Approximately 10% of patients acutely infected with HBV become chronic carriers and are at risk for other renal manifestations of HBV.

Table 3.11.1 Bacterial infection-related glomerular disease

Mycobacterium leprae
Amyloidosis (AA)
Glomerulonephritis
   Diffuse proliferative GN
   Focal proliferative GN
   MCGN
   Mesangial proliferative GN

Mycobacterium tuberculosis
Amyloidosis (AA)
MCGN type II

Treponema pallidum
Congenital syphilis
   Membranous nephropathy
Acquired syphilis
   Membranous nephropathy
   Diffuse endocapillary GN
   MCGN
   Mesangial proliferative GN
   Amyloidosis (AA)

Salmonella typhi
Mesangial proliferative GN
IgA nephropathy

Streptococcus pneumoniae
Mesangial proliferative GN
Diffuse proliferative GN

Others reported in association with GN
Brucella melitensis
E. coli
Klebsiella pneumoniae
Yersinia enterocolitica
Mycoplasma pneumoniae
Legionella
Bartonalla henselae

Polyarteritis nodosa (PAN)

Epidemiology:

The frequency of HBsAg in PAN is reported to be 17–52%.

It is observed primarily in men and does not occur if HBV is acquired at birth or during childhood.

It is also more common if infection is acquired through blood transfusion or drug abuse.

It tends to occur during recovery from an episode of mild hepatitis.

Clinical features:

It typically presents with signs of serum sickness (fever, rash, and arthralgia) during a mild or asymptomatic hepatitis.

Arteritis of small and medium-sized arteries can lead to myocardial/coronary ischemia, CNS alteration, peripheral neuropathy and mononeuritis multiplex.

Renal vasculitis is manifested by microscopic hematuria, proteinuria (nephrotic or non-nephrotic) and renal failure.

Diagnosis:

HBsAg positive, anti-HBc positive, anti-HBs negative.

Mildly elevated transaminases.

Biopsy of kidney, skeletal muscle, or peripheral nerves reveals transmural inflammation of small or medium-sized arteries characterized by fibrinoid necrosis, leukocyte infiltration, fibrin deposition and occasional aneurysm formation.

Angiography may show aneurysms of the celiac and renal arteries.

Prognosis:

Without treatment, almost all affected patients die within 2–5 years.

Treatment:

Combination therapy with corticosteroids and a cytotoxic agent (usually cyclophosphamide) is associated with good short-term outcome. However, this treatment is associated with accelerated progression of the liver disease.

Recent studies suggest an excellent survival and low relapse with combination treatment with corticosteroids, plasma exchange, and antiviral treatment (vidarabine, interferon-α, or lamivudine).

Membranous nephropathy (MN)
Epidemiology:

This is more common in children (peak incidence 2–12 years).

There is a male preponderance (male:female 8:1).

Pathogenesis:

It is thought to be due to passive trapping or *in situ* formation of immune complexes containing HBeAg, mainly in the subepithelial compartment of the glomerular capillary.

HBeAg is found in 80% of cases. Spontaneous remission is associated with appearance of anti-HBe antibodies.

Clinical features:

Nephrotic syndrome, microscopic hematuria, and renal failure (<10%).

A history of clinically apparent hepatitis is often absent.

Diagnosis:

HBsAg positive, anti-HBc positive, HBeAg positive (80% cases).

Reduced C3 and C4 levels are seen in 20–50% of cases.

Renal biopsy: membranous nephropathy with granular deposits of IgG, IgM and C3 in the capillary wall. Electron-dense deposits may be seen in the mesangial and subendothelial areas in contrast to idiopathic MN.

Prognosis:

In children, a favorable outcome with a high spontaneous remission rate is observed.

In adults, spontaneous remission is uncommon. 40% develop CKD and 10% develop ESRD within 5 years.

Treatment:

In children, treatment is not advocated due to the high spontaneous remission rate.

However, data suggest that sustained resolution of proteinuria is significantly more frequent in treated children.

Treatment is recommended for adults.

Steroid and cytotoxic agents may enhance viral replication and precipitate hepatitic flares.

Antiviral therapy:

- Interferon-α (5 MU daily for 6 months) was shown to be beneficial in children but had variable outcomes in adults.

- Oral lamivudine (100 mg daily for 52 weeks) is useful in inducing remission in nephrotic membranous nephropathy. However, resistance to lamivudine with long-term use is commonly reported.
- Combination treatment with lamivudine and interferon-α is currently being evaluated.

MCGN
This is more common in adults than in children and is the most common glomerular lesion in adults with HBV infection.

It results in nephrotic syndrome, microscopic hematuria, hypertension (80%) and renal insufficiency (50%).

There is often no history of liver disease but patients have abnormal transaminases and also chronic persistent or chronic active hepatitis on liver biopsy.

MCGN is induced by HBsAg and anti-HBs antibody-containing immune complexes.

Histologically an MCGN type I pattern is observed.

Antiviral treatment as described above should be considered.

Hepatitis C virus (HCV)
HCV typically causes MCGN with or without cryoglobulinemia.

Epidemiology
HCV is present in 60% of patients with MCGN in Japan and in 10–20% in the USA.

It predominantly affects adults in the fifth and sixth decades of life.

Pathogenesis
HCV infects circulating B-lymphocytes and stimulates them to synthesize polyclonal IgM rheumatoid factor (RF) responsible for type III cryoglobulinemia or monoclonal RF causing type II cryoglobulinemia.

Clinical features
Renal involvement in HCV infection may be asymptomatic. The most common presenting features are proteinuria, microscopic hematuria and renal insufficiency (50%). Nephrotic syndrome occurs in ~25% of cases.

Renal disease occurs in 50% of patients with mixed cryoglobulinemia associated with HCV. They present with palpable purpura, arthralgia, neuropathy and abdominal pain secondary to mesenteric vasculitis.

RPGN may occur.

Diagnosis
Reduced C4, C1q, CH50, with normal/reduced C3.

Cryoglobulin is present in 60–70% of cases.

Transaminases are elevated.

Anti-HCV antibody positive and HCV RNA positive.

Renal biopsy demonstrates MCGN type I, occasionally with cryoglobulin deposition.

Prognosis
The clinical course of renal disease is variable:
- 30% have partial or complete remission;
- 30% have an indolent course and do not progress to ESRF;
- 30% have intermittent flares of acute nephritis or nephrotic syndrome.

Most patients die of heart disease, liver disease or infection.

Treatment

There are several approaches available for the treatment of HCV-related GN:

1. Symptomatic treatment (BP control and RAS blockade).
2. Specific antiviral treatment:
   - pegylated interferon-α with ribavirin (ribavirin dose needs to be adjusted according to GFR and should not be used if GFR is <50 mL/min);
   - others: standard interferon-α therapy.
3. Immunosuppressive therapy should be considered if vasculitis or RPGN develops:
   - plasmapheresis to remove cryoglobulin;
   - corticosteroid (pulse IV followed by oral);
   - cyclophosphamide;
   - mycophenolate mofetil or rituximab (anti-CD20 monoclonal antibody) may also be helpful.

Human immunodeficiency virus (HIV)

HIV can induce a number of renal manifestations.

HIV-associated nephropathy

Epidemiology:

This affects 2–10% of untreated HIV-infected patients.

It predominantly affects African-Americans (>95%).

There is a male preponderance (male:female 10:1).

Over 95% patients are in the advanced stages of infection (CD4 count <200/μL).

Clinical features:

It typically presents with severe nephrotic syndrome and renal insufficiency.

Hypertension and edema are uncommon.

Pathogenesis:

A direct effect of HIV or viral protein on renal epithelial cells has been implicated.

Diagnosis:

USS demonstrates highly echogenic normal-sized or large kidneys.

Renal biopsy:

- Focal segmental glomerulosclerosis (FSGS) with hypertrophy and hyperplasia of visceral cell epithelium ('pseudo crescent'), capillary wall collapse leading to shrunken glomerular tuft (collapsing variant of FSGS).
- Tubules are focally enlarged with 'micro cystic' dilatation.
- Tubuloreticular inclusion bodies in the endoplasmic reticulum of the endothelial cells can be seen on electron microscopy.

Treatment:

- HAART (highly active antiretroviral therapy) is effective in slowing disease progression.
- Proteinuria reduction with renin–angiotensin system (RAS) blockade slows progression if the creatinine <176 μmol/L (2 mg/dL).
- Corticosteroids (reserved for patients at high risk of developing renal failure) may be helpful but relapse is common when they are stopped.

Prognosis:

Without treatment ESRD usually develops within 3–6 months.

The use of HAART has reduced the proportion of HIV patients who develop ESRD.

Dialysis survival is comparable to that of the general ESRD population.

Renal transplantation can be performed and the short-term outcome appears to be comparable to that of the general transplant population.

Lupus-like syndrome

This is found predominantly in African-Americans.

It is an immune-complex-mediated disease associated with complement activation and cryoglobulin formation in 30–50% of patients.

It presents with nephrotic syndrome or heavy proteinuria and microscopic hematuria. Renal insufficiency and hypertension are common.

The renal biopsy findings are similar to lupus nephritis with 'full house' deposition of IgG, IgM, IgA, C3 and C1q, and with subendothelial immune deposits and wire loop changes.

Typical SLE serology is not present.

70% of such patients progress to ESRD within 1 year of diagnosis.

The optimal treatment is unclear. It does not appear to be responsive to HAART or corticosteroids.

HIV-associated thrombotic microangiopathy

Most patients present with acute kidney injury, microscopic hematuria, non-nephrotic proteinuria, evidence of microangiopathic hemolysis and neurological manifestations.

Multiple organ involvement is frequent.

The mortality rate is high and survival beyond 2 years is unusual.

The incidence is falling with use of HAART.

Other viral causes of glomerular disease are listed in Table 3.11.2.

Table 3.11.2 Viral infection-related glomerular disease

Acute GN	
Parvovirus B19	MCGN and/or endocapillary GN
Hepatitis A virus	Mesangial proliferative GN
	IgA dominant GN
	Acute renal failure
Dengue fever	Mesangial proliferative GN
Measles	
Yellow fever	
Epstein–Barr virus	
Chronic GN	
Hepatitis B virus	Membranous GN – see text
	MCGN – see text
	Polyarteritis nodosa – see text
	Mesangial proliferative
	Minimal change disease
	IgA nephropathy
Hepatitis C virus	MCGN with or without cryoglobulinemia – see text
	Membranous GN
	Mesangial proliferative GN
	Focal glomerulosclerosis
	Fibrillary GN
	Immunotactoid glomerulopathy
HIV	See text
Parvovirus B19	Collapsing glomerulopathy
	Focal segmental glomerulosclerosis

Parasitic infections

Malaria

Epidemiology
Globally, there are 300–500 million cases of malaria per year.

90% occur in Africa, India, South East Asia and Central America.

Clinical features
Malaria is associated with a spectrum of renal involvement:

Malarial acute renal failure has a mortality of 15–45%.

Acute GN:

- This occurs with *P. ovale, P. vivax* and *P. falciparum* and is usually transient.
- Renal manifestations are microscopic hematuria and mild proteinuria.
- C3 and C4 levels are reduced and circulating immune complexes may be identified.
- Renal biopsy features are of a mesangioproliferative GN with fine deposition of IgM and C3 in mesangial and sub-endothelial regions.

Chronic GN:

This occurs with *P. malariae*.

It predominantly occurs in children and young adults.

It presents with the clinical features of quartan malaria, heavy proteinuria or overt nephrotic syndrome, and microscopic hematuria.

Renal biopsy features are of MCGN without cellular proliferation. Crescents are rare. Granular deposits of IgG, IgM and C3 are seen in the subendothelial region.

Prognosis: Chronic renal insufficiency progresses inspite of successful eradication of malaria, and steroids or immunosuppressive agents do not alter the course of the disease.

This topic is also covered in detail in Chapter 3.13.

Schistosomiasis
This topic is dealt with in detail in Chapter 7.4.

Filaria
Filarial infection can result in a variety of renal lesions.

Nephropathy can present with variable proteinuria and microscopic hematuria. In some patients the nephrotic or nephritic syndrome may develop.

Onchocerca volvulus is found in South America and tropical sub-Saharan Africa and is associated with minimal change nephropathy and MCGN.

Wuchereria bancrofti and *Brugia malayi* are found in Africa and South-East Asia and are associated with MCGN and diffuse proliferative GN.

Loa loa infection is prevalent in West Central Africa and is associated with membranous GN, MCGN, and FSGS (collapsing variant).

Pathologically, microfilariae can be identified in the capillary loops and in most instances filarial antigens can be identified in glomerular immune deposits.

Antifilarial treatment with diethylcarbamazine improves renal disease in those with subnephrotic proteinuria.

Nephrotic or nephritic patients tend not to improve with antifilarial treatment.

Others

Visceral Leishmaniasis (kala-azar) often presents with microscopic hematuria and proteinuria with either diffuse proliferative GN, membranous nephropathy, or interstitial nephritis on renal biopsy.

Trichinosis may present with microscopic hematuria and proteinuria caused by MCGN.

Trypanosomiasis and toxoplasmosis may occasionally be associated with glomerular disease.

Further reading

Bandi L. Renal manifestations of hepatitis C infection. *Postgraduate Med* 2003; **113**: 73–86.

Guillevin L, *et al.* Hepatitis B virus associated polyarteritis nodosa. *Medicine* 2005; **84**: 313–322.

Haas M, *et al.* HIV-associated immune complex GN with lupus like features. *Kidney Int* 2005; **67**: 1381–1390.

Jones R, *et al.* Renal complications in HIV. *Int J Clin Pract* 2007; **61**: 991–998.

Kamar N, *et al.* Treatment of hepatitis C virus-related glomerulonephritis. *Kidney Int* 2006; **636**: 436–439.

Khan S, *et al.* HIV-associated nephropathy. *Adv Chronic Kidney Dis* 2006;**13**:307–313.

Lai ASH. Viral nephropathy. *Nat Clin Pract* 2006; **2**: 254–262.

Rodriguez-Iturbe B. Post-infectious glomerulonephritis. *Am J Kidney Dis* 2000; **35**: xlvi–xlviii.

Internet resources

Review of nonstreptococcal infection-related GN:

www.emedicine.com/med/topic888.htm

Review of the pathology of infection-associated GN:

www.kidneyatlas.org/book2/adk2_04.pdf

Review about HIV-related renal disease:

www.emedicine.com/med/topic3203.htm

Review of infection-related renal disease in the tropics:

www.uninet.edu/cin2000/conferences/chugh/chugh.html

See also

Glomerular disease in the tropics, p. 138

Membranous nephropathy, p. 106

Acute endocapillary glomerulonephritis, p. 116

Systemic vasculitis, p. 168

Mixed cryoglobulinemia and hepatitis C infection, p. 176

Schistosomiasis, p. 260

Renal tuberculosis and other mycobacterial infections, p. 256

Malignancy-associated glomerular disease

The etiology of renal failure in the setting of malignancy can be quite diverse (Table 3.12.1).

Table 3.12.1 Renal involvement in malignant disease

Direct effects
Metastasis
Infiltration
Ischemia
Obstruction
Indirect effects
Electrolyte disorders
Hypokalemia, hyponatremia, hypercalcemia
Acute renal failure
Disseminated intravascular coagulation
Thrombotic microangiopathy
Renal vein thrombosis
Amyloidosis
Glomerular disease
Nephrocalcinosis
Treatment-related
Drug nephrotoxicity
Tumor lysis syndrome
Radiation nephritis

This chapter will focus on glomerular disorders associated with solid tumors and hematological malignancies (Table 3.12.2).

Renal disease resulting from plasma cell dyscrasias will be described in detail in Chapter 4.3.

Epidemiology

Urinary abnormalities such as proteinuria and microscopic hematuria are not uncommon in patients with cancer.

The prevalence of malignancy-associated glomerulonephritis is unknown.

The incidence varies substantially with the type of cancer. In most series it is estimated to be <2% of the population with a particular cancer.

Glomerulonephritis is a histological diagnosis that requires a renal biopsy. There is a paucity of renal biopsy data for a variety of reasons. This in turn has led researchers to depend on autopsy series. Many of the glomerulonephritides that occur with malignancy require immunological testing which may not be reliable on an autopsy tissue. Thus the accuracy of these series could be easily challenged.

The Danish Kidney Biopsy Registry was examined for rates of cancer in patients with glomerular disease, and these rates were compared with those of the general Danish population.

- 102 *de novo* cancers were found in 1958 patients.
- These cancer rates represent a two- to three-fold excess of the expected number at <1 and 1–4 but not ≥5 years after a biopsy.
- Non-Hodgkin's lymphomas were observed six to eight times more than expected.

This study suggests a strong association based on a possible common pathogenesis between glomerulonephritis and cancer.

Table 3.12.2 Glomerular disorders associated with malignant disease

Glomerular disease	Associated malignancy
Membranous nephropathy	Colon, breast, stomach, and lung cancer
Minimal change disease	Hodgkin's lymphoma, pancreatic cancer, mesothelioma, prostate cancer
Focal segmental glomerulosclerosis	Lymphoma, leukemia, lung cancer
AA amyloidosis	Carcinoma (especially renal)
AL amyloidosis	Myeloma
Crescentic GN	Lung carcinoma, renal cell carcinoma, stomach cancer, lymphoma, lung cancer
Mesangiocapillary GN	Chronic lymphocytic leukemia (CLL), lymphoma
IgA nephropathy	Lung carcinoma, lymphoma
Light chain nephropathy	Myeloma, lymphoma
Fibrillary GN	Lymphoma
Thrombotic microangiopathy	Stomach, prostate, pancreas and breast cancer

Pathogenesis

A number of mechanisms could potentially underlie the association between glomerulonephritis and malignancy.

- Immune-complex-mediated glomerular injury is thought to be a common mechanism. This is supported by the observation that in contrast to idiopathic membranous nephropathy (MN), mesangial and subendothelial electron-dense deposits are often detected in secondary MN. This implicates circulating immune complexes in the pathogenesis of disease.
- Re-expression of fetal antigens may be important for disease induction. In support of this concept, carcinoembryonic antigen (CEA) has been isolated from diseased glomeruli in patients with adenocarcinoma.
- Various cytokines that exhibit antitumor activity (e.g. IL-6) have also been implicated.

Clinical features

Glomerulonephritis is an intrinsic renal disease. The following features are commonly encountered with glomerular disorders.

- Nephrotic range proteinuria and the classical features of nephrotic syndrome (NS) may be the primary manifestation of the associated GN. However, non-nephrotic range proteinuria may also occur.
- Microscopic hematuria (in the absence of bladder pathology) with erythrocyte casts and dysmorphic red cells indicates the presence of glomerulonephritis.
- Macroscopic nonglomerular hematuria is of particular significance because it is much more likely than

microscopic hematuria to be associated with a urological malignancy.

- A bland urinary sediment (absent proteinuria, hematuria, erythrocyte casts) argues strongly against the diagnosis of glomerulonephritis. In the context of renal function impairment, alternative explanations such as obstructive uropathy and tubulointerstitial disease should be considered.
- Acute renal failure is more likely to occur with crescentic and membranoproliferative glomerulonephritis. The former may present with extrarenal symptoms such as skin rash or hemoptysis.

An elevated ESR is not uncommon in NS and by itself is not an indication to investigate for occult malignancy.

Immunological testing for ANCA and anti-GBM antibodies is indicated when there is a reasonable suspicion of rapidly progressive glomerulonephritis with the relevant features such as the characteristic vasculitic rash and active urinary sediment. Without such features, positive immunological testing carries little significance. False-positive ANCA has been reported with several malignancies such as lymphomas and lung cancer.

Ultimately the confirmation of the diagnosis and identification of the underlying glomerulonephritis requires a renal biopsy.

Renal biopsy is an invasive test, with potentially serious complications. The decision to carry out such a test is affected by the prognosis of the associated cancer. Although essential for diagnostic purposes, it may not always be technically possible due to concurrent coagulopathy and/or thrombocytopenia.

Specific glomerular disorders

Membranous nephropathy (MN)

This is the commonest malignancy-associated glomerulopathy. Up to 20% of patients, particularly those aged >60 years, who have MN are reported to have a malignancy.

Age, smoking, and the presence of glomerular leukocytic infiltrates strongly increase the likelihood of malignancy in MN patients.

Secondary MN will present with nephrotic syndrome with or without renal impairment.

It is associated with solid tumors particularly cancers of the lung, breast stomach and colon.

Histological findings in MN

The renal biopsy appearances, particularly the immunofluorescence and electron microscopy findings, will help differentiate idiopathic from secondary membranous nephropathy.

Diffuse thickening of the glomerular basement membrane without any hypercellularity is typical on light microscopy (Fig. 3.12.1).

In malignancy-associated MN, immunofluorescence shows a diffuse granular pattern of IgG1 and IgG2 rather than IgG4 (which is characteristic of idiopathic membranous nephropathy).

Tubular basement membrane positivity on IF is rare with idiopathic MN, but common in secondary forms of MN.

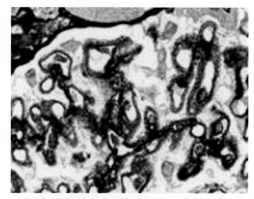
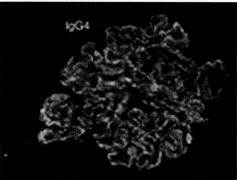

Fig. 3.12.1 Membranous nephropathy (MN). (*Upper*) Methanamine-silver stain showing extensive 'spikes' in a case of advanced MN. The 'spikes' represent basement membrane material laid down between the subepithelial immune complexes. The latter are eventually incorporated into the basement membrane and are resorbed. (*Lower*) Global coarsely granular positivity for IgG highlighting the capillary walls in a case of 'idiopathic' MN, which also showed a similar pattern of fluorescence with IgG and C3. IgG1 and IgG2 subtypes have been found to be more often associated with malignancy-associated MN, but these antibodies are not typically used in routine diagnostic practice. (Courtesy of Dr Nick Mayer, Consultant Histopathologist, University Hospitals of Leicester, UK.)

Minimal change disease (MCD)

This is the commonest glomerulonephritis encountered with Hodgkin's lymphoma.

MCD has also been reported less frequently with leukemias, other lymphomas, and rarely with mesothelioma, and prostate and pancreatic cancer.

In a review of 21 cases of MCD associated with Hodgkin's lymphomas:

- nephrotic syndrome appeared before the diagnosis of lymphoma in 38% of patients;
- nephrotic syndrome was frequently steroid resistant (50%) or steroid dependent (12.5%);
- curative treatment of the lymphoma resulted in remission of the nephrotic syndrome.

It has been reported that nephrotic syndrome due to MCD may be diagnosed up to a median of 2 years prior to the diagnosis of malignancy.

In the absence of features suggestive of an underlying neoplasm (e.g. fever, weight loss, lymphadenopathy), exhaustive investigation is not indicated.

Focal segmental glomerulosclerosis (FSGS)

This has been observed primarily with hematological malignancies although with a lower frequency than the association of MCD and Hodgkin's lymphoma.

It has also been reported with non small-cell lung cancer. In that case it presented with nephrotic syndrome and the proteinuria reduced dramatically during radiotherapy for the lung cancer.

Amyloidosis

Both primary and secondary amyloidosis may be associated with malignancies.

Primary amyloidosis (AL) occurs as a result of deposition of light chain fragments and may occur in association with multiple myeloma; these fibrils are derived from λ light chains in the majority of cases.

Secondary amyloidosis (AA) has been described in association with a number of malignancies, particularly renal cell carcinoma, Hodgkin's lymphoma and CLL.

- Presentation will typically be of nephrotic syndrome and less commonly renal failure.
- Extrarenal manifestations are not uncommon especially in primary amyloidosis (AL).
- Serum paraprotein and monoclonal urinary light chain may be detected in AL. This should be assessed further using serum free light chain assays.
- Tissue diagnosis can be obtained by biopsy of the abdominal fat pad, rectum, or the affected organ, e.g. liver or kidney (most sensitive and most specific).

Histological finding in amyloidosis

The renal biopsy will show the typical fibrillar arrangement on electron microscopy. These amyloid fibrils are characterized by their ability to bind Congo Red. This gives the typical apple green birefringence under polarized light. Immunohistochemical staining for λ or κ light chains, or serum amyloid A, can define the type of amyloidosis.

Crescentic glomerulonephritis

Crescentic GN commonly presents with acute renal failure.

Extra-renal manifestations such as pulmonary hemorrhage may be the initial manifestation of the vasculitic process.

Serological testing may demonstrate positive ANCA serology.

Patients with ANCA-positive vasculitis have an increased risk of simultaneous malignancy.

Crescentic GN has been reported with a number of cancers:

- Renal cell carcinoma (and following immunotherapy for renal cell carcinoma).
- Gastric adenocarcinoma.
- Carcinoma of the hypopharynx.
- Non-Hodgkin lymphoma.

A review of 80 patients with a renal biopsy diagnosis of crescentic GN revealed seven cases with a coexistent non renal malignancy.

- All of the malignancies occurred in patients aged >40 years.

- Light, immunofluorescence and electron microscopy revealed fibrin deposition in all cases and no evidence of anti-GBM or immune complex disease.
- Three patients experienced a rapidly progressive course while renal function improved in four patients following treatment of the underlying malignancy.

Treatment of crescentic GN requires immunosupression with steroids and other agents such as cyclophosphamide.

In addition plasma exchange may be required to alleviate both the renal and nonrenal manifestations of the vasculitis. However, this may increase the neoplastic burden.

Mesangiocapillary GN (MCGN)

When nephrotic syndrome presents in association with lung cancer, MCGN tends to be the most common glomerulonephritis.

Chronic hepatitis C virus infection has been linked to cryoglobulinemia, mesangiocapillary glomerulonephritis, and malignant B-cell lymphoproliferation.

However, this proposed linkage has been challenged in a case report where this clinical triad has occurred in the absence of hepatitis C infection.

This form of glomerulonephritis has a progressive nature and is usually associated with renal impairment.

IgA nephropathy

IgA nephropathy has been reported with small cell lung carcinoma, and lymphomas such as Hodgkin's disease.

Thrombotic microangiopathy

Thrombotic microangiopathy is characterized by the triad of acute renal failure, idiopathic thrombocytopenia and microangiopathic hemolysis.

Hemolytic uremic syndrome (HUS) commonly causes acute renal failure due to microthrombi formation within the glomerular capillaries and renal arterioles (Fig. 3.12.2).

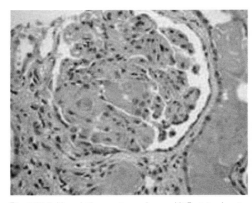

Fig. 3.12.2 Hemolytic uremic syndrome. H&E stain showing glomerular and arteriolar thrombosis. (Courtesy of Dr Nick Mayer, Consultant Histopathologist, University Hospitals of Leicester, UK.)

Patients with disseminated malignancy are at risk for developing HUS. The diagnosis must be differentiated from DIC, which may also be encountered in the context of malignancy.

HUS has been reported with mucin-producing gastric adenocarcinomas, and adenocarcinomas of the prostate, pancreas and breast.

It may present in its acute form with acute kidney injury or may have a more chronic indolent presentation.

Rarely occult disseminated malignancy may mimic TTP. This should be suspected when plasma exchange, the mainstay of treatment, is ineffective. In such situations the search for an underlying malignancy should be considered.

Treatment

Most of the common glomerulonephritides and the associated renal failure if present will respond to treatment of the associated malignancy.

However, conventional therapies, such as steroids for MCD and immunosuppression and plasma exchange in crescentic glomerulonephritis, have been shown to be effective.

Screening for malignancy

To date there is no consensus on cancer screening for patients with newly diagnosed secondary glomerulonephritides. This is certainly true when clinical features such anemia, fever, and weight loss are absent.

In cases of secondary MN and in the presence of the high-risk indicators, e.g. age >50 years and a heavy smoking history, following a detailed history and physical examination for evidence of neoplastic disease, relevant screening strategies may be employed.

In general there is a paucity of evidence and further research is needed to address the most appropriate screening strategies, if any, in such patients. A reasonable approach would include CXR, occult blood testing of the stools, mammography (in women), measurement of tumor markers (e.g. CEA and prostate-specific antigen (PSA)), and possibly colonoscopy and abdominal CT scanning if abdominal symptoms are present.

Conclusions

Urinary abnormalities are common in patients with malignant disease.

Malignancy-associated glomerulonephritis is rare but should be considered in the context of the appropriate clinical clues.

The confirmation of the diagnosis requires a renal biopsy.

The treatment should be aimed at the underlying malignancy.

Immunosuppression for selected glomerulonephritides increases the cancer burden and should be considered on an individual basis.

The prognosis of the GN is strongly linked to the natural history of the associated cancer.

Further reading

Birkeland SA, Storm HH. Glomerulonephritis and malignancy: a population based analysis. *Kidney Int* 2003; **63**: 716–721.

Brueggemayer CD, et al. Membranous nephropathy; a concern for malignancy. *Am J Kidney Dis* 1987; **9**: 23–26.

Burstein DM, et al. Membranous glomerulonephritis and malignancy. *Am J Kidney Dis* 1993; **22**: 5–10.

Cathen R, et al. Aetiology of membranous glomerulonephritis: a prospective study of 82 adult patients. *Nephrol Dialysis Transpl* 1989; **4**: 172–180.

Couser WG, et al. Glomerular deposition of tumour antigen in membranous nephropathy associated with colonic carcinoma. *Am J Med* 1974; **57**: 962–970.

Helin M, et al. Glomerular electron-dense deposits and circulating immune complexes in patients with malignant tumours. *Clin Nephrol* 1980; **14**: 23–30.

Kincaid-Smith P. The investigation of hemturia. *Semin Nephrol* 2005; **25**: 127–135.

Lefaucheur C, et al. Epidemiologic evidence and determinants of high-risk cancer association. *Kidney Int* 2006; **70**: 1510–1517.

Muthia P. New lung lesion in immunocompromised host-correct diagnosis despite a false positive ANCA. *Southern Med J* 2006; **99**: 701–702.

Ohtani H, et al. Distribution of IgG subclass deposits in malignancy-associated membranous nephropathy. *Nephrol Dialysis Transpl* 2004; **19**: 74–579.

Rihova Z, et al. Secondary membranous nephropathy – one center experience. *Renal Failure* 2005; **27**: 397–402.

Sawyer, N, Wadsworth J, et al. Prevalence, concentration and prognostic importance of proteinuria in patients with malignancies. *Br Med J* 1988; **296**: 295–298.

See also

Glomerular disease in the tropics

Glomerulonephritis (GN) accounts for 30–60% of all end-stage renal disease (ESRD) in the tropics.

Infection is the commonest cause of glomerular disease in this setting with hypertension and diabetes mellitus accounting for the majority of the remainder. Infectious causes of glomerular disease in the tropics are listed in Table 3.13.1.

Human immunodeficiency virus (HIV)-associated disease is becoming increasingly common.

Renal biopsy confirmation of the diagnosis is often difficult due to lack of diagnostic facilities and to late presentation when, in the face of advanced disease, renal biopsies become difficult to interpret.

Epidemiology

There is variability in the etiology of glomerular disease in different parts of the tropics due to differences in the epidemiology of infections, standards of living, and infrastructure development.

The high prevalence of chronic GN points to variety of etiological agents.

GN usually presents in one of four ways in the tropics: acute nephritic syndrome, nephrotic syndrome, asymptomatic urinary abnormalities, and ESRD.

This chapter focuses on causes of the nephrotic and nephritic syndromes, and incorporates asymptomatic urinary abnormalities and ESRD where appropriate.

Acute nephritic syndrome

Etiology

Post-streptococcal GN (PSGN) is the commonest cause of rapidly progressive renal failure in the tropics.

It is most common in children.

It may occur during epidemics of post-streptococcal skin (impetigo, pyoderma) and throat infections.

Different nephritogenic serotypes have been identified:
- skin: M types 47, 49, 55, and 57;
- throat: M types 1, 2, 4, and 12.

The risk of nephritis is 5% with throat infection and up to 25% for pyoderma.

GN occurs 1–3 weeks after the onset of a streptococcal infection.

Pathogenesis

PSGN is generally assumed to be due to deposition of circulating immune complexes in the glomeruli. However, this should result in activation of the classical complement pathway (with C3 and C4 activation), but C4 levels are normal and only C3 is found in the glomerular immune deposits (suggesting alternative pathway activation).

The following possibly contribute to inflammation and injury:
- activation of the alternative complement pathway by glyceraldehyde-3-phosphate dehydrogenase (GAPDH);
- cationic streptococcal antigen promoting development of subepithelial immune deposits ('humps');
- cytokines IL-6, TNF-α and vasoactive mediators such as platelet activating factors;
- in situ deposition of antigen followed by antibody formation;

- IgG rheumatoid factor initiating an autoimmune reaction in the glomerulus.

Table 3.13.1. Infections associated with glomerulonephritis in the tropics

Bacterial
Streptococus pyogenes
E. coli 0157 :H7 (HUS)
Salmonella typhi
Mycobacterium leprae
Mycobacterium tuberculosis
Staphylococcus epidermidis/aureus
Treponema pallidum
Streptococcus pneumoniae

Protozoal
Plasmodium falciparum
Plasmodium malariae
Leishmania donovani
Toxoplasma gondii
Trypanosoma cruzi

Viral
Hepatitis B
Hepatitis C
HIV
Epstein–Barr virus

Helminthic
Schistosoma mansoni
Schistosoma haematobium
Wuchereria bancrofti
Brugia malayi
Loa loa
Onchocerca volvulus

Clinical course

Most children (>90%) recover completely. Approximately 5% develop progressive acute kidney injury or acute GN.

In acute GN, there is rapid deterioration of renal function, oliguria, fluid overload from sodium and water retention, hypertension (80%), edema (80–90%), and pulmonary edema.

Approximately 20% have long-term sequelae with asymptomatic urinary abnormalities, nephrotic syndrome, hypertension, or very rarely progressive renal dysfunction.

Examination of renal histology of the nephrotic syndrome in nonmalarious parts of the tropical world would suggest that PSGN may be a cause in some patients. It may be the reason why minimal change disease is rarely seen in Black African children with nephrotic syndrome.

Chronic GN leading to progressive chronic kidney disease is more likely in adolescents than in children, especially in those with persistent proteinuria.

Elderly patients do less well (70% have azotemia, 40% heart failure, 25% early mortality). Longer-term prognosis is also less good than in children with up to 25% being left with abnormal renal function.

Diagnosis

This is usually easy to make from the clinical features and simple laboratory tests.

Oliguria may not be obvious in children, but 'coca-cola'-colored urine, due to macroscopic hematuria, is usually apparent.

Urinalysis
- Red blood cells and red cell casts.
- Variable degree of proteinuria.
- Some may have nephrotic range proteinuria.
- Leukocytes.

Serology

A positive antistreptolysin O (ASO) titer is seen in only ~30% of patients (perhaps because of early antibiotic use).

Serum C3 levels are reduced in >90% of patients in the first week, but return to normal within 2 months.

Serum C4 is typically normal.

Serum IgG and IgM are elevated in 75–80% of patients.

A low level of anti-DNA antibodies and ANCA may be seen.

Renal biopsy

This is rarely needed to confirm the diagnosis.

Indications:
- Nephrotic-range proteinuria.
- Acute kidney injury.
- Patients with sickle-cell anemia (a recognized cause of hematuria).

Light microscopy:
- Diffuse endocapillary, mesangial and endothelial prolif-eration. Neutrophil infiltration in glomeruli.
- Interstitial infiltration by monocytes and lymphocytes.

Immunofluorescence microscopy:
- C3, IgG, IgM deposition in capillary loops and the mesangium is invariable.

Electron microscopy:
- Classic subepithelial electron-dense deposits ('humps').

Differential diagnosis

Protein-energy malnutrition and nephrotic syndrome due to other causes.

Treatment

Treat ongoing streptococcal infection with appropriate antibiotics, e.g. benzathine penicillin (1.2 million U intra-muscularly as a single dose).

Restrict salt and water intake.

Diuretics (e.g. furosemide) for volume overload.

Antihypertensive agents which may also prevent hyper-tensive encephalopathy: nifedipine, hydralazine, Na nitroprusside.

Dialysis, although rarely needed in children, is a challenge in many tropical countries due to lack of dialysis infra-structure.

Prognosis

This is excellent in children who recover, but poor in ado-lescents who may progress to chronic GN.

Proteinuria may persist for months, and sometimes years.

Follow-up

It may be necessary to screen other family members – especially young children, who may have subclinical disease in epidemics of PSGN.

Nephrotic syndrome (NS)

NS is 2–10 times more common in the tropical countries than in Western Europe or North America.

It has recently been reported that NS accounts for 38% of nephrological admissions in the Democratic Republic of Congo.

Etiology

Even within the tropics, there are interracial differences. For example:

In South Africa minimal change disease is more common in Indian children than in Black children who have a prepon-derance of mesangiocapillary GN (MCGN). Minimal change disease is also common in India, suggesting a genetic predisposition.

MCGN predominates in Nigerian and Kuwaiti children. The disparities in histological features may suggest that NS may be a complication of PSGN and other forms of glomerular diseases. This may account for the rarity of minimal change disease as a cause of NS in African children.

The three main primary causes of NS are:
- MCGN.
- membranous GN.
- focal segmental glomerulosclerosis.

The most common secondary form of GN causing NS in the tropics is Quartan malarial nephrotic syndrome. Because this is peculiar to the tropics, it is discussed in more detail.

Quartan malarial nephrotic syndrome (QMNS)

Plasmodium malariae is the most important cause of sec-ondary GN causing NS in children and adolescents.

QMNS is probably due to deposition of soluble immune complexes in the glomerulus but it is characterized by the absence of specific antibody and antigen. This has raised questions about the exact pathogenetic mechanism.

Pathology:

The characteristic appearance is of MCGN with progressive mesangial sclerosis leading to obliteration of glomerular capillaries with eventual involvement of tubules.

Immunofluorescence microscopy demonstrates coarse granular deposits of IgG, IgM and C3 mainly within the glomerular capillary walls.

Electron microscopy shows subendothelial electron-dense deposits and thickened GBM.

Clinical features:

Fever peaking once every 72 h is the earliest feature.

Gross edema and ascites are the main symptoms which develop several weeks after the onset of fever. This may easily be confused with protein-energy malnutrition (kwashiorkor).

Other features are nonselective proteinuria, micro-scopic hematuria, normal blood pressure, anemia, and hepatomegaly.

Hypoalbuminemia may be severe (10–20 g/L). Due to associated malnutrition in the majority of cases, the serum cholesterol is characteristically normal.

P. malariae may be detected in 69–70% of cases. The pres-ence of parasites even when glomerular changes are present does not necessarily indicate cause and effect. Detection of a specific antigen has been demonstrated in only a few cases.

Clinical course:

Prognosis is poor, and spontaneous remission is rare. QMNS causes end-stage renal failure in <4 years.

Treatment:

There is a uniformly a poor response to corticosteroids, and to antimalarials. There are reports of remission of steroid-resistant patients with cyclophosphamide but this leads to no improvement in overall survival. Giving a therapeutic trial of corticosteroids before biopsy is therefore a practice that is increasingly being called into question.

Falciparum malaria

P. falciparum infection is mainly a disease of children in the tropics. Unlike QMNS, it is not progressive, and it resolves following eradication of *P. falciparum*. Indeed, GN may pass unnoticed especially with the widespread use of antimalarials.

There is nonselective proteinuria, microscopic hematuria and casts.

The typical pathological abnormalities are mesangial hypercellularity with mild matrix expansion changes without basement membrane involvement.

IgG, IgM and C3 can be identified in the mesangium. Immune deposits can be identified by EM in the mesangial and subendothelial areas.

The renal lesions recover with conventional antimalarial treatment.

Schistosoma mansoni-associated nephropathy (see Chapter 7.4 for more detail)

This is common in Brazil and Egypt, and patients often present with the nephrotic syndrome.

Glomerulonephritis is most common when there are hepatosplenic manifestations and chronic salmonella infection.

Males are twice more affected than females, probably due to outdoor activities in rivers and pools.

Clinical features include:
- overt peripheral edema and ascites;
- poorly selective proteinuria and, rarely, hematuria;
- low serum C3 with hypergammaglobulinemia;
- normal cholesterol.

Pathology:

Several patterns of glomerular pathology have been observed:
- class I mesangioproliferative lesions;
- class II diffuse proliferative GN;
- class III MCGN types I and III;
- class IV focal and segmental glomerulosclerosis (FSGS);
- class V amyloidosis.

Treatment:

Praziquantel 20 mg/kg body weight is effective in eradicating the parasites but this does not result in resolution of glomerular disease that has progressed beyond class II.

The treatment of chronic salmonella infection may cause resolution of glomerular disease (usually class II changes), suggesting a critical role for salmonella antigens in the pathogenesis of disease.

A good response to oxamniquine has been observed in class II disease.

The role of immunosuppression is unclear.

Hepatitis B virus (HBV)-associated GN

HBV infection is prevalent in certain tropical countries, and the kidneys may be affected by immune-complex-mediated disease.

Acute HBV infection is associated with a serum sickness-like syndrome characterized by fever, arthralgias/arthritis, hepatitis, rash (urticaria/maculopapular) and renal involvement (microscopic hematuria, sterile pyuria, and proteinuria)

Renal biopsy, if performed, shows mesangial proliferative GN.

GN resolves with remission of the acute phase of the disease.

Approximately 10% of patients acutely infected with HBV become chronic carriers and are at risk for other renal manifestations of HBV. These include membranous nephropathy, polyarteritis nodosa, MCGN, and IgA nephropathy.

This topic is covered in detail in Chapter 3.11.

The treatment of HBV-related renal disease is more effective for membranous GN than for MCGN.

Treatment regimens that have shown benefit usually include interferon-α and lamivudine.

However, since these agents are not widely available in the tropics, the management of HBV-mediated renal disease (and the other manifestations of HBV infection) can be suboptimal.

Steroids and cytotoxics are contraindicated since they enhance viral replication and may precipitate hepatitic flares.

Hepatitis C virus (HCV)-associated GN

Glomerular disease associated with HCV has not been well-described in the tropics, even though the pathological changes and clinical course are not expected to be different from those described in the Western world.

These include variable degrees of proteinuria, microscopic hematuria, and renal impairment.

Mesangiocapillary GN has been described.

HIV-associated renal disease

The tropical regions, especially sub-Saharan Africa currently bear the brunt of the HIV/AIDS pandemic. Therefore, occurrence of renal disease associated with HIV is on the increase, and impacting negatively on the outcome of HIV disease.

HIV is immunocytopathic, and it therefore can cause a variety of renal syndromes such as:
- HIV nephropathy (HIVAN) (in >60% it occurs with advanced disease).
- Immune complex GN ('lupus-like syndrome').
- Thrombotic microangiopathy.

In addition, chemotherapy can present a challenge because some antiretroviral (ARV) and adjunct medications can cause nephrotoxicity (pentamidine) or nephrolithiasis (indinavir).

HIVAN: Occurs in about 60% of patients with advanced disease, but may be subclinical in the majority of cases. It is rapidly progressive and may reach ESRD within 5 months.

HIVAN is a diagnosis of exclusion, and therefore other treatable causes such as hypovolemia from diarrhea should be excluded. In the tropics, a significant number of patients use herbal preparations for recurrent febrile illness, and this may cause nephrotoxicity.

Pathogenesis:

HIV infects tubular and glomerular epithelial cells and podocytes. This may explain the occurrence of NS in affected individuals.

Pathology:

This typically shows a preserved Bowman's space with collapsed/shrunken glomeruli ('collapsing glomerulopathy'), and focal dilatations of tubules presenting a 'microcystic' appearance.

Treatment:

RAS blockade can slow progression in those with moderate CKD (creat <176 μmol/L (2 mg/dL)).

HAART (highly active antiretroviral therapy) may cause remission of glomerulopathy.

Prednisolone may be beneficial in high risk patients.

Sickle cell-associated renal disease

Sickle cell disease is common in certain population groups in the tropics, particularly Black Africans and Africans in the Caribbean. It causes renal disease by one or all of the following mechanisms:

- hypoperfusion/ischemia;
- iron overload and deposition;
- intracapillary fragmentation and phagocytosis of sickled cells;
- immune complex formation;
- hyperfiltration and subsequent glomerular sclerosis.

Pathology:

The following appearances may be observed:

- congestion of capillary loops with sickled cells;
- FSGS ;
- MCGN ;
- tubular atrophy ;
- iron pigment deposits.

Clinical features:

- gross hematuria;
- acute kidney injury from renal papillary necrosis, pregnancy, multiple organ failure;
- nephrotic syndrome.
- ESRD.

Treatment:

RAS blockade improves proteinuria by reducing intra-glomerular pressure, but large-scale studies are required to prove their long-term benefit for prevention/resolution of glomerular sclerosis.

NSAIDs and immunosuppressive drugs (steroids and cyclophosphamide) are not of proven benefit.

Leprosy-associated GN

Mycobacterium leprae may cause immune complex disease, secondary amyloidosis, interstitial nephritis, and renal tubular disorders.

Glomerular lesions occur more commonly in the lepromatous form, and the histological lesions include: mesangio-proliferative, mesangiocapillary, and crescentic GN, especially when patient is being treated with rifampicin.

Clinical features:

Only a few patients present with nephrotic syndrome, nephritic syndrome and rapidly progressive GN. Most patients are asymptomatic with a variety of urinary abnormalities.

Treatment:

Early treatment of leprosy may prevent occurrence of renal involvement. Treatment with rifampicin and occurrence of erythema nodosum leprosum (ENL) may exacerbate glomerular lesions. Steroids have no proven benefit.

Other forms of secondary GN

The following organisms can cause GN, even though the prevalence varies from region to region depending on the level of preventive measures: filarial worms, helminths, protozoas, and fungi. They induce various forms of GN, e.g. MCGN, membranous GN.

Patients often present with asymptomatic proteinuria or hematuria, and sometimes nephrotic syndrome. Generally, glomerular lesions do not respond to treatment of causative organisms.

Further reading

Akinkugbe OO. Tropical nephropathy – an overview. *Afr J Med Med Sci* 1992; **21**: 3–7.

Asinobi AO, Gbadegesin, R. The predominance of membranoproliferative glomerulonephritis in childhood nephrotic syndrome in Ibadan, Nigeria. *W Afr J Med* 1999; **18**: 203–206.

Barsoum RS. Schistosomal glomerulopathies. *Kidney Int* 1993; **44**: 1–12.

Barsoum RS. Malarial nephropathies. *Nephrol Dial Transpl* 1998; **13**: 1588–1597.

Browne SG. Epidemioology and prevention of kidney disease in Africa. *Trans R Soc Trop Med* 1980; **74**: 8–16.

Hendrickse RG, Adeniyi A. Quartan malarial nephrotic syndrome in children. *Kidney Int* 1979; **16**: 64–74.

Hutt MSR. Renal disease in a tropical environment. *Trans R Soc Trop Med* 1980; **74**: 17–21.

Jha V, Chugh KS. Glomerular disease in the tropics. In: Davison AM, Cameron JS, Grunfield JP (eds), *Oxford textbook of clinical nephrology*, 3rd edn. New York: Oxford University Press; 2005.

Rodriguez-Iturbe B, Burdman EA, Ophascharoensuk V, Barsoum RS. Glomerular diseases associated with infections. In: Johnson RJ, Feehally J (eds), *Comprehensive clinical nephrology*, 2nd edn. Philadelphia: Mosby, Elsevier; 2003.

Pham PT, Pham PT, Wilkinson AH, *et al*. Renal abnormalities in sickle cell disease. *Kidney Int* 2000; **57**: 1–8.

Internet resources

Information on schistosomiasis:

www.who.int/ctd/schisto

See also

Infection-related glomerulonephritis, p. 128

Acute endocapillary glomerulonephritis, p. 116

Mesangiocapillary glomerulonephritis, p. 112

Mixed cryoglobulinemia and hepatitis C infection, p. 176

Sickle cell disease, p. 192

Renal tuberculosis and other mycobacterial infections, p. 256

Schistosomiasis, p. 260

Fungal infections and the kidney, p. 264

Chapter 4

The kidney in systemic disease

Chapter contents

Diabetes mellitus

Diabetic renal disease is the commonest cause of end-stage renal disease (ESRD) in the Western world and is rapidly becoming the leading cause in developing countries. Diabetes mellitus (mainly type 2) is present in 25–50% of new patients with ESRD.

The development of diabetic renal disease occurs both in type 1 and type 2 diabetes, with a similar evolution over time for both types of diabetes.

The quality of care of diabetes and its complications directly influences the occurrence and development of diabetic nephropathy.

In most cases, chronic kidney disease in diabetics results from diabetic nephropathy (diabetic kidney disease in the K/DOQI Guidelines) and does not require a renal biopsy for diagnosis.

Definitions

Microalbuminuria

Albumin excretion of 30–300 mg/24 h or 20–200 μg/min, (Table 4.1.1) is the first detectable sign of renal injury associated with diabetes.

Diabetic nephropathy (DN)

Typically presents with the constellation of:
- albuminuria (>300 mg/24 h or >200 μg/min, Table 4.1.1);
- high blood pressure;
- progressive renal failure.

In most patients with diabetes, CKD can be attributable to diabetes if:
- macroalbuminuria is present;
- microalbuminuria is associated with the presence of diabetic retinopathy in patients with type 1 diabetes of ≥10 years duration.

Diabetes and other forms of renal disease

Alternative presentations of renal disease may occur:
- ischemic nephropathy with little or no proteinuria;
- diabetes may also be associated with other causes of CKD (glomerulonephritis, polycystic kidney disease, etc.) and may worsen their evolution.

Other cause(s) of CKD should be considered in diabetic patients in the following circumstances:
- absence of diabetic retinopathy, particularly in type 1 diabetes;
- low or rapidly decreasing GFR;
- rapidly increasing proteinuria or nephrotic syndrome;
- refractory hypertension;
- presence of an active urinary sediment;
- symptoms or signs of other systemic disease;

- >30% reduction in GFR within 2–3 months after initiation of an angiotensin-converting enzyme inhibitor (ACEI) or angiotensin II receptor blocker (ARB).

Epidemiology

Type 1 diabetes

Microalbuminuria develops in 20–30% of patients after 15 years.

Overt DN develops in 50% of patients with microalbuminuria.

Intensive monitoring and treatment of diabetes prevents microalbuminuria and halts its progression to overt nephropathy.

After 30 years of type 1 diabetes, the prevalence of ESRD used to be >15%. With intensive monitoring and treatment regimens, this proportion may be reduced to <9%.

Type 2 diabetes

The renal risk in patients with type 2 diabetes is the same as for type 1, whatever stage of DN (see below) is considered.

The benefits of tight glycemic and blood pressure control are identical to those shown in type 1 diabetes. They have been demonstrated in the UKPDS (UK Prospective Diabetes Study) that included >5000 patients.

More than 90% of diabetic patients who enter dialysis programs have type 2 diabetes. This proportion has steadily increased over the last decade.

However, a trend towards stabilization of the number of diabetics who reach ESRD is observed in countries with programs of aggressive diabetes management such as Denmark.

Genetic and environmental factors

A higher incidence of DN is observed in countries of Northern Europe and in the USA than in Southern Europe. This may be the consequence of genetic and/or environmental factors.

DN occurs with a higher frequency in certain ethnic groups (e.g. African-Americans, Indo-Asians in the UK, Pima Indians).

DN is more likely to develop in diabetic patients who have relatives with DN.

The incidence of DN peaks ~15 years after the onset of type 1 diabetes. By contrast with other microangiopathic complications such as proliferative retinopathy, new cases then become rare, which suggests that some patients are protected from the development of nephropathy.

Table 4.1.1 Definitions of abnormalities in albumin excretion (from the K/DOQI guidelines)

Category	Spot collection (mg/mmol creatinine)	24 h collection (mg/24 h)	Timed collection (μg/min)
Normoalbuminuria	<3	<30	<20
Microalbuminuria	3–30	30–300	20–200
Macroalbuminuria	>30	>300	>200

Because of variability in urinary albumin excretion, at least two specimens, preferably first morning void, collected within a 3–6 month period should be abnormal.

Pathology

DN is characterized by three cardinal pathological glomerular features:

- mesangial expansion;
- glomerular (and tubular) basement membrane thickening;
- nodular glomerular sclerosis.

Thickening of glomerular and tubular basement membranes leads to the typical nodular glomerular intercapillary lesions described by Kimmelstiel and Wilson in 1936, in type 2 diabetic patients with heavy proteinuria and renal failure accompanied by arterial hypertension (Fig. 4.1.1).

Progressive mesangial matrix expansion leading to glomerular sclerosis.

Other features include:

- arteriolar sclerosis with early afferent and efferent glomerular arteriolar hyalinosis;
- tubular atrophy and interstitial fibrosis;
- nonspecific linear staining for IgG in the glomerular and tubular basement membranes, and in Bowman's capsule on immunofluorescence microscopy.

Nephrosclerosis may be the predominant feature, particularly in older patients with type 2 diabetes who have arteriosclerotic vascular lesions, and little proteinuria.

Nephrosclerosis includes arteriolar injury, focal and segmental glomerular sclerosis (with much lesser matrix expansion than in DN), and interstitial injury.

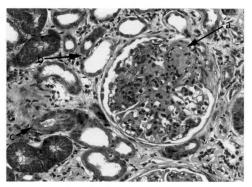

Fig. 4.1.1 Typical lesions of DN with (a) diffuse and nodular glomerulosclerosis, (b) interstitial fibrosis with tubular atrophy, and (c) arteriolar sclerosis with lumen narrowing.

Pathogenesis

The development of diabetic renal disease is a multifactorial process involving several mechanisms.

Metabolic consequences of diabetes

The magnitude of hyperglycemia correlates with the functional and structural changes of diabetic nephropathy.

Kidney enlargement, with glomerular enlargement is an early event in the course of diabetes-mediated renal injury. In animal models, it occurs as soon as 4 days after the initiation of diabetes.

Hyperglycemia stimulates mesangial cell matrix production and cell growth.

Hyperglycemia favors the formation of advanced glycation end-products (AGEs): glucose combines with free amino acids on circulating and tissue proteins to form AGEs. These products, which are normally excreted by the kidney, accumulate in diabetic patients, particularly in arteries and the kidneys where they promote matrix accumulation.

Glomerular hemodynamics

Glomerular hypertension and hyperfiltration are early events in the course of DN: a GFR 25–50% above normal is observed in 50% of patients with type 1 diabetes of <5 years duration.

Systemic hypertension leads to glomerular hypertension.

These glomerular hemodynamic alterations lead to arteriolar and glomerular sclerosis.

Activation of the renin–angiotensin–aldosterone system (RAAS)

Activation of components of the local renal RAAS in diabetes has been demonstrated in animal models and in humans, even though circulating levels of components of the RAAS may be low or normal.

Local RAAS activation promotes cell growth and matrix accumulation in all compartments of the kidney.

RAAS inhibition has been shown to be protective against the development and progression of DN. This is true at each level of the RAAS: renin inhibitors, ACEIs, ARBs, and antialdosterone agents have all been shown to be protective against the development of DN at some stage, either in humans or in experimental models.

Proteinuria

Initially, microalbuminuria arises from glomerular injury and evolves towards macroproteinuria.

As in other types of chronic kidney diseases, proteinuria has deleterious effects *per se*, inducing tubular injury and interstitial fibrosis.

Nephroprotection may be obtained by reducing proteinuria through lowering blood pressure (and therefore intraglomerular pressure) and antagonizing the RAAS.

Role of podocytes

Podocyte function is altered in diabetic patients, with reduced expression of nephrin, a glomerular slit-diaphragm protein which has a central role in the permeability of the glomerulus to proteins.

Natural history of diabetic nephropathy

Overview

Progressive renal injury from diabetes has been classified by Mogensen into five stages (summarized in Table 4.1.2).

In the early stages, glomerular hyperfiltration and kidney hypertrophy result from hyperglycemia.

Renal lesions develop during a clinically and biologically silent phase of several years.

Microalbuminuria and high blood pressure are the consequences of the glomerular and arterial lesions that develop during 10–20 years of diabetes-induced injury.

The evolution of DN with typical pathological features leads to macroalbuminuria and high blood pressure which result in decreasing GFR.

This evolution is observed preferentially in type 1 diabetes.

The evolution of DN in type 2 diabetes is less predictable, partly because DN develops later in life after a hypertensive

Table 4.1.2 Stages of diabetic nephropathy according to Mogensen

Stage	Duration of diabetes	Clinical, biological and pathological signs related to renal disease
1	At diagnosis	No clinical or biological signs of renal injury Hypertrophy of the kidneys Glomerular hyperfiltration
2	2–5 years	Clinically and biologically 'silent' nephropathy
3	5–10 years	Early nephropathy: • Microalbuminuria • High blood pressure • Normal GFR
4	10–20 years	Established diabetic nephropathy: • Macroalbuminuria • High blood pressure • Decreasing GFR • Pathology: mesangial expansion; GBM thickening; and glomerular sclerosis
5	>20 years	End-stage renal disease • Pathology: advanced fibrosis of the kidneys Need for: • Renal transplant (± pancreas) • Peritoneal dialysis • Hemodialysis

phase and in association with exposure to other cardiovascular risk factors, which are deleterious in themselves.

From microalbuminuria to macroalbuminuria

Type 1 diabetes
The prevalence of microalbuminuria ranges from 30 to 50%. The evolution from microalbuminuria to overt nephropathy is variable.

If microalbuminuria develops within the first 10 years of type 1 diabetes, progression to macroalbuminuria is very likely.

If microalbuminuria develops later in the course of type 1 diabetes, progression may occur in only ~20–50% of patients.

Patients who progress from normoalbuminuria to microalbuminuria or microalbuminuria to macroalbuminuria are more likely to have higher hemoglobin A1$_C$ (HbA1$_C$) values and higher blood pressure than nonprogressors.

Regression of microalbuminuria may be achieved in 50% of patients with good control of glycemia, blood pressure, and cholesterol levels, and in those with microalbuminuria of short duration.

Type 2 diabetes
The evolution from microalbuminuria to overt nephropathy occurs in 20–40% of patients over 10 years.

In both type 1 and 2 diabetes
Several factors favor the development and progression of microalbuminuria:
• hyperglycemia;
• onset of type 1 diabetes before the age of 20 years;
• hypertension;
• cigarette smoking;

• male gender;
• ethnicity (more frequent in Indo-Asians, African Americans and Pima Indians in the USA);
• familial clustering;
• socioeconomic factors (poverty) may compound ethnic factors, and lead to poor control of glycemia, blood pressure, and other determinants of the occurrence of microalbuminuria and DN.

Renal pathologic changes in microalbuminuric patients can range from relatively normal histologic findings to clear evidence of diabetic nephropathy.

Evolution of established diabetic nephropathy: from macroalbuminuria to CKD stage 5

Once established (i.e. at macroproteinuric stages), DN may progress with increasing proteinuria and a median GFR loss as great as 1 mL/min/month.

All factors cited as favouring the development and progression of microalbuminuria may contribute to a steeper progression of DN.

Most important factors are:
• blood pressure control;
• the magnitude of proteinuria;
• glycemic control (HbA1C).

Therapeutic interventions may slow or even halt the progression of DN (see below).

Diagnosis

Detection of renal injury in diabetics
In all patients with diabetes, dipstick urinalysis for protein should be performed yearly:
• if no protein is detected in the urine by dipstick, microalbuminuria should be measured;
• if proteinuria is present, the potential diagnosis of DN should be investigated.

Positive diagnosis of microalbuminuria
Microalbuminuria should be measured in at least two out of three consecutive sterile urine samples. Use of the albumin:creatinine ratio in an untimed urine sample is the preferred screening strategy (Table 4.1.1).

The magnitude of microalbuminuria can be variable in an individual because of confounding factors such as:
• exercise;
• infection;
• fever;
• marked hyperglycemia;
• pregnancy and menstruation;
• urinary tract infection.

These should all be excluded before interpretation of microalbuminuria is attempted.

Diagnosis of DN
The diagnosis of DN relies on clinical and simple biological criteria and does not require a renal biopsy in most cases.

Patients with type 1 diabetes
A diagnosis of DN can be made in the presence of:
• proteinuria;
• retinopathy;
• diabetes of >10 years duration.

If these criteria are not fulfilled, a renal biopsy may be necessary.

Patients with type 2 diabetes
A diagnosis of DN can be made if the above criteria are present. However, retinopathy may be absent, and the date of onset of type 2 diabetes is often uncertain.

Nephrosclerosis may present with the same clinical and biological features as DN. However, the distinction between these 2 types of renal insult has no significant influence on therapeutic goals (see below).

Indications for renal biopsy
Renal biopsy should be considered in the following circumstances:
- absence of retinopathy in patients with type 1 diabetes (type 2 diabetics can have DN without retinopathy);
- clinical and/or paraclinical signs which may suggest another cause of secondary glomerular disease (e.g. inflammatory joint disease, monoclonal gammapathy, positive lupus antibodies, etc.);
- rapidly progressing glomerular disease;
- active urine sediment containing red cells and cellular casts;
- massive proteinuria or proteinuria of rapid onset, as may be seen in amyloidosis or glomerular diseases such as minimal change disease and membranous nephropathy;
- increase of serum creatinine after administration of ACEI or ARB, after exclusion of renovascular disease;
- in proteinuric patients with type 1 diabetes of short duration (<10 years), renal biopsy might be discussed.

Special investigations
Ocular fundus examination
This should be performed in all diabetic patients with renal disease, since the presence of retinopathy demonstrates the presence of diabetes-related microangiopathy, and, therefore, supports a diagnosis of DN.

Duplex Doppler ultrasonography
Renal artery stenosis may be present in patients with diabetes, particularly type 2. It should be screened by Doppler ultrasonography or MR angiography if:
- serum creatinine increases by >20–30% after administration of ACEIs or ARBs.
- hypertension resolves dramatically after administration of ACEIs or ARBs.

Therapeutic management
Goals
In diabetics without albuminuria, glycemic control is the main therapeutic target

In patients with overt DN, blood pressure control and proteinuria reduction are the most important goals.

Glycemic control
Aim for $HbA1_C$ of 6.5%.

In type 1 diabetes, intensive insulin treatment is necessary when microalbuminuria or DN are present.

In type 2 diabetes:
- the benefits of intensive therapy are independent of the type of treatment administered;
- metformin should be discontinued when the GFR falls to <40 mL/min, because of the increased risk of metabolic acidosis;
- discontinuation of sulfonylureas should be considered when the GFR falls to <30 mL/min, because of the risk of hypoglycemia;

- meglitinides may be used in patients with impaired renal function, because of their hepatic elimination;
- thiazolidinediones may be used if the GFR is <30 mL/min, but there are limited data about their safety;
- insulin is often necessary to achieve optimal glycemic control.

Blood pressure control
Aim for ≤130/80 mmHg.

Avoid a systolic BP of <110 mmHg.

In type 1 diabetes, ACEIs should be used first.

In type 2 diabetes, ARBs should be used first.

If the target of 130/80 mmHg is not achieved, a combination of ACEIs and ARBs should be considered.

In all cases, start with a low dose (e.g. enalapril 2.5 mg/day, ramipril 1.25 mg/day for ACEIs, losartan 25 mg/day, irbesartan 75 mg/day for ARB), monitor renal function and serum K^+ after 5–10 days, and increase treatment progressively with monitoring.

Diuretics should be used as third-line therapy, either thiazides (if GFR >30 mL/min) or loop diuretics (if GFR <30 mL/min).

Other antihypertensive agents may be used, including calcium antagonists and β-blockers.

In some patients drugs from four to five different therapeutic classes will be required to achieve the target BP.

Reduction of proteinuria
In patients with microalbuminuria, the lowest albumin excretion rate is the best.

In patients with DN, aim for <0.5 g/24 h or 50 mg/mmol creatinine.

The magnitude of proteinuria is dependent on the level of blood pressure.

At similar levels of blood pressure reduction, inhibitors of the RAAS have a greater impact on proteinuria.

Moderate salt restriction (4–6 g/24 h (Na^+ <100 mmol/day)) increases the antiproteinuric effect of RAAS inhibitors.

Future therapies: additional inhibition of the RAAS using renin and aldosterone antagonists (aliskiren and eplerenone respectively) may be recommended in the near future depending on the results of ongoing clinical trials.

Cardiovascular risk
Diabetic patients with DN are at very high cardiovascular risk.

Aim for LDL-cholesterol of ≤3 mmol/L (≤100 mg/dL).

Dietary advice is necessary.

Statins need to be used in many patients to reach the target LDL-cholesterol.

Lifestyle modifications and diet
Smoking cessation should be strongly encouraged: The deleterious effect of active smoking on the progression of DN has been demonstrated in type 2 diabetes.

Moderate protein restriction (0.8 g/kg body weight/day) is recommended, although the effect of low protein diets to slow the progression of CKD and to decrease proteinuria is debated.

Moderate salt restriction (4–6 g/24 h (<100 mmol/day)) as stated above.

Increase dietary fruit and vegetable intake (at least five portions of either type per day).

Avoid malnutrition: The diet should provide ≥30 kcal/kg/day, unless weight reduction is needed.

Weight reduction should be encouraged in obese type 2 diabetics.

Regular exercise should be encouraged.

Follow-up

Patients with DN and CKD 1–3 can be followed up in primary care.

Patients with progressive renal decline and CKD 4/5 require ongoing nephrological review on a 2–6-monthly basis dependent upon their eGFR.

Pregnancy

As with other chronic glomerular diseases, pregnancy-related complications in diabetic nephropathy are increased when there is:

- renal impairment;
- proteinuria (>1 g/24 h);
- hypertension.

The risk of rapidly progressing retinopathy is a particular concern.

Patients with high risk clinical profiles should be offered preconception counselling and when pregnant careful monitoring in a combined renal–obstetric clinic.

Patient advice

General

As with all causes of chronic kidney disease patients with diabetic nephropathy and CKD 3–5 must pay close attention to cardiovascular risk and:

- monitor blood sugar and adapt insulin therapy as needed;
- stop smoking;
- eat a healthy and balanced diet (see above);
- take regular exercise.

Information and support

Resources and information for patients with diabetic nephropathy may be found at the following web sites:

UK Renal Association:

http://www.renal.org/

Diabetes UK:

http://www.diabetes.org.uk/

National Kidney Foundation (US):

http://www.kidney.org/patients/

American Diabetes Association:

http://www.diabetes.org/

Further reading

Brenner BM, Cooper ME, et al. Effects of losartan on renal and cardiovascular outcomes in patients with type 2 diabetes and nephropathy. N Engl J Med 2001; **345**: 861–869.

Genuth S, Eastman R, et al. Implications of the United kingdom prospective diabetes study. Diabetes Care 2003; **6**(Suppl 1): S28–32

K/DOQI Clinical Practice Guidelines and Clinical Practice Recommendations for Diabetes and Chronic Kidney Disease. Am J Kidney Dis 2007; **49**: S1–S179.

Lewis EJ, Hunsicker LG, et al. The effect of angiotensin-converting-enzyme inhibition on diabetic nephropathy. The Collaborative Study Group. N Engl J Med 1993; **329**: 1456–1462.

Lewis EJ, Hunsicker LG, et al. Renoprotective effect of the angiotensin-receptor antagonist irbesartan in patients with nephropathy due to type 2 diabetes. N Engl J Med 2001; **345**: 851–860.

Nathan DM, Cleary PA, et al. Intensive diabetes treatment and cardiovascular disease in patients with type 1 diabetes. N Engl J Med 2005; **353**: 2643–2653.

Internet resources

National Diabetes Support Team, UK, guidelines:

http://www.diabetes.nhs.uk/downloads/NICE_and_Diabetes.pdf

Canadian diabetes guidelines:

http://www.diabetes.ca/

UK Renal Association guidelines contain guidelines for diabetic patients with CKD:

http://www.renal.org/CKDguide/full/CKDprintedfullguide.pdf

United States National Kidney Foundation KDOQI guidelines:

http://www.kidney.org/professionals/kdoqi/guideline_diabetes/

Association de Langue Française pour l'étude du Diabète et des Maladies Metaboliques (in French):

http://www.alfediam.org

Amyloid and immunotactoid glomerulopathy

Amyloidosis is a multisystem clinical disorder caused by extracellular deposition of insoluble abnormal fibrils, derived from the aggregation of a misfolded, normally soluble, protein.

Amyloid is diagnosed on the basis of its pathognomonic red-green birefringence when an affected tissue biopsy is viewed under cross polarized light after staining with Congo Red.

Amyloid fibrils of all types are 8–12 nm in diameter and always express a ligand that binds the normal plasma protein, serum amyloid P component (SAP).

Renal amyloidosis can result from a number of amyloid precursors, most commonly:
- monoclonal Ig light chains (AL amyloidosis);
- serum amyloid A protein (SAA) (AA amyloidosis);

and less commonly:
- fibrinogen Aα chain;
- transthyretin;
- lysozyme;
- apolipoprotein AI;
- apolipoprotein AII;
- gelsolin.

The organized deposition of immunoglobulin components can also result in Congo Red-negative organized deposits that display two characteristic patterns on EM:
- fibrils that are randomly arranged (fibrillary glomerulopathy (FGN));
- microtubules that are usually larger, have a hollow core, and are ordered in parallel arrays (immunotactoid glomerulopathy (ITG)).

In ITG the microtubules are usually >30 nm in diameter and the glomerular Ig deposits are monoclonal, whereas in FGN the fibrils are usually 12–30 nm in diameter and are derived from polyclonal, subclass restricted IgG.

An overt B-cell proliferative disorder is evident in up to 50% of ITG cases.

Immunoglobulin-associated glomerulopathies

The recognized spectrum of renal diseases characterized by deposition or precipitation of monoclonal immunoglobulin (Ig) and related material has expanded dramatically in recent years.

The precise diagnosis can only be determined after detailed examination of renal tissue by both light and electron microscopy (EM), the latter defining two broad disease categories:

Organized deposits which include:
- systemic AL ('light chain') amyloidosis;
- fibrillary glomerulonephritis (FGN);
- immunotactoid glomerulopathy (ITG).

Nonorganized deposits referred to as:
- monoclonal immunoglobulin deposition diseases (MIDD) (discussed further in Chapter 4.3).

Epidemiology
AL amyloid deposits are identified in ~2% of native adult kidney biopsies compared to ITG which comprises <0.1%.

The peak age of diagnosis of AL amyloidosis and ITG is ~60 years.

Etiology
The fibrils in AL amyloid deposits and the microtubules in ITG deposits are derived from monoclonal immunoglobulins or fragments thereof.

The B-cell dyscrasias that underlie AL amyloidosis and ITG are frequently very subtle. In contrast, minor clinically insignificant AL amyloid deposits occur in 15% of patients with symptomatic myeloma.

AL amyloid may be deposited in almost any organ in the body, whereas the deposits in ITG are generally limited to the kidneys.

The propensity for certain monoclonal immunoglobulins to form either amyloid fibrils or microtubules is determined by their intrinsic physicochemical properties.

The pattern of organ involvement in AL amyloidosis is also, in part, governed by intrinsic properties of the particular monoclonal amyloidogenic light chain.

Clinical features
AL amyloidosis
Symptoms in AL amyloidosis depend on which organs are involved, and this varies enormously.

Weight loss and general malaise are common.

Involvement of the heart, liver, peripheral nerves and tongue causes restrictive cardiomyopathy, hepatomegaly, peripheral sensorimotor neuropathy, and macroglossia respectively.

There may be autonomic nerve involvement causing postural hypotension, gastrointestinal disturbances and erectile dysfunction.

Gut involvement may cause bleeding and occasionally bowel obstruction.

Approximately 50% of patients with AL amyloidosis have renal manifestations, usually nephrotic syndrome, which may be accompanied by varying degrees of chronic kidney disease (CKD).

Proteinuria can be >20 g/24 h and microscopic hematuria is not infrequent.

Occasionally, patients with predominantly tubulo-interstitial amyloid deposits progress to advanced CKD in the absence of heavy proteinuria.

The clinical signs of systemic AL amyloidosis are protean and the majority are not specific for the disease, including those of restrictive cardiomyopathy, nephrotic syndrome, hepatomegaly, splenomegaly and peripheral neuropathy.

Certain signs are almost pathognomonic of AL amyloidosis such as macroglossia and recurrent periorbital purpurae.

Immunotactoid glomerulopathy and fibrillary glomerulonephritis
ITG and FGN usually present with nephrotic syndrome and CKD.

Extra-renal involvement is rare but microtubular deposits have been reported in the skin, peripheral nerve, lung, liver, and in the cytoplasm of circulating or bone marrow lymphocytes in ITG associated with chronic lymphocytic leukemia or non-Hodgkin B-cell lymphomas.

Table 4.2.1 Comparison of histological features in immunoglobulin deposition diseases of the kidney

	Fibrillary GN	Immunotactoid glomerulopathy	AL (light chain) amyloid	Monoclonal immunoglobulin deposition diseases (MIDD)
Red-green birefringence with Congo Red staining	Negative	Negative	Positive	Negative
Light microscopy	MCGN Mesangial proliferation	Atypical membranous GN Lobular MCGN	Predominant mesangial deposits	Nodular glomerulosclerosis Tubular basement membrane deposits
Immunohistochemistry	Polyclonal IgG deposits of γ4 isotype	Coarse granular mono-typic IgG (IgG1, or IgG2, or IgG3) and C3 deposits	Monotypic light or heavy chain deposits, λ > κ	Monotypic light or heavy chain deposits, κ > λ
Electron microscopy	Organized but randomly arranged fibrils, usually ~20 nm in diameter	Hollow microtubules, usually >30 nm in diameter, ordered in parallel	Organized but randomly arranged fibrils, 8–12 nm in diameter	Nonorganized granular electron-dense deposits

GN, glomerulonephritis; MCGN, mesangiocapillary GN.

The signs of ITG and FGN are usually those of the nephrotic syndrome.

Renal biopsy

Histological diagnosis of amyloid requires staining of the tissue deposits with Congo Red and demonstration of pathognomonic red–green dichroism when viewed in cross-polarized light. The lesions of ITG and FGN are Congo Red negative.

A renal biopsy is the most frequent diagnostic test.

Renal AL amyloid deposits are typically found in the mesangium, along the glomerular basement membrane (GBM) and in the blood vessels but are also often present in the tubules and interstitium.

However, there is a significant rate of false-positive and false-negative diagnoses, owing to sampling errors and inadequate preparation, staining and interpretation.

The presence of SAP within deposits, identified by immunohistochemistry (optimally using frozen sections) and/or immunogold labelling, also distinguishes amyloid (including AA and hereditary forms) from ITG and MIDD.

The basis of a report of SAP within the deposits of FGN is unclear.

Amyloid deposits identified histologically must be further characterized immunohistochemically to identify the particular amyloid fibril type, of which there are ~20.

Renal involvement by amyloid occurs in amyloidosis associated with the following amyloid fibrils:
- AL;
- AA;
- fibrinogen Aα chain;
- transthyretin;
- lysozyme;
- apolipoprotein AI;
- apolipoprotein AII;
- gelsolin.

Commercially available antibodies to serum amyloid A protein (SAA), transthyretin (TTR) and β2-micro-globulin

generally yield definitive results, but AL deposits are stained with standard antisera to κ or λ light chains in only ~50% of fixed biopsies.

Confirmation of AL amyloidosis therefore commonly requires exclusion of other types through an immunohistochemical panel and sequencing of the genes associated with hereditary systemic amyloidosis.

Differentiating between the various immunoglobulin-related glomerulopathies can be difficult (Table 4.2.1).

Light microscopy

ITG and FGN are characterized by atypical membranous GN lesions or lobular mesangiocapillary GN but there may be mesangial proliferation, crescents or sclerosing GN.

MIDD is characterized by Congo Red-negative nodular glomerulosclerosis and deposition of periodic acid–Schiff (PAS) positive material in the tubular basement membrane.

Immunofluorescence (IF) microscopy

Immunofluorescence in ITG should include not only standard antisera to κ and λ light chains, but also antisera to IgG subclasses, in order to demonstrate clonality. IF will reveal coarse granular staining for IgG (IgG1, or IgG2, or IgG3) and C3 along the capillary basement membranes and in the mesangium. In both ITG and AL amyloidosis the Ig deposits are clonal and therefore always have a monotypic light chain (κ or λ), although this is not always demonstrable by immunohistochemistry.

In FGN, polyclonal IgG deposits of the κ4 isotype are typical.

In MIDD, IF reveals monotypic light or heavy chain deposits along glomerular and/or tubular basement membranes, more commonly κ than λ isotype.

Electron microscopy

In ITG there are typically large (>30 nm) (Fig. 4.2.1C) thick-walled microtubular (hollow) fibrils with hollow, lucent centers arranged in parallel arrays, compared with small (8–12 nm) organized solid fibrils without a lucent core in amyloidosis (Fig. 4.2.1A) and organized but randomly arranged fibrils of 12–30 nm in FGN (Fig. 4.2.1B).

Electron microscopy in MIDD shows nonorganized granular electron-dense deposits in the glomerulus and along tubular basement membranes.

Tests for cryoglobulins should be undertaken in all cases in which microtubular renal deposits are identified.

General investigations

Discovery of AL amyloid deposits should be followed by a careful assessment of renal, hepatic, cardiac and peripheral and autonomic nerve function. ITG and FGN almost always have renal-limited manifestations.

Imaging for soft tissue or lymph node involvement by amyloid may be indicated by the clinical features.

Special investigations

All patients with AL amyloidosis or ITG should undergo comprehensive investigation for an underlying clonal B-cell dyscrasia, which may be extremely subtle.

Electrophoresis and immunofixation of blood and urine are mandatory.

Serum free light chain assay

A high sensitivity serum free light chain assay has recently been developed which can quantify circulating free immunoglobulin light chains with a remarkable sensitivity of <5 mg/L.

The serum free light chain assay has increased identification of an underlying clonal B-cell dyscrasia from ~80% to >95% in patients with systemic AL amyloidosis, and it is frequently the only quantitative measure of clonal response to treatment.

[123I]SAP scintigraphy

This was developed and is routinely available at the National Amyloidosis Centre, UK. The scan identifies the presence, distribution and extent of amyloid deposits in systemic amyloidosis.

Serial SAP scans monitor progress, and have shown that amyloid deposits often regress when the supply of the respective amyloid fibril precursor protein is sufficiently reduced (Fig. 4.2.2).

SAP scans are negative in Congo Red-negative fibrillary glomerulopathies and nonorganized MIDD, providing valuable corroborative support of this diagnosis.

Natural history

Without treatment, AL amyloidosis is inexorably progressive and almost always fatal with a median survival of only 6–15 months.

Diagnosis of renal AL amyloidosis is associated with a median time to renal replacement therapy (RRT) of ~1 year in the absence of effective chemotherapy, and median survival on dialysis is only 8 months.

ITG and FGN are generally renal-limited and more slowly progressive diseases, with the median time from diagnosis to RRT >2 years and with a markedly better overall prognosis than AL amyloidosis.

Approximately 20% of patients with kidney dysfunction due to renal AL amyloid deposits eventually develop ESRD.

The outcome of AL amyloidosis can be dramatically improved by chemotherapy that suppresses monoclonal Ig production. This can halt disease progression and may facilitate regression of amyloid.

There may be complete resolution of the nephrotic syndrome following effective chemotherapy in AL

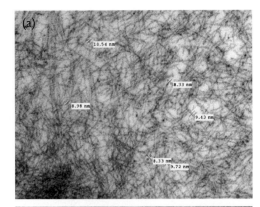

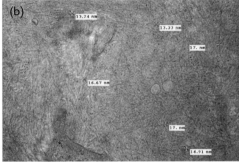

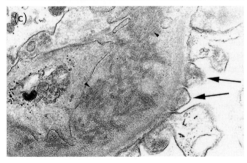

Fig. 4.2.1 Electron micrographs demonstrating the fibrils of (a) amyloidosis (randomly arranged 8–12 nm in diameter), (b) fibrillary glomerulonephritis (randomly arranged 12–30 nm in diameter), and (c) immunotactoid glomerulopathy (parallel arrays, hollow centred microtubules (arrowheads) >30 nm in diameter).

amyloidosis, and progression of CKD may be substantially retarded.

50% of patients with ITG or FGN reach ESRD. However, marked improvement in nephrotic-range proteinuria and renal excretory function have been reported following chemotherapy in patients with ITG (or FGN).

Recurrence after renal transplantation

Amyloid deposits may recur in the renal allograft.

Suppression of monoclonal light chain production by chemotherapy reduces the risk of graft amyloid.

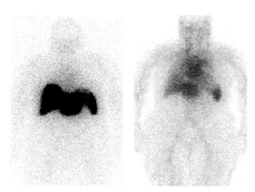

Fig. 4.2.2 Serial anterior whole body scintigraphs in a patient with AL amyloidosis treated with oral melphalan and corticosteroids: baseline scan (*left*) showed extensive amyloid deposits in the liver and spleen obscuring the signal from the kidneys; follow-up scintigraphy 6 months later (*right*) showed complete regression of amyloid from the liver and marked regression from the spleen with a reciprocal increase in the blood-pool signal.

Microscopic amyloid deposits frequently develop within the graft when monoclonal light chain production is not completely suppressed, but often these do not impair graft function.

Five-year patient and renal allograft survival among patients with AL amyloidosis visiting the UK National Amyloidosis Centre is ~70%, probably reflecting careful selection of patients for transplantation.

There is very little literature on renal transplantation in ITG or FGN. Early recurrence in a renal allograft with subsequent response to chemotherapy has been reported.

Risk stratification

Poor prognostic features in AL amyloidosis include:

- cardiac involvement;
- extensive liver involvement;
- peripheral neuropathy;
- symptomatic autonomic neuropathy.

Median survival with predominant cardiac disease is <1 year from diagnosis.

Creatinine clearance at the time of diagnosis of amyloidosis or ITG influence the renal prognosis.

Risk of treatment-related mortality (TRM) with high-dose melphalan and autologous stem cell transplantation (SCT) in AL amyloidosis is strongly influenced by:

- ECOG (Eastern Cooperative Oncology Group) performance status;
- the number of organs involved by amyloid;
- the extent of cardiac involvement.

Pharmacological treatment

In many patients with systemic AL amyloidosis, suppression of the B-cells producing amyloidogenic monoclonal immunoglobulin light chains through chemotherapy is associated with:

- reduction of new amyloid formation;
- regression of existing deposits;
- preservation of organ function;
- enhanced survival.

However, patients with AL amyloidosis often tolerate chemotherapy poorly, some are refractory, and clinical benefit after effective chemotherapy is always delayed.

Oral melphalan and prednisolone
This is well-tolerated but responses are slow and limited, and this treatment should be reserved for older, sicker patients.

Oral intermediate dose combinations
Includes cyclophosphamide, thalidomide and dexamethasone (CTD), and melphalan and dexamethasone (Mel Dex).

They induce swifter clonal responses in >50% of cases.

High-dose melphalan chemotherapy with autologous peripheral stem-cell rescue
This may achieve even higher clonal response rates, but at the expense of TRM of 12–25%, limiting its appeal as first line treatment to highly selected, fitter patients.

Other agents
Rituximab may be used in patients with CD20-positive (usually IgM) clones.

The proteasome inhibitor, bortezomib, and lenalidomide have also been used.

Frequent satisfactory responses to intermediate intensity chemotherapy indicate that high dose treatment is unnecessary in many patients. However, there been very few comparative trials of chemotherapy in AL amyloidosis.

The fundamental objective of treatment in AL amyloidosis is to adequately suppress production of amyloidogenic free light chains without unacceptable toxicity. This requires tailored individual treatment and close monitoring.

In ITG, chemotherapy aimed at suppressing the underlying B-cell clone is also rational although there is a much smaller body of evidence than in AL amyloidosis. Renal benefit has been reported when hematological remission is achieved.

Follow-up

The underlying clonal dyscrasia and amyloidotic organ function require regular monitoring following chemotherapy in patients with AL amyloidosis and ITG, with the expectation that the disease is likely to relapse at some stage.

AA amyloidosis

Epidemiology
The prevalence of AA amyloidosis in postmortem studies is 0.50–0.86%.

In developed countries ~70% of cases are found in patients with autoimmune inflammatory diseases (most commonly juvenile and adult rheumatoid arthritis).

Heredofamilial forms account for 10% of cases.

In developing countries chronic infection still accounts for the majority of cases.

Etiology
AA protein is a proteolytic fragment of serum amyloid A (SAA) protein.

SAA has several isoforms of which SAA1 and SAA2 are the acute phase isoforms. They are apolipoproteins that associate with HDL and are thought to enhance the affinity of HDL for macrophages during an acute phase response.

Persistence of an acute phase response causes persistent production and elevated serum levels of SAA1 and SAA2 (probably via proinflammatory cytokines IL-1, IL-6 and TNF-α).

Subsequent proteolytic cleavage of SAA by macrophages generates amyloidogenic peptides (AA) which then aggregate to form fibrils.

Although elevated serum SAA levels are required for the development of AA amyloidosis, it is unclear why only ~5% of patients with a persistent inflammatory response develop AA amyloidosis.

There is speculation that polymorphisms in SAA genes may determine the risk of developing AA amyloidosis. This may partially explain the geographical variability in AA amyloidosis risk in patients with chronic inflammatory disease. For instance the SAA1.3 allele has been shown to be associated with the development of AA amyloidosis and is a predictor of poor outcome for Japanese patients with rheumatoid arthritis.

The major causes of AA amyloidosis are listed in Table 4.2.2.

The heredofamilial forms of AA amyloidosis will be described later.

Table 4.2.2 Conditions associated with AA amyloidosis

Chronic inflammatory disease
Rheumatoid arthritis
Juvenile rheumatoid arthritis
Ankylosing spondylitis
Reiter syndrome
Behçet syndrome
Crohn's disease
Chronic infection
Tuberculosis
Leprosy
Osteomyelitis
Bronchiectasis
Cystic fibrosis
Malignant disease
Lymphoma
Castleman disease
Renal cell carcinoma
Hairy cell leukemia
Heredofamilial disease
Familial Mediterranean fever
Muckle–Wells syndrome
TRAPS

Clinical features

Renal

The kidney is affected in almost all patients with AA amyloidosis.

Approximately 95% of patients with renal AA amyloidosis will have glomerular involvement but amyloid deposition within the interstitium is equally common. The presentation may vary from low grade proteinuria to severe nephrotic syndrome.

Invisible hematuria is present in about one-third of patients.

A small minority have predominantly vascular deposits and present with progressive renal dysfunction and little proteinuria.

Extra-renal

Amyloid deposition in other sites can be clinically important.

These other sites include:
- spleen always involved first but usually asymptomatic (occasional functional hyposplenism);
- gastrointestinal tract 20% (diarrhea, constipation, malabsorption, GI bleeding). A feature of advanced disease;
- liver 15% (hepatomegaly) in advanced disease.
- adrenal glands 50–60% (abnormal synacthen test in ~50% of patients);
- heart (extremely rarely clinically significant).

Skin, tongue, and nerve involvement is rare in AA amyloidosis (in contrast to AL amyloidosis).

Investigations

The best approach for diagnosing AA amyloidosis remains controversial.

Renal biopsy is diagnostic in virtually all patients with renal manifestations. The renal biopsy features of amyloidosis have been described previously.

However, renal biopsy involves a small but definite risk and therefore less invasive biopsy options have been advocated.

Biopsies of salivary glands, abdominal fat, and rectal mucosa (full thickness biopsy is required) have a diagnostic yield of up to 80%.

The identification of amyloid on a biopsy requires further characterization to differentiate it from other forms of amyloidosis.

Immunohistochemical staining for SAA protein using commercially available antibodies is diagnostic in nearly all cases of AA amyloidosis.

[^{123}I]SAP scintigraphy can also be used to assess the distribution and extent of AA amyloid deposits, and to monitor the response to treatment.

Natural history

Patients with AA amyloidosis usually survive longer than those with AL amyloidosis (40% 3 year survival, median survival 24–50 months).

Causes of death include infection (currently the major cause accounting for 40–50% of deaths), dialysis-related complications, bowel perforation, GI bleeding, and myocardial infarction.

Poor prognostic factors include:
- low serum albumin;
- significant proteinuria;
- raised serum SAA;
- raised CRP.

The level of SAA predicts outcome.

Estimated 10 year survivals are:
- 90% if median serum SAA levels <10 mg/L;
- 40% if median serum SAA levels >10 mg/L.

Recurrence after renal transplantation

Renal transplantation is reasonably successful in those with AA amyloidosis.

Recurrent amyloid deposition can occur in up to 33% of cases, although graft loss due to recurrent disease is uncommon. Recurrent amyloid can be avoided if serum SAA concentration is maintained at <10 mg/L.

Graft survival is comparable to that seen with nonamyloid recipients, but patient survival at 3 years is reduced (50% versus 80%) mainly due to infectious and cardiovascular disease.

Treatment

The goal of treatment is suppression of SAA synthesis by treatment of the underlying cause of chronic inflammation. This prevents further amyloid deposition and may lead to regression of existing deposits.

As indicated above, suppression of SAA synthesis improves outcome.

For infectious and malignant causes definitive treatment of the underlying disease (where possible) is clearly the most appropriate treatment.

For chronic inflammatory disease a number of treatment options appear to be effective.

Alkylating agents
In juvenile and adult rheumatoid arthritis, cyclophosphamide and chlorambucil have been shown to improve patient survival. In general these studies have demonstrated a 5 year survival of >70% with treatment compared to <30% without.

Colchicine
This has become accepted treatment for patients with familial Mediterranean fever (FMF) (see below).

It has never been formally studied in nonfamilial inflammatory AA amyloidosis although anecdotal reports have suggested benefit in patients with ankylosing spondylitis, ulcerative colitis, and Behçet disease.

The benefit of colchicine is almost certainly due to its anti-inflammatory effect although there have previously been suggestions of a direct effect on fibril formation.

Anticytokine therapy
Given the role of cytokines in the induction of SSA protein synthesis, inhibition of IL-1 and TNF-α is an attractive therapeutic option.

Although not yet formally studied, small series suggest that biologics with activity against proinflammatory cytokines suppress SAA production thereby permitting amyloid regression.

Heredofamilial disease causing AA amyloidosis

Familial Mediterranean fever (FMF)
FMF causes AA amyloidosis and is the commonest familial amyloidosis.

It is an autosomal recessive disorder most commonly found in Sephardic Jews and Armenians, but has been identified in a wide variety of ethnic groups.

It is caused by mutation of the gene encoding pyrin/marenostrin. This is an intranuclear regulator of transcription of inflammatory mediators, and also appears to regulate the activity of the inflammasome (a complex of proteins that triggers the release of IL-1β). Inflammasome dysregulation also underlies other autoinflammatory diseases including Muckle–Wells syndrome.

Patients typically have their first attack before the age of 20 years.

Features of an attack include:
• severe pain (due to serositis (peritonitis, pleuritis, synovitis))'
• fever (which typically persists for 1–3 days).

Attacks are accompanied by a substantial increase in acute phase reactants.

Usually patients will have recurrent attacks although the frequency can be very variable.

FMF is complicated by AA amyloidosis in up to 60% of patients. There is a substantial ethnic influence on this risk (Turks 60%, non-Ashkenazi Jews 30%, Armenians 2%).

Amyloidosis predominantly affects the kidneys, spleen, liver and gut.

Colchicine is the mainstay of treatment for FMF.

Over 80% of patients respond to 1–2 mg/day (i.e. a reduction in the frequency of attacks), and it has been shown to substantially reduce the risk of developing AA amyloidosis. It may also permit amyloid regression and reversal of nephrotic syndrome and/or prevent renal function decline in patients with established AA amyloidosis.

Others
Other familial inflammatory diseases that can underlie AA amyloidosis include:
• TNF receptor-1-associated periodic syndrome (TRAPS);
• hyper IgD syndrome;
• Muckle–Wells syndrome;
• familial cold autoinflammatory syndrome.

Hereditary amyloidosis

Hereditary renal amyloidosis is rare.

Mutations in a number of precursor proteins can result in relatively selective renal amyloid deposition.

Fibrinogen A alpha-chain
This is the commonest type of hereditary amyloidosis associated with nephropathy.

Four mutations of this gene have been identified, all of which are associated with renal disease.

The renal disease is exclusively glomerular with sparing of the interstitium and vessels.

Patients have been successfully managed with combined liver and kidney transplantation.

Transthyretin
More than 100 mutations have been identified in the transthyretin gene and most of these produce an amyloidogenic protein.

Different mutations result in different phenotypes: predominantly cardiomyopathic, neuropathic, and ocular forms have been described. Clinically significant renal amyloid is unusual.

Successful treatment with orthotopic liver transplantation has been described.

Gelsolin
Mutations in the gelsolin gene produce familial amyloidosis, Finnish type, which classically presents with corneal dystrophy, cranial neuropathy, and cutis laxa.

Renal and cardiac involvement can also occur, but is rarely clinically significant.

Apolipoprotein AI and AII

Apo AI mutations produce dominant nephropathy and/or cardiomyopathy. Liver, skin laryngeal, and nerve involvement may also appear.

A successful outcome from combined liver and kidney transplant has been described.

Apo AII mutations result in slowly progressive renal disease with both glomerular and interstitial involvement.

Lysozyme

Mutations in this gene produce predominant renal and GI/liver disease. The renal phenotype can be very variable even within families.

The only available treatment is supportive care.

The diagnosis of hereditary amyloidosis can be difficult since monoclonal gammopathy can be identified in 3% and 5% of patients above the age of 50 and 70 years respectively. Such patients may therefore be labelled as having AL amyloidosis.

10% of patients with a diagnosis of AL amyloidosis have been shown to have hereditary forms of amyloidosis.

Characterization of the amyloid type is of paramount importance therefore. This often requires both immuno-histochemical and genetic analysis to rule out hereditary amyloidosis.

This potentially may allow unnecessary chemotherapy to be avoided.

Future prospects

Elucidation of aspects of the molecular pathogenesis of amyloid and amyloidosis is leading to the development of novel treatments.

A small molecule glycosaminoglycan analogue, eprodisate, designed to inhibit the amyloidogenic interaction between SAA and glycosaminoglycans, has lately been reported to delay the onset of ESRD in AA amyloidosis in a randomized placebo-controlled trial.

Small molecule ligands that stabilize amyloid precursor proteins in the blood and inhibit their propensity to form fibrils are in clinical trial.

Other approaches to destabilizing and disrupting established amyloid deposits using antibodies and small molecule drugs are poised for study in man.

Further reading

Bridoux F, Hugue V, Coldefy O, et al. Fibrillary glomerulonephritis and immunotactoid (microtubular) glomerulopathy are associated with distinct immunologic features. *Kidney Int* 2002; **62**: 1764–1775.

Ivanyi B, Degrell P. Fibrillary glomerulonephritis and immunotactoid glomerulopathy. *Nephrol Dial Transplant* 2004; **19**: 2166–2170.

Lin J, Markowitz GS, Valeri AM, et al. Renal monoclonal immunoglobulin deposition disease: the disease spectrum. *J Am Soc Nephrol* 2001; **12**: 1482–1492.

Markowitz GS. Dysproteinemia and the kidney. *Adv Anat Pathol* 2004; **11**: 49–63.

Pepys MB. Amyloidosis. *Annu Rev Med* 2006; **57**: 223–241.

Internet resources

Amyloidosis Support Network:

http://www.amyloidosis.org/

UK National Amyloid Centre:

http://www.ucl.ac.uk/medicine/amyloidosis/nac/

See also

Immunological investigation of renal disease, p. 36

Infection-related glomerulonephritis, p. 128

Plasma cell dyscrasias, p. 158

Mixed cryoglobulinemia and hepatitis C infection, p. 176

Plasma cell dyscrasias

Malignant plasma cells produce abnormal immunoglobulin proteins which cause renal injury by a number of mechanisms (Table 4.3.1).

Table 4.3.1 Mechanisms of immunoglobulin-related renal injury

Primary mechanism	Secondary mechanism	Example
Excess IgM	Hyperviscosity	Waldenstrom's macroglobulinemia
Abnormal LC binding to THP	Blockage of distal tubule	Cast nephropathy
Binding to BM	Glomerular injury	Monoclonal Ig Deposition disease
IgM RhF binding to IgG	Immune complex formation	Cryoglobulinemia
Aggregation and binding	Tissue deposition	AL amyloid

LC, light chain; THP, Tamm–Horsfall protein; BM, basement membrane; Ig, immunoglobulin; RhF, rheumatoid factor; AL, light chain amyloid.

Disease syndromes

There are four important disease states driven by plasma cell dyscrasias:
- myeloma kidney;
- light chain (AL) amyloid;
- cryoglobulinemia;
- monoclonal immunoglobulin deposition disease (MIDD) and immunotactoid glomerulopathy (ITG).

These clinical syndromes result from the combination of the tumor load of the underlying plasma cell malignancy, and the secondary effects of the abnormal immunoglobulin protein.

The contribution of each to the illness varies. In patients with myeloma the illness is dominated by the effects of the malignant plasma cell clone, whereas in the AL amyloid the clone may be hard to detect and the illness is largely a consequence of the tissue deposition of the amyloid protein containing the abnormal light chain (LC).

Myeloma kidney

Myeloma is characterized by expansion of a malignant clone of plasma cells which:
- occupy >10% of the bone marrow;
- produce a paraprotein >30 g/L;
- suppress the production of normal immunoglobulins;
- cause damage by local effects on the skeleton and the bone marrow, and distally on the kidney.

It is an incurable disease with an incidence of 40 cases pmp per year.

It is more common in the elderly, males and Blacks.

Effects on the kidney (Table 4.3.2)

10% of patients who develop myeloma will suffer severe renal injury but 50% of newly diagnosed cases will have a degree of transient and reversible renal dysfunction at the time of diagnosis.

Table 4.3.2 Renal effects of myeloma

Clinical presentation	Cause
Acute kidney injury	Dehydration
	Hypercalcemia
	Infection
	Cast nephropathy
Chronic kidney disease	Cast nephropathy
	AL amyloid
	MIDD
Proteinuria	AL amyloid
	MIDD

This is often a consequence of dehydration, hypercalcemia or infection.

Clinical presentation, investigation and immediate management

Patients may be found to have renal dysfunction at the time myeloma is first diagnosed or when it relapses.

They usually present with the systemic effects of the plasma cell malignancy (malaise, weight loss, anemia, symptoms of hypercalcemia, or bone pain).

A number will present with isolated acute renal failure without obvious manifestations of myeloma. The diagnosis is made on renal biopsy or from the routine tests performed in patients with unexplained acute renal failure.

The diagnostic and staging investigations should include:
- FBC to assess marrow failure;
- bone marrow to assess infiltration;
- skeletal survey to determine the sites and extent of bone deposits;
- serum paraprotein and immunoglobulin concentrations;
- serum free LC concentrations;
- urine LC concentration.

Immediate management should include:
- rehydration;
- antibiotics for infection;
- intravenous bisphosphonates for hypercalcemia;
- blood transfusion for anemia.

Severe renal failure (eGFR <30 mL/min)

This occurs in 10% of patients with myeloma and is usually an early manifestation.

The cause is almost always cast nephropathy (Fig. 4.3.1).

Cast nephropathy develops when the excessive load of filtered abnormal LCs reacts with Tamm–Horsfall protein (THP) in the distal tubule to produce an insoluble plug. This blocks tubular flow, disrupts the tubule, and leads to interstitial injury which is usually permanent and seldom reversible.

This reaction depends on the property of the LC (i.e. whether it has an affinity for THP), the LC concentration, and a trigger which favors the reaction, e.g. hypercalcemia and dehydration.

Although cast nephropathy can only be confirmed from a renal biopsy the investigation is not essential if the diagnosis

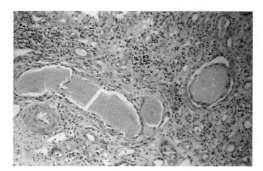

Fig. 4.3.1 Renal biopsy of cast nephropathy. The tubular casts have a 'fractured' appearance.

can be inferred and management decisions will not be affected by the lack of histological confirmation.

Initial treatment

The immediate aim is to reverse the renal failure or stop it progressing. This treatment is therefore urgent.

1. Counter the precipitants and aggravants.

- Rehydration.
- Treat hypercalcemia.
- Stop NSAIDs.

2. Reduce the load of light chains.

- Prescribe dexamethasone to suppress the malignant plasma cell clone.
- Consider plasma exchange. One clinical trial has shown no benefit but another is in progress.

Light chain concentrations can be reduced more effectively with a high flux dialysis technique. This treatment is being tested in a randomized trial.

Subsequent treatment

Once attempts at renal rescue have been made a medium and long-term management plan is needed.

1. Chemotherapy:

The treatment choice will be made by hematooncologists and will depend on whether the aim is palliation or remission induction. (Cure is rarely possible unless a bone marrow allograft is feasible.)

Melphalan doses should be reduced but cyclophosphamide and dexamethasone are used in conventional doses.

Thalidomide and its analogues can be used without dose reduction.

High dose chemotherapy with stem cell rescue is offered to selected, usually younger patients without major comorbidity but higher treatment-related mortality has to be expected.

2. Renal support:

Patients whose renal failure is complete and irreversible will require dialysis.

Because the presentation is usually acute, most patients will be treated by hemodialysis but there is no contraindication to peritoneal dialysis.

Both modalities carry an infection risk and myeloma patients are especially vulnerable because of hypogammaglobulinemia and leukopenia.

The issue of renal transplantation seldom arises but should only be undertaken if remission has been achieved. This will usually have required a stem cell autograft or a bone marrow allograft.

3. General support:

Anemia can be managed with ESAs (erythopoiesis-stimulating agents), there being no evidence that the plasma cell dyscrasias are 'driven' by erythropoietin. Response will be poor if there is marrow failure in which case regular blood transfusions will be needed.

Pain control, especially of skeletal deposits, requires careful administration of opiate analgesia and, in the absence of residual renal function, NSAIDs can be used.

Local myeloma deposits respond well to radiotherapy.

The prognosis of patients with myeloma and renal failure is poor – median survival is ~12 months so plans for palliative care should be put in place in advance of the inevitable irreversible complications or relapse.

AL amyloid

Amyloidosis is the disease caused by the systemic deposition of an insoluble protein consisting of a 'rogue' protein which has misfolded into fibrils and associated with serum amyloid P protein (SAP).

Certain LCs (λ in 70% of cases), produced by plasma cell dyscrasias have this rogue property and give rise to AL amyloid.

Renal biopsy will reveal abnormal glomeruli and/or blood vessels with featureless amorphous deposits that are Congo Red positive and have a fibrillary appearance on electron microscopy (Fig. 4.3.2).

Although AL amyloid is the most common form of systemic amyloid, 20% of cases have a different origin. A specific diagnosis is essential to plan appropriate management.

Unfortunately immunocytochemistry of renal biopsy material is unreliable in that the offending LC may not be stained. Similarly, the finding of a serum paraprotein is not diagnostic as the patient may have an incidental MGUS.

Amyloidosis is more common in the elderly (median age of presentation is ~60 years) and in men.

The most important affected systems are: kidney, heart, gut, liver, and peripheral nerves. Heart and gut involvement predict a poor prognosis.

Patients come to the attention of nephrologists when they develop heavy proteinuria or the nephrotic syndrome.

The plasma cell dyscrasia is not usually prominent and only a minority of patients have overt myeloma. Diagnosis should not therefore rely on bone marrow examination or conventional evidence of the presence of a paraprotein.

Diagnosis and monitoring of response to treatment now relies on estimates of serum free LC concentrations.

Treatment

This is generally aimed at neutralizing the abnormal plasma cell clone in the hope of reducing the amount of precursor LC available to produce further amyloid deposits.

Despite the insolubility of amyloid, tissue damage can be stabilized by halting the production of the offending LC.

Hematological remission is associated with an improved prognosis.

In practice the choice of treatment will be tailored to the individual patient depending on age, the number and extent of organ involvement and the presence or absence of myeloma. Indeed in some patients it is appropriate to do no more than provide support for organ failure.

In patients without extensive organ involvement the treatment choice is between high dose melphalan and PBSCT (peripheral blood stem cell support), or high dose combination chemotherapy, e.g. VAD (vincristine, adriamycin and dexamethasone).

Whether the higher treatment-related mortality of high dose melphalan is justified remains to be established.

Those patients who develop end-stage renal failure have a two-fold greater annual risk of death than the general dialysis population.

Renal transplantation is seldom a realistic option but there are cases of successful outcomes in individuals fortunate enough to receive both a marrow and a renal allograft.

Cryoglubulinemia

Cryoglobulins are so-called because of their tendency to precipitate at lower than body temperature: a dramatic *in vitro* phenomenon and a partial explanation of the microcirculatory problems that occur in the periphery.

They are classified according to their constituents (Table 4.3.3).

Types 1 and 2 are associated with plasma cell dyscrasias but the abnormal clone is recognized more from its product than its expansion.

It is type 2 that causes renal injury by the deposition of IgM/IgG complexes manifesting usually as a mesangiocapillary glomerulonephritis causing the nephritic and/or nephrotic syndromes.

The extrarenal manifestations are: lower limb purpura and ulceration, arthritis and a multifocal ischemic neuropathy (mononeuritis multiplex) caused by occlusion of the vasa nervorum.

The diagnosis will be suspected from the clinical presentation and confirmed by identification of the cryoglobulin in serum extracted from a blood sample allowed to clot at 37°C.

The constituents are identified by immunochemistry.

Table 4.3.3 Classification of cryoglobulins

Type	Constituent	Cause
1	Monoclonal IgG, IgM or IgA	Lymphoma Myeloma Waldenström's
2	Monoclonal IgM rheumatoid factor and polyclonal IgG	'Essential' Lymphoma Hepatitis C Sjögren's syndrome
3	Polyclonal IgM RhF and polyclonal IgG	SLE Rh arthritis Chronic infections Hepatitis B virus Hepatitis C virus Idiopathic

A quick screening test is the finding of a high titer rheumatoid factor and a low C4 level (evidence of activation of the classic complement pathway by the immune complexes).

A bone marrow examination may reveal clusters of monoclonal IgM (usually κ)-positive plasma cells.

Treatment is directed against the clone and the inflammation but because the condition is chronic and often indolent, corticosteroids, alkylating agents and plasma exchange/cryofiltration are only deployed during nephritic flares.

Patients with hepatitis C virus-associated disease are treated with interferon-α and those with underlying lymphomas with conventional chemotherapy.

Monoclonal Ig deposition disease and immunotactoid glomerulopathy

The deposition of monoclonal light or heavy chains on basement membranes is dependent on their particular physicochemical properties.

Monoclonal Ig deposition disease

LC deposition disease (LCDD), which is more common, is usually caused by an abnormal κ chain, and heavy chain deposition disease (HCDD) by either μ or γ chains.

The disease presents with the classic signs and symptoms of glomerular injury: proteinuria, hematuria, nephritic syndrome and renal impairment which often progresses rapidly.

The diagnosis is usually made with a renal biopsy.

The histological appearances are of a nodular glomerulosclerosis with both glomerular and tubular basement membrane thickening (Fig. 4.3.3).

The electron microscopic and immunohistochemical findings of ribbon-like deposits with chain-restricted reactivity are diagnostic (Fig. 4.3.3).

A plasma cell dyscrasia is obvious in ~50% of cases but the majority will have an identifiable paraprotein in the urine or blood.

The heart, liver and nerves can also be affected by the deposition of the abnormal light or heavy chains.

Treatment is directed against the plasma cell dyscrasia using the same regimens and criteria applied to myeloma. Some patients will respond but the majority are refractory.

Response to treatment is monitored by measurement of the serum concentration of the free LC in LCDD.

To avoid recurrent disease, transplantation should not be performed unless there is complete remission of the plasma cell dyscrasia.

Immunotactoid glomerulopathy

This is a rare condition caused by deposition of whole monoclonal IgG (κ or λ). Deposition is confined to glomeruli.

Patients present with proteinuria or renal impairment and may have an underlying lymphoma or chronic leukemia.

The light microscopic appearances are of an atypical membranous glomerulopathy but electron microscopy reveals microtubular deposits (Fig. 4.3.3). These are Congo Red negative.

The condition is refractory to treatment and patients progress rapidly to renal failure.

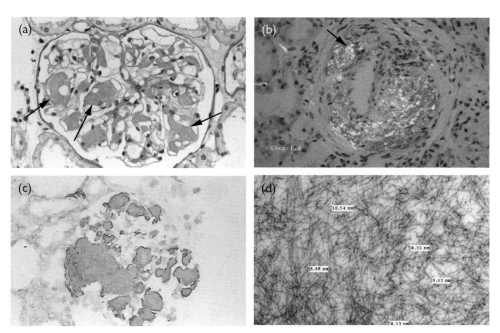

Fig. 4.3.2 AL amyloid. (a) Glomerular amyloid deposits (arrows) (periodic acid–Schiff). (b) Congo Red-stained medium-sized renal artery. Birefringence (Apple Green) can be seen under polarized light (arrow). (c) Anti-λ staining of glomerulus (immunoperoxidase). (d) Electron micrograph of amyloid deposit showing randomly orientated, nonbranching fibrils 8–15 nm in diameter.

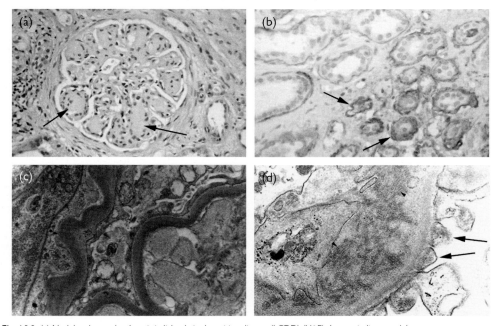

Fig. 4.3.3 (a) Nodular glomerulosclerosis in light chain deposition disease (LCDD) (H&E). Arrows indicate nodules. (b) Immunoperoxidase for κ light chain demonstrating staining of tubular basement membrane in LCDD (arrows). (c) Electron micrograph demonstrating ribbon-like deposits in the GBM in LCDD. (d) Elecron micrograph of a GBM deposit in immunotactoid glomerulopathy demonstrating microtubular substructure (arrowheads). Arrows indicate podocyte foot processes.

Further reading

Clark WF, *et al*. Plasma exchange when myeloma presents as acute renal failure. A randomised, controlled trial. *Ann Intern Med* 2005; **143**: 777–784.

Korbert SM, Schwartz MM. Disease of the month: multiple myeloma. *J Am Soc Nephrol* 2006; **17**: 2533–2342.

Rajkumar SV, Gertz MA. Advances in the treatment of amyloidosis. *New Engl J Med* 2007; **356**: 2413–2415.

Ronco P, Plaiseier E, Mougenot B, Aucouturier P. Immunoglobulin light (heavy)-chain deposition disease: from molecular medicine to pathophysiology-driven therapy. *Clin J Am Soc Nephrol* 2006; **1**; 1342–1350.

Internet resources

General information about myeloma:

http://myeloma.org

Multiple Myeloma Research Foundation. General information:

http://www.multiplemyeloma.org/about_myeloma/

See also

Amyloid or immunotactoid glomerulopathy, p. 150

Mixed cryoglobulinemia and hepatitis C infection, p. 176

Sarcoidosis

Sarcoidosis is a chronic multisystem granulomatous disorder that most commonly affects the lungs. Clinically significant renal involvement, although uncommon in sarcoidosis, may present in a number of different ways (Table 4.4.1).

Epidemiology

The prevalence of sarcoidosis is 10–20 per 100 000 population.

The exact prevalence of renal sarcoid is unknown.

Renal insufficiency only occurs in ~1% of sarcoidosis patients.

10–90% of cases present between 10 and 40 years of age.

There is worldwide distribution but the prevalence is higher in certain races and geographical locations (African-Americans, Scandinavians).

The incidence is increased among first- and second-degree relatives of affected patients.

Etiology

The etiology is unknown.

There is thought to be a genetic influence and various infectious agents have also been implicated.

Genetic
- A genetic predisposition is supported by familial clustering and variations in incidence amongst different races. Several studies have also shown associations (both positive and negative) with class II MHC alleles.

Infective
Mycobacteria and *Propionibacteria* have both been suggested to be involved in the pathogenesis but there is currently no firm evidence to support or refute either.

Renal involvement in sarcoidosis

Renal involvement can be broadly divided into conditions resulting from disordered calcium homeostasis, the classical granulomatous interstitial nephritis (GIN) and a few rare disorders (Table 4.4.1).

Table 4.4.1 Renal involvement in sarcoidosis

	Frequency
Functional (Disordered Ca^{2+} metabolism)	Common
• Hypercalcemia	
• Hypercalciuria	
• Tubular dysfunction	
Structural (Due to disordered Ca^{2+} metabolism)	
• Nephrolithiasis	
• Nephrocalcinosis	
Structural (Due to granulomatous infiltration or other mechanism)	
• Granulomatous interstitial nephritis	
• Glomerular disease	
• Retroperitoneal disease	Rare

Disordered calcium homeostasis
Problems related to disordered calcium homeostasis are far more common than interstitial nephritis.

It is caused by increased calcitriol production resulting from 1α-hydroxylase expression by granulomatous macrophages.

Hypercalciuria:
- This is defined as >300 mg/day.
- It occurs in up to 50% of sarcoidosis patients.

Hypercalcemia
This occurs in 10–20% of sarcoidosis patients. It is more common in:
- male patients;
- Caucasians;
- patients aged >40 years (cf. pulmonary sarcoidosis).

Tubular dysfunction
This occurs frequently with hypercalcemia and/or GIN.

Polyuria is the most common abnormality and is caused by a urinary concentrating defect (which may result in frank nephrogenic diabetes insipidus).

Other possible defects include the development of:
- renal tubular acidosis;
- glycosuria;
- salt wasting;
- Fanconi syndrome.

Nephrolithiasis
Hypercalciuria increases the incidence of calcium oxalate stone formation.

10–14% of sarcoidosis patients develop at least one symptomatic stone.

Nephrocalcinosis
This can result from persistent hypercalcemia.

It is the commonest cause of progressive renal impairment in sarcoidosis.

It is generally not visible on plain radiography but can be seen on histological examination.

Granulomatous interstitial nephritis (GIN)
This is more common in male patients.

50% of patients with GIN have a normal CXR and 50% have an elevated serum angiotensin-converting enzyme level (even in the absence of CXR changes).

Hypercalcemia is frequently observed with GIN and may contribute to the renal insufficiency.

Clinical features

Patients with renal sarcoidosis may present with polyuria or loin pain, or may present with symptoms relating to sarcoid involvement in another organ (malaise and dyspnea are the commonest symptoms).

There may be no specific findings on examination but a thorough physical examination should be carried out paying particular attention to the skin, lungs and eyes. Ophthalmic examination may reveal evidence of uveitis, retinal vasculitis, or keratoconjunctivitis.

Diagnosis

There is no definitive diagnostic test and other conditions can present in a similar way. Diagnosis is therefore one of exclusion and depends on:

• noncaseating granulomas on histological examination;
• compatible clinical and radiological signs;
• exclusion of other conditions.

Differential diagnosis

Consideration should be given to whether any of the following may explain the clinical findings:

• berylliosis: hilar lymphadenopathy and granulomata;
• tuberculosis: hilar lymphadenopathy and granulomata;
• fungal infection (e.g. histoplasmosis): hilar lymphadenopathy and granulomata;
• drug-induced interstitial nephritis: GIN;
• malignancy (lymphoma, breast, lung): GIN;
• foreign body reaction (e.g. cholesterol emboli): GIN;
• Wegener's granulomatosis: GIN.

It is therefore essential that a thorough history is taken when assessing any patient suspected of having sarcoidosis, paying particular attention to:

• occupational history (beryllium exposure);
• exposure to infections (TB);
• risk factors for immunodeficiency (fungal infection).

General investigations

Full blood count

This may be normal or may show an eosinophilia or leukopenia.

Serum biochemistry

This may be normal or may show hypercalcemia and/or renal impairment.

Immunology

This may reveal hypergammaglobulinemia.

Serum ACE

This is raised in 75% cases of sarcoidosis.

False positives are rare but can occur with advanced renal disease.

It may be more useful in monitoring the response to treatment rather than for diagnosis.

Parathyroid hormone

This is normal or low–normal in the presence of hypercalcemia.

Urinalysis

This may be bland, or show hematuria and/or proteinuria (usually <1 g/day).

Urinary calcium excretion

This is elevated in up to 50% of patients.

Chest X-ray

Hilar lymphadenopathy is the commonest abnormality and is classed as stage I pulmonary disease (Fig. 4.4.1).

Pulmonary function tests

A restrictive pattern on spirometry with reduced diffusing capacity for carbon monoxide (DLCO) is seen with lung involvement.

Consider also:

ECG to look for conduction defects.

Tuberculin skin test (no response in sarcoidosis).

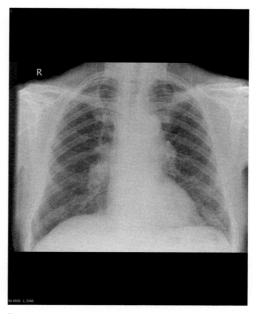

Fig. 4.4.1 Chest X-ray showing hilar lymphadenopathy. (Courtesy of Dr Nick Mayer, University Hospitals of Leicester, UK.)

Renal biopsy

Renal biopsy findings depend on which pathological process(es) is/are present. The commonest findings in sarcoidosis are GIN and/or nephrocalcinosis. Glomeruli are usually normal.

GIN is the classical lesion of sarcoidosis.

Noncaseating granulomas are formed from epithelioid macrophages surrounded by T cells (see Fig. 4.4.2).

GIN is seen in 7–40% of biopsy series of sarcoidosis (including autopsy studies).

Lesions may be scant and are often clinically silent, thus these numbers may underestimate the true incidence.

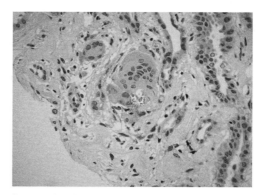

Fig. 4.4.2 Granulomatous interstitial nephritis showing a granuloma with multinucleate giant cell and calcinosis (H&E) (Courtesy of Dr Nick Mayer, University Hospitals of Leicester, UK.)

Nephrocalcinosis may be seen as calcium deposits within the renal parenchyma (see Fig. 4.4.2).

ATN can occasionally occur with GIN or hypercalcemia.

Treatment

Hypercalcemia

General measures

- Adequate oral hydration.
- Dietary calcium, vitamin D and oxalate (spinach, rhubarb, certain nuts) restriction.
- Avoidance of sunlight.
- Avoidance of thiazide diuretics (which can predispose to hypercalcemia in sarcoid patients).

Pharmacological treatment

Prednisolone 20–40 mg/day.

Calcium levels and renal function usually respond within a few days if sarcoidosis is the cause of the hypercalcemia. After an adequate response is obtained, tapering the dose while monitoring serum and urine calcium levels and calcitriol levels is advised.

Granulomatous interstitial nephritis

Pharmacological treatment

Prednisolone 1 mg/kg/day initially.

A prolonged course or steroids is required.

Treatment for <6 months frequently results in relapse.

One author suggests continuing the full dose for 2 months then tapering the dose gradually, but continuing steroid treatment for ≥1 year.

Consideration should be given toward gastric protection and prophylaxis against bone disease especially in at-risk groups.

Prognosis

Functional defects are generally fully reversible with prednisolone.

Recovery of renal function may be incomplete if fibrosis has occurred.

Nephrolithiasis and nephrocalcinosis do not regress following steroid treatment.

Internet resources

Renal Involvement in sarcoidosis:

http://www.kidneyatlas.org/book4/adk4-08.pdf

Sarcoidosis:

http://www.emedicine.com/PED/topic2043.htm

Further reading

Baughman RP, Lower EE, du Bois RM. Sarcoidosis. *Lancet* 2003; **361**: 1111–1118.

Berliner AR, Haas M, Choi MJ. Sarcoidosis: the nephrologist's perspective. *Am J Kidney Dis* 2006; **48**: 856–870.

Mery JP. The patient with sarcoidosis. In: Davison AM, *et al.* (eds), *Oxford textbook of nephrology*, 3rd edn. Oxford; Oxford University Press; 2005.

Systemic vasculitis

Classification of vasculitis

Inflammation and necrosis of blood vessels occurs in a number of disorders; classically these conditions have been categorized based on the predominant size and types of blood vessels involved.

The American College of Rheumatology has also produced classification criteria for most forms of vasculitis based on signs and symptoms. These are not meant to be used as diagnostic criteria.

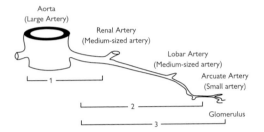

1. Large: giant cell arteritis, Takayasu's.
2. Medium: polyarteritis nodosa, Kawasaki's disease.
3. Small: without immune complex: Wegener's granulomatosis, microscopic polyangiitis, Churg–Strauss syndrome.
4. Small: with immune complex: Henoch–Schönlein purpura, SLE, rheumatoid, essential cryoglobulinemia.

ANCA-associated vasculitis

This group of vasculitides is associated with a circulating antineutrophil cytoplasmic antibody (ANCA) and includes:

- Wegener's granulomatosis;
- microscopic polyangiitis;
- Churg–Strauss syndrome.

Epidemiology

In the UK:

- incidence 20 pmp per year;
- prevalence 170 pmp.

Churg–Strauss syndrome is less common, with an incidence of 2.4/million population.

It occurs in all age groups with a peak age of onset of 55–70 years.

Wegener's granulomatosis is predominant in northern Caucasian populations with microscopic polyangiitis being predominant in southern Caucasian and non-Caucasian populations.

Etiology

It is an autoimmune disease of unknown etiology.
Both genetic and environmental factors are thought to be important.

Genetic

HLA associations have not been consistently reported in ANCA-associated vasculitis.

An association exists between α1-antitrypsin deficiency (the main inhibitor of proteinase-3 (PR3)) and Wegener's granulomatosis. Patients carrying the main deficiency allele, PiZ, have more severe disease and a poor prognosis. However, α1-antitrypsin deficiency *per se* is not sufficient to induce vasculitis, suggesting that it acts as a 'second-hit' amplifier of inflammation.

Polymorphisms that predispose to autoimmunity per se are also associated with ANCA-associated vasculitis. For example, Wegener's granulomatosis has been shown to be associated with polymorphisms of the protein tyrosine phosphatase PTPN22 (R620W allele which influences the signalling threshold of the T-cell receptor), and also polymorphisms in the CTLA4 gene.

Environmental

Infection: nasal carriage of *Staphylococcus aureus* is associated with an increased risk of relapse of Wegener's granulomatosis. No other infectious agents have been associated with disease.

Exposure to silica has been associated with an increased risk of disease.

Drug exposure may precipitate disease, including propylthiouracil, minocycline and penicillamine.

Pathogenesis

ANCA are pathogenic: murine models show that when antimyeloperoxidase (MPO) antibodies are transferred to naïve mice they develop disease.

Direct evidence in humans that ANCA are pathogenic was provided by a newborn in which the placental transmission of maternal anti-MPO antibodies resulted in the development of a pulmonary–renal syndrome.

ANCA activate cytokine-primed neutrophils and monocytes that express myeloperoxidase and PR3 on the cell surface.

ANCA-activated neutrophils generate a respiratory burst, degranulate and release proinflammatory cytokines.

Cytokine-activated endothelial cells, which express adhesion molecules, are important in localizing damage: ANCA promote neutrophil transmigration across endothelial cells.

Neutrophils are important in the induction of early damage, whereas T-cells and monocytes are important for chronic inflammation.

T-cells are thought to be important in pathogenesis; the phenotype of T-cells is altered with an expansion in effector memory T-cells which are a source of Th1 cytokines. ANCA are T-cell-dependent, class-switched IgG antibodies.

Pathology

The characteristic lesion is small vessel vasculitis with inflammation and necrosis of arterioles, venules and capillaries (although larger vessels may be affected).

Granulomatous lesions occur in Wegener's granulomatosis and Churg–Strauss syndrome, but not in microscopic polyangiitis.

In the lung, there are often large, ill-defined collections of inflammatory cells near affected vessels; these may present as cavitating nodules.

In the kidney, the process primarily affects glomeruli, leading to focal segmental necrotizing glomerulonephritis with crescent formation without immunoglobulin deposition; this is termed 'pauci-immune glomerulonephritis'. There is often associated interstitial inflammation.

Within the kidney there are no absolute differences in pathology between microscopic polyangiitis and Wegener's granulomatosis, although patients with microscopic polyangiitis tend to have more chronic lesions.

Granulomata are generally not found in the kidney.

Clinical features
The clinical differentiation between Wegener's granulomatosis and microscopic polyangiitis is often difficult. However, this distinction is not important clinically, because their treatment and prognosis are similar.

Systemic nonspecific symptoms such as malaise, flu-like symptoms and weight loss are common and may pre-date the development of other symptoms.

Wegener's granulomatosis – limited disease
Respiratory tract symptoms are common and may be present in 90% of patients at the time of diagnosis; symptoms include:
- sinusitis;
- epistaxis;
- otitis media;
- hoarseness.

Complications of granulomatous inflammation may cause mucosal ulceration, nasal septal perforation, and development of a saddle nose.

Subglottic stenosis occurs in up to 16% of adults and 48% of children. It often becomes fixed and irreversible and can cause life-threatening upper airways obstruction.

So-called limited disease may have an indolent course for many years before transforming into systemic disease.

Wegener's granulomatosis – systemic disease
This is characterized by:
- upper respiratory tract involvement;
- pulmonary disease;
- renal involvement with glomerulonephritis;
- ANCA directed against the neutrophil enzyme PR3.

Microscopic polyangiitis
This is characterized by:
- renal disease;
- pulmonary disease;
- ANCA directed against myeloperoxidase (MPO).

Specific organ involvement
This may occur in Wegener's granulomatosis or microscopic polyangiitis (Table 4.5.1).
- Pulmonary disease:
  This is recorded in 45–70% of patients at presentation. However, 85% of patients with Wegener's granulomatosis will have pulmonary involvement at some stage of the disease. Presentation may be with asymptomatic pulmonary infiltrates or cough, hemoptysis, pleuritis or dyspnea.
  Life-threatening alveolar hemorrhage may occur and is associated with a poor prognosis. Pulmonary disease is less common in microscopic polyangiitis but 30% of patients will have pulmonary hemorrhage.
- Renal disease:
  This can range from an active urinary sediment to rapidly progressive glomerulonephritis with severe damage.
  Renal involvement in microscopic polyangiitis is invariable. Hypertension occurs in 30% of patients. So-called idiopathic rapidly progressive glomerulonephritis, without immune deposits and with no systemic features of vasculitis, is now considered part of the spectrum of microscopic polyangiitis.
  Renal involvement is not a common presentation in patients with Wegener's granulomatosis (18%), but 77% of patients will develop glomerulonephritis at some stage.
- Disease of other organs:
  Ocular involvement is not uncommon and may present as conjunctivitis, scleritis or uveitis. In those with granulomatous inflammation, proptosis may occur and is commonly associated with extensive sinus disease. Optic nerve vasculitis and retinal artery thrombosis are rare but important complications. Loss of sight has been reported in 8% of patients.

  Myalgia and arthralgia are common. Nonerosive arthritis occurs in 28% of patients.

  Skin disease may manifest as palpable purpura, ulcers and subcutaneous nodules, and occurs in up to 50% of patients.

  The heart (pericarditis, coronary arteritis), nervous system (mononeuritis multiplex, peripheral neuropathy) and gastrointestinal tract (hemorrhagic ulceration, bowel perforation) may also be involved.

Table 4.5.1 Organ involvement in small vessel vasculitis

Organ involvement throughout disease course	Wegener's granulomatosis	Microscopic polyangiitis	Churg–Strauss syndrome
Upper respiratory tract	80%	Uncommon	55%
Lower respiratory tract	70%	30%	100%
Eye	46%	10%	6%
Kidney	80%	90%	33%
Peripheral nervous system	35%	20%	67%
Gastrointestinal system	5%	5%	17%
Heart	Uncommon	Uncommon	28%
Skin	50%	25%	44%
Constitutional symptoms	95%	90%	94%

Churg–Strauss syndrome
This is characterized by:
Hypereosinophilia with tissue infiltration, formation of granulomata and vasculitis.

Allergic rhinitis and/or asthma precedes the development of vasculitis, often in association with nonspecific symptoms.

Asthma is often more severe in the weeks preceding the development of vasculitis.

ANCA directed against MPO are identified in ~50% of patients, particularly in the vasculitic phase.

Rash and mononeuritis multiplex commonly occur at presentation.

Pulmonary involvement is characterized by dyspnea, alveolar hemorrhage or pleurisy and is associated with nonspecific pulmonary infiltrates on chest radiography.

Cardiac involvement, manifest by myocarditis with eosinophilic infiltration, coronary artery vasculitis and myocardial infarction carries a poor prognosis and is often a late manifestation.

Gastrointestinal involvement can present in various ways including abdominal pain, diarrhea and ascites.

Renal involvement is not uncommon but it is usually mild.

Investigations

Routine laboratory investigations
These will reveal nonspecific abnormalities.

Common abnormalities include:
- leukocytosis;
- thrombocytosis (>400 000/mm^3);
- normochromic, normocytic anemia;
- elevation of inflammatory markers including erythrocyte sedimentation rate (ESR) and C-reactive protein (CRP).

In addition, Churg–Strauss syndrome is usually associated with a blood eosinophilia (>1.5 × 10^9/L) and elevated IgE levels.

Urinalysis is a sensitive marker of renal involvement.

An active urinary sediment with red blood cells and casts indicates glomerular disease.

Proteinuria is often present although rarely in the nephrotic range.

Elevated urea and creatinine levels are common, though active renal disease may be present even if biochemical indices are normal.

Antineutrophil cytoplasmic antibodies
ANCA are a useful marker for diagnosis.

Wegener's granulomatosis is associated with ANCA directed against PR3 (PR3-ANCA), giving a granular cytoplasmic staining pattern on indirect immunofluorescence (IIF).

Combining IIF and ELISA is highly sensitive (>95%) and specific (>99%) in patients with active systemic disease.

Microscopic polyangiitis is associated with ANCA directed against MPO (MPO-ANCA) in 70% of patients, but PR3-ANCA can also occur.

MPO-ANCA give a perinuclear staining pattern on IIF.

The positive predictive value of a positive test for ANCA is dependent on the clinical situation.
- Wegener's granulomatosis: 85–90% ANCA positive in systemic disease, 73% PR3-ANCA or cANCA.
- Microscopic polyangiitis: 85–90% ANCA positive, 67% MPO-ANCA or pANCA.

- Churg–Strauss syndrome: 50% ANCA positive, majority MPO-ANCA particularly during vasculitis phase.

Chest radiography
Pulmonary hemorrhage is the most serious form of lung involvement and is seen as diffuse pulmonary shadowing associated with a reduced hemoglobin concentration, low arterial pO$_2$ and a raised corrected transfer factor.

In Wegener's granulomatosis, chest radiography commonly shows pulmonary nodules, which often cavitate. Other radiographic features include reticulonodular shadowing, pneumonic changes, collapse and pleural involvement with effusions.

Tissue biopsy
A tissue biopsy usually confirms disease.

The kidney is usually the best site for diagnosis.

In Wegener's granulomatosis nasopharyngeal or transbronchial biopsy often shows nonspecific inflammation.

Lung biopsy generally requires an open procedure, and special stains and cultures need to be undertaken to exclude the presence of infections that can produce granulomata, vasculitis and necrosis.

Differential diagnosis
The differential diagnosis of the pulmonary–renal syndrome is wide (Table 4.5.2).

A serological assessment for circulating autoantibodies is necessary and distinguishes primary small vessel vasculitis from other causes.

Management
Diagnosis and treatment should be made rapidly before permanent organ scarring occurs.

Treatment should be tailored to the stage and severity of disease: the level of immunosuppression should reflect the severity of disease (Table 4.5.3).

There are no treatment guidelines provided by NICE although the British Rheumatology Society have recently published guidelines on the management of systemic vasculitis (BSR & BHPR Guidelines for the Management of Adults ANCA Associated Vasculitis. *Rheumatology* 2007; 46: 1615–6).

Induction therapy: Wegener's granulomatosis and microscopic polyangiitis
Initial therapy in patients with ANCA-associated vasculitis and generalized or threatened vital organ loss should include cyclophosphamide and a reducing course of corticosteroids (Tables 4.5.4 and 4.5.5).

Cyclophosphamide can be administered using an oral or pulsed regimen. Preliminary results of a randomized controlled trial suggest that there is no difference in the relapse rate or safety using either regimen although with the pulsed regimen the total dose of cyclophosphamide is lower.

In those with limited disease, methotrexate in combination with a reducing course of steroids may be appropriate, although this may be at the expense of a higher relapse rate compared to when cyclophosphamide is used as an induction agent.

Maintenance therapy: Wegener's granulomatosis and microscopic polyangiitis
Cyclophosphamide should be discontinued after remission is achieved, usually after 3–6 months of treatment.

Table 4.5.2 Differential diagnosis of pulmonary–renal syndrome

Disease	Vasculitis	Granuloma	ANCA status	Features
Wegener's granulomatosis	Present	Present	PR3-ANCA	See text.
Microscopic polyangiitis	Present	Absent	MPO-ANCA	Primary small vessel vasculitis is the most common cause of pulmonary renal syndrome (~56% of cases).
Churg–Strauss syndrome	Present	Present	MPO-ANCA (50%)	See text.
Goodpasture's disease	Present	Absent	Seldom positive (10–38%)	Linear IgG deposition on glomerular basement membrane.
				Antiglomerular basement membrane antibody positive.
				In patients with ANCA, treatment should be as for primary small vessel vasculitis; prognosis may be better than in those with antiglomerular basement membrane antibody alone.
Systemic lupus erythematosus	Present	Absent	Seldom positive	Antinuclear factor and anti-dsDNA positive.
				Low C3 and C4.
Henoch–Schönlein purpura	Present	Absent	Negative	Lung involvement uncommon.
				IgA deposition in vessel walls and mesangium.
Behçet's disease	Present	Absent	Negative	Diagnosed on clinical criteria.
				Associated with recurrent oral and genital ulceration, eye lesions (including uveitis) and skin lesions; renal involvement usually mild.
Infection	Rarely present (e.g. subacute bacterial endocarditis)	Absent	Negative	Pneumonia may be associated with acute tubular necrosis or interstitial nephritis (rarely).
				Subacute bacterial endocarditis may be associated with ANCA-negative pauci-immune glomerulonephritis.
				Post-streptococcal glomerulonephritis.
				Blood cultures, atypical serology and antistreptolysin-O titre should be undertaken.

Patients should be maintained on immunosuppression therapy following remission to reduce the risk of relapse, e.g. azathioprine.

The optimum duration of maintenance therapy is unknown, but it should continue for ≥24 months following the induction of remission.

Cotrimoxazole may reduce upper respiratory tract relapses in Wegener's granulomatosis but it is not a substitute for conventional immunosuppression.

Methotrexate may be used as maintenance therapy in those with limited disease. It is contraindicated in those with creatinine >170 µmol/L.

Mycophenolate may be used as maintenance therapy in those who have contraindications to azathioprine or who have a disease relapse while on azathioprine.

Rescue therapy for relapsing and refractory disease
Standard induction therapy fails to induce remission in 10% of patients; patients who frequently relapse necessitating recurrent use of cyclophosphamide are also a difficult group to treat.

Newer therapies that may prove beneficial include B-cell depletion with rituximab, polyclonal antithymocyte globulin, deoxyspergualin and other newer immunosuppressant drugs that have shown promise in organ transplantation or other autoimmune diseases.

Churg–Strauss syndrome
Steroids are the mainstay of treatment; however, in those with more severe disease an induction maintenance regimen as for Wegener's granulomatosis or microscopic polyangiitis should be used.

Disease severity can be assessed using the five factor score, 1 point for each:
- creatinine >140 µmol/l;
- proteinuria >1 g/day;
- severe GI involvement;
- cardiomyopathy;
- CNS signs.

Cyclophosphamide improves survival in those with a five-factor score of >2.

Side-effects of therapy
- Corticosteroids:
  Diabetes, hypertension, gastritis, osteoporosis, mood disturbance, and infection.

Table 4.5.3 Disease stratification

Clinical subgroup	Constitutional symptoms	Typical ANCA status	Threatened vital organ function	Serum creatinine (µmol/L)
Localized/ early systemic	Yes	Positive or negative	No	<150
Generalized	Yes	Positive	Yes	<500
Severe	Yes	Positive	Yes	>500

Table 4.5.4 Management of primary small vessel vasculitis

Induction therapy	Continued for 3 months following remission.
	Prednisolone 1 mg/kg, maximum dose 80 mg; rapid reduction in corticosteroid dose: 50% over 2 weeks and to a dose of 0.25 mg/kg at week 8.
	Cyclophosphamide, 2 mg/kg/day PO, maximum dose 200 mg; age >60 years reduce by 25%, age >70 years reduce by 50%.
	Pulsed cyclophosphamide can also be given: 10 pulses over 25 weeks, 15 mg/kg IV; dose reductions must be made for age and creatinine.
	(See http://www.vasculitis.org/protocols/CYCLOPS.pdf for suggested dose reduction.)
Limited disease	Methotrexate 20–25 mg/week.
	Reducing dose of corticosteroid (Table 4.5.5).
	May be at expense of increased relapse rate compared with cyclophosphamide.
Adjuvant therapy for life-threatening disease	Life-threatening disease includes creatinine >500 μmol/L and/or pulmonary hemorrhage.
	Plasma exchange should be considered.
Maintenance therapy	Prednisolone 5–10 mg/day.
	Azathioprine 1.5 mg/kg/day, maximum dose 200 mg.
	Methotrexate 20–25 mg/week (contraindicated in patients with creatinine >170 μmol/L).
	Alternatives to azathioprine include mycophenolate mofetil, 1 g bd.
	Consider addition of cotrimoxazole.
Relapse therapy	Major relapse: return to initial induction therapy.
	Minor relapse: increase corticosteroid dose.

Prevent gastritis with an H2-blocker or proton pump inhibitor.

Consider bone prophylaxis (calcium and vitamin D, or bisphosphonates).

Consider TB prophylaxis in those at risk as suggested by British Thoracic Guidelines (http://www.brit-thoracic.org.uk/AntiTNFaTreatmentGuidline).

Patients should receive pneumococcal and influenza vaccines but avoid all live vaccines until immunosuppression is discontinued.

- Cyclophosphamide:
Infertility, opportunistic infection, bone marrow suppression, hemorrhagic cystitis, bladder cancer, lymphoma.

Monitor for leukopenia regularly.

If continuous oral cyclophosphamide is administered: check the white cell count (WCC) weekly for the first month, 2-weekly for the second and third month, and then monthly thereafter.

If the WCC falls to $<4 \times 10^9$/L cyclophosphamide should be discontinued temporarily. Restart with a dose reduced by ≥ 25 mg/day when WCC has recovered, thereafter monitor weekly for 4 weeks.

If neutropenia is severe ($<1 \times 10^9$/L) or leukopenia is prolonged (total WCC $<4 \times 10^9$/L for >2 weeks) then restart cyclophosphamide at 50 mg/day (when the WCC has recovered), increasing to target dose weekly if the WCC permits.

For a falling WCC ($<6 \times 10^9$/L and a fall of $>2 \times 10^9$/L from the previous count), reduce the dose by 25%.

If pulsed cyclophosphamide is administered: check the FBC on the day of the pulse or the day before.

If the WCC prior to the pulse is $<4 \times 10^9$/L, postpone the pulse until the WCC is $>4 \times 10^9$/L (check the FBC weekly). Reduce the dose of the pulse by 25%.

With any further episodes of leukopenia make an equivalent dose reduction.

Check the FBC between days 10 and 14 after a pulse.

If the leukocyte nadir is $<3 \times 10^9$/L, even if the WCC just before to the next pulse is $>4 \times 10^9$/L, reduce the dose of the next pulse according to:

- leukocyte nadir $1–2 \times 10^9$/L reduce cyclophosphamide pulse by 40% of previous dose.
- leukocyte nadir $2–3 \times 10^9$/L reduce cyclophosphamide pulse by 20% of previous dose.

Counsel for the risks of infertility and consider gamete storage.

Table 4.5.5 Suggested algorithm for reduction of prednisolone

Time from diagnosis (weeks)	Prednisolone dosage (mg/kg/day)	Prednisolone dosage (mg/day for 60 kg person)
0	1	60
1	0.75	45
2	0.5	30
3	0.4	25
4	0.4	25
6	0.33	20
8	0.25	15
	Prednisolone dosage (mg/day)	
12	15	15
16	12.5	12.5
6 months	10	10
During months 12–15	7.5	7.5
>15 months	5	5

Based on EUVAS trials: www.vasculitis.org/comptrials.htm

Consider prophylaxis for *Pneumocystis jiroveci* (previously known as *Pneumocystis carinii*) with cotrimoxazole (Septrin) or dapsone and for *Candida* with amphotericin lozenges.

Consider co-administration of mesna, which binds the cyclophosphamide metabolite acrolein that is toxic to the uroepithelium, to reduce risk of hemorrhagic cystitis.

Patients should be encouraged to drink unless fluid-restricted. In those receiving continuous therapy, cyclophosphamide should not be given last thing at night.

Regular urinalysis should be performed and unexplained microscopic or macroscopic hematuria should precipitate cystoscopy to exclude bladder cancer.

- Azathioprine:
Bone marrow suppression, infection, cutaneous malignancy, liver dysfunction.

Monitor the WCC weekly for 6 weeks then 2- and 4-weekly after any dose adjustment. There is a risk of marrow suppression, particularly in those with thiopurine methyltransferase enzyme deficiency.

Monitor liver function monthly until the dose is stable.

Assessment and monitoring of disease activity
ANCA-associated vasculitides are relapsing conditions; 50% of patients will relapse within 5 years of diagnosis. The risk of relapse is increased if patients:
- remain ANCA positive despite disease remission;
- are PR3-ANCA positive;
- have Wegener's granulomatosis;
- have lung or upper respiratory tract involvement.

Indicators of relapse:
- rising ANCA levels or reappearance of ANCA; however, the positive predictive value of a rising ANCA titer is not sufficient to alter immunosuppressive therapy;
- raised inflammatory markers.

Relapse is usually milder than the initial presentation.

Monitoring
Patients should be seen regularly to assess disease activity; the intensity of clinic visits will be dependent on disease phase (at least monthly until disease remission is achieved, 2–3-monthly for first 12 months following remission, and 3–6-monthly thereafter).

Investigations at each clinic visit should include:
- ANCA.
- CRP and/or ESR.
- Urinalysis.
- Assessment of renal function.

Clinicians should maintain a high index of suspicion for both disease relapse and the side-effects of therapy.

Prognosis
Survival is 70–80% at 5 years and is dependent on renal involvement.

Early mortality often results from opportunistic infection.

Poor prognostic indicators include greater age, pulmonary hemorrhage and severe renal disease.

End-stage renal disease occurs in 20–25% of patients.

With improved survival, long-term damage from disease and drug toxicity is associated with significant morbidity.

Polyarteritis nodosa (PAN)
PAN typically affects medium-sized arteries but not veins and is characterized by transmural inflammation.

The incidence is 4–9 pmp in Europe, which rises with age, peaking in the 6th decade.

The cause in most cases is unknown but 30% are associated with hepatitis B virus (HBV) infection, typically occurring early (within 1 year of infection), and occasionally in association with hairy cell leukemia.

Clinical features
PAN typically presents with systemic features:

Kidney disease: this is the most commonly affected organ. It is associated with chronic renal failure, an inactive urinary sediment, mild–moderate proteinuria, and hypertension.

Neurologic disease: mononeuritis multiplex occurs most commonly, but PAN may cause ischemic or hemorrhagic stroke in up to 10% of patients.

Gastrointestinal disease: weight loss and abdominal pain (which may be most prominent after meals) are typical. The disease may lead to frank bowel ischemia and perforation. It affects the small bowel more often than the large bowel.

Skin: livedo reticularis, ulcers, tender erythematous nodules.

It may cause myocardial ischemia although infarction is rare.

Orchitis.

Diagnosis
Mesenteric or renal arteriography demonstrates multiple aneurysms and irregular constrictions in larger vessels with occlusion of smaller penetrating arteries.

PAN is not associated with ANCA.

Treatment
Steroids are the mainstay of treatment in idiopathic PAN; however, as in Churg–Strauss syndrome cyclophosphamide should be added in those with a five-factor score >2.

Those with severe PAN should receive pulses of cyclophosphamide (0.6 g/m^2 monthly) for 1 year.

In those with HBV infection, treatment should include a short course of steroids initially (2 weeks), plasma exchange and antiviral therapy such as lamivudine.

PAN relapses infrequently.

Takayasu's disease
This is a chronic inflammatory condition of unknown etiology that results in a granulomatous arteritis, with marked intimal proliferation and fibrosis of the media and adventitia.

This causes arterial stenosis, occlusion, and occasionally post-stenotic dilations and aneurysms when the media is destroyed.

The disease typically affects the aorta and its main branches and may include the pulmonary vessels in 50–80% of patients.

It preferentially affects young Asian women, although the incidence in older patients may be rising. In middle-aged patients chronic vasculitis latently progresses with atherosclerosis.

The prevalence is reported as 2.6 pmp in Caucasians and 1 per 3000 in Japan.

Clinical features

There is a classic triphasic pattern of disease expression, with an early prepulseless phase with systemic features, a vascular inflammatory phase, and a quiescent occlusive phase. However, disease is recurrent and different phases may coexist.

Systemic symptoms, weight loss, fever, fatigue are common in the early phase.

Vascular symptoms are rare at onset but 98% will develop stenosis or occlusion causing ischemic symptoms, such as limb claudication, angina, stroke, vertebrobasilar insufficiency, and/or subclavian steal syndrome.

27% of patients will develop aneurysms.

Development of collateral circulations may minimize some ischemic symptoms.

There is often reduced blood pressure in one or more limbs.

Vascular bruits are present, especially in the subclavian and abdominal arteries.

50% develop renovascular hypertension which may be associated with renal failure and congestive cardiac failure.

Aortic regurgitation is common particularly if the ascending aorta is involved.

Diagnosis

Acute phase proteins may be elevated in the early phase and fall in response to therapy but they do not always correlate with disease activity.

Anemia of chronic disease is typical.

Autoantibodies are negative although antiendothelial cell antibodies may be positive.

Angiography should be performed for diagnosis. MR angiography has advantages over conventional angiography as it may provide information on active inflammation. Gadolinium enhancement of vessel walls is thought to be indicative of edema associated with active inflammation. Late phase findings include stenosis, typically of the proximal portion of vessels. Occlusions commonly are abrupt, often with abrupt change to collateral vessels and flame-shaped terminations. The disadvantages of MRA are that it may overestimate the degree of stenosis, and it is poor at demonstrating vascular calcification.

Treatment

Steroids are the mainstay of treatment but 50% of patients will relapse during the steroid taper requiring additional use of immunosuppressants.

There are no randomized controlled trials to guide therapy.

Responses have been seen with methotrexate, azathioprine and other immunosuppressants.

Anti-TNF therapy may be beneficial in cases that are resistant to these therapies.

Stenotic lesions are not reversible with immunosuppressant therapy. Hemodynamically significant stenosis may require revascularization using bypass grafting. However, 20–30% of grafts re-stenose.

Lesions are often not amenable to angioplasty, and re-stenose more often following angioplasty and stenting than grafting.

Regrafting of renal arteries may reduce blood pressure.

Sildenafil may be useful for ischemic symptoms such as digital ischemia.

Treatment should also include strict management of the traditional cardiovascular risk factors.

Prognosis

Sustained remission is uncommon. At least 75% of patients will relapse following steroid taper despite use of other immunosuppressants.

Patients tend to have considerable morbidity due to the chronic vascular damage.

Further reading

Chan AT, Flossman O, Mukhtyar C, Jayne DR, Luqmani RA. The role of biologic therapies in the management of systemic vasculitis. *Autoimmune Rev* 2006; **5**: 273–278.

Guillevin L, Cohen P, Mahr A, Arene JP, Mouthon L, Puechal X, et al. Treatment of polyarteritis nodosa and microscopic polyangiitis with poor prognosis factors: a prospective trial comparing glucocorticoids and six or twelve cyclophosphamide pulses in 65 patients. *Arthritis Rheum* 2003; **49**: 93–100.

Guillevin L, Mahr A, Callard P, Pagnoux C, Leray E, Cohen P. Hepatitis B. Virus-associated polyarteritis nodosa: clinical characteristics, outcome and impact of treatment in 115 patients. French Vasculitis Study Group. *Medicine (Baltimore)* 2005; **84**: 313–322.

Maksimowicz-McKinnon K, Clark TM, Hoffman GS. Limitations of therapy and a guarded prognosis in an American cohort of Takayasu arteritis patients. *Arthritis Rheum* 2007; **56**: 1000–1009.

Morgan MD, Harper L, Williams J, Savage C. Anti-neutrophil cytoplasm associated vasculitis. *J Am Soc Nephrol* 2006; **17**: 1224–1234.

Internet resources

European Vasculitis Study Group (EUVAS) website:

www.vasculitis.org/comptrials.htm

Paper describing steroid taper protocol:

http://www.vasculitis.org/protocols/CYCLOPS.pdf

National Kidney Federation vasculitis information:

http://www.kidney.org.uk/Medical-Info/kidney-disease/vasc.html

Cochrane Collaboration review of Treatment for renal vasculitis and Goodpasture's disease in adults:

http://www.cochrane.org/reviews/en/info_001400081113510954.html

The Stuart Strange Vasculitis Trust. Patient support group in the UK:

http://www.vasculitis-uk.org.uk/

See also

Mixed cryoglobulinemia and hepatitis C infection

Cryoglobulins (CG) are immunoglobulins that precipitate from both serum and plasma at temperatures <37°C and dissolve on rewarming.

Cryoglobulinemia refers to the presence of a CG in the blood, although often the term is used to describe the clinical syndrome that results from the presence of CG.

Cryoglobulinemia is commonly asymptomatic but may lead to features of hyperviscosity or systemic vasculitis.

Cryoglobulin classification

Type I

These are comprised of monoclonal immunoglobulin (usually IgG or IgM) and account for 5–25% of cases.

It usually results from plasma cell dyscrasias (usually Waldenström's macroglobulinemia and multiple myeloma) but can also rarely be associated with connective tissue diseases.

Type II

These are comprised of polyclonal IgG and a monoclonal IgM directed against the IgG (i.e. IgM rheumatoid factor (RhF)), and account for 40–60% of cases.

This is also known as essential mixed cryoglobulinemia although it is now recognized that most cases are due to persistent viral infection (typically with hepatitis C virus (HCV), although can also be seen with HIV, hepatitis B virus (HBV) and Epstein–Barr virus (EBV)). It can also be associated with chronic lymphocytic leukemia, and B-cell lymphoma.

Type III

These are comprised of polyclonal IgG and a polyclonal IgM rheumatoid factor, and account for 40–50% of cases.

Up to half of cases are due to HCV infection but it can also result from other infections (HBV, EBV, endocarditis, schistosomiasis etc.), chronic inflammatory conditions (e.g. systemic lupus erythematosus, rheumatoid arthritis), and lymphoproliferative disorders.

Occasionally CGs are identified that do not fit into either the type II or type III classification. It is thought that these represent a transition from type III to type II (i.e. polyclonal to monoclonal transformation).

60–75% of cryoglobulinemic patients have an identifiable underlying cause (connective tissue disease, lymphoproliferative disease, infection, hepatobiliary disease) and are known as secondary cryoglobulinemia. When an underlying cause is not identifiable, the term essential mixed cryoglobulinemia is used.

Epidemiology

Clinically significant cryoglobulinemia is found in ~1 per 100 000 of the general population.

In specific groups CGs can be detected in a significant proportion (2–15% in patients with HIV infection; 15–25% of patients with connective tissue diseases; 40–50% of patients with HCV infection).

Etiology and pathogenesis

Clinically significant cryoglobulinemia results from several events:

- chronic immune stimulation or lymphoproliferation resulting in production of CG;
- formation of immune complexes;
- defective immune complex clearance, leading to accumulation and disease induction.

Mechanism of cryoprecipitation

The mechanism of cryoprecipitation is not well understood. A number of factors that appear to be important for aggregation have been identified:

Antibody–antigen interaction-dependent mechanisms.

- Rheumatoid factor activity appears to be important.
- The individual components of CGs do not interact or aggregate.
- Intrinsic properties of the target antibody/antigen are critical since cryoprecipitation is optimal when the isolated RhF component is mixed with IgG isolated from the same patient, but not when mixed with IgG from normal serum.
- IgG3 is enriched in precipitates and anti-IgG3 RhF activity is prevalent in CGs. IgG3 is more able to self-aggregate via Fc–Fc interactions than other IgG subclasses.
- Fibronectin is invariably found in cryoprecipitates and IgM RhF found in CGs has strong affinity for immobilized fibronectin.

Immunoglobulin-dependent mechanisms.

- Some CGs do not have RhF activity (usually type I CGs).
- In these cases the intrinsic physicochemical properties of the immunoglobulin molecule determine its cryoprecipitability.
- The absence of sialic acid moieties has been described.
- Overall changes in physicochemical properties that render the immunoglobulin more hydrophobic increase cryoprecipitability.

Type I cryoglobulinemia

This results from an underlying lymphoproliferative disorder that produces high levels of monoclonal immunoglobulin that, due to its physicochemical properties, has CG activity. Clinically these cold-induced precipitates can induce vasculitis but more usually result in problems related to hyperviscosity.

Type II and III cryoglobulinemia

Mixed CGs result from the chronic activation and proliferation of CG-producing B-cell clones by chronic inflammatory disease and chronic viral infection, particularly HCV infection.

The mechanism of CG production has been best described in HCV infection.

Hepatitis C virus and cryoglobulinemia

There is now convincing evidence of a role for HCV in the production of B-cell clonal expansion and mixed CG production.

HCV-related CG usually contains IgMκ monoclonal antibody that associates with anti-HCV IgG. HCV RNA can also be identified in the cryoprecipitates.

B-cell stimulation may occur either by direct engagement of B-cell CD81 by HCV, or via chronic stimulation by anti-HCV–HCV virion complexes.

Clinical features

The majority of patients with circulating CGs are probably asymptomatic.

The clinical manifestations are often dependent on the underlying type of CG that is present.

Type I cryoglobulinemia

Symptomatic patients usually present with hyperviscosity-related problems (neurological symptoms of blurring or loss of vision, headache, vertigo, nystagmus, dizziness, sudden deafness, diplopia, ataxia, confusion, and signs of Raynaud's phenomenon, digital ischemia, livedo reticularis and purpura).

Type II and III cryoglobulinemia

This typically presents with features related to systemic vasculitis. Common symptoms and signs are palpable purpura (most common sign), arthralgias, myalgia, fatigue, and numbness and weakness related to peripheral neuropathy.

These symptoms often are present for several years before a diagnosis is made and over this time it is common for the symptoms to spontaneously wax and wane.

Cutaneous

Purpura is the commonest cutaneous manifestation (present in ~90% of patients).

It usually occurs on the extremities, less commonly on the buttocks and trunk, and very rarely on the face.

Skin biopsy usually demonstrates a leukocytoclastic vasculitis.

Other less common skin manifestations include an urticarial rash due to venulitis, a deep cutaneous vasculitis leading to necrotic lesions, and digital ischemia/gangrene.

Musculoskeletal

Arthralgia is present in >70% of patients.

It is typically symmetrical and involves knees, hips, shoulders, metacarpophalangeal, and proximal interphalangeal joints.

Arthritis is uncommon.

Exacerbation in cold conditions is described by some patients.

Neuropathy

Symptomatic neuropathy is seen in up to 40% of patients.

Subclinical disease can be detected in up to 80% of patients by electrophysiological studies.

Neuropathy may be more common in non-HCV-related disease.

Pulmonary

40–50% of patients will have respiratory symptoms (cough, dyspnea, pleuritic pain).

Severe pulmonary disease with bronchiolitis obliterans organizing pneumonia (BOOP), lung hemorrhage, pulmonary vasculitis is uncommon but can seen when patients present with fulminant CG-related disease.

Renal

This usually results from immune complex deposition in type II and III disease, or from hyperviscosity in type I disease.

Up to 60% of patients will have renal disease.

It usually develops after a systemic prodrome, but can be the presenting manifestation of disease in a minority of patients.

More than 50% have proteinuria and/or hematuria.

20% have nephrotic syndrome.

20% have an acute nephritic syndrome.

10% present with acute oliguric renal failure.

50% are hypertensive, and this may be malignant and associated with acute renal dysfunction.

Other manifestations

A variety of other symptoms/signs can be identified.

Raynaud's phenomenon is seen in 50% of patients (usually associated with connective tissue diseases).

Sjögren's syndrome is seen in up to 20%.

Hepatomegaly and/or abnormal liver function tests in up to 90%.

Lymphadenopathy in 20%.

Splenomegaly in up to 50%.

Vasculitic involvement of the heart, central nervous system, and eye is very uncommon.

Investigation

The following investigations should be undertaken when CG-related disease is suspected.

Cryoglobulins.

The identification of a CG is clearly of fundamental importance.

The detection of a CG requires care in blood sample collection, transport, and processing.

Blood must be collected into prewarmed syringes and bottles, and then transported to the laboratory at 37°C. The serum is separated by centrifugation at 37°C.

The serum is transferred to a graduated tube and placed at 4°C for 5 days.

The serum is centrifuged and the volume of the precipitate is reported as a percentage of the serum volume (cryocrit).

The precipitate is then rewarmed (it should redissolve) and then subjected to further investigation (e.g. immunofixation, ELISA) to determine the concentration and constituents of the CG.

False-negative results can be caused by mishandling of the sample. If it cools at any time before serum separation, the CG may be lost. A negative result therefore needs to be interpreted in the clinical context, and repeat testing with appropriate sample handling may be necessary.

Cryocrits vary between 1 and 70% (higher values typically seen with type I cryoglobulinemia).

There is poor correlation between the cryocrit and the severity of clinical disease.

Complements

Type I disease usually leads to no complement abnormality.

Type II and III disease is associated with reduced C1q, C4 and CH$_{50}$. C3 is usually unaffected.

Autoantibodies

Rheumatoid factor is typically present in type II and III disease.

Antinuclear antibodies with multiple specificities (e.g. smooth muscle, microsomal, Ro, La, Sm, mitochondrial) are often present reflecting the association with connective tissue diseases.

Viral studies
Serological studies for HCV, HBV, HIV, and EBV, should be undertaken.

Other investigations
If a lymphoproliferative disorder is suspected, bone marrow biopsy, CT scanning for lymphadenopathy, and lymph node biopsy may be necessary.

Histology
In the evaluation of patients with cryoglobulinemia, biopsy of an affected organ is appropriate. This may be skin, peripheral nerve, or kidney (in those with abnormal urinalysis or renal function).

Renal biopsy
In patients with type II or III cryoglobulinemia, the histological appearances are usually those of mesangiocapillary glomerulonephritis (MCGN) type I. Endocapillary proliferation is invariable and in two-thirds GBM thickening/reduplication is seen.

Less commonly a focal and segmental pattern of injury, or mesangial proliferative GN can be seen.

Findings that differentiate cryoglobulinemic GN from idiopathic MCGN are:

- hyaline thrombi in the subendothelial space or in capillary lumen (seen in 70% of cases) (Fig. 4.6.1);
- intense leukocytic (monocyte) infiltration of glomeruli;
- fibrinoid necrosis of extraglomerular arterioles/arteries (seen in up to 30% of cases).

Immunofluorescence microscopy demonstrates IgM, IgG and C3 in a granular capillary wall distribution.

Electron microscopy reveals subendothelial and mesangial electron-dense deposits. These deposits may have an organized substructure ('fingerprint-like' appearance). These are not specific and can be seen in others situations, e.g. lupus nephritis.

Management
The optimal management of CG-related disease has not been well-defined.

The disease tends to follow a relapsing and remitting pattern. Data suggest that prolonged immunosuppression has no effect on the risk of developing progressive renal dysfunction; therefore such treatment is usually reserved for acute flares.

Treatment of the underlying disease process (i.e. lymphoproliferative disorder, viral disease, connective tissue disease) is important, however.

The general management principles for patients with glomerular disease should be adopted, i.e. blood pressure control, treatment of hyperlipidemia, and reduction of proteinuria using renin–angiotensin system inhibition.

Type I cryoglobulinemia
Chemotherapy (and radiotherapy) for the underlying lymphoproliferative disease is required.

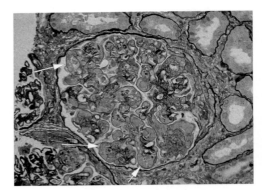

Fig. 4.6.1 Methanamine-silver-stained glomerulus showing hyaline deposits in capillaries and in the subendothelial compartment. Arrows indicate the position of the glomerular basement membrane. Endocapillary proliferation is also visible. (Courtesy of Dr Nick Mayer, University of Leicester Hospitals, UK.)

Corticosteroids and cyclophosphamide can be used for nonmalignancy-associated type I disease during acute flares.

Types II and III cryoglobulinemia
Mild symptoms (arthralgias, myalgia, fatigue) without evidence of end-organ damage can be treated conservatively with analgesia and cold avoidance. NSAIDs can be helpful, and low-dose corticosteroids can be used in those without symptomatic relief from NSAIDs.

Disease with evidence of end-organ damage requires immunosuppressive therapy.

Immunosuppression/plasmapheresis
For an acute flare with progressive renal dysfunction, severe neuropathy, or necrosis of extremities, the following regimen may be used:

- IV methylprednisolone 1 g/day for 3 days then 60 mg prednisolone/day followed by a slow taper over 2–3 months.
- Cyclophosphamide 2 mg/kg/day orally for 2 months.
- Plasmapheresis: 1 plasma volume exchange on alternate days for 2–3 weeks. Alternatively, cryofiltration (double filtration plasmapheresis with a cooling unit on the second filter) can be used in order to selectively remove the CG.

Improved renal function can be seen in 50–80% of patients with this regimen.

Monitoring of the cryocrit is not necessarily helpful given the poor correlation between the cryocrit and the severity of disease. Therefore the length of the course of plasmapheresis is determined by the clinical response.

Immunosuppression may theoretically be complicated by enhanced replication of underlying HCV, and exacerbation of low-grade non-Hodgkin lymphoma (in addition to the conventional risks of treatment, i.e. infection, bone marrow suppression, late malignancy, etc.).

Antiviral therapy

For HCV-related disease, antiviral therapy is appropriate.

Antiviral treatment should be delayed for 3–4 months after an acute flare that requires immunosuppressive treatment.

The treatment of choice is a combination of:
- Pegylated interferon-α 1 μg/kg weekly for 48 weeks.
- Ribavirin 1000 mg/day for 48 weeks.

This regimen should not be used in those with a GFR <50 mL/min (ribavirin is contraindicated and the prolonged half-life of pegylated interferon-α in this setting raises concerns about its use).

For those with renal impairment, nonpegylated interferon-α can be used alone. The optimal dose is unclear but interferon-α 3 million units 3 times a week for 12 months has been used with success.

This regimen is less effective than combination therapy, but can lead to a virological and clinical response in 60% of patients. Cessation of treatment almost invariably results in viral relapse.

Other treatments

Rituximab (monoclonal anti-CD20 antibody) has been evaluated in small studies with apparent clinical success, although at the expense of increased HCV RNA levels.

Its role remains to be determined but it can be considered in patients who do not respond to the treatments described above.

Dialysis and renal transplantation

The outcome on hemodialysis or peritoneal dialysis is similar to that seen in the matched dialysis population.

Renal transplantation should not be precluded in patients with CG-related disease even though 50–70% of renal allograft recipients develop clinically significant disease.

This is not usually a cause of graft failure.

The transplant immunosuppression appears to have no clinically significant effect on HCV replication.

Prognosis

Overall survival at 10 years after symptom onset and time of diagnosis is 70% and 50% respectively. Death is usually due to liver disease, cardiovascular disease or infection.

The risk of developing renal failure appears to be highest in those with HCV-related disease (up to 40%).

Approximately 5–10% of patients with type II cryoglobulinemia develop a lymphoproliferative disorder (usually B-cell non-Hodgkin lymphoma), usually 5–10 years after diagnosis. This risk is 35 times higher than that of the general population.

Risk factors for a poor outcome are: renal failure, infection, hypertension, and four or more extra-renal manifestations.

HCV-related renal disease (without cryoglobulinemia)

HCV infection can also cause MCGN type I without evidence of CG production. It has also been associated with membranous nephropathy in some patients.

In both conditions if there is evidence of severe, progressive glomerular disease (i.e. severe nephrosis, progressive renal function decline), antiviral therapy (as described above) should be considered (although in membranous nephropathy a causal role for HCV has not been established).

Further reading

Braun GS, Horster S, Wagner KS, Ihrler S, Schmid H. Cryoglobulinaemic vasculitis: classification and clinical and therapeutic aspects. *Postgrad Med J* 2007; **83**: 87–94.

Fabrizi F, Colucci P, Ponticelli C, Locatelli F. Kidney and liver involvement in cryoglobulinemia. *Semin Nephrol* 2002; **22**: 309–318.

Kamar N, Rostaing L, Alric L. Treatment of hepatitis C-virus-related glomerulonephritis. *Kidney Int* 2006; **69**: 436–439.

Meyers CM, Seeff LB, Stehman-Breen CO, Hoofnagle JH. Hepatitis C and renal disease: an update. *Am J Kidney Dis* 2003; **42**: 631–657.

Internet resources

Review article about cryoglobulinemia:

http://www.kidneyatlas.org/book4/adk4-09.pdf

See also

Immunological investigation of the patient with renal disease, p. 36

Proteinuria and/or hematuria, p. 76

Nephrotic syndrome, p. 80

Mesangiocapillary glomerulonephritis, p. 112

Infection-related glomerulonephritis, p. 128

Systemic lupus erythematosus

Systemic lupus erythematosus (SLE) is the most common multisystem autoimmune disease.

It has variable presentations and outcomes and can potentially be fatal.

Kidney involvement is the most frequent severe manifestation and it can lead to end-stage renal disease.

Definition

SLE represents a spectrum of disease characterized by:
- acute and chronic inflammation in multiple organs;
- circulating antinuclear autoantibodies (ANA);
- pathology featuring immune complex deposition and complement consumption.

Overlapping presentations with other autoimmune syndromes are common.

Persistence of inflammation results in tissue damage, loss of organ function and incapacity.

Epidemiology

Nine-fold female preponderance.

Five-fold preponderance among Blacks compared with Caucasians.

Peak age of diagnosis is 20–40 years but it may occur at any age. Diagnosis is often delayed in the elderly.

Prevalence of 40–200 per 100 000.

Etiology

There is a multifactorial genetic susceptibility including contributions from:
- C-reactive protein;
- Fc gamma receptor;
- complement components;
- Toll-like receptor 5;
- MHC class II and III;
- B-lymphoid tyrosine kinase.

Concordance rate for monozygotic twins is 25%, and 2% for dizygotic twins.

Drug-induced SLE (procainamide, hydralazine, quinidine) usually affects the skin and joints. Renal and CNS involvement is rare.

Infection often precedes the initial presentation or relapse. Patients have a higher prevalence of EBV and CMV infection than controls.

Ultraviolet radiation causes a photosensitive rash and increases the relapse risk.

Pathogenesis

The pathogenesis of SLE is complex with dysregulation of many levels of the immune system.

Autoantibody and immune complex formation

Antinuclear antibodies are present in the circulation in >97% of cases and pathogenic anti-dsDNA antibodies are deposited in the kidneys and other sites of inflammation.

Other pathogenic antibodies can occur:
- antibody-mediated cytopenias;
- fetal heart disease mediated by anti-Ro antibodies.

Immune complexes such as anti-dsDNA–nucleosome complexes, deposit in tissues and:
- activate complement;
- attract inflammatory cells;
- initiate acute inflammation.

Lymphocyte activation

There is increased T-cell:B-cell activation and interaction through co-stimulatory ligands (e.g. CD40:CD40 ligand), antigen presentation, and B-cell-stimulating cytokines (e.g. Blys, APRIL).

Apoptosis

There is excess apoptosis and defective removal of apoptotic debris. Autoantigens present on apoptotic blebs trigger antigen-driven immune responses.

Cytokine production

There is increased interferon-α and interleukin-10 activity with upregulation of interferon-dependent inflammatory genes.

The role of TNF-α remains controversial.

Natural history

SLE may resolve after one episode but it usually follows a relapsing-remitting course.

Outcomes are variable and depend on disease severity and treatment response.

Mortality is increased. In Europe (1990–2000) this was 5% at 10 years for nonrenal SLE and 12% at 10 years for lupus nephritis.

Chronic morbidity and incapacity is frequent as a result of chronic inflammation and organ damage, and the consequences of therapy, especially glucocorticoids.

There is a greatly increased risk of cardiovascular disease and possibly an increased risk of malignancy.

Quality of life is impaired due to chronic fatigue, fibro-myalgia, depression, neurocognitive dysfunction and incapacity.

Presentation

The presentation of SLE is very variable.

There is often a prodomal phase of several months or years of constitutional disturbance and other symptoms before the diagnosis is made.

Acute presentations are more common in younger patients.

Subacute or atypical presentations are more common in those aged >50 years.

Prodomal phase

Serological abnormalities can precede clinical manifestations by several years.

Organ-specific autoimmunity, e.g. idiopathic thrombocytopenic purpura, can precede SLE.

Acute presentation

Fever, rash, polyarthritis and organ-specific manifestations, such as nephritis.

Subacute presentation

Remitting, relapsing course with constitutional disturbance, especially fatigue and organ-specific features, such as polyarthralgia/polyarthritis, rash, pleuritic chest pain.

Differential diagnosis

The diagnosis of SLE first requires suspicion of the diagnosis, exclusion of other possible causes for the presenting symptoms, and then integration of the clinical features with the results of serological and other investigations.

There are no consensus diagnostic criteria for clinical practice but the American College of Rheumatology criteria for inclusion into clinical trials (4/11 required) are widely used (Table 4.7.1).

Table 4.7.1 American College of Rheumatology (ACR) criteria for inclusion into clinical trials (requires at least four)

Mucocutaneous (4)	1. Malar erythema
	2. Erythematous raised patches
	3. Photosensitivity
	4. Oral or nasopharyngeal ulceration
Organ-specific (4)	5. Arthritis
	6. Serositis
	7. Nephritis
	8. CNS
Hematology or serology (3)	9. Cytopenia
	10. Specific autoantibodies
	11. ANA

Limited and early lupus presentations may not meet these criteria – a diagnosis of SLE should not be ruled out in this setting.

Almost all SLE patients are ANA positive at diagnosis (except some with cutaneous SLE).

Some patients with antiphospholipid syndrome (APS) without ANA may have features of SLE.

In the absence of ANA a diagnosis of SLE should always be treated with suspicion and other conditions should be considered. These include:
* malignancy and paraneoplastic syndromes;
* other organ specific or multisystem autoimmune diseases, such as vasculitis.

Infections, especially chronic viral infections such as HIV, can cause multisystem chronic inflammation and ANA positivity.

Investigation

Serology

Antinuclear antibodies
Although sensitive, ANA has a low specificity for SLE.

Specificity is increased by:
* confirmation of ANA positivity by immunofluorescence on Hep 2 cells;
* anti-dsDNA or ENA positivity (e.g. Ro, La, Jo, Sm, RNP);
* specificity of anti-dsDNA assay is increased by the crithidia immunofluorescence test.

Complement
Usually there is reduced C3 or C4.

An isolated low C4 level can be a normal variant.

If complement is low and ANA is normal, consider an alternative cause of complement consumption, such as cryoglobulinemia or chronic infection.

Antiphospholipid antibodies
Antiphospholipid antibodies (aPL) comprise a family of antibodies reactive with epitopes on proteins which are themselves complexed with negatively charged phospholipid and include:
* β_2-glycoprotein I;
* annexin V;
* protein C;
* protein S;
* prothrombin.

The presence of aPL is determined using immunoassays that typically use cardiolipin as the antigen (and detect anticardiolipin antibodies (aCL)), but some methods use phosphatidylserine.

Anticardiolipin antibodies:

There is debate over the importance of the aCL isotype.

IgG antibodies may be more clinically significant, although IgM aCL appear to be associated with thrombotic events and miscarriage in some series.

Tests for IgA antibodies may not be clinically informative and their use is not currently recommended.

Anti-β_2-GP-I antibodies:

Many aPL require β_2-glycoprotein I (β_2-GP-I), a phospholipid-binding plasma protein with weak anticoagulant activity, for binding to acidic phospholipids such as phosphatidylserine and cardiolipin.

The precise relationships among β_2-GP-I, phospholipid and autoantibody are disputed.

β_2-GP-I antibody assays show higher precision and better correlation with the thromboembolic complications in APS and SLE than assays for aCL and are less likely to show transient positive results in association with infection.

Lupus anticoagulant
This is an *in vitro* anomaly where there is prolongation of phospholipid-dependent coagulation due to the presence of a phospholipid-dependent inhibitor (aPL).

A prolonged activated partial thromboplastin time (APTT) suggests the presence of a lupus anticoagulant.

The presence of a lupus anticoagulant is confirmed with the diluted Russell's viper venom test (DRVVT).

Immunoglobulins
Total IgG levels are often raised but are nonspecific.

ANCA
P-ANCA and myeloperoxidase (MPO)-specific ANCA can be 'false positive' in SLE and have no clinical significance in this setting.

Histology
Skin biopsy has characteristic features with immune complex deposition at the dermal–epidermal junction.

Renal biopsy: see below.

Treatment

Initial subclassification depends on the presence/absence of organ-threatening features.

Without organ-threatening features
Consider:
* hydroxycholoroquine;
* prednisolone.

Hydroxycholoroquine 200–400 mg/day, especially for skin and joint disease (mepacrine is an alternative). Long-term hydroxychloroquine reduces cardiovascular and SLE relapse risk. It is often continued despite the requirement for other agents.

Prednisolone, orally in doses of <0.5 mg/kg/day reduced to 5–10 mg/day. Consider immunosuppressive if dose cannot be reduced below 10 mg/day without relapse.

With organ-threatening features
Use a combination of:
- daily oral prednisolone with an immunosuppressive (see lupus nephritis treatment below).

Acute flare
Consider:
- IV methylprednisolone (e.g. 500 mg/day × 3 doses); or
- higher-dose oral prednisolone.

Refractory disease
Consider:
- IV methylprednisolone;
- an alternative immunosuppressive;
- rituximab;
- high dose IV immunoglobulin;
- plasma exchange.

The role of autologous stem cell transplantation is uncertain.

Hormonal therapy
Trials of dehydroepiandrosterone have been disappointing. Female hormone replacement therapy increases relapse risk.

The oral contraceptive pill appears safe.

Monitoring
This is multidimensional.

Disease activity
Can be guided by validated tools such as:

SLEDAI:
http://www.rheumatology.org/sections/pediatric/sledai.asp?aud=mem

BILAG index:
http://www.limathon.com/BLIPS%20Bilag.htm

Blood pressure and urine dipstick for blood and protein at every evaluation.

Treatment toxicity and infections
End-organ damage
Can be guided by validated tools such as:

The SLICC/ACR Damage Index:
http://www.rheumatology.org/publications/classification/guide4.asp?aud=mem

Comorbidity
Particular attention should be paid to:
- cardiovascular risk;
- malignancy;
- bone disease.

Quality of life and neurocognitive function
Laboratory studies should include:
- full blood count, ESR;

- urea and electrolytes, creatinine, liver function tests and C-reactive protein;
- anti-dsDNA, C3 and C4 levels.

Frequency of evaluation
At least every 3 months for organ-threatening disease and/or treatment with immune suppression.

At least every 6 months for mild/moderate disease.

Lupus nephritis
Classification
The 1982 WHO histological classification has been replaced by the 2003 ISN/RPS system (Table 4.7.2).

Table 4.7.2 The 2003 International Society of Nephrology/Renal Pathology Forum (ISN/RPF) classification of lupus nephritis

Class O	Normal.
Class I	Light microscopy normal, immune deposits on immunofluorescence.
Class II	**Mesangial** deposits and hypercellularity.
Class III	Focal **proliferative** glomerulonephritis (<50% glomeruli) with leukocyte infiltration. Immune deposits in the mesangium and subendothelium.
Class IV	Diffuse **proliferative** glomerulonephritis (>50% glomeruli). May also see glomerular crescents and fibrinoid necrosis.
Class V	**Membranous** nephropathy with uniform thickening of capillary walls and subepithelial immune complex deposition.
Class VI	**Glomerulosclerosis**

Classes III and IV are subdivided into active (a), chronic (c) or mixed (a/c). Class IV is also subdivided into segmental or global.
Mixed membranous and proliferative glomerulonephritis is termed class III + V or IV + V.

Membranoproliferative nephritis is now III + V or IV + V, instead of subsets of V.

Proliferative lesions (class III and IV) are now subclassified as active (a), chronic (c) or mixed (a/c), and segmental or global.

The prognostic significance of the 2003 system has not been determined.

Previous studies have found the worst prognosis with class VI, then class IV, then III, but there are conflicting data on the outcome of class V due to differences in definition.

The 2003 system only reflects proliferative and membranous glomerulonephritis.

Other important renal pathologies occur in SLE, including:
- tubulointerstitial nephritis;
- thrombotic microangiopathy;
- podocytopathy (presents as 'minimal change' glomerulopathy);
- arteritis;
- renal artery stenosis.

Presentation
Asymptomatic hematuria/leukocyturia or proteinuria.

Nephrotic syndrome.

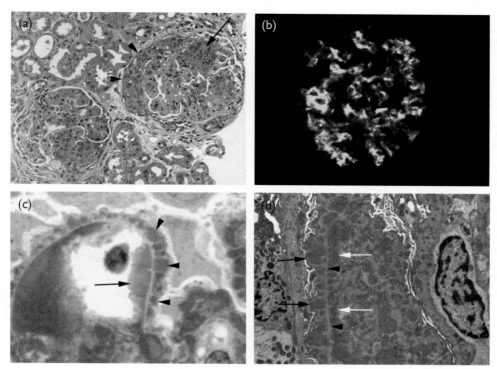

Fig. 4.7.1 (a) H&E-stained section showing two glomeruli from a biopsy with class IVa (g) nephritis. There is global proliferation, segmental necrosis with leukocyte infiltration (arrow), and crescent formation (arrowheads). (b) Immunofluorescence micrograph from a biopsy with class IVa (g) nephritis demonstrating C3 deposition in a mesangial and capillary loop distribution. (c) Photomicrograph of a Toluidine Blue-stained glomerulus from a biopsy demonstrating class IVa (g) lupus nephritis. Extensive deposits can be identified in the subendothelial (arrow) and intramembranous/subepithelial (arrowheads) compartments. (d) Electron micrograph of a tangentially sectioned glomerular basement membrane demonstrating multiple subendothelial (white arrows) and intramembranous/subepithelial (black arrows) electron-dense deposits. The line of the GBM is indicated by the arrowheads. (Courtesy of Prof. Peter Furness, Consultant Histopathologist, University Hospitals of Leicester, UK.)

Nephritic syndrome, often with declining renal function, 'rapidly progressive glomerulonephritis'.

Hypertension.

Treatment
Aims of treatment are to:
- induce a renal response or partial remission then a full remission (Table 4.7.3);
- prevent relapse.

Table 4.7.3 Renal response and remission criteria

Criterion	Partial remission (response)	Full remission
Proteinuria	<50% baseline	<500 mg/24 h
Hematuria	<30 rbc/hpf, no cellular casts	<5 rbc/hpf, no cellular casts
GFR	Stable, or <10% decrease from baseline	Stable and within 10% of normal

rbc/hpf, red blood cells per high-powered field; GFR, glomerular filtration rate.

Definitions of renal response and remission vary between consensus statements and between clinical trials. Definitions of full remission often require a period of observation, e.g. >1 month, and concomitant medication to be below a threshold, e.g. prednisolone ≤10 mg/day.

Induction of remission

The induction period necessary to induce remission is 6–24 months.

Class I and II lupus nephritis with proteinuria: glucocorticoids are used alone.

Class III, IV and V lupus nephritis: induction of remission requires the use of combination glucocorticoid/immunosuppressive therapy.

Glucocorticoids

There is no consensus on the optimum regimen.

Two common approaches are:
- IV methylprednisolone 500 mg/day × 3, followed by oral prednisolone 0.5 mg/kg/day reducing in steps (Eurolupus); or
- oral prednisolone 1 mg/kg/day reducing in steps with no IV glucocorticoid.

Immunosuppression

IV cyclophosphamide and oral mycophenolate mofetil are equally effective and have a similar early toxicity profile.

Cyclophosphamide causes ovarian failure and an increased malignancy risk.

Azathioprine is an alternative.

Calcineurin inhibitors are alternatives for class V lupus nephritis.

Methotrexate is also an alternative but avoid with renal impairment.

Cyclophosphamide:

Most clinicians use 'sequential' regimens with 3–6 months of cyclophosphamide followed by mycophenolate mofetil or azathioprine.

Two cyclophosphamide regimens are in common use:
- 500 mg every 2 weeks × 6 doses ('Eurolupus'); or
- 0.75 g/m²/month × 6 doses, adjusted to a neutrophil nadir of 3–4 × 10⁹/L ('NIH').

Consider bladder protection with prehydration and MESNA (sodium 2-sulfanylethanesulfonate).

Consider ovarian protection with gonadotrophin antagonism.

Mycophenolate mofetil:

The target dose is 2–3 g/day.

Lower doses may be effective for intolerant patients.

There is no effect of age, sex, weight or ethnicity on pharmacokinetics.

Treatment failure
20% of patients will be intolerant of either cyclophosphamide or mycophenolate mofetil and a further 20% will fail to achieve remission.

For these cases a switch between immunosuppressives or a switch to rituximab should be considered.

Consider azathioprine for intolerance.

Progressive disease
First, switch between immunosuppressive agents and administer IV methylprednisolone 500 mg/kg/day × 3 doses.

Then, consider rituximab or plasma exchange.

Prevention of relapse
There is no consensus on drugs or duration.

The typical duration of treatment is 3–5 years.

Relapse risk is increased by:
- hydroxychloroquine, glucocorticoid or immunosuppressive removal;
- shorter duration of therapy;
- persisting positive anti-dsDNA or low complement levels;
- infection.

Blood pressure control
Maintain good BP control and consider ACEIs or ARBs as long-term therapy for all patients.

Transplantation
There is a high risk of early thrombotic complications with APS.

There is an increased early infective risk due to SLE and prior treatment exposure.

Long-term outcomes are otherwise similar to other causes of ESRD.

Monitoring
As for general SLE above.

Proteinuria quantification (albumin/creatinine ratio or 24 h collection) at every visit.

Hematuria: look for dysmorphic erythrocytes and consider lower urinary tract origin.

Blood pressure rise can indicate renal relapse.

Role of repeat biopsy has not been determined but may be used:
- in relapse, for diagnosis, to identify change of pathology and score activity and chronicity;
- in remission, when there is poor association between urinary abnormalities and renal histology to score activity and chronicity and guide therapy.

Other organ manifestations
Skin
Assess using standardized classification.

Therapy with hydroxychloroquine, dapsone, topical tacrolimus, thalidomide, or as for general SLE.

Central nervous system
Assess with brain MR and diffusion-weighted imaging, CSF examination and neurology opinion. Psychiatric evaluation may be required.

Consider infection, APS, embolization, drug effects and hypertensive encephalopathy (especially in lupus nephritis).

Treat with high-dose glucocorticoid and immunosuppressive (current evidence supports cyclophosphamide). For treatment failure, consider an alternative immunosuppressive or rituximab.

Lung and heart
Pulmonary pathology includes the following.

Parenchymal disease:
- pneumonitis;
- alveolar hemorrhage;
- pulmonary fibrosis;
- shrinking lung syndrome.

Pulmonary vascular disease:
- thromboembolism;
- nonembolic pulmonary hypertension.

Assess with CT scanning, pulmonary function tests and, rarely, lung biopsy.

Cardiac pathology includes:
- pericarditis;
- myocarditis;
- endocarditis;
- valvular lesions;
- coronary atheroma.

'Libman–Sachs' endocarditis is associated with APS.

Assess with echocardiography and cardiac MR, angiography and right-heart catheterization when indicated.

Treat as for general SLE with 'organ-threatening' disease.

Antiphospholipid syndrome
APS is defined as:
- positive aCL and/or lupus anticoagulant (LAC) detected on two occasions;
- spontaneous arterial or venous thrombosis.

Primary APS is the disease occurring as a sole entity and secondary APS is the disease occurring in the context of SLE.

Thrombosis risk in SLE is increased without APS.

Positive aCL and/or LAC without thrombosis in SLE indicates further increased risk and is usually treated with aspirin.

A first thrombotic event then requires prolonged, possibly lifelong, anticoagulation.

Catastrophic APS is a clinical presentation of multiple and progressive thromboses. Treatment can include IV methyl prednisolone, plasma exchange and anticoagulation.

APS and the kidney
• Thrombotic microangiopathy.
• Renal artery thrombosis.
• Increased risk of renal biopsy due to hemorrhage and withdrawal of anticoagulation.
• Increased risk of early thrombotic complications post-transplantation.

Pregnancy
Preconception counselling is necessary to consider:
• fertility;
• risk of miscarriage;
• risk of pregnancy to the baby and to the mother;
• risk of lupus flare;
• preconception medication;
• medications during and after pregnancy and breast feeding.

The following drugs should be avoided at conception and during pregnancy:
• mycophenolate mofetil;
• cyclophosphamide;
• methotrexate;
• warfarin;
• ACEIs and ARBs.

Hydroxychloroquine, prednisolone and azathioprine can be continued during pregnancy.

Consider aspirin throughout pregnancy and low molecular weight heparin for patients with a history of:
• miscarriage;
• thrombosis;
• antiphospholipid syndrome;
• significant proteinuria.

Do not reduce the intensity of therapy during pregnancy as the lupus flare risk remains.

Use IV methylprednisolone or high dose IV immunoglobulin for flares.

Withdraw ACEIs and ARBs before or after conception and replace with labetolol or methyldopa until after delivery.

Monitor lupus activity, blood pressure, proteinuria, fetal growth and uterine artery Doppler during pregnancy.

If anti-Ro positive, monitor fetal heart rate. There is a 1 in 20 risk of fetal complete heart block.

Relapse risk is highest immediately after delivery, high-dose oral prednisolone or IV methylprednisolone should be considered as prophylaxis.

There is an increased risk of HELLP syndrome.

Patient advice
Areas to be considered when counselling patients:
• about SLE and outcomes;
• drug information and management of toxicity;
• fertility, conception and pregnancy counselling;
• management of cardiovascular and malignancy risk, e.g. smoking avoidance, cervical screening and mammography.

Encourage patient involvement in monitoring of disease, e.g. blood pressure, urine dipstick analysis.

Patient support groups, e.g. Lupus UK.

Further reading
Bertsias G, Ioannidis JP, Boletis J, et al. EULAR recommendations for the management of systemic lupus erythematosus. Report of a Task Force of the EULAR Standing Committee for International Clinical Studies Including Therapeutics. Ann Rheum Dis 2008; **67**: 195–205.

Flanc RS, Roberts MA, Strippoli GF, Chadban SJ, Kerr PG, Atkins RC. Treatment for lupus nephritis. Cochrane Database Syst Rev 2004; CD002922.

Ponticelli CB, Moroni G. Systemic lupus erythematosus (Clinical). In: Davison AC, Grunfeld J-P; Ponticelli C, Ritz E, Winearls C, van Ypersele C (eds), Oxford textbook of clinical nephrology. Oxford: Oxford University Press; 2006. 4.7.2.

Walsh M, James M, Jayne D, Tonelli M, Manns BJ, Hemmelgarn BR. Mycophenolate mofetil for induction therapy of lupus nephritis: a systematic review and meta-analysis. Clin J Am Soc Nephrol 2007; **2**: 968–975.

Walsh M, Jayne D. Rituximab in the treatment of anti-neutrophil cytoplasm antibody associated vasculitis and systemic lupus erythematosus: past, present and future. Kidney Int 2007; **72**: 676–682.

Weening JJ, D'Agati VD, Schwartz MM, et al. The classification of glomerulonephritis in systemic lupus erythematosus revisited. Kidney Int 2004; **65**: 521–530.

Yee CS, Farewell V, Isenberg DA, et al. British Isles Lupus Assessment Group index is valid for assessment of 2007. Arthritis Rheum 2004; **56**: 4113–4119.

Internet resources
British Society of Hematology Guidelines for Investigation and Management of Antiphospholipid syndrome:

http://www.blackwell-synergy.com/links/doi/10.1046/

j.1365-2141.2000.02069.x/full/

Lupus Foundation of America:

www.lupus.org/

Lupus UK:

http://www.lupusuk.com/

The lupus site:

http://www.uklupus.co.uk/

See also
Immunological investigation of renal disease, p. 36

Rheumatoid arthritis, connective tissue diseases and Sjögren's syndrome, p. 188

Glomerulonephritis, vasculitis, and nephrotic syndrome, p. 340

Scleroderma–systemic sclerosis

Systemic sclerosis (SSc) is a heterogeneous autoimmune rheumatic disease of uncertain etiology, characterized by inflammation and fibrosis in skin and other organs, and vascular abnormalities including Raynaud's phenomenon. It is classified into diffuse cutaneous systemic sclerosis (dcSSc: skin involvement proximal to the elbows and knees) and limited cutaneous systemic sclerosis (lcSSc: distal skin involvement only). These have distinct associations with organ involvement and outcomes.

Epidemiology
It is more common in women (female:male 5:1).

The onset peaks at 40–60 years of age.

There is an association with silica and solvent exposure.

The prevalence is estimated to be 3–24 per 100 000.

Autoantibodies and SSc
Autoantibodies associated with SSc are listed in Table 4.8.1. These are valuable for diagnosis and for identifying cases at risk of particular complications.

Renal disease in systemic sclerosis
This may be divided into:
- scleroderma renal crisis;
- other acute presentations;
- chronic kidney disease.

Renal function should be routinely monitored in all cases of SSc with estimated GFR determination and urinalysis at least every 6 months, and close home-monitoring of BP in dcSSc cases.

Scleroderma renal crisis

Definition
Scleroderma renal crisis (SRC) is a clinical syndrome of acute renal failure and accelerated hypertension in the presence of systemic sclerosis.

Frequency
It occurs in 5% of all SSc patients (15% of dcSSc cases, and 2% of lcSSc cases).

Risk factors
- Recent-onset diffuse scleroderma.
- Active, progressive skin disease.
- Tendon friction rubs.
- Anemia.
- New cardiac events.
- Steroid use (≥15 mg prednisolone/day).
- Presence of anti-RNA polymerase III.

Clinical features
Patients with SRC will typically have an acute or subacute presentation with fluid overload and/or symptoms of end-organ complications of hypertension. Often nonspecific systemic symptoms (malaise, exertional breathlessness) are present for weeks before presentation with:
- acute kidney injury.
- new-onset hypertension (>90%).
- pulmonary edema (>50%).
- encephalopathy (20%).
- seizures (10%).
- hypertensive retinopathy (>60%).

Table 4.8.1 Autoantibody associations with scleroderma

Autoantibody target	% of SSc	Clinical association
ACA[a] (anticentromere ab)	30%	lcSSc Pulmonary arterial hypertension
Scl-70[a] (topoisomerase-1)	20%	dcSSc Pulmonary fibrosis
RNA polymerase[a]	12%	High risk of renal crisis
PM-Scl[a]	4%	Overlap with myositis
Antifibrillarin[a] (U3-RNP)	5%	dcSSc PAH Myositis
U1-RNP	10%	Overlap with SLE, myositis, arthritis
Th/To	<5%	lcSSc with lung fibrosis

[a]Scleroderma-defining antibody.

lcSSc, limited cutaneous systemic sclerosis; dcSSc, diffuse cutaneous systemic sclerosis; PAH, pulmonary arterial hypertension.

Investigations
Urinalysis: non-nephrotic range proteinuria; microscopic hematuria.

Blood film: microangiopathic hemolytic anemia (MAHA) with schistocytes is found in 50%.

Renal biopsy shows intimal proliferation, thrombotic microangiopathy, and often fibrinoid necrosis. It also excludes other pathology (Fig. 4.8.1).

Echocardiography commonly demonstrates reduced left ventricular systolic function. This will usually resolve as afterload falls with successful treatment.

Pericardial effusions are common, but tamponade occurs infrequently (<5%).

Tachy- or bradyarrhythmias may occur and are associated with a poor prognosis.

Treatment
The target for antihypertensive treatment is to bring the systolic BP down by 20 mmHg and the diastolic by 10 mmHg per 24 h, into the normal range, while avoiding periods of hypotension. An arterial line and central venous catheter may aid in monitoring the response to treatment.

ACEIs must be instituted since they have been shown to reduce mortality. Captopril has a short half-life and may be easiest to titrate to the blood pressure initially, but longer-acting ACEI are usually more convenient in the long term.

Intravenous prostacyclin (0.2–2 ng/kg/min) increases renal perfusion, and also may help to normalize blood pressure.

ARBs can be safely added if required once ACEIs are at full dose. Alpha-blockers and calcium antagonists are also helpful for refractory hypertension.

Plasma exchange may be of use in profound MAHA.

Renal support with hemodialysis is required in approximately two-thirds of all cases.

Prognosis

Of the two-thirds of patients who require dialysis, one-half of these will be able to discontinue dialysis by 2 years after the onset of SRC.

A poor renal outcome is predicted by low blood pressure at presentation, and the presence of fibrinoid necrosis and mucoid intimal thickening on renal biopsy.

Mortality is significant (30% at 3 years) and is highest in those requiring permanent dialysis.

Renal transplantation may be considered in patients who still require dialysis at 2 years. Survival rates are similar to transplant recipients with other connective tissue diseases.

Recurrence of SRC is rare in patients concordant with medication, and uncommon (5%) following transplantation.

Prevention

There is no evidence that ACEI or ATII receptor blockade is effective in preventing SRC.

Patients at risk of SRC should avoid doses of steroid >10 mg prednisolone/day.

Further practical advice on the management of SRC is described in Table 4.8.2.

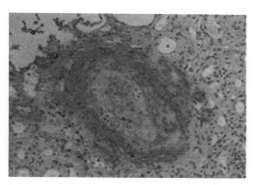

Fig. 4.8.1. Renal biopsy of scleroderma renal crisis artery: smooth muscle actin immunohistochemistry stain ×10. Note expansion of the vessel media, proliferation of the intima and obliteration of the lumen.

Other renal disease in systemic sclerosis

Acute disease

SSc patients with SLE overlap features can develop glomerulonephritis – suspect this in patients with red cell casts, and in those with serological features of SLE in the presence or absence of a scleroderma-defining antibody (Table 4.8.1).

Systemic vasculitis occurs in a small proportion (<2%) of SSc patients. It often affects the lungs in addition to the kidney, is accompanied by pANCA positivity, and responds to cyclophosphamide.

Chronic disease

CKD is common in patients without SRC. The fibrotic burden in SSc kidneys is significantly greater than in controls, with high levels of collagen in the interstitium, the mesangium, and around blood vessels.

Use of drugs such as NSAIDs, cyclosporin and penicillamine may also contribute to renal fibrosis.

Follow-up studies of SSc patients with CKD do not demonstrate significant rates of progression to dialysis however.

Table 4.8.2 Practical tips in scleroderma renal crisis

- Patients may present with normal BP/serum creatinine in the normal range.
- Fluid balance is difficult due to the high peripheral vascular resistance – use small volume fluid challenges.
- BP is often labile initially. ACEIs are first-line therapy but additional agents often also required.
- Manage in the HDU/ITU setting with central venous and arterial monitoring.
- Biopsy is safe when BP is controlled, and excludes alternative diagnoses.
- Anti-RNA polymerase III antibody is suggested by the presence of fine speckled pattern of ANA in the absence of other routine ENA positivity.
- Fistula formation is safe in those requiring long-term hemodialysis (despite secondary Raynaud's phenomenon).
- Line-related sepsis is a common complication in these patients due to abnormal skin function.
- Peritoneal dialysis is well-tolerated in those with sufficient intrinsic renal function.
- Recovery of renal function can occur up to 2 years after SRC and renal transplantation should only be considered after this time.

HDU, high dependency unit; ITU, intensive therapy unit.

References

Bunn CC, Denton CP, Shiwen X, *et al.* Anti-RNA polymerases and other autoantibody specificities in systemic sclerosis. *Br J Rheumatol* 1998; **37**: 15–20.

Gibney EM, Parikh CR, Jani A, *et al.* Kidney transplantation for systemic sclerosis improves survival and may modulate disease activity. *Am J Transplant* 2004; **4**: 2027–2031.

Penn H, Howie A, Stratton R, *et al.* Scleroderma renal crisis – patient characteristics and long term outcomes in 110 cases. *Q J Med* 2007; in press.

Steen V, Syzd A, Johnson JP, *et al.* Kidney disease other than renal crisis in patients with diffuse scleroderma. *J Rheumatol.* 2005; **32**: 649–655.

Steen VD, Costantino JP, Shapiro AP, *et al.* Outcome of renal crisis in systemic sclerosis: relation to availability of angiotensin converting enzyme (ACE) inhibitors. *Ann Intern Med* 1990; **113**: 352–357.

Internet resources

The Scleroderma Clinical Trials Consortium:

www.sctc-online.org

The EULAR scleroderma trials and research group:

www.eustar.org

Raynaud's and Scleroderma Association – for medical information and patient support:

www.raynauds.org.uk

Rheumatoid arthritis, connective tissue diseases, and Sjögren's syndrome

Rheumatoid arthritis

Clinical

Rheumatoid arthritis (RA) is a multisystem autoimmune disorder characterized by involvement of synovial joints, in which inflammation can lead to joint erosion.

Epidemiology

The prevalence of RA in the UK has recently been estimated to be 0.8% with a female predominance, particularly in younger age groups.

Treatment

A range of disease-modifying antirheumatic drugs (DMARDs) can be used (Table 4.9.1) but methotrexate has become the commonest first-choice DMARD.

Recently, the use of biologic drugs in patients resistant to or unable to tolerate treatment with standard DMARDs has become more common.

Supports diagnosis

The presence of rheumatoid factor and/or anti-CCP (cyclic citrullinated peptide) antibodies.

Renal manifestations

RA *per se* is rarely associated with clinically overt renal disease although longstanding RA, particularly if poorly controlled, may be associated with the development of amyloidosis (AA amyloid).

When renal disease does occur, it most commonly arises as a result of the treatments used (Table 4.9.1), but mesangioproliferative glomerulonephritis, membranous nephropathy and IgA nephropathy have all been reported in association with RA.

Mixed connective tissue disease

Clinical

Mixed connective tissue disease (MCTD) is characterized by overlapping features of systemic sclerosis, systemic lupus erythematosus (SLE) and polymyositis and is associated with antibodies to the U1 ribonuclear protein (U1RNP).

Clinical features include a high frequency of Raynaud's syndrome, swollen hands, sclerodactyly, polymyositis, fibrosing alveolitis and pulmonary hypertension.

Joint involvement can range from joint pain (arthralgia) through to an erosive arthritis.

Other clinical features reflect those of the diseases with which it overlaps.

Epidemiology

Like other connective tissue diseases, it shows a female predominance (9:1) and has a prevalence of ~10/100 000.

MCTD often evolves over time into systemic lupus erythematosis (SLE) or systemic sclerosis.

Pulmonary hypertension and scleroderma renal crisis are important causes of death, the former being the most frequent.

Diagnosis

This is dependent on the presence of high titer U1RNP antibodies.

Treatment

The treatment choice depends on the pattern of clinical involvement. For example, NSAIDs (Table 4.9.1) and anti-malarials (Table 4.9.1) are used for joint (arthralgia) and skin involvement, corticosteroids for arthritis, and high dose corticosteroids for myositis and fibrosing alveolitis.

Fibrosing alveolitis may also require more intensive treatment with cyclophosphamide (Table 4.9.1).

Azathioprine (Table 4.9.1) is often used as a steroid-sparing agent.

Renal manifestations

Clinically overt renal disease is said to be rare but biopsy studies have revealed that glomerular disease, particularly membranous nephropathy, does occur in 10–50% of patients.

As the disease evolves, the renal manifestations will also evolve into those of the underlying disease (i.e. lupus nephritis or scleroderma renal disease) and should be managed accordingly.

Overlap syndromes

Clinical

Overlap syndromes are defined as the overlap of clinical features of connective tissue diseases such as those listed above, but without anti-U1RNP antibody positivity.

As in MCTD, patients often evolve features more consistent with one connective tissue disease over time.

Treatment

As above, treatment will depend on the pattern of clinical involvement.

Renal manifestations

The renal manifestations will depend on the connective tissue disease features and should be managed as such.

For example, a patient with features of SLE and myositis may well develop lupus nephritis.

Polymyositis and dermatomyositis

Clinical

These conditions are characterized by an inflammatory myositis of skeletal muscles, often presenting as symmetrical weakness of proximal limb muscles.

Dermatomyositis is associated with characteristic skin involvement such as a heliotrope rash on the eyelids and Gottron's papules.

When it presents in the >50 year age group, dermatomyositis may be associated with underlying neoplasia.

Epidemiology

The prevalence of the disease is 50 per 100 000 and women are affected twice as commonly as men.

A bimodal pattern of age at onset is seen with a peak in childhood (5–15 years) and a second peak in middle age (50–70 years).

The incidence of renal disease is ~20%.

Supports diagnosis

Raised creatine kinase, abnormal electromyography, abnormal muscle biopsy, anti-aminoacyl-tRNA synthetase antibodies, e.g. anti-Jo-1.

Table 4.9.1 Potential renal complications of drugs used to treat rheumatoid arthritis

Drug therapy	Renal manifestation	Comment
NSAIDs	Hemodynamically mediated AKI. Presents with significant increases in plasma creatinine and reduced GFR.	Potentially reversible on drug withdrawal. Occurs as a result of renal ischemia caused by inhibition of prostaglandin production, which alters local glomerular arteriolar perfusion.
	Acute interstitial nephritis.	Presents with fever, rash and eosinophilia and is usually the result of an allergic reaction to the drug. Eosinophils are often present in the urine. Reversible with removal of drug.
Antimalarials (chloroquine/ hydroxychloroquine)	Very rare cases of chloroquine toxicity mimicking the appearance of Fabry disease have been reported in the literature.	Reversible on drug withdrawal.
Sulphasalazine	None reported in relation to treatment for RA.	When used as treatment for inflammatory bowel disease, interstitial nephritis has been reported to occur in 0.29 cases per 100 person-years.
Methotrexate	Decrease in GFR	Reversible on drug withdrawal. 90% of dose is cleared via kidneys.
Oral gold (auranofin) Rarely used now for treatment of RA.	Proteinuria in ~10% patients, usually mild.	Gradual improvement on drug withdrawal.
Parenteral gold (sodium aurothiomalate) Rarely used now for treatment of RA.	Affects ~10% of patients. Membranous nephropathy most common renal lesion. Presents with proteinuria (can be nephrotic range) and hematuria.	Usually gradual improvement on drug withdrawal. Can take up to 3.5 years (median 1 year).
D-Penicillamine Rarely used now for treatment of RA.	Affects ~15% of patients. Membranous nephropathy most common renal lesion. Presents with proteinuria (can be nephrotic range).	Usually gradual improvement on drug withdrawal but may persist for up to 1 year.
Ciclosporin	Hemodynamically mediated AKI. Presents with significant increases in plasma creatinine and reduced GFR.	CsA-induced renal afferent arteriolar constriction. Even at low doses, all patients show some degree of renal toxicity. Usually reversible on drug withdrawal. Drug is contraindicated in RA patients with renal dysfunction.
	Up to 10% may develop a nephropathy if treated with higher doses of CsA (>5 mg/kg/day).	
Leflunomide	None reported	
Azathioprine	None reported	
Cyclophosphamide	None reported	Used to treat renal complications of vasculitic disorders.
Anti-TNF biologics: Infliximab Etanercept Adalimumab	None reported None reported None reported	
Anti-B cell biologic: Rituximab	None reported	In small case series, used to treat renal manifestations of antibody-mediated diseases including Wegener's granulomatosis and idiopathic membranous nephropathy.

Treatment
Corticosteroids are the mainstay of treatment for the inflammatory manifestations of these conditions.

Azathioprine (Table 4.9.1) may be used as a steroid-sparing agent.

Renal manifestations
They most commonly present with microscopic hematuria and mild–moderate proteinuria.

The commonest patterns of renal involvement are:

Acute tubular necrosis with renal failure
This is related to myoglobinuria, occurring as a result of rhabdomyolysis.

Acute rhabdomyolysis occurs following inflammatory injury to the skeletal muscle with extravasation of intracellular toxic metabolites into the circulatory system.

This affects up to 15% of patients with polymyositis/dermatomyositis.

Hemodialysis may be required.

It is associated with a high mortality.

Chronic glomerulonephritis
This affects up to 5% of patients.

Membranous nephropathy, mesangial proliferative glomerulonephritis, and IgA nephropathy have been reported.

Sjögren's syndrome

Clinical

Sjögren's syndrome is a multisystem autoimmune disorder, which can be classified as primary or secondary to another autoimmune disease such as RA, SLE or systemic sclerosis.

The commonest presenting complaints are dryness of the eyes and mouth which arise as a result of lymphocyte-mediated infiltration of the exocrine glands, particularly the lachrymal and salivary glands.

Epidemiology

The prevalence of clinical Sjögren's syndrome is ~3%.

Renal involvement occurs in up to 20% of patients.

Supports diagnosis

The presence of antibodies to SS-A (anti-Ro) and SS-B (anti-La).

Treatment

Treatment is symptomatic as there are no drug therapies with proven efficacy for the underlying condition.

General recommendations include wearing glasses with side panels to minimize evaporation from the eyes, chewing sugar-free gum, sipping water frequently and emphasizing the importance of good dental hygiene.

Artificial tears and saliva replacements may be used.

Prednisolone or ciclosporin eye-drops or surgical ablation of the nasolachrymal ducts is sometimes necessary.

Renal manifestations

Distal renal tubular acidosis
This may be complete or incomplete.

It is usually clinically silent but results in a tendency to form stones.

The diagnosis is confirmed by an abnormal fasting urine acidification test (pH >5.5) and the presence of a metabolic acidosis.

Ammonium chloride loading may be required to exclude the diagnosis.

It is more common in autoantibody-positive patients: ANA, anti-SS-A or -SS-B.

Hyposthenuria
Abnormalities of urine-concentrating ability are reported in up to 30% of cases.

Renal impairment
Glomerular disease is rare.

Interstitial nephritis is the most commonly reported lesion on renal biopsy.

In patients with interstitial nephritis, high dose corticosteroids may substantially improve renal function.

Renal dysfunction tends to progress slowly over time but ESRD is rare.

Further reading

Rheumatoid arthritis

Gisbert JP, González-Lama Y, Maté J. 5-Aminosalicylates and renal function in inflammatory bowel disease: a systematic review. *Inflamm Bowel Dis* 2007; **13**: 629–638.

Helin HJ, Korpela MM, Mustonen JT, Pasternack AI. Renal biopsy findings and clinicopathologic correlations in rheumatoid arthritis. *Arthritis Rheum* 1995; **38**: 242–247.

Salama AD, Pusey CD. Drug Insight: rituximab in renal disease and transplantation. *Nature Clin Pratice* 2006; **2**: 221–230.

Schiff MH, Whelton A. Renal toxicity associated with disease-modifying antirheumatic drugs used for the treatment of rheumatoid arthritis. *Semin Arthritis Rheum* 2000; **30**: 196–208.

Suarez-Almazor ME, Belseck E, Shea B, Wells G, Tugwell P. Cyclophosphamide for treating rheumatoid arthritis. *Cochrane Database Syst Rev* 2000; (**4**): CD001157.

Guidelines published by the British Society for Rheumatology:

Chakravarty K, McDonald H, Pullar T, et al. on behalf of the British Society for Rheumatology and British Health Professionals in Rheumatology Standards, Guidelines and Audit Working Group in association with the British Association of Dermatologists (BAD). (2006) BSR & BHPR guideline for disease-modifying anti-rheumatic drug therapy (DMARD) in consultation with the British Association of Dermatologists. *Rheumatology (Oxford)*; 2006(Sep 27). [Epub ahead of print]

Mixed connective tissue disease

Venables PJW. Mixed connective tissue disease. *Lupus* 2006; **15**: 132–137.

Polymyositis and dermatomyositis.

Yen TH, Lai PC, Chen CC, Hsueh H, Huang JY. Renal involvement in patients with polymyositis and dermatomyositis. *Int J Clin Pract* 2005; **59**: 88–193.

Sjögren's syndrome

Aasarod K, Haga HJ, Berg KJ, Hammerstrom J, Jorstad S. Renal involvement in primary Sjögren's syndrome. *Q J Med* 2000; **93**: 297–304.

Venables PJ. Management of patients presenting with Sjogren's syndrome. *Best Pract Res Clin Rheumatol* 2006; **20**: 791–807.

Internet resources

Patient information leaflets about various aspects of rheumatoid arthritis and its management:

http://www.arc.org.uk/arthinfo/patpubs/6033/6033.asp -

National Rheumatoid Arthritis Society:

www.rheumatoid.org.uk

Information on the biologics register on which patients treated with a biologic agent should be included. Publications arising from the register are also referenced:

www.medicine.manchester.ac.uk/arc/BSRBR/

MCTD information:

http://www.patient.co.uk/showdoc/40001176/

Arthritis Research Campaign information:

http://www.arc.org.uk/arthinfo/patpubs/6009/6009.asp

Myositis Support Group:

http://www.myositis.org.uk/

Sjögren's patient-based website:

http://www.sjogrens.com

Information leaflet aimed at patients with Sjögren's:

http://www.arc.org.uk/arthinfo/patpubs/6041/6041.asp

Arthritis Research Campaign; useful resource for information about all the above:

http://www.arc.org.uk/

See also

Systemic lupus erythematosis, p. 180

Scleroderma–systemic sclerosis, p. 186

Membranous nephropathy, p. 106

Renal tubular acidosis, p. 208

Sickle cell nephropathy

Introduction

Sickle cell hemoglobinopathies (sickle cell anemia (SCA) and sickle cell carrier/trait (SCT)) are a group of genetic disorders characterized by the production of an abnormal sickle hemoglobin (Hb) that irreversibly polymerizes at low oxygen saturations resulting in crescent-shaped red blood cells (sickle cells) which block the microcirculation.

Changes in both red and white blood cell adherence to vascular endothelium are also found and together these changes result in ischemic damage to organs.

Anemia arises due to the premature removal of the abnormal sickle cells by the reticuloendothelial system.

SCA classically presents with acute painful crises (e.g. bone pain and acute chest syndrome).

Recurrent splenic infarction is associated with increased susceptibility to infection, particularly with encapsulated organisms (e.g. pneumococci). Early vaccination and antibiotic prophylaxis are essential to reduce infection and the risk of childhood death.

End-organ damage includes renal failure, pulmonary hypertension, cardiac failure, avascular necrosis, cholelithiasis, leg ulceration, priapism, retinopathy and stroke.

SCT patients do not suffer from acute, painful crises but are susceptible to sickle cell nephropathy albeit less frequently and usually at an older age.

Genetics of sickle cell disorders

SCA arises most frequently from homozygosity for a single point mutation in the β-globin gene (HbSS). Other sickle disorders occur with compound heterozygosity for HbS and other globin mutations and tend to be less severe (SC (most common), SOarab, SDpunjab, SE and Sβ-Thal).

Considerable variation in severity of disease is also seen between individual patients, influenced by factors such as associated S gene-cluster haplotype, HbF concentration, white cell count, level of Hb and the coinheritance of α-thalassemia.

SCT occurs when the patient has one normal β-globin gene and one affected gene generating Hb AS.

Definition

Sickle cell nephropathy can affect the whole length of the nephron from the glomerulus to the papillary tip.

In particular, the high oxygen demands and relatively slow blood flow rate within the renal medulla create a hypoxic, hyperosmolar and acidotic environment which predisposes to red blood cell sickling within the vasa recta and the development of ischemia/infarction.

Epidemiology

Studies in Western populations indicate that:
- 20–30% of adults with SCA have an eGFR <90 mL/min (28% HbSS and 6% non-HbSS having CKD 3 or worse);
- ESRD develops in 4–5% of patients with SCA; mean age at onset 41 ± 14 years;
- ESRD is rare in SCT.

Risk factors for ESRD include:
- HbSS (4.2% HbSS vs 2.4% HbSC);
- S gene-cluster haplotype;
- proteinuria;
- anemia;
- hypertension.

Clinical features

Glomerular involvement

This is manifest by microscopic hematuria, increasing proteinuria and a progressive decline in GFR.

This is less common with non-HbSS sickling disorders.

Sickle cell anemia
By age 40 (HbSS):
- 79% have an abnormal ACR;
- 40% have overt proteinuria.

Median age at which ACR is increased is 11–14 years, but can be as early as 5 years.

Nephrotic syndrome is seen in 4–5% of cases; 2/3 of nephrotic patients develop ESRD with a 50% mortality at 2 years despite renal replacement therapy.

Sickle cell trait
Proteinuria and nephrotic syndrome is uncommon.

Tubular involvement

Hyposthenuria
This is associated with childhood enuresis (up to 40% of patients aged 2–20 years) and nocturia.

There is also a risk of rapid dehydration with water deprivation, which may precipitate or prolong a sickling crisis.

It is reversible with an exchange transfusion programme until age ~10 years.

It is more pronounced in SCA than SCT.

Impaired potassium excretion and impaired acidification of urine
This is not normally clinically apparent.

Hyperkalemia is more likely to be seen with progressive CKD and when drugs such as ACEI/ARB and K⁺-sparing diuretics are used.

Patients are rarely acidotic unless there is concomitant multiple organ dysfunction.

Hyperkalemia and acidosis are rarely seen in SCT.

Hematuria
This is usually painless micro- or macroscopic hematuria; rarely massive hematuria may occur.

It can be associated with renal 'clot' colic and obstruction (renal papillary necrosis).

Bleeding is mostly unilateral (~80% arises from the left kidney).

Common causes:
- glomerulopathy;
- renal papillary necrosis;
- renal medullary carcinoma.

It is commonly seen in SCA, but is less common in SCT (up to 4% admission rate for hematuria with SCT).

Renal papillary necrosis
This occurs in both SCA and SCT as a result of sickling and ischemia in the renal medulla.

It is found as an incidental finding in up to two-thirds of patients undergoing urography.

It is most commonly asymptomatic but may be associated with hematuria or rarely urinary tract obstruction due to sloughing of infarcted papillae.

Acute kidney injury

This occurs in 10% of patients hospitalized with acute crises (associated with multiple organ failure).

No specific treatment is required and renal recovery is usual with supportive management.

Acute crisis can rarely be associated with renal vein thrombosis.

AKI is also rarely seen with nontraumatic and exertional rhabdomyolysis (SCT).

Renal medullary carcinoma

This is rare (incidence 1.74 per 1000 patient-years).

It is almost exclusively seen in patients with SCT.

The average age at diagnosis is 21 years, but it has also been described in children.

The male:female ratio is 2:1.

It presents with gross hematuria and flank pain.

The majority have metastatic disease at diagnosis therefore the median survival is 4 months.

Investigations

The assessment of GFR is inaccurate in SCA due to increased proximal tubule secretion of creatinine and low muscle mass leading to overestimation of GFR by both creatinine clearance and derived eGFR. Cockcroft–Gault and MDRD formulae have not been validated in SCA.

Therefore, there must be a low threshold for investigation of even a mild increase in creatinine.

In SCA patients <25 years, the suggested upper limit of Cr:
- males   80 µmol/L;
- females   68 µmol/L.

Treatment

Glomerular disease

Consider ACEI or ARB if the ACR is increased: small, short term studies suggest benefit but it is unclear if progression to ESRD is slowed.

Tubular disease

Ensure adequate hydration particularly during acute crises and have a low threshold to check for hyperkalemia and metabolic acidosis during intercurrent illness.

Hematuria

Conservative management is usually sufficient; exclude UTI; angiography + embolization/nephrectomy is rarely required; consider renal medullary carcinoma if macroscopic hematuria is persistent.

Hypertension

In SCA the BP is lower than age-/sex-matched African-American controls.

The difference is most marked in HbSS patients >45 years.

'Relative' hypertension (120–139/70–89 mmHg) is associated with an increased risk of CKD, stroke, pulmonary hypertension, and all-cause mortality.

Little data is available to guide treatment decisions.

NIH advises introducing antihypertensive treatment if:
- systolic/diastolic increases 20/10 mmHg above baseline;
- >130/85 mmHg and nephropathy/cardiovascular disease;
- >120/75 mmHg and proteinuria >1 g/24 h.

ACEI, ARB, and calcium antagonists are preferred agents; β-blockers and diuretics can be used with caution (Table 4.10.1).

Erythropoiesis stimulating agents (ESAs)

Erythropoietin levels are usually lower than expected for the degree of anemia.

ESAs can be used cautiously in individual patients; precipitation of sickle crisis has been reported (Table 4.10.1).

ESA requirements are much higher than in other CKD patients.

Target Hb is 8–10 g/dL.

Renal replacement therapy

Hemodialysis and peritoneal dialysis

Very few data are available in the literature. There is no evidence for superiority of HD or PD although an increased risk of dialysis-related septicemia has been reported.

There is an increased incidence of hepatitis B and C virus infection in some areas of the world due to transfusion requirements.

Transplantation

Patients with SCA are less likely to be listed for transplantation or be transplanted compared to other ESRD patients (due to coexistent end organ damage).

For those transplanted (mainly HbSS) 1 year survival is similar to that of the general transplant population.

However, at 3 years, when compared to the general transplant population, there is:
- reduced allograft survival (48% vs 60%);
- significantly reduced patient survival (59% vs 81%).

Despite this there is a trend to better survival with transplantation compared to remaining on dialysis and therefore transplantation should always be considered in patients with SCA and ESRD.

The observed morbidity and mortality is largely due to improved post-transplantation hemopoiesis which increases plasma viscosity and the likelihood of acute crises.

Recurrent sickling is also associated with recurrent sickle cell nephropathy, renal vein thrombosis and rarely acute allograft loss. Therefore venesection should be considered if Hb is >10 g/dL.

Preparation of patients with SCA for surgery

A multidisciplinary approach (hematologist, anesthetist surgeon, nephrologist) is essential and a protocol outlining perioperative management should be written in the patient's notes prior to surgery.

Patients may require preoperative transfusion (top-up or exchange transfusion).

Postoperatively, careful attention to fluid balance and tissue oxygenation is required.

Follow-up

All patients with SCA require annual review of renal function and measurement of proteinuria. Once renal disease

Table 4.10.1 Therapeutic considerations in patients with SCD and CKD

Therapy	Comment
Hydroxycarbamide (hydroxyurea)	Used to treat sickle cell hemoglobinopathies (increases HbF synthesis and reduces likelihood of sickling).
	Caution in patients with nephropathy as hydroxycarbamide is predominantly cleared by the kidney.
Analgesics	Frequently used during painful acute crises.
NSAIDs	SCA patients more susceptible to glomerular hemodynamic effects of NSAIDs as more dependent on prostaglandins derived from ischemic renal medulla to maintain glomerular blood flow.
	Avoid in patients with nephropathy. If necessary, carefully monitor renal function and limit to 5 days of treatment.
Opiates	Caution in patients with nephropathy as these drugs (e.g. pethidine) are predominantly cleared by kidney.
EPO	**Consider EPO if:** Hb <8 g/dL.
	Cautious escalation of EPO dosing Commence with 100 U/kg twice a week increasing by 100 U/kg/dose every 4–6 weeks until Hb rises.
	Stop if Hb >10.5 g/dL, if rise is >1.5 g/dL over 4 weeks or Hct >0.33
	Close monitoring is essential FBC, reticulocyte count and BP should be monitored weekly after any dose change.
Hypertension	
Diuretics	Caution due to tubular dysfunction and susceptibility to dehydration.
β-Blockers	Caution due to tubular dysfunction and susceptibility to hyperkalaemia particularly in progressive CKD.
ACEIs/ARBs	Caution due to tubular dysfunction and susceptibility to hyperkalaemia particularly in progressive CKD.

becomes apparent the frequency of follow-up will be determined by the stage of CKD.

Prognosis
The median survival for patients with ESRD is 4 years despite RRT. Poor outcome is linked to coexistent end-organ damage and refractory anemia.

However, survival is similar to matched ESRD controls when the low transplantation rate is taken into account.

Further reading
Ataga KI, Orringer EP, et al. Renal abnormalities in sickle cell disease. Am J Haematol 2000; **63**: 205–211.

Guasch A, Navarrete J, et al. Glomerular Involvement in adults with sickle cell haemoglobinopathies: prevalence and clinical correlates of progressive renal failure. J Am Soc Nephrol 2006; **17**: 2228–2235.

Little JA, McGowan VR, et al. Combination erythropoietin hydroxyurea therapy in sickle cell disease: experience from the National Institutes of Health and a literature review. Haematologica 2006; **91**: 1076–1083.

Ojo AO, Govaerts TC, et al. Renal transplantation in end stage sickle cell nephropathy. Transplantation 1999; **67**: 291–295.

Thompson J, Reid M, et al. Albuminuria and renal function in homozygous sickle cell disease. Arch Intern Med 2007; **167**: 701–708.

Internet resources
Sickle Cell Disease in Childhood: Standards and Guidelines for Clinical Care (NHS):

http://www.sickleandthal.org.uk/Documents//DETAILED_CLIN_Oct19.pdf

Management of Sickle Cell Disease (NIH NHLBI):

http://www.nhlbi.nih.gov/health/prof/blood/sickle/index.htm

BCSH Guideline. Management Of Acute Painful Crisis In Sickle Cell Disease:

http://www.bcshguidelines.com/

Sickle Cell Society:

http://www.sicklecellsociety.org/index.htm

Sickle Cell Disease Association of America:

http://www.sicklecelldisease.org/

The Sickle Cell Information Center:

http://www.scinfo.org/

Standards for the clinical care of adults with Sickle Cell disease in the UK

http://www.sicklecellsociety.org/CareBook.pdf

See also

Tumors of the kidney p. 668

Urinary tract obstruction, p. 652

Hematological disorders in CKD, p. 426

Cancer and the kidney

Etiology of renal impairment in cancer patients

Renal dysfunction is relatively common in patients with cancer as a result of complications related to their cancer or treatment (see below) and concomitant comorbidities such as diabetes mellitus and hypertension. The causes include:

- pre-renal failure secondary to fluid depletion;
- anticancer drug-related nephrotoxicity;
- metabolic causes, e.g. hypercalcemia;
- mechanical obstruction;
- paraneoplastic glomerulonephropathies;
- paraprotein-related disease;
- amyloidosis;
- radiation nephropathy;
- renal metastasis.

Hypercalcemia of malignancy

Hypercalcemia is a common metabolic problem occurring in 10–20% of patients with cancer. In the hospital population an underlying malignancy is the most frequent cause of hypercalcemia. Cancers of the lung and breast and multiple myeloma are most frequently implicated. Hypercalcemia often develops in the later stages of cancer, and is not often the isolated presenting feature of malignancy in the absence of other symptoms and/or signs.

Hypercalcemia is a result of increased bone resorption and release of calcium from bone. The mechanisms are discussed below although it is often multifactorial.

Mechanisms of hypercalcemia

Osteolytic metastases

Hypercalcemia results from direct induction of local osteolysis by tumor cells.

This is common in solid tumors metastatic to bone (especially lung and breast).

Cytokines (e.g. IL-1 and TNF) stimulate osteoclast differentiation and activity.

PTH-related protein

This is often called humoral hypercalcemia of malignancy.

It is the commonest cause of hypercalcemia in patients with nonmetastatic solid tumors and some patients with non-Hodgkin's lymphoma.

PTH-related peptide (PTHrP) is expressed in non-neoplastic tissues and is required for normal function and development.

It is structurally similar to PTH at the amino-terminal end which permits binding to PTH receptors.

PTHrP has physiological effects similar to PTH, but is structurally distinct and can be measured with antibody-based assays.

Osteoclast-activating factors

These mediate the hypercalcemia in multiple myeloma and some cases of lymphoma.

Various osteoclast-activating factors (e.g. IL-1, IL-6, TNF and vascular cell adhesion molecule (VCAM-1)) are released by adjacent tumor cells.

Coexisting primary hyperparathyroidism

A higher incidence of primary hyperparathyroidism is seen in patients with cancer.

Calcium levels >3.25 mmol/L are rarely due to primary hyperparathyroidism.

Investigations in the hypercalcemic patient

Measure serum urea, creatinine, calcium, chloride, and phosphate.

Measure vitamin D and PTH.

CXR (for evidence of malignancy or sarcoidosis).

Perform isotope bone scan if not known to have bone metastases.

Management of hypercalcemia of malignancy

Saline

Saline is administered to produce volume expansion and increase urinary calcium excretion.

Give 3–4 L of 0.9% saline/day. Adjust infusion rate to maintain a urine output of 100–150 mL/h. This alone rarely normalizes serum calcium.

Bisphosphonates

These are nonhydrolyzable analogues of inorganic pyrophosphate.

They inhibit bone resorption by adsorbing to the surface of bone hydroxyapatite, thereby interfering with the metabolic activity of osteoclasts.

Third-generation bisphosphonates (e.g. zoledronic acid) have been shown to be superior to second generation bisphosphonates (e.g. pamidronate).

Third-generation bisphosphonates normalize the corrected calcium level in almost 90% of patients by day 10 with a median duration of calcium control of 32–43 days.

Calcitonin

Consider for severe or symptomatic hypercalcemia.

It decreases bone calcium resorption and increases urinary excretion.

It has a rapid onset of action beginning 4–6 h post administration although only lowers calcium by 0.3–0.5 mmol/L.

Mechanical obstruction

Hydronephrosis is particularly common in patients with bladder or cervical cancer, and may be acute or chronic.

Ureteric obstruction may be due to primary or secondary disease.

Acute edema can precipitate mechanical obstruction in patients undergoing pelvic radiotherapy.

Management

The stage and prognosis of the disease, and the potential reversibility of the obstruction, need to be taken into account when planning treatment.

Intervention may be unnecessary since the disease may regress with treatment or be inappropriate in patients with advanced or terminal cancer.

Following isotope renogram assessment of residual renal function, ureteric stenting or insertion of uni- or bilateral nephrostomies is often appropriate to facilitate treatment. These may be removed if there is adequate tumor regression.

Tumor lysis syndrome (TLS)

Tumor lysis syndrome is a condition which may occur following massive cell death after treatment of neoplastic conditions. It is most frequently seen just after the commencement of chemotherapy treatment for very chemosensitive disease, classically high grade lymphomas (particularly Burkitt's lymphoma) and high leukocyte count leukemias.

The mainstay of treatment is to predict which patients are at risk and institute measures to prevent TLS from developing.

It should be suspected in patients who develop AKI with marked hyperuricemia and/or hyperphosphatemia.

Pathophysiology

Massive cellular lysis releases metabolites into the circulation. Cellular breakdown of nucleic acids leads to the production of uric acid. Uric acid becomes insoluble and precipitates in the renal tubules at low pH causing obstruction and a decreased GFR.

Acute nephrocalcinosis can occur as a result of hyperphosphatemia and precipitation of calcium phosphate crystals.

Risk factors for TLS

- Chemosensitive tumor with high proliferation index.
- Large tumor burden.
- Renal dysfunction.
- Hyperuricemia.
- Hypovolemia.

Metabolic abnormalities

TLS will result in severe hyperuricemia. hyperphosphatemia, hyperkalemia, hypocalcemia, and biochemical evidence of AKI.

Prevention of TLS in at-risk patients

Allopurinol 300 mg/day for at least 2 days prior to commencing treatment of cancer.

Aggressive IV fluid prehydration for 24–48 h before treatment.

The role of urinary alkalinisation is unclear (target pH 6.5–7; give sodium bicarbonate or acetazolamide)

Management of TLS

Give IV fluids and loop diuretics to 'wash out' obstructing uric acid crystals.

Give rasburicase (recombinant urate-oxidase) 200 µg/kg IV once daily for 5–7 days. Consider in severe cases

Treat the metabolic abnormalities including hyperkalemia and symptomatic/profound hypocalcemia.

Consider transfer to high dependency/intensive care unit and consider hemodialysis if the response to the above measures is poor.

Para-neoplastic conditions and the kidney

Syndrome of inappropriate ADH secretion (SIADH)

Ectopic secretion of ADH by malignant cells is a common cause of hyponatremia in patients with cancer, e.g. small cell lung carcinoma. SIADH also occurs in patients with primary or secondary brain tumors.

Glomerulonephropathies

Glomerular disease occurs in 6–10% of patients with cancer. There have been associations reported between many glomerulonephropathies and a variety of solid and hematological malignancies.

Membranous nephropathy (MN)

- 6–22% of patients with (MN) have an underlying malignancy.
- It is associated with carcinomas; especially breast, lung and gastrointestinal tract.
- The diagnosis of MN may be made before or after cancer diagnosis.
- It presents with hypertension, nephrotic syndrome, and microscopic hematuria.

Minimal change nephropathy

- This is associated with Hodgkin disease and lymphomas although the prevalence is low (<1%).

Glomerular amyloidosis

- AL amyloid glomerulopathy is the renal deposition of free monoclonal chains from a benign or malignant clonal expansion of plasma cells, e.g. myeloma.
- AA amyloid is the deposition of a variety of proteins including the acute phase reactant, serum amyloid A protein, in extracellular tissue. Cancers associated with AA amyloid glomerulopathy include renal cell carcinoma and Hodgkin disease.

IgA nephropathy

- This is associated with tumors of the mucosal immune system (especially in upper respiratory tract).

Management of glomerulopathies

Associated malignancies should be considered in adults aged >50 years presenting with a glomerulopathy with no apparent cause.

Management of the underlying malignancy is the primary objective with regression of the glomerulopathy frequently observed with successful treatment.

Patients with untreatable malignancies may benefit from standard management of the nephrotic syndrome including control of blood pressure (with ACEIs and ARBs) and fluid balance to minimize the progressive decline in GFR.

Radiation nephropathy

This can develop 6 months to several years following exposure to radiotherapy; it does not tend to occur acutely.

It is an uncommon complication, provided recognized radiation tolerance doses are not exceeded (see below).

It is defined as renal injury and loss of function following ionizing radiation. Clinical radiation nephropathy has become less common because of the routine use of kidney shielding during radiotherapy and the increased use of chemotherapy.

Etiology

- Bone marrow transplant nephropathy: total body irradiation with partial kidney shielding is used as conditioning regimen for the bone marrow transplant.
- Parenteral radioisotope therapy: e.g. yttrium 90 conjugated to somatostatin is filtered and reabsorbed in the proximal tubule.
- Upper abdominal radiotherapy.

Kidney tolerance

Studies suggest that 10 Gy as a single dose or >23 Gy in fractionated doses can lead to radiation nephropathy.

Pathophysiology

Ionizing radiation causes radiochemical injury to cells. Studies suggest that glomerular endothelial cell injury is the start of a cascade leading to glomerular sclerosis and later tubulo-interstitial fibrosis.

Presentation

Findings include hypertension, proteinuria, azotemia, anemia, and hyperkalemia.

Management

There is strong experimental data to support the use of ACEIs or angiotensin II blockers in the treatment and prevention of experimental radiation nephropathy.

Anemia is driven by low blood erythropoietin levels and responds to erythropoietin replacement therapy.

Further reading

Cohen EP. *Cancer and the kidney*. Oxford: Oxford University Press; 2005.

Souhami RL, Tannock I, Hohenberger P, Horiot J-C. *Oxford textbook of oncology*. Oxford: Oxford University Press; 2002.

See also

Malignancy-associated glomerular disease, p. 134

Hypo-/hypercalcemia, p. 52

Uric acid and the kidney, p. 232

Chapter 5

Tubular disease

Chapter contents

Isolated defects of tubular function

This chapter briefly covers the miscellaneous isolated defects of tubular function: renal glycosuria, phosphaturia and aminoaciduria.

Renal glycosuria

Renal glycosuria (or glucosuria) is the excretion of glucose in the urine in detectable amounts in the absence of hyperglycemia.

The underlying defect is an abnormally low renal threshold for glucose reabsorption.

Renal glycosuria needs to be differentiated from glycosuria associated with more complex tubular disorders like the renal Fanconi syndrome, cystinosis, Wilson's disease, hereditary tyrosinemia, interstitial nephritis and heavy metal poisoning, which can all affect the proximal tubule; it can also occur in myeloma, transiently following renal transplantation, and in the nephrotic syndrome (Table 5.1.1).

Isolated hereditary renal glycosuria is a benign autosomal recessive disorder that does not require treatment. It just needs to be recognized and is usually detected on routine urine testing.

Plasma glucose and serum insulin concentrations, glucose tolerance test and glycosylated hemoglobin level are all normal; although there is a rare association with late onset diabetes mellitus of the young (MODY3) caused by a mutation in the gene for hepatocyte nuclear factor-1.

Renal glycosuria is also seen in familial glucose–galactose malabsorption, another rare autosomal recessive disorder, which presents in the neonate with severe diarrhea.

Epidemiology

In the USA the incidence is estimated to be 0.16–6.3% (~1 in 20 000).

There is no gender difference.

Pathophysiology and clinical features

Glucose is freely filtered at the glomerulus and then almost completely reabsorbed along the proximal tubule: fractional excretion is normally <0.1%.

Reabsorption of glucose occurs mainly in the first (S1) and second (S2) parts of the proximal tubule. Most glucose enters the proximal tubule cell via the sodium-dependent glucose cotransporters SGLT1 and SGLT2, and leaves the cell via the facilitated transporters GLUT1 and GLUT2.

SGLT2 is a low affinity–high capacity glucose transporter that reabsorbs the bulk of filtered glucose in S1.

SGLT1 is a high affinity–low capacity glucose transporter that 'scavenges' the remaining glucose in S2 (and S3). Glucose reabsorption is age-dependent and in premature infants of <30 weeks gestation glycosuria, is a common finding.

Glucose–galactose malabsorption is due to mutations of SGLT1, which is also the transport protein responsible for glucose and galactose reabsorption in the small intestine (in which there is no SGLT2). Treatment consists of eliminating these sugars from the diet, including their disaccharide, lactose.

About 90% of cases of isolated renal glycosuria are due to mutations in SGLT2 (SLC5A2). It is usually an incidental finding and there are no clinical features or sequelae, in particular there is no polyuria or polydipsia.

Renal glycosuria has been divided clinically into three types (A, B and O) according to measured changes in the renal threshold for, versus the maximal rates of, glucose reabsorption. However (similar to the original clinical classification of cystinuria – see below), this separation into types is of limited clinical use and it almost certainly only reflects differences in the effects of different SGLT2 mutations.

Diagnosis and treatment

Both are straightforward. Benign renal glycosuria must be distinguished from other causes of glycosuria with or without hyperglycemia:

- diabetes mellitus;
- gestational diabetes;
- any cause of a renal Fanconi syndrome, inherited or acquired (see Table 5.1.1).

There is no specific treatment and none is required.

Table 5.1.1. Causes of a renal Fanconi syndrome

Idiopathic renal Fanconi syndrome	Autosomal dominant
	X-linked (e.g. Lowe syndrome)
Inherited renal Fanconi syndrome associated with inborn errors of amino acid or carbohydrate metabolism	Cystinosis
	Galactosemia
	Hereditary fructose intolerance
	Tyrosinemia
	Glycogen storage diseases
	• Fanconi–Bickel syndrome
	• Glucose-6-phosphatase deficiency
Wilson's disease	
Mitochondrial disease	
Acquired renal Fanconi syndrome:	
Toxic	Exposure to heavy metals (Pb, Hg, Cd)
	Chinese herbs
	Aminoglycoside antibiotics and outdated tetracyclines
	Antiretrovirals (HIV)
	Ifosfamide
Dysproteinemias	Multiple myeloma, amyloidosis, light chain nephropathy, and benign monoclonal gammopathy
Immune-mediated	Sjögren's syndrome, interstitial nephritis, renal transplantation

Hypophosphatemia and phosphaturia

Maintaining a normal plasma phosphate concentration depends on normal renal function and phosphate excretion.

Reabsorption of phosphate in the renal proximal tubule is regulated and it can adjust rapidly in response to changes in parathyroid hormone (PTH), which inhibits phosphate reabsorption, and 1,25-$(OH)_2$ vitamin D (renal production of which is increased by PTH and hypophosphatemia), which stimulates phosphate reabsorption.

Phosphate reabsorption is mediated by two sodium-dependent phosphate transporters (cf. glucose), NaPi-2a and NaPi-2c; NaPi-2a is the more important and is regulated under normal conditions (although mutations in both transporters have been linked to isolated hypophosphatemia and phosphaturia in some patients with recurrent renal stone disease).

Abnormal renal losses of phosphate are evident when there is hypophosphatemia, which may be due to increased PTH secretion or a primary defect in phosphate reabsorption (mainly via NaPi-2a) in the proximal tubule.

In adults, hypophosphatemia is defined as a fasting plasma phosphate concentration <0.75 mmol/L, and in children <1.35 mmol/l.

Urinary phosphate wasting is likely to be present when the urine phosphate concentration is >2 mmol/L and the plasma phosphate concentration is <0.5 mmol/L, or the tubular maximum for phosphate reabsorption (TmPi/GFR; see Chapter 5.2) is reduced to <0.8 mmol/L (in adults), or the fractional excretion of phosphate is >20%.

Causes of hypophosphatemia (Table 5.1.2):
Hyperparathyroidism
- Primary hyperparathyroidism with hypophosphatemia and hypercalcemia due to a parathyroid adenoma or hyperplasia, or inactivating mutations of the calcium-sensing receptor (in the parathyroid gland and kidney).
- Secondary hyperparathyroidism with hypophosphatemia and hypocalcemia due to vitamin D deficiency or resistance to vitamin D.

Renal tubular defects
- Renal Fanconi syndrome (with associated glycosuria, uricosuria, aminoaciduria and tubular proteinuria) (Table 5.1.1).
- X-linked hypophosphatemic rickets and autosomal dominant hypophosphatemic rickets (with reduced intestinal absorption of calcium and phosphate, rickets or osteomalacia, and inappropriately low or normal $1,25\text{-}(OH)_2$ vitamin D levels).
- Osteogenic (tumor-induced) osteomalacia (due to mesenchymal tumors secreting a 'phosphatonin' like FGF-23, which inhibits phosphate reabsorption in the proximal tubule and synthesis of $1,25\text{-}(OH)_2$ vitamin D).
- In diabetic patients with ketoacidosis, phosphate is released from cells and lost in the urine; treatment with insulin can unmask the deficit in phosphate by stimulating anabolism and shifting phosphate back into cells

(which can also occur in severe malnutrition during re-feeding).
- Renal losses of phosphate have been described in association with hypokalemia, hypomagnesemia (particularly in alcoholics), chronic metabolic acidosis, hypothyroidism, humoral hypercalcemia of malignancy, and after severe burns.

Intestinal
- Decreased intake.
- Phosphate binders.

Symptoms and signs
The important ones are:
- bone pain with rickets or osteomalacia;
- muscle weakness;
- myocardial and respiratory depression, coma and rhabdomyolysis. These only occur in severe cases of hypophosphatemia (plasma or serum phosphate concentration <0.35 mmol/L).

Investigations
Key investigations include:
- measurement of plasma phosphate and calcium concentrations, and (fasting) urinary phosphate excretion; estimate GFR to calculate TmPi/GFR (see Chapter 5.2) and fractional excretion of phosphate;
- measurement of PTH, 25-(OH) vitamin D (assay of $1,25\text{-}(OH)_2$ vitamin D is not always widely available) and alkaline phosphatase, and urinary screening for glycosuria, aminoaciduria and low molecular weight proteinuria (e.g. retinol binding protein);
- bone X-rays for signs of osteomalacia.

Management
This will depend on the underlying cause, but if supplements are required, oral phosphate can be given in divided doses of up to 3 g/day. Too much oral phosphate will stimulate PTH secretion.

Aminoaciduria
As with glucose, amino acid transport occurs in the proximal tubule, although the variety of transporters involved is more diverse than for glucose (or phosphate).

Approximately 50 g of filtered amino acids are recovered by the proximal tubule each day. This is important for the maintenance of normal nitrogen balance.

Uptake into proximal tubule cells is by sodium- or proton-dependent cotransport, or exchange with another (neutral) amino acid; exit from the cell is via a group of less-well-defined unidirectional transporters and exchangers (Table 5.1.3).

Table 5.1.2 Biochemical features of the main causes of renal phosphate wasting

	Plasma/serum calcium	PTH	25-(OH) vitamin D	$1,25\text{-}(OH)_2$ vitamin D	Other signs of proximal tubular dysfunction
Primary hyperparathyroidism	↑	↑	→	→, ↑	No
Secondary hyperparathyroidism	→, ↓	↑	→, ↓	→, ↓	No
Renal Fanconi syndrome	→	→	→, ↓	→, ↓	Yes
Hereditary hypophosphatemic rickets	→	→	→	→, ↓	No
Tumor-induced osteomalacia	→	→	→	↓	No
Diabetic ketoacidosis	→	→	→	↑	No

→, normal; ↓, reduced; ↑, increased.

Table 5.1.3 Amino acid transporters

Amino acids	Apical (luminal) transporter	Basolateral transporter	Clinical aminoaciduria
Acidic (anionic) amino acids (glutamic acid)	Na$^+$-dependent cotransporter EAAT3 (*SLC1A1*)		
Imino-amino acids (proline, hydroxyproline, glycine, alanine, serine)	H$^+$-dependent cotransporter PAT1 (*SLC36A1*)		Iminoglycinuria
Neutral amino acids (leucine, valine) and **aromatic neutral** amino acids (phenylalanine, tryptophan, tyrosine, histidine)	Na$^+$-dependent cotransporter B^{0}AT1 (*SLC6A19*)		Hartnup disease
Basic (cationic) amino acids (lysine, arginine, ornithine) and **cystine**	Heterodimeric exchanger rBAT† (*SLC3A1*) and b^{0+}AT† (*SLC7A9*)	Heterodimeric exchanger y+LAT1‡ (*SLC7A7*) and 4F2hc (*SL33A2*)	Cystinuria† Lysinuric protein intolerance‡

The amino acid transporters shown are only those that have been linked (so far) to an aminoaciduria.
†,‡Shared superscripts: transporter defects matched with clinical outcomes.

These transporters are shared with the small intestine and so any defect in amino acid transport is usually present in both the gut and kidneys.

Cystinuria

Cystine is formed by oxidation of the neutral sulfur-containing amino acid cysteine, which has a thiol group and can pair through a disulfide bond.

In cystinuria, there is increased excretion of cystine and the basic (cationic) amino acids lysine, arginine and ornithine.

It is an autosomal recessive disorder with a reported incidence ranging from 1 in 10 000 to 1 in 20 000.

Originally, three types were described according to the amount of cystine excreted by those affected and their parents. Two gene defects have since been identified as the underlying cause: *SLC3A1* (rBAT) on chromosome 2 and *SLC7A9* on chromosome 19, which together form a heteromeric amino acid transporter (Table 5.1.3).

The degree of cystinuria in an affected individual depends on which gene is mutated: heterozygotes versus homozygotes, or if both genes are mutated (compound heterozygotes) (Table 5.1.4).

Symptoms and signs

Cystine stones form and can present in childhood or adulthood. They make up ~1–2% of renal stones in adults and up to 8% in children.

Cystine stones are orange in colour, radio-opaque (though less so than calcium-containing stones) and composed of hexagonal crystals, which have a characteristic appearance on urine microscopy.

Investigations

Cystine can be screened for qualitatively and then quantified in a 24 h urine collection.

Urinary cystine excretion can be >4 mmol/24 h, although treatment should begin with levels >0.8 mmol/24 h, as its solubility is low (0.7 mmol/L).

If possible, family screening should be arranged.

Management

In order for cystine to remain in solution, the urine must be dilute and alkaline.

Initial treatment measures are to increase fluid intake to ≥3 L per day and in severe cases to continue drinking overnight, despite the inconvenience of nocturia.

Alkali therapy, usually given as sodium bicarbonate, is titrated to maintain a urine pH of >7, and dietary sodium intake is restricted as much as possible.

Cystine is a reversible dimer of cysteine (see above), which is more soluble than cystine; drugs with thiol groups, like penicillamine and tiopronin, can combine with cysteine to form a more soluble compound and so reduce the concentration and urinary excretion of cystine.

Pencillamine (0.25–2 g/day), although widely used, has important side-effects (skin rashes and proteinuria) that prevent many patients from taking it.

Table 5.1.4 Classification of cystinuria

Old (descriptive) classification of cystinuria	New (genetic) classification of cystinuria	Corresponding pattern of cystine excretion
Type I/II: parents have no cystinuria*	**Type I** (60% of cases) is homozygous mutation in *SLC3A1* (rBAT)	1–3 mmol/24 h
	(*SLC3A1* heterozygote is *not* cystinuric)	<0.01 mmol/24 h*
Type II/II: parents have heavy cystinuria**	**Nontype I** (types II and III) is a homozygous mutation in *SLC7A9* or a compound heterozygote with mutations in *SLC7A9 and SLC3A1*	1–3 mmol/24 h**
	(*SLC7A9* heterozygote is cystinuric)	>0.5 mmol/24 h***
Type III/III: parents have modest cystinuria***		

*,**,***Shared superscripts: quantity of cystinuria matched with the clinical phenotype.

Though similar to penicillamine, tiopronin (10–40 mg/kg/day, maximum 2 g/day) is better tolerated, but less readily available in the UK. It is used more in pediatric practice.

The thiol-containing ACEI captopril has been proposed as a safe alternative to penicillamine, but it is ineffective at conventional (antihypertensive) doses.

Ascorbic acid (5 g/day) can also be tried, but its effect on cystine excretion is small (and too much may increase oxalate excretion).

Hartnup disease

Hartnup disease is another autosomal recessive disorder, this time due to a mutation in *SLC6A19*, which encodes a neutral amino acid transporter (Table 5.1.3); although this gene defect does not account for all cases.

Many of those affected have no signs or symptoms, but typical cases have a pellagra-like rash and ataxia. These complications arise not from the renal losses of amino acids, but from impaired intestinal absorption of tryptophan, the precursor of nicotinic acid (niacin, vitamin B3), and can be treated with nicotinamide.

Iminoglycinuria

This is a benign aminoaciduria due to a defect in PAT1 (*SLC36A1*) (Table 5.1.3).

Lysinuria

This is a defect in basic (cationic) amino acid transport, with protein intolerance and hyperammonemia, leading to coma. It affects intestinal absorption and kidney reabsorption. It is due to a mutation in the gene *SLC7A7* (Table 5.1.3).

Further reading

Pontoglio M, Prie D, Cheret C, *et al*. HNF1alpha controls renal glucose reabsorption in mouse and man. *EMBO* Rep 2000; **1**: 359–365.

Santer R, Kinner M, Lassen CL, *et al*. Molecular analysis of the SGLT2 gene in patients with renal glucosuria. *J Am Soc Nephrol* 2003; **14**: 2873–2882.

Wright EM, Hirayama BA, Loo DF. Active sugar transport in health and disease. *J Intern Med* 2007; **261**: 32–43.

Internet resources

International Cystinuria Foundation:

http://www.cystinuria.org/

See also

Fanconi syndrome, p. 204

Hypo-/hyperphosphatemia, p. 56

Medical management of stone disease, p. 270

Renal and urinary tract stone disease in children, p. 282

Fanconi syndrome

Definition

The renal Fanconi syndrome (FS) (also known as Fanconi renotubular syndrome and Lignac–de Toni–Debré–Fanconi syndrome, and not to be confused with Fanconi's anemia) refers to a set of clinical features resulting from a generalized loss or disturbance of the normal transport processes in the proximal renal tubule (PT) of the nephron.

Originally described in the 1930s by the Swiss pediatrician Guido Fanconi, its characteristic features are glycosuria, aminoaciduria and phosphaturia (hypophosphatemia) in affected children (or adults).

FS is recognized by urinary losses of substances normally reabsorbed by the PT, such as glucose, amino acids and phosphate (as already mentioned).

It also includes loss of bicarbonate (leading to metabolic acidosis – a form of renal tubular acidosis (RTA)) and low molecular weight proteins (LMWPs) (for example vitamin D binding protein which affects vitamin D metabolism, leading to phosphate wasting and rickets or osteomalacia).

Urinary loss of LMWPs (a commonly measured example of which is retinol-binding protein, RBP) is a consistent feature of FS and a hallmark of the disorder, making it a useful screening test.

Hypercalciuria is also commonly present, though the mechanism is not clear.

Prevalence and pathophysiology

There is no overall estimate for the prevalence of FS, because there are several different genetic and toxic causes (Tables 5.2.1 and 5.2.2).

It was previously thought of as a rare disease, particularly in adults. Development and wider use of assays for urinary LMWPs in urine ('tubular proteinuria') have made it possible to detect milder forms of PT dysfunction. However, the clinical significance of mild PT dysfunction and tubular (LMW) proteinuria remains unclear, although it is possible that some LMWPs are toxic to the renal tubule and this may partially explain the common association of FS with progressive renal impairment.

Various drugs and toxins (Table 5.2.2) can cause renal FS, especially heavy metals (cadmium, uranium, lead and mercury), aminoglycoside antibiotics, some antiretroviral drugs (e.g. azidothymidine (AZT)), and certain cytotoxic drugs (ifosfamide), many of which seem to affect mitochondrial function (which might explain their predilection for the PT).

Myeloma affecting the kidney and also some autoimmune diseases (e.g. lupus nephritis or Sjögren's) are important causes in adults.

Inherited forms of FS include autosomal recessive diseases such as cystinosis, tyrosinemia, fructose intolerance, galactosemia, glycogen storage disease type I, and cytochrome c oxidase deficiency; an autosomal dominant idiopathic form of FS; and various inherited mitochondrial diseases.

Dent's disease and Lowe syndrome are X-linked Fanconi-like disorders in which glycosuria is often absent.

The prevalence of FS is difficult to estimate, though most inherited cases are rare: even for the more common cystinosis there is a wide range of estimates (from 0.03 to 0.4 per 10 000 live births), depending on the population studied.

The underlying pathogenic mechanisms that unite the different causes of FS are still not fully understood.

FS can be mild, with only tubular proteinuria, or severe, with all the classical features listed above.

Unlike the monogenic tubular disorders, such as Gitelman's or Bartter's syndromes, whatever the underlying defect in FS may be, it leads to disturbed transport (reabsorption) of more than one solute/ion.

Originally thought to be a nonspecific cell toxic effect due to disturbed cell metabolism, it is now emerging that altered cell trafficking of proteins is a significant consequence of any underlying defect.

Transport in the PT is coupled to sodium (Fig. 5.2.1) and depends on the gradient for sodium generated by the basolateral ATP-dependent sodium pump: Na^+/K^+-ATPase. As mentioned before, tubular proteinuria is an important early finding in FS. LMWPs (<70 kDa, the size of albumin) are filtered at the glomerulus and are normally reabsorbed (together with small amounts of filtered albumin) – 'reclaimed' – in the PT.

The reabsorptive mechanism is not completely clear, but it does involve binding of LMWPs to two large receptor proteins called megalin and cubilin, which seem to be associated and interdependent. Following binding, the receptor–LMWP complex is internalized (endocytosed) by the PT cell and transported into the cytoplasm in endosomes (Fig. 5.2.1). Acidification of these endosomes then dissociates the receptor–ligand complex and the receptor (megalin) is recycled to the apical membrane for re-use. The LMWP is either broken down in lysosomes or transported to the basolateral membrane of the cell.

Dent's disease and Lowe syndrome have shown us that this process is disturbed, which explains the presence of tubular proteinuria, but exactly how the other transport processes are dependent on this mechanism and are affected in FS is less clear.

FS is a heterogeneous disorder and its natural history varies, depending on the underlying cause. Cases due to drug toxicity are often reversible on stopping the offending drug. However, many patients with FS can develop chronic renal failure, although this is not universal and it is difficult to predict.

Clinical features

Symptoms

Children with FS may present with polyuria, polydipsia, rickets, or failure to thrive.

In adults, the main clinical symptom and presenting feature of FS is bone pain and muscle weakness due to osteomalacia and phosphate wasting. Hypokalemia and metabolic acidosis can also occur, but in less severe cases of FS there may be no symptoms or clinical signs.

Patients often present with other symptoms or signs of the underlying disease, for example, renal stones or unexplained renal impairment in Dent's disease, or cardiac and neurological complications in mitochondrial disorders.

Table 5.2.1 Genetic causes of the renal Fanconi syndrome

Disorder	Defective gene	Encoded Protein	Inheritance
ADIF (autosomal dominant idiopathic Fanconi)	Unknown	Unknown	Autosomal dominant
Cystinosis	CTNS	lysozymal cystine transporter	Autosomal recessive
Cytochrome c oxidase deficiency	COX	Cytochrome c oxidase	Autosomal recessive
Fructose intolerance	ALDOB	Fructose-bisphosphate aldolase B	Autosomal recessive
Galactosemia	GALT	Galactose-1-phosphate uridyl transferase	Autosomal recessive
Glycogen storage disease type Ia (von Gierke disease)	G6PC	Glucose-6-phosphatase	Autosomal recessive
Tyrosinemia	fahA	Fumarylacetoacetase	Autosomal recessive
Wilson's disease	ATP7B	Copper-transporting ATPase 2	Autosomal recessive
Dent's disease	CLCN5	Chloride channel 5	X-linked recessive
Lowe syndrome	OCRL	Inositol polyphosphate 5-phosphatase (PIP2 5-phosphatase)	X-linked recessive

Table 5.2.2 Drugs commonly known to cause a renal Fanconi syndrome

Nucleoside reverse transcriptase inhibitors (NRTIs)
Aminoglycosides
Sodium valproate
Ifosfamide
Suramin
Tetracyclines (outdated)
Ethanol (chronic alcoholism)

A thorough family history is required in all cases, especially in those without an obvious cause.

A complete drug and occupational history is also important, particularly with regard to herbal remedies obtained from unknown or unapproved sources, and exposure to heavy metals or industrial solvents.

Signs

In children, short stature, volume depletion, and rickets are the main signs of FS.

There are no specific signs in adults, as volume depletion is generally less striking.

Patients may have signs of the underlying disease causing FS (e.g. stones in Dent's disease and cataracts in Lowe syndrome).

Diagnosis of FS

The diagnosis is commonly made in childhood.

The combination of hypophosphatemia, glycosuria (in the absence of hyperglycemia), aminoaciduria, a hyperchloremic metabolic acidosis with hypokalemia, and signs of vitamin D deficiency is very suggestive of FS.

If there is multisystem involvement, as in glycogen storage disease, detection may be prompted by the primary disorder.

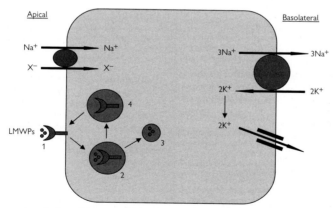

Fig. 5.2.1 The basic transport mechanisms of the proximal tubule (PT). Substances (X) such as glucose, amino acids and phosphate are cotransported at the luminal (apical) cell membrane with sodium (Na). The gradient for sodium entry is maintained by the basolateral sodium pump (Na^+/K^+-ATPase) with recycling of potassium across the basolateral cell membrane via a potassium channel. In the case of bicarbonate (not shown), its reabsorption depends indirectly on the apical Na/H exchanger (also not shown) that secretes protons (H^+). LMWPs (<70 kDa) are bound by two large nonselective receptors (megalin and an associated protein cubilin) at the luminal membrane (1). They bind LWMPs and the complex is internalized (receptor-mediated endocytosis) and packaged into early endosomes (2). Acidification of the endosomes then dissociates the receptor–ligand complex and the protein cargo is either transferred to lysosomes, where it is degraded, or transported to the basolateral membrane and into the blood (3). The megalin receptor is recycled to the luminal membrane (4).

In adults, a high index of suspicion is often necessary in the context of unexplained renal impairment, renal stone disease or unexplained hypokalemia with other fluid and electrolyte disorders.

In some cases an 'incomplete' form of FS can occur: for example in carriers of X-linked disorders such as Dent's disease or Lowe syndrome, tubular proteinuria may be present in isolation.

Milder forms of FS can lead to isolated abnormalities such as hypophosphatemia, and this needs to be differentiated from other causes like malabsorption from the gastrointestinal tract or primary hyperparathyroidism.

Tubular proteinuria can be either primary, due to a defect of the PT (FS), or secondary, due to glomerular disease. If in doubt, these two possibilities can be distinguished by comparing the relative amounts of albumin and LMWP (e.g. RBP) in urine (see below). However, it must be noted that when glomerular proteinuria is heavy, tubular proteinuria will also be present.

Investigations

Initial screening

Urine dipstick testing (for glycosuria without hyperglycemia) and spot urine total protein/creatinine are useful initial screening tests in the clinic for tubular and glomerular disease, but isolated tubular proteinuria is not usually detectable by these routine methods.

Plasma or serum creatinine may be raised (and eGFR reduced), either because of impaired PT secretion of creatinine, or because of glomerular disease with reduced filtration.

Hypophosphatemia and hyperchloremic metabolic acidosis are common in full-blown FS. The latter is a proximal form of renal tubular acidosis (type 2 RTA) and can be distinguished from distal (type 1) RTA, because patients with proximal RTA are able to acidify their urine to pH <5.5 following an acid load (e.g. with NH_4Cl), whereas patients with distal RTA cannot (see Chapter 5.3).

Hypokalemia is a feature of more severe cases; it is secondary to the loss of bicarbonate, which behaves as an osmotic diuretic, and to sodium losses, which stimulate aldosterone release and increase potassium secretion in the collecting duct.

To confirm that the PT is the site of the defect:

1. Screen for tubular proteinuria by assaying for RBP (or other LMWPs such as $\alpha1$- or $\beta2$-microglobulin).
2. Screen for aminoaciduria.
3. Renal handling of phosphate can be assessed by calculating the tubular maximum for phosphate reabsorption normalized for GFR; TmPi/GFR = PPi − (UPi × Pcreat/Ucreat) from a spot urine (ideally a fasting and early morning sample). The normal range changes with age and in adults is 0.8–1.6 mmol/L. An alternative is to calculate the fractional excretion of phosphate ([UPi × P_{creat}]/[U_{creat} × PPi] × 100), which is normally <20%.
4. Renal biopsy (see below).

To identify the underlying cause of FS:

In children, appropriate screening tests for 'inborn errors of metabolism' are necessary.

Exclude cystinosis as it is the commonest cause of FS in childhood.

Exclude myeloma in adults by serum protein electrophoresis and urine testing for Bence–Jones protein.

If a mitochondrial cytopathy is suspected, measure plasma creatine kinase (CK) and blood lactate:pyruvate ratio. Investigate further by undertaking a skeletal muscle biopsy, an assay of respiratory chain enzyme activities, and an analysis of the more common mitochondrial DNA mutations.

Renal biopsy

There are no characteristic or diagnostic findings of FS, except in mitochondrial disease, in which mitochondria (on EM) in the proximal tubule are enlarged and dysmorphic.

Management

Advice to patients

Patients will need to be counselled about the more specific complications of FS, the need for vitamin and mineral supplements, the features of any underlying and associated disease, and the genetic implications of any inherited form of disease.

Treatment

Specific treatment may be available for a particular form of FS (e.g. cysteamine in cystinosis, penicillamine in Wilson's disease, and diet in fructose intolerance).

In general, treatment of FS involves replacing electrolyte losses, including bicarbonate for acidosis, and preventing osteomalacia/rickets:

- Vitamin D (calcitriol) and calcium supplements – but ensure that endogenous vitamin D (25-(OH) vitamin D) levels are also adequate – and also phosphate supplements, if hypophosphatemia is severe and is not responding to vitamin D and diet.
- Oral bicarbonate supplements (as sodium or potassium salt) for metabolic acidosis. Give 1–2 mmol/kg aiming to maintain plasma or serum bicarbonate concentration >20 mmol/l.
- Oral potassium (as bicarbonate or chloride salt) supplements sufficient to maintain plasma or serum potassium concentration >3.0 mmol/L.

In addition, if there is evidence of chronic kidney disease (CKD): blood pressure control, antiproteinuric therapy if there is significant glomerular proteinuria, and treatment of any cardiovascular risk factors that are present (e.g. use of statins for hyperlipidemia).

Follow-up

This depends on the underlying disease, but in most forms of FS, patients need long-term follow-up to monitor treatment and renal function, particularly if there is associated renal stone disease.

Exceptions may be reversible causes of FS, for example following drug-induced toxicity, when PT function has recovered after the withdrawal of the relevant drug (e.g. antiretroviral drugs).

Many patients who have developed FS following chemotherapy are young and should be monitored long-term as part of the 'late effects of cancer chemotherapy' follow-up, because we do not yet know enough about the natural history of this form of nephrotoxicity.

Further reading

Christensen EI, Gburek J. Protein reabsorption in renal proximal tubule-function and dysfunction in kidney pathophysiology. Pediatr Nephrol 2004; **19**: 714–21.

Guggino SE. Mechanisms of disease: what can mouse models tell us about the molecular processes underlying Dent disease?. Natl Clin Pract Nephrol 2007; **3**: 449–455.

Malik A, Abraham P, Malik N. Acute renal failure and Fanconi syndrome in an AIDS patient on tenofovir treatment – case report and review of literature. *J Infect* 2005; **51**: E61–65.

Hau Am, Unwin R. The not so 'mightychondrion'. Emergence of renal diseases due to mitochondrial dysfuction. *Nephron Physiol*, 2007; **105**: 1–10.

Skinner R, Cotterill SJ, Stevens MC. Risk factors for nephrotoxicity after ifosfamide treatment in children: a UKCCSG Late Effects Group study. United Kingdom Children's Cancer Study Group. *Br J Cancer* 2000; **82**: 1636–1645.

Internet resources

Galactosaemia Support Group:

http://www.galactosaemia.org/

The Association for Glycogen Storage Diseases UK:

http://www.agsd.org.uk/

UK Lowe Syndrome Trust:

http://www.lowetrust.com/

See also

Renal tubular acidosis

Background

Systemic acid–base balance is maintained by the lungs (short-term via carbon dioxide loss or retention) and the kidneys (long-term via bicarbonate reabsorption or excretion, and net acid excretion).

The kidneys reabsorb (reclaim) filtered bicarbonate, and synthesize the important urinary buffer ammonia/ammonium, in the proximal tubule, and secrete acid in the distal tubule and collecting duct:

Net urinary acid excretion = Titratable acid (TA, mainly phosphate) + Ammonium (NH_4^+) − Bicarbonate (usually negligible).

Renal tubular acidosis (RTA) is a generic term that can be used to describe several disorders in which there is a failure of normal (and appropriate) renal acid excretion.

Acid retention due to impaired renal function occurs in chronic kidney disease (CKD), but in this setting the problem is due to a reduction in nephron number and the availability of urinary buffer (TA: less filtered phosphate; NH_4^+: reduced proximal tubular capacity to synthesize ammonia, NH_3), rather than a primary defect in renal tubular function and proton (H^+) secretion.

In 'true' RTA there is usually a hyperchloremic normal anion gap acidosis and normal (relatively) glomerular filtration rate (GFR). Ammonium excretion may be reduced, but this reflects (probably) decreased conversion of NH_3 to NH_4^+, because of impaired H^+ secretion, rather than reduced synthesis of NH_3 (cf. CRF; see also type 4 RTA).

In CKD, the acidosis is usually of the increased anion gap type (due to retention of weak organic acids), and the GFR is significantly reduced.

Classification of RTA

The classification of RTA can be based on the main sites and mechanisms of renal tubular acid and base transport along the nephron:

1. The proximal tubule is responsible for reclaiming filtered bicarbonate and generating 'new' bicarbonate as a by-product of NH_3/NH_4^+ synthesis from glutamine.
   - Impaired bicarbonate reabsorption is the hallmark of proximal RTA (or type 2 RTA), but this usually occurs as part of a renal Fanconi syndrome. There is, however, a very rare genetic form due a mutation of NBC1, the sodium bicarbonate cotransporter (SLC4A4) in the basolateral membrane of the proximal tubule.
2. As already mentioned, the distal tubule and collecting duct are responsible for the net acid excretion that is necessary for normal acid–base balance (~1 mmol of H^+/kg on a typical Western diet).
   - A characteristic feature of distal RTA (or type 1 or classical RTA), the more commonly encountered clinical form of RTA, is low urinary citrate excretion. This is not seen in proximal RTA.
   - Nephrocalcinosis, renal stone disease, and bone loss are also more common in distal RTA than in proximal RTA.
   - Hypokalemia can be present in both forms of RTA. In the variant of distal RTA associated with hyperkalemia (type 4 RTA), the primary cause is usually reduced aldosterone secretion (or its action). The associated hyperkalemia suppresses ammonia synthesis and impairs acid excretion.

- Clinically, type 1 distal RTA commonly occurs in patients with autoimmune disease, especially in those with hypergammaglobulinemia.

The numbered classification of RTA is not easy to remember or to use:

- type 1: distal renal tubular acidosis (dRTA);
- type 2: proximal renal tubular acidosis (pRTA);
- type 3: a rare autosomal recessive form due to a deficiency of the enzyme carbonic anhydrase 2 (CAII), which can lead to a mixture of types 1 and 2;
- type 4: hyperkalemia and hypoaldosteronism.

Distal RTA (dRTA)

Definition

This form of RTA is best thought of as a failure of acid secretion by the acid-secreting α-intercalated cell (αIC) (see Fig. 5.3.1) of the distal nephron (distal tubule and collecting duct).

Measuring urine pH alone cannot diagnose RTA, although a urine pH >5.5 (conventionally) in the setting of a systemic acidosis (as indicated by a low plasma bicarbonate concentration) with a near normal GFR, and in the absence of urine infection, makes a diagnosis of RTA likely and appropriate investigations should be undertaken.

The best confirmatory test is a urinary acidification test with either oral ammonium chloride (NH_4Cl) or oral furosemide plus fludrocortisone, which should normally reduce urine pH to <5.3.

In dRTA urine pH cannot reach this threshold, but in proximal RTA, if the plasma bicarbonate concentration is low and the filtered bicarbonate load is reduced, urine pH can fall to <5.3 (see below and Fig. 5.3.2).

Etiology

Inherited

Mutations in either of the two key acid–base transport proteins in the αIC (Fig. 5.3.1):

1. AE1 (or 'band 3'), the chloride/bicarbonate exchanger located in the basolateral membrane of the αIC. AE1 mutations can be autosomal dominant (in European cases) or autosomal recessive (in South-East Asian cases).
2. vH+-ATPase is the proton pump located in the apical membrane of the αIC. vH+-ATPase mutations are autosomal recessive and can be associated with sensorineural deafness, as some mutations also affect the proton pump (a subunit) present in the inner ear.

Acquired

The pathogenesis in these cases is unclear:

1. Autoimmune disease (Sjögren's syndrome, SLE, rheumatoid arthritis, hypergammaglobulinemia).
2. Obstructive uropathy.
3. Nephrocalcinosis (secondary dRTA, e.g. medullary sponge kidney).
4. Renal transplantation (often transient in the postoperative period).
5. Toxins (amphotericin, toluene ('glue sniffing'), ifosfamide, lithium).
6. Sickle cell anemia.

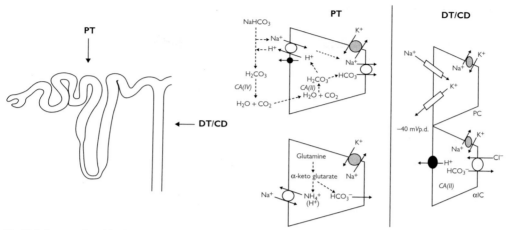

Fig. 5.3.1 Current cell models of tubular acidification. Schematic of the nephron illustrating the main sites of acidification in the proximal and distal segments, and the cellular transport processes involved in bicarbonate (HCO_3^-) reabsorption and proton (H^+) secretion. PT, proximal tubule; DT, distal tubule; CD, collecting duct; PC, principal cell; αIC, α-intercalated cell; CA, carbonic anhydrase.

Epidemiology

This is unknown because of the different causes of dRTA:

- Inherited dRTA due to AE1 mutations is rare in Europe, but more common in South-East Asia, where it is endemic in parts of Thailand and Papua New Guinea.
- vH$^+$-ATPase mutations are rare and most cases have been reported from Middle Eastern countries or isolated communities where consanguinity is frequent.
- Acquired dRTA is more common and is probably underdiagnosed in patients with autoimmune disease,

especially in Sjögren's syndrome in which up to 40% of patients may be affected.

Clinical features

The natural history of dRTA can vary from asymptomatic to symptoms and signs of renal stone disease and nephrocalcinosis, rickets and growth retardation in children, osteomalacia and weakness in adults, and even (rarely) renal failure.

Its main clinical features are:

- variable metabolic acidosis with a normal anion gap;
- renal calculi (typically almost pure calcium phosphate) due to hypocitraturia, hypercalciuria and alkaline urine;
- nephrocalcinosis due to deposition of calcium salts in

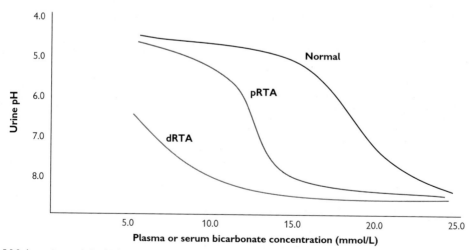

Fig. 5.3.2 Approximate relationship between urine pH and plasma or serum bicarbonate concentration in response to an acid load (acidosis) in normal subjects and in patients with proximal (pRTA) and distal (dRTA) RTA. Note that in pRTA the essentially normal curve is displaced to the left, whereas in dRTA the curve is flattened.

the renal medulla, which also leads to a urinary concentrating defect and nocturia;

- bone demineralization due to bone buffering in chronic acidosis and urinary calcium losses causing rickets in children and osteopenia in adults;
- hypokalemia due to (incompletely explained) urinary losses causing muscle weakness and sometimes paralysis.

Diagnosis

Distal RTA needs to be distinguished from proximal RTA and other causes of a normal anion gap metabolic acidosis from losses of bicarbonate (e.g. gastrointestinal).

The response to an acid load will identify dRTA and can distinguish it from proximal RTA (see Figure 5.3.2).

An underlying diagnosis of dRTA should always be considered in patients with recurrent renal stone disease, particularly if nephrocalcinosis is present, and in patients with autoimmune disease, especially if there is hypokalemia.

Investigations

- The acidosis is usually compensated and arterial blood pH normal, but plasma or serum bicarbonate concentration is reduced and the anion gap is normal. Plasma bicarbonate concentration is often much lower in dRTA than in pRTA, but is usually <20 mmol/L and the urine pH >5.5. However, many patients with dRTA have what is known as 'incomplete dRTA', in which the plasma bicarbonate concentration is normal.
- Hypokalemia is common, but not invariable.
- A plain abdominal X-ray (AXR) often shows (medullary) nephrocalcinosis, which may also be detected on ultrasound scan.
- Urinary pH is >5.5 (in the absence of a urinary tract infection).
- Urinary potassium losses are increased.
- Urinary citrate excretion (and citrate:creatinine ratio) is low.
- Urinary ammonium excretion is low (urine anion gap or net charge is positive (it is normally negative) = $[Na^+]$ + $[K^+] - [Cl^-]$) (see Table 5.3.1).
- Urine osmolality may be reduced (due to a concentrating defect).

Special investigations

In patients with 'incomplete' dRTA the diagnosis can be more difficult because there is no metabolic acidosis.

An acidosis can be provoked by giving oral ammonium chloride (100 mg/kg) and monitoring the urine pH over the subsequent 8 h. In dRTA the urine pH should not fall to <5.3 (see Fig. 5.3.3).

An alternative is to use oral furosemide (40 mg) plus fludrocortisone (1 mg) and to monitor the urine pH over 4 h; again, failure to generate a urine pH <5.3 suggests dRTA.

Renal biopsy

Renal biopsy is not required or usually justified to make a diagnosis of dRTA. Findings differ depending on the etiology of dRTA: widespread tubular damage with calcium deposition and scarring, tubulo-interstitial cellular infiltration, loss of αICs, and reduced immunostaining for AE1 and vH$^+$-ATPase may be observed.

Table 5.3.1 Indirect measures of urinary ammonium in RTA and the use of urine pCO_2

Urine anion gap or net charge

Normally negative ([Na] + [K] < [Cl]), because of unmeasured NH_4^+ (~80 mmol/L) and so it is *positive* when urinary ammonium is *low*.

Urine osmolal gap

Excretion of NH_4^+ with an anion other than Cl$^-$ will *increase* the difference between the measured and the calculated ($2[Na^+]$ + $[K^+]$ + glucose + urea) urine osmolalities.

~ $[NH_4^+]$ = urine osmolal gap/2; however, the urine net charge (above) will be positive.

Urine pCO_2

H$^+$ secretion along the collecting duct generates CO_2 in urine, because unlike in the proximal tubule there is no carbonic anhydrase in the apical membrane to hydrate it; therefore, when the urine is alkaline and rich in bicarbonate the CO_2 is high (>70 mmHg) and the difference from blood is >30 mmHg.

Treatment and management

Those with renal stone disease are advised to maintain a high fluid intake (3 L per day), as well as to comply with their alkali-based replacement therapy:

- Correction of acidosis with oral alkali (1–2 mmol/kg) is given to achieve a plasma bicarbonate concentration >20 mmol/l. It is given to protect the bones and to promote urinary citrate excretion. A drawback is that by further alkalinizing the urine (without a commensurate increase in citrate excretion), calcium phosphate stone precipitation can be exacerbated.
- Correction of hypokalemia is important for any symptoms of weakness, but also because it increases urinary citrate excretion. Thus, alkali therapy is often given as a combination of potassium and sodium bicarbonate (citrate salts can be given, but they are converted in the liver to bicarbonate).

Long-term follow up consists of ensuring the adequacy of replacement therapy and monitoring patients with evidence of nephrocalcinosis and renal stone disease for disease progression.

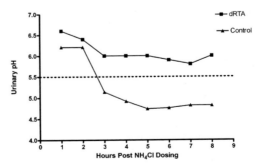

Fig. 5.3.3 Ammonium chloride urinary acidification test: typical changes in urine pH over time following an oral ammonium chloride load in a normal subject and in a patient with dRTA. Note the flattened response in dRTA (cf. Fig. 5.3.2).

Proximal RTA (pRTA)

Definition

Proximal RTA is due to a failure of the proximal tubule to reabsorb filtered bicarbonate, which results in urinary bicarbonate wasting and (initially) an alkaline urine.

Proximal RTA is usually, though not always, part of a renal Fanconi syndrome with generalized proximal tubular dysfunction.

Etiology

Inherited:

- autosomal recessive pRTA;
- Dent's disease;
- Lowe syndrome;
- idiopathic (autosomal dominant) renal Fanconi syndrome;
- cystinosis;
- type 1 galactose deficiency;
- Wilson's disease;
- tyrosinemia;
- paroxysmal nocturnal hemoglobinuria.

Acquired:

- myeloma;
- amyloidosis;
- interstitial nephritis;
- chemotherapy (ifosfamide, cisplatin);
- antiretrovirals (adefovir, tenofovir);
- carbonic anhydrase inhibitors;
- heavy metal poisoning.

Epidemiology

The genetic forms are rare. The acquired forms are more common and determine the incidence and prevalence of pRTA.

Clinical features

Isolated inherited pRTA is associated with ocular defects when due to mutations of *SLC4A4*, and with osteopetrosis, cerebral calcification and mental retardation when due to mutations of the gene for carbonic anhydrase. Both may have a phenotype similar to dRTA with renal stones, nephrocalcinosis and hypokalemia.

Systemic acidosis in pRTA is less severe than in dRTA, but the bone effects can be more significant when it is part of a renal Fanconi syndrome, because of the associated phosphate wasting and vitamin D deficiency. In this setting there may also be aminoaciduria, glycosuria, uricosuria and tubular proteinuria.

Clinical features can include renal stones and nephrocalcinosis, but these are less common than in dRTA, in part because of increased urinary citrate excretion.

Rickets and osteomalacia are more common, because of vitamin D deficiency and phosphate wasting.

Diagnosis

Proximal RTA must be distinguished from dRTA as well as other causes of a normal anion gap acidosis.

Signs of a renal Fanconi syndrome can be helpful, but in some patients there is a mixture of pRTA and dRTA, for example in Dent's disease, and in some autoimmune diseases (as well as type 3 RTA – see below).

If the plasma bicarbonate concentration is low and the filtered bicarbonate load is reduced, patients with pRTA can acidify their urine normally in response to an NH_4Cl acid load (Fig. 5.3.2).

Investigations

- Plasma or serum bicarbonate concentration is typically in the range 15–20 mmol/L, though not as low as 10 mmol/L, which can occur in dRTA.
- Hypokalemia does occur, but it is more usually seen, or becomes worse, when bicarbonate replacement therapy is given.
- Plain AXR may show nephrocalcinosis.
- Urinary potassium losses can be high, especially with bicarbonate therapy.

Special Investigations

To demonstrate the renal bicarbonate leak, a bicarbonate loading test may be necessary. This consists of giving sufficient IV bicarbonate to normalize the plasma bicarbonate concentration and then to measure the fractional excretion of bicarbonate, which will be >15%.

The difference between urine and blood pCO_2 (during a bicarbonate loading test) is a way of detecting reduced H^+ secretion along the collecting duct (see Table 5.3.1) and thus dRTA, but it is unreliable in the presence of nephrocalcinosis.

Renal biopsy

There are generally no specific features to indicate proximal RTA. Mitochondrial cytopathies are sometimes evident on electron microscopy (EM) in some cases of the renal Fanconi syndrome.

Treatment and management

Again, alkali therapy is the mainstay of treatment, but the more bicarbonate that is given, the more is lost in the urine. This can cause, or worsen, hypokalemia.

Large amounts of bicarbonate (10–15 mmol/kg/day) may be required.

Additional potassium supplements are usually necessary.

A thiazide diuretic can also be used to (indirectly) increase (paracellular) bicarbonate reabsorption in the proximal tubule, but again this will increase urinary potassium losses.

Regular follow-up is required, but this usually does not need to be more than once a year in the absence of complications.

Other forms of RTA

Type 3 RTA

Although this was originally thought to be due to 'immaturity' of the acidification mechanisms along the nephron, it is now defined as a rare autosomal recessive disorder that is due to deficiency of the enzyme carbonic anhydrase. This is present in proximal tubules and catalyses the intracellular reaction that generates bicarbonate from CO_2 (Fig. 5.3.1).

This enzyme is also present in the distal nephron and so type 3 RTA is often a mixture of pRTA and dRTA.

Complications are osteopetrosis, cerebral calcification and mental retardation.

Most cases are in Arab families from the Middle East and the Maghreb, where rates of consanguinity are high.

Type 4 RTA

This form of RTA is not really a primary tubular disorder; it is therefore distinct from the other forms of RTA.

It is due to a lack of aldosterone and its actions on the collecting duct, which results in reduced potassium and H^+ secretion.

This leads to hyperkalemia, which suppresses ammonia synthesis in the proximal tubule and thus excretion of ammonium. This diminishes net acid excretion, resulting in a metabolic acidosis.

Causes are:
- primary adrenal insufficiency;
- congenital adrenal hyperplasia;
- aldosterone synthase deficiency;
- potassium-sparing diuretics;
- heparin and low molecular weight heparin.
- hyporeninemic hypoaldosteronism (in diabetic nephropathy);
- ACEIs or angiotensin receptor blockers (less likely);
- nonsteroidal inflammatory drugs;
- cyclosporin;
- HIV infection;
- drugs (amiloride, spironolactone, triamterene, trimethoprim, pentamidine);
- tubulointerstitial disease.
- pseudohypoaldosteronism (types 1 and 2).

The presence of hyperkalemia and mild metabolic acidosis can suggest the diagnosis of type 4 RTA.

Its treatment depends on the underlying cause, but is mainly aimed at correcting the hyperkalemia. This may include a loop diuretic, but in most cases it will also mean mineralocorticoid supplementation.

Summary

The treatment of RTA remains empirical and mainly involves oral alkali supplementation, which is best given as potassium citrate or bicarbonate, especially when hypokalemia is present.

In hyperkalemic dRTA, treatment is of the underlying mineralocorticoid defect.

The aim of correcting the acidosis in RTA has more to do with preserving growth in children and protecting the bones in adults; it seems to have a limited effect on the progression of nephrocalcinosis or renal stone disease.

As yet the recent and important genetic advances and insights in RTA have not translated into any new therapies, but they have highlighted the wider prevalence of RTA – 'presby-RTA' – and its earlier recognition and treatment.

Further reading

Laing CM, Unwin RJ. Renal tubular acidosis. *J Nephrol* 2006; **19**(Suppl 9): S46–52.

Laing CM, Toye AM, Capasso G, Unwin RJ. Renal tubular acidosis: developments in our understanding of the molecular basis. *Int J Biochem Cell Biol* 2005; **37**: 1151–1161.

Walsh SB, Shirley DG, Wrong OM, Unwin RJ. Urinary acidification assessed by simultaneous furosemide and fludrocortisone treatment: an alternative to ammonium chloride. *Kidney Int* 2007; **71**: 1310–1316.

See also

Clinical acid–base disorders, p. 64

Hypo-/hyperkalemia, p. 46

Fanconi syndrome, p. 204

Hypokalemic tubular disorders, p. 214

Hypokalemic tubular disorders

Definition

Hypokalemia is conventionally defined as a serum or plasma potassium concentration <3.5 mmol/L.

The distribution of body potassium contrasts strikingly with that of sodium; whereas Na^+ is predominantly extracellular, K^+ is intracellular (~98%; ~3500 mmol) and is the most abundant intracellular cation (Fig. 5.4.1).

A high intracellular fluid (ICF) K^+ concentration is necessary for regulation of cell volume, pH, enzyme function, DNA and protein synthesis, and growth.

A low extracellular fluid (ECF) K^+ concentration, and the associated steep K^+ gradient across the cell membrane, is largely responsible for the membrane potential of excitable and nonexcitable cells; any change in this gradient can disturb cell excitation and contraction – a doubling or halving of plasma potassium concentration will have this effect.

Chronic potassium depletion causes an impaired urinary concentrating ability, a tendency to metabolic alkalosis and increased ammonium excretion.

Normal potassium homeostasis depends on extrarenal balance: intake (80–120 mmol/day) versus excretion (kidney ~95%; colon ~5%); and intrarenal balance: distribution of K^+ between ICF (most in skeletal muscle cells) and ECF (Fig. 5.4.2).

Note that a shift of as little as 1% of ICF K^+ into or from the ECF would cause a ~50% change in plasma potassium concentration (Fig. 5.4.1). Indeed, a good steak meal could potentially double plasma potassium concentration if there were no mechanisms to modulate extrarenal K^+ distribution acutely. The important ones are hormonal (insulin, α-adrenergic agonists, e.g. epinephrine) and they promote the rapid transfer of K^+ from ECF to ICF via the ubiquitous 'sodium pump': Na^+/K^+-ATPase (Fig. 5.4.1). (Aldosterone's action is slower and it increases renal K^+ excretion.)

As predicted by the Nernst equation ($E_m = -61.5 \log [K^+]_i/[K^+]_0$), the ratio of intracellular to extracellular potassium ($[K^+]_i/[K^+]_0$) is critical in maintaining the resting membrane potential (E_m) of all cells. Hypokalemia increases $[K^+]_i/[K^+]_0$ and causes membrane hyperpolarization.

Neuromuscular excitability can be defined as the arithmetic difference between E_m and the membrane potential required to trigger an action potential (its threshold). Hyperpolarization reduces excitability (which can cause muscle paralysis) by increasing this difference, because the E_m is shifted further away (is more negative) from the threshold potential (which is unaffected); thus, a larger depolarization is required to activate the action potential.

Pathophysiology

The kidneys are the major route of potassium excretion, excreting ~90% of the daily dietary intake (Fig. 5.4.2).

At the glomerulus, potassium is freely filtered and its concentration in Bowman's space matches that in plasma.

The daily filtered load is ~720 mmol/day.

As fluid moves along the nephron, potassium is reabsorbed and secreted (Fig. 5.4.3).

The proximal tubule

The proximal tubule (PT) reabsorbs ~70% of the filtered load.

In the early PT, sodium-dependent electrogenic reabsorption of solutes drives passive reabsorption of water via the paracellular pathway. The movement of water molecules 'entrains' (by solvent drag) movement of K^+.

In the late PT, potassium reabsorption continues by solvent drag, but also by diffusion driven by the reversal of the transepithelial potential difference (V_{te}) in this nephron segment.

Although hypokalemia can result from proximal tubular disorders (see renal Fanconi syndrome), it is more usually associated with diuretics, overactivity of the renin–angiotensin–aldosterone system (RAAS) or autosomal recessive disorders causing dysfunction along the thick ascending limb (TAL) of the loop of Henle (Bartter's syndrome) and distal tubule (Gitelman's syndrome).

The thick ascending limb of the loop of Henle

Salt reabsorption in the TAL is critical to urinary concentrating ability; ~10% of the filtered load of potassium is reabsorbed in this segment.

There is a lumen-positive V_{te} in the TAL due to the differences in potassium and chloride permeabilities of the apical and basolateral membranes (Fig. 5.4.3).

Potassium enters cells of the TAL by secondary active transport via NKCC2, the loop diuretic-sensitive $Na^+/K^+/2Cl^-$ cotransporter. The driving force for sodium and chloride entry is maintained by the action of the basolateral Na^+/K^+-ATPase and by chloride exit across the basolateral membrane via ClC-Ka and ClC-Kb channels, the activity of which is modulated by an accessory protein subunit 'Barttin'.

The apical membrane potential difference favors exit of potassium via secretory potassium channels known as 'SK'.

SK channels are composed of various isoforms of the ROMK (Kir1.1) potassium channel family.

'Recycling' of potassium across the apical membrane (from its absorption via NKCC2 and its secretion via ROMK) maintains adequate levels of luminal potassium to sustain NKCC2 function.

This process also maintains the electrical (lumen-positive V_{te}) driving force for paracellular reabsorption of cations, including the divalent cations calcium and magnesium.

The activity of ROMK is inhibited by activation of the extracellular calcium-sensing receptor (CaSR) that is located in the basolateral membrane. In this way, increases in peritubular (but not luminal) calcium concentration (hypercalcemia) reduce TAL sodium and potassium reabsorption and increase their delivery to more distal nephron sites.

Maintenance of V_{te}, and reabsorption of sodium and potassium by the TAL, is critical for paracellular reabsorption of calcium and magnesium through selective tight junctional pores composed of members of the claudin (CDN 16 and 19) family of membrane proteins.

K⁺ gradient across the cell membrane sets its membrane potential

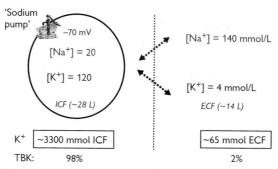

Fig. 5.4.1 Distribution of total body potassium (TBK) between intracellular (ICF) and extracellular (ECF) fluid spaces, and the key role of the 'sodium pump' (Na⁺/K⁺-ATPase). Note that dietary intake of potassium can range from 80 to 120 mmol/day and that this could easily double the plasma potassium concentration, unless there is a 'buffering' mechanism, which involves rapid transfer into the ICF (see text for details).

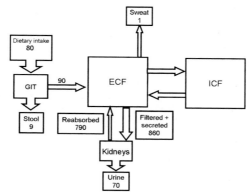

Fig. 5.4.2 Pathways and contributions to normal potassium balance. The numbers refer to the amount of potassium (in mmol) per day. ECF, extracellular fluid; ICF, intracellular fluid; GIT, gastrointestinal tract.

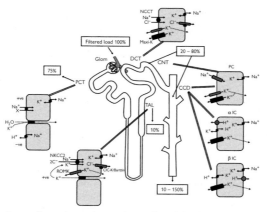

Fig. 5.4.3 Main sites of potassium reabsorption and secretion, and models of potassium movement across cell membranes (see text for details). Basolateral exit of potassium also occurs to varying degrees along the nephron, but the molecular identity of the channels involved is not yet completely resolved. PCT, proximal convoluted tubule; DCT, distal convoluted tubule; CNT, connecting tubule; TAL, thick ascending limb; CCD, cortical portion of collecting duct; α/β IC, intercalated cells.

Approximately 20% of filtered calcium is reabsorbed in the TAL. Therefore, like chronic loop diuretic therapy, loss of function of these key TAL ion channels and transporters (or gain of function of the CaSR) in Bartter's syndrome (Bartter's types I–V; see Table 5.4.1) results not only in impairment of urinary concentrating ability and losses of sodium and potassium, but also in hypercalciuria.

Although the TAL is responsible for reabsorption of the major fraction (>70%) of filtered magnesium, in Bartter's syndrome, perhaps surprisingly, hypomagnesemia is not usually present.

The distal nephron

The distal nephron is an anatomically complex structure that can exhibit net reabsorption or secretion of potassium, depending on potassium balance.

In addition, the overlapping expression of some channels from TAL to distal convoluted tubule (DCT) (Table 5.4.1) makes genotype–phenotype correlations in Bartter's and Gitelman's syndromes difficult, because the degree of 'upstream' compensation can vary according to the underlying gene defect.

The DCT consists of early (DCT1) and late (DCT2) segments.

The activity of the basolateral Na^+/K^+-ATPase maintains the driving force for sodium and chloride entry via the thiazide-sensitive sodium chloride (NaCl) cotransporter (NCCT).

Chloride exits across the basolateral membrane via Barttin–ClC–Kb channels.

Although ROMK channels are expressed in both DCT1 and DCT2, there is little evidence for significant net potassium secretion in DCT1.

Loss of function mutations in NCCT results in the symptoms and signs of chronic thiazide diuretic treatment (Gitelman's syndrome). In marked contrast to Bartter's syndrome, Gitelman's syndrome is accompanied by hypocalciuria and severe hypomagnesemia.

These contrasting effects on divalent cation handling result from incompletely understood differences in the handling of calcium and magnesium between cells of DCT1 and DCT2. The late DCT, the connecting tubule (CNT) and the cortical portion of the collecting duct (CCD) are all primary sites of net potassium secretion (Fig. 5.4.3). In these segments there are two distinct types of cell:

1. *Principal cells (PCs)* reabsorb sodium via an amiloride-sensitive sodium channel (ENaC) by an electrogenic process that creates a lumen-negative Vte favoring secretion of potassium through SK channels (thus coupling indirectly sodium reabsorption with potassium secretion).

A second potassium-conducting channel known as 'maxi-K' or 'Slo' is also present in the apical membrane of PCs.

These channels have a higher electrical conductance than SK channels, but unlike SK channels, they are not open at normal resting membrane potentials. However, they are activated by an increase in tubular fluid flow rate, which increases potassium secretion and loss in the urine.

In the distal nephron, as sodium delivery increases, so does sodium reabsorption. As a result, potassium secretion also increases.

In the CCD, any factor that increases sodium delivery and reabsorption (e.g. aldosterone) will increase potassium secretion.

2. *Intercalated cells (ICs)* are a minority cell population that consists of two subtypes (α and β) that participate in the regulation of acid–base balance and the reabsorption of potassium when dietary intake is restricted, or in metabolic acidosis.

Acid secretion by α-ICs takes place via an electrogenic H^+-ATPase in the apical membrane.

Reabsorption of potassium by acid-secreting α-ICs and bicarbonate-secreting β-ICs takes place via an H^+/K^+-ATPase present in the apical membrane of these cells: potassium reabsorption is coupled to proton (H^+) secretion.

Both types of IC might also secrete potassium when tubular flow rate is increased because, like PCs, they also express maxi-K channels.

Aldosterone increases potassium secretion due to its stimulatory effect on sodium reabsorption (via ENaC and increased Na^+/K^+-ATPase activity).

Aldosterone also increases acid secretion by direct stimulation of H^+-ATPase in α-ICs, and indirectly by stimulating sodium reabsorption in PCs and increasing the lumen-negative Vte (favoring H^+, as well as K^+, secretion).

Hypokalemic alkalosis in Bartter's and Gitelman's syndromes

In Bartter's syndrome, inhibition of sodium and chloride reabsorption in the TAL leads to an increase in delivery of these ions, as well as an increase in tubular flow, to the distal nephron.

Increased delivery of sodium, combined with activation of the RAAS following salt and water losses, augments secretion of both potassium and protons in the collecting duct, leading to their increased urinary excretion and a hypokalemic alkalosis.

The hypokalemia of type II Bartter's (Table 5.4.1) is less severe than in the other types, because of reduced K^+ secretion in the CCD via ROMK.

Indeed, neonatal type II patients can display transient and severe hyperkalemia, reflecting a reduction in potassium secretion in the CCD. These individuals go on to develop more modest levels of hypokalemia in the postneonatal period, because of the emergence of flow-dependent potassium secretion via the maxi-K channel (see earlier).

Loss of NCCT activity in the DCT in Gitelman's syndrome results in a milder and delayed onset of hypokalemia, consistent with a less marked increase in tubular flow rate compared with a defect in the TAL.

Etiology and clinical features

Lack of dietary potassium alone does not cause hypokalemia.

Hypokalemia can arise because of:

- potassium shift into the cells (ICF);
- extrarenal losses of potassium;
- renal losses of potassium.

Hypokalemia due to potassium shifts

Since most potassium is in the ICF, a small shift from the ECF to the ICF can cause significant hypokalemia.

Table 5.4.1 The genes and their proteins causing hypokalemic metabolic alkalosis in Bartter's syndrome (BS) and Gitelman's syndrome (GS)

Gene name	Ensemble cytogenetic band	Protein	Disease	Nephron segment affected
SLC12A1	15q21.1	NKCC2	BS I	TAL
KCNJ1	11q243	Kir1.1 (ROMK)	BS II	TAL
CLCNKA	1p36.13	CLC-Ka	BS VI[a]	tAL + TAL
CLCNKB	1p36.13	CLC-Kb	BS III	TAL + DCT
BSND	1p32.3	Barttin	BS IV	TAL + DCT
CASR	3q21.1	CaSR	BS V	TAL
SLC12A3	16q13	NCCT	GS	DCT

[a] BS VI is a digenic disorder resulting from loss of function of both ClC-Ka and ClC-Kb.

tAL, thin ascending limb of Henle; TAL, thick ascending limb.

Insulin, catecholamines, alkalosis, barium poisoning, and hypokalemic periodic paralysis can all cause hypokalemia due to a reversible shift in potassium from ECF to ICF.

Extrarenal potassium loss
Potassium is reabsorbed in the small intestine and secreted in the colon (which is aldosterone-dependent).

Diarrhea is the main cause of extrarenal potassium loss.

Protracted vomiting and the associated metabolic alkalosis lead to secondary renal losses of potassium due to increased renal bicarbonate excretion, which increases renal potassium excretion, and activation of the RAAS as a result of volume deletion.

Renal potassium loss
Renal potassium wasting is suggested by losses in urine of >20 mmol per day in the presence of hypokalemia.

Once an extrarenal cause for hypokalemia has been excluded, it is generally sufficient to think of clinical situations that:

(a) increase the delivery of Na^+ to the K^+-secreting distal nephron (and its PCs);

(b) increase the mineralocorticoid status (primary hyperaldosteronism with hypertension, with or without hyperreninism or secondary hyperaldosteronism); or

(c) directly affect distal nephron (TAL, DCT and CCD) function (genetic tubulopathies).

As already alluded to, the rare genetic tubulopathies presenting with hypokalemia and normotension are Bartter's and Gitelman's syndromes (autosomal recessives).

Genetic forms of hypokalemia presenting with hypertension are Liddle's syndrome (autosomal dominant), the syndrome of apparent mineralocorticoid excess (AME, autosomal recessive) and glucocorticoid-responsive aldosteronism (GRA, autosomal dominant).

Diagnosis
Bartter's syndrome (BS) (Table 5.4.1)
Antenatal neonatal Bartter's and hyperprostaglandin E syndromes (BS I and II)

These are the most severe forms of Bartter's syndrome and are associated with hypercalciuria and nephrocalcinosis, which can lead to renal failure.

Polyhydramnios in pregnancy is an important clue. It is due to fetal polyuria, which continues in the neonatal period and usually lasts up to 6 weeks; it may cause severe and life-threatening fluid and electrolyte depletion.

Mutations have been described in two genes; *SLC12A1* and *KCNJ1* (Table 5.4.1).

Familial hypomagnesemia with nephrocalcinosis can be confused with this form of antenatal Bartter's syndrome.

Classical Bartter's syndrome (BS III)

This presents in infancy or early childhood with a variety of clinical features ranging from severe volume depletion and failure to thrive (as in BS I and II) to only mild muscle weakness.

It usually presents before the age of 6 years and symptoms include polyuria (manifest as nocturia and bedwetting), polydipsia, vomiting, constipation, salt-craving and chronic fatigue. Muscle weakness and cramps are also common.

BS III is caused by mutations in the basolateral chloride channel ClC-Kb (Table 5.4.1 and Fig. 5.4.3).

Nephrocalcinosis is not a feature.

Antenatal Bartter's syndrome with deafness (BS IV and VI)
This form of Bartter's syndrome is rare and particularly disabling.

It is caused by loss of function of the protein Barttin, which regulates the two chloride channels ClC-Ka and ClC-Kb; both also present in the inner ear, hence the association with deafness.

Bartter's syndrome type VI is similar to type IV, but is due to a digenic mutation affecting the genes for ClC-Ka and ClCKb.

Hypocalcemia with Bartter's syndrome (BS V)
This is a very rare form of Bartter's syndrome due to heterozygous activating mutations of the calcium-sensing receptor, CaSR. Clinical features include hypocalcemia and hypoparathyroidism.

Gitelman's syndrome (GS)
Gitelman's syndrome was originally described as a variant of Bartter's syndrome.

It has similar clinical features to Bartter's syndrome, except for hypomagnesemia, which is common, and hypocalciuria, which is characteristic.

Gitelman's syndrome is often not diagnosed until adolescence or early adulthood; it is frequently detected on routine blood testing.

Hypokalemia in Gitelman's is typically milder than in Bartter's syndrome: 2.5–3.0 vs 1.5–2.5 mmol/L, respectively.

Diagnosis can be difficult and delayed, though many patients are symptomatic and complain of fatigue, muscle cramps and in some cases tetany with carpo-pedal spasm.

They are often intolerant of alcohol and exercise, which can worsen their symptoms.

Diuretic or laxative abuse and eating disorders can all mimic Gitelman's syndrome or worsen its clinical signs and symptoms.

Unlike Bartter's syndrome, so far only one gene defect has been shown to cause the Gitelman phenotype, *SLC12A3* (Table 5.4.1).

A large number of different mutations have been described, but most patients are compound heterozygotes; so unlike

Bartter's syndrome, in which first-cousin marriages are more common, there is usually no consanguinity.

Another complication that is characteristic of Gitelman's syndrome is chondrocalcinosis, which has been linked to reduced activity of the magnesium-dependent enzyme pyrophosphatase.

Other normotensive hypokalemic tubulopathies

As already mentioned, some proximal tubular disorders, including the renal Fanconi syndrome, can have Bartter's-like features.

Other specific examples are patients with the mitochondrial disorder Kearn–Sayre syndrome and patients with a form of familial hypokalemic alkalosis known as Gullner's syndrome.

Treatment

Despite the new genetic knowledge about these syndromes, and our improved understanding of the underlying pathophysiology, treatment and management remain empirical.

Treatment is based on oral potassium (1–3 mmol/kg/day in children) and magnesium (beware of causing diarrhea) supplements, as required, and are guided by symptoms rather than a target blood level for potassium or magnesium.

For hypokalemia, ACE inhibitors and angiotensin receptor blockers can be used (in low doses) to block the activated RAAS, and spironolactone (10–15 mg/kg/day in children) can be used to antagonize hyperaldosteronism. Potassium-sparing diuretics such as amiloride can be added, and where prostaglandin excretion is high, NSAIDs such as indomethacin (2–5 mg/kg/day in children) can be given.

These treatments have to be tried and tailored to suit individual patients. The main problem is compliance with what is often a large number of tablets to be taken life-long, and which are prescribed 'off label'.

Advice about a potassium- and magnesium-rich diet is also important.

Above all, supportive care and long-term follow-up are required.

Genetic screening is still not widely available, but it may help in diagnosis and eventually improve tailored management; moreover, many of these patients appreciate having a definite diagnosis.

Further reading

Giebisch G, Krapf R, Wagner C. Renal and extrarenal regulation of potassium. *Kidney Int* 2007; **72**: 397–410.

Reinalter SC, Jeck N, Peters M, *et al.* Pharmacotyping of hypokalaemic salt-losing tubular disorders. *Acta Physiol Scand* 2004; **181**: 513–521.

Unwin RJ, Capasso G. Bartter's and Gitelman's syndromes: their relationship to the actions of loup and thiazide diuretics. *Curr Opn Pharmacol* 2006; **208**: 208–213.

Internet resources

The Bartter Site (Bartter's and Gitelman's syndrome resource):

http://www.barttersite.org/

Online Mendelian Inheritance in Man (online catalogue of genes and diseases):

http://www.ncbi.nlm.nih.gov/sites/entrez?db=omim

Gitelman's: http://www.ncbi.nlm.nih.gov/entrez/dispomim.cgi?id=263800

Bartter's: http://www.ncbi.nlm.nih.gov/entrez/dispomim.cgi?id=241200

See also

Hypo-/hyperkalemia, p. 46

Hypo-/hypermagnesemia, p. 60

Nephrogenic diabetes insipidus

Definition
Nephrogenic diabetes insipidus (NDI) is defined as the kidney's inability to concentrate urine, despite the presence of adequate levels of circulating vasopressin (antidiuretic hormone (ADH)); it is an endocrine example of end-organ failure.

Almost all cases are diagnosed in childhood.

The kidneys continue to excrete dilute urine independent of a raised plasma or serum osmolality, resulting in polydipsia and predisposing to hypernatremic dehydration if water intake is impaired (e.g. loss of physical access or vomiting) or if there are additional fluid losses (e.g. from diarrhea).

Pathophysiology
Blood (plasma or serum) osmolality is centrally monitored by the hypothalamus: in response to a rise in osmolality, arginine vasopressin (AVP or ADH) is secreted.

In the kidney, AVP binds to a receptor (AVPR2) in the final (distal) part of the nephron, the collecting duct.

The urine entering the collecting duct is dilute and has an osmolality that is much lower than that of plasma (~100 vs ~300 mOsm/kg), because of active solute removal (transport) in the thick ascending limb (TAL) of Henle's loop.

In the absence of circulating AVP, the collecting duct is water impermeable and the final urine will remain dilute.

However, binding of AVP to its receptor (and through a series of intermediate steps) leads to the insertion of water channels (aquaporin 2 or AQP2) in the luminal (urine-facing) membrane of collecting duct (principal) cells, making them water permeable.

Since the osmolality in the interstitium of the renal medulla is high (because of the counter-current multiplier mechanism), water is reabsorbed, which concentrates the urine (to a maximum of ~1000 mOsm/kg).

Thus, AVP regulates water permeability of the collecting duct so that the final urine concentration can vary between the osmolality of the urine entering the collecting duct (~100 mOsm/kg) and that of the interstitium (~1000 mOsm/kg).

In NDI, the kidney's ability to respond to AVP is impaired and the urine remains maximally dilute (with an osmolality <100 mOsm/kg).

Aetiology
Congenital
This presents in the first weeks to months of life:
- X-linked recessive due to mutations in AVPR2 (90%);
- autosomal recessive due to mutations in AQP2 (10%);
- (autosomal dominant DI due to mutations in AQP2 is very rare; autosomal dominant DI is more likely to be of the central rather than nephrogenic type).

Acquired
This presents at any age:
- obstructive uropathy ('post-obstructive diuresis');
- renal failure/tubular dysfunction (e.g. nonoliguric acute kidney injury, tubulo-interstitial nephritis, renal dysplasia, nephronophthisis, cystic kidney diseases);
- lithium (in ~20% of patients treated with lithium);

- hypokalemia (chronic);
- hypercalciuria (acute and chronic).

Clinical features
Congenital NDI
Patients with congenital NDI typically present in the first few weeks of life with polyuria, dehydration, fever, irritability, constipation and a failure to thrive.

Often parents report that the child is always thirsty and suckling vigorously, but vomiting shortly after feeds; vomiting may be due to reflux from the large volume of fluid ingested.

Interestingly, breast-fed infants with NDI typically do better than those given formula feeds; probably because breast milk contains a lower osmolar load than most standard formula feeds (see below).

It is worth noting that in pregnancy with a fetus with NDI, polyhydramnios does not occur (cf. classical Bartter's syndrome), because the AVP-dependent mechanism of urine concentration is not fully developed until after birth, and any osmolar load is cleared by the placenta.

Symptoms typically improve with increasing age, especially once food has changed to solids and there is free access to water, allowing self-regulation of plasma osmolality.

However, patients remain polyuric and problems such as constipation and bedwetting often continue.

The frequency and volume of voiding and drinking, particularly at night, is useful information in assessing the severity of NDI.

Parents often also report problems with the attention span and mental concentration of an affected child, which may be partly due to the constant interruptions needed to drink and to void.

With adequate treatment patients with NDI can function well. In contrast, untreated patients typically have a persistent failure to thrive, as the constant intake of fluid limits their appetite.

Mental retardation used to be an almost invariable feature, probably as a result of repeated episodes of hypernatremic dehydration, but it is rarely seen in patients who have been diagnosed and treated early.

Some patients develop dilatation of the lower urinary tract from the high urine flow rate ('functional outflow tract obstruction') especially if they have poor voiding habits and they are not encouraged to 'double micturate' to ensure bladder emptying.

Acquired NDI
The presenting symptom in acquired NDI is typically polyuria and frequency, including nocturia, but the onset is usually much later than in congenital NDI and there is usually no family history.

Diagnosis of DI
An inappropriately dilute urine in the face of a raised plasma osmolality defines DI.

A large urine volume in a dehydrated patient should always raise the possibility of a urinary concentrating defect.

The diagnosis is easily made by obtaining plasma and urine biochemistries, particularly osmolalities.

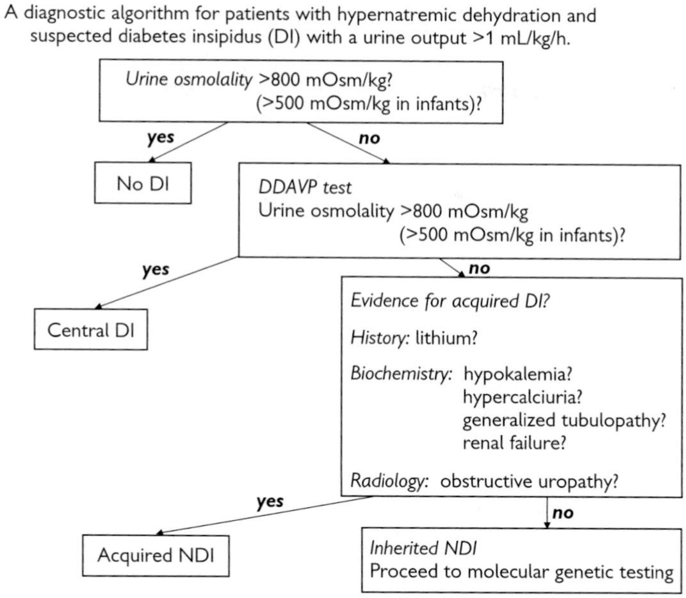

A diagnostic algorithm for patients with hypernatremic dehydration and
suspected diabetes insipidus (DI) with a urine output >1 mL/kg/h.

Fig. 5.5.1 A diagnostic algorithm for patients with hypernatremic dehydration and suspected diabetes insipidus (DI) with a urine output > 1 ml/kg/h.

Maximal urinary concentrating ability increases during the first year of life, but a urine osmolality <500 mOsm/kg (infant) or <800 mOsm/kg (adult) in the presence of hypernatremia indicates DI.

In classic inherited NDI the urine osmolality is always <200 mOsm/kg (and typically ~100 mOsm/kg). A diagnostic algorithm for a child or adult presenting with hypernatremic dehydration is given in Fig. 5.5.1.

Diagnostic procedures

DDAVP test

A DDAVP test is used to discriminate central (cranial) from nephrogenic DI.

The effects of AVP are mediated by two different receptors:
• AVP receptor type 1 (AVPR1) mediates vasoconstriction;
• AVP receptor type 2 (AVPR2) mediates antidiuresis.

The AVP analogue 1-desamino-8-D-arginine vasopressin (DDAVP) has a high specificity for AVPR2 and can be used to assess the renal response, while avoiding the systemic effects mediated by AVPR1.

DDAVP can be given intranasally (20 µg), intramuscularly (0.4 µg if <10 kg, 2 µg if >10 kg), intravenously (0.3 µg/kg) or orally (200 µg).

While intranasal DDAVP is less invasive, absorption is less reliable; if the result of the test is inconclusive, it may need to be repeated using injected DDAVP.

DDAVP given intravenously or orally requires a shorter observation period (2–4 h) than when given by the other routes (4–6 h).

Interestingly, intravenous DDAVP at high doses (0.3 µg/kg) can cause systemic side-effects: a mild decrease in blood pressure and an increase in heart rate via AVPR2.

Patients with mutated AVPR2 (X-linked recessive NDI) do not experience these hemodynamic effects, while patients with intact AVPR2, but mutated AQP2 (autosomal recessive and dominant NDI), do. Thus, the intravenous DDAVP test can help to discriminate between these two forms of NDI.

A typical protocol for the DDAVP test is given in Table 5.5.1.

A rare complication of the DDAVP test is hyponatremia.

Patients with an intact thirst mechanism and who respond normally to DDAVP will stop drinking water as their plasma osmolality falls.

Hyponatremia may develop in those patients with psychogenic polydipsia who keep on drinking, despite lowered plasma osmolality, and in infants who continue to be fed by their parents or carer during the test. Therefore, close observation and limitation of fluid intake to a volume equal to the amount of urine excreted during the test period is necessary to avoid this potentially serious complication.

DDAVP test interpretation (see also Fig. 5.5.1)

If urine osmolality after DDAVP in the test period is:
• <200 mOsm/kg: the diagnosis of NDI is established;
• >800 mOsm/kg: normal renal concentrating ability: NDI is excluded;
• 200–800 mOsm/kg: this is an intermediate response, arising because:
   The test is invalid and needs to be repeated.

Table 5.5.1 Typical protocol for the DDAVP test

Time (min)	−30	−15	0	10	15	20	30	40	50	60	75	90	110	130	150
Actual time (e.g. 09:00)	_:_	_:_	_:_	_:_	_:_	_:_	_:_	_:_	_:_	_:_	_:_	_:_	_:_	_:_	_:_
dDAVP infusion															
BP (mmHg)															
HR (beats/min)															
Fluid intake (mL)															
Urine volume (mL)															
Urine osmolality															
Urine Na+															
Plasma osmolality															
Plasma urea, creat, Na+															

The kidneys are immature (renal concentrating ability is diminished in infants).

The patient has partial NDI. (This is physiologic in children aged <1 year if >500 mosm/kg. It is more common in acquired forms of NDI, but rare in inherited forms.)

Water deprivation test
A water deprivation test is used to discriminate central DI from psychogenic polydipsia.

The aim of the water deprivation test is to produce mild dehydration to challenge the kidney's concentrating ability.

A simple water deprivation test can be undertaken by determining the osmolality of the first morning urine sample (ideally the second void, as there may be some carryover from the evening before). A concentrated urine excludes a diagnosis of DI.

In those patients with dilute first-morning urine, and who are suspected of having psychogenic polydipsia, a formal water deprivation test may be necessary.

Water is withheld until the plasma osmolality rises to just above the upper limit of normal (>295 mOsm/kg).

A water deprivation test carries the risk of hypernatremic dehydration, especially in infants, as there may be delays in obtaining (and reacting to) laboratory results.

It should only be done with close monitoring of body weight, vital signs and biochemistry.

Some useful (adult) guideline values are summarized below:

1. Early morning urine: osmolality >700 mOsm/kg and [Na$^+$] <80 mmol/L is normal.
2. Eight-hour water deprivation test:
   • Normal response. Urine volume <1 L, and urine osmolality >700 mOsm/kg.
   • Diabetes insipidus. Urine volume >1.5 L, urine osmolality <400 mOsm/kg (if urine [Na$^+$] >100 mmol/L, there may be a salt-wasting disorder), and plasma osmolality >295 mOsm/kg.

Congenital NDI
Treatment in the outpatient setting
Diet
The importance of proper treatment of NDI is highlighted by the fact that mental retardation used to be a common complication, but can be completely prevented by early and proper treatment.

Treatment should be provided by a specialist physician and a dietician with experience of the condition, and consists mainly of osmotic load reduction.

The osmotic load consists of salts and protein (urea), which the kidney must excrete and can be roughly estimated using the following formula:

Osmotic load = ×2 amount of sodium and potassium (to account for the accompanying anions) in millimoles plus protein (in grams) ×4.

Since lipids and sugars are metabolized without products that require renal excretion, only protein intake needs to be restricted, but it should still meet the recommended daily allowance.

A reasonable goal is a diet containing ~15 mOsm/kg/day: a child with a urine osmolality of 100 mOsm/kg will need a fluid intake of 150 mL/kg/day to be able to excrete this load.

Diuretics
The use of a diuretic in a polyuric disorder seems counterintuitive, but it does make physiological sense.

Thiazide diuretics inhibit reabsorption of sodium and chloride in the distal convoluted tubule (DCT; part of the urinary diluting mechanism – see above) and so increase the NaCl concentration and osmolality of the urine.

The increased loss of NaCl in the urine decreases intravascular volume, which increases proximal tubular reabsorption of sodium and fluid (in this nephron segment). As a result, less fluid is delivered to the collecting duct and the urine volume decreases.

An example is hydrochlorothiazide at a dose of 2 mg/kg/day in two divided doses. The more long-acting bendroflumethiazide (50–100 µg/kg/day) can be given as a single daily dose.

Hypokalemia is a complication of thiazide diuretic administration, but supplementation with potassium salts can increase the osmolar load and is best avoided. Combining a thiazide diuretic with a potassium-sparing diuretic such as amiloride (0.1–0.3 mg/kg/day) is a better choice, although amiloride can cause gastrointestinal side-effects.

Prostaglandin synthesis inhibitors
Prostaglandin synthesis inhibitors can help to decrease polyuria.

Indomethacin (1–3 mg/kg/day in three or four divided doses) is most widely used.

However, the long-term use of this drug risks impairing renal function, and is associated with hematological and gastrointestinal side-effects, which include life-threatening hemorrhage.

A histamine H2-antagonist (e.g. ranitidine 2–4 mg/kg/dose twice daily) and a prokinetic drug (e.g. domperidone 250–500 µg/kg three to four times daily) can help with the vomiting often seen in infants with NDI, and may also help to reduce the gastrointestinal side-effects of indomethacin.

A combination of a thiazide diuretic and indomethacin is useful during the first years of life, with or without amiloride.

Close monitoring of a patient with NDI for side-effects and for any changes in urine output or growth are key components of management.

Future perspective: molecular chaperones
The vast majority of mutations identified in the *AVPR2* gene lead to improper folding of the protein product, its entrapment in the endoplasmic reticulum (ER), and failure to reach the plasma membrane.

Small membrane-permeable AVP-receptor antagonists ('vaptans') can induce correct folding and transport the protein to the plasma membrane.

Pilot studies in NDI patients have shown a significant decrease in urine output when given these antagonists.

Treatment in the hospital setting
Patients are always prone to the development of dehydration, especially if they are without free access to fluids (infants are at greatest risk) or if there are extrarenal fluid losses (vomiting and diarrhea).

There should be a low threshold for admission to hospital for intravenous hydration to prevent dehydration.

Hypotonic fluids that match the osmolality of the urine, such as dextrose in water or 0.2% saline, are standard solutions for intravenous hydration in NDI.

Hypotonic fluids should never be given in boluses, since any acute lowering of plasma sodium concentration risks causing cerebral edema.

Fluid administration should be calculated to meet maintenance requirements and to correct fluid deficits over 48 h, while keeping in mind any ongoing losses – a tonicity balance (see below).

Replacement fluids that have a higher osmolality than urine osmolality can worsen hypernatremia.

For example, 0.9% normal or isotonic saline contains ~150 mmol Na^+ with an osmolality of ~300 mOsm/kg; if water balance is maintained and the input volume is matched to the output volume of urine, 3 L of this solution will give 900 mOsm (450 mmol Na^+) intravenously; if urine output is also 3 L over the same time period, but with an osmolality of ~100 mOsm/kg (maximally dilute), only 300 mOsm (150 mmol Na^+) will be excreted, resulting in retention of 600 mOsm (or 300 mmol Na^+).

By contrast, if there are increased salt losses, as can occur with diarrhea, or if hypotonic fluids are administered at a rate higher than urinary losses, hyponatremia may occur.

Therefore, close monitoring of the patient – weight, fluid balance, clinical symptoms and biochemistry – is essential to avoid these complications.

Further reading

Bernier V, Morello JP, Zarruk A, et al. Pharmacologic chaperones as a potential treatment for X-linked nephrogenic diabetes insipidus. *J Am Soc Nephrol* 2006; **17**: 232–243.

Bockenhauer D. Diabetes insipidus. In: Geary DF, Schaefer F (eds), *Comprehensive Pediatric Nephrology*. St Louis, MO: Mosby; 2008; **11**: 489–98.

Fujiwara TM, Bichet DG. Molecular biology of hereditary diabetes insipidus. *J Am Soc Nephrol* 2005; **16**: 2836–2846.

Nielsen S, Frokiaer J, Marples D, et al. Aquaporins in the kidney from molecules to medicine. *Physiol Rev* 2002; **82**: 205–244.

Sands JM, Bichet DG. Nephrogenic diabetes insipidus. *Ann Intern Med* 2006; **144**: 186–194.

Internet resources

The Diabetes Insipidus Foundation:

http://www.diabetesinsipidus.org/

The NDI Foundation:

http://www.ndif.org/

See also

Chronic interstitial disease

Chapter contents

Analgesic nephropathy

Analgesic nephropathy is the commonest drug-induced chronic kidney disease.

It is characterized by renal papillary necrosis and chronic tubulointerstitial nephritis.

Papillary necrosis is an ischemic lesion of the inner medulla secondary to a decrease in blood flow, in combination with inflammation.

Analgesic abuse accounts for >25% of cases of papillary necrosis in the USA, and 75% in Australia.

Epidemiology

Early recognition of analgesic abuse is important as it causes a completely preventable form of renal disease and renal failure.

There is wide variation in the geographic incidence, based on differences in the annual *per capita* consumption of phenacetin. The incidence is highest in Australia (20%) and Sweden, and lowest in Canada (2–5%).

Pathogenesis

It results from the habitual consumption of combination analgesics, particularly those containing phenacetin, aspirin and caffeine.

Dependence on these combination mixtures is encouraged by the caffeine component.

This risk of developing renal disease is dependent on the cumulative dose. Renal injury begins after consumption of 2–3 kg of both phenacetin and aspirin, and is clinically evident after 5–7 kg is consumed over a period of 5–8 years.

The principle site of damage is in the medulla, which is vulnerable due to the higher concentration of toxic metabolites in this region.

Injury is enhanced by the countercurrent mechanism and the associated low oxygen content in that area.

- Phenacetin is converted to acetaminophen, depleting the cells of glutathione, resulting in the generation of oxidative and alkylating metabolites.
- Aspirin and other NSAIDs decrease vasodilatory prostaglandins, resulting in the unrestricted influence of vasoconstrictors.
- Caffeine is metabolized to adenosine, which further promotes vasoconstriction in the kidney.

In combination these effects cause oxidant and ischemic injury to the medulla, which is compounded by volume depletion.

This leads to coagulative necrosis of the medulla with renal papillary necrosis and overlying interstitial nephritis.

Risk factors include increasing age, volume depletion, hypertension and recurrent urine infection.

Clinical features

Females are more commonly affected than males, with a ratio of 5:1.

Analgesic abuse and nephropathy is more common in the middle-aged to elderly population.

Median age of onset is 53 years.

Affected patients have a typical psychiatric profile with a tendency to addictive behavior.

Prolonged consumption of combination analgesics for migraine, low backaches and menstrual pain is common.

Renal manifestations

Polyuria and nocturia (secondary to concentrating defect), and urinary acidification defects.

Low–moderate grade proteinuria (<2 g/day). More severe proteinuria suggests associated focal segmental glomerulosclerosis and predicts a poor prognosis.

Sterile pyuria.

Occasional episodes of hematuria may be due to papillary necrosis causing sloughed papilla to be shed in the urine, or due to recurrent urinary tract infections. Persistent hematuria suggests the possibility of urinary tract malignancy.

Papillary necrosis may present as an acute devastating illness with early mortality secondary to sepsis. It may have a protracted course extending from months to years, with recurrent urinary tract infection and tubular dysfunction. It also may be totally asymptomatic in ~75% of cases, and may be detected incidentally on IVP or CT scan.

The risk of uroepithelial carcinoma is 8–10%.

Early cessation of analgesic abuse arrests progression of renal dysfunction in 50% of cases and leads to an improvement in renal function in a further 20%. In the remaining 30%, progression to end-stage renal disease occurs.

Factors that predict progressive renal function deterioration include severe hypertension, persistent proteinuria, and the presence of small kidneys on presentation.

Extra-renal manifestations

Peptic ulcer disease is seen in more than one-third of the patients.

Microcytic anemia due to chronic blood loss is more common and severe than expected for the level of renal dysfunction.

Hypertension is seen in >70% of patients, and is severe in 6–10%.

Ischemic heart disease and renal artery stenosis are seen occasionally.

Pathology

The characteristic lesions include renal papillary necrosis and chronic tubulointerstitial nephritis.

Damage starts with focal coagulative necrosis of the medulla, followed by overlying interstitial nephritis.

Golden-brown lipofuchsin like pigment in the tubular cells is characteristic.

The earliest changes are at the papillary tip, which is the site of highest tissue concentration of analgesics.

The classical lesion is capillary sclerosis in the vessels of the renal pelvis and the ureteral mucosa. It is the earliest detectable pathological lesion and can be demonstrated in 80–90% of analgesic abusers.

The severity of the pathological lesions increases from the pelvis to the pyeloureteral transition.

Initially, the kidneys are normal in size with unchanged cortex. With continued damage, the patchy lesions coalesce, the entire papilla becomes necrotic, and is sequestrated and sloughed into the urine.

This is associated with prominent tubulointerstitial nephritis in the cortical labyrinth over the necrotic papilla.

Retraction of the affected tissue, with compensatory hypertrophy of the unaffected medullary rays, gives the classic nodular kidneys of papillary necrosis.

Renal papillary necrosis may be *medullary,* when focal areas involving innermost medullary regions are necrotic, but the fornices and papillary tips are viable, or *papillary,* when the calyceal fornices and the entire papillary tip are destroyed.

Diagnosis

The lack of specific features makes the diagnosis difficult.

The history of analgesic abuse has to be sought by asking leading questions for chronic pain (headaches, backache and menstrual pains).

Intravenous urography has historically been the investigation of choice. Depending on the stage of the kidney disease, the changes include (Fig. 6.1.1):

- atrophic asymmetrical kidneys;
- clubbed calyces that result from contrast penetrating the spaces that develop following parenchymal necrosis;
- early cavitation and sinus formation;
- arc shadows that result from contrast trapping in the sinus and reflect separation of the sequestrum;
- ring shadows that are due to the sloughed papilla lying in the pool of contrast;
- cavities that develop after the sloughing of the sequestrum. medullary cavities are round or oval, and the papillary cavities are triangular;
- hydronephrosis may be seen following obstruction by the sloughed sequestrum;
- caliectasis that is secondary to the shrinkage of the papillary cavities and enlarged medullary cavities;
- Radio-opaque concretions due to calcification.

Ultrasound shows a classic garland pattern of papillary calcifications surrounding the renal sinus.

Hydronephrosis, secondary to obstruction by the sloughed papilla, may also be seen. The kidneys have an irregular outline with increased echogenicity.

Noncontrast CT is the new 'gold standard' in patients with renal failure.

It is superior to other methods in the detection of papillary calcifications. In patients with moderate renal failure (serum creatinine of 130–350 μmol/l), papillary calcifications were detected with a sensitivity of 92% and a specificity of 100%.

Diagnostic features include decreased renal mass with bumpy contours and papillary calcifications.

The differential diagnosis of analgesic nephropathy will include all forms of slowly progressive kidney diseases.

Renal papillary necrosis has many other etiologies including:

- diabetes mellitus;
- chronic pyelonephritis;
- sickle cell nephropathy;
- transplant rejection;
- reflux nephropathy;
- dehydration and hypoxia (children).

Analgesic Nephropathy [IVU]

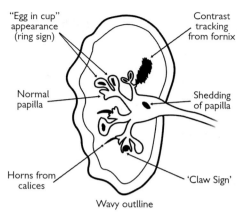

Fig. 6.1.1 Diagrammatic representation of papillary changes in analgesic nephropathy (IVU).

Management

Stop further exposure to analgesics.

Maintain a daily urine output of >2 L. This decreases the medullary hypertonocity, and the concentration of the analgesics at the papillary tip.

Identify and treat urinary tract infection promptly. Correct anemia.

Urologic intervention for relief of ureteral obstruction due to shed papillae.

Regular follow-up for detection and control of hypertension and proteinuria, according to current recommendations for the mangement of CKD.

Regular surveillance for hematuria. If it develops, a full urological work-up is usually required to identify uroepithelial malignancy. Screening may be undertaken with yearly urinary cytology.

Further reading

De Broe ME, Elseviers MM. Analgesic nephropathy. *N Engl J Med* 1998; **388**: 446–452.

Gault MH, Barrett BJ. Analgesic nephropathy. *Am J Kidney Dis* 1998; **32**: 351–360.

Nanra RS. Analgesic nephropathy in the 1990s – an Australian perspective. *Kidney Int* 1990; **42**: S86–92.

See also

NSAIDs and the kidneys, p. 228

Sickle cell disease, p. 192

Drug-induced nephropathies, p. 698

Tumors of the renal pelvis and ureter, p. 676

Tumors of the bladder, p. 680

Nonsteroidal anti-inflammatory drugs and the kidney

Nonsteroidal anti-inflammatory drugs (NSAIDs) are one the most widely prescribed groups of drugs and in addition are available for sale over-the-counter. They can be associated with significant gastrointestinal and renal toxicity.

The therapeutic and adverse effect profile is mediated via inhibition of prostaglandin (PG) synthesis from arachidonic acid by nonspecific blockade of the enzyme cyclo-oxygenase (COX).

A variety of renal side-effects can be observed including salt and water retention, acute tubular necrosis, acute interstitial nephritis, hyperkalemia, and chronic kidney disease.

NSAIDs reported to induce kidney damage include aspirin, ibuprofen, fenoprofen, indomethacin, naproxen, diclofenac and mefenamic acid.

Pharmacokinetics

The liver is the site of metabolism for most NSAIDs. Since they are protein-bound, in hypoalbuminemic states such as liver failure and nephrotic syndrome, the free drug levels increase and can cause nephrotoxicity.

Role of prostaglandins

Renal prostaglandins are autacoids that are synthesized on demand and exert their physiologic effects locally.

PGI2 (prostacyclin) is the most abundant prostaglandin synthesized in the renal arterioles and the glomerulus. It regulates renal blood flow and GFR by causing vasodilatation of the renal vasculature and relaxation of mesangial cells. It induces a preferential increase in medullary blood flow.

PGE2 is found mainly in the tubules and medullary interstitial cells, where it modulates sodium and chloride transport in the loop of Henle, and inhibits vasopressin-mediated water transport in the collecting duct.

In the presence of hypovolemia prostaglandins have an important role in maintaining the glomerular filtration rate.

Consumption of NSAIDs causes inhibition of prostaglandin synthesis, which permits unopposed vasoconstrictive actions of leukotrienes, angiotensin II, vasopressin, and catecholamines.

In salt- and water-replete subjects, this has no major effects. However, in states of renal hypoperfusion, this is associated with a decline in GFR, and can precipitate renal failure (Table 6.2.1).

Elderly patients are more susceptible to NSAID-induced renal failure because of:

- Decreased albumin levels causing decreased protein binding and increased free NSAID levels.
- Decreased total body water and hepatic metabolism, which increases the total concentration of the drug.
- Age-related decrease in GFR and RBF.

Diuretics increase the dependence of renal blood flow and GFR on vasodilatory prostaglandins. The use of NSAIDs in this situation may precipitate renal failure.

The degree of renal disturbance depends on the combination of NSAIDs and the diuretic used. Triamterene is the most commonly implicated.

Table 6.2.1 Risk factors for NSAID-associated AKI

Congestive cardiac failure
Nephrotic syndrome
Cirrhosis with ascites
Hemorrhage
Drugs, e.g. ACEIs, diuretics, calcineurin inhibitors, gentamicin
Underlying renal disease
Diabetes mellitus
Hypertension
Sepsis
Anesthetic agents
Renal artery stenosis

Renal syndromes

The spectrum of nephrotoxicities seen with NSAIDs includes:

- AKI/acute tubular necrosis;
- acute tubulointerstitial nephritis;
- renal papillary necrosis;
- salt and water retention;
- hyperkalemia;
- hypertension.

Acute kidney injury (AKI)

NSAIDs (and aminoglycosides) are the leading causes of drug-induced AKI.

AKI associated with NSAIDs account for 15.5% of all cases of drug-induced renal failure.

All groups of NSAIDs are implicated, although indomethacin is the most commonly associated with AKI.

Short-acting NSAIDs are more harmful than long-acting NSAIDs.

Deterioration in renal function may be related to the dose and duration of exposure. Rechallenge with the same or any another NSAID can result in recurrence of the toxicity.

Under conditions of circulatory stress, use of NSAIDs shifts the balance towards vasoconstriction, causing a decline in the GFR. Patients with underlying chronic kidney disease are highly susceptible, with up to 30% of them developing worsening of renal function on exposure to NSAIDs. In severe cases ATN may ensue.

Affected individuals are usually oliguric with unremarkable urinalysis, significant hyperkalemia, and a fractional sodium excretion (FENa) of <1%, reflecting avid sodium retention.

AKI typically develops within the first week, and is usually reversible within 24–h of stopping the offending agent. Dialysis support is rarely required.

Acute tubulointerstitial nephritis (AIN)

This is much less common than hemodynamically mediated AKI, and usually develops after an average of several months of NSAID therapy.

It has been reported with all types of NSAIDs, although it is most strongly associated with propionic acid derivatives, with >50% of cases occurring with fenoprofen.

It is characterized by a nephrotic presentation in ~75% of cases, is often seen in an elderly population, with a mean age of 65 years, and after a longstanding exposure to the drug.

An increased risk is seen in patients with diabetes, hypertension, increasing age, diuretic use, and a past history of interstitial nephritis.

The reaction is renal-limited, with systemic features (fever, rash, eosinophilia) present in <10% of patients.

The pathogenesis of NSAID-induced AIN is unclear.

The underlying mechanism may be a hypersensitivity reaction, which is milder than that seen with other drugs, since the offending drug itself inhibits the inflammatory reaction.

A primary T-cell disorder or delayed hypersensitivity reaction may be responsible.

Arachidonic acid metabolism may be altered such that leukotrienes are preferentially synthesized. These are proinflammatory, they increase vascular permeability, and they are chemotactic, directing an influx of inflammatory cells into the interstitium.

Heavy proteinuria may be due to the lymphokines produced as a response to the immunological activity.

The clinical presentation may be determined by the severity of the immune response: a robust immune reaction produces acute renal failure with less proteinuria; and a weak immune reaction permits immunocompetent cells to produce lymphokines that result in heavier proteinuria.

The lack of fever, rash or arthralgia suggests that an allergic etiology is unlikely (Table 6.2.2).

Table 6.2.2 Comparison of clinical features of NSAID-associated tubulo-interstitial nephritis (TIN) and typical drug-induced TIN

Feature	NSAID-induced	Drug-induced
Exposure time	Days to months	<1 month
Nephrotic	>90%	<10%
Eosinophilia	<20%	>80%
Eosinophiluria	<5%	>80%
Fever and rash	<10%	>80%

A typical presentation is with acute onset of edema, and rarely oliguria. Urinalysis shows proteinuria, microscopic hematuria, and sterile pyuria.

Diagnosis requires a renal biopsy. Pathologically NSAID-associated AIN is characterized by a focal or diffuse lymphocytic infiltrate (Fig. 6.2.1). Glomeruli typically have changes of minimal change disease (foot process effacement).

Other less common presentations include:
- nephrotic syndrome without tubulointerstitial disease. Histology typically shows features of minimal change disease or membranous nephropathy;
- interstitial nephritis with non-nephrotic proteinuria which resembles a more typical allergic interstitial nephritis.

Resolution of the disease on withdrawal of the drug is common. Time to recovery varies.

Occasionally dialysis support is necessary, and in this situation recovery of renal function may be incomplete.

The use of steroids in this situation is controversial, although they may shorten the duration of the illness.

Papillary necrosis
This is associated with a history of ingestion of an NSAID during a period of severe volume depletion or infection.

In the presence of volume depletion, renal blood flow is dependent on local PG production. NSAIDs, by decreasing local PG production, cause medullary ischemic necrosis.

It is limited to the distal segment of the involved pyramid.

Histology reveals coagulative necrosis, consistent with infarction.

The presentation can be acute with an episode of a renal colic associated with hematuria, or the passage of the slough causing obstruction, or it can be subtle with features of impaired urine concentration.

Though more commonly seen with combination analgesics, it has also been reported with the use of NSAIDs alone, especially propionic acid derivatives.

Elderly men appear to be more susceptible.

Electrolyte imbalance
Sodium retention secondary to inhibition of prostaglandin-induced natriuresis is very common. It is usually transient and insignificant, except when associated with diuretic resistance.

The extent to which salt retention becomes clinically manifest depends on the degree of baseline prostaglandin production and the presence of sodium-retaining states (e.g. heart failure).

Hyperkalemia is secondary to inhibition of renin release, with secondary hypoaldosteronism. It is more often seen in patients with underlying renal disease and diabetes mellitus, and in the elderly.

Hyponatremia results from NSAID-induced impairment of solute-free water excretion. This is caused by increasing both the hydro-osmotic effect of any given level of circulating ADH, and the interstitial tonicity.

Hypertension
The combination of salt and water retention, with a decrease in vasodilatory prostaglandins, causes a rise in the blood pressure, which is more pronounced in known hypertensives. An average increase in the mean blood pressure of 6–8 mmHg is seen.

Patients taking diuretics and β-blockers, the elderly, and blacks with low-renin hypertension are more susceptible.

Subclinical renal dysfunction
There have been a few reports describing subclinical renal dysfunction in the form of functional abnormalities.

Safe NSAIDs – a myth
Sulindac is a prodrug requiring hepatic conversion of an inactive sulfoxide to an active sulfide. This active metabolite is then oxidized and inactivated in the kidney.

Because of this it is suggested to be less likely to inhibit renal prostaglandins. However, it has been associated with renal toxicity in some patients and therefore its use still needs to be closely monitored.

COX-2 inhibitors are a group of drugs which inhibit only the damaging COX-2 enzyme, with no effect on the COX-1 enzyme.

COX-2 enzyme is constitutively expressed in the visceral epithelial cells of the glomerulus, and is upregulated by salt depletion.

In a study of >5000 subjects receiving the COX-2 inhibitor, celecoxib, for >2 years, renal adverse events were more common than with a placebo, and similar in frequency to that seen with other NSAIDs.

Thus, although initially theoretically appealing, recent reports indicate that COX-2 inhibitors are not devoid of renal side-effects.

Therapeutic use of NSAIDs in renal disease.

The therapeutic uses of NSAIDs in renal disease are listed in Table 6.2.3.

Table 6.2.3 Therapeutic use of NSAIDs in kidney disease

Bartter's syndrome

Characterized by hyperreninemic hyperaldosteronism with hypokalemia secondary to NaCl wasting in the loop of Henle. It is also associated with exaggerated renal prostaglandin synthesis.

Several manifestations of this condition are corrected by NSAID therapy. See Chapter 5.4.

Nephrotic syndrome

NSAIDs reduce proteinuria by decreasing renal blood flow and GFR.

NSAID therapy in this setting involves a risk of irreversible renal failure.

Further reading:

Ejaz P, Bhojani K, Joshi VR. NSAIDs and kidney. *J Assoc Physns Ind* 2004; **52**: 632–640.

Gault MH, Barrett BJ. Analgesic nephropathy. *Am J Kidney Dis* 1998; **32**: 355–360.

Klienknecht D. Interstitial nephritis, the nephrotic syndrome, and chronic renal failure secondary to nonsteroidal anti-inflammatory drugs. *Semin Nephrol* 1995; **15**: 228–235.

See also

Uric acid and the kidney

Uric acid is a water-insoluble end-product of purine metabolism. It is a weak acid, therefore at a physiological pH, 98% of uric acid is in the ionized form as urate. By contrast, in collecting tubules where the pH is ≤5.0, the majority is in the form of undissociated uric acid.

In humans, the fractional excretion of uric acid is ~10%. Net reabsorption is greater in males (92%) than in females (88%) and children (70–85%). Gout is therefore most common in males.

Race also influences uric acid excretion: Polynesians (both males and females) have much higher plasma urate concentrations than Caucasians, and therefore a greater prevalence of gout.

Pathophysiology

Renal excretion of uric acid involves four processes: filtration, reabsorption, secretion, and postsecretory reabsorption.

Increasing tubular fluid flow and urine pH decreases uric acid precipitation in the collecting ducts while increasing renal blood flow regulates secretion.

Decreased urate clearance results from:
- Drugs (ciclosporin, NSAIDs, pyrazinamide, and vasoconstrictors such as adrenaline, noradrenaline, and angiotensin).
- Overproduction of lactate (starvation and status epilepticus).
- Plasma volume contraction (inadequate salt and water intake, loss of fluid from diarrhea, or diuretics).

Increased urate clearance is seen with:
- Circulatory volume expansion (e.g. in pregnancy).
- Drugs (probenicid and sulphinpyrazone, warfarin, corticosteroids, and X-ray contrast media) (Table 6.3.1).

Table 6.3.1 Factors affecting renal handling of urates

Decreased clearance	Increased clearance
Volume contraction	Volume expansion
Renal vasoconstrictors	Pregnancy
Increased lactate	Drugs (e.g. probenicid, sulphinpyrazone, warfarin, steroids)
Chronic lead toxicity	X-ray contrast
Drugs (e.g. pyrazinamide)	

Renal deposition of urate causes three types of kidney injury:
- Acute uric acid nephropathy.
- Chronic urate nephropathy.
- Uric acid nephrolithiasis.

These disorders all result from excess uric acid or urate deposition, although the clinical features may vary (Fig. 6.3.1).

Acute uric acid nephropathy

Renal tubular obstruction by urate and uric acid crystals results in acute oligoanuric renal failure.

It usually occurs in a setting of rapid cell turnover and lysis, as seen in leukemia and lymphoma (usually after treatment). There is release of large quantities of

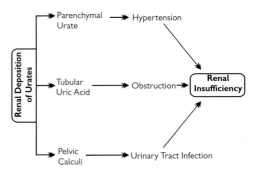

Fig. 6.3.1 Urate and renal disease.

intracellular nucleotides causing hyperuricemia (tumor lysis syndrome).

Risk factors include: volume depletion, lymphoma, rapid response to chemotherapy, pre-existing renal failure, urine pH <5, and high lactate dehydrogenase (LDH) levels.

Volume contraction, leading to reduced urine flow and an acidic pH will decrease the solubility of the uric acid within the tubular lumen.

Uric acid crystals precipitate and cause blockage of tubules and collecting ducts. Elevated tubular pressure and decreased renal blood flow cause a decline in the GFR, and AKI.

Uptake of uric acid crystals by tubular epithelial cells leads to tubular necrosis and inflammation.

Gross overproduction of urate with hyperuricemia is also seen in Lesch–Nyhan syndrome (HGPRT (hypoxanthine guanine phosphoribosyl transferase) deficiency, an X-linked disorder), rhabdomyolysis, phencyclidine toxicity, and metabolic muscle disorders.

In this setting serum urate levels are usually very high (in the range of 900–3000 µmol/L (15–50 mg/dL)). There is progressive renal impairment with a disproportionate rise in the serum phosphate and LDH levels.

A random urine uric acid:creatinine ratio of >0.7 (for mmol/L, or >1 for mg/dL) is highly suggestive of acute uric acid nephropathy.

Ultrasound typically demonstrates large echogenic kidneys.

Birefringent needle-shaped uric acid crystals may be identified on urine microscopy.

Treatment

Volume expansion and diuresis to maintain a high urine flow rate is the cornerstone of prevention and treatment of acute urate nephropathy.

Alkalinization of the urine increases the solubility of uric acid. The urine pH should be maintained at >7.0, until the hyperuricemia has resolved.

Allopurinol inhibits the conversion of xanthine and hypoxanthine to uric acid, thereby reducing both the serum uric acid concentration and the urinary excretion of urate (Fig. 6.3.2). It may, however, induce acute xanthine nephropathy, since xanthine is more insoluble than uric acid.

The dose of allopurinol has to be adjusted according to the creatinine clearance.

If dialysis support is required, hemodialysis is preferable because urate is less efficiently cleared by peritoneal dialysis.

Rasburicase (US Food and Drug Administration- and European Medicines Agency-approved drug for tumor lysis syndrome (only pediatric cases in USA)) is recombinant urate oxidase, which converts uric acid to the non-nephrotoxic product, allantoin. The dose used in children and adults is 0.15–0.2 mg/kg/day IV for 5 days.

Chronic urate nephropathy

Chronic kidney disease (CKD) has been associated with persistently high uric acid levels, as seen in patients with longstanding gout.

Sodium urate deposits in the renal medullary interstitium and induces a foreign body reaction.

The typical pathological appearance is of central accumulation of crystalloid monosodium urate surrounded by an inflammatory infiltrate that includes inflammatory giant cells. Within this lesion neutrophil activation releases oxidants and protease enzymes that activate platelets and the coagulation cascade, which leads to chronic inflammation, and ultimately interstitial fibrosis and tubular atrophy.

Hyperuricemia can also induce hypertension which may cause or promote the subsequent development of albuminuria and progressive CKD.

Lesch–Nyhan syndrome causes chronic uric acid overproduction with hyperuricemia, uricosuria and CKD.

Familial juvenile hyperuricemic nephropathy (FJHN) is an autosomal dominant disease characterized by hyperuricemia (due to underexcretion), with gout and CKD. Mutation of the uromodullin gene is seen in the majority of Japanese families with FJHN.

There is now increased recognition of subclinical lead intoxication in the renal disease associated with hyperuricemia and tubulointerstitial nephritis. Lead probably has both a direct toxic effect on renal epithelia, and an effect of increasing tubular uric acid reabsorption.

The renal biopsy features of chronic urate nephropathy are tubulointerstitial fibrosis, arteriosclerosis and glomerulosclerosis. Uric acid crystals may be seen in the tubules and the interstitium.

The functional associations include mild tubular dysfunction causing minimal proteinuria and renal impairment. A disproportionate increase in the serum uric acid concentration relative to the degree of the renal dysfunction is seen.

The response to allopurinol is variable. Early administration may prevent the progression of the disease, but it is ineffective when renal insufficiency is established.

Uric acid nephrolithiasis

Uric acid stones account for 5–10% of all renal calculi in the USA and UK, and 75% in Israel. It may manifest as crystalluria, stone formation or urinary tract obstruction.

Stone formation is promoted by increased serum urate levels, and increased urate excretion in the urine.

However, the risk of stone formation is affected more by the urine pH than by the daily excreted load of uric acid. For example, a urine pH change from 5 to 6 increases the

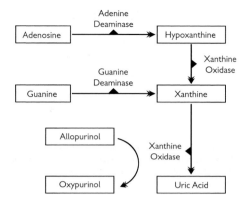

Fig. 6.3.2 The purine degradation pathway and the role of allopurinol.

dissociated acid concentration six-fold and promotes the solubilization of anionic urate.

Acidic pH oversaturates the urine with undissociated uric acid and promotes the formation and precipitation of crystals in the collecting system.

The male to female ratio is 4:1.

Risk factors for uric acid nephrolithiasis are: gout, acute diarrheal states with acidic urine, purine-rich diets (meat, fish (particularly salmon and tuna), vegetables such as cauliflower, beans and spinach), and drugs like aspirin and probenicid.

In addition a variety of disorders involving genetic disorders of purine metabolism, defective renal handling, and altered urinary pH predispose to uric acid stone formation.

Idiopathic

These patients will have normal serum urate levels, but a consistently low urine pH keeps the urine saturated with uric acid. Cases may be sporadic or familial. Sporadic disease begins in middle age, and may be due to low urine pH secondary to decreased ammonium excretion. They recur until the underlying disorder is treated.

Familial forms are autosomal dominant, with an ethnic predilection for Jews and Italians.

Hyperuricemic

In patients with gout, ~22% will develop uric acid nephrolithiasis. It is due to the overproduction of endogenous purines.

Lesch–Nyhan syndrome causes gout and uric acid calculi in childhood. Acute leukemia in childhood and myeloproliferative diseases in adults increase uric acid excretion, causing precipitation and obstruction of the urinary tract.

Gastrointestinal diseases

Salt, water and bicarbonate loss from the GI tract results in reduced urine volumes and decreased urine pH which both promote uric acid stone formation.

Clinical features

Patients present with flank pain and hematuria. Recurrent pyelonephritis is common. Acute ureteral obstruction secondary to uric acid sludge may occur as a part of tumor lysis syndrome.

Uric acid stones are radiolucent, and have a characteristic yellow-cream appearance, and crush with great difficulty. They may be identified by a positive response to uricase and by chemical analysis using high-performance liquid chromatography, or mass spectrometry.

Treatment

The goals include regression in the size of preformed stones, and prevention of new stone formation.

The urine volume should be increased to 3 L per day.

Urine pH should be maintained at 6.0–6.5 with the use of urinary alkalinizers like citrate (1 meq/kg/day in divided doses), or a nocturnal dose of acetazolamide (250 mg).

Decreasing animal protein in the diet helps to reduce the excreted load of uric acid.

Allopurinol may be used in resistant cases with urinary uric acid levels of >60 mmol/day (1000 mg/day), or in cases with gout. It is used prior to chemotherapy to prevent increased serum uric acid levels, and in the dissolution of large nonobstructive stones in the pelvis.

Further reading

Conger JD. Acute uric acid nephropathy. *Med Clin North Am* 1990; **74**: 859–871.

Kudo E, Kamatani N, Tezuka O, *et al.* Familial juvenile hyperuricemic nephropathy: detection of mutations in the Uromodullin gene in five Japanese families. *Kidney Int* 2004; **65**: 1589–1597.

Nickeleit V Mihatsch MJ. Uric acid nephropathy and end stage renal disease – a review of a non disease. *Nephrol Dial Transplant* 1997; **12**: 1832–1838.

Internet resources

Lesch–Nyhan Disease Registry:

http://www.lndinfo.org/

See also

Medical management of stone disease, p. 270

Surgical management of stone disease, p. 274

Renal and urinary tract stone disease in children, p. 282

Cancer and the kidney, p. 196

Inherited disorders of purine metabolism and transport, p. 636

Nephrotoxic metals

The toxic effects of chronic exposure to heavy metals are far more common than acute poisoning. Many Chinese and Ayurvedic herbal products contain lead, mercury and arsenic that are considered to have medicinal properties themselves.

Metals cause injury by combining with sulfhydryl groups in proteins, thereby altering structure and function (e.g. enzymatic activity).

Children are more susceptible to the toxic effects of metals.

Acute metal toxicity causes acute tubular necrosis due to selective damage to the proximal tubule, while low dose chronic exposure leads to chronic tubulointerstitial nephritis which may be confused with changes caused by aging and other disorders, e.g. hypertension.

Urinary biomarkers used to characterize the early stages of toxic renal injury are classified as follows:
- proximal tubular injury: low molecular weight proteins and intracellular enzymes;
- distal tubular injury: Tamm–Horsfall glycoprotein and kallikrein;
- increased glomerular permeability: high molecular weight proteinuria;
- vascular injury: eicosanoids.

The specificity of tubular injury tends to disappear once significant renal damage has occurred. These urinary markers should be determined in freshly voided spot samples and expressed relative to the creatinine concentration. They should ideally be collected at 08:00, when both GFR and biomarker excretion are highest (Table 6.4.1).

Table 6.4.1 Urinary biomarkers in toxic nephropathies

Metal	Markers
Lead	TXB2 , NAG
Cadmium	HIAP, NAG, RBP
Mercury	HIAP, THG
Perchloroethylene	TNAP

TXB2, thromboxane B2; NAG, N-acetyl-D-glucosaminidase; HIAP, human intestinal alkaline phosphatase; RBP, retinol binding protein; THG, Tamm–Horsfall glycoprotein; TNAP, total nonspecific alkaline phosphatase.

Lead

Early reports were from Queensland in Australia, where lead nephropathy was seen in young adults following exposure to lead-based paint in childhood, and from the southeastern USA where Moonshiners drank contaminated illicit liquor.

The different patterns of renal toxicity seen with lead include:
- acute lead poisoning from sudden massive exposure associated with Fanconi syndrome;
- chronic progressive interstitial nephritis associated with hypertension and gout;
- lead-induced hypertension without renal failure.

Pathophysiology
Lead exposure can occur in occupational and environmental settings, and when engaged in hobbies.

Absorption is via the skin, gut and lungs, and is indirectly proportional to the particle size. It is increased with iron and calcium deficiency, and low calorie and high fat diets.

Children are more susceptible to lead toxicity.

Absorbed lead binds to the red blood cells with a half-life of 30 days, diffuses into soft tissues, and is later deposited in bone.

Low socioeconomic status is a risk factor for both lead exposure and the coexisting conditions that increase the susceptibility to lead toxicity. In susceptible populations such as those with hypertension, diabetes and chronic kidney disease (CKD), lead can contribute to nephrotoxicity at blood levels as low as 5 µg/dl.

Mean blood lead levels are decreasing in the developed nations. NHANES III reported a drop in the mean blood lead level to 0.075 µmol/L (1.56 µg/dL), compared to 0.63 µmol/L (13.1 µg/dL) in NHANES II. However, blood lead levels are higher in developing nations due to the continued use of leaded gasoline and paints.

Laboratory features
Anemia with basophilic stippling in red blood cells, reduced erythrocyte aminolevulinic acid dehydratase (ALAD) activity, Fanconi syndrome, hypophosphatemia, raised urea and creatinine, and hyperuricemia.

Blood lead levels
They reflect acute poisoning, and are a very insensitive indicator for assessing the cumulative lead stores in the body. They tend to fall rapidly once acute exposure is completed.

Blood lead levels >3.9 µmol/L (80 µg/dL) in adults and >1.95 µmol/L (40 µg/dL) in children are considered high. Sustained levels of >0.48 µmol/L (10 µg/dL) may be associated with lead-induced nephropathy.

EDTA test
Chronic lead load is estimated using a lead mobilization test. This is performed by parenteral administration of two doses of 1 g of calcium disodium edetate, 12 h apart in adults (20–30 mg/kg in children) with subsequent collection of 24 h urine samples. In the presence of renal failure, the collection should be done for ≥3 days. Normal adults excrete <650 µg of lead chelate in urine.

Bone lead content is a cumulative dose measure of endogenous exposure. Lead in trabecular bone is more bioavailable with a shorter half-life than lead in the cortical bone, which has a half-life of >10–30 years.

Tibial K X-ray fluorescence (XRF)
Diagnostic monitoring of body lead burden is done by a new noninvasive technique using XRF. K-line XRF permits detection of lead molecules from the full thickness of bones, and allows accurate assessment of the lead:calcium ratio.

Acute lead nephropathy
Children are predisposed by their habits like pica, and adults are prone to high dose respiratory exposure. Acute toxicity causes multisystem involvement with symptoms

of colic, vomiting, tremor, convulsions, and features of Fanconi's syndrome. Gingival red line is seen in adults. On renal biopsy, lead/protein complexes are seen as acid-fast nuclear inclusion bodies in proximal tubular epithelial cells.

Chronic lead nephropathy

It is usually a diagnosis of exclusion. The classic presentation is with a benign urinary sediment with <2 g/day of proteinuria, hyperuricemia, hypertension and gout.

It should be suspected in all cases of CKD and gout. New-onset hypertension is seen, and the CKD may eventually progress to ESRD.

Grossly the kidneys appear contracted with a granular surface, and microscopically show features of acellular interstitial nephritis, with dilated tubules alternating with atrophic tubules. Arteriolar nephrosclerosis suggests a role for hypertension in the progression of the disease.

Lead and hypertension

Lead industry workers have been shown to have higher systolic and diastolic blood pressure. NHANES III data showed an increase in the mean SBP and DBP of 7 mmHg and 5 mmHg respectively, with an increase in the blood lead levels from 0.67 to 1.5 µmol/L (14–30 µg/dL).

Treatment

Since no effective therapy reverses the long-term consequences of lead poisoning, the best therapy is to prevent further exposure.

Individuals should be removed from the work place if a single blood lead level is >1.5 µmol/L (30 µg/dL), or if two successive blood lead levels, measured over a 4 week interval are >1 µmol/L (20 µg/dL).

Chelation is preferred if levels are >2.2 µmol/L (45 µg/dL) in children and >3.4 µmol/L (70 µg/dL) in adults.

Succimer (DMSA) (and penicillamine) are used as oral drugs in children, and calcium edetate (and dimercaprol (BAL; British anti-lewisite)) are used as parenteral drugs in adults. The aim of treatment is a lead chelate product that is normal.

Such treatment is effective in reversing acute toxicity, but there is no evidence that it reverses chronic tubulointerstitial disease.

It should also be considered that the toxicity of chelating agents in the presence of renal dysfunction has not been fully evaluated.

Cadmium

This is found in plastics, alloys and electrical equipment (e.g. rechargeable batteries). Cigarette smoking is a major source of toxicity. After absorption, it binds to albumin, and is then complexed with metallothionein in the liver. This complex is filtered in the glomerulus, pinocytosed by proximal tubular epithelial cells, and stored in lysosomes. This accumulation promotes interstitial injury.

Cadmium toxicity is known to be associated with low molecular weight proteinuria. Persisting Fanconi syndrome, and hypercalciuria leads to kidney stones and osteomalacia. Chronic interstitial nephritis occurs rarely but is progressive.

Blood levels >0.089 µmol/L (1 µg/dL), and urine levels >10 µg/g creatinine are suggestive of toxicity.

Urinary excretion is a reliable indicator of total body cadmium burden. The American Conference of Government Industrial Hygienists recommends a value of 5 µg/g creatinine in urine as the occupational limit.

'Itaï-Itaï' or 'ouch-ouch' disease, seen in Japanese women after World War II, was due to consumption of rice contaminated with cadmium. Postmenopausal multiparous women developed a waddling gait, with anemia, osteomalacia with pseudofractures, and glucosuria.

Since binding of cadmium to metallothionein makes disodium edetate ineffective as a chelating agent, there is no effective treatment.

Arsenic

Exposure to a toxic dose causes a dry burning sensation in the mouth, cramping abdominal pain, diarrhoea with rice-water stools, and circulatory collapse leading to hepatic and renal failure.

Hemolysis occurs within 4–6 h followed by jaundice, anemia and hemoglobinuria. Acute oliguric renal failure secondary to acute tubular necrosis is seen.

Treatment includes volume expansion, gastric lavage with warm water, and in severe cases whole bowel irrigation using a solution of polyethylene glycol has been recommended. Occasionally hemodialysis, and chelation therapy with dimercaprol is necessary. Exchange transfusion removes the arsenic–hemoglobin complex.

Incomplete recovery may lead to chronic tubulointerstitial nephritis.

Mercury

Mercury is primarily a neurotoxin, although an association with nephrotic syndrome (membranous nephropathy) has been described.

It resolves with exposure control, and rarely requires chelation therapy.

Acute exposure with <0.5 g of mercuric chloride causes erosive gastritis, hematemesis, and acute tubular necrosis, causing rapidly developing oliguric renal failure. Early chelation therapy with dimercaprol helps.

Other rare metal-induced nephropathies

Uranium can induce ATN.

Copper sulphate can lead to hemolysis/hemoglobinuria.

Gold can cause membranous nephropathy.

Further reading

Ekong EB, Jaar BG, Weaver VM. Lead related nephrotoxicity: a review of the epidemiologic evidence. *Kidney Int* 2006; **70**: 2074–2084.

Sanchez-Fructuoso AI, Torralbo A, *et al.* Occult lead intoxication as a cause of hypertension and renal failure. *Nephrol Dial Transplant* 1996; **11**: 1775–1780.

Internet resources

Poisons information monographs:

http://www.inchem.org/pages/pims.html

Balkan nephropathy

Balkan nephropathy (BN) is a chronic tubulointerstitial nephropathy, geographically limited to people living in the alluvial plains along the tributaries of the Danube River in Bosnia, Bulgaria, Croatia, Romania and Serbia (Fig. 6.5.1).

BN has a familial predisposition. In a single household, several members of one or several generations may be affected.

Within the same village, affected and spared households may be found in close proximity.

Affected villages are sometimes separated from disease-free villages by only a few kilometres.

So far the disease has been identified in:
- 142 villages in Bosnia, Croatia, and Serbia with a local prevalence ranging between 0.5 and 4%;
- 40 settlements in Bulgaria with a local mean morbidity rate of 3%;
- 40 villages and small towns clustered in a limited south-western territory of Romania (districts of Mehedinti and Caras–Severin), where the prevalence of manifest disease was >2%.

A high prevalence of tumors of the renal pelvis and ureter has been described in patients with BN and in affected families.

The geographic correlation between BN and urinary tract tumors supports the speculation that these diseases share a common etiology.

Etiology

The etiology is unknown.

However, accumulated evidence indicates that BN is an environmentally induced disease produced by chronic intoxication with aristolochia, ochratoxin A, or caused by a long-term exposure to polycyclic aromatic hydrocarbons and other toxic organic compounds leaching into the well drinking water from low rank coals in the vicinity of the endemic settlements.

Moreover, the risk of developing BN is influenced by inherited susceptibility factors.

The impact of environmental triggers on individuals genetically predisposed to BN was demonstrated by the higher frequency of folate-sensitive fragile sites, and spontaneous and radiation-induced chromosome breakages in blood samples of BN patients compared to controls.

Moreover, structural changes were described in the third chromosome at 3q25-3q26 in patients and in some healthy relatives with initial morphological changes peculiar to BN. Some of the rearranged chromosome bands contain oncogenes.

Clinical features

BN is a chronic tubulointerstitial disease with insidious onset, slow progression to end-stage renal failure, and an association with urothelial malignancies.

The disease usually affects adults in their fifth decade with the eventual development of end-stage renal failure in their sixth decade.

Its clinical presentation is that of chronic interstitial nephritis of any cause (Table 6.5.1): it is asymptomatic for years or decades, and becomes clinically apparent only when advanced renal failure ensues.

Proteinuria is initially intermittent and mild (up to 1 g/day).

In the early stages, patients have tubular proteinuria, which includes β2-microglobulin, the most readily recognizable low molecular weight protein.

Urinary β2-microglobulin excretion increases not only in patients but also in some clinically healthy relatives and can thus serve as a marker for early tubular damage in BN.

The urinary sediment is usually normal although a few red and white blood cells per high power field may be seen.

Macroscopic hematuria usually indicates an associated urinary tract tumor.

Urate and some other crystal formations are frequent, especially during summer months.

Imaging studies demonstrate normal-sized kidneys in the early stages. When renal failure develops, the kidneys are bilaterally, symmetrically small with a smooth outline.

BN is characterized by diffuse cortical interstitial fibrosis, which is hypocellular in the majority of cases, and by tubular atrophy with both features decreasing from the outer to the inner cortex.

In the early stages the lesions are focal and associated with interstitial edema as well as proximal tubule epithelial cell degeneration.

Table 6.5.1 Epidemiological, clinical and functional characteristics of Balkan nephropathy

Epidemiological characteristics
Residence in an endemic settlement
Family history of renal disease and of renal deaths
Urothelial tumors
Occupational history of farming

Clinical characteristics
Slowly progressive renal insufficiency
Anemia: normochromic or slightly hypochromic
Edema absent
Hypertension: rare in early stages of disease, common in advanced renal failure
Urothelial tumors: common
Abnormalities on urinalysis
Reduced kidney size, normal size in early stages

Functional changes
Impaired concentrating capacity
Decreased glomerular filtration rate
Impaired urinary acidification
Glycosuria, aminoaciduria
Increased uric acid excretion
Renal salt wasting
Proteinuria of the tubular type

Modified from Stefanovic (1983). Stefanovic V. (1983): Diagnostic criteria for endemic (Balkan) nephropathy. In: Strahinjic S, Stefanovic V, editors. Current research in endemic (Balkan) nephropathy. Nis University Press, p 351–63.

Diagnosis

The diagnosis of BN is made in inhabitants from endemic settlements using:
1. Epidemiologic criteria.
2. Demonstration of:
   - reduced GFR;
   - proteinuria (generally <1 g/24 h);
   - microalbuminuria;

- bland urinary sediment;
- tubular markers of injury (renal glucosuria, increased urinary excretion of β2-microglobulin or α1-microglobulin, and N-acetyl-D-glucosaminidase);
- typical renal histology showing hypocellular cortical interstitial fibrosis decreasing from the outer to the inner cortex (if renal biopsy feasible).

3. Exclusion of other kidney disease (chronic pyelonephritis – obstructive and atrophic, adult dominant polycystic kidney disease, glomerulonephritis, etc.).

Kidney disease outside of the Balkans

BN may not be confined exclusively to the Balkans but could probably have spread elsewhere in Europe and the world.

Outside of the endemic regions, in Europe and overseas, BN should be suspected in any case of chronic interstitial nephritis of unknown etiology.

An increased incidence of both BN and urothelial tumours not associated with analgesic abuse should draw attention to the possibility of BN.

However, only once the etiological factor(s) underlying the development of BN have been identified will it be possible to make a firm diagnosis of BN through the use of specific laboratory tests.

Screening

BN is still a major problem in several endemic regions in Bosnia, Croatia and Serbia.

Many patients are not diagnosed until the late stages of disease have developed, since early kidney disease may be asymptomatic.

Ideally all adults in endemic villages should be routinely screened for evidence of early BN and associated risk factors.

Members of a working party for the management of CKD have identified several recommendations for the screening of patients at risk of CKD.

These could be used for the screening of patients at risk of BN, with addition of tubular markers. Renal ultrasonography is usually needed.

Treatment

In the absence of an identified etiological factor, effective prevention of BN is not yet possible.

As with all causes of CKD, patients with BN must pay close attention to cardiovascular risk and stop smoking, eat a healthy and balanced diet, and take regular exercise.

Treatment of BN is similar to that of all chronic interstitial nephropathies.

Hypertension should be treated with ACEIs or ARBs.

Volume depletion from salt wasting should be avoided, particularly during the summer months.

A low protein diet can be used in CKD stages 3 and 4 .

Hemo- and peritoneal dialysis as well as kidney transplantation have been used with success. BN does not recur after renal transplantation.

With longer survival on renal replacement therapy, patients develop tumors of the renal pelvis, ureter, and urinary bladder and long-term surveillance is required for this.

Further reading

Djukanovic L, Radovanovic Z. Balkan endemic nephropathy. In: De Broe ME, Porter GA, Portner WM, Ver Poten GA (eds), *Clinical nephrotoxins – renal injury from drugs and chemicals*. 2nd edn. Dordrecht: Kluwer Academic Publishers; 2003. pp. 587–601.

Stefanovic V, Cosyns JP. Balkan Nephropathy. In: Davison AM, Cameron JS, Grunfeld JP, Ponticelli C, Van Ypersele C, Ritz E, Winearls CG (eds), *Oxford textbook of clinical nephrology*, 3rd edn. Oxford: Oxford University Press; 2004. pp. 1095–1102.

Stefanovic V, Toncheva D, Atanasova S, Polenakovic M. Etiology of Balkan endemic nephropathy and associated urothelial cancer. *Am J Nephrol* 2006; **26**: 1–11.

Stefanovic V, Jelakovic B, Cukuranovic R, et al. Diagnostic criteria for Balkan endemic nephropathy: Proposal by an international panel. *Ren Fail* 2007; **29**: 867–880.

Voice TC, Long DT, Radovanovic Z, et al. Critical evaluation of environmental exposure agents suspected in the etiology of Balkan endemic nephropathy. *Int J Occup Environ Health* 2006; **12**: 369–376.

See also

Aristolochic acid nephropathy ('Chinese herb nephropathy') and other rare causes of chronic interstitial nephritis, p. 240

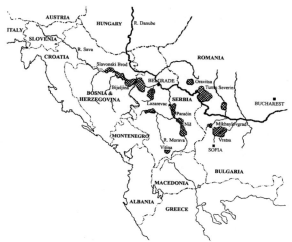

Fig. 6.5.1 Map of Balkan nephropathy distribution.

Aristolochic acid nephropathy ('Chinese herb nephropathy') and other rare causes of chronic interstitial nephritis

Chinese herbs

A chronic interstitial nephritis has been reported in patients taking Chinese herbal medicine. Subsequent investigation has shown that aristolochic acids contained in the Chinese plants are the nephrotoxic agent and there is now general agreement that this condition should be named 'Aristolochic acid nephropathy' instead of 'Chinese herb nephropathy'.

Aristolochic acid nephropathy

Aristolochic acid nephropathy (AAN) is a chronic interstitial nephritis that may be complicated by urothelial carcinoma.

Aristolochic acids (AA) are botanical compounds contained in various plants (*Aristolochia* sp. and others) that are used mainly in traditional Chinese medicine but also in other forms of herbal medicine such as Japanese Kampo or Ayurvedic medicine.

Experimentally AA are nephrotoxic and carcinogenic.

The typical clinical presentation of AAN includes renal failure of variable severity, profound anemia, normal blood pressure, normal urine sediment, mild tubular proteinuria, glucosuria and small and shrunken kidneys on ultrasound examination. Some cases present with Fanconi syndrome.

Histologically AAN is characterized by a dense paucicellular interstitial fibrosis extending from the outer to the inner cortex. The tubules are atrophic and the glomeruli are generally preserved.

Despite withdrawal of AA exposure, generally renal function progressively declines to end-stage renal disease (ESRD).

Exposure of the patient to AA may be demonstrated either by phytochemical analysis of the ingested herbs or by the identification of specific AA-DNA adducts in kidney tissue.

In patients with ESRD, systematic histological examination of the urinary tract has demonstrated a prevalence of urothelial carcinoma of ~40%.

Therefore, in dialysed or transplanted patients with AA-related ESRD, it is recommended that the native kidneys and ureters are removed, and the bladder is examined by cystoscopy every 6 months.

Reports have indicated a worldwide distribution of AA nephropathy.

AA-containing products have been banned in some countries but are still available in others and may be obtained over-the-counter or from the internet. Therefore, in a case of chronic interstitial nephritis of unknown origin, especially when associated with a urinary tract carcinoma, nephrologists should always search for an exposure to AA (herbal medicine).

Recent evidence seems to indicate that AA (*Aristolochia clematitis*)-contaminated cereals cultivated in Balkan regions may be the causal agent (as well as ochratoxin) of the so-called Balkan nephropathy (BN).

Ochratoxin nephropathy (and Balkan nephropathy)

Ochratoxin is a mycotoxin produced by various species of *Aspergillus* and *Penicillium*.

Ochratoxin may contaminate foods (mainly cereals) destined for humans as well as for cattle.

Experimentally, ochratoxin is oncogenic and nephrotoxic.

Ochratoxin is responsible for chronic nephropathy in pigs.

High blood levels of ochratoxin have been reported in association with chronic interstitial nephritis in Tunisia and in France.

Ochratoxin has been incriminated in BN as well as in BN-associated urothelial carcinoma.

Currently the relative contribution of AA and ochratoxin to the development of BN is a matter of debate.

Metals

Comparison of the occupational histories of patients with CKD with those of matched controls having normal renal function has shown exposure to mercury, tin, chromium, copper, lead and cadmium can be associated with an increased risk of CKD.

Lead

Lead nephropathy is a chronic interstitial nephritis associated with diverse routes of chronic lead exposure: children eating lead paint or drinking lead-contaminated water at home; ingestion of lead-contaminated flour; drinking of illegal moonshine whiskey; occupational exposure in lead-producing industries.

Clinical manifestations of lead nephropathy are arterial hypertension, gout and renal dysfunction.

Hyperuricemia is an early prominent feature in lead nephropathy and may explain the confusion between lead nephropathy and gout nephropathy.

The EDTA lead mobilization test (EDTA calcium disodium acetate, 2 g intramuscularly in divided doses 12 h apart, followed by the measurement of 24 h urinary lead excretion over 3 consecutive days) facilitates the identification of lead nephropathy: persons without excessive lead exposure excrete <0.6 mg of lead over a 3 day period.

Cadmium ('ouch-ouch' or 'itaï-itaï' disease)

Chronic cadmium intoxication leads to hypocellular interstitial renal fibrosis.

Endemic renal failure (complicated by a severe painful osteomalacia), was described in Japanese villages after the contamination of rice fields by cadmium-containing industrial discharge ('ouch-ouch' or 'itaï-itaï' disease).

Injury of the renal proximal tubular epithelium has been documented by an increase in urinary neutral endopeptidase 24.11 (an enzyme of the proximal tubule brush border), as well as by an increase in microproteinuria in workers chronically exposed to cadmium.

Germanium nephropathy

Germanium is contained in soil, plants, and animals as a trace metal.

It is widely used in industry because of its semiconductive properties.

Increased use of natural remedies and trace elements has led to supplementation with germanium either through addition to food or by the means of elixirs and capsules.

Chronic supplementation with germanium salts was associated with the development of chronic interstitial nephritis (focal tubular atrophy and interstitial lymphocyte infiltration) with renal tubular epithelial cells showing typical small dark inclusions.

Drugs

Chronic exposure to various drugs may lead to chronic interstitial nephritis.

The drugs most commonly associated with chronic interstitial nephritis are: analgesics, NSAIDs, lithium, calcineurin inhibitors and some antineoplastic agents. This subject is covered in more detail in Chapter 18.2.

Further reading

Debelle FD. Vanherweghem J-L, and Nortier JL. Aristocholic acid nephropathy: A worldwide problem. *Kidney Inf.* 2008; **74**: 158–169.

Internet resources

US Food and Drug Administration. Dietary supplements: Aristolochic acid:

`http://www.cfsan.fda.gov/ ~dms/ds-bot.html`.

See also

Balkan nephropathy, p. 238

Nephrotoxic metals, p. 236

Drug-induced nephropathies, p. 698

Urinary tract infection

Chapter contents

Lower and upper urinary tract infection in adults

Urinary tract infection (UTI) is a common condition result-ing in significant morbidity and occasional mortality. UTI may be divided into several categories:
- asymptomatic bacteriuria;
- uncomplicated lower UTI;
- uncomplicated upper UTI;
- complicated UTI;
- recurrent uncomplicated UTI.

Definitions

Asymptomatic bacteriuria is the isolation of a specific quantitative count of bacteria, in an appropriately collected sample, in an asymptomatic patient.

Uncomplicated lower UTI is a symptomatic bladder infec-tion (cystitis) in a woman with a normal genitourinary tract.

Uncomplicated upper tract infection is a renal infection (acute pyelonephritis) in a woman with a normal genitouri-nary tract.

Complicated UTI is a symptomatic infection of any part of the urinary tract, in a patient with functional, metabolic or structural genitourinary tract abnormalities.

Reinfection is recurrent UTI with the same or a different organism following clearance of the organism from the genitourinary tract.

Relapse is recurrent UTI with the same organism that has not been cleared from the genitourinary tract.

Epidemiology

UTI is one of the most common medical conditions.

50–60% of women will have at least one UTI in their life-time.

Young sexually active woman have an incidence of UTI of 0.5–0.7 episodes per person-year.

Approximately 10% of postmenopausal women have a UTI each year.

Males have a far lower incidence of UTI (5 per 10 000 per year).

Microbiology

Causative organisms are detailed in Table 7.1.1.

Similar organisms cause uncomplicated upper and lower UTIs.

Escherichia coli is by far the most common organism.

Staphylococcus saprophyticus is a common cause of UTI in young women.

Proteus, Klebsiella and Enterococci spp. are less common pathogens.

Complicated UTIs are caused by a broad range of patho-gens.

E. coli remains the most common pathogen.

Proteus, Klebsiella, Citrobacter, Pseudomonas aeruginosa, Enterococci, Group B streptococci and Staphylococci account for a higher proportion of cases.

Pathogenesis

In women UTIs occur when uropathogens from fecal flora colonize the periurethral area, enter the bladder via the urethra and stimulate a host response.

Table 7.1.1 Bacterial etiology of urinary tract infections

Organism	Urinary tract infection (%)	
	Uncomplicated	Complicated
Gram-negative organisms		
Escherichia coli	70–95	21–54
Proteus mirabilis	1–2	1–10
Klebsiella pneumoniae	1–2	2–17
Citrobacter spp.	<1	5
Enterobacter spp.	<1	2–10
Pseudomonas aeruginosa	<1	2–19
Other	<1	6–20
Gram-positive organisms		
Coagulase-negative staphylococci (S. saprophyticus)	5–20 or more	1–4
Enterococci	1–2	1–23
Group B streptococci	<1	1–4
Staphylococcus aureus	<1	1–2
Other	<1	2

Adapted with permission from: Hooton (2003).
Data for complicated infections from: Nicolle (1997).

Upper tract infections almost always occur as an ascending infection from the lower urinary tract.

Multiple host factors predispose young, healthy women to UTIs. These include:
- sexual intercourse;
- use of a spermicidal agent;
- previous recurrent UTI;
- recent antimicrobial use;
- nonsecretion of ABH blood group antigens;
- P1 blood group phenotype (pyelonephritis).

The lower incidence of UTI in males is likely due to a com-bination of:
- a greater distance between the anus and the urethral orifice;
- a drier periurethral environment leading to less frequent colonization;
- increased urethral length;
- antibacterial substances in prostatic fluid.

Bacterial factors also play an important role.
- Bacteria and urothelial cells are both negatively charged.
- Bacteria are unable to overcome the negative–negative repulsion away from the urothelial cell, unless they have fimbriae or other adhesion systems.
- Uropathogenic E. coli have been demonstrated to be associated with a small group of O-serotypes.
- These serotypes account for most cases of E. coli acute pyelonephritis.
- Adhesins (lectins) on bacterial fimbriae or the bacterial surface can recognize specific urothelial cell receptors.

- This is demonstrated by the PAP adhesin which recognizes P blood group determinants on urothelial cells.
- Nonsecretors of these blood group antigens have an increased incidence of recurrent UTIs.
- In addition, different adhesins induce different chemokine repertoires, leading to different host responses.
- Multiple other bacterial virulence factors have been identified.

Complicated infections are associated with urinary obstruction, altered urinary flow (stasis), a nidus of infection (renal calculi or foreign body) not readily treatable with antimicrobials, or mechanisms that alter host defenses (immunosuppression). Bacterial virulence factors are probably less important in these cases.

Urine microscopy and dipstick

In most cases the identification of bacteriuria is required to confirm a diagnosis of a UTI.

However, collected urine may be contaminated with bacteria from periurethral areas.

Urine aspirated suprapubically is normally sterile and does not contain leukocytes. A positive culture from a suprapubic aspirate is the gold standard for diagnosis of UTI.

Clean-catch specimens are usually used in clinical practice. Some degree of contamination with urethral organisms must be accepted with specimens collected in this way. The technique for taking a clean-catch midstream urine is detailed in Table 7.1.2.

Table 7.1.2 Clean-catch urine technique

Start with a full bladder
Stand with legs either side of the toilet
Women hold labia apart with one hand
Cleanse penis tip or vulva area with a sterile swab or soapy water (front to back)
Pass urine into toilet until half finished
Catch sample in a sterile pot (don't stop)
Finish passing urine into the toilet

Noncommunicating collections in the kidney or perinephric tissues, obstructed pyonephrosis or bacterial prostatitis may not necessarily result in bacteriuria.

Traditionally a bacterial count of 10^5 cfu/mL of urine is considered significant bacteriuria.

However, low count bacteriuria (10^2–10^5 cfu/mL) is common particularly with *Staphylococcus saprophyticus* or with increased urinary frequency.

A bacterial count of $\geq 10^2$ cfu/mL in association with pyuria, with suggestive symptoms, almost always represents UTI.

Contamination of carefully collected specimens is less common in men and a count of 10^3 cfu/mL is considered significant bacteriuria.

White cell counting is now the preferred method for assessing pyuria. Most infections will have >10^4 leukocytes/mL of urine. Bacteriuria in the absence of pyuria is usually due to contamination.

Causes of sterile pyuria include:
- leukocytes from other sources
- interstitial nephritis
- stone disease
- uroepithelial tumor
- *Chlamydia trachomatis*
- *Ureaplasma urealyticum* infection
- tuberculosis.

Enterobacteriaceae convert urinary nitrate to nitrite which may be detected on dipsticks.

Other dipsticks detect leukocyte esterase which implies the presence of significant pyuria. These tests may be useful in confirming a clinical diagnosis, but have high false-positive or false-negative rates depending on diagnostic criteria.

Using a cut-off of 10^5 cfu/mL, dipstick testing for both leukocytes and nitrites has a positive predictive value of ~66% and a negative predictive value of ~90%.

Asymptomatic bacteriuria

Asymptomatic bacteriuria is a common condition with a range of definitions dependent on patient gender and method of urine collection.

By definition patients have no symptoms attributable to the urinary tract.

Asymptomatic bacteriuria may be defined as:
- in women, two consecutive voided urines, with isolation of the same bacterial strain, with quantitative counts of $\geq 10^5$ cfu/mL;
- in men, a single clean-catch urine with isolation of a single bacterial strain, with a quantitative count of $\geq 10^5$ cfu/mL;
- a single catheterized urine with isolation of a single bacterial strain, with a quantitative count of $\geq 10^2$ cfu/mL in men or women.

Epidemiology
The prevalence of asymptomatic bacteriuria increases with age:
- 1% in schoolgirls vs 20% in women aged >80 years;
- it is rare in young men vs 15% in men aged >75 years.

It is strongly associated with:
- sexual activity
- diabetes in women (but not men)
- impaired urinary voiding
- indwelling urinary devices
- residence in a long-term care facility.

Natural history
Pregnant women with asymptomatic bacteriuria have an:
- increased risk of pyelonephritis;
- increased risk of premature delivery;
- increased risk of low birth weight infants.

In patients with asymptomatic bacteriuria undergoing urological intervention:
- traumatic procedures associated with mucosal bleeding have a high rate of bacteremia and sepsis.

All others with asymptomatic bacteriuria have:
- an increased risk of symptomatic UTI;
- no increased risk of hypertension, chronic kidney disease, proteinuria or genitourinary malignancy;
- no proven survival disadvantage.

Microbiology

E. coli remains the most common organism (generally strains with fewer virulence characteristics).

Recommendations

The Infectious Disease Society of America has recently reviewed asymptomatic bacteriuria and made a number of recommendations. These include:

- Screening and treatment is not appropriate except for pregnant women and patients about to undergo traumatic urological procedures.
- Pregnant women should be screened at least once in early pregnancy and if results are positive treated with a 3–7 day course of antimicrobial therapy. Periodic screening for recurrent bacteriuria should be undertaken following therapy.
- Patients about to undergo traumatic urological procedures should be screened beforehand. If positive, appropriate antimicrobial therapy should be given shortly before the procedure. Antimicrobial therapy should not be continued unless an indwelling catheter remains in place.
- The role of screening and treatment is not established in patients with a renal allograft or in severely neutropenic patients.

Uncomplicated lower urinary tract infection

Cystitis is very common.

Urinary tract infections are considered complicated if there are features which suggest a higher risk of treatment failure.

Risk factors for treatment failure are detailed in Table 7.1.3.

A pragmatic approach is to consider cystitis in healthy young nonpregnant women as uncomplicated and in all others as complicated.

Table 7.1.3 Complicated vs uncomplicated urinary tract infection

Uncomplicated	Infections considered complicated
Young healthy non-pregnant females	Other conditions with an increased incidence of complicated infection (male gender, pregnancy, elderly, recent urinary tract instrumentation, children, recent antimicrobials, diabetes mellitus, immunosuppression).
	Obstruction or other structural abnormalities of the urinary tract (nephrolithiasis, malignancy, strictures, bladder diverticuli, cysts, fistulae, ileal conduits, and other urinary diversions).
	Functionally abnormal urinary tract (neurogenic bladder, vesicoureteric reflux).
	Foreign bodies (urinary catheters, ureteric stents, nephrostomy tubes)
	Multiresistant organisms.
	Others (e.g. renal failure, renal transplantation, nosocomial infection, prostatitis-related infection).

Adapted with permission from: Hooton T. Urinary tract infections in adults. In: Johnson RJ, Feehally J (eds) Comprehensive clinical nephrology, 2nd edn. Baltimore: Mosby; 2003. Table 53.1, p. 695.

Epidemiology

As for UTIs as a whole, 50–60% of women will have at least one episode of cystitis in their lifetime.

Young sexually active women have an incidence of cystitis of 0.5 episodes/person/year.

Natural history

Antimicrobial therapy hastens the resolution of symptoms.

Most women will improve without antibiotic therapy, but at a higher risk of upper tract or complicated infections.

Cure rates of 85–95% are achieved with antimicrobial therapy.

It is not associated with an increased risk of chronic kidney disease.

Clinical features

Acute onset of dysuria, frequency and urgency of micturition, and/or suprapubic pain.

Usually there are no specific physical signs.

Differential diagnosis

Complicated infection is suggested by other conditions as detailed in Table 7.1.3.

Fever, flank pain and systemic symptoms suggest infection of the upper tract.

Acute urethritis due to Chlamydia trachomatis, Neisseria gonorrhoeae or herpes simplex.

Vaginitis due to Candida or Trichomonas.

Diagnosis

Definitive diagnosis is made by demonstration of bacteriuria (traditionally this is $\geq 10^5$ cfu/mL).

This may miss 'low count cystitis' which may account for up to one-third of cases of cystitis.

Counts of $\geq 10^3$ cfu/mL in young women with typical symptoms achieves reasonable sensitivity and specificity.

Urine dipstick positivity for leukocytes and nitrites may be a useful diagnostic adjunct.

Microbiology

As detailed in Table 7.1.1, E. coli and Staphylococcus saprophyticus are the most common causative organisms.

Other investigations

No other investigations are required in most women.

Pharmacological therapy

Three-day courses of trimethoprim, trimethoprim-sulfamethxazole (TMP-SMX) and fluoroquinolones are as effective as longer courses of these antimicrobials (in most cases).

Fluoroquinolones may not be as effective against Staphylococcal saprophyticus when administered as a 3 day course.

The optimal duration of nitrofurantoin therapy is not well established.

Beta-lactam antibiotics are less effective when given for 3 days and longer courses of these agents are probably required.

The efficacy of single dose regimens remains controversial.

Single dose regimens of TMP-SMX, flouroquinolones and other agents, while highly effective, may not be as effective as three day regimens.

Empiric therapy
- Narrow range of causative organisms.
- Relatively predictable antimicrobial sensitivities.
- Bacterial culture and sensitivities are generally not available until most patients are cured.
- Urine culture is usually unnecessary in cases with a typical presentation.
- Presence of leukocytes or nitrites on urine dipstick may aid clinical decision-making in this situation (a recent study suggests, however, that treatment should be offered whatever the dipstick result).
- Empiric therapy should reflect local antimicrobial sensitivities.
- Antimicrobial sensitivity data may overestimate resistance levels, due to the disproportionate quantity of cultures obtained in treatment failures and more serious infections.
- An arbitrary level of 20% resistance has been suggested as a cut-off for empiric antimicrobial choice.
- Trimethoprim is as effective as TMP-SMX.
- Fluoroquinolone resistance is increasing.

Alternative therapies
- There is no evidence supporting urinary alkalinization.
- There is no evidence for cranberry products in the treatment of cystitis (see 'Prevention').
- There is no evidence for or against increasing fluid intake to increase urine volumes and micturition frequency.

Follow-up
Post-treatment urine cultures in patients whose symptoms have resolved are not indicated.

Prevention
Avoid spermicidal agents.

Cranberry products may prevent recurrence.

Maintaining a high urine output with frequent micturition as well as voiding after intercourse are often recommended but are of unproven benefit.

Recommendations
Healthy nonpregnant women with a typical presentation of cystitis, with no risk factors for complicated UTI, can be treated empirically, without a urine culture.

Antibiotic choice should be based on local sensitivities.

Trimethoprim or TMP-SMX is an appropriate choice in most areas.

Unless there is a specific reason to use a fluoroquinolone, the use of these agents as empiric therapy should be avoided.

The optimum duration of therapy with these agents is probably 3 days.

If nitrofurantoin or β-lactams are used, a longer course of treatment is advisable.

Uncomplicated upper urinary tract infection
It is important to recognize the difference between acute pyelonephritis and chronic pyelonephritis (a misnomer) associated with urinary tract obstruction or vesicoureteric reflux.

The spectrum of acute pyelonephritis ranges from cystitis with mild flank pain to severe sepsis with multiple organ dysfunction syndrome.

Epidemiology
It is much less common than cystitis.

Incidence 20–80 per 10 000 people per year.

Natural history
Acute uncomplicated pyelonephritis, when effectively treated, does not cause chronic damage.

Acute renal failure is an uncommon complication. It is usually associated with complicated infection in an abnormal urinary tract.

Clinical features
Acute onset of flank pain, nausea, vomiting, myalgia and fever with or without lower tract symptoms.

Lower tract symptoms (when present) may occur before, after or at the same time as upper tract symptoms.

The kidney(s) may be exquisitely tender.

Differential diagnosis
Complicated upper tract infection is suggested by the presence of another condition as detailed in Table 7.1.3.

Severe pain, insidious onset or severe sepsis suggests the presence of a complicated infection.

Other causes of flank/back/abdominal pain with fever include:
- pneumonia/lung abscess/empyema;
- intra-abdominal sepsis (pancreatitis, appendicitis, cholecystitis);
- pelvic inflammatory disease;
- vertebral osteomyelitis/discitis;
- obstructive uropathy;
- other renal disease (acute glomerulonephritis, renal infarction, renal vein thrombosis).

Diagnosis
Urine microscopy and culture is required in all suspected cases.

Almost all patients have pyuria and a bacterial count of $\geq 10^4$ cfu/mL.

Blood cultures are not usually required (the demonstration of bacteremia does not alter the management or outcome).

Microbiology
As for cystitis, *E. coli* is by far the most common causative organism.

Most other cases are caused by *Staphylococcus saprophyticus* or other Enterobacteriaceae.

Other investigations
Imaging is not usually performed but would generally demonstrate an enlarged kidney with decreased opacity of the affected parenchyma on CT.

Indications for imaging (ultrasound or CT) of the urinary tract are:
- no clinical improvement after 72 h of treatment;
- two recurrences of acute pyelonephritis;
- the presence of any complicating factor (Table 7.13).

Histology is characterised by an acute interstitial nephritis with neutrophilic infiltration and oedema (Fig. 7.1.1).

Treatment
Mild–moderate cases may be managed in the community with oral antimicrobials with or without a single parental dose.

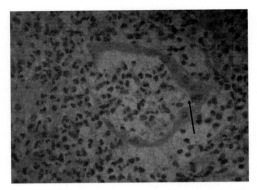

Fig. 7.1.1 Acute pyelonephritis. High power view of renal medulla with prominent neutrophilic infiltrate and visible bacteria (arrow). (Courtesy of Dr Alex Dempster, Southern Community Laboratories, Dunedin, New Zealand.)

Indications for admission to hospital are:
- inability to take oral medications or maintain hydration;
- compliance concerns;
- diagnostic uncertainty;
- severe illness.

Empiric antimicrobial choice should be guided by local antimicrobial sensitivity.

Certain antimicrobials, such as some fluoroquinolones (ciprofloxacin) and aminoglycosides, achieve high concentrations in the renal medulla.

Fluoroquinolones such as ciprofloxacin or levofloxacin are the oral agents of choice.

Aminoglycosides or third-generation cephalosporins such as ceftriaxone are effective parental agents.

Oral agents should be substituted when the patient is improving and can tolerate oral medications and hydration.

If there is suspicion of *Enterococci*, amoxicillin should be added until culture results are available.

Two weeks of therapy is as effective as 6 weeks.

Shorter treatment regimens (5–7 days) are often effective in patients with mild disease who respond rapidly, but these regimens have not been evaluated in well-controlled trials.

Alternative therapy
As for cystitis, no alternative therapies have been proven to be effective.

Follow-up
Post-treatment urine cultures are not cost-effective in patients whose symptoms have resolved.

Recommendations
Parental therapy with an aminoglycoside, fluoroquinolone or an extended spectrum cephalosporin.

Amoxicillin if infection with *Enterococci* is suspected.

Oral therapy with fluoroquinolones.

Shorter courses of therapy (5–7 days) for mild cases with a rapid response to therapy.

Complicated urinary tract infection

UTIs are considered complicated if they occur in the setting of a structurally, functionally or metabolically abnormal urinary tract or in association with a condition which is associated with risk of treatment failure (Table 7.1.3).

At initial presentation it may be difficult to identify a complicated infection. Longer-lasting symptoms, more prominent systemic features and known abnormalities of the urinary tract suggest complicated infection.

Complicated infections are associated with a wider range of causative organisms, with a higher rate of antimicrobial resistance. All patients with a suspected complicated infection must have their urine cultured.

Due to the wide range of organisms it is difficult to make specific treatment recommendations beyond this: that most complicated infections require a longer course of therapy (≥7 days), based on microbial culture and sensitivity.

Infections related to conditions such as an obstructing stone are unlikely to improve without correction of the underlying pathology. Similarly, if the underlying structural or functional abnormality is not corrected, there is a high chance (50%) of recurrent infection in the subsequent 6 weeks.

Urinary tract infections in males
UTIs are much less common in men than in women.

Urethritis is the main differential diagnosis in sexually active men.

Prostatitis must be considered in those with recurrent infection.

Lower UTI in healthy young men, with no features of a complicated infection, may be treated with a 3 day course of antimicrobials.

In others, empiric therapy should be broad spectrum (e.g. a fluoroquinolone), for ≥7 days and rationalized according to culture and sensitivity testing.

If there is no clinical response at 48–72 h, consider repeat cultures and urinary tract imaging.

If there is no obvious cause for the infection, urological evaluation should be considered.

Young healthy males, with a single episode of cystitis, do not need urological evaluation.

Urine should be cultured 2 weeks after treatment is completed.

Persistent bacteriuria suggests the presence of prostatitis or another underlying abnormality of the urinary tract.

Pregnant women
Asymptomatic bacteriuria and UTI in pregnancy are associated with an increased incidence of premature delivery and reduced infant birth weight.

About 1% of pregnant women will have cystitis.

There is an increased risk of acute pyelonephritis in pregnancy associated with asymptomatic bacteriuria.

The clinical presentation is as for nonpregnant women.

Treatment of cystitis is with a 3–7 day course with an agent that is safe in pregnancy.

Acute pyelonephritis is associated with a higher complication rate and is traditionally managed as an inpatient.

Acute pyelonephritis has a recurrence rate of 6–8% and antimicrobial prophylaxis should be considered.

Following treatment, urine should be screened intermittently for the remainder of the pregnancy.

Diabetes mellitus, emphysematous pyelonephritis and papillary necrosis

Most forms of urinary tract infection are more common in diabetics.

In general, all diabetics with infective urinary tract symptoms require urine culture and empiric broad spectrum antimicrobials.

Emphysematous pyelonephritis

- This occurs most commonly in diabetic patients (90%).
- It is caused by gas-producing Enterobacteriaceae.
- It presents as fulminant pyelonephritis.
- Urine culture is usually positive.
- Gas is seen on plain X-ray and CT (Figure 7.1.2).
- CT is required to confirm the diagnosis.
- Treatment is with emergency nephrectomy and broad spectrum antimicrobials (mortality 60% without and 20% with nephrectomy).

Papillary necrosis

- This occurs most commonly in diabetics, almost always in association with infection, and is due to a combination of infection and ischemia.
- Presentation is as for upper UTI, with possible obstructive symptoms in addition (if a sloughed papilla lodges in the urinary tract).

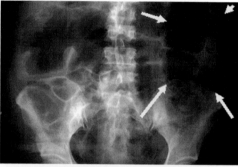

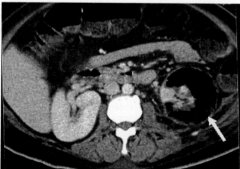

Fig. 7.1.2 Emphysematous pyelonephritis with gas visible in the left kidney on plain film and abdominal CT scan (arrows). (Courtesy of Gabriel Lau, Dunedin Hospital, Dunedin, New Zealand.)

Urinary tract infection in renal transplant recipients

UTIs are the most common infection in renal allograft recipients.

Infections are associated with graft dysfunction and an increased risk of rejection.

Prophylactic TMP-SMX given for other reasons effectively reduces the incidence of UTI.

Indwelling urinary catheter

Bacteriuria occurs in 3–10% of patients with an indwelling urinary catheter (IDUC) per day.

The best prevention for bacteriuria associated with an IDUC is to avoid catheterization and to remove catheters as soon as possible.

A sterile insertion technique, good catheter care, and use of a closed system reduce the rate of infection.

Intermittent self-catheterization may reduce the risk of infection when long-term catheterization is required.

All other strategies are either unproven or have conflicting evidence.

Urine samples are preferably taken following exchange of the catheter and are taken directly from the catheter (not from the urine drainage bag).

Signs and symptoms of IDUC-associated infection may be subtle.

Pyuria is not a reliable marker of infection.

Initial treatment should be broad spectrum and rationalized according to culture and sensitivity testing.

Optimal duration of therapy is unknown but a minimum of 7 days is usually appropriate.

Biofilm on urinary catheters represents a reservoir of infection which antimicrobial therapy may not penetrate, therefore an IDUC associated with infection should be changed.

There is no role for screening or treatment of asymptomatic patients.

Renal calculi

Infection plays an important role in the formation of renal stones and is also an important complication of renal stones.

Prostatitis

Acute bacterial prostatitis

This is likely due to the reflux of infected urine into the prostatic ducts.

Presentation is with symptoms of lower tract infection, associated with fever, myalgia and occasionally urethral obstruction.

On rectal examination the prostate is tender and swollen.

Urine testing demonstrates pyuria and bacteriuria.

Prostatic massage may precipitate bacteremia and should be avoided.

Treatment of ≥4 weeks duration is required.

Fluoroquinolones are the best choice for empiric oral therapy.

Prostatic abscess is uncommon and is suggested by failure to respond to therapy.

Chronic prostatitis

This is characterized by recurrent single pathogen UTIs with intervening asymptomatic periods.

Diagnosis is based on the presence of inflammatory cells on split urines before and after prostatic massage.

Treatment is with a 1–3 month course of an antimicrobial (usually a fluoroquinolone).

Renal and perinephric abscesses

These are uncommon.

The majority are secondary to ascending infection with pyelonephritis followed by liquefaction and walling off. They usually occur in the setting of an abnormal urinary tract.

They are usually caused by Gram-negative Enterobacteriaceae.

The medulla is characteristically involved.

Hematogenous spread (*Staphylococcus aureus*) is less common and typically causes a renal cortical abscess (renal carbuncle).

The presentation is as for acute pyelonephritis, but the response to antimicrobial therapy is either slow or absent.

Systemic features are usually prominent.

Urine culture is usually positive unless there is no communication with the urinary tract (more common with hematogenous spread).

Ultrasound or CT demonstrates a fluid-filled cavity.

Aspiration may be required to distinguish an abscess from other mass lesions.

Antimicrobial therapy, guided by culture and sensitivity testing, is required for 1–2 months.

Cortical abscesses usually respond to antimicrobials and may not require drainage.

If the underlying abnormality is corrected, ascending infection may also respond to antimicrobials.

Drainage may hasten recovery and is required for large or nonresponding collections.

Perinephric collections typically occur with obstruction or other complicating factors. They can occur secondary to an ascending infection with rupture of the renal capsule or due to hematogenous spread.

The symptom onset may be insidious.

Antimicrobials are administered according to culture and sensitivity results.

Drainage of the collection is usually required.

Infected cysts

These most commonly occur in patients with adult polycystic kidney disease.

They may result from ascending infection or hematogenous spread.

Cyst infection may be difficult to distinguish from cyst hemorrhage.

Ultrasound may demonstrate the appearances of a 'complicated' cyst.

Urine culture is positive if secondary to ascending infection.

Antimicrobials are administered according to urine culture and sensitivity results.

The optimal duration of therapy has not been established, but ≥4 weeks of treatment is usually required.

Large infected cysts may need external drainage.

Renal malacoplakia

This is an uncommon chronic granulomatous disorder of unknown etiology.

It involves the genitourinary, gastrointestinal, skin and pulmonary systems.

Genitourinary disease is secondary to urinary tract infection.

It presents with recurrent UTI or obstructive symptoms.

Intravesical plaques on cystoscopy with submucosal aggregates of macrophages containing bacterial debris (Michaelis–Gutman bodies) are characteristic.

It may involve the kidneys and present as flank pain and fever with lower urinary tract symptoms.

Renal insufficiency may occur if both kidneys are involved.

It is probably due to a monocyte–macrophage bactericidal defect.

Treatment is with prolonged courses of appropriate antimicrobials.

Xanthogranulomatous pyelonephritis

This is an uncommon chronic infection associated with obstruction.

The renal parenchyma is replaced by lipid-laden macrophages.

It is usually seen in women and causes flank pain and fever.

It is usually diagnosed on imaging studies.

Antimicrobials are used but nephrectomy is usually required.

Recurrent uncomplicated urinary tract infection

Around a quarter of healthy women with an episode of cystitis will have a second confirmed episode within 6 months.

Fewer than 5% will have a third episode.

Most episodes are reinfection with a different organism or with the same organism which has persisted in the gastrointestinal tract.

Risk factors are the same as for other uncomplicated UTIs.

Recurrence needs to be confirmed on carefully collected urine samples.

Prevention strategies (not well validated) include:
- avoidance of spermicidal agents;
- postcoital voiding;
- liberal fluid intake to maintain frequent micturition.

Cranberry products may reduce recurrence, but further trials are required.

Prophylactic antimicrobials, both continuous and postcoital (when UTIs can be shown to be temporally related to coitus) are effective at reducing recurrence.

Prophylaxis should be considered in women with two or more infections in a 6 month period. The optimal antimicrobial regimen has not been established.

Intermittent self-treatment, with pre-prescribed antimicrobials, is effective in rapidly improving symptoms.

There is conflicting evidence regarding the benefit of topical vaginal estrogen in postmenopausal women. It does not appear to be as effective as antimicrobial prophylaxis.

Routine urological investigation seldom finds underlying abnormalities and is usually unnecessary.

Further reading

Baerheim A. Empirical treatment of uncomplicated cystitis. *Br Med J* 2001; **323**: 1197–1198.

Hooton TM, Scholes D, Hughes JP, *et al.* A prospective study of risk factors for symptomatic urinary tract infection in young women. *New Engl J Med* 1996; **335**: 468–474.

Hooton T. Urinary tract infections in adults. In: Johnson RJ, Feehally J (eds) *Comprehensive clinical nephrology*, 2nd edn. St Louis, MO: Mosby; 2003. Table 53.3 p. 697 (permission pending).

Nicolle LE. A practical guide to the management of complicated urinary tract infection. *Drugs* 1997; **53**: 583–592.

Nicolle LE. A practical guide to antimicrobial management of complicated urinary tract infection. *Drugs and Ageing* 2001; **14**: 243–254.

Nicolle LE, Bradley S, Colgan, *et al.* Infectious Diseases Society of America guidelines for the diagnosis and treatment of asymptomatic bacteriuria in adults. *Clin Infect Dis* 2005; **40**: 643–654.

Scottish Intercollegiate Guidelines Network. *Management of suspected bacterial urinary tract infections in adults.* 2006.

Warren JW, Abrutyn E, Hebel JR, *et al.* Infectious Disease Society of America guidelines for antimicrobial treatment of uncomplicated acute bacterial cystitis and acute pyelonephritis in women. *Clin Infect Dis* 1999; **29**: 745–758.

Internet resources

Patient information:

www.patients.uptodate.com

Patient information from NHS Direct in the UK:

http://www.nhsdirect.nhs.uk/articles/article.aspx?articleId=384&sectionId=1

Patient information from the National Institute of Diabetes and Digestive and Kidney Diseases in the USA:

http://kidney.niddk.nih.gov/Kudiseases/pubs/utiadult/

See also

Urinary tract infections in infancy and childhood, p. 252

Urinalysis and microscopy, p. 8

Imaging in renal disease, p. 20

Urinary tract infection in children

This is an important problem because a urinary tract infection (UTI) not only causes morbidity (and rarely mortality from septicemia) but it may also be the clue to an underlying abnormality of the urinary tract that requires urological attention, or be associated with reflux-associated damage leading to hypertension and chronic renal impairment.

However, the vast majority of children presenting with UTI have normal urinary tracts. Hence there is a need to avoid over-investigation with tests which can be traumatic to children, such as cystograms and radionuclide scans.

Definition

UTI is defined as symptoms plus the detection of a significant growth of organisms in the urine.

- Any growth on culture of a suprapubic aspirate (this technique is usually confined to children <1 year of age and is ideally undertaken with ultrasound guidance).
- >10^5 organisms/mL in pure growth from a carefully collected urine sample (midstream urine from a continent child, or clean-catch or bag/pad urine from other children). Ideally two consecutive growths of the same organism with identical sensitivities should be obtained, but this is not always possible in practice.
- Bacteriuria in the absence of symptoms does not necessarily need treatment but needs to be considered in the clinical context, e.g. predisposing urinary tract abnormalities or previous UTI.

Epidemiology

It is estimated that at least 1% of boys and 3% of girls experience a UTI during their first decade of life.

The prevalence is uncertain since children may be treated for febrile episodes without urine being collected in both primary and secondary care settings.

During first 12 months of life both symptomatic UTI and asymptomatic bacteriuria affect males more than females. Thereafter UTI is more common in females.

Nosocomial UTIs, associated mainly with urinary catheters, are an important cause of hospital morbidity in children undergoing catheterization that is not covered with prophylactic antibiotics.

Circumcision is associated with a decreased risk of symptomatic UTIs and may be justified in male infants with major abnormalities of the urinary tract when combined with other procedures.

Breastfeeding reduces the risk of UTI.

Etiology

Escherichia coli is responsible for ≥80% of UTIs.

Other organisms include *Proteus, Enterococcus, Pseudomonas* and *Klebsiella* spp.

Staphylococcus aureus and *Staph. epidermidis* can be urinary pathogens in small children.

Inflammation of the urinary tract may be related to virulence factors, particularly P-fimbriae in *E. coli*.

Clinical presentation

In general, the younger the child the more nonspecific the symptoms tend to be.

Therefore one of the biggest problems is that the diagnosis is not thought of, especially in the prime target groups, i.e. infants.

UTI should be excluded in any febrile child with unexplained fever.

Neonatal jaundice is the classical association of bacteriuria in the newborn, but a high index of suspicion is required in any baby that is nonspecifically deteriorating.

Infants may present with vomiting, diarrhea, poor feeding, failure to thrive or fever. Suprapubic aspiration should be attempted as part of the septic work-up.

When infection occurs in an abnormal urinary tract, infants may present with AKI and also electrolyte abnormalities.

Cystitis-like symptoms such as frequency and dysuria are common in the older child.

Pyelonephritis with high fever, abdominal/loin pain, and rigors are uncommon presentations in children with upper urinary tract involvement.

History and examination

Always enquire about any abnormality on antenatal ultrasound or a family history of urinary tract problems (vesicoureteric reflux (VUR) has a 30% familial incidence).

Try to distinguish upper tract (fever and pyelonephritis) from lower tract (cystitis-like) symptoms.

Enquire about urinary stream in boys (posterior urethral valves) or incontinence.

Palpate for abdominal masses and fecal loading as there is a strong association between UTI and constipation.

A palpable bladder combined with poor urinary stream suggests obstructive uropathy or posterior urethral valves in the male infant, or a neurogenic bladder.

Examine the spine and lower limb reflexes especially in children with incontinence.

The genital area should be examined for foreskin problems in boys and local irritation and infection in females (sexual abuse is a rare cause of UTI).

Measure blood pressure using a cuff of the appropriate size.

Plot the growth centiles.

Handling of urine specimens

Inappropriate handling and culture of the urine can cause difficulties for the management of UTI.

An enquiry must be made as to how the urine was collected as previously mentioned.

Urine should be stored at 40°C in the refrigerator during any delay in transferring to the lab.

Urine microscopy is no longer routinely requested since the urine needs to be fresh and up to 50% of patients with significant bacteriuria demonstrate an insignificant number of white cells (<5 white cells per high power field in a centrifuged urine specimen) and pyuria may occur in 9% of febrile infants without a UTI.

If available, phase contrast microscopy may demonstrate bacteria and white cells in the acute situation.

Urine dipstick testing

Strips which detect leukocyte esterase and nitrite are usually favored for the diagnosis of UTI.

Nitrite may on occasion be falsely negative since nitrate might not be reduced to nitrite with frequent bladder emptying, production of a dilute urine, inadequate dietary nitrate, or infection with enzyme-deficient bacteria.

A positive nitrite and leukocyte result (usually with positivity for blood and protein) is a strong indicator of UTI in the symptomatic child and justifies empirical treatment with antibiotics while the urine culture result is awaited.

Outpatient follow-up of the asymptomatic child with a negative dipstick does not require urine to be sent for laboratory culture.

Management

Acute infection

If the child is not unwell enough to require hospitalization, oral therapy with an antibacterial drug chosen from Table 7.2.1 can be used.

The best choice of empiric antibiotic should be based upon information available from the local microbiology laboratory. Antibiotic resistance is high for ampicillin alone and increasing for trimethoprim. A cephalosporin is probably best first choice at present.

Parenteral antibiotic therapy is recommended in the unwell child with vomiting but oral therapy has recently been shown to be as effective. Therapy in neonates is usually IV ampicillin and gentamicin but in the older child cephalosporins such as cefotaxime are used.

There is no firm evidence for the optimal duration of treatment but usually 10 days of oral or IV/oral antibiotics in those with vomiting appears equally effective in children with suspected pyelonephritis.

A 2–4 day course of oral antibiotics for the child with lower tract symptoms who is systemically well is adequate and supported by meta-analysis data.

For children who have had an abnormal early ultrasound, prophylactic therapy should be continued until investigations are completed. In all groups, a urine culture should be taken to ensure resolution of infection.

Treatment and investigation of UTI in children go hand-in-hand. Children who are hospitalized with severe illness and recurrent or atypical UTI should have an ultrasound performed during the acute admission to rule out underlying obstructive uropathy such as posterior urethral valves or other congenital abnormalities. Such patients should be managed in centres where there is both urology and nephrology expertise.

Prevention of UTI recurrences

Recurrence of UTI is common with ~30% of girls having another UTI within 1 year (mainly lower urinary tract in nature).

A good fluid intake needs to be encouraged with regular voiding (school toilets are often a problem!).

Enquire about constipation which has a strong association with voiding dysfunction and recurrent UTI.

Ensure that personal hygiene is stressed with proper wiping, and avoidance of bubble bath and tight-fitting underwear.

Antibiotic prophylaxis with trimethoprim or nitrofurantoin (Table 7.2.1) is usually only employed in patients

Table 7.2.1 Antibiotics used to treat UTI in childhood

Antibiotic	Treatment (mg/kg/day)	Prophylaxis (mg/kg/day)
Coamoxiclav	Check BNF as depends upon age and drug concentration	Not recommended
Trimethoprim	4 mg/kg orally 12-hourly	2 mg/kg 24-hourly (at night)
Cefuroxime	20 mg IV (max 750 mg) 8-hourly	NR
Cefradine	12.5–25 mg/kg orally 12-hourly	3 mg/kg 24-hourly (at night)
Nitrofurantoin	0.75 mg/kg orally 6-hourly	1 mg/kg 24-hourly (at night)
Ciprofloxacin	Not licensed but refer to BNF	Not recommended

demonstrated to have Grades 3–5 VUR (reflux distending the pelvis and calyces). Prophylaxis is usually maintained for ≥2 years in this situation.

There are no formal trials comparing prophylactic antibiotics vs urine culture when symptoms develop (a point which needs to be stressed to parents/carers even if the child is on antibiotics). However, some recent evidence indicates that prophylaxis may not significantly decrease the risk of recurrent UTI and may increase the risk of antibiotic resistance.

Shorter courses of prophylactic antibiotics (6 months) may be employed in children (usually girls) with recurrent UTIs and normal urinary tracts along with continued emphasis on general preventative measures. Dysfunctional voiding can be assessed by monitoring bladder emptying on ultrasound or occasionally urodynamics if symptoms are severe.

Investigation

This is a surprisingly controversial area previously with a lot of focus on detecting VUR because of its known association with scarring (reflux nephropathy), CKD, and hypertension.

There is increasing recognition from antenatal studies that VUR without infection may be associated with abnormal renal development giving rise to 'global scarring' without UTI (dysplasia).

A significant dissociation between the presence of scars on DMSA and the presence of VUR has been recognized.

In younger children VUR can only be defined by micturating cystourethrography (MCUG) which is a potentially traumatic examination in children.

For continent children aged >4 years, one can assess reflux by using MAG3 scans with indirect micturating cystograms (see below).

Algorithms for the investigation of UTI have not distinguished between those who have upper tract symptoms from those with lower tract (dysuria and frequency) symptoms. Until recently, the consensus was that all children (both boys and girls) should undergo appropriate investigation after the first proven UTI. However, there is often difficulty interpreting urine cultures, particularly in young children where the risk of renal damage is probably greatest.

Ultrasound scan (USS) is the primary investigation and will reveal anatomical information even in nonfunctioning kidneys. Kidney size should be recorded and interpreted with reference to centile charts based on the child's height. USS will also reveal problems with bladder obstruction and other abnormalities such as stones (plain AXR is no longer routinely performed). USS is operator dependent and can demonstrate scarring of kidneys in experienced hands. One important caveat is that significant VUR may be present with a normal USS, particularly in the newborn period.

Recent NICE guidance suggests restricting MCUG to those aged <6 months who have severe, atypical, or recurrent UTI (Table 7.2.2(a)).

MCUG is only required in older children if operative intervention is being considered.

MCUG is the most traumatic of the imaging investigations for a UTI and children require prophylactic antibiotics for 48 h to cover the procedure. In addition information for the family and play preparation for the child is required.

A DMSA scan is the best technique for detection of scars and determination of differential renal function. This should be delayed for 6 months after the UTI if permanent renal damage following an episode of pyelonephritis is being sought.

Isotope renography (MAG3) is used to determine the presence of obstruction as well as for calculating differential kidney function. In the co-operative child aged >4 years the scanning can be continued until the child empties his or her bladder (indirect micturating cystography). Direct nuclear cystography has less radiation burden but still requires catheterization.

IVU, CT or MRI should be used after consultation at the nephrouroradiology meeting.

The majority of children with UTI have lower tract cystitis-like symptoms and no demonstrable abnormality on imaging. However, it can be difficult to distinguish between upper and lower tract symptoms and there is always the concern regarding the presence of rare abnormalities of the urinary tract. NICE guidelines (2007) suggest that in children with UTI who are systemically well it is only those who are aged <6 months who need a routine ultrasound. In older children it should only be done in those with atypical or recurrent UTI (Table 7.2.2(b,c)).

Vesicoureteric reflux

This is classified grades 1–5; grade 1 into ureter only and grade 5 gross dilatation of pelvis and calyces involving tortuosity of the ureter.

Although ~30% of children investigated for symptomatic UTI have VUR, in most it is of minor grade.

Table 7.2.2(b)

Children aged ≥6 months but <3 years	Responds well to treatment within 48 h without any features for atypical and/or recurrent UTI	Atypical UTI	Recurrent UTI
USS during the acute infection	No	Yes[a]	No
USS within 6 weeks	No	No	Yes
DMSA 4–6 weeks following the acute infection	No	Yes[b]	Yes[b]
MCUG	No	No[c]	No[c]

[a] In a child with a non-E.coli UTI, responding well to antibiotics and with no other features of atypical infection, the USS can be requested on a nonurgent basis to take place within 6 weeks.

[b] A detailed USS by an experienced operator can detect renal scarring.

[c] While MCUG should not be performed routinely it should be considered if the following features are present: dilatation on USS; poor urine flow; non-E.coli infections; family history of VUR.

Table 7.2.2(c)

Children aged ≥3 years	Responds well to treatment within 48 h without any features for atypical and/or recurrent UTI	Atypical UTI	Recurrent UTI
USS during the acute infection	No	Yes[a,b]	No
USS within 6 weeks	No	No	Yes[a]
DMSA 4–6 weeks following the acute infection	No	No	Yes[c]
MCUG	No	No[a]	No[d]

[a] USS in toilet-trained children should include repeat scan after bladder emptying if bladder very full.

[b] In a child with a non-E.coli UTI, responding well to antibiotics and with no other features of atypical infection, the USS can be requested on a nonurgent basis to take place within 6 weeks.

[c] A detailed USS by an experienced operator can detect renal scarring.

[d] MAG3 scan with indirect cystogram may be considered in continent child aged >4 years if USS is abnormal.

Table 7.2.2(a) Scheme for investigation of children following UTI based on recent NICE guidance

Children aged <6 months	Responds well to treatment within 48 h without any features for atypical and/or recurrent UTI	Atypical UTI	Recurrent UTI
USS during the acute infection	No	Yes[a]	Yes[a]
USS within 6 weeks	Yes[b]	No	No
DMSA 4–6 weeks following the acute infection	No	Yes[c]	Yes[c]
MCUG	No	Yes	Yes

[a] In a child with a non-E. coli UTI, responding well to antibiotics and with no other features of atypical infection, the USS can be requested on a nonurgent basis to take place within 6 weeks.

[b] If abnormal consider MCUG.

[c] A detailed USS by an experienced operator can detect renal scarring.

Hence there is reluctance to perform routine MCUG except in young, febrile children with proven UTI since it is potentially traumatic and involves a high radiation dose.

Evidence indicates that clinical management for VUR (antibiotic prophylaxis) and reimplantation surgery have similar outcomes in terms of incidence of renal scarring, renal function and recurrent UTI.

Controlled trials of prophylactic antibiotics versus urine culture and treatment of UTIs on an expectant basis in children with VUR have not yet been reported.

Children who suffer recurrent febrile UTIs despite prophylaxis (also consider compliance issues) require discussion with urologists for consideration of reimplantation surgery or more likely endoscopic correction (injection of a bulking substance around the entry of the ureter into the bladder: STING procedure).

Long-term follow-up of children with VUR

If antibiotic prophylaxis is used it is usually given for a 2 year period and discontinued if the child has been infection-free.

After 2 years the kidneys can be checked with ultrasound for growth and scarring. If the quality of ultrasound is inadequate, a DMSA scan may be required.

Discharge to primary care is appropriate if there is no evidence of scarring with referral back if recurrent infections develop.

If scarring is identified in one kidney an annual review for 5 years is required to check for recurrence of infections and measurement of the blood pressure, since there is a small risk (<2%) of developing hypertension as a result of renal scarring. The child can then be referred back to primary care for annual blood pressure measurements and urinalysis until growth is completed.

Bilateral renal scarring puts children at high risk for developing CKD and/or hypertension. Review in a pediatric nephrology or shared renal clinic for monitoring of blood pressure, urinalysis (for proteinuria), and estimated GFR at intervals may be appropriate depending upon the stage of CKD.

If the child develops recurrent UTI, discuss with urologist about operative intervention. In older children this is likely to be an endoscopic STING procedure.

When adult, depending on the GFR, the patient should either be transferred to an adult centre or followed up in primary care with provision of clear guidance on the criteria for subsequent referral.

References

Barry BP, Hall N, Cornford E, et al. Improved ultrasound detection of renal scarring in children following urinary tract infection. *Clin Radiol* 1998; **53**: 747–751.

Bloomfield P, Hodson EM, Craig JC. Antibiotics for acute pyelonephritis in children. *Cochrane Database Syst Rev* 2005; (**1**): CD003772.

Conway PH, Cnaan A, Zaoutis T, et al. Recurrent urinary tract infections in children: risk factors and association with prophylactic antimicrobials. *J Am Med Assoc* 2007; **298**: 179–186.

Gordon I, Barkovics M, Pindoria S, et al. Primary vesicoureteric reflux as a predictor of renal damage in children hospitalised with urinary tract infection: a systematic review and meta-analysis. *J Am Soc Nephrol* 2003; **14**: 739–744.

Hodson EM, Wheeler DM, Vimalchandra D, et al. Interventions for primary vesicoureteric reflux. 2007. *Cochrane Database Syst Rev* 2007; (**3**): CD001532.

Jodal U, Smellie JM, Lax H, Hoyer PF. Ten-year results of randomised treatment of children with severe vesicoureteral reflux. Final report of the International Reflux Study in Children. *Pediatr Nephrol* 2006; **21**: 782–792.

Michael M, Hodson EM, Craig JC, et al. Short versus standard duration oral antibiotic therapy for acute urinary tract infection in children. 2003. *Cochrane Database of Systematic Reviews* 2003; (**1**): CD003966.

Montini G, Toffolo A, Zucchetta P, et al. The IRIS 1 study of antibiotic treatment of pyelonephritis in children: a multicentre randomised controlled non inferiority trial. *Br Med J* 2007; **335**(7616): 386.

Internet resources

National Kidney Federation:

http://www.kidney.org.uk/

NICE Clinical Guideline CG54. Urinary tract infection in children: diagnosis, treatment and long-term management. Aug 2007:

http://guidance.nice.org.uk/CG34

See also

Renal and urinary tract stone disease in children, p. 282

Lower and upper urinary tract infection in adults, p. 244

Imaging in renal disease, p. 20

Renal tuberculosis and other mycobacterial infections

The members of genus *Mycobacterium* have characteristic acid-fastness due to their elaborate lipid-rich cell walls.

They are comprised of two major pathogens: the *Mycobacterium tuberculosis* complex (*M. tuberculosis, M. bovis, M. africanum M. microti* and *M. canetti*); and *Mycobacterium leprae*.

In addition there are many mycobacterial species which live freely in the environment as saprophytes and cause opportunistic human disease (environmental mycobacteria (EM)). These are divided into two main groups: rapid and slow growers. Slow growers are mainly responsible for human disease. Major pathogenic EM are *M. avium-intracellulare, M. kansasii, M. xenopi, M. malmoense, M. fortuitum, M. chelonei, M. ulcerans* and *M. marinum*.

Renal involvement is mainly seen with *M. tuberculosis, M. leprae* and a small number of EM as discussed below.

Renal tuberculosis

Epidemiology

Globally, tuberculosis is a common disease, with 8–10 million new cases annually with 95% of these occurring in developing countries.

The genitourinary system is involved in 15–20% of cases of extrapulmonary tuberculosis.

Approximately 4–8% of patients with pulmonary tuberculosis will develop clinically significant genitourinary infection.

Approximately 25% of patients who present with genitourinary tuberculosis (GUTB) have a background of pulmonary tuberculosis and an additional 25–50% of patients will have radiographic evidence of previous subclinical pulmonary infection.

GUTB occurs later than other forms of TB (age 20–40 years), and is more common in males (other UTIs are more common in females) and in the right kidney.

Predisposition to genitourinary TB is increased by medical conditions such as: HIV, diabetes mellitus, analgesic abuse, and a number of urinary tract abnormalities such as vesicoureteral reflux, neurogenic bladder, urinary obstruction, and congenital anomalies.

Pathogenesis

M. tuberculosis reaches the kidney by hematogenous spread.

Granulomata (tubercles) develop in the glandular and cortical arterioles near glomeruli.

Tubercles may remain dormant for several years after infection (up to 15–20 years) before rupturing and releasing live bacilli into the proximal tubule. These then reach the loop of Henle and lead to the formation of medullary granulomata and eventually papillary necrosis.

Granulomata may coalesce into large, necrotic, irregular cavities which usually communicate with the renal collecting system. This may progress to a pyonephrosis-like lesion (cement or putty kidney).

Renal calcification occurs in 24% of cases and is associated with renal or ureteric stones in up to 19% of cases.

Ureteric involvement with strictures and segmental dilatation can lead to obstruction and/or vesicoureteric reflux.

Urinary bladder involvement starts with interstitial cystitis and mucosal ulceration. Later, thickening of the bladder wall with a diminished capacity ('thimble' bladder) may result.

Clinical features

Classical renal tuberculosis

Early features:
- symptoms of cystitis;
- microscopic or macroscopic hematuria;
- pyuria with negative bacterial culture ('sterile pyuria');
- constitutional symptoms.

Late features:
- nephrolithiasis and ureteral colic;
- intractable frequency and urgency;
- refractory hypertension;
- renal insufficiency due to obstructive nephropathy.

Tuberculous interstitial nephritis

Tuberculosis can affect the kidney more insidiously. For example in three patients with advanced renal failure and normal-sized kidneys, a renal biopsy demonstrated chronic tubulointerstitial nephritis with granuloma formation and caseation. Evidence of pulmonary tuberculosis was seen in two patients and one had tuberculous peritonitis.

Tuberculosis and glomerular disease

Chronic tuberculosis may be complicated by amyloidosis and in areas where tuberculosis is endemic it can be a common cause of amyloidosis. Mesangiocapillary glomerulonephritis type II and focal proliferative glomerulonephritis have also been reported in patients with tuberculosis; however, a causal link has not been established

Hyponatremia

Mild hyponatremia (plasma sodium concentration usually between 125 and 135 mmol/L) may develop in patients with active pulmonary or miliary tuberculosis. Most patients appear to have the syndrome of inappropriate ADH secretion, with approximately one-third having a reset osmostat. Hyponatremia resolves after effective therapy of the infection.

Tuberculosis causing end-stage renal disease (ESRD)

Progressive renal failure due to tuberculosis, although uncommon, is potentially preventable and treatable. Since most of the tuberculosis patients are in developing countries with inadequate registries and diagnostic facilities, there is little information on the contribution of tuberculosis to the burden of renal disease.

In 1991, European Dialysis and Transplant Association registry data revealed that 195 of 30 064 new patients (0.65%) had renal failure caused by renal tuberculosis, an incidence similar to that of previous years.

Tuberculosis in patients with chronic renal insufficiency and ESRD

Tuberculosis is more common in patients with renal dysfunction than in the general population.

There is evidence for a state of relative immunological anergy in uremia as indicated by skin testing.

Commonly, the patient presents with fever, anorexia, and weight loss, and usually is either known to have had pulmonary or other forms of tuberculosis or is a member of a high risk ethnic or social group.

The recrudescence is extrapulmonary in most cases and hence it is likely that the disease is due to reactivation of past disease rather than a primary infection.

Tuberculosis in transplant recipients

Tuberculosis is a serious complication in solid organ transplantation, with an incidence, depending on geographic region, from ~0.3% in the USA to as high as 15% in the Indian subcontinent.

In most cases, the disease involves the lung, but it is disseminated in one-third of cases.

Patients who had tuberculosis while on dialysis are at increased risk.

Immunosuppression can obscure the diagnosis (false-negative tuberculin tests) and mask the common symptoms of the disease. The diagnosis is therefore often delayed and the mortality is high (~30%).

Laboratory diagnosis

- Three early morning urine samples: acid-fast bacilli (AFB) may be demonstrated by Ziehl–Neelsen (ZN) staining of the sediment after centrifugation.
- Definitive proof by urine culture on Löwenstein–Jensen medium (may take 2–8 weeks).
- More rapid radiometric culture system (BACTEC)-mycobacterial growth within 2–10 days.
- Nucleic acid amplification techniques, e.g. polymerase chain reaction.

Histopathology

Tuberculosis may involve the kidney as part of generalized disseminated infection or as localized genitourinary disease.

The morphology of the lesions depends on the type of infection, the virulence of the organism, and the immune status of the patient.

Histological findings include:

- Miliary tubercles (up to 3 mm in diameter) seen throughout the renal cortex. Histologically, they consist of epithelioid granulomata, with or without caseation, and often contain Langhans-type giant cells (Fig. 7.3.1). Organisms may be demonstrated microscopically within these lesions.
- In immunosuppressed patients more diffuse and poorly formed granulomas are seen. These contain histiocytic cells with abundant pale cytoplasm packed

with organisms ('multibacillary histiocytosis'). Caseous necrosis is not a feature.

- In some patients with pulmonary or disseminated tuberculosis, there is evidence of renal failure without typical miliary involvement or localized genitourinary lesions. In such cases, biopsy demonstrates interstitial nephritis, usually with granuloma formation.
- Healing produces scarring and usually calcification.

The differential diagnosis of necrotizing granulomata in the renal tract includes fungal infections and Wegener's granulomatosis. Noncaseating granulomata may be seen in sarcoidosis, leprosy, and brucellosis.

Imaging

Plain radiology

Signs of extrarenal tuberculosis may be apparent, for example osseous or paraspinal changes, and old healed calcified splenic, hepatic, lymph node, and adrenal granulomata.

Chest radiographs may show evidence of active or healed tuberculosis in 50% of patients.

A plain KUB radiograph may show a variety of patterns of calcification: punctate, speckled, or hazy.

Intravenous urography

A variety of radiologic abnormalities may be demonstrated:

- Smudged papillae with surface irregularity and a moth-eaten calyx (early sign).
- Papillary necrosis (Fig. 7.3.2).
- Hydrocalycosis without pelvic dilatation, an atrophic pelvis, and cephalic retraction of the inferior medial margin of the renal pelvis ('the hiked-up renal pelvis') are highly suggestive of tuberculosis.
- There may be no calyceal filling and the infundibulum shows a typical 'pinched-off' appearance. The whole pelvicalyceal system and ureter may be outlined by calcification ('tuberculous autonephrectomy').
- Ureters may show asymmetrical involvement (mainly upper and lower thirds): Intraluminal filling defects due to mucosal granulomata; and irregularity in outline of contrast-filled ureter resulting in a beaded or corkscrew configuration.

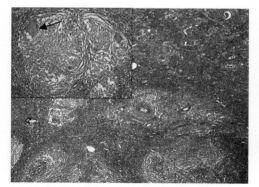

Fig. 7.3.1 Photomicrograph of H&E-stained renal biopsy showing multiple epithelioid cell granulomata in the tubulointerstitium (magnification: ×200). *Inset:* Granuloma with Langhans-type giant cell (arrow). (Courtesy of Dr Ritambra Nada, Postgraduate Institute of Medical Education and Research, Chandigarh, India.)

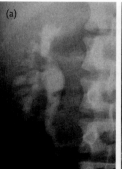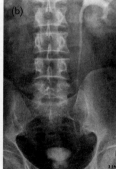

Fig. 7.3.2 (a) Intravenous urogram image showing papillary necrosis and contrast-filled cavities communicating with pelvicalyceal system. (b) Multiple calcified lymph nodes in the mesentery and markedly reduced capacity of urinary bladder ('thimble bladder'). (Courtesy of Dr Anupam Lal, Postgraduate Institute of Medical Education and Research, Chandigarh, India.)

- Thickened bladder wall with reduced bladder volume ('thimble bladder') (Fig. 7.3.2), trabeculations, incompetence of the vesicoureteric junction (VUJ) orifice, or VUJ narrowing with hydroureter and hydronephrosis. Bladder wall calcification is rarely seen.

CT scan

CT scans clearly reveal changes of renal tuberculosis (calcification, calyceal dilatation without hydropelvis, parenchymal loss, and extrarenal spread) particularly in advanced disease.

MRI

MRI with contrast enhancement is good at demonstrating tuberculous cavities, sinus tracts, fistulous communications, and extrarenal and extraprostatic spread. Multiplanar MRI allows evaluation of the disease extent in the prostatic bed and the presence of sinuses and fistulae. MRI is also useful in the evaluation of peritoniteal involvement and adnexal masses.

Ultrasound

Ultrasonography is not as sensitive as intravenous urogram or CT scanning because of problems with identifying calyceal, pelvic, or ureteric abnormalities.

Nuclear medicine

Radionuclide imaging is confined to assessment of relative renal function when surgery or nephrectomy is contemplated.

Treatment of tuberculosis

Most modern regimens are based on an intensive phase, usually lasting 2 months, during which time virtually all the tubercle bacilli in the lesions are killed, followed by a 4 month less-intensive phase designed to kill any remaining organisms.

The drugs used in the intensive phase are rifampicin, isoniazid, pyrazinamide, and ethambutol.

Rifampicin is the principal drug used in the continuation phase (unique ability to kill near-dormant organisms), in combination with isoniazid (kills rifampicin-resistant mutants that may arise).

Multidrug-resistant tuberculosis, (disease caused by bacilli resistant to rifampicin and isoniazid, with or without resistance to other drugs) is becoming increasingly common.

Therapy requires the use of at least four drugs that are selected on the basis of drug susceptibility tests. Options include: ethionamide, prothionamide, quinolones (e.g. ofloxacin), newer macrolides (e.g. clarithromycin), cycloserine, kanamycin, viomycin, capreomycin, thiacetazone, and para-aminosalicylic acid. These are less effective, often more toxic, and often more expensive than the first-line drugs. Therapy may need to be prolonged (18 months or longer).

Treatment of tuberculosis in patients with impaired renal function

Rifampicin, isoniazid, pyrazinamide, ethionamide, and prothionamide may be given in normal doses.

Streptomycin and other aminoglycosides should be avoided if possible in patients with impaired renal function, especially those on ciclosporin, because of the high risk of nephrotoxicity.

Ethambutol is renally excreted and a reduced dose is therefore used (according to the GFR) to minimize the risk of optic neuritis.

Isoniazid-induced encephalopathy is an uncommon complication and is usually prevented by pyridoxine (25–50 mg/day). Pyridoxine-resistant isoniazid-induced encephalopathy has rarely been reported in hemodialysis patients. Recovery occurs with isoniazid withdrawal.

Rifampicin can cause interstitial nephritis and rarely crescentic glomerulonephritis.

Rifampicin increases the rate of metabolism of a wide range of drugs, including corticosteroids, cyclosporin, and tacrolimus, therefore close drug level monitoring is required.

In HIV-positive patients, rifampicin interacts with HAART, therefore rifabutin may be used in preference. The duration of therapy can be extended to 9 months.

Surgical intervention

This is undertaken in the following circumstances:

- to correct obstruction caused by fibrosis;
- to remove large foci of infection that can be difficult to treat medically. Surgery should be performed after 8–12 weeks of antituberculous treatment;
- partial/total nephroureterectomy and/or cystectomy may be required in extensive disease.

TB prophylaxis in transplant patients

Many renal transplant units give isoniazid prophylaxis for 1 year to patients at high risk of developing active tuberculosis.

The European Best Practice Guidelines for Renal Transplantation (2002) recommend that all renal transplant candidates and recipients considered as having latent tuberculosis be treated with isoniazid 300 mg daily for 9 months.

Such patients are defined as those with one or more of the following:

- induration after Mantoux testing of 5 mm (transplant recipients) or 10 mm (transplant candidates on dialysis);
- a history of inadequately treated tuberculosis;
- a CXR suggestive of old tuberculosis; and
- close contact with a person with tuberculosis.

Preventive therapy should also be given to tuberculin-negative patients who receive a kidney from a tuberculin-positive donor.

Leprosy and renal disease

Direct involvement of the kidney by *M. leprae* is unusual but leprosy patients may have a large spectrum of renal manifestations. These include interstitial nephritis, amyloidosis, and most forms of glomerulonephritis.

Between 11 and 38% of leprosy patients die because of renal failure due to glomerulonephritis or amyloidosis and therefore renal disease may be the main cause of death in such patients.

Organ dysfunction seems to correlate with the quantity of bacilli and/or the presence of coexistent disease, amyloid infiltration, concomitant infections, leprosy reactions and side-effects of drugs.

The incidence of the various forms of renal disease varies geographically. In an autopsy study in Brazil of 199 leprosy patients dying between 1970 and 1986, renal lesions were found in 144 (72%). The renal lesions were: amyloidosis 43%, glomerulonephritis 20%, nephrosclerosis 15%, tubulointerstitial nephritis 12%, granulomata in 1%, and other lesions in 6%. In the Indian subcontinent and Japan renal amyloidosis is less frequent.

Glomerulonephritis and amyloidosis are associated with multibacillary (lepromatous and borderline lepromatous) leprosy.

Glomerulonephritis appears to be related to immune complex deposition (containing IgG, IgM and C3) although mycobacterial antigen has not been identified in the immune complexes or renal lesions.

Episodes of erythema nodosum leprosum (ENL) may be associated with reversible acute kidney injury. It is unclear whether ENL is associated with glomerulonephritis.

Amyloidosis occurs more frequently in patients with recurrent flares of ENL and trophic ulcers.

More severe proteinuria (may be nephrotic range), hematuria, and renal dysfunction are found in multibacillary patients.

Distal tubular dysfunction (urinary acidification and concentration defects) have also been documented in leprosy patients.

Treatment of leprosy
Treatment is with standard antileprosy drugs (rifampicin, dapsone and clofazimine (for multibacillary leprosy)), making allowance for the degree of renal dysfunction.

Environmental mycobacterial (EM) disease
Disease of the genitourinary system due to EM is exceedingly rare.

Because EM are commonly found in the urine as harmless contaminants, making a diagnosis of EM-mediated disease can be difficult. Six diagnostic criteria have therefore been proposed:

1. Symptoms of chronic or recurrent genitourinary infection.
2. Radiological or endoscopic evidence of genitourinary disease.
3. Abnormalities on urinalysis.
4. Failure to isolate other urinary tract pathogens.
5. Repeated isolation of the same mycobacterial species.
6. Histological demonstration of granulomata and, preferably, AFB.

The first four criteria should alert the clinician to the possibility of a mycobacterial etiology, the fifth strongly suggests the diagnosis, but only the sixth is confirmatory.

A retrospective application of these criteria showed a high false-negative rate for diagnosis.

Only few cases of renal tract disease caused by EM have been documented in immunocompetent hosts. These include renal disease caused by *M. avium–intracellulare* (MAC), epididymitis due to *M. xenopi* and *M. kansasii*, and prostatitis caused by *M. xenopi* and *M. fortuitum*.

EM disease in end-stage renal disease
There have been number of reports of EM causing disease in dialysis and transplant patients.

Hemodialysis
Small clusters and isolated cases of disseminated disease due to *M. chelonae* have occurred in patients on hemodialysis (probably due to contamination of the dialysis machine by EM).

Peritoneal dialysis (PD)
A number of EM have been implicated as rare causes of PD peritonitis. These include: *M. chelonae*, *M. fortuitum*, *M. kansasii* and *M. gordonae.*

Renal transplantation
The incidence of mycobacterial disease following renal transplantation is much higher than in the general population and in 25–40% of cases an EM is the cause.

EM disease in transplant patients may be disseminated, localized to the lungs, or most commonly confined to the skin. Typical causative organisms include: *M. haemophilum, M. marinum, M. chelonae*, and *M. fortuitum.*

Treatment of EM disease
Owing to their rarity, there are no good data on the optimal therapy of genitourinary disease caused by EM.

The therapeutic choices depend on the causative species and specialist reference centres should be consulted.

Broadly, treatment regimens are based on those that have been evaluated for pulmonary and disseminated disease. These include (azithromycin, 600 mg daily or clarithromycin, 500 mg twice daily), in combination with ethambutol for disease due to MAC-complex infections.

Further reading
Ahsan N, Wheeler DE, Palmer BF. Leprosy-associated renal disease: case report and review of the literature. *J Am Soc Nephrol* 1995; 5: 1546–1552.

Altintepe L, Tonbul HZ, Ozbey I, Guney I, *et al*. Urinary tuberculosis: ten years' experience. *Ren Fail* 2005;**27**:657–661.

Corbishley, CC, Grange, JM. Tuberculosis and the kidney. *J Am Soc Nephrol* 2001; **12**: 1307–1314.

da Silva Júnior GB, Daher Ede F. Renal involvement in leprosy: retrospective analysis of 461 cases in Brazil. *Braz J Infect Dis* 2006; **10**: 107–112.

Eastwood JB, Abdelrahman M, Sinha AK, Karkar A. Tuberculosis in end-stage renal disease patients on hemodialysis. *Hemodial Int* 2006; **10**: 360–364.

Glassroth J. Pulmonary disease due to nontuberculous mycobacteria. *Chest* 2008; **133**: 243–251.

John GT, Shankar V, Abraham AM, Mukundan U, *et al*. Risk factors for post-transplant tuberculosis. *Kidney Int* 2001; **60**: 1148–1153.

Mallinson WJW, Fuller RW, Levison DA, *et al*. Diffuse interstitial renal tuberculosis – an unusual cause of renal failure. *Q J Med* 1981; **50**: 137–148.

Mapukata A, Andronikou S, Fasulakis S, *et al*. Modern imaging of renal tuberculosis in children. *Australas Radiol* 2007; **51**: 538–542.

Muttarak M, ChiangMai WN, Lojanapiwat B. Tuberculosis of the genitourinary tract: imaging features with pathological correlation. *Singapore Med J* 2005; **46**: 568–574.

Nakayama EE, Ura S, Fleury RN, Soares V. Renal lesions in leprosy: a retrospective study of 199 autopsies. *Am J Kidney Dis* 2001; **38**: 26–30.

Youmbissi JT, Malik QT, Ajit SK, *et al*. Nontuberculous mycobacterium peritonitis in continuous ambulatory peritoneal dialysis. *J Nephrol* 2001; **14**: 13213–13215.

Internet resources
Centers for Disease Control and Prevention document on the treatment of tuberculosis:

http://www.cdc.gov/mmwR/preview/mmwrhtml/rr5211a1.htm

World Health Organization Tuberculosis information:

http://www.who.int/topics/tuberculosis/en/

World Health Organization Leprosy information:

http://www.who.int/lep/en/

See also
Infection-related glomerulonephritis, p. 128

Glomerular disease in the tropics, p. 138

Nephrocalcinosis, p. 278

Schistosomiasis

Schistosomiasis is a parasitic disease, acquired by contact with contaminated fresh water, that causes significant morbidity and mortality in >20 million inhabitants of 76 countries.

While its prevalence is decreasing in a few endemic foci owing to effective eradication programs (e.g. China), it is still increasing in most other areas (e.g. Africa), as well as in nonendemic regions owing to the exchange of immigrants and expatriates.

The disease is caused by a blood fluke that belongs to the family *Schistosomidae*, of which three species are responsible for the bulk of human infection:
- *S. hematobium* which causes lower urinary tract morbidity and upstream consequences, in Africa;
- *S. japonicum* which causes hepatosplenic disease often complicated by neurological sequelae, in the Far East;
- *S. mansoni* which causes hepatosplenic disease occasionally complicated by glomerular pathology, in Africa, South and Central America, and certain parts of Asia.

Pathology

All pathological lesions in established schistosomiasis (Fig. 7.4.1) are attributed to two types of host immune response.
- Type IV delayed hypersensitivity to soluble egg antigens is the prototype of the supervening granulomatous response (Fig. 7.4.2) at the sites of oviposition in the lower urinary and intestinal tracts, as well as in distant metastatic sites in most organs.
- Type-III immune-complex-mediated response to adult worm gut antigens is responsible for the less common

glomerular lesions (Fig. 7.4.3) mostly seen with hepatosplenic schistosomiasis.

Clinical features

The clinical profile of schistosomal infection passes through four phases:

Phase I

This occurs at the time of first acquisition of infection, and is attributable to the immune response to the infective cercariae. The site of entry may form a small itchy skin papule or blister, which resolves spontaneously in <48 h. A couple of weeks later, a serum-sickness-like syndrome (Takayama disease) may occur, particularly in expatriates, which resolves in a few days.

Phase II

This occurs several weeks later after the parasite has matured and the females have started laying eggs. While the majority of ova are passed with respective excreta, some are deposited in the lower urinary tract, sigmoid or rectum. The local inflammatory response caused by tissue oviposition is responsible for the symptoms which hallmark this phase. These are:
- Terminal hematuria and dysuria in *S. hematobium* infection, which can mimic calculus disease, tuberculosis, or severe bacterial cystitis. The diagnosis is confirmed by finding live ova in the urinary sediment. Failing this, a cystoscopic examination can confirm the diagnosis, by showing the typical lesions (Fig. 7.4.2).
- Tenesmus, diarrhea and the passage of red blood in stools with *S. mansoni* or *S. japonicum* infection. This presentation may be confused with amebic or bacillary dysentery,

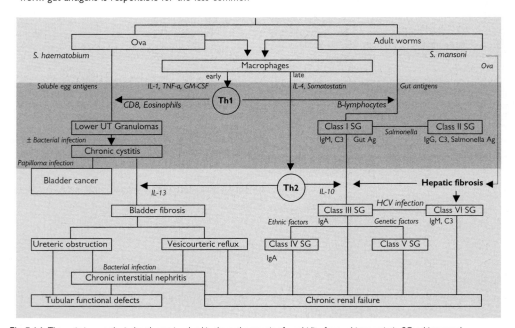

Fig. 7.4.1 The main immunological pathways involved in the pathogenesis of morbidity from schistosomiasis. SG, schistosomal glomerulopathy.

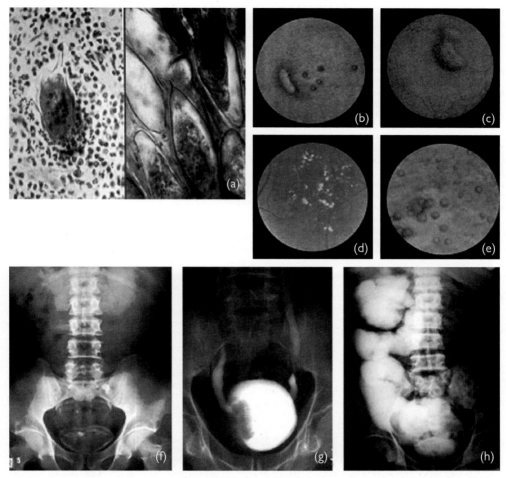

Fig. 7.4.2 Profile of schistosomiasis of the urinary tract, usually caused by *S. haematobium*. (a) Schistosomal granuloma (left panel) with sheets of *S. haematobium* eggs in the bladder mucosa (right panel). (b–e) Cystoscopic appearances in phase II: pseudotubercles (b), sessile mass (c) and phase IV: sandy patches (d), cystitis cystica (e). (f–h) Radiological appearances: linear calcifications (f), bladder cancer (g) and grade V vesicoureteric reflux (h).

inflammatory bowel disease, or malignancy. Diagnosis is confirmed by finding ova in the stools, or by endoscopic examination and biopsy of suspicious lesions.

Phase III

This is a quiescent period that extends for many years, often to the end of the patient's life, without any symptoms. In contrast to cure, which may follow effective therapy in phase II, the disease in phase III is active but clinically dormant, as a result of balanced host–parasite concomitant immunity.

Evidence of asymptomatic disease may be obtained by:

- examination of the urine or stools for evidence of ovishedding;
- examination of the urine for microalbuminuria or microhematuria which indicates early glomerular pathology;
- serological tests, including hemagglutinin inhbition, circumoral precipitin, ELISA, or others, which may provide evidence of recent (<3 months) release of schistosomal antigens;

- radiological examination of the lower urinary tract which may show typical bladder calcifications (Fig. 7.4.2);
- liver ultrasonography which may show evidence of periportal fibrosis.

Phase IV

This is the cause of chronic morbidity from schistosomiasis. Its incidence varies from <10% to >40% of infected individuals, depending on parasite, host and environmental factors. Any organ can be simultaneously or sequentially involved, particularly the urinary, gastrointestinal, cardiopulmonary and central nervous systems.

There are three domains of late schistosomal involvement of the urinary system:

Lower urinary tract
Chronic cystitis, with dysuria, scalding, frequency and hematuria may result from the advanced schistosomal

lesions of chronic ulcers, cystitis cystica or sandy patches (Fig. 7.4.2).

- The bladder capacity may be either reduced due to detrusor fibrosis or increased due to bladder neck obstruction.
- Secondary bacterial infection very often confounds the pathology, symptomatology and response to therapy.
- Bladder malignancy may further complicate this situation. It should be suspected when there is worsening or change in the pattern of symptoms, passage of necrotic tissue in the urine (necroturia), or when a bladder mass is palpated on rectal examination.

Upper urinary tract
Distal ureteric obstruction and vesicoureteric reflux are the two major consequences of late bladder pathology. (Both can also be transiently seen in phase II, but at that time are reversible with antiparasitic treatment).

- Chronic obstruction results from fibrosis at the ureterovesical junction. The ureter usually compensates for distal obstruction by dilatation hypertrophy of its spindle, without further upstream consequences. Failing this, back pressure eventually leads to hydronephrosis.
- Vesicoureteric reflux may result from schistosomal bladder fibrosis *per se*, but more often results from attempted instrumental dilation for obstruction.
- Secondary bacterial infection may complicate the picture of obstruction or reflux and is often the underlying cause of secondary stone formation.
- Interstitial fibrosis eventually develops, leading to impairment of tubular function, particularly with regards to salt conservation and urine acidification. Finally end-stage renal failure supervenes.

Glomerular disease
Glomerular pathology (Table 7.4.1, Fig. 7.4.3) is mostly seen with *S. mansoni*, although class I lesions may occur with any species, and class V lesions have been more often associated with mixed infections.

It is noteworthy that the lesions are nonspecific, which may lead to confusion with primary or other secondary glomerulopathies with similar pictures.

With the exception of a few patients (usually class I), in whom schistosomal antigens are demonstrated by immunofluorescence, the diagnosis of schistosomal glomerulopathy (SG) is usually made on circumstantial evidence, such as having lived in an endemic area, with historic or current evidence of schistosomal infection, the presence of schistosomal hepatosplenomegaly, and compatible renal histopathology.

Management

Active schistosomal infection must be eradicated by specific treatment. The drug of choice is Praziquantel in a dose of 40 mg/kg body weight as a single dose for *S. haematobium* and *S. mansoni* and 60 mg/kg body weight in two divided doses for *S. japonicum*.

Associated *Salmonella* infection in class II SG should be simultaneously treated with ampicillin and cotrimoxazole.

Concomitant hepatitis C virus infection may be treated with interferon and ribavirin in accordance with the general indications for such therapy.

Associated bacterial infection in urinary schistosomiasis should be treated; long term, low dose chemotherapy may be needed in chronic or relapsing infections.

Complicated upper urinary tract schistosomiasis may need surgical treatment.

Little can be done for SG beyond class II. Class I may respond to antiparasitic treatment and there are conflicting reports on the benefit of corticosteroids and immunosuppression.

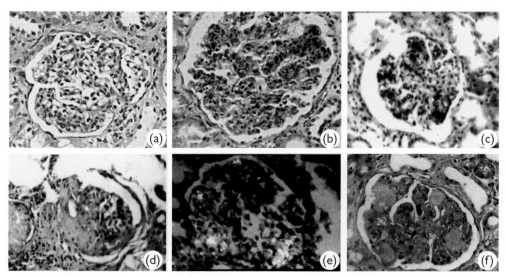

Fig. 7.4.3 Profile of glomerular disease in schistosomiasis, usually caused by *S. mansoni*. (a) Class I, mesangial proliferative; (b) class II, exudative; (c) class III, type I mesangiocapillary (membranoproliferative); (d) class IV, focal segmental sclerosis; (e) class V, amyloidosis (apple-green birefringence under polarized light); (f) class VI, cryoglobulinemic.

Table 7.4.1 Classification of schistosomal glomerulopathies

Class	Histology	IF	Etiologic agent	Prevalence	Clinical findings	Treatment of renal disease
I	Mesangiopro-liferative	IgM, C3. Schistosomal gut antigens	S. haematobium S. mansoni S. Japonicum	27–60% of asymptomatic patients, 10–40% of patients with renal disease	Microhematuria Proteinuria	Anti-parasitic treatment
II	Diffuse proliferative exudative	C3. Salmonella antigens	S. haematobium S. mansoni + Salmonella spp.	Salmonella infections. Reduced serum C3	Acute nephritic syndrome Toxemia	Combined treatment of schistosomal and salmonella infection
III	Mesangiocapillary	IgG, IgA, C3. Schistosomal antigens	S. mansoni (S. haematobium?)	7–20% of asymptomatic patients and in 80% of patients with overt renal disease	Hepatosplenomegaly nephrotic syndrome hypertension, renal failure	No
IV	Focal segmental glomerulosclerosis	IgM, IgG (occasionally IgA)	S. mansoni	11–38%	Hepatosplenomegaly, nephrotic syndrome, hypertension, renal failure	No
V	Amyloid	AA protein	S. mansoni S. hematobium	16–39%	Hepatosplenomegaly, nephrotic syndrome, hypertension, renal failure	No
VI	Cryoglobulinemic	IgM, C3	S. mansoni + HCV	Unknown	Hepatosplenomegaly nephrotic syndrome, purpura, vasculitis, arthritis, hypertension, renal failure	? Interferon + ribavirin Corticosteroids. Immunosuppression Plasmapheresis

Patients with end-stage kidney disease may pose certain problems with renal replacement therapy.

- Hemodialysis may constitute a risk for bleeding from esophageal or gastric varices associated with advanced liver disease.
- Peritoneal dialysis may not be possible in the presence of ascites.
- Transplantation may be technically difficult in the presence of significant lower urinary tract pathology, and the metabolism of immunosuppressive drugs may be altered in those with significant hepatocellular dysfunction. However, the overall outcome of renal transplantation in patients without these limitations is satisfactory. Recurrence may occur in transplanted kidneys if the disease is still active in the recipient.

Further reading

Abdel-Wahab, MF *Schistosomiasis in Egypt*. Boca Raton: CRC Press; 1982.

Barsoum, RS. Schistosomal glomerulopathy: selection factors. *Nephrol Dialysis Transplant* 1987; **2**: 488–497.

Barsoum RS: Schistosomiasis. In: Davison AM, Cameron JS, Grunfeld JP, Ponticelli C, Ritz E, Winearls CG, Van Ypersele (eds): *Oxford textbook of clinical nephrology*, 3rd edn. Oxford: Oxford University Press; 2005. Vol. II, Chap. 7-4, pp. 1173–1184.

Barsoum R. The kidney in schistosomiasis. In: Feehally J, Floege J, Johnson R (eds), *Comprehensive clinical nephrology*, 3rd edn. St Louis, MO: Mosby/Elsevier; 2007. pp. 631–639.

Mostafa MH, Sheweita SA, O'Connor PJ. Relationship between schistosomiasis and bladder cancer. *Clin Microbiol Rev* 1999; **12**: 97–111.

Internet resources

World Health Organization:

http://www.who.int/topics/schistosomiasis/en/

CDC Division of Parasitic Diseases:

http://www.cdc.gov/ncidod/dpd/parasites/schistosomiasis/

Schistosomiasis Control Initiative:

http://www.schisto.org/

See also

Infection-related glomerulonephritis, p. 128

Glomerular disease in the tropics, p. 138

Fungal infections and the kidney

The incidence of invasive fungal infections (IFIs) has risen dramatically in the last 20 years with the increased survival of patients with immunocompromised states.

These infections are often insidious and their diagnosis is usually delayed because of coexisting illnesses.

There are many fungi which may involve deeper tissues including the kidneys (Table 7.5.1).

Candida and *Aspergillus* species are common causes but *Zygomycetes*, *Cryptococcus* and Dimorphic fungi (e.g. *Histoplasma*, *Coccidioides*, *Blastomyces* and *Penicillium*) species may also rarely involve the kidneys.

Table 7.5.1 Pathogenic fungi affecting the genitourinary system

Common	Rare and unusual
Primary pathogens	*Geotrichum candidum*
Histoplasma capsulatum	*Paracoccidioides brasilensis*
Coccidioides immitis	*Penicillium glaucum*
Blastomyces dermatidis	*Penicillium ciftrinum*
	Trichosporon
Opportunistic pathogens	*Fusarium*
Candida albicans	*Pseudallescheria boydii*
Aspergillus species	*Cunninghamella*
Cryptococcus neoformans	*Rhinosporidium seeberi*
Zygomycetes fungi	*Sporothrix schenckii*

Pathogenesis

Most IFIs are caused by hematogenous spread.

Animal experiments have shown that fungi injected intravenously are usually cleared from the bloodstream. In the immunocompromised host, however, bloodborne fungi infect the kidneys by attachment to endothelial surfaces followed by penetration into the interstitium, and multiplication.

Ascending infection of the kidneys may also be important in a minority of individuals.

Risk factors for the multiplication of the organisms in renal tissue include: AIDS, diabetes, lymphoma, leukemia, burns, renal failure, organ transplantation, and immunosuppressive drugs.

Opportunistic infections

Candidiasis

Candidiasis refers to the range of infections caused by species of the genus *Candida* which includes >160 species.

The five most frequent human pathogens are *C. albicans*, *C. krusei*, *C. parapsilosis*, *C. tropicalis*, and *C. glabrata* (also called *Torulopsis glabrata*).

Candida can exist in two morphological states: yeast (cellular form) and filaments (hyphal or mycelial form).

Torulopsis (Candida) glabrata, which does not develop pseudohyphae or produce germ tubes, represents 5–21% of the isolates from positive fungal cultures and is the second most common genitourinary fungal pathogen. It has a worse prognosis than other *Candida* species.

Clinical features

Candidal urinary tract infections can cause a variety of clinical symptoms and signs.

Patients may be asymptomatic or have features of bladder irritability (pyuria, hematuria or pneumaturia) suggesting candida cystitis.

Cystoscopy reveals grey-white patches on the bladder wall, mucosal edema and erythema, and also on occasion a 'snow storm effect' that obscures visualization.

Urinary colony counts of >10 000–15 000/mL, and urinary casts containing fungal material (Papanicolaou stain) suggest bladder infection rather than colonization.

Classical pyelonephritis with flank pain, renal tenderness and fever may also develop.

Pathological findings may include evidence of multiple abscesses in the interstitium and glomeruli, with budding yeast and pseudomycelia in peritubular vessels and collecting tubules.

Emphysematous pyelonephritis, pyelitis and renal papillary necrosis have also been described.

Flank pain and symptoms of renal colic may also be caused by the passage of fungal balls that obstruct the collecting system. Fungal accretions may develop in the collecting system without overt clinical findings. Oliguria and anuria have also been known to occur.

Zygomycosis

Zygomycosis (previously known as phycomycosis and mucormycosis) is a rare mycotic infection caused by angio-invasive fungi belonging to the class *Zygomycetes*.

The most common pathogenic species include *Rhizopus oryzae*, *Rhizomucor pusillus*, and *Absidia corymbifera*. They usually cause serious disease in immunocompromised patients.

Rarely apparently healthy subjects may also be affected.

The list of predisposing conditions continues to grow, the latest additions being desferrioxamine therapy for iron/aluminium overload in dialysis patients.

The organisms invade blood vessels leading to ischemia and necrosis associated with acute inflammation in the affected organ.

The four main presentations of zygomycosis in man are the rhinocerebral, pulmonary, gastrointestinal and disseminated forms.

Rarely infection of isolated organs such as bones, kidney or heart may occur.

Renal involvement occurs both as part of disseminated infection, or in apparent isolation probably due to hematogenous dissemination from subclinical pulmonary infection (similar to renal tuberculosis).

Clinical features

Renal zygomycosis causes fever, flank pain and oligoanuria.

Renal failure (occurs in up to 95% of patients with bilateral involvement) results from the near total occlusion of the renal arteries and/or their branches.

Pathologically the kidneys may be enlarged with extensive cortical and medullary involvement, evidence of vasculitis with infarction, and parenchymal neutrophil infiltration.

Fungal hyphae can often be seen in the infiltrate with granulomata and Langhans-type multinucleated giant cells. Hyphae may be seen invading both glomeruli and tubules.

Imaging studies

Radiographic studies demonstrate poor excretory renal function and obstructive uropathy caused by fungal hyphae occluding the vascular and collecting systems respectively.

Characteristic findings on CT scanning include diffuse enlargement of the kidneys, the absence of contrast excretion, and the presence of multiple low density areas in the renal parenchyma (fungal abscesses). Abscess rupture may result in perinephric collections.

MRI scanning may be preferred in diabetic patients in order to avoid the use of nephrotoxic contrast agents.

Aspergillosis

Invasive aspergillosis is caused by fungi of the genus *Aspergillus*.

Twenty aspergillus species are said to be pathogenic to human beings including *A. fumigatus, A. flavus, A. terreus, A. nidulans* and *A. niger* species.

They have characteristic septate hyphae with dichotomous branching which readily distinguishes them from the hyphae of *Mucor*.

Aspergillosis is primarily a pulmonary infection, which can present with allergic alveolitis and bronchopulmonary aspergillosis.

Disseminated infection can occur following hematogenous spread in patients with debilitating diseases.

Renal involvement has been reported in 8–13% of patients with disseminated disease. Most (80%) have unilateral involvement.

Clinical features

Clinically proteinuria, pyuria, hematuria and sometimes oliguric renal failure is present.

Most have fungal bezoars producing hydronephrosis and less frequently they may have single or multiple parenchymal abscesses.

The fungi are angioinvasive, therefore vascular thrombosis and patchy infarction in the kidney may develop (less severe than with zygomycosis).

Renal papillary necrosis may also occur.

Renal aspergillosis may present in the following ways:

1. Disseminated aspergillosis with renal involvement. It results from hematogenous spread of fungi to the kidneys leading to formation of multiple focal abscesses.
2. Aspergillus cast of the renal pelvis. It results in obstructive uropathy which may present with urinary retention or anuria.
3. Ascending panurothelial aspergillosis. This refers to ascending infection involving the urethra, bladder, ureters and the kidney.

Cryptococcosis

Cryptococcosis, also known as torulopsis, is caused by the basidiomycetous encapsulated yeast, *Cryptococcus neoformans*, which is found in bird excreta, decaying organic matter and soil.

The initial focus of infection is usually the respiratory tract which occurs following inhalation of the fungal spores.

Dissemination may occur with involvement of the CNS, bone, spleen, gastrointestinal system, and kidneys (in 50% of cases).

Cystitis, pyuria, hematuria, moderate proteinuria and mild renal insufficiency may develop. Cryptococcal infection has never been reported to cause renal failure.

The pathological changes can range from sparse lymphocytic infiltration to an intense granulomatous reaction in the renal parenchyma with caseation and microabscess formation.

In the medulla, abscesses may be accompanied by interstitial inflammation, fibrosis and papillary necrosis. Tubular obstruction, dilatation and atrophy may result, associated with intense interstitial and glomerular fibrosis.

Endemic infections

Histoplasmosis

Histoplasma capsulatum, a dimorphic fungus, is found worldwide in soil contaminated by bird excreta.

Infection often develops in city dwellers exposed to construction excavations.

Approximately 90% of these infections result in mild and clinically insignificant respiratory infection.

Approximately 1:2000 individuals exposed to *H. capsulatum* develops disseminated disease involving the lungs, the reticuloendothelial system (liver, spleen and bone marrow), and the genitourinary system.

The kidneys are involved in ~20% of cases of disseminated disease. The renal lesions include noncaseating granulomata, microabcesses, and rarely cutaneous fistulae. These are usually not associated with significant renal symptoms.

Histoplasmosis in transplant recipients may lead to graft loss, and sometimes obstructive uropathy secondary to sloughed papillae.

Blastomycosis

Blastomycosis is a systemic pyogranulomatous infection, caused by the fungus, *Blastomyces dermatidis*.

It primarily involves the lungs and frequently disseminates to other organs.

It exhibits thermal dimorphism, with a mycelial phase at 25°C and a yeast phase at 37°C. Humidity is important in promoting growth of the organism.

Pulmonary infection may be followed by hematogenous dissemination in adult males, pregnant women and their unborn children, and immunocompromised patients with end-stage AIDS and organ transplants.

Skin, bone, and the CNS are common sites of extrapulmonary blastomycosis.

Genitourinary disease has also been reported in as many as 20–30% of patients with disseminated disease.

Involvement of the prostate, epididymis and testes is common whereas kidney and ureteric involvement is less frequent.

Patients may present with symptoms of prostatitis. Pyuria and hematuria are found in the majority.

Infections of the female genital tract are uncommon.

Coccidiomycosis

Coccidioidomycosis is the infection caused by the dimorphic fungus, *Coccidioides immitis*, which is endemic to the semi-arid sub-Sonoran regions of the western USA.

The saprophytic mycelial phase of this fungus exists in the soil and under proper environmental conditions is highly infectious.

Following inhalation, an asymptomatic and transient pulmonary infection ensues.

60% of infected individuals have subclinical disease while the remainder will have a mild–severe respiratory illness with complete resolution.

Approximately 5% will have residual pulmonary infection and <1% develop extrapulmonary multiple organ dissemination (to the meninges, bone, joints, skin, and soft tissues).

Renal involvement occurs in 46–60% of cases of disseminated disease.

Microabcess or granulomata formation typically develops. Bladder infection may present with hematuria, pneumaturia (caused by a vesicocolic fistula) and concomitant bacilluria.

Prostate infection may present with symptoms suggestive of a bladder outflow tract obstruction.

Laboratory diagnosis of renal mycosis

Conventional microbiologic methods
Direct microscopy (Gram, Giemsa, and KOH/calcofluor stains), culture, identification and susceptibility testing.

Histopathologic methods
Conventional microscopy, direct immunofluorescence and *in situ* hybridization.

Immunologic and biochemical methods
Histoplasma antigen test, cryptococcal antigen test, galactomannan test (for Aspergillosis with 67–100% sensitivity and 81–98% specificity), and (1,3)β-D-glucan test (for *Candida* and *Aspergillus* spp.).

Molecular methods
Direct detection and identification, e.g. peptide nucleic acid fluorescence *in situ* hybridization (PNA FISH) for *Candida* spp. Polymerase chain reaction, although promising for the diagnosis of IFI, has not been widely used.

Fungal infections following renal transplantation

Fungal infections remain a significant challenge after transplantation. Their incidence varies according to the organ transplanted.

In renal transplant recipients an incidence of 1–14% has been reported and these infections are associated with a very high mortality. This is related to environmental exposure and the degree of immunosuppression.

In an analysis of 850 renal transplant recipients from a tertiary care center in North India, Gupta (2001) described fungal infections in 83 patients (9.8%). These were candidiasis in 25 (2.8%), cryptococcosis in 16 (1.9%), aspergillosis in 20 (2.3%), zygomycosis in 17 (2.0%) and rare fungal infections in five others including pheohyphomycosis in three and disseminated histoplasmosis in two patients.

The role of prophylaxis or pre-emptive therapy in subsets of solid organ transplant patients is still being defined, but evidence supports the use of fluconazole prophylaxis in liver transplant recipients.

Emerging fungal pathogens may be resistant to conventional antifungal agents, and specific microbiological diagnosis is important.

Treatment of fungal infections

The treatment of invasive deep-seated fungal infections can be difficult due to the limited number of drugs available and the undesirable toxicity of some of them.

Amphotericin B, fluconozole and itraconozole have been the mainstay of therapy for IFI, but recent advances in therapy are described below.

Lipid formulations of amphotericin B
Whereas the continuous 24 h infusion of amphotericin B has been found to have less overall infusional toxicity and nephrotoxicity than conventional 4 h infusion, there is a clear benefit with the use of lipid formulations. These allow higher doses of amphotericin B to be administered before toxicity develops. The three available lipid formulations are liposomal amphotericin B (AmBi-some), amphotericin B lipid complex (Abelcet), and amphotericin B colloidal dispersion (Amphocil).

Triazoles
Voriconazole, a new triazole, has activity against yeasts, including those intrinsically resistant to fluconazole, as well as moulds such as *Aspergillus* spp., some *Fusarium* spp. and, importantly, *Scedosporium* spp., which are often resistant to amphotericin B.

However, voriconazole specifically causes transient visual disturbance and interacts with various drugs including rifampicin, erythromycin, ciclosporin, and cyclophosphamide through inhibition of the hepatic enzymes CYP2C9 and CYP2C19.

The newer triazoles, posaconazole and ravuconazole, also have broad spectrum *in vitro* activity against filamentous fungi. Posaconazole, in particular, has found clinical utility as salvage therapy in zygomycosis.

Echinocandins
Echinocandins inhibit the synthesis of β-1,3-D-glucan in the fungal cell wall.

They have most activity in the growing ends of fungal hyphae and rapidly cease hyphal growth and replication.

Although caspofungin has activity against *Aspergillus* and *Candida*, it is not active against *Cryptococcus*, *Fusarium* or *Zygomycetes*.

Micafungin and anidulafungin are the two other Echinocandins approved by the US Food and Drug Administration.

Combination therapy
With the availability of antifungal agents acting on different targets in the fungal cell, the possibility of combination therapy exists.

In vitro testing suggests combination therapy (e.g. caspofungin + fluconazole or flucytosine + amphotericin) produces synergy which is particularly useful in difficult-to-treat infections such as scedosporiosis and aspergillosis as well as candidiasis and cryptococcosis.

The drug management of various renal mycoses is described in Table 7.5.2.

Surgery
Surgical measures may also be necessary to treat the fungal balls as well as to remove infected tissue.

Debulking of bezoars in patients with candidiasis and aspergillosis may be carried out by percutaneous nephrostomy, endoscopic removal, or open pyelotomy. In addition, it may be combined with local irrigation with amphotericin B.

Table 7.5.2 Treatment of invasive fungal infections

Infection	Drugs and dosage
Candiduria[a]	Fluconazole 200 mg/day (loading 400 mg) for 14 days
	Amphotericin B 0.3–0.7 mg/kg/day for 1–7 days
Candidemia[a]/ invasive candidiasis	Fluconazole 200–400 mg/day or
	Caspofungin 70 mg on day 1, 50 mg/day thereafter or
	Amphotericin B 0.5–1 mg/kg/day or Lipid-AmB 5 mg/kg/day
	Comments
	C. krusei, C. glabrata are fluconazole resistant; treat with an echinocandin, voriconazole or posaconazole
Invasive aspergillosis	Voriconazole 6 mg/kg IV×2 doses, then 4 mg/kg/day twice daily IV, can convert to 200 mg twice daily orally.
	Caspofungin 70 mg on day 1, 50 mg/day thereafter
	Amphotericin B 1–1.5 mg/kg/day or Lipid-AmB 5 mg/kg/day
	Itraconazole 400 mg/day
Cryptococcosis	Fluconazole 200–400 mg/day or itraconazole 200–400 mg/day; or
	Lipid-AmB 5 mg/kg/day with flucytosine 100 mg/kg/day for 2 weeks followed by fluconazole 400 mg/day
Zygomycosis	Posaconazole 800 mg/day
	Lipid-AmB 5–15 mg/kg/day

[a] Infectious Diseases Society of America (IDSA) published guidelines for the treatment of candidiasis (2004).

For extensively damaged tissues in patients with angioinvasive infections such as mucormycosis, debridement and excision of the tissue (which may include nephrectomy) may be necessary.

Immune therapy

Adjunctive immune therapy with interferon-γ, granulocyte-macrophage colony-stimulating factor and granulocyte colony-stimulating factor can be considered for severe IFI refractory to conventional antifungal treatment.

Further reading

Almyroudis NG, Sutton DA, Linden P, et al. Zygomycosis in solid organ transplant recipients in a tertiary transplant center and review of the literature. *Am J Transplant* 2006; **6**: 2365–2374.

Chayakulkeeree M, Ghannoum M, Perfect J. Zygomycosis: the re-emerging fungal infection. *Eur J Clin Microbiol Infect Dis* 2006; **25**: 215–229.

Chugh KS, Sakhuja V, Gupta KL, et al. Renal mucormycosis: computerized tomographic findings and their diagnostic significance. *Am J Kidney Dis* 1993; **22**: 393–397.

Gabardi S, Kubiak DW, Chandraker AK, et al. Invasive fungal infections and antifungal therapies in solid organ transplant recipients. *Transpl Int* 2007; **20**: 993–1015.

Gupta KL. Fungal infectons and the kidney. *Ind J Nephrol* 2001; **11**: 147–154.

Meersseman W, Lagrou K, Maertens J, et al. Invasive aspergillosis in the intensive care unit. *Clin Infect Dis* 2007; **45**: 205–216.

Pappas PG, Rex JH, Sobel JD, et al. Infectious Diseases Society of America. Guidelines for treatment of candidiasis. *Clin Infect Dis* 2004; **38**: 161–189 [Revised in 2008: see journal website.]

Pappu LD, Purohit DM, Bradford BF, et al. Primary renal candidiasis in two preterm neonates. Report of cases and review of literature on renal candidiasis in infancy. *Am J Dis Child* 1984; **138**: 923—926.

Scheinfeld NA. Review of the new antifungals: posaconazole, micafungin, and anidulafungin. *J Drugs Dermatol* 2007; **6**: 1249–1251.

Internet resources

Infectious Diseases Society of America. Guidelines for treatment of candidiasis. 2008 update:

`www.idsociety.org/WorkArea/downloadasset.aspx?id=7818`

Information about aspergillus and apergillo-sis:

`http://www.aspergillus.org.uk/`

Information about human mycoses:

`http://www.doctorfungus.org/`

See also

Infection-related glomerulonephritis, p. 128

Renal stone disease

Chapter contents

Medical management of stone disease

Definition
Nephrolithiasis is the formation of stones in the renal tubules or collecting system.

Epidemiology and incidence
The incidence of nephrolithiasis varies geographically.

In industrialized nations the incidence is ~1 in 1000.

The peak age is the third decade and the prevalence is higher in men.

A prevalence of 10% occurs in industrialized nations but is higher in areas such as the Middle East.

The recurrence rate for nephrolithiasis ranges from 50 to 80%.

Etiology
Stones form when the urinary concentration of the stone constituents rises above the supersaturation level. The supersaturation level reflects the product of free ion activities. It is not solely dependent on the concentration of constituents but also on the presence of promoters and inhibitors of stone formation such as urine pH and citrate concentration.

The common types of renal stones are listed in Table 8.1.1.

Table 8.1.1 Types of renal stones (listed in order of decreasing prevalence)

Combination of calcium oxalate and calcium phosphate
Calcium oxalate
Struvite
Calcium phosphate
Uric acid
Cystine

Clinical presentation
Pain is the commonest presenting feature. Stones passing through the renal pelvis or ureter cause colicky loin pain with or without radiation to the groin, testis or labia.

Macroscopic or microscopic hematuria is a common finding but its absence does not exclude stone disease. Hematuria may occur with or without associated pain.

Stones can be an incidental finding in asymptomatic patients undergoing imaging for other reasons.

History
Assessing risk factors
- Age.
- Family history.
- History of stone disease (age at presentation, frequency, surgical history).
- History of urinary tract infections.
- History of neoplastic disease, sarcoidosis, endocrine disease (risk factors for hypercalcemia).
- Diseases of the gastrointestinal tract.
- Gout.
- Obesity.
- Diabetes mellitus.

Environmental factors
- Occupation.
- Fluid intake.
- Diet.
- Exercise intensity.
- Urine volume.

Drug history
Drugs that may precipitate into stones
- Triamterene.
- Aciclovir.
- Indinavir.

Drugs that increase the risk of stone formation
- Loop diuretics.
- Calcium and vitamin D supplements.
- Glucocorticoids.
- Antacids.
- Theophylline.
- Acetozalamide.
- Salicylates.
- Probenecid.
- Vitamin C.

Examination
Physical examination should be undertaken to identify other possible causes for pain and hematuria.

Investigations
Following formation of a single stone
Stone analysis
If the stone is not captured ask the patient to sieve the urine to collect any remaining stone fragments.

Urine analysis
- Urine microscopy to identify crystals.
- Urine culture.
- Cystine concentration on a 'spot' urine sample.

Venous blood analysis
- Calcium.
- Parathyroid hormone (if hypercalcemic).
- Phosphate.
- Uric acid.
- Bicarbonate.
- Sodium, potassium, chloride, urea and creatinine.

Table 8.1.2 Imaging techniques for the investigation of renal stones

Noncontrast enhanced helical CT	Highest specificity and sensitivity. Investigation of choice at first presentation.
Plain KUB radiograph	If history of radio-opaque stones.
Intravenous urogram	Time-consuming. In practice now used only if CT is not available.
Ultrasound	Poor at detecting ureteric stones. Useful in pregnant patients and in detecting hydronephrosis. Use if cholecystitis or gynecological cause of pain is suspected.

Imaging

The imaging modalities used in the evaluation of patients with suspected stone disease are listed in Table 8.1.2 and discussed in Chapter 1.6.

Following the formation of second or multiple stones

In addition to the above investigations at least two 24 h urine collections 'on a normal day, on a normal diet' should be made to allow measurement of the items listed in Table 8.1.3.

Table 8.1.3 Components to be measured in a 24 h urine collection in recurrent stone disease

Volume	
Calcium	Usually requires an acid preservative
Phosphate	
Oxalate	Usually requires an acid preservative
Uric acid	Usually a plain or alkaline solution
Sodium	
Citrate	
Creatinine	To ensure complete collection
pH	

General management of stone disease

The general principles of management that apply to all types of stone disease are listed in Table 8.1.4. The management of specific risk factors and individual stone types is described in the remainder of this chapter.

Management of calcium stone disease

Several risk factors for calcium stone formation are discussed in this section (Table 8.1.5).

Table 8.1.4 General advice for prevention of recurrent stone formation of all stone types

Maintain sodium intake of <100 meq/day (5 g).
Maintain urine output >2 L/day with drinking at bedtime to induce nocturia.
Reduce animal protein intake.
Encourage potassium intake.
Review medication use and where possible avoid drugs that increase risk of stone formation.

Table 8.1.5 Summary of risk factors for calcium stone formation

Hypercalciuria
Renal tubular acidosis
Hypocitraturia
Hyperoxaluria
Hyperuricosuria

However, in some patients no risk factors can be identified. Management of these patients relies upon general stone prevention advice (Table 8.1.4).

Excess excretion of urinary calcium

Idiopathic hypercalciuria

This is commonly familial, affects males more than females, and typically presents in the third decade of life.

The mechanism of hypercalciuria is unclear but is likely to be a combination of increased intestinal absorption and abnormal handling of calcium by the kidney.

Management: Advise the general management measures (Table 8.1.4) plus:

Dietary:
- Restrict sodium intake to reduce renal calcium excretion.
- Maintain a normal calcium diet, but avoid additional calcium supplementation. There is no benefit to restricting dietary calcium and this may lead to bone demineralization and reduce oxalate binding in the gut leading to hyperoxaluria (see below).

Pharmacological (Table 8.1.7):
- Long-acting thiazide (e.g. chlorthalidone 25–50 mg/day) to reduce urinary calcium excretion.
- Potassium supplements, potassium-sparing diuretic or potassium citrate to maintain serum potassium *at normal levels* and increase urinary citrate (use potassium citrate liquid or urocit-K wax tablet 20–40 mmol/day). Hypokalemia leads to intracellular acidosis resulting in hypocitraturia. Oral potassium supplementation and a diet rich in fruit has been shown to increase urinary citrate excretion.

Hypercalcemic hypercalciuria

The common causes are:
- hyperparathyroidism;
- granulomatous disease, e.g. sarcoidosis;
- neoplastic disease;
- lithium therapy.

Management:
- treat underlying cause;
- general stone prevention advice.

Distal renal tubular acidosis

This causes mainly calcium phosphate stone formation.

Hypercalciuria, hyperphosphaturia and high urinary pH leads to urinary calcium phosphate supersaturation, and the metabolic acidosis causes hypocitraturia.

Management:
- Alkalinize the serum and when possible treat the underlying cause of RTA.
- Avoid a urine pH >6.5 as this encourages calcium phosphate precipitation.

Dent's disease (see Chapter 8.3)

Decreased citrate excretion

Citrate binds with urinary calcium forming a soluble complex which inhibits its crystallization.

Metabolic acidosis results in an increase in citrate reabsorption and therefore hypocitraturia.

Other causes include hypokalemia, hypomagnesemia, urinary tract infection, and acetozalamide therapy. In one study urinary potassium levels were the strongest predictor of urinary citrate levels.

Most laboratories will not measure urinary citrate.

Management

- Reduce animal protein content of diet.
- Supplement with oral potassium citrate or bicarbonate (Table 8.1.7).

Hyperoxaluria

Urinary oxalate excretion is normally ~20% that of calcium excretion. Hyperoxaluria increases the risk of calcium oxalate stone formation. However, these stones can form and precipitate even in the absence of hyperoxaluria.

Causes of hyperoxaluria

Three causes of hyperoxaluria have been described.

Dietary hyperoxaluria

Management involves restricting dietary oxalate (Table 8.1.6) while maintaining the balance between calcium and oxalate ultimately to reduce the urinary supersaturation of calcium oxalate.

Restriction of dietary oxalate may reduce calcium binding in the gut, leading to increased calcium absorption and hypercalciuria. Dietary oxalate should not therefore be restricted in the presence of a high calcium diet or calcium supplementation.

Restriction of dietary calcium is not recommended for the reasons discussed above. There is some evidence to suggest that a high calcium diet in the absence of calcium supplements may reduce oxalate absorption from the gut, thereby reducing the risk of hyperoxaluria. Usually, a normal calcium diet is recommended.

Table 8.1.6 Oxalate-rich foods

High bioavailability of oxalate	Moderate bioavailability of oxalate
Spinach	Peanuts
Rhubarb	Instant tea
	Almonds
	Chocolate
	Pecans

Enteric hyperoxaluria

This is caused by excessive colonic absorption of oxalate. It is seen in disorders that result in fat malabsorption such as Crohn's disease, chronic pancreatitis and short bowel syndrome.

Increased fatty acid delivery to the colon increases oxalate absorption.

Malabsorption may also lead to reduced urine volume, hypokalemia and hypocitraturia, which will all promote stone formation.

Management includes treating the underlying cause, increasing dietary calcium (as part of the diet and not with additional supplements) to enhance oxalate binding in the gut and reduce its absorption, and using pharmacological agents such as cholestyramine to bind fatty acids.

Increased systemic production of oxalate

This can occur in several situations:

- Primary hyperoxaluria I and II. These are inherited liver enzyme deficiencies (alanine-glyoxylate amino-transferase and glyoxylate reductase/hydroxypyruvate reductase (GRHPR) respectively) which lead to increased oxalate formation. Treatment is with pyridoxine and liver transplantation if multiple organ involvement occurs. Alkalinization of the urine and use of orthophosphate (if GFR is well preserved) may reduce stone formation.
- Ethylene glycol (EG) intoxication. EG is metabolized to glycolate, glyoxylate and oxalate. Its metabolism is catalyzed by alcohol dehydrogenase (AD) and other enzymes. Management consists of urinary alkalinization to reduce the risk of stone formation, and prevention of formation of EG metabolites by inhibition of AD using ethanol or fomepizol.
- Excessive intake of ascorbic acid which is oxidized to form oxalate.

Hyperuricosuria

Calcium stone formers are more likely to have increased urinary uric acid excretion.

Furthermore, uric acid crystals can form a nidus for calcium oxalate crystal aggregation.

A reduction in the intake of dietary animal protein and the use of allopurinol reduces uric acid excretion and may reduce the risk of calcium stone formation.

Uric acid stones

Uric acid stones are radiolucent and therefore not detectable on a plain KUB X-ray.

Risk factors for stone formation are low urine volume, low urine pH, and a high urine uric acid concentration.

Low urine volumes can be a feature of gastrointestinal disease, for example in patients with a high output ileostomy.

Uric acid solubility increases with rising pH.

Increased levels of urinary uric acid can result from:

- gout;
- tumor lysis syndrome;
- inherited disorders of metabolism such as Lesch–Nyhan syndrome;
- high dietary purine intake from animal protein;
- drugs that increase urinary uric acid excretion, e.g. salicylates.

Management

- Increase the fluid intake to increase urine volumes (>3 L/day).
- Reduce dietary animal protein intake.
- Alkalinize the urine with bicarbonate or citrate aiming for a pH between 6 and 7. Sodium salts should be avoided as the volume expansion will enhance sodium urinary excretion and with it passive calcium excretion from the proximal tubule.
- Encourage patients to test the urine pH at home.
- Allopurinol may be of benefit (Table 8.1.7).

Struvite stones (magnesium ammonium phosphate)

These occur in patients with urine infection due to urea-splitting organisms (e.g. Proteus).

The breakdown of urea generates excess ammonium leading to a rise in urinary pH. The excess ammonium and the reduction in phosphate solubility caused by the increased urinary pH lead to an increase in the concentration of insoluble magnesium ammonium phosphate and stone formation.

These stones can increase to a large size forming a staghorn calculus.

Risk factors include female gender, indwelling urinary catheters, neurogenic bladder and alkaline urine.

Occasionally special culture medium is required to isolate urea-splitting organisms such as *Mycoplasma* and the lab will need to be alerted if this is suspected.

Management

- Struvite stones are difficult to eradicate. Any residual fragments form a nidus for new stone formation and make eradication of infection difficult.
- Surgical or percutaneous nephrolithotomy may be required to remove the stones.
- Continuous cyclical antibiotic therapy may be beneficial.
- Urease inhibitors have not been useful clinically due to a high side-effect profile.

Cystine stones

Cystine stone disease presents typically in the fourth decade in patients with cystinuria. This is a rare hereditary disorder in which dibasic amino acid transport is impaired.

The diagnosis is made by measuring the urine cystine concentration on a 'spot' urine sample and then quantifying cystine excretion in a 24 h urine collection.

Management

To keep cystine in solution the urine must be very dilute and alkaline. The treatment therefore includes:

- maintaining very large urine volumes (>3 L/day);
- alkalinization of the urine;
- D-penicillamine 250 mg to 2 g/day, or tiopronin (10–40 mg/kg/day, max. 2 g/day) to reduce the urinary supersaturation of cystine (Table 8.1.7).

Table 8.1.7 Pharmacological agents used in the management of stone disease

Drug	Indication/mode of action
Thiazides or indapamide	Reduce urinary calcium excretion.
Potassium citrate	Increase urinary citrate and urinary pH. Not advisable in the presence of urinary tract infection.
Allopurinol	Reduce uric acid formation.
D-Penicillamine or tiopronin	Bind cystine.

Complications of nephrolithiasis

- Stones can lead to obstruction at the level of the pelviureteric junction (PUJ) or ureter causing hydronephrosis or pyonephrosis.
- Staghorn calculi increase the risk of urinary infection.
- Progressive renal failure may occur. A report from France suggests that 2.2% of patients on an end-stage renal disease program had nephrolithiasis as the underlying cause.

Further reading

Bushinsky D. Nephrolithiasis. *J Am Soc Nephrol* 1998; **9**: 917–924.

Domprongkitchaiporn S, Sticharntrakul W, Kochakarn W. Causes of hypocitraturia in recurrent calcium stone formers: focusing on urinary potassium excretion. *Am J Kidney Dis* 2006; **48**: 546–554.

Goldfarb DS, Coe FL. The medical mangement of stone disease. 2005. In: Davison AM, Cameron JS, Grunfeld J-P, Kerr DNS, Ritz E, Winearls CG (eds), *The Oxford textbook of nephrology*, 3rd edn. Oxford: Oxford University Press; 2005. pp. 1225–1242.

Heilberg I. Update on dietary recommendations and medical treatment of renal stone disease. *Nephrol Dial Transplant* 2000;**15**:117–123.

Jungers P, Joly D, Barbey F, *et al*. ESRD caused by nephrolithiasis: prevalence, mechanisms, and prevention. *Am J Kidney Dis* 2004; **44**: 799–805.

Monk R, Bushinsky D. Nephrolithiasis and nephrocalcinosis. In: Johnson RJ, Feehally J (eds), *Comprehensive clinical nephrology*, 3rd edn. Amsterdam: Elsevier; 2003. pp. 641–655.

Pak C. Medical management of urinary stone disease. *Nephron Clin Pract* 2004; **98**: c49–c53.

Pak CY, Poindexter JR, Adams-Huet B, *et al*. Predictive value of kidney stone composition in the detection of metabolic abnormalities. *Am J Med* 2003; **115**: 26–32.

Tiselius H-G. Aetiological factors in stone formation. In: Davison AM, Cameron JS, Grunfeld J-P, Kerr DNS, Ritz E, Winearls CG (eds), *The Oxford textbook of nephrology*, 3rd edn. Oxford: Oxford University Press; 2005. pp. 1199–1224.

See also

Imaging in renal disease, p. 20

Hypo-/hypercalcemia, p. 52

Renal tubular acidosis, p. 208

Uric acid and the kidney, p. 232

Surgical management of stone disease, p. 274

Nephrocalcinosis, p. 278

Inherited disorders of purine metabolism and transport, p. 636

Isolated defects of tubular function, p. 200

Surgical management of stone disease

Demographics and incidence

Symptoms caused by urinary tract stone disease are common. The estimated lifetime risk of a stone episode is 1 in 10 for men and 1 in 25 for women.

The costs associated with stones are considerable and in the USA in 1993 were estimated at $1.7 billion.

Much of the cost is due to the fact that stone episodes tend to afflict the most financially productive age groups with the peak incidence occurring in the 20s to 40s.

There is no clear relationship between stone incidence and geography, but there is a relationship between environmental temperature and stone episodes: the highest incidence of stone-related episodes occurs 2 months after the maximum mean annual temperature.

Pathophysiology of stone formation

Stone production and composition is dictated by environmental factors, the anatomy of the urinary tract, and the constituents of the urine, and not by cellular processes.

Three basic phenomena are critical to stone formation, irrespective of the composition of the stone:

- *Supersaturation of the urine*
  In this situation urine has in solution the maximum amount of dissolved solute. This is a reflection of the product of free ion activities rather than the absolute molar concentrations, and the supersaturation level can be altered by stone promoters and inhibitors.
- *Particle formation*
  The addition of extra solute to the urine or changes in the contents of the urine may cause solute to precipitate as crystals, a process known as nucleation. In urine, crystal nuclei usually form on a surface, such as cell debris, casts or red blood cells.
- *Particle retention*
  Individual crystals are small and cannot grow large enough to occlude tubules in the 5–7 min it takes to pass into the renal pelvis. Aggregation of many individual crystals into a clump is required to produce a large enough particle to be retained by obstruction of a collecting duct.

Promoters of stone formation include:

- excess urinary solute caused by cystinuria, oxaluria, hypercalciuria, uricosuria;
- slow tubular transit for example in chronic volume depletion and medullary sponge kidney.

Inhibitors of stone formation include:

- water diuresis which speeds tubular transit and prevents particle formation;
- citrate which binds with calcium to form a soluble compound which inhibits nucleation;
- magnesium which also inhibits crystal aggregation.

Aggregated crystals/early stones may be seen during endoscopic procedures in the pelvicalyceal system. These aggregates develop beneath the epithelium on the tips of renal papillae and are called Randall's plaques. Ulceration through the mucosa releases the stone into the pelvicalyceal system.

Clinically, the risk factors for stone formation may be considered as:

- congenital: cystinuria, medullary sponge kidney.
- malignant: hyperuricosuria following treatment of malignancy, particularly myeloproliferative disorders.
- idiopathic: calcium oxalate stones.
- metabolic: the hypercalciuria of hyperparathyroidism, hyperuricosuria.
- social: inadequate fluid intake, excess fluid losses particularly bakers and foundry workers.

Stone composition subtypes

The common types of renal stones are listed in Table 8.2.1.

Table 8.2.1 Stone composition subtypes

Calcium oxalate (± calcium phosphate)	80%
Struvite	6–14%
Uric acid	5–10%
Calcium phosphate and others	5%
Cystine	1–2%

Calcium oxalate stones

These are common stones and are radio-opaque.

They form in association with:

- hypercalciuria (idiopathic or with hypercalcemia);
- primary or secondary hyperoxaluria;
- hyperuricosuria and hypocitraturia.

Struvite stones

These are composed of a mixture of magnesium ammonium phosphate and calcium carbonate–apatite.

These almost always fill the pelvicalyceal system to form a staghorn stone.

Urine infection with a urease-producing bacterium (e.g. *Proteus*, *Klebiella*, *Pseudomonas* spp.) results in ammonia production and a urine pH of >7.2. This promotes the precipitation of struvite.

They can be potentially life-threatening because of septicemia if left untreated.

Uric acid stones

These are radiolucent stones.

They have a strong geographical distribution. They are particularly common in Israel.

They are associated with the production of an acidic urine (pH 5) and low urine volumes over prolonged periods.

There is an association with the presence and therapy of myeloproliferative disorders in which nucleic acid conversion to uric acid is increased.

They may be dissolved *in situ* by alkalinizing the urine to a pH of 6.5–7.0.

Cystine stones

Cystinuria is an autosomal recessive disease characterized by defective transport of dibasic amino acids (cystine, ornithine, arginine and lysine).

This defect leads to decreased cystine absorption from the intestine and reabsorption from the proximal tubule.

Only homozygotes form cystine stones.

Cystine is poorly soluble at normal urinary pH, but much more soluble at pH 7–8.

Cystine stones are very hard and do not respond to shock wave lithotripsy.

Clinical presentations

Acute ureteric colic
This presents with loin-to-groin colic with associated nausea and vomiting. Dipstick urinalysis usually reveals evidence of nonvisible hematuria.

Urinary frequency and penile tip or clitoral pain may develop with stones impacted at the vesicoureteric junction.

Hematuria
Stone disease is a common cause of both visible and nonvisible hematuria. Although usually associated with colicky pain, it may also be painless.

Pyonephrosis
This is suppuration within an obstructed pelvicaly-ceal system. This combination of infection and obstruction results in septicemia, usually with Gram-negative bacilli.

Failure to relieve the obstruction begins to irreversibly damage nephrons within hours and a nonfunctioning kidney may result.

Gram-negative septicemic shock is a life-threatening complication.

Chronic loin pain
Vague loin pain, which may occur in the absence of other urinary symptoms, may also be present.

Relapsing urine infections
Organisms may be found within the crystalline structure of some stones, especially struvite stones.

Antibiotics eradicate the organisms that are free in the urine, but penetrate the stone structure poorly. Therefore when the antibiotics are stopped, the urine is rapidly repopulated from organisms residing within the stone.

Asymptomatic
Stones may be identified on imaging studies that are undertaken for other indications.

Clinical assessment and investigation
The evaluation of acute colic and chronic loin pain should include:

The assessment of vital signs for evidence of fever, septicemia, and shock.

Dipstick urinalysis for the urine pH, the presence of hematuria, and evidence of infection (leukocyte esterase and nitrite).

Measurement of full blood count, renal function, serum calcium and uric acid.

Culture of a midstream urine sample.

Diagnostic imaging. The diagnosis of a ureteric stone can only be made by imaging.
- Plain X-ray of the abdomen. This has little role in establishing the initial diagnosis. Uric acid stones are radiolucent and are not detected on plain films; radio-opaque stones in the middle third of the ureter may not be detectable against the background of the sacroiliac joint.
- Intravenous urogram (IVU). Historically this was the first-line investigation, but there are concerns about the nephrotoxic effects of the contrast and the potential for rare but fatal anaphylaxis in 0.9 per 100 000 cases.
- Noncontrast enhanced spiral CT scan. This is now the standard of care. All stones (except indinavir stones) are detected by CT. Stones as small as 1 mm diameter may be identified. The presence of ureteric dilatation and/or perinephric stranding indicates ureteric obstruction.

Principles of management

Relief of pain
The pain of acute ureteric colic is described by many patients as the worst pain imaginable.

NSAIDs work well. Administration by suppository avoids the difficulty of administering oral drugs to nauseated patients.

Parenteral opiates and antiemetics may also be required.

Relief of obstruction
The diagnostic imaging will indicate if the ureter or renal pelvis is obstructed.

In the absence of infection a short period of obstruction (i.e. 2–4 weeks) probably does not result in permanent renal damage.

In the presence of infection and obstruction (pyonephrosis) urgent relief of obstruction (within hours) is mandatory.

Insertion of a percutaneous nephrostomy under local anesthesia, or a ureteric stent under general anesthesia (although it can be inserted under local anesthesia if necessary) are the initial treatment choices.

Treatment of associated sepsis
Where there is fever or other evidence of infection, antibiotics should be used.

The selected agent should have excellent activity against Gram-negative bacilli, including *Pseudomonas* spp., and for this reason gentamicin has traditionally been used. This should, however, be avoided when there is renal impairment.

The insertion of a nephrostomy to treat pyonephrosis is commonly followed shortly afterwards by profound septicemia and this should be anticipated.

Treatment of the stone
The options available are:
- conservative management with observation and analgesia;
- extracorporeal shock wave lithotripsy;
- ureteroscopy and *in situ* fragmentation ± extraction of fragments usually using holmium laser energy;
- percutaneous nephrolithotomy for larger renal stones or stones in the proximal ureter;
- open surgery; this is now rarely required, but the open techniques may now be replicated by laparoscopic surgeons and the future may see a growing role for laparoscopic ureterolithotomy and pyelolithotomy.

Treatment of stones in the pelvicalyceal system

Chemical dissolution therapy for uric acid stones
This can be achieved noninvasively using a combination of:
- high fluid intake (>2–2.5 L/day);
- urine alkalinization using potassium citrate 6–10 mmol 2–3 times a day to achieve a urine pH of >6.5;
- allopurinol 300 mg/day (particularly if urinary urate excretion is >1000 mg (6 mmol)/day).

Alternatively percutaneous dissolution can be achieved by the infusion of an alkaline solution (e.g. trihydroxymethyl aminomethan (THAM)) through a percutaneous nephrostomy. To prevent either the chemolysis solution draining into the bladder, or an increase in intrarenal pressure, a second nephrostomy tube is usually required for drainage of the irrigation fluid.

Extracorporeal shock wave lithotripsy (ESWL)
Fragmentation of stones needs to be followed by clearance of the fragments. The likelihood of fragment clearance is determined by the pelvicalyceal anatomy.

A dependent calyx with a long infundibulum may retain fragments which then form a nidus for further stone formation.

The passage of multiple large fragments may obstruct the ureter as a Steinstrasse or 'stone street'.

For stones >2 cm diameter a ureteric stent should be placed prior to ESWL to prevent this complication.

Flexible ureterorenoscopy and in situ laser lithotripsy
The flexible ureteroscope can carry a flexible laser fiber to a stone in any part of the collecting system.

Lithotripsy by contact with holmium laser energy is very effective but the technique is limited by the very small size of the instruments (200 μm diameter laser fiber) and the view down the ureteroscope which is obscured by even trivial bleeding.

Percutaneous nephrolithotomy
A sheath is delivered into the pelvicalyceal system through the skin of the loin via the renal parenchyma.

The stone is removed under direct vision using instruments passed down the sheath.

The main complications relate to the puncture and include hemorrhage, which rarely requires embolization of the kidney or even emergency nephrectomy, and septicemia.

Excellent stone-free rates are achievable, but other less invasive techniques may subsequently be required to treat residual fragments ('sandwich therapy').

Treatment of ureteric stones

In ureteric colic, encouraging patients to drink plenty of fluid to induce a forced diuresis is of no benefit.

An increased urine output reduces the rate of ureteric peristalsis, which is the mechanism by which stones are expelled.

As obstruction of the ureter becomes chronic (>18 h), afferent arteriolar vasoconstriction causes a decrease in glomerular filtration and effectively diverts urine production to the contralateral kidney.

Conservative, observational management
Many ureteric stones may be safely left to pass spontaneously.

Stones ≤5 mm in diameter will pass in ~68% of cases, and stones 5–10 mm in diameter will pass in only 47% of cases.

Medical expulsive therapy
α-adrenoceptor blockers have recently been shown to increase the proportion of patients with ureteric stones who pass their stone spontaneously.

The increase in stone passage rate is ~29%.

Some studies also show a decrease in both the number of hospital readmissions and interventions that are required.

Most studies have restricted themselves to distal ureteric stones and it should be noted that the use of α-blockers for this indication is not licensed.

Patients who elect conservative observation or medical expulsive therapy should have well-controlled pain and no evidence of sepsis.

These patients should be monitored with periodic imaging studies to monitor stone position, and to identify developing hydronephrosis or obstruction.

Management of ureteric obstruction
Persistent or marked obstruction with gross hydronephrosis warrants intervention.

Obstruction may be relieved by insertion of a percutaneous nephrostomy under radiological guidance, or by insertion of a ureteric stent.

The nephrostomy drains an obstructed system more reliably, but necessitates an external drainage bag.

Ureteric stents drain internally but give rise to lower urinary symptoms of frequency and urgency.

Ureteric stone removal
This is indicated in the presence of persistent obstruction, failure of stone progression, or recurrent or uncontrolled pain.

ESWL and ureteroscopy are both acceptable first-line treatments for ureteric stones. The success rates for each treatment modality are listed in Table 8.2.2.

Ureteroscopy is associated with a higher stone-free rate after a single treatment in all cases except for larger stones in the proximal one-third of the ureter.

However, this advantage comes at the cost of greater risks of ureteric injury and sepsis, and the requirement for anesthesia.

Use of ESWL for stones in the middle third of the ureter may be restricted by the bones of the pelvis which prevent penetration of the shock wave.

Ureterolithotomy
Open ureterolithotomy should be required only rarely.

A small number of series describe good results when laparoscopic ureterolithotomy is used to treat large impacted stones in the proximal ureter.

Table 8.2.2 Stone-free rate after single treatment for ureteric stone

	ESWL	Ureteroscopy
Proximal	82%	87%
Mid-ureter	73%	86%
Distal ureter	74%	94%

Prevention of recurrence

In high risk patients or recurrent stone-formers a formal metabolic screen may be useful. Identification of the likely stone composition can facilitate targeted therapy.

This involves analysis of a 24 h urine collection for volume, and the quantity of calcium, oxalate, phosphate, uric acid and sodium (and citrate if available). A spot urine test for the presence of cystine (followed by a 24 h collection for cystine excretion if the spot urine is positive) should also be undertaken.

The composition of the stone should also be analysed when possible.

In all cases and irrespective of the stone subtypes, maintenance of a large output of dilute urine (minimum 2 L, ideally more) is the most important intervention. This should also include drinking at bed-time to induce nocturia.

Calcium oxalate stones

Following an initial stone episode ~50% of patients will have another episode within 10 years. After a second episode the risk rises to ≥75%.

The risk of further stone formation can be minimized with the following approach.

Maintain a large urine output.

Treat hypercalcemia if present.

Restrict dietary sodium intake to <100 mmol/day.

Restrict dietary oxalate by avoidance of oxalate-rich foods (coffee, chocolate, nuts, strawberries, green leafy vegetable).

Avoid purine gluttony to decrease uric acid excretion.

Increase citrus fruit consumption to increase urinary citrate excretion.

It is well-established that calcium restriction is not helpful. Indeed a calcium-rich diet may bind dietary oxalate in the gut and thereby reduce urinary oxalate excretion.

Consider thiazide diuretics. Thiazides stimulate calcium reabsorption from the distal tubule and so decrease calcium excretion. However, there is little evidence of benefit compared with placebo and side-effects mean long-term compliance is poor.

Consider the administration of allopurinol to patients with recurrent calcium oxalate stones and hyperuricosuria.

Uric acid stones

Recurrent uric acid stones may be prevented by the following approach.

Maintain a large urine output, ideally 3 L per day.

Uric acid stones may be dissolved by alkalinization of the urine to a pH of 6.5–7.0.

Potassium citrate is the preferred alkalinizing agent, but many patients are intolerant of the taste.

Allopurinol is useful if the patient is hyperuricemic or if the urinary uric acid excretion is >1000 mg (6 mmol)/day.

Cystine stones

The risk of forming recurrent cystine stones can be minimized by the following approach.

Forced diuresis is essential. Patients should aim for a urine output >3 L per 24 h and this requires the patient to wake at night to drink.

Alkalinization of the urine to a pH of 7–8.

Use of cystine complexing agents: cystine forms soluble complexes with D-penicillamine, tiopronin or captopril.

These oral agents reduce urinary cystine excretion but many patients experience intolerable side-effects.

Further reading

Auge BK, Preminger GM. Surgical management of urolithiasis. *Endocrinol Metab Clin North Am* 2002; **31**: 1065–1082.

Miller NL, Lingeman JE. Management of kidney stones. *Br Med J* 2007; **334**: 468–472.

Teichman JM. Acute renal colic from ureteral calculus. *N Engl J Med* 2004; **350**: 684–693.

Wen CC, Nakada SY. Treatment selection and outcomes: renal calculi. *Urol Clin North Am* 2007; **34**: 409–419.

Internet resources

Detailed guidelines on the management of stone disease from the European Association of Urology:

`http://www.uroweb.org/fileadmin/user_upload/Guidelines/Urolithiasis.pdf`

General stone information for patients:

`http://www.kidney.niddk.nih.gov/kudiseases/pubs/stonesadults`

National Kidney Foundation information on stone disease:

`www.kidney.org/atoz/atozTopic.cfm?topic=13`

See also

Nephrocalcinosis

Nephrocalcinosis is defined as calcification within the renal parenchyma.

This can be microscopic or macroscopic and be in a cortical or medullary distribution. Medullary nephrocalcinosis is the commonest form.

The prevalence of nephrocalcinosis is not known but a small study of nephrectomy specimens (removed for renal tumors) found that interstitial calcification is a common finding.

Microscopic nephrocalcinosis is sometimes detected incidentally on renal biopsy.

It is caused predominantly by metabolic disorders affecting calcium metabolism such as Bartter's syndrome, distal renal tubular acidosis, primary hyperoxaluria, and secondary hyperparathyroidism.

The clinical implication of microscopic nephrocalcinosis has not been extensively studied in man but is likely to be similar to that seen with macroscopic nephrocalcinosis.

This chapter will focus on macroscopic nephrocalcinosis that is detectable on imaging as discussed below.

Etiology

Cortical nephrocalcinosis
Cortical nephrocalcinosis generally follows tissue destruction and tends to have an asymmetric distribution.

Underlying causes include:
- trauma (e.g. following lithotripsy);
- renal infarction;
- renal neoplasms;
- chronic pyelonephritis;
- vesicoureteric reflux;
- renal transplant rejection;
- granulomatous disease;
- chronic glomerulonephritis;
- acute cortical necrosis (e.g. following severe postpartum hemorrhage);
- oxalosis.

Medullary nephrocalcinosis
Medullary nephrocalcinosis is usually symmetrical and bilateral in its distribution. The list of causes is extensive.

Excess urinary constituents that may precipitate (calcium, phosphate, oxalate):
- primary hyperparathyroidism;
- milk-alkali syndrome;
- vitamin D toxicity;
- sarcoidosis;
- idiopathic hypercalciuria;
- oxalosis;
- type 1 renal tubular acidosis (RTA);
- rapidly progressive osteoporosis.

Hereditary and congenital disorders
- Dent's disease. This is an X-linked recessive disorder caused by a mutation in voltage-gated chloride channels with a Fanconi syndrome phenotype, hypercalciuria, medullary nephrocalcinosis, renal impairment and variable urinary acidification defects.

75% of patients with Dent's disease develop nephrocalcinosis but the extent of this does not correlate with the progression of the renal impairment.
- Type 1 renal tubular acidosis.
- Hypomagnesemia–hypercalciuria syndrome.
- Bartter's syndrome.
- Amelogenesis imperfecta.
- Congenital hypothyroidism.
- Primary hyperoxaluria (cortical nephrocalcinosis in this setting carries a worse renal outcome than medullary nephrocalcinosis).
- X-linked hypophosphatemic rickets.

Structural kidney disease
Medullary sponge kidney. Calcified deposits form in the malformed collecting ducts in the pericalyceal region of the medullary pyramids.

Medullary sponge kidney disease generally follows a benign course and rarely causes progressive CKD.
- Papillary necrosis (e.g. caused by NSAIDs) can lead to nephrocalcinosis in the damaged papillae and gives a characteristic radiological appearance.

Drugs
- Acetazolamide (probably by interfering with urinary acidification).
- Furosemide. This inhibits the sodium–potassium–chloride channel in the ascending loop of Henle. This leads to reduction in the luminal electropositivity and reduces the paracellular reabsorbtion of calcium leading to hypercalciuria. Furosemide is particularly implicated in the nephrocalcinosis seen in severely premature babies.
- NSAIDs (as discussed above).
- Oral sodium phosphate solution used as bowel preparation. Several case reports have described widespread calcium phosphate deposition in the renal medulla on renal biopsy. This is seen particularly in patients with pre-existing renal disease. In some reports the renal biopsy findings included acute tubular necrosis but whether this is caused by the calcium phosphate deposition or by intercurrent volume depletion is not clear.
- Amphotericin. This causes renal tubular injury and may lead to a clinical picture similar to that seen in distal RTA including nephrocalcinosis. Lipid and colloidal preparations of amphotericin B appear to have a less nephrotoxic profile.
- Total parenteral nutrition (TPN). The mechanism of this is unclear but is probably related to the calcium:phosphate ratio required for maintaining a neutral or positive calcium balance to prevent bone disease. This may be compounded by the acidosis which results from a catabolic state.

Other conditions associated with medullary nephrocalcinosis
- Hyperaldosteronism and apparent mineralocorticoid excess syndromes. This is likely related to chronic hypokalemia influencing calcium handling by the kidney.
- Recurrent pyelonephritis.
- Severe prematurity (see below).

Clinical presentation
- The extent of calcification does not correlate with disease activity.
- Medullary calcification is more likely to have clinically relevant consequences than cortical calcification.
- The symptoms and signs are caused by several mechanisms:
  - damage to the tubular epithelium leading to loss of concentrating ability and therefore polyuria and thirst;
  - erosion of the papillary epithelium causing symptoms and signs of nephrolithiasis;
  - distal tubular dysfunction leading to salt wasting and hypovolemia;
  - erythrocytosis: the mechanism is unclear but may be related to capillary damage and hyperreninism caused by salt wasting.

Investigations
To confirm the diagnosis of nephrocalcinosis
Imaging
Macroscopic nephrocalcinosis can be detected by plain KUB radiography, ultrasonography and noncontrast enhanced helical CT.

The specificity and sensitivity are increased if two imaging techniques are used one of which is a noncontrast enhanced helical CT.

Intravenous urography has a higher sensitivity for demonstrating medullary sponge kidney.

Renal biopsy
As proteinuria is not commonly present in nephrocalcinosis unless the underlying cause produces Fanconi's syndrome, renal biopsy is not usually performed as part of the diagnostic evaluation.

When nephrocalcinosis is suspected, imaging and metabolic evaluation are commonly used to confirm the diagnosis.

Nephrocalcinosis can be seen on biopsies performed for other indications, however, and has been reported in association with focal segmental glomerulosclerosis.

To identify the causes and complications of nephrocalcinosis
Detailed family and drug history.

History of skeletal disease.

Serum metabolic evaluation:
- calcium (if elevated investigate as described in Chapter 2.3);
- phosphate;
- magnesium;
- bicarbonate;
- sodium;
- potassium;
- chloride;
- thyroid function tests.

Urine metabolic evaluation:
24 h urine collection (refer to Chapter 8.1 for details) to measure:
- calcium;
- phosphate;
- oxalate;
- sodium;
- protein;
- creatinine (to confirm complete collection).
- Spot urine sample to measure:
- pH;
- amino acids;
- β2-Microglobulin (as a measure of low molecular weight proteinuria);
- glucose;
- bacterial culture (inflammatory pyuria is common).

Natural history and management
Potential long-term complications
- Distal RTA can develop secondary to medullary nephrocalcinosis. It is therefore difficult to diagnose primary dRTA in patients with nephrocalcinosis in the absence of a family history of the disease.
- Progressive CKD can occur and is more likely to be associated with metabolic disorders such as primary hyperoxaluria and Dent's disease than with medullary sponge kidney.
- Reports of the likelihood of progression vary. In one series 15% of patients evaluated for nephrocalcinosis had a creatinine clearance of <50 mL/min.
- Osteopenia was reported in 15 of 23 patients with nephrocalcinosis in a small study. This may be related to an underlying calcium metabolism disorder rather than to nephrocalcinosis *per se*.

Pharmacological management
Management of the underlying cause may halt the precipitation of further deposits.

Nephrocalcinosis lesions are no longer visible radiologically in most severely premature infants by the age of 7 years.

In adults resolution of established lesions is not widely described but thiazides have been reported to arrest progression.

Another report suggests that sodium thiosulphate could play a role in halting or reversing progression. The beneficial effect may be mediated by generation of calcium thiosulphate that is a soluble compound, and/or stabilization of glutathione which may protect the renal parenchyma from free radical-induced injury.

Nonpharmacological management
In patients with hypercalciuria, salt and animal protein restriction may reduce progression and the risk of nephrolithiasis.

Depending on the underlying cause, metabolic derangements may occur and dietary supplementation may become necessary such as in hypomagnesemia–hypercalciuria syndrome.

Surveillance
If a familial disease is suspected, family members should be counselled and evaluated.
Regular monitoring should include:
- renal function and proteinuria;
- serum and urinary electrolytes;
- bone chemistry;
- bone density.

Further reading

Beyea A, Block A, Schned A. Acute phosphate nephropathy follow-ing oral sodium phosphate solution to cleanse the bowel for colonoscopy. *Am J Kidney Dis* 2007; **50**: 151–154.

Cheidde L, Ajzen SA, Tamer Langen CH, Christophalo D, Pfeferman, Heilberg I. A critical appraisal of the radiological evaluation of nephrocalcinosis. *Nephron Clin Pract* 2007; **106**: c119–124.

Kummeling MT, de Jong BW, Laffeber C, et al. Tubular and intersti-tial nephrocalcinosis. *J Urol* 2007; **178**(3 Pt 1): 1097–1103.

Manley P, Somerfield J, Simpson I, Barber A, Zwi J. Bilateral uraemic optic neuritis complicating acute nephrocalcinosis. *Nephrol Dial Transplant* 2006; **21**: 2957–2958.

Monk R, Bushinsky D. Nephrolithiasis and nephrocalcinosis. In: Johnson and Feehally (eds), *Comprehensive clinical nephrology*, 2nd edn. Amsterdam: Elsevier; 2003. pp. 731–741.

Müller D, Eggert P, Krawinkel M. Hypercalciuria and nephrocalcino-sis in a patient receiving long-term parenteral nutrition: the effect of intravenous chlorothiazide. *J Pediatr Gastroenterol Nutr* 1998; **27**: 106–110.

Porter E, McKie A, Beattie TJ, McColl JH, Aladangady N, Watt A, White MP. Neonatal nephrocalcinosis: long term follow up. 2007. *Arch Dis Child Fetal Neonatal Ed* 2006; **91**: F333–336.

Seikaly MG, Baum M. Thiazide diuretics arrest the progression of nephrocalcinosis in children with X-linked hypophosphatemia. *Pediatrics* 2001; **108**: E6.

Wrong, O. Nephrocalcinosis. In: Davison AM, Cameron JS, Grunfeld J-P, Kerr DNS, Ritz E, Winearls CG (eds), *The Oxford textbook of nephrology*, 3rd edn. Oxford: Oxford University Press; 2005. pp. 1257–1280.

See also

Renal stone disease in children

Renal stones are still very rare in children. However, as the age of onset of stone disease in adults reduces, there is an increasing number of young people, especially females, with stones.

The presentation and etiology of stone disease differs considerably from adults, with a greater burden of inherited metabolic stone disorders.

Similarly, the management of stones, especially in infants, reflects the technical limits of lithotripsy and minimally invasive techniques.

Pathogenesis

In the UK and developed countries, ~25% of cases are related to previous urinary tract infection (UTI), 50% have an underlying metabolic abnormality, and in 25% no cause is identified.

However, such a definition of abnormality (e.g. higher than 95% centile for age-related normal ranges) is scientifically not useful since there is overwhelming evidence in adult stone-formers that the risk of stone formation increases steadily with increasing urinary oxalate and calcium excretion (even within the 'normal range').

Infective stones are commonest in young children, especially in uncircumcized boys. Infection with urea-splitting bacteria produces ammonium ions, alkalinizes the urine and leads to supersaturation of magnesium ammonium phosphate.

Most children with infective stones do not have underlying congenital urological abnormalities but children with reconstructed bladders, ileal conduits, urinary stasis or obstructive lesions are at increased risk of stone formation.

The commonest type of stone is calcium oxalate, usually as dihydrate and often with a minor component of calcium phosphate.

Hypercalciuria is a common finding in such situations although usually this is unrelated to renal tubulopathy (such as distal RTA or hypomagnesemia–hypercalciuria syndrome) or hypercalcemia. Primary hyperparathyroidism is extremely rare in children. Hypocitraturia is a common finding.

Children with hyperoxaluria (either primary or secondary) will produce calcium oxalate stones. The finding of monohydrate crystals suggests a need to exclude hyperoxaluria.

Cystine stones are diagnostic of cystinuria.

Uric acid stones require further investigation to exclude specific metabolic disorders.

Presentation

Stones can develop at any age, and as young as the first weeks of life (grit or 'putty-like' material in nappies).

Typical symptoms (pain, hematuria, persistent UTI) may be present but pain is not reported in 50% of children with stones.

Nonspecific symptoms may occur in infants: poor feeding, vomiting, poor weight gain (mean weight and height of children presenting with stones are below 50% centile).

A family history is common (~20% of first degree and 40% of second degree relatives have stones).

Groups at higher risk for stone formation include ex-premature infants and children with severe neurological disability.

Management

Initial management

After analgesia, rehydration and treatment of infection, the first aim is to confirm the stone burden and plan for stone removal (delay metabolic evaluation until stones are cleared).

Ultrasound is the first-line investigation in children (it is much more sensitive than in adults).

Obtain a plain radiograph of the abdomen (KUB) to check for the presence of ureteric stones (ultrasound will miss these due to overlying bowel gas).

Following diagnosis, it is essential to liaise with clinicians with specific expertise in the management of renal stones in the pediatric age group (for example a regional pediatric stone service).

Usually further imaging is required to define split renal function and identify pre-existing renal damage (e.g. DMSA renogram), and calyceal anatomy to plan stone removal (e.g. limited IVU). This may be undertaken at a specialist unit.

Metabolic evaluation should usually be postponed until after stone clearance is achieved.

Stone clearance

Single stones may require one or two treatments with the newer minimally invasive techniques.

Clearance rates are comparable to those in adults, with clearance rates of 85–90% for each of the modalities listed below.

Children with a significant stone burden (e.g. bilateral and multiple stones) will need several sessions over a number of months to clear the calculi.

Lithotripsy

- Very successful for many pediatric stones but it usually requires a general anesthetic, and may need several sessions for complex (staghorn or multiple) stones.
- Less successful for lower pole stones and cystine calculi.
- Associated with transient renal 'injury' e.g. enzymuria, but there is currently no evidence of long-term complications.

Percutaneous nephrolithotomy

- Very good success rate.
- Technically very demanding in small children.
- Main complications are bleeding, infection and urine leakage.

Ureteroscopy and laser disintegration of stones

- Useful for ureteric and mobile renal stones.
- Main complications are infection and ureteric damage.

Open surgery

- This is rarely required but still has a limited role.

Metabolic evaluation

Stone analysis. This may suggest the etiology:
- Magnesium ammonium phosphate/calcium apatite (struvite). This suggests urinary infection.
- Calcium oxalate dihydrate (weddellite) and monohydrate (whewellite). This is suggestive of idiopathic stone formation, and is also seen in hyperoxaluria (primary or secondary).
- Calcium phosphate (usually hydroxyapatite, rarely brushite, tricalcium phosphate (whitlockite) or octocalcium phosphate). It is often a minor component of other calcium or struvite stones. It suggests alkaline urine and hypercalciuria, so if it is a major component of the stone consider distal renal tubular acidosis and primary hyperparathyroidism.
- Cystine. This indicates cystinuria.
- Uric acid. Magnesium ammonium phosphate is seen in endemic stone areas; other uric acid stones are rare (see below)

Plasma biochemistry (including bicarbonate, urate).

Urine biochemistry. Measure urine specific gravity, calcium, oxalate, citrate, urate and cystine excretion:
- Screen with spot urine samples in young children.
- Confirm results with 24 h urine collections.
- Specialist laboratory analysis.
- Reference data for children rather than adults.

Further metabolic studies as indicated.

Ongoing management and prevention

The principles of medical management are similar to those in adult stone disease.

Hydration
- The mainstay of stone prevention is good hydration to maintain high urine flow rates.

Diet
- Dietary review is useful but in general protein and calorie intake should be maintained to permit good growth.
- In contrast to adult stone disease where a significant proportion of patients are overweight, growth parameters are below average in children with stones.
- Sodium intake should be reviewed but restriction of calcium intake is counterproductive (as well as impractical in young children).

Hypercalciuria
- This alone is not necessarily an indication for specific therapy other than increased fluid intake and salt restriction. The risk of further stone formation in hypercalciuric children is low.
- In those with a significantly damaged kidneys, or recurrent symptoms or stones, consider firstly potassium citrate, and then a thiazide diuretic.

Cystinuria
- Children with cystinuria should all receive a high fluid intake (>1.5 L/m^2/day), salt restriction and potassium citrate.
- Urinary cystine concentrations should be maintained at <1000 μmol/L.
- Tiopronin or penicillamine act as sulfhydryl-chelating agents and are effective but have significant adverse effects (rash, bone marrow suppression, nephropathy and other systemic effects). They are therefore reserved for those with recurrent stones or kidney damage.

Hyperoxaluria and purine disorders
- The specific management of hyperoxaluria and purine disorders is detailed in later Chapters 15.13 and 15.14.

Prognosis

Most children have a single stone episode but a significant number have a potential biochemical abnormality that increases stone risk and a small number have monogenic metabolic disorders that cause recurrent stones and can lead to CKD. All children therefore should receive prompt stone clearance and thereafter undergo a metabolic evaluation.

Further reading

Coward RJM, Peters CJ, Duffy PG, *et al*. Epidemiology of paediatric renal stone disease in the UK. *Arch Dis Child* 2003; **88**: 962–965.

Rizvi SA, Naqvi SA, Hussain Z, *et al*. Pediatric urolithiasis: developing nation perspectives. *J Urol* 2002; **168**: 1522–1525.

VanDervoort K *et al*. Urolithiasis in pediatric patients: a single center study of incidence, clinical presentation and outcome. *J Urol* 2007; **177**: 2300–2305.

van't Hoff W. Renal and urinary tract stone disease in children. In: Davison AM, Cameron S, Grunfeld J-P, Ponticelli C, Ritz E, Winearls C, van Ypersele C (eds), *Oxford textbook of clinical nephrology*, 3rd edn. Oxford: Oxford University Press. Chapter 8.3, pp. 1281–1291.

Internet resources

Information on kidney stones aimed at teenagers:

`http://www.childrenfirstforhealth.co.uk/teens/health/conditions/k/kidney_stones.html`

Information on childhood stone disease:

`http://www.pediatriconcall.com/forpatients/CommonChild/Urinary_renal.asp`

See also

Primary hyperoxalurias, p. 632

Inherited disorders of purine metabolism and transport, p. 636

Isolated defects of tubular function, p. 200

Medical management of stone disease, p. 270

Surgical management of stone disease, p. 274

Hypertension

Chapter Contents

Clinical approach to hypertension

Introduction
Hypertension (HTN) is one of the most common conditions encountered in medical practice. For the majority of patients, the etiology is unknown and the treatment is straightforward. This chapter provides an overview of the clinical assessment of a hypertensive patient with particular reference to the less common etiologies, its complications and initial treatment options.

Definition
British, European and WHO guidelines define the categories of HTN based on clinic blood pressure (BP):

Blood pressure

Optimum: <120/80 mmHg
Normal: <130/85 mmHg
High–normal: 130–139/85–89 mmHg.

Hypertension

Mild (grade 1):   140–159/90–99 mmHg
Moderate (grade 2):   160–179/100–109 mmHg
Severe (grade 3):   >180/110 mmHg.

Isolated systolic hypertension

Grade 1:   140–159/<90 mmHg
Grade 2:   >160/<90 mmHg.

Epidemiology
The prevalence of HTN increases with age.

Data from the Health Survey for England 1998 revealed 72% of men and 68% of women aged >75 years had HTN (defined by a BP >140/90 mmHg).

This compares to 17% and 4% in men and women aged 16–24 years respectively.

However, the number of patients prescribed treatment for HTN is much less.

Data from primary care (Key Health Statistics from General Practice 1998) revealed that <2.5% of patients aged under 35 years (men: 1.7%; women: 2.4%) and <30% of patients aged ≥85 years (men: 20.1%; women: 29.1%) were taking antihypertensive drugs.

It is not known whether these patients were treated to target BP.

Etiology
The cause of HTN in the vast majority of cases, even in young people, is not clear.

About 90% of people with newly diagnosed HTN are given the diagnosis 'primary' (or 'essential') HTN and the etiology is likely to reflect a multifactorial genetic predisposition and/or lifestyle factors such as obesity and poor diet.

Secondary HTN accounts for the remaining 10% of cases and the causes are listed in Table 9.1.1.

Renal disease
This is the cause of HTN in ~5% of newly diagnosed hypertensive subjects.

Diabetic renal disease accounts for the majority of cases and this is increasing both in terms of absolute numbers and as a proportion of all CKD.

Renovascular HTN is a relatively uncommon cause of HTN (<1% of newly diagnosed patients) and can present as fibromuscular dysplasia in the young or atherosclerotic renal artery stenosis in older people.

Endocrine disease
This is the cause of HTN in ~5% of cases.

Hyperaldosteronism (e.g. Conn's syndrome, adrenal hyperplasia) accounts for the majority of cases.

The combined oral contraceptive pill increases BP by an average of 5/3 mmHg; in ~1% of women, severe HTN may be seen.

Other causes
Other causes are rare and combined account for ~1% of all HTN.

Single gene disorders affecting renal tubular function are very rare and usually present in childhood.

Pregnancy-induced HTN affects 8–10% of pregnancies and pre-eclampsia affects a further 8% of pregnancies.

Blood pressure returns to normal in most women with pregnancy-related HTN after 3–6 months, but is a risk factor for the development of HTN later in the woman's life.

Assessment of the patient
History
Hypertension is often asymptomatic, hence its description as the 'silent killer'.

The history from a hypertensive patient should:
- attempt to establish an etiology;
- identify complications/end organ damage;
- put the HTN into the context of overall cardiovascular risk.

Baseline features to assess:
- duration of HTN and BP values;
- treatment history and concordance with treatment;
- any adverse drug reactions.

Establishing an etiology
A family history of HTN.

In women a history of pregnancy-related HTN.

A history of any recent 'over the counter' and/or prescribed drug therapy:
- NSAIDS;
- combined oral contraceptives;
- corticosteroids;
- sympathomimetics.

A history of renal or urological disease.

A pheochromocytoma might be suggested by:
- episodic palpitations;
- sweating;
- chest pain;
- paroxysmal HTN.

Identifying complications/end-organ damage
Common complications to specifically enquire about:
- ischemic heart disease;
- heart failure;

Table 9.1.1 Causes of secondary hypertension

Renal
- Diabetic renal disease
- Chronic pyelonephritis
- Renovascular hypertension
- Obstructive nephropathy
- Renal parenchymal disease
- Renin-secreting tumors

Endocrine
- Mineralocorticoid hypertension
  - Conn's syndrome
  - Bilateral/(unilateral) adrenal hyperplasia
  - Glucocorticoid-remediable aldosteronism
  - Adrenal carcinoma
- Deoxycorticosterone excess
  - Congenital adrenal hyperplasia
  - 11β-Hydroxylase deficiency
  - 17β-Hydroxylase deficiency
  - Glucocorticoid receptor resistance
- Cortisol excess
  - Cushing's syndrome
  - 11β-Hydroxysteroid dehydrogenase deficiency
- Apparent mineralocorticoid excess
  - Glycyrrhetinic acid (licorice)
- Pheochromocytoma
- Oral contraceptive and estrogen replacement
- Hypothyroidism/hyperthyroidism
- Acromegaly
- Hyperparathyroidism/hypercalcemia
- Carcinoid

Genetic diseases of renal tubular function
- Liddle's syndrome
- Gordon's syndrome
- Gain of function mutation of the mineralocorticoid receptor

Other
- Coarctation of the aorta
- Neurologic disorder
- Psychogenic
- Sleep apnea
- Drug-induced (e.g. cocaine)
- Pregnancy

- cerebrovascular disease;
- peripheral vascular disease;
- renal impairment.

Assessing overall cardiovascular risk:
- obesity;
- high salt intake;
- excess alcohol;
- lack of exercise;
- diabetes mellitus;
- hyperlipidemia;
- smoking.

Examination
Apart from elevated BP readings, the clinical examination may be normal.

Measurement of blood pressure
BP should be measured after the patient has been seated for 5 min.

At the initial assessment, the BP should be measured three times, a minute between each reading, and in both arms.

The BP for each arm should be recorded as the average of the 2nd and 3rd readings.

A standing BP should be recorded in:
- patients with a history of postural hypotension;
- the elderly;
- those at risk of autonomic dysfunction (e.g. diabetics);
- those taking multiple antihypertensive drugs.

Physical examination
A full examination with particular reference to the heart and circulatory system should always be undertaken.

The general appearance of the patient may give clues towards an endocrine diagnosis such as acromegaly or Cushing's disease.

Signs of tar staining on the hands, obesity or hyperlipidemia (e.g. corneal arcus, xanthelasma) would suggest additional cardiovascular risk.

Radio-femoral delay or weak peripheral pulses may suggest a coarctation of the aorta.

A palpable kidney would raise the suspicion of hydronephrosis or polycystic kidney disease.

Abdominal (renal) bruits are rarely heard in patients with renovascular disease, but their presence is highly indicative.

Complications of HTN may be evident from signs of heart failure, peripheral vascular disease (femoral or carotid bruits) or a neurological deficit.

Fundoscopy
Fundoscopy is useful in assessing for end-organ damage.

Type 2 hypertensive retinopathy (copper wiring, arteriovenous nipping) is very common in middle-aged/elderly patients with longstanding HTN.

Patients with recently elevated severe high BP and type 3 hypertensive retinopathy (hard exudates, flame-shaped hemorrhages), and all patients with type 4 hypertensive retinopathy (type 3 abnormalities and papilloedema) are, by definition, hypertensive urgencies and require immediate treatment.

Conversely, normal fundoscopy in a patient with a longstanding history of high BP readings would cast doubt on the diagnosis of severe HTN, suggesting an alternative diagnosis of 'white-coat HTN'.

Initial investigation
Routine investigations in the initial evaluation of a patient will HTN must include:
- urinalysis for protein and blood;
- serum electrolytes;
- serum creatinine providing an estimated GFR;
- fasting blood glucose and lipid profile;
- electrocardiogram.

Renal disease may be identified by a reduced eGFR and/or abnormal urinalysis.

The presence of hematuria without other evidence of renal dysfunction should be confirmed by microscopy and investigated for disease of the bladder and urinary system.

Hypokalemia may be a pointer towards hyperaldosteronism (even without hypernatremia).

A previous history of diuretic-induced hypokalemia should not be ignored.

Thiazide diuretic-induced hypokalemia in patients with hyperaldosteronism can be severe.

Hypokalemia may be seen in renovascular disease.

Other investigations such as thyroid and liver function tests should be taken as clinically indicated.

In those patients with ECG evidence of increased ventricular voltages, echocardiography is advised to confirm (or refute) the presence of left ventricular hypertrophy.

Cardiovascular risk assessment
Hypertension is one of several factors that can be used to calculate an individual's cardiovascular disease (CVD) risk.

Risk can be calculated using:
- age;
- smoking history;
- pretreatment BP;
- lipid profile (total cholesterol:HDL-cholesterol ratio).

The Cardiovascular Risk Prediction Charts published in the British National Formulary provide an easy reference guide.

These charts are designed to support clinical decisions about the use of antihypertensive, antiplatelet and lipid-lowering therapy in primary prevention.

Diabetes mellitus is no longer included in the risk calculation – all patients with diabetes should be offered primary prevention.

Measurement of BP outside the clinic
Investigator-led clinical studies that have generated the evidence for BP targets and thresholds have almost exclusively used clinic BP readings.

About 30% of hypertensive subjects have 'white-coat HTN' or a pronounced 'white-coat effect' at the time of BP measurement that prevents a reliable estimation of BP for these individuals. Home BP monitoring can reduce this 'white-coat effect'.

Ambulatory 24 h BP monitoring allows frequent BP measurements to be made automatically at intervals of 20–30 min throughout the day and night. The patient wears a small device around their waist which is connected to a BP cuff.

Self-monitoring of home BP readings is easy with the use of digital BP monitors. Home BP readings should be taken for a fixed period of time (e.g. 5–7 days) and patients should record their BP three times after being seated for 5 min. The average BP is calculated taking the mean of the 2nd and 3rd readings at each sitting, excluding the first day's readings.

Patients should be advised to use BP monitors that have been validated by the British Hypertension Society.

Upper arm devices are recommended in preference to wrist monitors.

Blood pressure thresholds and targets
The decision to treat high BP with drug therapy is usually determined when the BP rises above a set threshold.

Once treatment is indicated, drug therapy is initiated and escalated until the BP falls below a defined target.

Thresholds and target BPs differ between different patient populations.

Even in the same population, the target BP may be lower than the threshold BP.

Thresholds for treatment
Antihypertensive drug treatment should be initiated in patients with:
- sustained systolic BP ≥160 mmHg; or
- diastolic BP ≥100 mmHg.

A lower threshold exists for patients with:
- diabetes;
- an elevated 10 year CVD risk (>20%);
- end-organ damage;
- cardiovascular complications of HTN.

For these patients treatment should be initiated for:
- sustained systolic BP 140–159 mmHg; or
- sustained diastolic BP 90–99 mmHg.

For patients with established CKD and/or proteinuria, the threshold for treatment is identical for those with diabetes or target-organ damage.

Target blood pressure
The usual recommended BP target is ≤140/90 mmHg.

For patients with established cardiovascular disease and/or diabetes, a lower target of ≤130/80 mmHg is advised.

For patients with CKD, a BP target of ≤130/80 mmHg is recommended.

For patients with proteinuria (>1 g /24 h), a more stringent target of ≤125/75 mmHg is advised.

The concept of a lower BP target than those currently recommended for patients with CKD has yet to be proven in clinical trials.

Treatment
The effective management of HTN continues to lag behind guidelines from clinical trial data.

Although the 'rule of halves' (*half of patients with HTN are diagnosed, of whom half are treated, and of those, half are treated to target*) is no longer applicable, many patients with HTN remain undertreated.

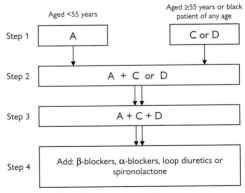

Fig. 9.1.1 'ACD rule' for the treatment of newly diagnosed hypertension. A: angiotensin-converting enzyme inhibitor (or ARB). C: calcium channel blocker. D: thiazide diuretic. (Adapted from the British Hypertension Society and NICE.)

Nonpharmacological treatment

All patients with raised BP should be advised about appropriate lifestyle regimens that could reduce their BP and/or reduce their cardiovascular risk.

There is robust evidence that lifestyle modifications can significantly reduce BP including:
- maintaining an ideal body weight;
- dietary salt restriction;
- a diet high in fruit and vegetables;
- physical exercise;
- limiting alcohol consumption (if applicable).

This advice is particularly pertinent for patients with borderline HTN (140/90 to 159/99 mmHg) who do not require drug therapy.

Smoking cessation does not reduce BP, but significantly reduces cardiovascular risk.

Drug treatment

Previously, thiazide diuretic and β-blocker drugs were considered the mainstay of BP treatment.

Newer drug classes, angiotensin-converting enzyme inhibitors (ACEIs), angiotensin receptor blockers (ARBs) and dihydropyridine calcium channel blockers (CCBs) are increasingly prescribed.

As a general rule, there is no class of drug more effective than others in either reducing BP or reducing the risk of cardiovascular events associated with HTN.

The key determinant of cardiovascular risk reduction appears to be the BP target attained rather than the drugs prescribed.

There are several caveats.

Firstly there are age and ethnicity factors that influence the initial drug treatment and secondly β-blockers have recently been shown to be less effective at preventing cardiovascular events despite similar BP reduction when compared to other drug classes.

The British Hypertension Society and NICE guidelines propose the 'ACD' rule based on an individual's age and ethnicity (Fig. 9.1.1). Younger (<55 years) Caucasian subjects have a greater serum renin level compared with older or Black (African/Caribbean) subjects. Therefore those drugs (ACEIs or ARBs) which have greater activity against the renin–angiotensin system (RAS) are likely to provide greater BP reduction in younger patients and thus are more effective first-line drugs.

CCBs and thiazide diuretics have less activity against the RAS and are consequently first-line agents for older or Black patients.

If additional drug treatment is required, combining a drug that would not have been considered as first-line therapy with the initial therapy is preferred; for example a young Caucasian patient initially taking an ACEI and requiring further treatment would be prescribed a CCB or thiazide diuretic.

Further up-titration of therapy to triple therapy would result in all populations taking an ACEI, CCB and thiazide diuretic.

If required, fouth-line therapy options include:
- β-blockers;
- α-blockers;
- loop diuretics;
- spironolactone.

For some patients, there are overriding factors that may influence the initial prescription of antihypertensive therapy.

For example, β-blockers are first-line therapy for patients with angina and there is good clinical evidence for the early prescription of ACEI (or ARB) in patients with diabetes.

In many proteinuric renal diseases ACEIs (or ARBs) are considered first-line therapy as they afford renal protection in addition to BP reduction.

A slight fall in GFR should be expected (<15% fall in GFR requires no further investigation) on commencement of ACEI and ARB and this is not a reason to stop treatment.

Treatment with ACEI should be up titrated to the maximum tolerated dose and if significant proteinuria remains (>1 g/24 h), combination ACEI–ARB therapy should be considered.

BP targets for patients with CKD are lower than other patient groups and additive therapy can be based on the 'ACD' rule.

An underlying diagnosis of renovascular disease is a relative contraindication to ACEI and ARB as these drugs preferentially dilate the efferent renal arterioles and can cause a profound reduction in glomerular BP and lead to AKI.

Primary and secondary prevention

Primary prevention is indicated for hypertensive patients with:
- diabetes;
- evidence of end-organ damage (i.e. left ventricular hypertrophy, renal impairment);
- an estimated 10 year risk of developing cardiovascular disease >20%.

Secondary prevention is treatment for any patient with established cardiovascular disease.

Antiplatelet therapy

Unless contraindicated, antiplatelet therapy with aspirin is indicated for all patients requiring secondary prevention.

The evidence for antiplatelet therapy as primary prevention only supports treatment of those hypertensive patients with good BP control (<150/90 mmHg) and aged >50 years.

Statin therapy

Statin therapy should be considered in all hypertensive patients aged ≤80 years.

Based on clinical trial evidence, the Joint British Societies suggest:
- a total cholesterol target of <4.0 mmol/L and
- low density lipoprotein (LDL)-cholesterol <2.0 mmol/L,

or
- a 25% reduction in total cholesterol and
- 30% reduction in LDL-cholesterol,

whichever provides the lower value.

Follow-up

It is usual practice to monitor patients monthly after initiating therapy and to increase drug therapy as required.

Patients with severe HTN should be reviewed more frequently.

Once BP is controlled, review of BP should take place every 6 months with an annual assessment of renal function and lipid parameters.

Those subjects with 'high–normal' BP readings should be reassessed annually.

All adults with a 'normal' BP should have their BP measured every 5 years.

Prognosis

The cardiovascular and renal risks associated with HTN are related directly to the level of BP.

At one extreme, untreated malignant HTN has a life expectancy of <25% at 12 months and <1% at 5 years.

Observational studies comparing risk of stroke or ischemic heart disease with diastolic BP show a linear relationship from 75–105 mmHg, suggesting that a J-shaped relationship between BP and outcome is unlikely to exist.

Well-controlled HTN is still associated with a very small increased risk of cardiovascular events.

It is important to remember that BP alone does not determine the overall prognosis, but is one of several key factors that also include smoking status, glycemic control, lipid profile and age.

Further reading

British Hypertension Society. Guidelines for management of hypertension: report of the fourth working party of the British Hypertension Society, 2004—BHS IV. *J Hum Hypertens* 2004; **18**: 139–185.

Joint British Societies' Guidelines on Prevention of Cardiovascular Disease In Clinical Practice. *Heart* 2005; **91**(Suppl V): v1–v52:

Recent major clinical trials

ALLHAT Officers and Coordinators for the ALLHAT Collaborative Research Group. Major outcomes in high-risk hypertensive patients randomized to angiotensin-converting enzyme inhibitor or calcium channel blocker vs diuretic: the antihypertensive and lipid lowering treatment to prevent heart attack trial (ALLHAT). *J Am Med Assoc* 2002; **288**: 2981–2997.

Brenner BM, et al., for the RENAAL Study Investigators. Effects of Losartan on renal and cardiovascular outcomes in patients with type 2 diabetes and nephropathy. *N Engl J Med* 2001; **345**: 861–869.

Dahlof B, et al. Cardiovascular morbidity and mortality in the Losartan Intervention for endpoint reduction in hypertension study (LIFE): a randomised trial against atenolol. *Lancet* 2002; **359**: 995–1003

Dahlof B, et al. Prevention of cardiovascular events with an antihypertensive regimen of amlodipine adding perindopril as required versus atenolol adding bendroflumethiazide as required, in the Anglo-Scandinavian Cardiac Outcomes Trial – Blood Pressure Lowering Arm (ASCOT-BPLA): a multicentre randomised controlled trial. *Lancet* 2005; **366**: 895–906.

Hansson L, et al., for the HOT Study Group. Effects of intensive blood pressure lowering and low-dose aspirin in patients with hypertension: principal results of the Hypertension Optimal Treatment (HOT) randomised trial. *Lancet* 1998; **351**: 1755–1762.

Lewis EJ, et al. Renoprotective effect of the angiotensin-receptor antagonist Irbesartan in patients with nephropathy due to type 2 diabetes. *New Engl J Med* 2001; **345**: 851–860.

Sacks FM, et al. Effects on blood pressure of reduced dietary sodium and the Dietary Approaches to Stop Hypertension (DASH) diet. DASH – Sodium Collaborative Research Group. *N Engl J Med* 2001; **344**: 3–10.

Internet resources

British Hypertension Society:

www.bhsoc.org/

NICE CG34 Hypertension guideline:

www.nice.org.uk/nicemedia/pdf/Hypertension Guide.pdf

Hypertension Education Foundation:

http://www.hypertensionfoundation.org/

European Society of Hypertension:

http://www.eshonline.org/

The London Hypertension Society (an excellent link to many of the national guidelines on management of hypertension):

http://www.lhs.sgul.ac.uk/links/guidelines.htm

Joint British Societies' Guidelines on prevention of cardiovascular disease in clinical practice:

www.bcs.com/download/651/JBS2final.pdf

The British National Formulary:

http://bnf.org/bnf/

See also

History and clinical examination of renal disease, p. 2

Renovascular disease, p. 292

Malignant hypertension, p. 300

Hypertensive children, p. 304

Hypertensive disorders in pregnancy, p. 310

Renovascular disease

Introduction

Narrowing of the main renal arteries, renal artery stenosis (RAS), is very common and can lead to clinical presentations of hypertension (HTN), mild–severe renal failure and cardiac failure. The most common condition leading to renovascular narrowing is atheromatous RAS (ARAS) change, which accounts for >90% of the renovascular disease in the Western world. Fibromuscular disease (FMD) accounts for most of the remaining cases. As the etiology, clinical presentations and responses to treatment of these two conditions can be quite different they are considered separately in this chapter. Takayasu's arteritis may be responsible for >50% of RAS cases in the Indian subcontinent and there are other rare causes of RAS such as middle aortic syndrome and antiphospholipid antibody syndrome; these are briefly considered below.

Definition and terminology

As complete occlusions of the renal artery (renal artery occlusion, RAO) are often seen the term atherosclerotic renovascular disease (ARVD) is preferable to ARAS.

Ischemic nephropathy is the term used when reduced renal function occurs in association with renovascular disease.

The strict definition of renovascular HTN requires an improvement or cure (i.e. no further need for antihypertensive therapy in the setting of normal BP) of the HTN following interventional treatment of a RAS lesion.

Takayasu's arteritis

A disease of large arteries.

In some parts of the world such as Japan and India it is the most important cause of RAS.

It has a predominance in female patients.

Diagnosis is based on the presence of inflammation and disease in a number of vascular territories.

Renal presentation is usually with HTN but patients may also have signs and symptoms due to arterial narrowing elsewhere in the body (e.g. cerebral or limb ischemia).

Treatment depends on suppression of local inflammation followed by improvement in kidney blood flow with surgery or angioplasty.

Antiphospholipid syndrome

Renal artery narrowing is common

There is typically coexistent HTN.

Individual case studies have shown that anticoagulation can cure the HTN.

At present the benefit of any other intervention is unclear.

Middle aorta syndrome

This is a rare condition that presents in childhood.

It is a non-inflammatory process leading to narrowing of the aorta at the level of the renal arteries at the aortorenal junction (Fig. 9.2.1).

Treatment is difficult and involves percutaneous interventions and surgical procedures.

The therapeutic approach must take account of the fact that the patients will grow and so any definitive intervention may need to be delayed until growth is completed.

Fibromuscular disease of the renal arteries

The renal arteries are affected in 60–75% of all cases of FMD but other major arteries can be involved, e.g. the carotids (in 15%), vertebral, mesenteric, celiac axis, hepatic, iliac and coronary vessels.

Epidemiology

FMD can be found in 5% of the normotensive population who wish to be a living kidney donor.

Just how common it is as a cause of HTN is uncertain, but it is likely to be <1%.

Predisposing factors

The pathogenesis of FMD is unknown.

It has been suggested that female hormones may play an important role and this would explain the female preponderance.

An association with α1-antitrypsin deficiency and smoking have also been observed in some cases.

Genetics

A familial autosomal dominant pattern has been observed in a few cases of FMD.

Clinical features

The typical presentation is with HTN in young adults, usually female, who have well-preserved renal function.

FMD should always be considered in young patients who present with severe or accelerated phase HTN.

Examination may reveal an abdominal bruit.

Carotid involvement can be associated with a range of neurological features.

Mesenteric angina or claudication may be manifestations of extrarenal FMD.

Investigations

See the section on ARVD below.

As some important FMD lesions occur in the distal renal circulation these may require spiral CT or intrarenal angiography for precise evaluation.

The value of MRA is more limited to proximal disease.

Pathology

There are three main subtypes of FMD:

Intimal fibroplasia
Seen in 5–10% of FMD.

There is circumferential deposition of collagen in the intima resulting in smooth tubular stenoses.

Medial fibroplasia
This is the commonest form of FMD.

It typically affects women in their 4th decade.

There are areas of arterial wall media thinning leading to aneurysm formation; these alternate with regions of fibrosis resulting in a 'string of beads' appearance at angiography (Fig. 9.2.2).

Perimedial fibroplasia
10% of FMD.

Fibrous tissue replaces the outer medial muscle layer leading to severe stenoses.

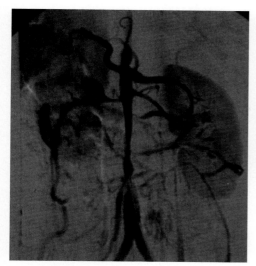

Fig. 9.2.1 Middle aorta arch syndrome.

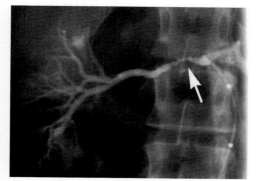

Fig. 9.2.2 Fibromuscular disease. Classical 'string of beads' appearance (arrowed) within the non-ostial segment of the left renal artery.

Treatment

Although the correct management of many ARVD cases is still uncertain, this is not the case for renal FMD.

Where there is significant HTN associated with a RAS >50%, percutaneous renal angioplasty (PTRA) is the intervention of choice.

RAS lesions in the distal renal arteries, as well as complicated or lengthy lesions, may not be amenable to PTRA and thus require surgery.

Follow-up

As progressive narrowing of the renal arteries occurs in a third of patients, the majority of stable patients should be seen annually.

Repeat imaging would only be indicated for those with clinical change, such as worsening control of HTN.

Prognosis

The overall prognosis is excellent.

Unlike atherosclerotic RAS, very few patients develop RAO and renal failure is almost unheard of.

The outcomes after PTRA are favorable with a low rate of restenosis (20%); 36% of patients are cured of HTN with most other patients having a reduced drug burden and improved BP.

The older the age at diagnosis of FMD, the less likely the possibility of cure.

Atherosclerotic renovascular disease

ARVD is the commonest cause of RAS. It is a disease of aging and may present to many different specialties including cardiology, vascular surgery, radiology, elderly care medicine as well as nephrology.

Epidemiology

Post-mortem studies have found an increased prevalence of incidental ARVD with increasing age.

ARVD is present in >40% of patients aged >75 years, irrespective of their cause of death.

The prevalence of ARVD in an elderly (>65 years) unselected general population in the USA was ~7%.

Large epidemiologic studies report an incidence of 3.9 cases per 1000 patient-years, in patients >65 years.

ARVD is frequently found in patients with other atheromatous macrovascular disease.

ARVD is found in ≥10% of outpatients investigated for CKD and 11% of US dialysis patients have a diagnosis of ARVD. However, as will be discussed later, ARVD is likely to be an association and not causative in many of these cases, and this has implications for treatment.

RAS is found in up to 2% of all cases of HTN but, as with CKD, it is unlikely to be causal in many of these cases.

Predisposing factors

Risk factors for development of ARVD, which is an 'inflammatory' disease, are the same as for all atheromatous vascular disease, and include:

- age
- hypertension
- smoking
- hyperlipidemia
- diabetes
- renal failure.

Genetics

Currently the only genetic association reported in ARVD is an association with the DD polymorphism of the *ACE* gene.

Clinical features

ARVD can present with one or more of several syndromes.

Hypertension

ARVD may be found in ~2% of all cases of HTN and >90% of all patients with ARVD are hypertensive.

Despite this frequent association it is often questionable whether a given RAS lesion actually causes the HTN.

In many patients the pattern is often that of severe systolic HTN resistant to medical therapy.

It is likely that in many patients essential HTN more often contributes to the development of ARVD, rather than the latter being important in the pathophysiology of the HTN.

It is this hypertensive renal damage which is also thought to be a major contributor to the CKD seen in many patients with ARVD.

Acute kidney injury

ARVD may present with AKI for a variety of reasons:

- severe bilateral RAS or occlusion (an indication for revascularization therapy);
- accelerated-phase HTN (an indication for revascularization therapy);
- cholesterol atheroembolization (seen in patients with severe aortic atheroma who undergo angiographic procedures or anticoagulation; Fig. 9.2.3);
- damage caused by radiocontrast agents during intra-arterial or CT angiography;
- acute tubular necrosis (ATN) due to a general fall in perfusion pressure;
- in association with use of ACEIs or ARBs (see below).

There should be a high clinical suspicion of underlying RAS if a significant deterioration in renal function occurs after initiation of ACEI or ARB therapy (e.g. >30% increase in serum creatinine).

AKI is not uncommon in patients treated with these drugs and is most often associated with volume depletion during intercurrent illness rather than the effects of a RAS lesion.

Although ACEIs and ARBs can usually be reintroduced safely after stabilization of the patient's circulation, renal artery imaging should be considered as a minority of patients will have significant RAS that might require a revascularization procedure to allow uncomplicated use of these beneficial drugs.

Chronic kidney disease

Many patients with newly identified CKD referred to nephrology clinics are found to have ARVD after further investigation, and this incidental presentation is by far the commonest.

Hypertension is usually also present.

A recent report of the US dialysis population showed that 11% had ARVD.

In most cases HTN rather than ischemia is thought to be the most important factor in the pathogenesis of CKD and ESRD.

ARVD is more often an association of, rather than the cause of, the majority of these cases of CKD and ESRD.

The few histopathological studies in ARVD have shown a pattern of intrarenal injury that is non-specific and hard to distinguish from hypertensive damage.

This has implications for treatment and it is also reflected in the outcomes after renal revascularization procedures.

Cardiac failure

Significant RAS lesions can be detected in patients presenting with cardiac failure.

'Flash pulmonary edema' refers to a life-threatening presentation of acute heart failure with no evidence of significant myocardial ischemia. There is usually severe HTN, and patients have significant bilateral RAS. This is considered a definite indication for revascularization.

More than 35% of elderly patients with congestive cardiac failure (CCF) will have ARVD, and this association is now of growing interest because of the potential for revascularization to improve cardiac function and patient survival.

Non-renal atheromatous macrovascular disease

Many patients have asymptomatic, clinically silent ARVD that is detected incidentally during investigation for other extrarenal atheromatous conditions.

Atherosclerotic RAS can be detected in:

- 30–50% of patients with peripheral vascular disease;
- 10–15% of patients with coronary artery disease;
- 30% of patients undergoing investigation of aortic aneurysm;
- 10% of patients with cerebrovascular disease.

Physical signs and other suggestive features of ARVD

The presence of audible vascular bruits (epigastric, renal or ilio-femoral) in a patient with unexplained HTN and/or CKD is suggestive of ARVD.

Patients with unilateral significant RAS or RAO may have an atrophic kidney.

An unexplained 1.5 cm disparity in bipolar renal length on USS is also an indication to investigate for ARVD.

Investigation

Random cholesterol need not be elevated.

Urinary protein:creatinine ratio (PCR) or albumin creative ratio (ACR) should be assessed. Proteinuria is commonly present in ARVD and is usually reflective of the degree of underlying renal parenchymal damage, as is the case in CKD from other causes.

Two-dimensional USS may show renal asymmetry.

There are a number of options for imaging of the renal arteries.

Magnetic resonance angiography (MRA)

This is non-invasive.

Sensitivity and specificity for detection of RAS are >90% (Fig. 9.2.4).

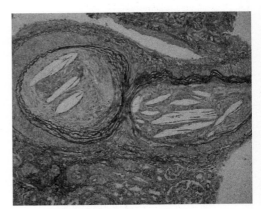

Fig. 9.2.3 Cholesterol embolization within renal arterioles. Atheromatous material is seen blocking the arteriolar lumen, containing several cholesterol clefts.

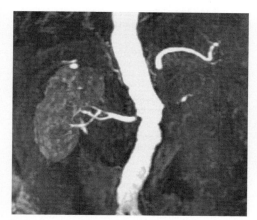

Fig. 9.2.4 Magnetic resonance angiogram showing significant right ostial RAS and left renal artery occlusion.

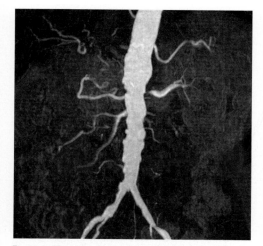

Fig. 9.2.5 CT angiography showing significant left ostial RAS. Note the heavily calcified aorta and left renal artery.

It is of limited usefulness for defining distal disease.

Although the contrast agent was previously thought to be non-toxic there are now concerns over use of gadolinium-enhanced MRA in patients with advanced CKD.

Over 250 cases of nephrogenic fibrosing dermopathy have accompanied use of certain preparations of gadolinium although the majority of cases have occurred in dialysis patients.

Computed tomography angiography or multislice CT
This has a similar sensitivity and specificity to MRA for detection of RAS. CT will demonstrate calcification (Fig. 9.2.5) which, if present at the renal ostium, can make assessment of the degree of RAS difficult.

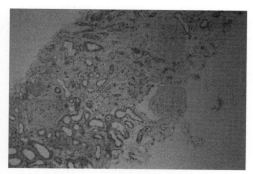

Fig. 9.2.6 Histopathological changes in ARVD. Non-specific tubular atrophy, interstitial fibrosis and glomerulosclerosis; features are often indistinguishable from hypertensive injury.

The main limitation is the risk of contrast nephropathy in patients with advanced CKD.

Duplex ultrasonography
Although time-consuming and operator dependent, this technique is non-invasive and can be very accurate for detection of significant RAS.

Key measurements are peak velocity of renal arterial blood flow and intrarenal vascular resistive index (RI).

Renal scintigraphy
It is often important to assess the function of each kidney in ARVD. This can be performed accurately by use of DMSA and isotopic GFR techniques in combination.

The demonstration of a non-functioning/poorly functioning RAS kidney with scintigraphy can also be useful.

Captopril renography is now rarely used to detect functionally significant RAS as its diagnostic usefulness is limited in CKD.

Renal angiography
Conventional angiography is now reserved to confirm the presence of RAS at the time of a revascularization procedure, or in diagnosis of more complicated/uncertain cases.

Selective renal angiography provides the best means of defining distal RAS lesions.

Limitations of angiography include:
- provides only 2-D images;
- no functional information;
- invasive with a risk of atheroembolism following instrumentation of aorta and renal artery;
- associated risk of contrast nephropathy.

Pathology
Atherosclerotic RAS lesions occur most commonly (90%) at the renal ostia, at or within 1 cm of the aortorenal junction.

It is likely that sheer stress injury contributes to development of atheromatous plaques at these sites in predisposed individuals.

Calcification is commonly seen in association with the plaques.

Bilateral ARVD is present in ~30% of individuals at presentation, and at this stage 25% already have at least one RAO.

The intrarenal 'parenchymal' injury that occurs in association with CKD is non-specific (Fig. 9.2.6), with variable contributions from:

- ischemia;
- hypertensive damage;
- cholesterol atheroemboli.

The natural history of RAS is usually one of slowly progressive stenosis of the renal arteries.

In one study examining the epidemiology of renal atrophy in ARVD, ~20% of kidneys supplied by an artery with a high grade RAS were seen to atrophy (here defined as reduction in length >1 cm) by 2 years, but atrophy was also seen in 5.5% of kidneys supplied by a normal vessel. Systolic hypertension was independently associated with a risk of renal atrophy.

Pathogenesis of renal dysfunction in ischemic nephropathy

Renal dysfunction is frequently seen in patients with ARVD.

There is often an assumption that reduced renal blood flow always accompanies severe RAS lesions and that this is responsible for the renal functional changes.

This is not supported by data on outcome following renal revascularization.

The majority of patients (~75%) who undergo renal revascularization for severe RAS lesions show no improvement in renal function despite restoration of renal artery patency.

There is a poor correlation between severity of RAS lesions and renal function either in groups of patients with different degrees of RAS, or in individual kidneys when GFR is measured isotopically.

Although few would argue that RAS lesions >75% are likely to be functionally significant, it does not necessarily follow that renal function will improve after revascularization – this depends on the degree of irreversible damage that has occurred in the kidney supplied by the narrowed vessel.

For RAS lesions of 50–75% the situation is even less clear; many of these will be functionally insignificant, although some kidneys do improve after angioplasty.

Several pieces of evidence suggest that intrarenal 'parenchymal' injury is most likely due to longstanding hypertension in the majority of ARVD patients who have CKD.

The hypertension likely pre-dates RAS development in most cases.

Pre-existing hypertensive injury would explain why the majority of patients with RAS fail to show an improvement in renal function after revascularization.

Proteinuria is a key marker of intrarenal injury, as it is in CKD from other causes, and it is strongly linked to renal function at diagnosis as well as long-term outcome in patients with ARVD.

Histopathological studies have been limited in ARVD, but changes identified in patients with RAS have demonstrated a picture which can be indistinguishable from hypertensive damage, the exception being those patients with cholesterol atheroembolism, or severe ischemic lesions such as focal segmental or global sclerosing glomerulopathy. The latter are occasionally seen with nephrotic presentations.

Treatment

Historically, repeat angiographic studies indicated that medically managed RAS lesions were at increased risk of progressing to more severe stenoses or to RAO (~10% of cases per year).

This led to the increased use of revascularization procedures in an effort to reduce the risk of loss of functioning renal mass.

This view has been challenged during the last decade and there are a number of ongoing RCTs which will hopefully address this question.

Medical treatment

ARVD is part of a diffuse vascular disease process.

Strategies aimed at slowing progression will reduce ischemic complications and should include:

- lifestyle modification;
- statins;
- antihypertensives;
- antiplatelet therapy.

Lifestyle modification: reduced dietary intake of salt and increased exercise; cessation of smoking.

Statins: can slow progression and may induce regression of atherosclerotic coronary and renal artery lesions. They may also have beneficial effects independent of lipid-lowering including:

- stabilization of atherosclerotic plaque;
- reduction of proteinuria.

Antihypertensive therapy: combinations of several antihypertensive drugs may be required for effective BP control (target <130/80, or 125/75 in those with significant proteinuria). As many ARVD patients have coronary artery disease, left ventricular dysfunction, proteinuria and a tendency to progressive renal parenchymal damage, both ACEIs and ARBs should be the antihypertensive drugs of choice for these patients. Renal function needs to be carefully monitored in case it deteriorates acutely with these drugs.

Antiplatelet therapy: although no evidence exists for a beneficial effect of aspirin in the treatment of ARVD, most clinicians would advocate its use.

Renal revascularization

Renal revascularization refers to a procedure that restores renal artery patency.

During the course of the last 15 years percutaneous treatments have been favored, and now >95% of revascularizations are with angioplasty/stenting.

The remainder are direct surgical revascularization procedures such as renal endarterectomy, bypass with saphenous vein or artificial grafting, or autotransplantation.

There are specific clinical situations where there is almost unanimous agreement for the value of revascularization in ARVD:

- patients with AKI secondary to severe RAS;
- control of severe HTN, when resistant to several (e.g. >4) antihypertensive drugs in combination;
- serious comorbid cardiac disease (e.g. 'flash' pulmonary edema).

There are several other clinical scenarios where there is uncertainty over the benefit of revascularization:

- preservation of renal mass (preventing RAO in patients with significant RAS);
- slowing or halting progressive CKD;
- allowing the use of ACEIs/ARBs (performing revascularization in those patients who need these therapies but in whom renal function deteriorated when they were previously prescribed);
- clinically stable patients with high grade RAS;

Currently, there is no evidence to support the use of revascularization in this second group of patients.

Percutaneous procedures are not without risk:

- arterial dissection, rupture or thrombosis;
- cholesterol embolization;
- contrast nephropathy.

Arterial damage occurs in ~1% of those treated with stenting while cholesterol embolization and contrast nephropathy is seen in a slightly greater proportion.

High quality large randomized trial evidence is required to help guide the clinician with regard to optimal application of interventional therapy.

None of the four published clinical trials addressing this issue has shown a beneficial improvement in renal function or mortality after angioplasty, but each of these trials was small.

One trial has established that ostial RAS lesions should be treated with stent placement, as the rate of restenosis is high with angioplasty alone.

There have been many retrospective studies of revascularization reported from individual centres, and in most of these a definite improvement in renal function is reported in ~25% of patients.

Large scale RCTs are essential in order to determine the overall effects of revascularization, and to help identify which subgroups will benefit from the procedure.

The UK-based ASTRAL trial (completed recruitment of 806 patients in October 2007) reported its initial findings in April 2008 (see below).

A US-based study, CORAL, will recruit a similar number of patients and should publish in several years' time.

Follow-up

All patients with ARVD should be followed up to assess clinical progress, especially as they are at high risk of vascular events.

Monitoring should occur on a 6-monthly basis and will involve assessment of:

- BP control;
- renal function;
- cholesterol;
- urinary PCR;
- new vascular events.

Any significant changes will necessitate review of medications but may also indicate the need for repeat renal artery imaging.

Development of significant proteinuria should trigger consideration of ACEI or ARB therapy, if not already prescribed.

Onset of new vascular events (e.g. intermittent claudication) will necessitate referral to other specialist services.

There is no indication for routine repeat renal artery imaging in these patients.

Prognosis

Patients with ARVD have a high mortality, and this is largely conferred by the influence of their macrovascular comorbidities.

Progression to ESRD only occurs in a minority of patients presenting with CKD.

A recent retrospective study has shown that statin therapy in conservatively managed ARVD patients was associated with a 72% reduction in likelihood of progression of RAS lesions.

Although statin therapy may reduce the risk of progression of atherosclerotic lesions, studies which might show a survival benefit have not been performed..

In a large US epidemiological study the risk of death in patients with ARVD was almost six times that of developing ESRD.

Factors associated with reduced survival are:

- greater extrarenal macrovascular disease burden;
- poor renal function at the time of diagnosis of ARVD.

Dialysis patients with ARVD have an annual mortality rate approaching 33%.

While renal artery revascularization will improve renal function in selected individuals, no trial has shown an overall benefit of intervention in terms of renal function or survival in ARVD populations. The ASTRAL trial unequivocally demonstrates this (see below).

Future prospects

There is a major need to increase the evidence base relating to the management of ARVD, and two large multicentre international trials have either just completed or are still recruiting.

The ASTRAL trial

ASTRAL has recently reported its initial results. In this trial 806 patients with ARVD, in whom the referring clinician was uncertain of whether or not to perform revascularization, were randomized on a one-to-one basis to:

- medical therapy; or
- renal revascularization (angioplasty plus stenting).

The primary outcome measure was to assess whether revascularization affected change in renal function with time, and secondary outcomes were BP control, effects upon cardiovascular events and death.

The initial results encompassed a mean follow-up period of 27 months. At 12 months after randomization, change in renal function, systolic and diastolic BP control, combined renal or cardiovascular end-points and survival were identical in the two arms of the study. Hence, conclusively, at 12 months after treatment there is no benefit of performing revascularization in ARVD patients with auotomically significant but asymptomatic lesions. Whether any longer term benefits might result from intervention will be determined after further follow-up of study patients.

The ASTRAL cardiac substudy is investigating whether renal revascularization beneficially affects cardiac structure and function in a subgroup of ~60 patients who have undergone baseline and 1 year cardiac MRI. The results should be available by the end of 2008.

The CORAL study

This US-based study seeks to recruit 1080 ARVD patients, and is designed to investigate:

- whether renal artery angioplasty + stenting will improve survival;
- the occurrence of major cardiovascular events.

Recruitment is ongoing, and the trial should report in 2011.

As well as providing guidance on the overall outcome of RAS patients treated with revascularization, it is hoped that subgroup analyses within these RCTs may help to identify those patients who are most likely to benefit from revascularization, in terms of renal function as well as cardiac events and survival.

Further reading

Cheung CM, Hegarty J, Kalra PA. Dilemmas in the management of renal artery stenosis. *Br Med Bull* 2005; **73**: 35–55.

Greco RA, Breyer-Lewis J. Atheromatous renovascular disease. In: Johnson RJ, Feehally J (eds), *Comprehensive clinical nephrology.* London: Harcourt; 2007: pp. 725–744.

Moss JG, Kalra PA, Cleveland T, Hamilton G. Renal and intestinal vascular disease. In: Beard JD, Gaines PA (eds), *Vascular and endovascular surgery. A companion to specialist surgical practice.* Elsevier, Edinburgh; 2005: pp. 265–283.

Internet resources

ASTRAL trial site:

http://www.astral.bham.ac.uk

CORAL trial site:

http://www.coralclinicaltrial.org/

The Renovascular Forum:

http://www.renovascularforum.org

Journal of Renovascular Disease:

http://www.journalrenovasculardisease.com

See also

Clinical approach to hypertension, p. 286

Ischemic acute kidney injury, p. 356

Hypertension in CKD, p. 406

Malignant hypertension

Introduction
The term 'malignant' hypertension (or malignant nephrosclerosis) was appropriately coined ~80 years ago. At that time the only available treatment was phenobarbital or other potent sedatives. Life expectancy was <25% at 12 months and <1% at 5 years with uremia as the common mode of death.

Definition
Malignant hypertension (HTN) is defined as:
- acute severe elevation of BP (often >220/120 mmHg)

with
- evidence of grade 3 (flame-shaped hemorrhages and exudates) or grade 4 (papilloedema) hypertensive retinopathy.

There may be other symptoms or signs reflecting end-organ damage, but these are not necessary for the diagnosis.

In those who were normotensive previously and who develop severe HTN (e.g. eclampsia or acute glomerulonephritis), malignant HTN can develop at lower levels of BP (diastolic BP of ~100 mmHg).

There are several other overlapping terms to describe severe HTN.

Accelerated HTN refers to those with severe HTN and a recent increase in BP, but hypertensive retinopathy is at worst grade 3.

At presentation, patients with severe HTN can be classified as:
- hypertensive emergencies.
- hypertensive urgencies; or

Hypertensive emergencies present with acute complications (e.g. AKI, pulmonary edema, stroke, Table 9.3.1).

Hypertensive urgencies may be asymptomatic or present with headache, visual disturbances, nausea and vomiting.

This classification will determine treatment options.

Epidemiology
Before modern antihypertensive drugs became available, ~7% of hypertensive subjects were diagnosed with malignant HTN; nowadays this accounts for <1%.

The average age of onset is 40 years.

Predisposing factors
The risk of malignant HTN is increased in:
- blacks;
- males;
- tobacco smokers;
- nonconcordance with antihypertensive drugs;
- catecholamine crises (pheochromocytoma/cocaine);
- monoamine-oxidase inhibitor interaction with tyramine-containing food; combined oral contraceptive pill (OCP);
- eclampsia;
- secondary HTN (e.g. acute glomerulonephritis, renovascular disease, hyperaldosteronism);
- acute β-blocker withdrawal.

Etiology
The precipitating event is an increase in peripheral vascular arterial resistance.

Such changes usually occur over years in patients with essential HTN, but in malignant HTN they occur over weeks to months and lead to severe HTN.

The rise in peripheral vascular resistance leads to an increased release of circulating vasoconstrictors and other neuro-humoral factors including:
- renin;
- angiotensin II;
- noradrenaline (norepinephrine).

This further fuels the rise in BP.

Other key pathological changes include:

Widespread endothelial damage in arterioles and small arteries with fibrinoid necrosis (microangiopathy). This results in a loss of the normal endothelial control of BP regulation (e.g. nitric oxide synthesis).

Endothelial damage is particularly marked in the kidney microcirculation with histological changes similar to those seen in other thrombotic microangiopathies such as scleroderma and hemolytic uremic syndrome.

Microangiopathic hemolytic anemia develops as a consequence of red blood cell fragmentation by fibrin strands in the microcirculation.

Arteriolar dilation will occur when BP exceeds the normal autoregulatory range. Dilation of cerebral arteries can result in cerebral edema and thus papilloedema.

Clinical features
A thorough assessment of the patient is important, as it will ultimately determine the appropriate method of treatment.

The assessment should answer three key questions:
- Does the patient have an acute complication as a result of severe HTN?
- Is there evidence of long-term end-organ damage?
- Is secondary HTN a possibility?

History
Baseline features to assess:
- duration of HTN and BP values;
- treatment history and concordance with treatment;
- any adverse drug reactions.

Identifying complications/end-organ damage
Symptoms suggesting an acute complication (Table 9.3.1):
- headache;
- chest pain;
- breathlessness;
- confusion;
- neurological deficit.

Symptoms related to long-term end-organ damage:
- ischemic heart disease;
- heart failure;
- cerebrovascular disease;
- peripheral vascular disease;
- renal impairment.

Table 9.3.1 Acute complications of severe hypertension

Acute pulmonary edema
Acute kidney injury
Aortic dissection
Catecholamine crisis
Cerebral infarction
Eclampsia
Encephalopathy
Intracerebral hemorrhage
Microangiopathic hemolytic anemia
Myocardial ischemia/infarction
Subarachnoid hemorrhage

Identifying causes of secondary hypertension
History of any recent 'over-the-counter' and/or prescribed drug therapy:
- NSAIDS;
- combined oral contraceptives;
- corticosteroids;
- sympathomimetics.

History of recreational drug use (e.g. cocaine).

History of renal or urological disease.

Pheochromocytoma might be suggested by:
- episodic palpitations;
- sweating;
- chest pain;
- paroxysmal HTN.

Assessing overall cardiovascular risk
As with any case of HTN the patient's overall cardiovascular risk should be assessed:
- obesity;
- high salt intake;
- excess alcohol;
- lack of exercise;
- diabetes mellitus;
- hyperlipidemia;
- smoking.

Examination
Blood pressure should be measured in both arms, lying and standing.

Clinical signs suggesting an underlying cause include:
- general appearance: Cushing's syndrome/acromegaly;
- reduced peripheral pulses: coarctation of the aorta;
- abdominal bruit: renovascular disease;
- abdominal masses: polycystic kidneys.

Clinical signs suggesting end-organ damage:
- cardiomegaly;
- retinopathy.

Clinical signs suggesting an acute complication:
- neurological deficit: cerebral infarction, cerebral hemorrhage or subarachnoid hemorrhage;
- pulmonary edema: heart failure;
- confusion or coma: hypertensive encephalopathy;
- unequal BP in right and left arms: aortic dissection.

Investigations
Investigations will both support the findings from clinical examination and highlight other complications, such as microangiopathic hemolytic anemia, which may not be apparent clinically.

The following are the essential investigations on admission:
- full blood count and blood film;
- urea, creatinine and electrolytes;
- glucose;
- ECG;
- urinalysis.

Other investigations necessary at the time of admission will depend on the patient's clinical status but may include:
- CXR;
- CT or MRI scan of the brain;
- ECG.

Although the majority of patients presenting with malignant HTN will have essential HTN, there is a greater prevalence of an underlying cause in these patients.

Unless the cause is obvious, further specialist tests are advised as follows:
- serum renin and aldosterone (hyperaldosteronism/ Conn's syndrome);
- renal USS (underlying renal disease);
- MR renal angiogram (renovascular disease);
- urinary catecholamines (pheochromocytoma).

The serum lipid profile is an important additional test as it will help to assess overall cardiovascular risk.

Treatment
When a patient presents with a sudden increase in BP resulting in severe HTN, it is the clinical status of the patient, not the level of BP *per se*, that dictates therapeutic management.

After assessing the patient, it will be clear if the patient has an acute complication of severe HTN or evidence of end-organ damage. There may be some evidence suggesting a secondary HTN cause.

The next stage of the patient's management is determined by the answer to the following two questions.

Does the patient require hospital admission?
Only those hypertensive patients without an acute complication or grade 3 or 4 hypertensive retinopathy can be safely managed as outpatients (this is also dependent on normal blood results).

In these cases, oral treatment can be initiated with regular follow-up at intervals of 2–3 days by the patient's primary care physician.

A further assessment in a specialist HTN or nephrology clinic within a week is mandatory.

Does the patient require intravenous or oral antihypertensive treatment?
Patients presenting with an acute complication (Table 9.3.1) are, by definition, hypertensive emergencies and require IV drug therapy.

These patients should be managed in a monitored environment with continuous ECG recording and regular BP monitoring.

An intra-arterial line for BP monitoring may be useful but is not essential.

In contrast, those patients presenting as a hypertensive urgency can be admitted to a less intensively monitored environment and oral drug therapy will suffice.

Treatment goals in patients with malignant hypertension
The goal of antihypertensive therapy is to reduce the BP to a 'safe' level rather than to normalize it.

More aggressive BP lowering may exceed the ability of the brain to maintain cerebral blood flow.

Intravenous drug therapy for patients with a hypertensive emergency should ideally reduce the mean BP by 25% over the course of 2–4 h.

Oral treatment can be introduced early to allow weaning of IV therapy after 24–48 h.

For those patients presenting with a hypertensive urgency, oral treatment should aim to reduce mean BP by 25% over 24 h.

Choice of antihypertensive medication
There is no definitive study that has highlighted a drug of choice, either IV or oral, in the management of hypertensive emergencies or urgencies.

The only exception is a comparison of nitroprusside and fenoldopam in patients with renal impairment. Fenoldopam was shown to improve natriuresis, diuresis and renal function. Fenoldopam is not licensed in the UK.

Intravenous treatment
In general, nitroprusside is the IV drug of choice in patients without significant renal impairment or myocardial ischemia. In patients with these conditions labetolol or nitroglycerine are preferable.

If one agent is not effective, sensible combinations would include nitroprusside and labetolol or nitroglycerine and labetolol.

The available IV antihypertensive drugs are summarized in Table 9.3.2.

Oral treatment
Oral treatment requires drug therapy of rapid onset (<12 h).

Nifedipine and atenolol are the drugs of choice.

ACEIs (or ARBs) are reserved for patients with scleroderma. These drugs are also effective in severe HTN, but their use in a nonscleroderma population is cautioned especially if renovascular disease is suspected.

The use of sublingual or oral liquid nifedipine is dangerous as the fast absorption of these formulations can result in sudden and large falls in BP.

Intravascular volume assessment
After BP correction some patients may develop intravascular volume depletion and require IV fluid.

Volume depletion can occur as a consequence of prior excessive vasoconstriction or pressure-related diuresis: high BP can lead to an increased GFR and a reduction in renal tubular sodium reabsorption.

This is particularly relevant in the management of patients with acute pulmonary edema as a hypertensive emergency where first-line treatment is often with a loop diuretic.

Follow-up
Patients can be safely discharged once their clinical status has improved and their BP is stable.

Table 9.3.2 Summary of IV antihypertensive drugs

Drug	Mode of action and indications
Nitroprusside	Causes relaxation of vascular smooth muscle.
	Used in most hypertensive emergencies.
	Caution cyanide toxicity and severe metabolic acidosis in renal failure.
Fenoldopam	Agonist action via selective peripheral DA1-receptors, which produces: • vasodilatation • increased renal perfusion • enhanced natriuresis.
	Used in most hypertensive emergencies (no UK licence) especially in renal insufficiency.
Labetolol	Blocks β1-adrenergic receptor sites, α1-adrenergic receptor sites, and β2-adrenergic receptor sites.
	Alternative to nitroprusside.
	Not used in heart failure or catecholamine crisis.
Hydralazine	Causes direct vasodilation of arterioles.
	Only indicated in pregnancy/eclampsia as it improves uterine blood flow.
Nitroglycerine	Preferred agent for patients with myocardial ischemia/infarction complicating hypertension.
Phentolamine	Blocks α1- and α2-adrenergic receptor sites.
	Used exclusively as first-line treatment for catecholamine crises.

The BP does not need to be ideally controlled, but the patient will need regular review every 2 weeks for BP measurement and adjustment of treatment if required.

Further investigations (see above) will need to be planned.

Prior to discharge, a specialist with an interest in HTN should ideally review the patient, or an early appointment made in a dedicated specialist clinic (within 2 weeks).

In the longer term, cardiovascular risk assessment, to take into account primary or secondary prevention, should be undertaken.

Prognosis
With successful early management of malignant HTN life expectancy is similar to patients with uncomplicated HTN.

Further reading
Anonymous. Treatment of hypertensive urgencies and emergencies. *European Society of Hypertension Scientific Newsletter: Update on Hypertension Management* 2006; **7**(28): http://www.eshonline.org/education/newsletter/2006_28_agabiti_rosei.pdf

Elliott WJ. Management of hypertension emergencies. *Curr Hypertens Rep* 2003; **5** 486–492.

Kaplan NM. Management of hypertensive emergencies. *Lancet* 1994; **344**: 1335.

Lip GY, Beevers M, Beevers DG. Does renal function improve after diagnosis of malignant phase hypertension? *J Hypertens* 1997; **15**: 1309.

Murphy MB, Murray C, Shorten GD. Fenoldopam: a selective peripheral dopamine-receptor agonist for treatment of severe hypertension. *N Engl J Med* 2001; **345** 1548–1557.

van den Born BJ, Honnebier UP, Koopmans RP, van Montfrans GA. Microangiopathic hemolysis and renal failure in malignant hypertension. *Hypertension* 2005; **45**: 246.

Internet resources

British Hypertension Society:

www.bhsoc.org/

NICE C G34 Hypertension guideline:

www.nice.org.uk/nicemedia/pdf/Hypertension
Guide.pdf

Hypertension Education Foundation:

http://www.hypertensionfoundation.org/

European Society of Hypertension:

http://www.eshonline.org/

London Hypertension Society (an excellent link to many of the national guidelines on management of hypertension):

http://www.lhs.sgul.ac.uk/links/guidelines.htm

See also

Clinical approach to hypertension, p. 286
Renovascular disease, p. 292
Hypertensive children, p. 304
Hypertensive disorders in pregnancy, p. 310

Hypertensive children

Introduction

Hypertension in childhood is an uncommon clinical problem. When it occurs, its investigation and management is often quite protracted and requires a specialist approach. Although it is increasingly recognized that 'adult' hypertension often has its roots in adolescence, the assumption in children should be that it is likely to be secondary to a specific cause until shown otherwise.

Definitions in children

The definition of hypertension in children is not simple.

BP is directly related to size (both height and weight) in growing individuals.

Tables and charts are available with ranges of systolic and diastolic BPs according to gender, age, height and weight. These are expressed as BP percentiles.

They are an important resource when evaluating BP in both population samples (for research), and individually in clinical practice.

Hypertension is defined as an average systolic and/or diastolic BP above the 95th percentile for these parameters of growth, with measurements on three or more separate occasions.

BP between the 90th and 95th percentiles is now known as 'prehypertension'.

Within the hypertensive range, severity can be categorized into two stages: significant and severe hypertension.

BP >5 mmHg above the 99th percentile requires urgent evaluation.

Table 9.4.1 gives approximate values for 'significant' and 'severe' hypertension and may be used as a very rough guide to BP levels that should be investigated and managed effectively.

Blood pressure measurement

The principles of BP measurement are the same as those for adults. There are major practical considerations, particularly in younger children and infants.

Auscultation is the standard means of taking BP, but automated oscillometric devices are increasingly employed, some of which have been 'validated' by appropriate organizations.

Several cuff sizes must be available to cope with upper arm sizes, whichever method is used. The inner bladder should cover ≥70% of the length and circumference of the upper arm.

In infants it is often necessary to use a Doppler probe to 'hear' the Korotkoff sounds. Even with this method, the 5th sound (disappearance) is commonly absent down to zero and systolic BP is in practice a better indicator.

Blood pressure should be measured on several separate occasions to clarify that it is truly elevated. 'White-coat hypertension' exists in children, and children do not usually remain quiet and physically relaxed for long.

Ambulatory BP monitoring

Ambulatory BP monitoring can be achieved even on quite small children, but requires appropriate devices and expertise to perform and interpret; the results must be evaluated in terms of appropriate normal data obtained using comparable methods.

Invasive BP monitoring

In sick and premature neonates BP is often measured invasively using umbilical or peripheral arterial catheters. This must be compared with appropriate normal values for mean BP.

Indications for measuring BP in children

In older children it is appropriate to take BP routinely in any medical consultation.

In children younger than ~3 years this is less easily recommended but certainly it should be considered if there are any relevant concerns such as renal tract problems.

Screening the pediatric population for hypertension cannot yet be advised, but this may be a future proposal, particularly in adolescence.

Causes of hypertension

Renal diseases predominate as secondary causes of hypertension in children.

Transient hypertension

Blood pressure can be transiently raised in acute nephropathies.

Conditions relatively commonly encountered in childhood include:

- postinfectious glomerulonephritis;
- Henoch–Schönlein purpura;
- hemolytic–uremic syndrome.

Paradoxically BP can also be raised in hypovolemic states, such as seen in nephrotic relapse, associated with vasoconstriction.

Sustained hypertension

In sustained hypertension, it is helpful to distinguish neonates from older age groups.

Coarctation of the aorta and other vascular problems including renal artery stenosis and thromboses relating to umbilical arterial catheterization are important causes in the very young.

The range of conditions associated with sustained childhood hypertension is very broad (Table 9.4.2). These problems can present at any age, but it should be noted that many of the processes are developmental in origin. The most important are discussed below.

'Scarring' nephropathy

The terminology for this group of conditions remains confusing, and this is mainly due to continuing uncertainty as to the fundamental cause of the processes leading to renal scarring in early life (Fig. 9.4.1).

Previously, it was assumed that urinary tract infections in the presence of vesicoureteric reflux led directly to chronic pyelonephritis and permanent scarring ('reflux nephropathy').

This may be the case in some individuals, but more recently it has been recognized that many of these patients are born with renal dysplasia or hypoplasia, without ongoing evidence of vesicoureteric reflux, urinary tract infection or upper urinary tract obstruction.

Table 9.4.1 Rough guide of hypertension values in childhood

Age	Significant hypertension		Severe hypertension	
	Systolic (mmHg)	Diastolic (mmHg)	Systolic (mmHg)	Diastolic (mmHg)
7 days	96		106	
<1 month	104		110	
<2 years	112	74	118	82
3–5 years	116	76	124	84
6–9 years	122	78	130	86
10–12 years	126	82	134	90
13–15 years	136	86	144	92
16–18 years	142	92	150	98

Table 9.4.2 Causes of hypertension in children

Renal
  Acute kidney injury
  Acute glomerulonephritis
  Hemolytic uremic syndrome
  Chronic glomerulonephritis
  Renal scarring and dysplasia
  Chronic kidney disease
  Renal transplantation
  Polycystic kidney disease (recessive and dominant)
  Renal tumors
  Renovascular

Endocrine
  Cushing's
  Conn's
  Mineralocorticoid dysregulation
  Pheochromocytoma

Primary hypertension

Others
  Coarctation of aorta

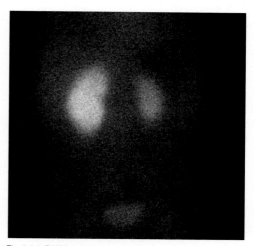

Fig. 9.4.1 DMSA radioisotope scan from a child with a small, scarred left kidney, probably congenital in origin.

The condition can be familial.

Abnormalities of early bladder development may be implicated in some cases, and fetal USS has been useful in delineating progress *in utero*.

Although the onset of renal scarring is a phenomenon of early life, it is often several years before clinical effects are evident, so that the associated hypertension is more likely seen in late childhood or in adults.

Increased renin secretion can be detected before this stage, and hypertension usually pre-dates significant renal impairment.

Renovascular hypertension

This is relatively uncommon as a cause of hypertension in children. Within this group, renal arterial stenosis is the commonest cause and often associated with fibromuscular dysplasia. Neurofibromatosis and other genetic conditions may also be responsible. Worldwide, Takayasu's disease is an important cause.

Endocrine causes

As well as acquired conditions including Cushing's syndrome (often iatrogenic) and pheochromocytoma, there are a number of specific genetic diseases now recognized as responsible for hypertension in a small proportion of children including:

• Liddle syndrome;

• glucocorticoid-remediable hyperaldosteronism;

• syndrome of apparent mineralocorticoid excess.

Liddle syndrome is a disorder of epithelial sodium channel tubular transport and responds to amiloride. Glucocorticoid-remediable hyperaldosteronism (GRH) and the syndrome of apparent mineralocorticoid excess (AME) are further examples of 'low renin state' inheritable conditions.

Primary hypertension

This is increasingly being recognized as an important issue in older children and adolescents.

Blood pressure can be seen to 'track' growth percentile lines in individuals from an early age, and there is also a familial influence on BP that can be detected in childhood.

It is accepted that growth *in utero* and early infancy affects later cardiovascular risk factors. How important these various factors are relative to morbidity and mortality later in life is still incompletely understood.

The rise of obesity in the youth of many societies and its associated morbidity has highlighted environmental factors in the development of hypertension, particularly food and exercise. Weight has now become the major factor in determining BP in this age group.

However, the clinical recognition of primary hypertension in individual children is still uncommon.

Clinical features

Often there are no symptoms or signs even in severe hypertension. If present, these are mainly neurological:

- visual symptoms;
- convulsions;
- hemiplegia;
- frank hypertensive encephalopathy.

The clinician should be particularly aware of facial palsy as a sign in severe hypertension.

Skilled fundoscopy may also alert the clinician to severe hypertension.

Cardiac failure is more commonly found in very young children in whom neurological complications are relatively rare.

There may be specific clues as to the cause of the hypertension from the history and physical examination.

Neurofibromatosis is an important diagnosis not to miss — ask about family history and look for early signs including café-au-lait spots.

Always assess clinically for coarctation, and listen for abdominal bruits.

Poor growth can indicate a chronic cause.

Investigations

Once it is considered that a child has significant hypertension, using the principles discussed in previous sections and in particular taking the BP on several separate occasions, further evaluation focuses on:

- looking for a cause;
- assessing the pathophysiological effects of the raised BP itself on target organs.

Because of the diverse nature of the causes of secondary hypertension, a structured and selective approach to investigation is indicated, depending on the severity of the hypertension. Secondary hypertension should still be considered in even mild cases in children.

Assessment of left ventricular function: echocardiography

An echocardiogram to assess left ventricular function has been shown to be sensitive in children and should be routine in this situation. This can also examine for coarctation as a possible cause.

Assessment of renal structure and function

First-line investigation will always include assessment of renal function and structure.

Because of the relatively high incidence of renal scarring/dysplasia, radioisotope scanning is often performed at an early stage as well as the less-invasive renal USS.

Assessment of the renin–angiotensin system

Routine biochemistry may give further clues, particularly whether plasma potassium is high or low, reflecting the activity of the renin–angiotensin system.

Measurement of plasma renin activity (PRA) itself is more sensitive but the normal range is strongly age-dependent (with much higher normal activity in young children particularly).

PRA may be high in renovascular hypertension, but, when depressed, it can be especially useful indicating a possible mineralocorticoid-mediated cause.

Assessment for endocrine causes of hypertension

More complex biochemistry tests are indicated if hormonal causes are suspected. The diagnosis of the various mineralocorticoid syndromes demands specialist steroid profiling, now also followed by genetic testing for conditions with known gene defects (including Liddle syndrome and GRH). Pheochromocytoma is assessed with plasma and urine catecholamines.

Assessment for renovascular hypertension

The further investigation of possible renovascular hypertension has traditionally been by direct angiography together with renal vein sampling for renin.

Renal isotope scans before and after ACE inhibition have also been helpful.

Newer techniques including MRI angiography and spiral computed tomography have not been extensively evaluated in children but are less invasive.

Assessment for other cardiovascular risk factors

Even when secondary causes are suspected, routine evaluation for the comorbidities associated with primary hypertension is now recommended in older children and adolescents.

These include, particularly in those overweight:

- abnormal glucose tolerance;
- blood lipid abnormalities;
- sleep disorders leading to obstructive sleep apnea.

The presence of acanthosis nigricans on examination is also a strong marker for insulin resistance.

A family history of hypertension, type 2 diabetes and cardiovascular disease will further influence the extent of investigation for diabetes and other comorbidities.

Treatment

Nonpharmacological measures

Lifestyle changes should be considered in the general management of hypertension in all cases of secondary as well as primary hypertension, if relevant.

Weight reduction is usually the most important objective. However, increasing exercise and dietary modification are goals difficult to achieve for many individuals.

In adults it has long been recognized that factors such as sodium intake, healthy diet and exercise are part of the public health scope of BP modulation. This is now increasingly being accepted as a priority in children.

Hypertensive emergencies

The principles of the management of hypertensive emergencies are at least as important as the specifics of the drugs used.

Consideration of the length of time over which the hypertension has developed is very important.

Cerebral autoregulation maintains cerebral blood flow relatively constant within systemic BP limits but over time this range is altered in hypertension. If BP is lowered too rapidly there is a real danger of relative hypotensive damage to water-shed areas, particularly visual cortex, cerebellum and end-arteries. Visual loss may be permanent.

Thus, the principle of slow reduction of severe, chronic hypertension is paramount.

Assessment of fluid balance and renal function is critical.

Beware of hypovolemia, which can cause or exacerbate hypertension.

Neurologic status (conscious level, irritability, fits) will often determine the level of medical and nursing care required.

Also, it can be difficult to decide whether fits in the presence of hypertension are the cause or an effect.

Treatment must be based on the cause of the hypertension if known or suspected.

In renal disease, intravascular fluid overload is often underestimated. Thus, the drug of choice may be a diuretic in the infant or child whose main problem is systemic fluid overload, with hypertension as part of the clinical picture.

Urine output should be monitored.

If serum creatinine is outside the normal (age-related) range, caution is needed in the use of drugs excreted by the renal route.

Hemodialysis or hemofiltration may be required when renal function is severely impaired.

The specific drugs most widely recommended for initial emergency management are:
• sodium nitroprusside;
• labetalol.

Other drugs that have also been recommended include nifedipine, nicardipine and diazoxide (Table 9.4.3).

Start with the lowest dose and titrate upwards.

These drugs have rapid onset, and short duration of action (except labetalol which is therefore not capable of such sensitive BP regulation as nitroprusside.).

Table 9.4.3 Drug doses for hypertensive emergencies

Drug	Route	Dose
Sodium nitroprusside	IV	0.5–8 µg/kg/min
Labetalol	IV	0.25–1.5 mg/kg/h
Nifedipine	Oral	0.1–0.25 mg/kg/dose
Nicardipine	IV	1–3 µg/kg/min
Diazoxide	IV	1–3 mg/kg/dose

The use of nifedipine in the acute phase is controversial.

In adults its use has been associated with extreme hypotension and neurological effects, but in children this has rarely been reported and many centres use this drug in an otherwise well child in small, frequent doses.

In the second phase of management, there is a slow reduction of short-acting drugs and gradual introduction of oral longer-acting drugs.

At this stage it is still important not to reduce BP too quickly.

Usually more than one drug is used, for example a β-blocker, diuretic and vasodilator.

Mild–moderate hypertension
At the other end of the spectrum are children in whom lifestyle interventions have not influenced BP sufficiently to avoid consideration of drug therapy.

In children there is no distinction between drugs used for primary or secondary hypertension.

Single drug therapy should be used if possible, and the general aim should be to reduce BP to the 95th percentile for age.

However, in the presence of ongoing concurrent conditions, particularly CKD and diabetes, there is growing evidence of the importance of lowering BP to well within the normal range to minimize progression.

Data are gradually accumulating about specific drugs in children, but the evidence base, particularly regarding long-term effects, is severely lacking compared to older age groups.

β-Blockers and diuretics are amongst the commoner drug classes used, as they have been available for longer than others.

There has been little experience in children of the use of ARBs until recently.

Within drug groups, newer drugs are usually avoided in favor of those with a greater knowledge base.

Drug combination formulations are best avoided as the relative doses are not necessarily suited to children.

Younger children may be particularly compromised by the relative nonavailability of suitable drug preparations for this age group.

The prescribing situation is now improved with specific drug formularies being available for children.

Specific situations
Renovascular HTN deserves special attention, especially when unilateral. ACE inhibition may precipitate renal infarction and should be avoided at least initially.

ACEIs are the drug class of choice in chronic glomerulonephritis associated with significant proteinuria.

Certain conditions respond to specific treatment:
• amiloride for Liddle syndrome;
• dexamethasone for glucocorticoid-remediable hyperaldosteronism (GRH).

Surgical management can be definitive in a number of conditions, including:
• coarctation;
• renovascular disease;
• tumor-associated hypertension (including pheochromocytoma and neuroblastoma).

Catecholamine-driven hypertension needs specialist advice regarding both α-adrenergic and β-blockade, with particular attention to problems that can occur around surgery for pheochromocytoma.

Follow-up and prognosis

Children with hypertension require continuity of medical care as they reach adulthood, but this is a period of psychosocial change and growth of independence. Medical practice is not traditionally equipped to provide seamless provision of care at such a time, although the development of adolescent and young adult services should help to address this. Because of these factors and others, prognosis in individual cases is often difficult to assess in childhood. More data are accumulating regarding later added cardiovascular risk from conditions in childhood such as nephrotic syndrome, as well as from hypertension itself.

Future prospects

The existence of databases containing BPs and growth parameters for large groups of children reaching adulthood should in time lead to a greater understanding of the possible relevance of interventions in pregnancy and childhood for later cardiovascular disease, but this will depend on social factors as much as on medical knowledge.

In terms of treatment of hypertension in children and young adults, this has thus far been studied only to a limited extent, and it is hoped that the substantial information about drug efficacy and side-effects in older age groups will in the future be mirrored by similar direct evidence in the young.

From a pediatric perspective, hypertension as a significant public health problem in adults has much of its roots in early life.

Further reading

Anonymous. *British National Formulary for children*. London: BMJ Publishing Group; 2006.

Webb NJA, Postlethwaite RJ (eds). *Clinical paediatric nephrology*, 3rd edn. Oxford: Oxford University Press; 2003.

Houtman PN. Management of hypertensive emergencies in children. In: Jacqz-Aigrain E, Choonara I (eds), *Paediatric clinical pharmacology*. London: Taylor & Francis; 2006. pp. 719–725.

National High Blood Pressure Education Working Group on High Blood Pressure in Children and Adolescents. The fourth report on the diagnosis, evaluation and treatment of high blood pressure in children and adolescents. *Pediatrics* 2004; **114**: 555–576.

Internet resources

The childrens British National Formulary:

http://www.bnfc.org

Hypertension Education Foundation:

http://www.hypertensionfoundation.org/

European Society of Hypertension:

http://www.eshonline.org/

The London Hypertension Society (an excellent link to many of the national guidelines on management of hypertension):

http://www.lhs.sgul.ac.uk/links/guidelines.htm

See also

Isolated defects of tubular function, p. 200

Chronic kidney disease in children, p. 462

Renal dysplasia, p. 646

Vesicoureteric reflux and reflux nephropathy, p. 648

Urinary tract infections in infancy and childhood, p. 252

Hypertensive disorders in pregnancy

Introduction

Hypertension is the commonest medical complication of pregnancy and affects ~10% of all pregnancies. BP may be raised before conception or become raised during pregnancy.

Hypertension in pregnancy may be due to:
- chronic hypertension (essential hypertension or secondary causes);
- pre-eclampsia;
- pregnancy-induced hypertension.

The relative incidences of each will depend on the study population.

Women who were born growth-restricted after a normotensive pregnancy are more likely to develop pregnancy-induced HTN in later life.

Hypertensive disorders of pregnancy are classified as shown in Table 9.5.1.

Definition

Hypertension in pregnancy is defined as a BP >140/90 mmHg.

The kidney in normal pregnancy

In normal pregnancy systemic hemodynamics are dramatically altered with:
- increased circulating volume;
- increased cardiac output;
- reduced systemic vascular resistance.

This leads to a high output state with a reduction in BP in early pregnancy.

The GFR increases progressively in the first half of pregnancy reaching a peak of 40–60% above nonpregnant levels which is maintained to the end of pregnancy. This increase is due to increased renal plasma flow due to dilatation of the afferent and efferent glomerular arterioles. The renal plasma flow increases by ~45–50% at 9 weeks gestation and by up to 70% later in pregnancy.

Increased GFR also results in:
- increased sodium filtration and reabsorption;
- increased urate reabsorption;
- glycosuria (due to increased filtered load which exceeds the tubular reabsorbtive capacity).

There is no increase in intraglomerular pressure in normal pregnancy.

Blood pressure in normal pregnancy

Blood pressure falls in the early stages of normal pregnancy and subsequently climbs back to prepregnancy baseline level by term.

There is a reduction in systemic vascular resistance in early normal pregnancy due to increased synthesis of vasodilatory prostaglandins and resistance to vasoconstrictor effects of angiotensin II and noradrenaline.

Measurement of blood pressure

The Royal College of Obstetricians and Gynaecologists (RCOG) guidelines state that the following factors need to be considered when measuring BP in pregnancy (grade A evidence):

Instrument
Mercury/aneroid sphygmomanometer or validated automated device.

Cuff size
It is imperative that the appropriate cuff size is used; it is better to use one that is too big than one that is too small.

Setting
Relaxed, quiet environment, preferably after rest.

Position
Lying at a 45° angle or sitting (cuff at heart level).

Arm
Left or right (use higher value if difference is >10 mmHg).

Dependent arm, if in a lateral position.

Korotkoff sounds
First (systolic) and fifth (diastolic).

If diastolic is persistently <40 mmHg use muffling or fourth sound and make a note.

Chronic hypertension in pregnancy

This is defined as HTN diagnosed before conception or before 20 weeks gestation.

The risk of pre-eclampsia is ~30% in women with chronic HTN.

Advice on antihypertensives preconception
Antihypertensive medication should be changed to a regime which is safe in pregnancy, ideally prior to conception or as soon as pregnancy is recognized.

BP should be stabilized on new medications before conception.

ACEIs and ARBs should be stopped (see below).

Combined renal–obstetric care
Pregnant women with chronic HTN should be managed as stated by the RCOG guidelines.

Combined renal–obstetric care is not required unless there is concern regarding underlying renal disease.

Pregnancy-induced hypertension

This is defined as an elevation of BP >140/90 mmHg in pregnancy, detected after 20 weeks gestation in the absence of proteinuria.

BP returns to normal postpartum (by 3 months).

There is a high risk of pre-eclampsia ~15–25% patients.

Pre-eclampsia

Introduction
Pre-eclampsia (PeT) is a multisystem disorder.

PeT is characterized by:
- vasoconstriction;
- endothelial dysfunction;
- metabolic changes;
- activation of the coagulation cascade;
- increased inflammatory response.

It can be very difficult to distinguish PeT from worsening renal disease in pregnancy.

Table 9.5.1 Classification of hypertensive disorders of pregnancy[a]

Pregnancy-induced hypertension (gestational)
Raised blood pressure >140/90 mmHg
Detected after 20 weeks gestation in the absence of proteinuria
Blood pressure returns to normal postpartum (by 3 months)
Pre-eclampsia
Raised blood pressure >140/90 mmHg *and* proteinuria >300 mg/L or 1+ on dipstick
Detected after 20 weeks gestation
Chronic hypertension
Hypertension diagnosed before conception or before 20 weeks gestation
Chronic hypertension with superimposed PeT (30% of women with chronic hypertension will develop PeT)

[a] National High Blood Pressure Education Programme 1990 and Australasian Society for the Study of Hypertension in Pregnancy.

15–25% of women with gestational HTN will develop PeT.

PeT may occasionally occur with HTN in the absence of proteinuria but with other features such as eclampsia, renal impairment, thrombocytopenia, liver dysfunction or fetal compromise. Occasionally PeT may present with proteinuria without HTN.

Epidemiology

PeT complicates 2–3% of all pregnancies and 5–7% of first pregnancies.

PeT is a major cause of maternal and perinatal morbidity and mortality worldwide with >4 million women developing PeT each year, mainly in developing countries.

Maternal morbidity and mortality
PeT is responsible for 25% of maternal deaths in the USA although in developed countries the absolute rate of maternal death is quite small.

In the UK, PeT accounts for 12 per 100 000 maternal deaths but the risk is up to 20 times higher in developing countries.

2% of women with PeT will develop eclampsia.

Women with PeT have a doubling of risk of death from cardiovascular disease in later life. This risk is highest in women with PeT who deliver preterm and those with recurrent PeT.

Perinatal morbidity and mortality
Fetal mortality and morbidity is considerable and related to the effects of the disease on the fetus and associated early delivery and prematurity

PeT accounts for 15% all preterm births.

Genetics

There is some evidence to support the role of maternal and paternal genetic factors in the pathogenesis of PeT.

A number of genetic polymorphisms have been reported to be more common in women with PeT.

Genes involved include those related to:
- coagulation (5,10-methylene-tetrahydrofolate reductase and factor V);
- folate metabolism;
- oxidative stress;
- components of RAS system.

However, findings are inconsistent.

An increased frequency of the M235T angiotensinogen polymorphism has been reported in women with PeT in some but not all studies.

Polymorphisms in the lipoprotein lipase gene have also been associated with an increased risk of PeT.

Etiology

There are several factors which are recognized to increase the risk of developing PeT in pregnancy (Table 9.5.2).

PeT is characterized by:
- vasoconstriction (increased peripheral vascular resistance);
- maternal volume contraction;
- platelet activation and intravascular coagulation;
- generalized dysfunction of the endothelium (the hallmark of the systemic syndrome of PeT).

PeT can be considered as a two-stage disorder.

Stage I:
There is placental hypoperfusion due to inadequate trophoblast invasion leading to reduced placental blood flow.

Stage II:
In some but not all women this progresses to the multisystem disorder of PeT and HELLP syndrome.

The clinical presentation of PeT depends upon the extent of involvement of different organ systems.

Table 9.5.2 Factors associated with an increased risk of pre-eclampsia (PeT)

Primigravida
Previous PeT
Family history of PeT (mother or sister)
High body mass index (>35 kg/m^2 at booking)
Older maternal age >40 years
>10 years since previous pregnancy
Multiple pregnancy
Underlying medical conditions:
• diabetes
• renal disease
• chronic hypertension
• connective tissue diseases (SLE, especially in presence of antiphospholipid antibodies)
Smoking: reduced risk of PeT

Pathogenesis of reduced placental perfusion

- Clinical observations:

  Reduced placental perfusion and placental hypoxia are important early features of pregnancies complicated by PeT and intrauterine growth retardation.

  PeT is more common in conditions associated with larger placentas, e.g. twin pregnancies.

  There is an increased incidence of PeT in women with medical diseases associated with microvascular disease (e.g. diabetes).

- Remodelling of spiral arteries:

  Normally, the spiral arteries in the intervillous space reduce their muscular coat and become capacitance vessels, thereby enabling greater blood flow in pregnancy.

  This remodelling of spiral arteries fails to occur in PeT and consequently there is increased resistance in these intervillous space vessels.

  The physiological control of trophoblast endovascular invasion depends on interactions between maternal decidua and fetal trophoblast. In PeT a number of abnormalities in trophoblast invasion have been described.

  These changes involve both ambient local oxygen tensions and local immune reactions.

  The oxygen tension increases in the intervillous space at 10–12 weeks and is associated with an increase in concentration of reactive oxygen species.

  The maternal antioxidant capacity is believed to be an important factor in the regulation of trophoblast invasion and defects in antioxidant capacity may impair remodelling of intervillous space vessels.

- Uterine natural killer cells:

  Uterine natural killer cells (uNK) reside within the decidua and interact with fetal trophoblasts through specific receptor–ligand interactions and influence trophoblast invasion.

  Normal placentation requires a balance of inhibition and activation of uNK cells that is mediated by maternal and fetal factors.

  It has been suggested that this balance is defective in PeT.

Pathogenesis of the maternal systemic disorder of PeT
Numerous factors have been implicated in the pathogenesis of PeT (Table 9.5.3).

Several of the more recently reported factors are considered in more detail below.

- Endothelial dysfunction:

  In PeT there is generalized dysfunction of the endothelium.

  Alteration in the normal functions of the endothelium in pregnancy can lead to:
  - vasoconstriction;
  - increased sensitivity to pressor agents including angiotensin II;
  - activation of the coagulation cascade.

  The activated endothelium also induces the production of inflammatory mediators, growth factors and cytokines which can influence vascular tone.

Table 9.5.3 Factors implicated in the pathogenesis of pre-eclampsia

Increased activity of the sympathetic nervous system
Increased responsiveness to angiotensin II and noradrenaline
Decreased activity of the nitric oxide system
Increased levels of:
• endothelin
• proinflammatory cytokines
• circulating microparticles
• circulating antiangiogenic proteins
Reduced levels of:
• relaxin
• antioxidants
Increased ratio of thromboxane:prostacyclin (increased urinary thromboxane B2 in pregnancy-induced hypertension)
Abnormalities in the coagulation cascade with thrombophilia
Hypocalciuria and abnormalities in PTH

Many factors have been suggested as potential triggers for this endothelial dysfunction including:
- the renin–angiotensin system;
- circulating antiangiogenic proteins;
- circulating microparticles;
- oxidative stress.

- The renin–angiotensin system (RAS):

  There are changes in the decidual and maternal RAS in pregnancy.

  Progesterone regulates the RAS and is increased in PeT which may stimulate activation of decidual RAS.

  In PeT there is a reduction in plasma renin levels and to a lesser degree aldosterone levels suggesting increased adrenal gland sensitivity to angiotensin II.

  This increased sensitivity to angiotensin II is important in generating the increased tendency to vasoconstriction in PeT.

  Increased heterodimerization of the angiotensin I receptor AT1 and bradykinin B2 receptor has been proposed as a mechanism for the increased sensitivity to angiotensin II in PeT.

  In addition, antibodies may develop against the AT1 receptor in PeT.

  These antibodies may play a role in enhancing vascular sensitivity to angiotensin II.

- Circulating antiangiogenic proteins:

  Normal placentation involves both angiogenesis and vasculogenesis.

  There are several receptor–ligand systems that are vital to this process including:

  vascular endothelial growth factor (VEGF);

  placental growth factor (PGF).

  VEGF and PGF are proangiogenic growth factors and bind to the receptor Flt-1 (fms-like tyrosine kinase 1) in target tissues.

  Interaction of VEGF and PGF with Flt-1 can be antagonized by the presence of a soluble form of the Flt-1 receptor, sFlt-1.

sFlt-1 is a secreted splice variant of Flt-1 that binds VEGF and PGF and therefore acts as an antiangiogenic factor.

The normal placenta induces a 20-fold increase in circulating sFlt-1 levels by the end of the third trimester of pregnancy.

Increased circulating levels of sFlt-1 are found in PeT and infusion of sFlt-1 in pregnant rats induces a PeT-like syndrome which can be reversed by VEGF administration.

Soluble endoglin (sENG) is another antiangiogenic protein which along with sFlt-1 can induce a severe PeT-like syndrome in pregnant rats.

In human pregnancy it is hypothesized that sENG could act with sFlt-1 to amplify endothelial dysfunction in PeT.

Rising circulating levels of sENG and ratios of sFlt1:PGF have been shown in some studies to herald the onset of PeT.

It is possible that if used together these markers could be of predictive value for development of PeT.

However, it is not clear if they are markers of the systemic syndrome of PeT or are involved in the pathogenesis of the syndrome.

- Circulating microparticles:

Small membrane vesicles released from apoptotic syncytiotrophoblast or endothelial cells have been found to circulate in excess in PeT and to impair endothelial function.

Microparticles have also been found to be procoagulant, inducing disturbances in the coagulation cascade.

- Oxidative stress:

There are many reports of increased oxidative stress in PeT.

In general, therapeutic interventions to reduce oxidative stress have not reduced risk of PeT except in one small study of combined vitamin C and vitamin E therapy after 20 weeks gestation.

Clinical features
Raised BP >140/90 mmHg and proteinuria after 20 weeks gestation.

Persistent severe headache.

Visual disturbances (blurred vision, diplopia).

Epigastric pain, tenderness and vomiting.

Hyper-reflexia.

Edema.

Bleeding diathesis.

Jaundice.

Placental abruption.

Reduced fetal movements.

Intrauterine death.

HELLP syndrome
Hemolysis, Elevated Liver enzymes, Low Platelets.

This is a severe form of PeT in which liver and platelet abnormalities are predominant.

The kidney in PeT
In the systemic syndrome of PeT there is a reduction in GFR caused by:
- decreased renal blood flow due to vasoconstriction;
- volume contraction;
- decreased cardiac output.

In addition, abnormal glomerular morphology leads to a reduction in ultrafiltration capacity, further reducing the GFR.

Renal biopsy features
- Light microscopy:

There is marked swelling of the glomerular endothelial cells which is sufficient to occlude the capillary lumen and result in hypoperfusion, so-called 'glomerular endotheliosis'. This change is not seen in any other form of hypertension and points to the endothelium as the primary target for the disorder.

There may also be mesangial expansion and interposition, thickening of capillary walls and diffuse 'double contours'.

Subendothelial 'fibrinoid' deposits and endothelial and mesangial fat vacuoles may also be seen.

These changes may progresses to acute tubular necrosis or cortical necrosis in severe cases of PeT.

- Immunofluorescence:

There may be IgM and fibrin deposition but no evidence of other immunoglobulin or complement deposition.

- Electron microscopy:

Thickening of glomerular capillary walls due to mesangial cell interposition is commonly seen.

Endothelial cell hyperplasia and hypertrophy, exudation of foamy macrophages, lymphocytes and polymorphonuclear cells and increased glomerular volume have all been reported.

Other systemic manifestations of PeT
In PeT there may also be:
- generalized vasoconstriction leading to hypoperfusion of numerous organs;
- activation of the coagulation cascade and formation of occlusive microthrombi in small vessels;
- loss of fluid from the intravascular compartment, leading to hypovolemia;
- metabolic syndrome with dyslipidemia;
- hyperuricemia.

Investigations
It is important to assess for:
- thrombocytopenia;
- microangiopathy (blood film: fragmented red blood cells);
- abnormal renal function;
- abnormal liver function tests;
- raised urate level (values >270 μmol/L suggestive of PeT);
- proteinuria on either dipstick, spot PCR or 24 h urine protein estimation;
- disseminated intravascular coagulation.

Treatment of hypertensive disorders in pregnancy

Delivery
The only definitive treatment for PeT is delivery.

If PeT presents after 32 weeks this is relatively straightforward. However, PeT presenting at earlier stages of gestation requires a difficult balance between delivery and medical management of HTN and maternal and fetal well-being.

Indications for delivery
Difficulty in controlling BP.

Reduced fetal growth, reversed end-diastolic flow on fetal ultrasound.

Evidence of maternal organ dysfunction:
- deteriorating renal function;
- deteriorating liver function;
- thrombocytopenia.

Antihypertensive medication in pregnancy
Antihypertensive drugs are used for the treatment of mild–moderate and hypertensive emergencies HTN in pregnancy.

The aim is to smoothly reduce BP to levels safe for mother and fetus, avoiding sudden falls.

The ideal target BP remains controversial:
- treatment is mandatory when BP >160/100 mmHg.

The ideal BP target in pregnant women with chronic HTN and underlying renal disease is unknown.

Concerns have been reported about the impact of lowering BP upon fetal growth, although evidence is conflicting.

One meta-analysis demonstrated that lowering maternal BP resulted in an increased incidence of small-for-gestational-age infants whereas a separate analysis showed no overall risk of a small baby in women taking antihypertensive medication.

Treatment of high BP in pregnancy probably has maternal benefits.

Treatment may reduce the risk of severe HTN compared to placebo or no treatment but it is not clear whether it delays the progression or the development of PeT.

Treatment may reduce the risk of fetal or neonatal morbidity (respiratory distress syndrome).

Management of hypertensive emergencies in pregnancy
When a patient has seizures or is at risk of stroke or eclampsia from acutely raised or very high BP in pregnancy (>170/110 mmHg) then IV treatment may be required as an emergency.

Intravenous medication should be given in a high dependency care setting with the aim to reduce the BP over a period ranging from minutes to 1–2 h.

Drug dosage should be titrated against the BP.

Aim for a target diastolic BP of 90 mmHg.

The patient will require intensive monitoring of cardiovascular, neurological, obstetric status and careful monitoring of urine output.

Labetolol
This is given as an IV infusion at 2 mg/min.

It should be stopped when target BP is reached and oral therapy commenced.

It can also be given as a 50 mg IV dose repeated every 10–20 min to a maximum dose of 200 mg.

Hydralazine
This is given as a slow IV injection of 5–10 mg repeated after 30 min to maximum of 20 mg.

This can be followed by an IV infusion if required (50–100 μg/min).

Magnesium sulphate
In women at high risk of seizures magnesium sulphate is the anticonvulsant of choice for both prevention and treatment of eclampsia.

Management of mild–moderate hypertension in pregnancy

Methyldopa
This is generally recommended as first-line treatment for mild–moderate HTN in pregnancy (0.5–2.0 g/day).

Side-effects of drowsiness and depression may occur.

The safety of methyldopa has been established in case control studies.

Long-term follow-up studies of children of mothers taking methyldopa have identified no adverse effects.

β-Blockers
A Cochrane Review demonstrated an increase in small for gestational age infants in association with atenolol treatment and this should be avoided in pregnancy.

Labetolol 0.2–1.2 g/day orally may be used.

Calcium channel blockers
These are frequently used in pregnancy.

E.g. nifedipine 40–80 mg/day orally.

Diuretics
These should be avoided in pregnancy.

Hypovolemia secondary to diuretics may compromise placental blood flow.

Some women with severe edema due to nephrotic syndrome or PeT at an early stage of pregnancy may require diuretic therapy for treatment of severe fluid retention or pulmonary edema.

Angiotensin-converting enzyme inhibitors (ACEIs) and angiotensin receptor blockers (ARBs)
These are contraindicated in pregnancy and should be avoided.

Previously, ACEIs/ARBs were not considered teratogenic in the first trimester. However, a recent study reported a 2.7-fold greater risk of serious congenital malformation with exposure to ACEIs in the first trimester of pregnancy.

Malformations were reported in the cardiovascular and central nervous systems (and in renal tract on post hoc analysis).

Exposure in the 2nd and 3rd trimesters of pregnancy is associated with ACEI fetopathy.

Fetuses with this syndrome have had:
- oligohydramnios;
- intrauterine growth retardation;
- hypocalvaria;
- renal dysplasia;
- renal failure with anuria;
- intrauterine death.

Prevention of PeT

Dietary calcium supplementation
Initial reports showed that supplementation with 1 g daily reduced risk of PeT.

However, subsequent trials produced conflicting results.

Secondary analyses have shown that calcium supplements may be beneficial in women with extremely low dietary calcium intake.

Antioxidants
Vitamin C and E: there is some evidence of reduced risk of PeT and several large trials are underway.

Low dose aspirin
Trials have shown conflicting results.

A meta-analysis in 1991 demonstrated that low dose aspirin reduced the risk of PeT but two subsequent larger multicenter studies reported minimal effects.

Secondary analyses identified that certain groups may derive some benefit from low dose aspirin.

Further studies have shown that a large number of women require treatment to prevent one case (need to treat 69 women to prevent one case of PeT and to treat 227 women to prevent one neonatal death).

Low dose aspirin may be prescribed to women at high risk of PeT:

• previous history of severe PeT;
• diabetes;
• chronic hypertension.

Aspirin should be started after 12 weeks if there are no contraindications.

Follow-up

It is important that women with *de novo* HTN during pregnancy or PeT are followed postnatally to determine whether ongoing medication or further investigation are required.

Investigation may be required to identify secondary or pre-existing HTN.

The BP should be monitored and antihypertensive medications reduced as BP falls.

When the BP is stable, antihypertensive medication should be converted back to the most appropriate regime for the nonpregnant women, i.e. restart ACEI/ARB, diuretic, etc.

Advice regarding safety of antihypertensive medication in breastfeeding women should be sought from a pharmacist.

Proteinuria following PeT can persist for a prolonged period, frequently ≥3–6 months. In this situation referral to a nephrologist should be made as a renal biopsy may be considered to exclude an underlying renal pathology.

Counselling for future pregnancies

Women with a history of PeT are at increased risk of PeT in future pregnancies and should be warned of this postnatally.

The presence of underlying medical conditions should be considered (Table 9.5.1).

The exact risk of PeT in future pregnancies is difficult to determine but is generally lower in a second pregnancy with the same partner. However, in the presence of an underlying medical condition such as CKD the risk may increase with disease progression and increasing age.

Further reading

Atallah A, *et al.* Calcium supplementation during pregnancy for preventing hypertensive disorders and related problems. *Cochrane Database Syst Rev* 2002; (**1**): CD001059.

Broughton-Pipkin F, Roberts JM. Hypertension in pregnancy. *J Hum Hypertens* 2000; **14**: 705–724.

Cooper WO, Hernandez-Diaz S, Arbogast PG, *et al.* Major congenital malformations after first trimester exposure to ACE inhibitors. *N Engl J Med* 2006; **354**: 2443–2454.

Duley L, Meher S, Abalos E. Management of pre-eclampsia. *Br Med J* 2006; **332**: 463–468.

Levine RJ, Lam C, Qian C, *et al.* Soluble endoglin and other circulating antiangiogenic factors in pre-eclampsia. *N Engl J Med* 2006; **355**: 992–1005. [Erratum: **355**: 1840.]

Shah D. Pre-eclampsia: new insights. *Curr Opin Nephrol Hypertens* 2007; **16**: 213–220.

Ventakatesha S, Toporsian, Lam C, *et al.* Soluble endoglin contributes to the pathogenesis of pre-eclampsia. *Nat Med* 2006; **12**: 642–649.

Von Dadelszen P, *et al.* Fall in mean arterial pressure and fetal growth restriction in pregnancy hypertension. *Lancet* 2000; **355**: 87–92.

Wolf M, Shah A, Lam C, *et al.* Circulating levels of the antiangiogenic marker sFlt-1 are increased in first versus second pregnancies. *Am J Obstet Gynecol* 2005; **193**: 16–22.

Internet resources

Cochrane Library, sets of reviews on pre-eclampsia:

http://www.thecochranelibrary.com

Geneva Foundation for Medical Education and Research:

http://www.gfmer.ch/guidelines/pregnancy_newborn

Royal College of Obstetricians and Gynaecologists. Pre-eclampsia Study Group recommendations September 2003:

http://www.rcog.org.uk

Action on Pre-eclampsia:

http://www.apec.org.uk

Pre-eclampsia Foundation:

http://www.Preeclampsia.org

See also

Acute kidney injury in pregnancy, p. 378

CKD in pregnancy, p. 476

Acute kidney injury (AKI)

Chapter contents

Clinical approach to acute kidney injury

Introduction

The term acute kidney injury (AKI) has been introduced to make clinicians aware of developing renal injury, and therefore potentially allow interventions designed to prevent the development of renal failure requiring dialysis. AKI is associated with a rapid reduction in renal function, characterized by a fall in glomerular filtration rate (GFR), with corresponding increases in serum urea, creatinine and cystatin C.

Definition

One of the major difficulties in studying AKI has been the lack of a consensus definition of AKI.

The Acute Dialysis Quality Initiative (ADQI) has proposed that for clinical research purposes AKI be defined as an 'abrupt (1–7 days) and sustained (>24 h) decrease in GFR, urine output or both'.

They have produced a classification system divided into three levels of severity (risk, injury and failure) and two clinical outcomes ('loss' and 'end-stage renal failure') (RIFLE Classification, Table 10.1.1). However these criteria are not intended to guide clinical management of individual patients.

More recently the Acute Kidney Injury Network (AKIN), simplified the RIFLE criteria to use just the first three grades of RIFLE: risk, injury and failure (Table 10.1.2).

Epidemiology

In the USA, the recorded incidence of AKI requiring dialysis has been steadily increasing from 14 per 1000 Medicare hospital discharges in 1992 to 35 per 1000 in 2001. The annual incidence of AKI in the UK has been reported to be 500 per million population (pmp), with some 200 pmp requiring dialysis.

Risk factors for developing AKI include:

- age (more than doubling in patients aged >85 compared with those <65 years);
- male sex;
- ethnicity (more common in African-Americans than in other racial groups in the USA).

Following the introduction of the modified MDRD equation, used to estimate GFR from serum creatinine, it is now generally recognized that many patients who develop AKI do so on a background of pre-existing CKD.

Traditionally the causes of AKI are divided into prerenal, intrinsic and postrenal etiologies (Fig 10.1.1).

AKI in the hospital setting:

- 40–70% prerenal;
- 10–50% intrinsic;
- 10% obstruction.

In the community, obstruction is a much more common cause of AKI (Fig. 10.1.2).

Genetics

Recent work has shown that single point mutations, typically in the promoter region of various genes, can influence mortality in AKI.

There is evidence that mortality in AKI is much higher in those patients with a high TNF-α and low IL-10 producer phenotype, whereas there is a survival advantage for those who are low TNF-α and high IL-10 producers.

Other studies have observed that the risk of developing AKI severe enough to require dialysis, plus failure to recover residual renal function following AKI, is greater in those patients who generate more free radical-derived nitrosotyrosine in response to inflammation and who also have reduced catalase, one of the enzymes involved in limiting hydrogen peroxide activity.

Clinical features

History

Clinical history is vital in helping to differentiate intrinsic AKI from CKD, in terms of obstruction, prerenal causes and also its time course (Fig. 10.1.3).

Prerenal AKI is due to a reduction in renal perfusion, either in terms of renal artery blood flow and/or renal perfusion pressure, or due to intrarenal ischemia (Table 10.1.3).

Similarly the history may reveal causes of intrinsic renal disease: drug-induced toxic or interstitial renal injury, pyelonephritis, and/or underlying vasculitis (Table 10.1.4). Some drugs predispose to AKI, such as tenovir in HIV patients, due to its mitochondrial effects, intravenous immunoglobulins due to osmotic damage, and some herbal remedies.

Total anuria and loin pain may suggest obstructive causes of renal failure (Table 10.1.5). Although obstruction can cause AKI, typically it causes acute on chronic kidney damage.

Clinical assessment

Thorough physical examination is required, not only to assess volume status (see below), but also to look for signs of small vessel vasculitis and/or systemic disorders:

- nail-fold infarcts;
- skin vasculitis;
- arthritis;
- oral ulceration;
- retinopathy;
- atrial fibrillation;
- hypo- and/or hypertension;
- cardiac murmurs;
- hemoptysis;
- abdominal distension;
- organomegaly and/or ascites.

A pelvic examination is mandatory to exclude an enlarged bladder, abnormal prostate and/or gynecological malignancy.

Bedside urine dipstick testing may detect:

- hematuria (due to excess red blood cells, hemolysis and/or myoglobin);
- protein (glomerular, tubular or overflow);
- leukocytes and nitrites (indicating infection).

Volume assessment

In the early stages of AKI due to prerenal etiologies, appropriate fluid resuscitation may well prevent progression to established AKI, and similarly minimize AKI in cases of myeloma/light chain disease, rhabdomyloysis, and post-tumor lysis syndrome.

Table 10.1.1 RIFLE[a] grading of AKI

RIFLE grade	GFR	Serum creatinine	Urine output
Risk	>25% ↓	×1.5 ↑	<0.5 mL/kg/h for 6 h
Injury	>50% ↓	×2.0 ↑	<0.5 mL/kg/h for 12 h
Failure	>75% ↓	×3.0 ↑ or Cr >350 with acute ↑ >45 µmol/l	<0.3 mL/kg/h for 24 h or anuria for 12 h
Loss		Persistent loss of kidney function >4 weeks	
ESRD		Dialysis dependent >3 months	

[a]Risk, injury, failure; loss, end-stage renal disease.

Table 10.1.2 Acute Kidney Injury Network (AKIN) grading of AKI

AKI stage	Serum creatinine criteria	Urine output criteria
1	Absolute ↑ Cr ≥25 µmol/l or ↑ Cr ≥150–200% above baseline	<0.5 mL/kg/h for >6 h
2	↑ Cr >200–300% above baseline	<0.5 mL/kg/h for >12 h
3	↑ Cr >300% above baseline or Cr ≥350 µmol/l with an acute rise of ≥45 µmol/l	<0.3 mL/kg/h for 24 h or anuria for 12 h

* refers to increase in serum creatinine within a 48 h period

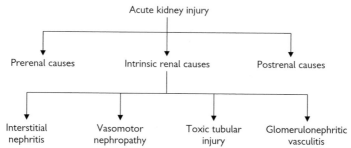

Fig. 10.1.1 Broad categories of AKI.

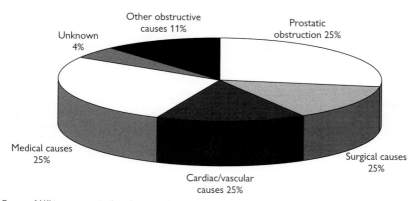

Fig 10.1.2 Causes of AKI in a community-based survey.

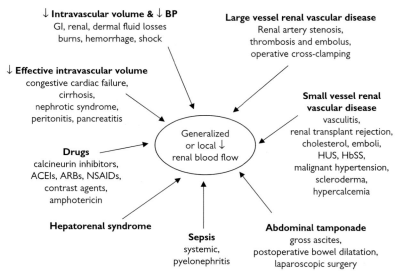

↓ Intravascular volume & ↓ BP
GI, renal, dermal fluid losses
burns, hemorrhage, shock

Large vessel renal vascular disease
Renal artery stenosis,
thrombosis and embolus,
operative cross-clamping

↓ Effective intravascular volume
congestive cardiac failure,
cirrhosis,
nephrotic syndrome,
peritonitis, pancreatitis

**Small vessel renal
vascular disease**
vasculitis,
renal transplant rejection,
cholesterol, emboli,
HUS, HbSS,
malignant hypertension,
scleroderma,
hypercalcemia

Drugs
calcineurin inhibitors,
ACEIs, ARBs, NSAIDs,
contrast agents,
amphotericin

Generalized
or local ↓
renal blood flow

Hepatorenal syndrome

Sepsis
systemic,
pyelonephritis

Abdominal tamponade
gross ascites,
postoperative bowel dilatation,
laparoscopic surgery

Fig. 10.1.3 AKI due to causes of reduced renal blood flow.

Table 10.1.3 Causes of prerenal AKI

Reduced renal artery blood flow
Volume losses
Hemorrhage
GI fluid losses: vomiting/diarrhea
Burns
Excessive diuresis
Renal arterial obstruction
Renal artery thrombosis/embolus
Renal artery stenosis
Aortic aneurysm
Intra-renal ischemia
Cardiogenic shock
Systemic sepsis
Hepatorenal failure
Anaphlyactic shock
Nephrotic syndrome
Abdominal compartment syndrome
Page kidney
Renal vein thombosis
Drugs
• COX-1 and -2 inhibitors
• ACEIs and ARBs
• Calcineurin inhibitors

However, in cases of established AKI, rapid fluid administration may well result in pulmonary edema. Review of clinical fluid balance charts and daily weights aids assessment along with history of fluid losses and reduced fluid intake.

Young patients can compensate for volume depletion to a far greater extent than the elderly, and may well maintain a 'normal' brachial arterial pressure with no demonstrable postural hypotension. However, the pulse pressure may be narrowed due to increased sympathetic nervous activity.

Typically hypovolemic patients have cooled peripheries, but patients with septic shock and/or liver failure, who may also have renal hypoperfusion, may have warm peripheries. The capillary refill test is a quick bedside test used to assess volume status; a normal refilling of the nail-bed capillaries takes <2 s after release of pressure.

In hypovolemic patients the jugular venous pulse (JVP) may well be depressed, and patients may need to be tilted head-down before it becomes visible. However, the JVP is an assessment of right atrial filling pressure, and not a measurement of cardiac output. Thus although a low JVP is associated with circulatory underfilling, an elevated JVP does not equate with adequate cardiac output and renal perfusion, particularly in cases of systemic sepsis, liver failure, hypoalbuminemia, severe metabolic acidosis and cardiac failure.

Fluid resuscitation should be designed to restore tissue perfusion (Fig. 10.1.4) and maintain tissue viability (Table 10.1.6). In clinical practice, it can be very difficult to assess the adequacy of the circulating volume, as this depends upon both vasomotor tone (systemic vascular resistance) and cardiac contractile performance.

In a previously normotensive patient, tissue organ flow, including renal perfusion, should be maintained with a mean arterial pressure of ≥65 mmHg, with fluid and/or vasopressors.

If patients are preload (volume) responsive (Table 10.1.3), then fluid resuscitation will be beneficial, by increasing cardiac output and renal perfusion, whereas if they are not, then vasopressors should be tried, as additional fluids may well be detrimental (treatment algorithm Fig. 10.1.4).

In the nonventilated patient, preload responsiveness can be assessed by monitoring the dynamic CVP during spontaneous respiration, and also by assessing the change in pulse density of the finger oxygen saturation probe (a change in CVP of >1 mmHg and a change in pulse

Table 10.1.4 Causes of intrinsic AKI

Small vessel vascular disease

Occlusion
- Cholesterol emboli
- Cryoglobulinemia
- HUS/TTP
- DIC
- Plasmodium malaria
- Sickle cell crisis
- Eclampsia

Vasculitis
- Microscopic polyangiitis

Wegeners granulomatosis
- SLE
- Henoch–Schönlein purpura
- Hyperacute renal transplant rejection

Hypertension
- Malignant hypertension
- Scleroderma

Acute glomerulonephritis

Crescentic rapidly progressive GN
- Anti-GBM disease
- Postinfectious GN
- Idiopathic

Interstitial nephritis

Drug-associated
- Antibiotics
- NSAIDs

Post-infection
- Leptospirosis
- Epstein–Barr virus

Drug toxicity
- Aminoglycosides
- Tenovir

Toxins
- Radiocontrast media
- Myoglobin
- Hemolysis
- Myeloma/light chains
- Snake/spider venom

Heavy metals
- Cisplatin

Poisons
- Plant
- Drugs
- Chemical (e.g. ethylene glycol)

Crystals
- Urate
- Indinavir
- Oxalate

Infiltration
- Sarcoid
- Lymphoma

Infection

Acute pyelonephritis
- Bacterial infection

Immunological

Renal transplant
- Cellular rejection

Table 10.1.5 Causes of post-renal (obstructive) AKI

Intrinsic

Intraluminal
- Calculus
- Blood clot
- Sloughed papilla

Intramural
- Ureteric malignancy
- Ureteric stricture (TB)
- Post-irradiation fibrosis
- Bladder cancer
- Prostatic hypertrophy

Extrinsic

Extramural
- Retroperitoneal fibrosis
- Pelvic malignancy
- Ureteric ligation

density >10% suggests that the patient will be preload responsive).

Volume loading in patients with CVP >12 mmHg is unlikely to increase cardiac output.

During mechanical ventilation, the variation in cardiac stroke volume, or finger pulse pressure variability during the ventilatory cycle, can also predict preload responsiveness.

In patients predicited to be volume responsive, a fluid bolus of 2 mL/kg of colloid or 3 mL/kg of crystalloid over 10 min should be given, and then the patient should be reassessed.

Investigations

All patients should have urine stick testing performed to detect blood, protein, glucose and nitrites. Depending upon the history and physical examination other investigations may be required (Table 10.1.7).

Urinary electrolytes

Urinary electrolytes may be helpful in determining those patients with reversible prerenal AKI.

Spot urinary sodium

Urinary sodium excretion can be affected by pre-existing CKD and prior treatment with diuretics.

Urinary sodium concentration on a spot urine sample may not be discriminant if normal or increased, but would suggest possible volume responsive in AKI if:
- <10 mmol/L in a healthy young adult;
- <20 mmol/L in an elderly patient.

Importantly, following relief of urinary obstruction, the patient may be intravascularly volume-depleted but still have a normal or increased spot urine sodium concentration.

Spot urine osmolality

Spot urine osmolality may be increased in volume responsive AKI, but is also normally increased in the immediate postsurgical period, due to changes in vasopressin release and renal free water clearance.

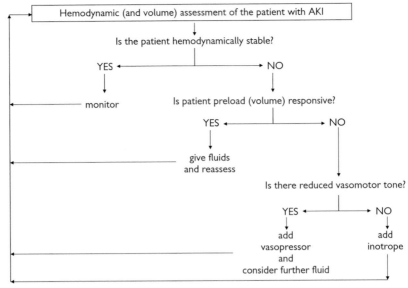

Fig. 10.1.4 Clinical approach to volume and vasopressor management in the patient with AKI.
After each step, reassess patient. Typical vasopressor: noradrenaline. Typical inotrope: dobutamine. Vasomotor tone typically assessed invasively as SVR (systemic vascular resistance).

Table 10.1.6 Assessment of tissue perfusion

Measured variable	Desired range
Mean arterial blood pressure	>65 mmHg
S_VO_2 mixed venous oxygenation	>70% sat. (4–6 kPa)
$S_{CV}O_2$ central venous oxygenation	>65% sat.
Arterial/venous lactate	<2 mmol/L(A) or <2.5 mmol/L (V)
Metabolic acidosis – base excess	± 2 mmol/L
Capillary refill time	<2 s
Tachycardia	<100 beats/min

Fractional excretion of sodium and urea

To try and improve the diagnostic accuracy of urine biochemistry in AKI, ratios of sodium and urea excretion relative to creatinine have been evaluated.

The fractional excretion of sodium (FE_{Na}) and fractional excretion of urea (FE_{Urea}) are useful parameters.

$$FE_{Na} = \frac{\text{urinary Na} \times \text{plasma Cr} \times 100}{\text{plasma Na} \times \text{urinary Cr}}$$

The normal FE_{Na} is >1% and FE_{Urea} is >45%.

In those patients with prerenal AKI:
- FE_{Na} <1%;
- FE_{Urea} <35%.

Other causes of a FE_{Na} <1% include:
- cardiac failure;
- contrast nephropathy;
- heme pigment nephropathy.

The FE_{Urea} is a better discriminant of prerenal AKI than FE_{Na}, as even when patients have been given diuretics the FE_{Urea} will be <35%, whereas the FE_{Na} is often >2%. In established AKI, both are elevated.

In the hepatorenal syndrome the FE_{Urea} is low, and the urinary sodium concentration is typically 10 mmol/L.

Novel biomarkers of AKI

Traditionally urea and creatinine have been used to assess renal function. However, following AKI, serum creatinine does not increase for some 24–72 h, and similarly there is a delay between the recovery of residual renal function and a fall in serum creatinine. This has led to the search for other biomarkers to detect AKI at an earlier stage. For example, cystatin C tends to increase ≥24 h prior to creatinine rises.

Other urinary biomarkers investigated include:
- neutrophil gelatinase-associated lipocalin;
- IL-18;
- kidney injury molecule-1;
- N-acetyl-β-(D)-glucosinidase.

Table 10.1.7

Investigation	Comment
Urine	
Urine stick testing	
Blood	Renal or lower urinary tract inflammation/myoglobin
Protein	Glomerular or renal tubular proteinuria
Nitrites	Urinary infection
Urine culture	Urinary infection
Microscopy/cytology	Red cell casts in glomerulonephritis and vasculitis
	Oxalate/indinavir/uric acid stones
	Malignant cells
	Eosinophiluria in interstitial nephritis
Biochemistry	
Serum	Urea, creatinine, cystatin C raised in AKI
	Hyperkalemia and metabolic acidosis
	Hypocalcemia and hyperphosphatemia in rhabdomyolysis
	Hypercalcemia in myeloma, sarcoid, malignancy
	Hypoalbuminemia in nephrotic syndrome, cirrhosis
	Bilirubin raised in liver disease, leptospirosis
	LDH raised in malignancy and hemolysis
	CPK raised in rhabdomyloysis, sickle cell crisis
	Haptoglobins reduced in hemolytic uremic syndrome
	ACE raised in sarcoid
	CRP raised in inflammation and sepsis
	Uric acid raised in tumor lysis syndrome, sickle cell crisis
Urine	Fractional excretion of sodium and urea
	Proteinuria; quantitation: protein/creatinine ratio
Hematology	
Full blood count	Eosinophilia in vasculitis, cholesterol emboli
	Thrombocytopenia in hemolytic uremic syndrome
Blood film	Red cell fragments in hemolytic uremic syndrome
	Malaria
Coagulation studies	Disseminated intravascular coagulation in sepsis, burns, fat embolism, eclampsia, amniotic fluid embolism, severe heat stroke, liver failure and neoplasia
Immunology	
Immunoglobulins	Immunoparesis, paraprotein/light chains in myeloma
Autoantibodies	ANA and dsDNA in SLE
	RhF in cryoglobulimemia
	ANCA in vasculitis, WG, MPA
	Proteinase 3 (PR-3) in WG, MPA
	Myeloperoxidase (MPO) in WG, MPA
	Antiglomerular basment membrane in Goodpasture's syndrome
Complement	Low C3 and/or C4 in SLE
	Low C4 in cryoglobulinemia
	Low serum complement activity (CH_{50}) acute post-streptococcal GN, type II MPGN, subacute bacterial endocarditis, 'shunt' nephritis, and cryoglobulinemia
Cryoglobulins	Cryoglobulin in hepatitis C, SLE and lymphoma
Serum amyloid A	Serum amyloid A protein in AA amyloid
Urine free light chain	Bence Jones protein/free light chain in urine in myeloma and AL amyloid
Microbiology	
Blood	Cultures to exclude bacteremia
Specific infections	Leptospirosis, legionella, viral hemorrhagic fevers
Virology	HIV (FSGS, increased risk of prerenal AKI in patients taking HAART)
	HBV/HVC (cryoglobulinemia and GN, also risk of transmission on hemodialysis)

Investigations to consider in the patient with AKI. The investigations required will vary in individual cases depending upon history and physical examination: systemic lupus erythematosis (SLE); Wegener's granulomatosis (WG); membranoproliferative glomerulonephritis (MPGN); microscopic polyangiitis (MPA); human immunodeficiency virus (HIV); hepatitis B and C viruses (HBV/HCV); glomerulonephritis (GN); HAART (highly active antiretroviral therapy).

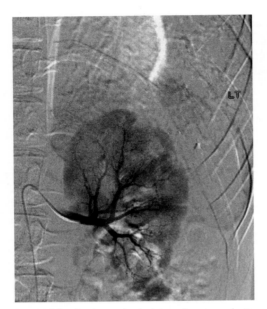

Fig. 10.1.5 Renal angiogram showing intrarenal aneurysms due to polyarteritis nodosa.

Some of these biomarkers can increase within 24 h of AKI, and similarly some have been shown to predict requirement for dialysis. However, in adult practice these biomarkers are not as helpful as in pediatric practice, as many adult patients have underlying CKD.

Renal imaging

Ultrasound

Ultrasound scanning (USS) is a key investigation and provides valuable information on renal size and intrarenal echogencity.

Small kidneys suggest pre-existing CKD.

USS can help to exclude obstruction by detecting bladder, prostate and pelvic pathology, and hydronephrosis. In acute obstruction, the renal pelvis may not have had time to dilate.

CT scan

CT-KUB (kidney ureters and bladder) scanning without contrast is now used to image renal/ureteric calculi, sloughed papillae.

Contrast CT is used to investigate extrinsic obstruction. The risk of contrast nephropathy can be reduced by choosing a hypo-osmolar contrast agent. Preloading the patient with isotonic bicarbonate (3 mL/kg/h for 1 h precontrast, and then 1 mL/kg/h for 6 h post CT scan) may also be beneficial.

Nephrostomy and contrast studies

In cases of obstruction, it is often easier and quicker to relieve obstruction by antegrade nephrostomy, and then subsequently perform appropriate retrograde investigations, and/or stenting.

Renal vascular imaging

Color Doppler USS may be helpful in assessing major renal arterial and venous flow, but MRI with contrast may be required. However, gadolinium contrast media may occasionally cause nephrogenic fibrosing dermopathy.

In AKI, renal function may not be sufficient for nuclear medicine imaging.

Occasionally formal renal angiography is required in cases of larger vessel vasculitis, such as polyartertis nodosa (Fig. 10.1.5).

Indications for renal biopsy

Renal biopsy should be performed when the history, examination, or laboratory tests suggest the possibility of an underlying systemic disorder amenable to specific treatment. It may also be indicated in those cases where there is doubt as to the cause of AKI (no convincing history or documentation of vasomotor renal injury), when renal recovery has been unusually delayed, or when there is the possibility of a second pathology, such as a drug-induced interstitial nephritis.

Treatment

Specific measures to reverse AKI

Despite years of research, no specific pharmacological treatment has been proven to prevent or shorten AKI. Loop diuretics and dopamine should not be routinely administered.

Patients with prerenal AKI should be appropriately resuscitated with fluids and/or vasopressors as outlined above.

Nephrotoxic drugs should be discontinued.

Renal obstruction and abdominal tamponade should be relieved.

The abdominal compartment syndrome should be considered in postoperative patients, and in those with a distended abdomen. The intra-abdominal pressure (IAP) can be measured by transducing the intravesical pressure. A compartment syndrome is present when the absolute IAP is ≥20 mmHg, or the difference between the mean systemic arterial pressure and the IAP is <60 mmHg.

Specific pharmacological treatments are appropriate in special circumstances to prevent or reduce AKI, including rasburicase in tumor lysis syndrome, and fomepizole in ethylene alcohol poisoning. Mannitol and sodium bicarbonate have been advocated in the management of rhabdomyolysis, but there is no evidence to support any additional benefit from aggressive fluid resuscitation alone.

More recently, in the intensive care setting, it has been suggested that strict blood glucose control can reduce the incidence of AKI.

Potential nephrotoxins, such as aminoglycosides, should be avoided, and iodine-based contrast studies minimized. If contrast studies are necessary then potential nephrotoxicty should be minimized by using the smallest volume of hypo-osmolar contrast required for the study. There may be an additional benefit of using sodium bicarbonate prophylaxis. Recently phosphate-containing enemas have been described causing AKI due to acute nephrocalcinosis.

Sepsis should be actively sought and aggressively treated.

Drugs known to potentially reduce renal perfusion, including as NSAIDs, ACEIs, ARBs and calcineurin inhibitors should be avoided if at all possible.

Nutrition

Nutritional support for patients with AKI must take into account not only the specific metabolic disturbances associated with AKI, but also the underlying disease process. Enteral nutrition is preferred, and as a general rule patients with AKI should receive 20–35 kcal/kg/day, with up to a maximum of 1.7 g amino acids/kg/day if catabolic and receiving continuous renal replacement therapy. The majority of enteral and parenteral supplements designed for patients with AKI are low in sodium. Electrolytes should be closely monitored to avoid hyper- and hypokalemia, and hypophosphatemia. Trace elements and water-soluble vitamins should be supplemented where appropriate.

Treatment of the complications of AKI

Hyperkalemia

Hyperkalemia in AKI may lead to cardiac arrest, due to alteration in the cardiac action potential resulting in characteristic ECG changes (Fig. 10.1.6).

ECG changes occur when the plasma potassium concentration increases to ~5.5 mmol/L or more. These include:
- 'tenting' of the T waves;
- prolongation of the QT interval.

More severe hyperkalemia causes:
- widening of the QRS complex;
- suppression of the P wave;
- lengthening of the PR interval.

Calcium administration (10 mL of 10% calcium gluconate, for patients aged >60 years) is the standard medical management of hyperkalemia in patients with ECG changes beyond simple T-wave 'tenting'. This should be repeated until the ECG changes reverse.

As calcium does not affect the serum potassium concentration, other treatments are required to reduce hyperkalemia. These include:
- IV insulin and glucose (10 U rapidly acting insulin + 50 mL 50% dextrose);
- salbutamol (10 mg via nebulizer);
- isotonic sodium bicarbonate (volume depending upon patient volume assessment);
- cation exchange resins (sodium or calcium polystyrene sulphonate 15 g by mouth 6-hourly or 15–30 g per rectum 6-hourly, with lactulose 20 mL qds).

In refractory cases dialysis is required.

Pulmonary edema

Salt and water overload in AKI leads to pulmonary edema. In some cases this is iatrogenic due to overzealous fluid administration.

Patients should be treated with:
- supplemental oxygen (CPAP +5 to +10 mmHg, or a rebreathing mask may be required);
- opiates;
- parenteral nitrate infusion;
- loop diuretics (furosemide infusion 5–10 mg/h).

In patients with oligoanuric AKI, dialysis may be required.

Postobstructive diuresis

Following relief of renal obstruction, and also in the polyuric phase of recovering AKI, fluid balance may be problematic, due to the loss of water and electrolytes. As well as loss of sodium and potassium, patients may develop tetany and/or fits due to profound hypocalcemia/hypomagnesemia. Careful monitoring of daily weights and electrolytes is mandatory to determine appropriate replacement.

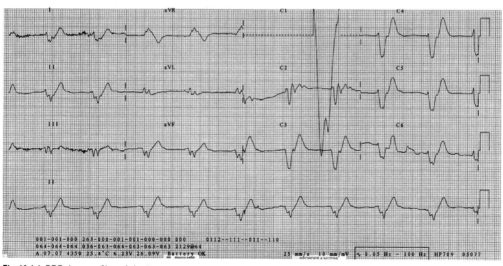

Fig. 10.1.6 ECG changes of hyperkalemia.

Table 10.1.8 Indications for renal replacement therapy in patients with AKI

Biochemical indications	
Potassium	Refractory hyperkalemia >6.5 mmol/L
Urea	Serum urea >30 mmol/L
Creatinine	×3.0 ↑ baseline serum creatinine
	or an absolute SCr >355 μmol/l
	or acute↑ SCr >44 μmol
Metabolic acidosis	Refractory metabolic acidosis pH ≤7.1
Other electrolyte disturbances	Refractory hypo- or hypernatremia, hypercalcemia
Tumor lysis syndrome	Hyperuricemia and hyperphosphatemia
Urea cycle defects and organic acidurias	Hyperammonemia, methylmalonic acidemia
Clinical indications	
Urine output	Urine output <0.3 mL/kg for 24 h or
	or absolute anuria for 12 h
Multiple organ failure	AKI with multiple organ failure
Volume overload	Refractory volume overload
	Create intravascular space for plasma and other blood product infusions and nutrition
End-organ damage	Pericarditis, encephalopathy, neuropathy, myopathy, uremic bleeding
Poisoning	Severe poisoning or drug overdose
Thermoregulatory disturbance	Severe hypothermia or hyperthermia

Initiation of renal dialysis

The decision to start renal replacement therapy depends on the clinical assessment of the individual patient. However, general guidelines are set out in Table 10.1.8.

Follow-up

Earlier studies demonstrated that renal function may continue to improve following AKI, for up to 6 months or even longer in some cases, such as in scleroderma renal crisis. Thus following recovery of renal function from AKI, patients should have their renal function checked at 6 months. If the patient is left with CKD, continued follow-up is required as patients may progress to ESRD.

Prognosis

Survival and renal recovery following AKI

For hospital inpatients an increase in serum creatinine is associated with a stepwise increased risk of mortality.

The relative risk of mortality increases:
- ×4 for a 27 μmol/L rise in creatinine;
- ×14 for a 180 μmol/L increase in creatinine.

Despite the increased risk of death associated with AKI, the overall survival of patients with AKI and of those requiring dialysis has improved over time. Mortality fell from ~40% in 1988 to 20% in patients with AKI and to 27% in patients with AKI requiring dialysis in 2002.

Traditionally renal recovery following severe AKI with acute tubular injury takes around 21 days, although this varies according to the severity of the original insult, pre-existing kidney disease and subsequent clinical course.

As more patients are surviving AKI, it is now becoming clearer that renal recovery is often only partial. Some 7% of survivors become dialysis dependent within 3 years of the AKI event, and this rises to 28% in those patients with pre-existing CKD.

Summary

The incidence of AKI is increasing in the hospital setting, and is more common with increasing age, male sex, and pre-existing CKD. The majority of cases result from multiple insults: dehydration, drugs in conjunction with inflammation and/or sepsis. Patients should be appropriately resuscitated to achieve a mean arterial BP >65 mmHg, and fluids to maximize cardiac preload responsiveness, without overloading the patient. Depending upon the individual history and examination, obstruction may need to be excluded by renal imaging, and other investigations obtained to establish the cause of AKI.

Future prospects

Changes in serum creatinine measurements are a relatively late feature of AKI. Although the introduction of urinary biomarkers has been shown, to precede changes in creatinine, particularly in pediatric practice, the current biomarkers cannot predict the severity of the insult. However, newer biomarkers are being investigated, and in the future we will probably use a panel of urinary biomarkers to detect both glomerular and tubular injury. This will have important applications in cancer chemotherapeutic regimens, to aid dose adjustments in those patients developing AKI. Biomarkers may also be used to predict the severity of renal injury, and thus the need for renal replacement therapy.

Further reading

Bellomo R, Kellum JA, Ronoc C. Defining acute renal failure: physiological principles. *Intens Care Med* 2004; **30**: 33–37.

Bellomo R, Ronco C, Kellum JA, Mehta RL, Palevsky P, and the ADQI workgroup. Acute renal failure – definition, outcome measures, animal models, fluid therapy and information technology needs. The second international consensus conference of Acute Dialysis Quality Initiative (ADQI) Group. *Crit Care* 2004; **8**: R204–R212.

Briguori C, Airoldi F, D'Andrea D, *et al*. Renal Insufficiency Following Contrast Media Administration Trial (REMEDIAL). A randomized comparison of 3 preventive strategies. *Circulation* 2007; **115**: 1211–1217.

Cano N, Fiaccadori E, Tesinsky P, *et al*. ESPEN guidelines on enteral nutrition: adult renal failure. *Clin Nutr* 2006; **25**: 295–310.

Druml W. Nutritional management of acute renal failure. *J Renal Nutr* 2005; **15**: 63–70.

Feest TG, Round A, Hamad S. Incidence of severe acute renal failure in adults: results of a community based study. *Br Med J* 1993; **306**: 481–483.

Ho KM, Sheridan DJ. Meta-analysis of frusemide to prevent or treat acute renal failure. *Br Med J* 2006; **333**(7565): 420–425.

Mehta RL, Kellum JA, Shah SV, Molitoris BA, Ronco C, Warnock DG, Levin A. AKIN: acute kidney injury network: report of an initiative to improve outcomes in acute kidney injury. *Ind J Nephrol* 2007; **17**: 1–3.

Metcalfe W, Simpson M, Khan IH, *et al*. Acute renal failure requiring renal replacement therapy: incidence and outcome. *Q J Med* 2002; **95**: 579–583.

Kreymann KG, Berger MM, Deutz NEP *et al*. ESPEN guidelines on enteral nutrition: intensive care. *Clin Nutrition* 2006; **25**: 210–223.

Mishra J, Ma Q, Prada A, *et al*. Identification of neutrophil gelatinase-associated lipocalin as a novel early urinary biomarker for ischemic renal injury. *J Am Soc Nephrol* 2003; **14**: 2534–2543.

Nash K, Hafeez A, Hou S. Hospital-acquired renal insufficiency. *Am J Kidney Dis* 2002; **39**: 930–936.

Internet resources

The Acute Dialysis Quality Initiative:

`http://www.ADQI.net`

The Acute Kidney Injury Network:

`http://akinet.org/index.php`

See also

Assessment of renal disease, p. 1

Urinary tract obstruction, p. 652

Crescentic glomerulephritis, p. 120

Antiglomerular basement membrane disease, p. 124

Systemic vasculitis, p. 168

Renal replacement therapies in acute kidney injury

Introduction

There are many potential modes of renal replacement therapy (RRT) now available for treating the patient with acute kidney injury (AKI) who has developed renal failure:

- peritoneal dialysis;
- intermittent hemodilaysis/hemofiltration;
- continuous renal replacement therapy;
- hybrid techniques.

Rather than trying to provide all possible modalities, units should become proficient in a limited number of options.

When to initiate renal replacement therapy

RRT is often initiated based on the clinical assessment of the patient coupled with the most recent biochemical data. Over the years the trend has been to start RRT earlier, particularly in those with multiple organ failure and sepsis, compared to those with AKI alone.

Peritoneal dialysis

In patients with an intact abdominal cavity, peritoneal dialysis (PD) remains an option.

PD catheter insertion

Hard PD catheters have generally been superseded by silastic soft catheters, which can still be inserted at the bed side under local anesthesia.

Insertion tends to be 'blind', typically inserting the catheter in the midline, one-third of the distance from the umbilicus to the symphysis pubis. The peritoneal membrane should be penetrated during inspiration, when tensed. Prefilling the peritoneal cavity with PD fluid using a venous cannula introduced at McBurney's point reduces the risk of bowel perforation with the PD catheter insertion stylet. Vascular and intestinal injury remain a possible complication of insertion.

Alternative methods of PD catheter insertion include use of peritoneoscopy, full laparoscopy and open surgical insertion. The method chosen will depend on the local expertise and the clinical state of the patient.

PD prescription in AKI

Small solute clearance

In cases of hyperkalemia, rapid cycles are required. Typically 1 L of dialyzate should run into the peritoneal cavity in 5 min, 2 L in 10 min. In severe hyperkalemia 30 min cycles may be required, although generally 1 h cycles will suffice.

For an hourly cycle of 2 L, 10 min will be required for the inflow, 12–15 min for the outflow, limiting the dwell time to 45–48 min. To compensate for the shortened dwell times, the fill volume has to be increased. For adults 2–2.5 L cycles with a dwell time of a 90 min may be required.

In many studies the clearances achieved with PD in AKI are similar to those of CKD patients regularly treated by PD, but are much less than other techniques. However, PD remains a viable option, particularly in infants and small children in whom vascular access problems preclude blood purification techniques, and in those patients who are not hypercatabolic.

Ultrafiltration

Ultrafiltration occurs due to the high glucose content of the fresh dialyzate causing an osmotic gradient:

- 1.36% = 64 mmol/L glucose;
- 2.27% = 120 mmol/L glucose.

Considerations for PD treatment in AKI

In patients with shock and in those on vasopressors, the mesenteric blood flow may be reduced. This will affect solute clearances and ultrafiltration volumes. Higher glucose concentrations may then be required to obtain effective ultrafiltration.

Glucose is absorbed, and this may result in hyperglycemia, particularly in diabetic patients. In addition peritoneal dialyzates are hyponatremic, and therefore should be avoided in patients with brain injury and/or cerebral edema.

Continuous flow PD has recently been introduced, using one catheter for dialyzate inflow, and a second for dialyzate outflow in an effort to increase the efficiency of solute clearances. Regeneration of the dialyzate using sorbents allows a limited volume of PD dialyzate to be continuously recycled.

Intermittent hemodialysis/hemofiltration

The key to prescribing intermittent hemodialysis (IHD) or hemofiltration (IHF) to the patient with AKI is to avoid intradialytic hypotension and further renal injury.

Intermittent hemodialysis

Compared with regular IHD for the patient with ESRD the following changes should be made:

- dialyzate cooled to 35°C or set at isothermic;
- dialyzate calcium of 1.35–1.5 mmol/L;
- dialyzate sodium of 10 mmol/L above plasma sodium (up to a maximum of 150 mmol/L);
- dialyzate potassium highest possible;
- minimize ultrafiltration rate.

Each of the first three strategies has been independently shown to reduce intradialytic hypotension. Similarly the highest possible potassium concentration should be chosen to minimize cardiac arrhythmias. As the rate of fluid removal during dialysis is also an important determinant of hypotension, then the ultrafiltration rate should be minimized by extending the duration of the treatment session, above the standard 4 h treatment of chronic dialysis patients, and increasing the frequency of treatments to alternate days or daily. The minimum dose of intermittent HD should exceed a Kt/V > 12 per thrice weekly session.

With the development of dialysis technology, there are now HD machines capable of assessing relative blood volume, as a surrogate of the difference between ultrafiltration rate and plasma refilling rate; the most sophisticated can vary the ultrafiltration rate to maintain the relative blood volume.

If at all possible the most sophisticated HD machine should be used for the treatment of the patient with AKI.

When IHD has been carefully delivered to minimize intradialytic hypotension, then patient outcomes have been reported to be similar to those of continuous renal replacement therapies (CRRTs).

Intermittent hemofiltration

Whereas the main driving force during IHD is diffusion along concentration gradients, during hemofiltration, hydrostatic pressure drives a bulk water movement across the hemofilter, known as convection (Fig. 10.2.1).

Intermittent HD is much more effective in clearing small solutes such as potassium, urea and creatinine than IHF, but IHF preferentially removes larger molecular weight solutes, and also drugs such as vancomycin.

During HF, the replacement/substitution fluid can be replaced pre, mid or postfilter (Fig. 10.2.2).

Small solute clearances are greater with:
• post > mid > prefilter fluid replacement.

Conversely, middle molecular weight solute clearances, are greater with:
• pre > mid > postfluid replacement.

However, to achieve the same small solute clearances much more fluid (and therefore a higher cost) is required with pre and mid compared with postdilutional replacement.

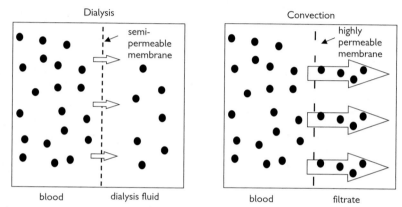

Fig. 10.2.1 Dialysis and convection. Dialysis occurs by diffusion down a concentration gradient and across a semipermeable membrane. Convection occurs down a hydrostatic pressure gradient with solutes moving with bulk water movement.

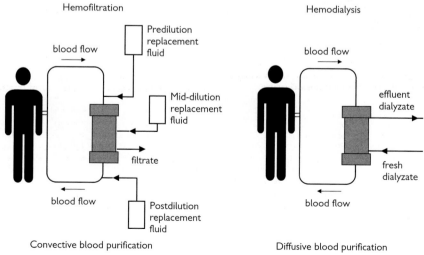

Fig. 10.2.2 Convective and diffusive blood purification.

Intermittent HD vs intermittent HF

Initially it was thought that IHF provided greater cardiovascular stability than IHD. However, it is now established that postdilutional IHF causes greater cooling than IHD, and the predilutional mode even more cooling.

In addition there are differences in sodium exchange between IHD and IHF. There is an obligatory sodium loss with any ultrafiltration. During IHF, plasma water passes across the hemofilter membrane due to a hydrostatic pressure gradient (convection). However, not all sodium in plasma water is freely available to move, as it may be associated with negatively charged proteins and other compounds. Thus for the same dialyzate/replacement fluid sodium concentration, patients treated by IHF will have a greater sodium gain than those by IHD, and this is greatest in the postdilution mode. This is compounded by the fact that compared to healthy dialysis patients, patients with AKI have a low dietary sodium intake.

Hemodiafiltration

Hemodiafiltration (HDF) is a technique in which there is both dialysis and filtration (convection).

Membranes

Hemodialysis

Diffusion is increased by having a large surface area, with a short distance for solutes to move, and thus dialyzer membranes designed for diffusion typically have long fiber lengths of narrow diameter. Typically dialyzer membranes restricted the passage of small solutes, and were therefore termed low flux, but over time the membranes have changed, so that many IHD treatments in AKI use high flux membranes.

Hemofiltration

For convective therapies, hydrostatic pressure is better maintained by shorter, wider diameter fibers. To allow convection, high flux membranes are required. Inappropriate use of a dialyzer designed for dialysis as a hemofilter, will result in excessive clotting problems.

Pure unadulterated cellulosic membranes have been shown to reduce renal recovery in patients with AKI. However, these membranes have generally been replaced by modified cellulose, and such membranes compare favorably with the synthetic membranes.

Septic patients and those with liver failure may have increased nitric oxide levels, and can be more prone to hypotension when first connected to the dialysis circuit, due to the generation of bradykinin. This can be minimized by priming the dialyzer with isotonic sodium bicarbonate, rather than 0.9% saline (pH 5.4).

Continuous renal replacement therapies

Continuous renal replacement therapies (CRRT) include:
- continuous arteriovenous hemofiltration (CAVH);
- continuous venovenous hemofiltration (CVVH);
- continuous venovenous hemodialysis (CVVHD);
- continuous venovenous hemodiafiltration (CVVHDF).

CAVH was the first CRRT, but often did not provide adequate clearances, so IHD was still required. CAVH has now been superseded by pumped venovenous systems which provide adequate clearances (Fig. 10.2.3).

Typically CRRT provides greater cardiovascular stability than conventional IHD. This is most likely due to the increased patient cooling associated with CRRT, despite warming of replacement fluids and dialyzates.

While no study to date has shown an improved patient survival with CRRT compared to IHD, there are data to show that recovery of renal function is greater with CRRT when compared to standard IHD.

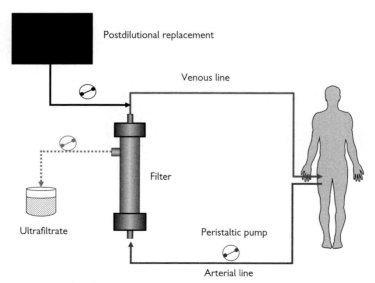

Postdilutional replacement

Venous line

Filter

Ultrafiltrate

Peristaltic pump

Arterial line

Fig. 10.2.3 Continuous venovenous hemofiltration.

Although there are differences between CVVH and CVVHD in terms of solute removal, it does not appear that one modality is superior to the other in clinical practice.

Whereas there are guidelines as to the dose of RRT required for patients with CKD, it was unknown until relatively recently whether the dose of CRRT impacted on patient survival. However, it has now been shown that the dose of treatment delivered has an impact on outcome, with greater patient survival during postdilutional CVVH with a delivered dose of >20 mL/kg/h or an equivalent dose of CVVHDF.

Although CRRT generally provides an effective RRT, with cardiovascular stability, it must be recognized that drugs, particularly antibiotics, may have a substantial clearance, and therefore dosages need adjusting, and that water-soluble vitamins and trace elements such as selenium are lost and may need replacing.

Replacement fluids and/or dialyzates
Whereas dialyzates for IHD have been bicarbonate-based for some time, the original fluids used for CRRT, as both replacement fluids and/or dialyzates, were derived from peritoneal dialyzates, containing high concentrations of glucose, and were lactate-based. Over time, specialized fluids have been developed, nevertheless there is a marked range in electrolyte composition, particularly lactate and chloride concentrations.

For the same blood flow, hematocrit and ultrafiltration volume, the filtration fraction is greater for postdilutional hemofiltration. (Fig. 10.2.4)

A hemofiltration replacement fluid containing a relatively high lactate and low chloride concentration will, after several days of CRRT, result in a hypochloremic alkalosis, and conversely a relatively low lactate–high chloride solution

will produce a hyperchloremic acidosis. These changes will occur more rapidly if high volumes are exchanged, and if predilutional fluid replacement is used during CRRT, as chloride mass balance is more positive when compared to postdilutional replacement.

Latterly bicarbonate-based, of buffer-free solutions have been developed, and although more costly have been shown to improve acid–base status and cardiovascular stability in critically ill patients with AKI, compared to standard lactate-based fluids. The advent of citrate as an anticoagulant for CRTT has again required further fluid development, as trisodium citrate leads both to sodium gain and to metabolic alkalosis, as each citrate molecule is indirectly metabolized to three bicarbonates. Thus fluids for citrate-based CRRT not only need to be calcium free, but also lower in both sodium and bicarbonate.

Anticoagulation for CRRT
Although unfractionated heparin (UFH) remains the most common anticoagulant used worldwide, CRRT systems can be run anticoagulant free. In AKI the platelet count may be reduced, and baseline clotting studies abnormal.

Simple measures to reduce clotting in the circuit
Adequate vascular access is required, using large French gauge catheters, preferably with no side port-holes. Femoral access is more reliable than internal jugular or subclavian, but the femoral catheters need to be long enough for the tips to lie in the inferior vena cava.

A hemofilter rather than a dialyser membrane is required, and the filtration fraction should be <30% (Fig. 10.2.4).

Predilutional fluid replacement prolongs circuit survival compared to postdilutional CVVH, by preventing hemoconcentration and limiting protein deposition on the hemofilter membrane, and increasing cooling.

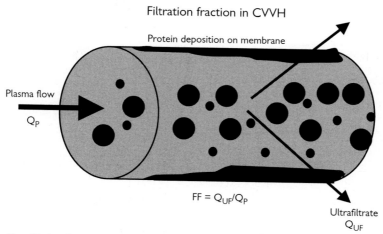

Filtration fraction in CVVH

Protein deposition on membrane

Plasma flow

Q_P

$FF = Q_{UF}/Q_P$

Ultrafiltrate
Q_{UF}

Postdilutional
Blood flow rate = 100 mL/min
HCT 30%
Ultrafiltration rate = 1500 mL/h
FF = 1500/[6000 × (1 − 0.30)] = 0.36%

Predilutional
Blood flow rate = 100 mL/min
HCT 24%
Ultrafiltration rate = 1500 mL/h
FF = 1500/[7500 × (1 − 0.24)] = 0.26%

Fig. 10.2.4 Filtration fraction in continuous venovenous hemofiltration (CVVH).

Anticoagulation

Unfractionated heparin. The main disadvantage of anticoagulation with UFH is an increased risk of hemorrhage especially when aPTT >65 s, while there is an increased risk of circuit clotting when aPTT <55 s.

A typical regime would be a bolus dose of UFH of 15–30 IU/kg followed by a maintenance infusion of 5–15 IU/kg/h.

Heparin is negatively charged and may adsorb onto the plastic tubing of the infusate line. To avoid this problem, and to achieve better mixing, UFH should be administered in a dilute rather than a concentrated solution.

Higher doses of UFH are required for hemoperfusion due to adsorption to the sorbent, and similarly some UFH may be lost in predilutional HDF.

In the ICU, particularly with septic patients, antithrombin (AT) levels may be reduced, and therefore heparin may not be as effective an anticoagulant when compared to its use in the chronic dialysis patient, with an increased risk of circuit clotting once AT levels have fallen to <60%.

Low molecular weight heparins (LMWHs). Although LMWHs are easier to administer when used for intermittent therapies in patients with AKI (single bolus of enoxaparin 0.5 mg/kg and/or tinzaparin 2500 IU), they require antiXa monitoring when used for CRRT, and with their increased half-life have no clinical advantage over UFH.

As LMWHs are smaller than UFH, some may be lost when hemofiltration is used, and therefore higher initial bolus doses may be required.

The other major problem that can occur with UFH, and to a lesser extent LMWHs, is the development of autoimmune thrombocytopenia. In this case, all heparin administration must be withdrawn, including LMWHs. Thrombocytopenia occurs due to platelet activation, and patients are at risk of thrombosis, so require an alternative systemic anticoagulant.

Alternative anticoagulants include:
1 Synthetic heparinoids: danaparoid.
2 Direct thrombin inhibitors:
   • hirudin (from the medicinal leech *Hirudo medicinalis*);
   • lepirudin (recombinant hirudin);
   • argatroban (synthetic molecule, available in the USA).
3 Citrate.

Danaparoid. Although the half-life of danaproid is increased in AKI, following a bolus dose of 1500 IU, studies have shown that a similar maintenance dose of 140 IU/h is required for both CVVH and CVVHD, thereafter adjusted according to antiXa level (target: 0.3–0.4). For IHD or HDF, a bolus dose of 2500 IU for patients >55 kg is recommended, with a lower dose of 2000 IU for smaller patients.

Hirudin. The half-life of hirudin is extensively elongated in AKI. Hirudin dosing is problematical for CRRT, as there is some hirudin clearance during CVVH, and antihirudin antibodies may develop after a few days, which reduce clearance and prolong biological activity even further. The plasma hirudin concentration is not linearly related to the aPTT, and once the aPTT ratio is >2.0, hirudin concentrations increase the aPTT ratio exponentially, so increasing the risk of hemorrhage. Thus a special test of thrombin activation, the ecarin clotting time, is required to monitor hirudin. Many centers give a single bolus dose

of 5–10 mg for CRRT, and then repeat when the aPTT ratio falls back to <1.2. For IHD of HDF, a bolus dose of 02–0.3 mg should suffice in AKI.

Lepirudin. This drug is used in a similar manner to hirudin. There is no antidote in cases of hemorrhage due to lepirudin (or hirudin) overdosage. There are reports that the combination of activated factor VIIa and tranexamic acid may help reduce bleeding, and high flux IHD or predilutional HDF may increase lepirudin clearance.

Argatroban. Argatroban has to be given by continuous infusion, and is mainly hepatically cleared, so dose reduction is required in patients with hepatic disease.

Citrate. Due to the problems with heparin in the critically ill patient with AKI, citrate has become a favored regional anticoagulant for CRRT, as it has minimal risk of hemorrhage, and is an effective anticoagulant (Fig. 10.2.5). However, citrate requires a degree of complexity, with low or zero calcium dialyzates/replacement solutions. The rate of citrate is adjusted according to blood flow (Table 10.2.1), and both the total and ionized calcium must be measured. If citrate accumulates then total plasma calcium rises due to the presence of an unmetabolized calcium citrate complex, and the rate of citrate should be reduced.

High volume CRRT

Animal experiments have shown improved cardiovascular stability during CVVH, when high volumes of ultrafiltrate were obtained. This could have been due to the high volume of fluid replacement (6 L/h), resulting in additional cooling, and positive sodium and calcium balances. However, the studies also showed that injection of the ultrafiltrate into healthy animals caused hypotension, suggesting that the improvement was due to the removal of a vasodilatory or inflammatory substance.

CVVH can remove cytokines, both pro-inflammatory, such as IL-6, and anti-inflammatory, including IL-10. A study showed that patients with the highest levels of cytokines, whether inflammatory IL-6 or anti-inflammatory IL-10, had the greatest mortality. The question arose as to whether high dose hemofiltration, often given in pulses of 6–8 h, could alter the inflammatory milieu, and thereby improve patient survival by reducing the peak cytokine levels.

Several uncontrolled studies reported improved patient hemodynamics and survival in those patients with AKI and severe hypotension refractory to vasopressors. Currently several multicenter prospective trials are underway to investigate the role of high volume hemofiltration on patient outcomes and to test the validity of the 'peak cytokine hypothesis'.

Superflux membranes for CRRT

High volume hemofiltration requires high volume fluid exchange, which is expensive, increases the risks of circuit clotting due to hemoconcentration and requires accurate fluid balance assessment. Thus those centers with experience of this technique usually perform pulses of therapy lasting 6–8 h.

An alternative method of removing inflammatory mediators is to use a superflux membrane.

Whereas the typical hemofiltration membrane will allow the passage of molecules up to 30 kDa in clinical practice, superflux membranes will allow molecules up to 100 kDa to pass into the ultrafiltrate.

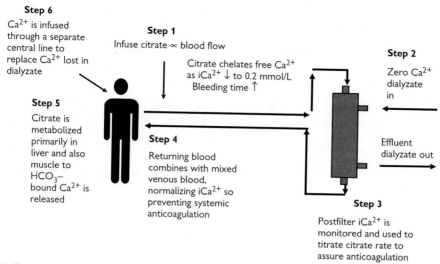

Step 6
Ca^{2+} is infused through a separate central line to replace Ca^{2+} lost in dialyzate

Step 1
Infuse citrate ∝ blood flow

Citrate chelates free Ca^{2+} as iCa^{2+} ↓ to 0.2 mmol/L
Bleeding time ↑

Step 2
Zero Ca^{2+} dialyzate in

Step 5
Citrate is metabolized primarily in liver and also muscle to HCO_3^- bound Ca^{2+} is released

Step 4
Returning blood combines with mixed venous blood, normalizing iCa^{2+} so preventing systemic anticoagulation

Effluent dialyzate out

Step 3
Postfilter iCa^{2+} is monitored and used to titrate citrate rate to assure anticoagulation

Fig. 10.2.5 Citrate anticoagulation for continuous renal replacement therapy (CRRT). iCa2+: ionized calcium.

Table 10.2.1 Citrate dose for varying blood flows

Blood flow (mL/min)	4% trisodium citrate (mL/h)	Acid citrate dextrose (mL/h)
100	175	210
125	218	262
150	262	315
200	350	420

The advantage of the superflux membranes is that other cytokines, such as TNF-α which exist as a trimer (51 kDa), can be removed using standard exchange volumes. One disadvantage of such permeable membranes is the potential loss of albumin- and protein-bound hormones.

Hybrid techniques

Optimal clearances with CRRT depend upon the therapy continuing for 24 h.

CRRT may be interrupted, and solute clearances compromised, for many reasons including:
- clotting of the extracorporeal circuit;
- patients having to leave the ICU to go to theatre, or for radiological investigations, e.g. CT scanning.

Also, during CRRT the patient is bed-bound and therefore may be at greater risk of developing nosocomial pneumonia, disuse atrophy and be less able to participate in physical therapy.

To overcome these problems a series of hybrid techniques was introduced, ranging from simply slowing down conventional hemodialysis – slow low efficiency daily dialysis (SLEDD), extended daily dialysis (EDD) – to specially designed systems, such as the Genius Batch dialysis system.

Essentially these treatments were designed to produce a very effective dialysis treatment lasting 8–16 h (Fig. 10.2.6),

using slower blood and dialyzate flows compared to standard IHD (Table 10.2.2). When not on the hybrid technique, patients could sit out of bed, go for scheduled scans, etc.

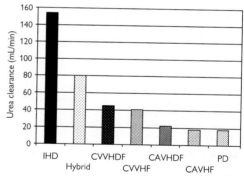

Fig. 10.2.6 Relative urea clearances for the different modalities of renal replacement therapy in AKI.

Table 10.2.2 Comparison of different modalities used for treating patients with AKI

Modality	Intermittent HD/HF/HDF	CRRT	Hybrid
Blood flow (mL/min)	200–300	75–150	100–150
Dialysate flow (mL/min)	500–800	16–40	200
Filtration flow (mL/min)	75–250	16–40	40–100
Treatment duration (h)	4–5	24	8–12
Treatment frequency	Alternate day – daily	Daily	Daily

Adjunctive therapies

Plasma exchange/immunoadsorption

For some conditions, including hemolytic uremic syndrome, plasma exchange (PE) is the treatment of choice. For other conditions such as the pulmonary renal syndromes, anti-GBM nephritis, Wegner's granulomatosis, and other vasculitic and/or crescentic glomerulonephritides, immunoadsorption with a staphylococcal A adsorption column may be equally effective as PE.

Plasma exchange has not been shown to improve outcome in septic patients with AKI.

Plasma exchange can be performed by either a centrifugal spinning bowl technique, or using a PE hemofilter. Typically 30–45 mL/kg of plasma is removed during a treatment session and replaced with a composite of both colloid and crystalloid including fresh frozen plasma, albumin, or colloid substitute and 0.9% saline.

Approximately 30% of PE treatments using fresh frozen plasma are associated with adverse reactions, ranging from anaphylaxis, and adult respiratory distress syndrome, to fevers, chills and rigors. Patients who are IgA deficient can react to IgA in pooled plasma. A pulmonary leak syndrome is relatively common due to the combination of the underlying condition, administration of fresh frozen plasma which contains both inflammatory cytokines and chemokines, coupled with the oncotic load of the colloid replacement solutions if not diluted with 0.9% saline. Thus it is important to achieve a negative fluid balance during PE, to prevent pulmonary leak syndrome, provoking pulmonary hemorrhage.

Immunoadsorption is an alternative technique for those conditions which do not require the addition of plasma factors. This avoids the use of plasma products which may potentially be contaminated with prions.

Albumin dialysis

Albumin binds not only hormones and drugs, but also many toxins, and scavenges nitric oxide. Patients with hepatorenal syndrome may benefit from vasopressor therapy in combination with albumin infusions. Unfortunately the number of potential binding sites is markedly reduced in stored albumin. More recently a number of dialysis systems which use albumin in the dialyzate have been developed, particularly for treating patients with liver failure. These include single pass albumin dialysis (SPAD) and two systems that regenerate albumin by passage of the spent dialyzate through charcoal and resin cartridges: MARS and Prometheus. Although MARS has been shown to improve outcome in a small series of patients with hepatorenal failure, further prospective studies with the Prometheus system are currently in progress to determine whether these systems have a beneficial role to play in the management of patients with combined liver and kidney failure.

Hemoperfusion

Dialysis and filtration techniques essentially remove water-soluble compounds, whereas hemoperfusion (HP) cartridges remove lipophilic substances. The earlier HP cartridges were associated with increased clotting, thrombocytopenia and leukopenia.

Today HP is predominantly used in Japan to remove endotoxin and peptidoglycans in Gram-negative and Gram-positive sepsis respectively, whereas in Europe HP is usually used in combination with other forms of RRT (see combination therapies).

Combination therapies

In an effort to remove inflammatory mediators in patients with sepsis and AKI, combination therapies have been developed, using a PE hemofilter, and the ultrafiltrated plasma is then passed over an HP cartridge before returning to the patient. These systems are currently in phase III clinical trials, as the initial phase I and II studies suggested improved patient survival.

The MARS and Prometheus albumin dialysis treatments are also examples of combination therapies, both using a conventional hemofilter in the extracorporeal circuit.

The bioartificial kidney

David Humes in Michigan has developed a bioreactor coated with proximal tubular cells, and this is currently being assessed in phase II and III clinical trials.

Further reading

Bellomo R, Tetta C, Brendolan A, Ronco C. Coupled plasma filtration adsorption. *Blood Purif* 2002; **20**: 289–292.

Davenport A. Replacement and dialysate fluids for patients with acute renal failure treated by continuous veno-venous haemofiltration and/or haemodiafiltration. *Contrib Nephrol* 2004; **144**: 317–328.

Fliser D, Kielstein JT. Technology Insight: treatment of renal failure in the intensive care unit with extended dialysis. *Nat Clin Pract Nephrol* 2006; **2**: 32–39.

Honore PM, Joannes-Boyau O. High volume hemofiltration (HVHF) in sepsis: a comprehensive review of rationale, clinical applicability, potential indications and recommendations for future research. *Int J Artif Organs* 2004; **27**: 1077–1082.

Morgera S, Haase M, Kuss T, et al. Pilot study on the effects of high cutoff hemofiltration on the need for norepinephrine in septic patients with acute renal failure. *Crit Care Med* 2006; **34**: 2099–2104.

Ronco C, Bellomo R, Homel P, et al. Effects of different doses in continuous veno-venous haemofiltration on outcomes of acute renal failure: a prospective randomised trial. *Lancet* 2000; **356**: 26–30.

Swartz R, Pasko D, O'Toole J, Starmann B. Improving the delivery of continuous renal replacement therapy using regional citrate anticoagulation. *Clin Nephrol* 2004; **61**: 134–143.

Tiranathanagul K, Brodie J, Humes HD. Bioartificial kidney in the treatment of acute renal failure associated with sepsis. *Nephrology (Carlton)* 2006; **11**: 285–291.

VA/NIH Acute Renal Failure Trial Network. Intensity of renal support in critically all patients with acute kidney injury. *N Engl J Med* 2008; **359**: 7–20.

Internet resources

Acute Dialysis Quality Initiative:

http://www.ADQI.net

Acute Kidney Injury Network:

http://akinet.org/index.php

See also

Dialysis and hemoperfusion treatment of acute poisoning

Introduction

The standard treatment of intoxications and acute poisonings is based on symptomatic and supportive therapy, coupled where appropriate with specific measures designed to remove toxins including:

- gastric lavage;
- instillation of adsorbents, such as activated charcoal;
- stimulation of endogenous pathways of elimination (typically a forced diuresis);
- administration of antidotes and/or chelating agents;
- extracorporeal circuits;

Extracorporeal circuits commonly used are:

- hemodialysis (HD);
- hemodiafiltration (HDF);
- hemoperfusion (HP).

All can be used to treat patients suffering from drug intoxication and/or poisoning when the clinical condition fails to respond to maximum supportive care, particularly when patients have developed hypoventilation, hypotension and hypothermia.

Extracorporeal therapies can also be used when patients have serum levels of drugs and/or poisons which are known to result in significant risk of patient mortality and/or organ failure, and the rate of extracorporeal clearance exceeds that of endogenous hepatic and/or renal clearance (Tables 10.3.1 and 10.3.2).

Volume of distribution

Although extracorporeal therapies are most effective when treating drugs and toxins with a small volume of distribution, e.g. confined to the plasma volume, they may have a role in treating tissue/protein-bound compounds: although only a small fraction of the total body load will be removed, a temporary reduction in plasma concentration may be useful in reversing life-threatening toxic effects.

Peritoneal dialysis

Peritoneal dialysis (PD) is not an effective therapy for drug/toxin removal from the blood, as it is only ~10% as efficient as high flux HD. However, in small children, due to vascular access difficulties, PD may have an adjunctive role. The efficiency of PD can be increased by using rapid cycles and maximizing the dwell volume, and also by using continuous flow-through techniques.

As peritoneal dialysis drug clearances are less than those with hemodialysis, peritoneal dialysis patients are more at risk of developing neurotoxicity with acyclovir, ganciclovir and high doses of penicillins and cephalosporins.

Hemodialysis

Hemodialysis is the modality of choice for removal of drugs and toxins that:

- are water soluble;
- are low molecular weight;
- have a small volume of distribution.

Examples of compounds for which there is virtually no protein binding include:

- alcohols;
- organic acids (which accumulate in urea cycle defects of metabolism);

- aminoglycosides;
- atenolol;
- lithium.

Alcohols, such as methanol and ethylene glycol, are readily removed by HD. However, alcohol dehyrodgenase can also be blocked by the administration of ethanol, and fomepizole. Thus HD should be reserved for cases which have not responded to conservative therapy, with clinical deterioration, metabolic acidosis and methanol or ethylene glycol levels >500 mg/L (Table 10.3.2).

Larger molecular weight drugs such as amphotericin (9241 Da) can be cleared using high flux dialyzers and adding in predilutional hemodiafiltration (HDF).

HDF has advantages over HD, in terms of clearing higher molecular weight drugs and toxins, and is the preferred choice for overdoses of valproate, vancomycin, amphotericin and hirudin.

Hemoperfusion

During hemoperfusion blood passes through a cartridge containing a sorbent. Commonly used sorbents include:

- charcoal;
- ion exchange resins;
- nonionic exchange macroporous resins.

These sorbents can bind drugs and toxins which are normally protein-bound. Examples of toxins with high protein binding are:

- arsenic;
- calcium channel blockers;
- benzodiazepines;
- phenytoin;
- tricyclic antidepressants.

Hemoperfusion will also remove lipophillic drugs and toxins more effectively than HD. There are no data comparing one manufacturer's hemoperfusion column with another in terms of drug and toxin removal. HP columns differ not only in the sorbent used, but also the amount and volume of the cartridge. Compared with HD, much more heparin is required to prevent clotting in the HP circuit, due to heparin absorption to the sorbent.

Albumin dialysis

More recently a variety of albumin dialysis-based systems have been introduced, ranging from single pass albumin dialysis (SPAD) to regeneration of the albumin-based dialyzate, using sorbents such as the MARS and Prometheus systems. These albumin dialysis systems can also be used to remove protein-bound and lipophillic drugs and/or toxins, and have been reported to improve the prognosis following *Amanita phalloides* (the deathcap mushroom) poisoning.

Plasma exchange

Plasma exchange (PE) can speed up the elimination of digoxin in severe cases where digoxin-specific antibodies have been administered, by removing the digoxin–antibody complexes. If the digoxin–antibody complexes are not endogenously cleared, then there is a risk of later digoxin toxicity, as digoxin is subsequently released from the antibody complex.

Table 10.3.1 Drugs and toxins preferentially removed by hemodialysis and hemoperfusion

Classes of drugs and toxins amenable to removal by extracorporeal circuits	Hemodialysis more effective	Hemoperfusion more effective
Barbiturates	Lithium	Barbiturates
Sedatives	Bromide	Sedatives
Hypnotics	Ethanol	Tranquillizers
Tranquillizers	Methanol	Theophyline
Antimicrobials	Ethylene glycol	Paraquat
Anticancer drugs	Salicylates	Deathcap mushroom
Antidepressants	Antimicrobials	Phenytoin
Cardiovascular	Antivirals	Trichloroethanol
Plant toxins	Valproate	Disopyramide
Animal toxins	Carbamazepine	
Solvents and gases	Metformin	
Herbicides		
Insecticides		
Metals		

Table 10.3.2 Serum drug and poison concentrations at which extracorporeal removal may be beneficial

Drug	Serum concentration	
	mg/L	mmol/L
Phenobarbital	100	0.43
Glutethimide	40	0.18
Methaqualone	40	0.16
Salicylates	800	4.4
Theophylline	40	0.22
Paraquat	0.1	0.5
Methanol	500	16
Ethylene glycol	500	8.1
Meprobamate	100	0.46
Lithium		
acute	4.0	4.0
chronic	>2.5	>2.5
Phenytoin	30	120
Valproate	1000	7.0

Continuous extracorporeal therapies

Most extracorporeal therapies for drug intoxications and poisonings have been used as intermittent therapies.

Once the HP cartridge has become saturated, typically between 4 and 6 h, the treatment is terminated.

However, for some drugs such as lithium, with a large volume of distribution, a continuous or extended form of HD would potentially prevent a rebound in drug serum concentration following a standard intermittent HD.

Continuous methods are useful for intoxicants such as:
* paraquat;
* thallium;
* methotrexate;
* procainamide.

They can be useful even if initiated many hours or days after exposure.

Clearances of 70–170 mL/min can be achieved during intermittent HD. During continuous renal replacement therapies (CRRT) as currently practiced on the intensive care unit, clearances typically only average ~40 mL/min; however, these can be increased with faster blood and dialyzate flows.

Intermittent HD is more efficient at clearing water-soluble toxins and drugs. In the cardiovascularly unstable patient intermittent HD may not be possible and continuous modes or hybrid dialysis techniques may be required.

When treating patients with drug toxicity due to a drug with a large volume of distribution, such as methotrexate, then in cases which have not responded to leucovorin, clearances can be improved by extending the duration of the intermittent HD session to 8–12 h. This can be done by slowing down either the blood or dialyzate flow rate to ~200 mL/min respectively, a procedure sometimes termed hybrid therapy. An alternative is to perform two consecutive 4–6 h intermittent HD treatments.

Complications of extracorporeal circuits

In addition to complications associated with vascular access and anticoagulation, many patients will have normal renal function, and therefore HD can result in electrolyte abnormalities, including hypokalemia and hypophosphatemia, which may need to be corrected.

HD also results in bicarbonate gains, which may be beneficial in patients with a metabolic acidosis, but could exacerbate a metabolic alkalosis, as in cases of salicylate toxicity.

HP is associated with transient leukopenia and thrombocytopenia. Hypoglycemia may also occur during HP and the albumin dialysis therapies.

Hypocalcemia may develop during PE due to calcium complexing with citrate.

Future prospects

Only a minority of self-poisonings and drug toxicities are with low molecular weight water-soluble agents with a small volume of distribution. So in many cases after an initial reduction in plasma concentrations with intermittent HD, there is redistribution and a rebound in the plasma concentration. To overcome this rebound, some centers use an initial intermittent HD treatment, followed either by a hybrid therapy or continuous RRT.

Future developments are underway to combine plasma filters within the dialysis/filtration circuit, so that the filtered plasma is passed across sorbent columns, and then returned to the patient. This technology will potentially help remove even protein-bound toxins.

Further reading

Godman JW, Goldfarb DS. The role of continuous renal replacement therapy in the treatment of poisoning. *Semin Dial* 2006; **5**: 402–407.

Goldfarb DS. Principles and techniques applied to enhance the elimination of toxic compounds. In: Goldfarb LR, Flomenbaum NE, Lewin NA, Howland MA, Hoffman RS, Nelson LS (eds), *Goldfrank's toxico-logical emergencies*, 7th edn. New York: McGraw-Hill; 2002. pp. 58–68.

Haddad LM, Shanon MW, Winchester JF (eds). *Clinical management of poisoning and drug overdosage*, 3rd edn. Philadelphia: WB Saunders; 1998.

Winchester JF. Dialysis techniques: haemoperfusion. In: Horl WH, Koch KM, Lindsay RM, Ronco C, Winchester JF (eds), *Replacement of renal function by dialysis*, 5th edn. Dordrecht: Kluwer; 2004. pp. 725–738.

Zimmerman JL. Poisonings and overdoses in the intensive care unit: General and specific management issues. *Crit Care Med* 2003; **12**: 2794–2801.

Internet resources

International Program on Chemical Safety (IPCS) INTOX databank:

http://www.intox.org/databank/index.htm

IPCS directory of poison centres: European Region:

http://www.intox.org/databank/documents/supplem/supp/european.htm

National Institutes of Health information resource:

http://www.nlm.nih.gov/medlineplus/poisoning.html

American Association of Poison Control Centers:

http://www.aapcc.org/

See also

Clinical approach to acute kidney injury, p. 318

Renal replacement therapies in acute kidney injury, p. 328

Handling of drugs in kidney disease, p. 690

Drug-induced nephropathies, p. 698

Glomerulonephritis, vasculitis, and nephrotic syndrome

Introduction

Acute glomerulonephritis (GN) is an important cause of AKI (Table 10.4.1). Early recognition and treatment is essential in order to preserve renal function. Small vessel vasculitis and systemic lupus erythematosus (SLE) are common causes of AKI whereas primary glomerular diseases are less commonly associated with AKI.

Epidemiology

The incidence of AKI due to GN is poorly defined but it is estimated that ~10% of cases of AKI are due to GN.

In Europe and North America the most common GN-causing AKIs are:
- small vessel vasculitis;
- lupus nephritis.

Worldwide, GN secondary to infection is the most common cause of AKI.

Etiology

The development of AKI in GN is multifactorial with variable contributions from each of the following depending on the cause.

Glomerular injury

Compression of the glomerular tuft and occlusion of glomerular capillaries by the influx of inflammatory cells (crescentic GN).

Local generation and release of the potent vasoconstrictor endothelin secondary to vascular inflammation.

Reduced production of the vasodilator nitric oxide secondary to vascular inflammation.

Tubulointerstitial injury

Direct tubular epithelial cell toxicity from the contents of lysed red blood cells (free iron, Hb).

Tubular obstruction by red blood cells.

Prerenal AKI due to hypovolemia (nephrotic syndrome, NSAIDs, overdiuresis).

Increased intrarenal pressure due to interstitial edema (nephrotic syndrome).

It has been proposed that an imbalance between endothelin and nitric oxide secretion potentiates the relative hypoxia that exists in the outer medulla, which may lead to acute tubular necrosis.

Vascular injury

Large vessel vasculitis with distal ischemia.

Renal vein thrombosis in nephrotic syndrome (hypercoagulable state).

Fibrinoid necrosis of afferent arterioles resulting in glomerular ischemia (systemic sclerosis).

Clinical features

Generalized clinical features will be dependent upon the degree of AKI.

More specific clinical features will be dependent upon the primary disease process causing the GN.

AKI associated with vasculitis

There may be clinical features of a multisystem disease:
- fever;
- purpuric rash;
- uveitis;
- arthralgia;
- epistaxis;
- conductive hearing loss;
- sinusitis;
- mouth ulcers;
- hemoptysis;
- mononeuritis multiplex;
- hypertension;
- reduced pulsation over temporal artery (giant cell arteritis);
- reduced pulsation in brachial arteries (Takayasu's arteritis);
- erythema nodosum (Behçet's disease).

The presence of hemoptysis usually signifies pulmonary hemorrhage and is associated with:
- ANCA-associated vasculitis;
- anti-GBM disease;
- SLE.

AKI associated with infectious glomerulonephritis

This may be associated with:
- fever;
- sore throat (typically 10–21 days preceding post-streptococcal GN);
- rash;
- loin pain;
- heart murmur (infectious endocarditis);
- peripheral emboli (infectious endocarditis).

AKI associated with primary glomerulonephritis

This may present with:
- synpharyngitic hematuria (IgA nephropathy);
- hypertension;
- nephrotic syndrome.

AKI associated with systemic sclerosis

Clinical features that may be present include:
- sclerodactyly;
- arthralgia;
- severe hypertension.

Differential diagnosis

The differential diagnosis can be difficult due to multisystem involvement.

Many of the clinical features have common causes.

A careful clinical evaluation should elicit evidence of:
- recent infection;
- foreign travel;
- drug use.

Intercurrent disease such as sepsis and hypovolemia may precipitate AKI.

Table 10.4.1 Glomerulonephritides associated with acute kidney injury

Vasculitis

Small vessel vasculitis

ANCA-associated vasculitis
- Wegener's granulomatosis
- Microscopic polyarteritis
- Churg–Strauss syndrome

Immune-complex-associated
- Henoch-Schönlein purpura
- Anti-GBM disease
- Mixed essential cryoglobulinemia
- Systemic lupus erythematosus
- Rheumatoid arthritis
- Relapsing polychondritis
- Behçet's disease

Infection-induced
- Hepatitis B and C
- HIV

Paraneoplastic
- Carcinoma-induced
- Lymphoproliferative neoplasm-induced
- Myeloproliferative neoplasm-induced

Medium vessel vasculitis
- Polyarteritis nodosa
- Kawasaki disease

Large vessel vasculitis
- Takayasu's arteritis
- Giant cell arteritis

Infection-associated glomerulonephritis

Postinfectious
- *Streptococcus* spp.
- *Staphylococcus* spp.
- Hepatitis B

Associated with active infection
- HIV
- Hepatitis C
- Infective endocarditis
- Shunt nephritis (ventricular shunt infection)

Primary glomerulonephritis
- IgA nephropathy
- Membranous nephropathy
- Minimal change nephropathy
- Focal segmental glomerulosclerosis
- Mesangiocapillary glomerulonephritis

Collagen–vascular disease
- Systemic sclerosis

Treatment prior to presentation with NSAIDs and antibiotics may cause an acute interstitial nephritis.

The precise diagnosis will require appropriate investigations which will usually include a renal biopsy.

Investigations

Blood tests

Full blood count, expect:
- anemia;
- neutrophilia (vasculitis);
- eosinophilia (Churg–Strauss syndrome);
- lymphopenia (SLE);
- thrombocytopenia (SLE);
- thrombocytosis (vasculitis).

Blood film, expect:
- fragmented red blood cells/schistocytes (systemic sclerosis).

Urea and electrolytes, expect:
- elevated urea and creatinine;
- elevated LDH (systemic sclerosis);
- elevated CRP (vasculitis, not SLE unless intercurrent infection).

Liver function tests, expect:
- elevated alkaline phosphatase (vasculitis).

Immunology screen:
- ANCA (ANCA-associated vasculitis);
  PR3-ANCA (Wegener's granulomatosis);
  MPO-ANCA (microscopic polyarteritis);
- anti-GBM antibody; (anti-GBM disease)
- anti-dsDNA antibody (SLE);
- reduced C4, normal C3 (SLE, mixed essential cryoglobulinemia (MEC));
- reduced C4, reduced C3 (SLE, MEC, mesangiocapillary GN type I);
- normal C4 reduced C3 (postinfectious GN, mesangiocapillary GN type II);
- elevated IgG and IgM (SLE, vasculitis, postinfectious GN);
- elevated IgE (Churg–Strauss syndrome);
- elevated IgA (IgA nephropathy, Henoch–Schönlein purpura);
- cryoglobulins (MEC);
- paraprotein (MEC, myeloma/lymphoma/amyloid);
- ASO titer (post-streptococcal GN).

Urine

Urinalysis, expect:
- hematuria (GN, vasculitis);
- proteinuria (GN, vasculitis).

Urine microscopy, expect:
- red-cell casts (GN, vasculitis);
- granular casts (ischemic AKI).

Microbiology

Blood cultures:
- positive with infection-associated GN.

Virology:
- hepatitis B (polyarteritis nodosa, membranous GN, mesangiocapillary GN);
- hepatitis C (membranous GN, mesangiocapillary GN, MEC);
- HIV (focal and segmental glomeruloscerosis).

Radiology

CXR:
- pulmonary infiltrates (pulmonary edema, hemorrhage, infection);
- cavitating lesions (Wegener's granulomatosis).

CT chest:
- may demonstrate smaller granulomatous lesions

Ultrasound, expect
- normal sized kidneys;
- ± increased cortical echogenicity;
- renal vein thrombosis (GN associated with nephrotic syndrome).

Renal angiography:
- arterial aneurysms (polyarteritis nodosa).

Arch angiogram:
- narrowing or occlusion of the aorta and its primary branches (Takayasu's arteritis).

Lung function tests
Carbon monoxide transfer factor coefficient:
- increased transfer factor coefficient (pulmonary hemorrhage).

Echocardiography
Transthoracic (ideally transoesophageal) echocardiogram:
- valve vegetations (infective endocarditis).

Renal biopsy
The renal biopsy findings will be dependent upon the primary pathology and is important in:
- establishing the diagnosis (Figs 10.4.1–10.4.3);
- assessing disease activity;
- assessing the degree of chronic damage.

Together these will determine the likely potential for recoverability with and without treatment.

Temporal artery biopsy
This may be indicated if giant cell arteritis is suspected.

Management
General treatment measures should include:
- fluid and electrolyte imbalance may necessitate renal replacement therapy;
- prompt treatment of infection;
- antimicrobial prophylaxis if the patient is immunocompromised or if immunosuppression is planned;
- stress ulcer prophylaxis with proton pump inhibitors;
- early enteral or parenteral nutrition;

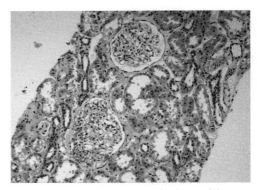

Fig. 10.4.2 Acute kidney injury associated with minimal change nephropathy. Minimal change nephropathy occurred secondary to mercury poisoning. There is acute tubular injury with apical cytoplasmic projections and normal glomeruli. EM confirmed foot process effacement and no immune deposits.

Specific treatment is dependent upon the underlying diagnosis.

In the case of immunologically mediated diseases including the vasculitides, early diagnosis and commencement of immunosuppression is essential to preserve renal function.

In patients with pulmonary hemorrhage it is important to maintain very careful fluid balance and avoid precipitating pulmonary oedema which may exacerbate the pulmonary hemorrhage.

Close attention must be paid to intercurrent infection, with a low threshold for removing hemodialysis catheters.

Patients who have developed AKI will require appropriate dose adjustments to their medications.

Prevention of AKI is particularly important in patients who have nephrotic syndrome. In patients receiving diuretics the dose must be carefully titrated with regular clinical review. The patient's weight should be measured daily and it is advisable not to diurese >3 kg/day. NSAIDs should be

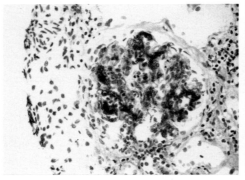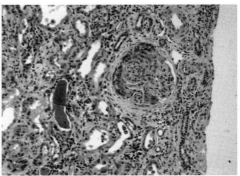

Fig. 10.4.1 Acute kidney injury secondary to crescentic IgA nephropathy. (*Right panel*) The glomerulus is hypercellular with a cellular crescent. There are red-cell casts present in the tubules. (*Left panel*) Immunohistochemistry demonstrates brown granular deposits of IgA in the mesangium.

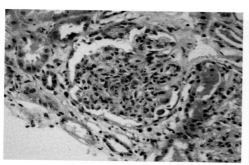 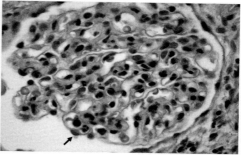

Fig. 10.4.3 Acute kidney injury secondary to post-streptococcal glomerulonephritis. (*Left panel:*). There are red-cell tubular casts and the glomerulus displays global endocapillary hypercellularity with neutrophils. (*Right panel:*) MSB stain of a glomurulus demonstrating intracapillary neutrophils and a subepithelial hump-like deposit. (All images courtesy of Dr D. Leitch, St James's University Hospital, Leeds, UK.)

avoided in patients with nephrotic syndrome as they can precipitate AKI.

Prognosis

The prognosis is dependent upon the underlying diagnosis and the response to therapy.

If there is significant secondary acute tubular necrosis on the renal biopsy, this can indicate a potential for reversibility of renal function.

Further reading

Furuya R, Kumagai H, Ikegaya N, *et al.* Reversible acute renal failure in idiopathic nephrotic syndrome. *Intern Med* 1993; **32**: 31–35.

López-Gómez JM, Rivera F. Spanish registry of glomerulonephritis. Renal biopsy findings in acute renal failure in the cohort of patients in the Spanish registry of glomerulonephritis. *Clin J Am Soc Nephrol.* 2008; **3**: 674–681.

Haas M, Spargo BH, Wit EJ, *et al.* Etiologies and outcome of acute renal insufficiency in older adults: a renal biopsy study of 259 cases. *Am J Kidney Dis* 2000; **35**: 433–447.

Smith JD, Hayslett JP. Reversible renal failure in the nephrotic syndrome. *Am J Kidney Dis* 1992; **19**: 201–203.

Internet resources

Acute Dialysis Quality Initiative:

`http://www.ADQI.net`

Acute Kidney Injury Network:

`http://www.akinet.org`

See also

Clinical approach to acute kidney injury, p. 318

Renal replacement therapies in acute kidney injury, p. 328

Crescentic glomerulonephritis, p. 120

Infection-related glomerulonephritis, p. 128

Systemic vasculitis, p. 168

Systemic lupus erythematosus, p. 180

Scleroderma–systemic sclerosis, p. 186

Acute tubulointerstitial nephritis

Introduction

Acute tubulointerstitial nephritis or acute interstitial nephritis (AIN) is an inflammatory condition affecting the interstitium. The inflammatory infiltrate consists of lymphocytes and monocytes with or without eosinophils and is most commonly secondary to drugs.

Epidemiology

Acute tubulointerstitial nephritis is an important cause of unexplained AKI that occurs in males and females with equal incidence.

It most commonly occurs in the 5th and 6th decades.

Etiology

The inflammatory cell infiltrate is triggered by a number of different provoking factors.

Drug-induced AIN is the most common cause accounting for 70–90% of cases and is not dose dependent (Table 10.5.1).

Many drugs have been reported to cause AIN. To determine a causative role for a specific drug, the patient must not be on any other drug or have any other condition that might cause the disease, and must undergo a confirmatory renal biopsy.

Clinical features

Classically presents as AKI associated with:
- fever;
- rash;
- arthralgia.

This presentation is now less common (10% of cases).

The classic triad is typically absent with NSAID-induced AIN.

Often there are nonspecific symptoms related to:
- uremic symptoms ± oliguria reflecting AKI;
- loin pain secondary to swelling of renal capsule.

A thorough drug history is essential.

A history of drug ingestion up to 18 months before presentation with AIN can occur.

The nephrotic syndrome can occur with NSAID-induced AIN.

There may be clinical features of an infective process or an underlying disease process:

Leptospirosis
The associated AIN may rarely be associated with multiple organ involvement with hemolytic anemia, liver failure and AKI.

Legionellosis
The associated AIN may be associated with multiple organ involvement with pneumonia, liver enzyme abnormalities and AKI.

Hantavirus
AIN may be associated with multiple organ involvement with respiratory symptoms, liver enzyme abnormalities, thrombocytopenia and AKI.

Severe hantavirus infection is mainly seen in Asia with milder forms of infection more usual in Europe.

Investigations

Blood tests
Full blood count:
- differential may reveal eosinophilia (25% cases);
- eosinophilia is typically absent in NSAID-induced AIN.

Urea and electrolytes, expect:
- elevated urea and creatinine.

Liver function tests:
- may be abnormal if AIN secondary to Legionella spp. or Leptospirosis spp. infection.

Bone profile:
- ↑ Ca^{2+} if AIN secondary to sarcoidosis.

Autoantibody screen:
- only required if autoimmune disease suspected;
- anti-Ro and -La, if Sjögren's syndrome suspected.

Serum ACE:
- if sarcoidosis suspected.

Urine
Urinalysis, expect:
- hematuria;
- proteinuria (<1 g/day);
- proteinuria (>1 g/day if concurrent nephrotic syndrome (NSAIDs and minimal change disease) or existing underlying renal disease);
- can be normal in a few patients.

Urine microscopy, expect:
- eosinophiluria (low sensitivity, also seen in RPGN and atheroembolic renal disease);
- white cell casts.

Microbiology
Specific tests dependent upon suspected underlying diagnosis:
- blood cultures;
- urinary legionella antigen;
- urine culture.

Serology:
- Legionella spp.;
- Leptospirosis spp.;
- hantavirus.

Radiology
CXR, may show signs consistent with:
- respiratory infection;
- sarcoidosis.

Ultrasound, expect:
- swollen or normal-sized kidneys.

Gallium scan:
- rarely performed;
- diffuse, intense uptake secondary to inflammatory infiltrate;
- positive scan suggests AIN;
- differentiates AIN from acute tubular necrosis (negative scan).

Table 10.5.1 Common causes of acute tubulointerstitial nephritis

Drugs
NSAIDs
Antibiotics
- penicillins
- cephalosporins
- rifampicin
- sulphonamides (including cotrimoxazole)
- ciprofloxacin

Allopurinol
Proton pump inhibitors
Indinavir
Diuretics (sulphur containing)
- furosemide
- bumetanide

Infections
Bacteria
- *Staphylococcus* spp.
- *Streptococcus* spp.
- *Tuberculosis* spp.
- *Legionella* spp.
- *Leptospirosis* spp.
- *Chlamydia* spp.
- *Mycoplasma* spp.

Viruses
- cytomegalovirus
- Epstein–Barr virus
- hantavirus
- hepatitis A and B
- herpes simplex virus
- HIV

Parasites
- toxoplasma

Autoimmune disease
Sarcoidosis
Sjögren's syndrome
TINU (tubulointerstitial nephritis and uveitis syndrome)

Renal biopsy
A renal biopsy is indicated in a patient with unexplained AKI and normal-sized kidneys on renal tract USS (Fig. 10.5.1).

However, renal biopsy may not be required in the absence of severe disease, clinical presentation highly suggestive of drug-induced AIN, and prompt improvement in renal function on discontinuing the offending drug.

Light microscopy
Glomerular morphology:
- normal.

Interstitium:
- inflammatory infiltrate:
  - T-lymphocytes;
  - monocytes;
  - eosinophils;
- giant cells and granulomata if:
  - TB;
  - sarcoidosis;
- interstitial edema.

Immunofluorescence and electron microscopy:
- nonspecific findings.

Management
This is dependant upon the underlying disease process.

Drug-induced AIN
Identify and stop offending drug.

A recent retrospective study has demonstrated that early steroid treatment improves the recovery of renal function with drug-induced AIN.

Therefore consider corticosteroids if worsening renal function or requiring renal replacement therapy:
- prednisolone 1 mg/kg/day, orally;
- taper over a period of 1 month dependent upon response;
- consider bone and GI protection;
- monitor blood glucose.

NSAID-induced AIN is less responsive to corticosteroid therapy.

Mycophenolate mofetil has been used in patients with steroid-resistant AIN.

Prognosis
This is dependant upon underlying disease process.

Good prognosis with drug-induced AIN:
- majority recover renal function;
- 5% mortality rate.

The prognosis is poorer if the AIN is not drug-induced.

There is a worse prognosis if interstitial fibrosis is present on the biopsy.

Tubulointerstitial nephritis and uveitis syndrome (TINU)
Introduction
Tubulointerstitial nephritis and uveitis syndrome (TINU) is a distinct entity occurring in a subset of patients who have tubulointerstitial nephritis and uveitis. The majority of the reports of this syndrome have been small descriptive case series or single case reports.

Epidemiology
Female preponderance, 3:1.

Median age at presentation is 15 years but has been diagnosed in the elderly.

Various HLA associations have been described but there is no consistent haplotype across studies.

Etiology
The underlying cause is unclear.

Concurrent infection with *Chlamydia* spp. and Epstein–Barr virus has been described.

There are reported associations with a number of auto-immune diseases.

Clinical features
Uveitis
- Typically bilateral.
- Anterior uveitis is most common:
  - painful eye or redness;
  - photophobia and decreased visual acuity.

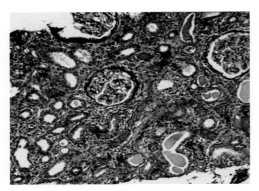

Fig. 10.5.1 Silver-stained renal biopsy demonstrating acute interstitial nephritis. The renal biopsy shows tubular injury with a mononuclear cell interstitial infiltrate and normal glomerular morphology. (Courtesy of Dr D. Leitch, St James's University Hospital, Leeds, UK.)

- Reported to occur between 2 months prior and up to 14 months after the onset of AIN.

Acute interstitial nephritis
- Anorexia and weight loss.
- Fever.
- Fatigue, malaise.
- Arthralgia, myalgia, headache.
- AKI.

Investigations
There are no specific laboratory investigations for TINU.

There are associations reported with hypocomplementemia and positive serology for autoantibodies, including ANCA, ANA and rheumatoid factor.

Renal biopsy findings are as per AIN.

Differential diagnosis
There is a broad differential diagnosis which includes a number of renal diseases associated with ocular disease:
- sarcoidosis;
- Sjögren's syndrome;
- systemic lupus erythematosus;
- Wegener's granulomatosis;
- Behçet's disease;
- Infectious disease (TB, toxoplasmosis, brucellosis).

The ocular disease manifestations are usually distinct from uveitis and there will be evidence of other organ involvement. However, it can be difficult to differentiate TINU from sarcoidosis and Sjögren's syndrome.

Management
Acute interstitial nephritis
This is usually self-limiting and resolves spontaneously.

In patients with progressive AKI consider:
- prednisolone 1 mg/kg/day, orally;
- taper over 3–6 months, dependent upon response;
- consider bone and GI protection;
- monitor blood glucose.

Most patients recover renal function.

Relapses are more likely to occur.

Uveitis
Early referral to ophthalmologist is required.

Topical or systemic corticosteroids may be indicated.

Relapses are common.

Rarely steroid sparing immunosuppression required.

Prognosis
This is dependent upon the degree of tubulointerstitial fibrosis on renal biopsy.

Further reading
Clarkson MR, Giblin L, O'Connell FP, *et al.* Acute interstitial nephritis: clinical features and response to corticosteroid therapy. *Nephrol Dialysis Transpl* 2004; **19**: 2778–2783.

Joss N, Morris S, Young B. *et al.* Granulomatous interstitial nephritis. *Clin J Am Soc Nephrol* 2007; **2**: 222.

Rossert J. Drug-induced acute interstitial nephritis. *Kidney Int* 2001; **60**: 804–817.

Takemura T. Okada M. Hino, S. *et al.* Course and outcome of tubulointerstitial nephritis and uveitis syndrome. *Am J Kidney Dis* 1999; **34**: 1016–1021.

Internet resources
Acute Dialysis Quality Initiative

http://www.ADQI.net

Epocrates® ONLINE provides continually updated information on brand and generic drugs (dosing, drug–drug interactions, adverse reactions and mode of action:

http://www.epocrates.com

A patient-friendly US-based site with drug information:

http://drugs.com

Ocular Immunology and Uveitis Foundation:

http://www.uveitis.org/

See also
Clinical approach to acute kidney injury, p. 318

Drug-induced nephropathies, p. 698

NSAIDs and the kidney, p. 228

Hemolytic uremic syndrome and thrombotic thrombocytopenic purpura

Introduction

The thrombotic microangiopathies (TMA) describe a group of systemic disorders characterized by the presence of microangiopathic hemolytic anemia (MAHA), thrombocytopenia and tissue ischemia secondary to platelet thrombosis in the microcirculation (Table 10.6.1).

Hemolytic anemia occurs secondary to mechanical fragmentation of erythrocytes during their passage through narrowed vessels.

Thrombotic thrombocytopenic purpura (TTP) and hemolytic uremic syndrome (HUS) are both well-recognized causes of TMA and present with very similar clinical features.

HUS associated with diarrhea is also known as diarrhea-positive (D^+) HUS or typical HUS and is the most frequent form of HUS.

HUS not associated with diarrhea is known as diarrhea-negative (D^-) HUS or atypical HUS.

Epidemiology

D^+/typical HUS:

- incidence of 2 cases per 100 000 per year;
- peak incidence is in children aged <5 years;
- most frequently seen in summer months.

TTP secondary to acquired deficiency of vWF-cleaving protease:

- incidence of 0.4 cases per 100 000 per year;
- occurs more commonly in females;
- peak incidence in third decade.

Etiology

D^+ hemolytic uremic syndrome

This occurs most commonly due to infection with enteropathogenic E. coli of different serotypes, usually O157:H7, or sometimes by shigellosis. These strains produce an enterotoxin called VT (verocyte toxin).

The source may be contaminated meat or milk or contact with infected animal or human excretions.

E.coli O157:H7 binds to the gastrointestinal mucosa; the VT translocates across the colon and disseminates through the circulation.

The VT binds to vascular endothelial cells and platelets, particularly those of the glomerular capillaries.

Activated endothelial cells produce large von Willibrand factor (vWF) multimers facilitating platelet adhesion through the glycoprotein 1b (GP1b) receptor, resulting in thrombosis and glomerular ischemia.

D^- hemolytic uremic syndrome

Over the last decade in the UK, pneumococcal-related HUS has become the second most common cause of HUS, accounting for 10–15% of all cases. The reason for this recent increase is not known.

HUS in the absence of diarrhea may also be associated with:

- factor H deficiency (complement regulatory protein);
- membrane cofactor protein (MCP) abnormalities;
- numerous drugs.

Factor H is a plasma protein mainly of liver origin that binds to endothelial cells in glomerular capillaries and other resident glomerular cells and regulates complement activation in the glomerulus.

Similarly, membrane cofactor protein is expressed in the kidney and regulates glomerular C3 activation.

Reduced expression of either factor H or MCP leads to excessive complement activation on glomerular endothelial cell surfaces with endothelial cell damage and thrombosis.

Thrombotic thrombocytopenic purpura

TTP has been associated with genetic and autoimmune-mediated deficiency of the vWF cleaving metalloproteinase ADAMTS13.

Inherited mutations or IgG autoantibodies (directed against ADAMTS13) lead to defective cleavage of vWF and the presence in the circulation of abnormally large vWF multimers.

These large vWF multimers bind and activate platelets which can result in the formation of platelet-rich thrombus in the microcirculation and tissue ischemia.

Clinical features

The clinical features of both HUS and TTP are very similar.

HUS and TTP secondary to genetic mutations can cluster in families and recur.

Hemolytic uremic syndrome

HUS may present with:

- diarrhea (± bloody);
- fever;
- hypertension;
- fluid overload;
- microangiopathic hemolytic anemia;
- thrombocytopenic purpura;
- AKI.

Postpartum HUS can occur up to 6 months post delivery.

Thrombotic thrombocytopenic purpura

CNS involvement is more typically associated with TTP, although one-third of patients with TTP have no CNS abnormalities.

TTP generally has more widespread organ involvement.

Autoimmune-mediated TTP may follow exposure to specific drugs (e.g. clopidogrel).

TTP may present with:

- fever;
- microangiopathic hemolytic anemia;
- thrombocytopenic purpura;
- CNS involvement (confusion, fits);
- AKI;
- pancreatitis;
- cardiomyopathy.

Pregnancy-associated TTP usually occurs before 28 weeks.

Differential diagnosis

Careful clinical evaluation and appropriate investigations will help to make the diagnosis and identify the cause (Table 10.6.1).

Table 10.6.1 Classification of thrombotic microangiopathies

Thrombotic thrombocytopenic purpura

Genetic
- ADAMTS13 deficiency

Autoimmune
- IgG directed against ADAMTS13 (e.g. post clopidogrel)

Hemolytic uremic syndrome

Infection
- *Eschericia coli* 0157:H7
- *Shigella dysenteriae* serotype 1
- *Salmonella* spp.
- *Campylobacter* spp.
- *Streptococcus pneumoniae* (neuraminidase)
- HIV

Genetic
- factor H deficiency
- membrane cofactor protein abnormalities

Autoimmune
- IgG directed against factor H

Drugs
- quinine
- ciclosporin
- tacrolimus
- oral contraceptive pill

Pregnancy-associated TMA
- Pre-eclampsia
- HELLP syndrome
- Postpartum TTP and HUS

Systemic disease-associated TMA
- Accelerated hypertension
- Antiphospholipid syndrome
- Systemic sclerosis
- Malignancy

A diagnosis of TTP or HUS can be made provisionally if there is thrombocytopenia and MHA in the absence of any other apparent cause.

Diagnoses to exlcude include:
- vasculitis (additional clinical features: rash and arthralgia, and presence of autoantibodies: ANCA);
- systemic sclerosis with renal crisis (additional clinical features: sclerodactyly, and presence of autoantibodies: Scl-70);
- accelerated hypertension (history of high blood pressure and retinopathy);
- disseminated intravascular coagulation (associated with sepsis and multiple organ failure, associated with an elevated PT and aPTT);
- hantavirus infection (associated with fever, AKI and thrombocytopenia but not MHA);
- HELLP syndrome (occurs late in 3rd trimester of pregnancy, has features of TMA along with liver dysfunction).

Investigations

Blood tests

Full blood count, expect:
- anemia;
- elevated WBC (D$^+$ HUS);
- thrombocytopenia;
- reticulocytosis.

Blood film:
- fragmented red blood cells/schistocytes.

Clotting screen:
- normal PT, aPTT, fibrinogen levels;
- reduced haptoglobin;
- Coombs' test negative (except in pneumococcal-associated HUS).

Urea and electrolytes, expect:
- elevated urea and creatinine;
- elevated LDH.

Liver function tests, expect:
- elevated bilirubin.

Autoantibody screen:
- dsDNA (if SLE considered);
- complement (if SLE considered);
- ANCA (if a small vessel vasculitis considered);
- Scl-70 (if systemic sclerosis considered);
- antiphospholipid antibody (if APL syndrome considered).

Other:
- ADAMTS13 activity (in TTP this will be < 5% normal);
- factor H mutations (atypical HUS);
- βhCG (if pregnancy-associated TTP suspected).

Urine tests

Urinalysis, expect:
- hematuria;
- proteinuria (usually mild);
- bilirubinuria (from hemolysis).

Urine microscopy, expect:
- few casts.

Microbiology

Stool culture (in D$^+$ HUS *E. coli* is shed for several weeks).

Other cultures depending on clinical suspicion (Table 10.6.1).

Virology

Consider HIV testing if there is a clinical suspicion.

Radiology

Ultrasound, expect:
- normal sized kidneys.

Renal biopsy

A renal biopsy is only performed if the platelet count normalizes.

The histology is similar for all causes of TMA.

Fibrin thrombi are present in the glomerular capillaries with surrounding ischemic damage (Fig. 10.6.1).

In HUS microthrombi are predominantly present in the kidneys.

Microthrombi are more extensively distributed in TTP and found mainly in the cerebral circulation but may also be seen in the kidneys, heart, adrenals and pancreas.

Management

Supportive treatment

Renal replacement therapy may be required dependent upon the degree of AKI.

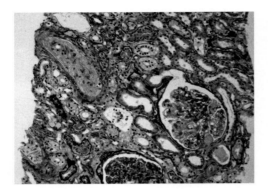

Fig. 10.6.1 Silver stain demonstrating features of thrombotic microangiography in glomeruli and a small interlobular artery. Glomeruli are bloodless with capillary thrombosis. The interlobular artery shows mural fibrinoid necrosis and luminal occlusion. (Courtesy of Dr D. Leitch, St James's University Hospital, Leeds, UK.)

Blood transfusions are required for symptomatic anemia.

Avoid platelet transfusions unless there is life-threatening hemorrhage or an urgent need for surgery.

D⁺ hemolytic uremic syndrome

Initial management is supportive.

Antibiotics should be avoided in cases of diarrhea (unless there is systemic bacteremia), due to the increased risk of precipitating HUS.

Plasma exchange should be commenced if there is any doubt concerning diagnosis (TTP or D⁻ HUS).

There is no proven benefit for treatment with plasma exchange in D⁺ HUS.

D⁻ hemolytic uremic syndrome

Plasma exchange can be effective but for most it is a relapsing and remitting disease.

Unlike D⁺ HUS, D⁻ HUS can recur following renal transplantation. A recurrence rate of up to 50% has been reported in adults.

The risk of recurrence is less with mutations in the membrane cofactor protein gene.

Combined liver and kidney transplantation following intensive plasma exchange has been performed successfully in HUS secondary to factor H deficiency.

Liver transplantation restores normal factor H synthesis.

Postpartum HUS requires supportive care. The role of plasma exchange is unproven.

Thrombotic thrombocytopenic purpura

TTP requires prompt treatment which is aimed at:
- removing vWF multimers;
- restoring the ability to cleave vWF multimers.

Plasma exchange should be performed daily with FFP until normalisation of platelets and LDH.

Cryosupernatant (devoid of vWF multimers and fibrinogen) should be used in patients resistant to plasma exchange with FFP.

Monitoring levels of ADAMTS13 autoantibodies may be useful in assessing patient response to therapy.

Rituximab (anti-CD20 monoclonal antibody) has been used for resistant TTP.

In pregnancy-associated TTP, delivery is recommended for those who fail to respond to plasma exchange.

HELLP syndrome

HELLP syndrome requires supportive therapy and delivery of the baby. Plasma exchange is ineffective during pregnancy but may help recovery of disease following delivery.

Prognosis

In childhood D⁺ HUS, expect:
- a good initial recovery (~90%);
- ~3% mortality;
- ~40% to develop hypertension and progressive CKD.

Factors associated with a poor renal prognosis in HUS:
- age <2 years;
- high white cell count;
- D⁻ (atypical HUS);
- anuria at presentation;
- HUS secondary to *S. pneumoniae* infection;
- HUS secondary to *Shigella* infection.

Postpartum HUS:
- ~50% mortality;
- most survivors will have CKD and hypertension.

In TTP you should expect:
- 90% patient survival if treatment is commenced early;
- relapse rate of ~30%.

Future prospects

Advances in the understanding of the etiology of HUS/TTP will improve the prospects for specific therapy and assessing patient prognosis. Most recently the complement factor H R1210C mutation has been demonstrated to be linked with development of D⁻ HUS.

Further reading

George JN. Clinical practice. Thrombotic thrombocytopenic purpura. *N Engl J Med* 2006; **354**: 1927–1935.

Gutterman L, Kloster B, Tsai H. Rituximab therapy for refractory thrombotic thrombocytopenic purpura. *Blood Cells Mol Dis* 2002; **28**: 385–391.

Noris M, Remuzzi G. Haemolytic uraemic syndrome. *J Am Soc Nephrol* 2005; **16**: 1035–1050.

Zipfel PF, Skerka C. Complement dysfunction in haemolytic uraemic syndrome. *Curr Opin Rheumatol* 2006; **18**: 548–555.

Internet resources

Acute Dialysis Quality Initiative:

http://www.ADQI.net

Acute Kidney Injury Network:

http://www.akinet.org

HUSH (Haemolytic Uraemic Syndrome Help); UK E. Coli Support Group:

http://www.ecoli-uk.com/

About TTP website:

http://www.about-ttp.com/

See also

Clinical approach to acute kidney injury, p. 318

Acute kidney injury in infants and children, p. 372

Acute kidney injury in pregnancy, p. 378

Hepatorenal syndrome

Introduction

Hepatorenal syndrome (HRS) is the development of AKI in the setting of advanced liver disease most commonly secondary to cirrhosis, but can also occur in patients with fulminant liver failure from any cause.

The AKI is initially entirely prerenal secondary to renal hypoperfusion with normal renal histology and preserved tubular cell integrity and function. HRS may progress to acute tubular necrosis (ATN).

Acute kidney injury can complicate the postoperative course of patients with obstructive jaundice or those undergoing liver transplantation. Acute kidney injury may also occur secondary to IgA nephropathy associated with liver disease and also secondary to cryoglobulinemia associated with hepatitis C.

Definition

HRS has been classified into two types dependent upon the rapidity of onset, the severity of AKI and prognosis.

Type I HRS
- AKI is the dominant clinical feature.
- Rapid fall in GFR <20 mL/min in <2 weeks.
- Progressive oligoanuria.
- Median survival 2 weeks.

Type II HRS
- Ascites is the dominant clinical feature.
- Protracted clinical course.
- AKI is less acute and severe.
- Potential to convert to type I HRS.
- Median survival 6 months.

Epidemiology

HRS is reported to occur in 20% of patients with liver cirrhosis and ascites at 1 year.

The incidence increases to 40% at 5 years.

Etiology

With progressive liver disease there is a rise in cardiac output and a fall in systemic vascular resistance (SVR).

Falling SVR results from the splanchnic vasodilatation that occurs in association with liver disease and has been proposed to be secondary to an increased secretion of a number of mediating factors including:
- vasoactive gut peptide secretion;
- glucagon;
- prostacyclin;
- nitric oxide (NO) secretion locally;
- bacterial translocation.

Low SVR in turn results in renal vasoconstriction and a fall in renal blood flow (RBF) secondary to secretion of:
- catecholamines (α-agonism);
- angiotensin ($2°$ hyperaldosteronism);
- endothelin;
- ADH (nonosmotic stimulation).

A resultant fall in RBF results in a parallel fall in GFR and prerenal AKI.

The onset of HRS is generally insidious but can be precipitated in patients with advanced liver disease and ascites by a number of different insults including:
- gastrointestinal hemorrhage;
- sepsis (e.g. spontaneous bacterial peritonitis);
- overdiuresis;
- nephrotoxins (aminoglycosides, NSAIDs, ACEIs, ARBs, contrast).

Clinical features

Stigmata of chronic liver disease:
- jaundice, spider nevi, etc.;
- ascites;
- wasting (secondary to poor nutritional intake);
- edema (sodium and water retention);
- hypotension ($\downarrow$ effective circulating volume and systemic vascular resistance).

Signs of the precipitating factor may also be present:
- GI hemorrhage (portal hypertension and coagulopathy);
- sepsis ($\uparrow$ susceptibility, spontaneous bacterial peritonitis and pneumonia).

A diagnosis of HRS is based upon the presence of predetermined major criteria. These include the demonstration of a markedly reduced GFR and the exclusion of other causes of AKI in the setting of acute or chronic liver disease with advanced liver failure and portal hypertension (Table 10.7.1).

It is important to recognize that:

Urine Na <10 mmol/L (off diuretics) is only a minor criteria.

Fractional excretion of sodium (FE_{Na}) may remain <1% in patients with ATN superimposed on HRS secondary to persistent vasoconstriction.

Patients with liver cirrhosis have reduced muscle mass and therefore serum Cr may underestimate GFR.

Serum urea will also be affected by:
- GI hemorrhage;
- $\downarrow$ production by the liver;
- $\downarrow$ dietary intake.

Differential diagnosis

Distinguishing HRS from other causes of AKI in patients with liver disease presents a diagnostic challenge.

The diagnosis of HRS is essentially one of exclusion and must be distinguished from other causes of combined liver disease and AKI.

Other common causes include:
- sepsis leading to relative hypovolemia and ATN;
- GI hemorrhage leading to hypovolemia and ATN;
- overdiuresis leading to hypovolemia and ATN;
- nephrotoxins leading to ATN;
- glomerulonephritis (suspect if active urinary sediment with red cell casts);
- mesangiocapillary glomerulonephritis and hepatitis C;
- IgA nephropathy and alcoholic liver disease.

Establishing the correct diagnosis is important clinically as patients with HRS have a poor prognosis. Most patients die

Table 10.7.1 Criteria for the diagnosis of hepatorenal syndrome

Major criteria

Acute or chronic liver disease with advanced liver failure and portal hypertension.

Progressive AKI over days to weeks (CrCl <40 mL/min).

Absence of other causes of AKI including:
- shock
- GI fluid losses
- overdiuresis
- sepsis (exclude spontaneous bacterial peritonitis)
- nephrotoxins (NSAIDs, aminoglycosides)
- obstruction or parenchymal disease on ultrasound.

No sustained recovery of renal function ($\uparrow$ CrCl >40 mL/min) following adequate fluid resuscitation and discontinuation of potential nephrotoxins.

Proteinuria <500 mg/dL (no evidence of renal parenchymal disease).

Minor criteria

Urine output <500 mL/day.

Urine Na <10 mmol/L (off diuretics).

Urine osmolality > plasma osmolality.

Urine red blood cells <50/HPF.

Serum Na <130 mmol/L.

within weeks of the onset of AKI, usually from a complication of their liver disease, e.g. GI hemorrhage, unless they receive effective treatment.

Other causes of AKI such as ATN or prerenal disease are usually reversible.

Investigations

Blood tests

Full blood count, expect:
- anemia (GI hemorrhage);
- neutrophilia (sepsis).

Urea and electrolytes, expect:
- elevated urea and creatinine;
- hyponatremia (dilutional).

Liver function tests, expect:
- $\uparrow$ bilirubin;
- hypoalbuminemia;
- $\uparrow$ INR.

Autoantibody screen:
- only required if autoimmune liver disease suspected.

Urine

Urine biochemistry, expect:
- urine Na <10 mmol/L;
- urine osmolality > plasma osmolality.

Urinalysis, expect:
- bland urinary sediment;
- no hematuria;
- proteinuria (<500 mg/day).

Urine microscopy, expect:
- red blood cells <50/HPF.

Microbiology

It is essential to exclude sepsis with:
- blood cultures;
- urine culture;
- cultures of ascitic fluid.

Radiology

CXR:
- to aid volume assessment;
- to detect pneumonia.

Ultrasound, expect:
- normal sized kidneys.

Renal biopsy

A renal biopsy is not usually required and may represent a significant risk in a patient with liver disease and coagulopathy.

Renal biopsy findings in patients with HRS are normal initially but prolonged renal hypoperfusion will result in ATN.

Management

Prevention

It is important to identify patients at risk of developing HRS; usually these are those with liver cirrhosis and ascites:
- check medications;
- beware of over diuresis;
- beware of esophageal varices → GI hemorrhage;
- prompt diagnosis and treatment of sepsis;
- increased risk associated with surgery.

Ensure adequate volume replacement with 100 mL 20% salt poor human albumin solution (HAS) per 1.5 L paracentesis.

If spontaneous bacterial peritonitis is suspected:
- IV salt poor HAS 1.5 g/kg at diagnosis and 1 g/kg at 48 h;
- antibiotic treatment.

In alcoholic hepatitis:
- consider pentoxifylline (TNF-α inhibitor) 400 mg PO tds.

Treatment

It is important to establish the diagnosis of HRS early and exclude other causes of liver disease and AKI.

Recovery of renal function is dependent upon prompt treatment of precipitants and recovery of liver function through the resolution of the primary liver disease or liver transplantation.

Improvement in the primary liver disease is most dramatic in patients with:
- alcoholic liver disease when patients abstain from alcohol consumption;
- decompensated liver cirrhosis secondary to hepatitis B virus infection treated with antiviral therapy.

General measures

Volume assessment and fluid resuscitation:
- IV 20% salt-poor human albumin solution (HAS).

Stop nephrotoxic medications.

Septic screen:
- culture blood, urine and ascitic fluid;
- consider prophylactic antibiotic treatment with cefotaxime 1 g bd or piperacillin/tazobactam 4.5 g tds.

Exclude intra-abdominal hypertension:
- check intra-abdominal pressure if there is tense ascites;
- if intra-abdominal pressure is >30 cm H_2O paracentesis is indicated.

Specific measures
Vasoconstrictors should be administered in combination with salt-poor HAS to improve systemic hemodynamics and improve renal perfusion. However, these drugs should be avoided in patients with ischemic heart disease, peripheral arterial disease and/or cerebrovascular disease due to the risk of precipitating an ischemic event.

Midrodine in combination with octeotide.
A small number of studies support the efficacy and safety.

Midrodine:
- selective α1-agonist;
- systemic vasoconstrictor;
- dose: 7.5–12.5 mg PO tds.

Octreotide:
- somatostatin analogue;
- inhibitor of endogenous vasodilator release;
- dose: 100–200 μg SC tds.

Both drugs are titrated to increase MAP by >15 mmHg.

Administer for 3–15 day trial with daily IV salt poor HAS (20–40 g).

Studies suggest they significantly improve renal function and reduce mortality.

Minimal side-effects have been reported.

A trial of therapy should be considered in selected patients.

Terlipressin.
There are a small number of studies with variable outcomes.
- Vasopressin analogue acts via V1 receptors.
- Dose: 0.5–1 mg IV 4–6 times per day.
- Daily IV salt poor HAS (20–40 g/day) for 3–15 days.

Responders appear to have a better prognosis.

Repeat courses can be given and are effective in selected patients.

It is not recommended as routine practice.

Transjugular intrahepatic portosystemic shunt (TIPS).
This is used in combination with vasoconstrictors when pharmacotherapy alone has failed.

There is little data available on outcomes.

Many patients are considered too unwell to undergo the procedure.

There is improved short-term survival in selected patients.

N-Acetylcysteine.
There are few data available on effectiveness in HRS.

Dose: 100 mg/kg IV bd.

It is not recommended as routine practice.

Renal replacement therapy.
This has no effect on outcome.

It should only be considered if:
- liver transplantation is awaited;
- there is a possibility of recovery of liver function.

Continuous renal replacement therapy is preferred due to hemodynamic instability.

Molecular adsorbent recirculating system (MARS).
This removes inflammatory cytokines.

There is a lack of convincing data regarding effect on outcome.

Liver transplantation.
This is an effective therapy.

There is an improvement in GFR following transplantation, but the majority do not regain normal renal function.

There is a 10% incidence of ESRD.

Long-term mortality is increased when pre-transplant renal dysfunction is present.

Prognosis
Patients with liver disease who develop HRS have a significantly worse prognosis.

Type I HRS:
- median survival 2 weeks.

Type II HRS:
- median survival 6 months.

Obstructive jaundice and acute kidney injury
Obstructive jaundice secondary to intra- or extrahepatic biliary system obstruction is the most commonly encountered form of jaundice.

Surgery performed in the setting of obstructive jaundice is associated with an 8% incidence of AKI.

The cause of AKI in such patients is multifactorial and includes:
- hypovolemia;
- endotoxinemia;
- hyperbilirubinemia;
- release of renal prostaglandins;
- activation and endothelin system.

There is no specific or effective therapy.

Preoperative optimization of fluid balance is essential preventative therapy.

The use of mannitol (osmotic diuretic) is controversial and cannot be routinely recommended.

Liver transplantation and acute kidney injury
Acute kidney injury is one of the most common postoperative complications of liver transplantation with an incidence reported between 21–70%.

Pretransplant renal function has an impact on the immediate and longer-term outcome post liver transplantation.

Patients undergoing liver transplantation are at risk of developing AKI in the setting of:
- pre-existing renal dysfunction (prevalence of 10–20%);
- intraoperative hypotension;
- postoperative sepsis and exposure to nephrotoxic medications (calcineurin inhibitors).

A significant proportion of patients will have HRS prior to surgery.

Therefore preoperative optimization of fluid balance is essential.

10–18% of patients require renal replacement therapy following liver transplantation and the mortality in these patients is high (40–90%).

Glomerulonephritis and acute kidney injury

IgA nephropathy

This is the glomerulonephritis most commonly associated with liver disease, invariably alcoholic liver disease.

IgA containing complexes are normally removed by the liver. Failure to remove these complexes in liver disease results in persistence of complexes in the circulation and mesangial IgA deposition.

Most patients are asymptomatic and present with microscopic hematuria, mild proteinuria and varying degrees of renal dysfunction.

Management is as for idiopathic IgA nephropathy.

Mesangiocapillary glomerulonephritis

Cryoglobulins can be found in up to 40% of patients with chronic liver disease.

It is associated with viral hepatitis, particularly hepatitis C.

Most commonly type II cryoglobulinemia is found.

Patients with chronic liver disease and cryoglobulinemia may present with an acute nephritic syndrome and AKI.

The clinical presentation is characterized by:
- arthritis;
- purpuric skin rash;
- lymphadenopathy;
- splenomegaly;
- liver dysfunction;
- peripheral neuropathy;
- microscopic hematuria;
- mild proteinuria (20% have nephrotic range).

Investigations demonstrate hypocomplementemia and circulating cryoglobulins.

Renal biopsy reveals a mesangiocapillary glomerulonephritis.

In the setting of severe AKI treatment with corticosteroids, cyclophosphamide with or without plasmapheresis may be considered.

Further reading

Arroyo V, Gines P, Gerbes AL, et al. Definition and diagnostic criteria of refractory ascites and hepatorenal syndrome in cirrhosis. International Ascites Club. *Hepatology* 1996; **23**: 164–176.

Pouria S, Barratt J. Secondary IgA nephropathy. *Semin Nephrol* 2008; **28**: 27–37.

Salerno F, Gerbes A, Gines P, et al. Diagnosis, prevention and treatment of hepatorenal syndrome in cirrhosis. *Gut* 2007; **56**: 1310.

Wadei HM, Mai ML, Ahsan N, et al. Hepatorenal syndrome: pathophysiology and management. *Clin J Am Soc Nephrol* 2006; **1**: 1066.

Internet resources

Acute Dialysis Quality Initiative:

http://www.ADQI.net

Acute Kidney Injury Network:

http://akinet.org/index.php

Cochrane Review of Terlipressin in hepatorenal syndrome:

http://www.cochrane.org/reviews/en/ab005162.html

US government register of clinical trials in hepatorenal syndrome:

http://clinicaltrials.gov/ct2/results?cond=%22Hepatorenal+Syndrome%22

See also

Clinical approach to acute kidney injury, p. 318

Renal replacement therapies in acute kidney injury, p. 328

IgA nephropathy and Henoch–Schönlein purpura, p. 100

Mesangiocapillary glomerulonephritis, p. 112

Ischemic acute kidney injury

Introduction

Ischemic AKI may result from either systemic hypotension (causing ATN) or disease of the renal vasculature. This chapter will discuss AKI due to arterial occlusive disease (atheromatous, thromboembolic and atheroembolic) and renal vein thrombosis.

Atheromatous renovascular disease (ARVD) may involve large, medium-sized and small renal vessels and can be associated with both slowly progressive CKD and AKI.

Thromboembolic AKI refers to occlusion of the renal artery or branch vessel secondary to a thrombus originating in the heart or aorta.

Atheroembolic AKI refers more specifically to renal arterial occlusive disease secondary to cholesterol emboli. Cholesterol crystals may break off from atherosclerotic plaques either spontaneously or following manipulation of the vascular tree and embolize resulting in occlusion of distal small vessels.

Epidemiology

The incidence of atheroembolic AKI has been estimated at 1.4% of the general population based on postmortem studies.

Factors associated with an increased incidence include:
- Caucasian males >60 years;
- diabetes mellitus;
- hypertension;
- peripheral vascular disease;
- ischemic heart disease;
- cerebrovascular disease.

The incidence of thromboembolic AKI has been estimated at 2%. It is most commonly secondary to atrial fibrillation and associated with underlying atherosclerotic disease.

Etiology

A number of different diseases may be associated with the development of ischemic AKI (Table 10.8.1).

Atheroembolic AKI

Most commonly occurs following:
- arterial instrumentation such as vascular surgery;
- angiography;
- renal angioplasty, and stent placement.

The procedures may result in arterial dissection or cholesterol embolization.

Cholesterol embolization results in partial or total occlusion of multiple small arteries due to the nondistensible nature of the crystals.

Thromboembolic AKI

The kidneys are at increased risk of thromboembolism originating from the heart or aorta because of their relatively high blood flow. The left renal artery is more commonly involved due to the angle at which it joins the aorta.

Thromboembolism is most commonly secondary to atrial fibrillation but can also occur secondary to emboli from valvular vegetations in infectious endocarditis and rarely tumour and fat embolization.

Renal artery occlusion

In situ renal artery (and vein) thrombus formation may occur in patients with a hypercoagulable state.

Renal artery occlusion can occur following direct trauma or following a deceleration injury when patients land on their feet following a fall from a height. On impact the renal arteries are acutely stretched and recoil resulting in acute thrombosis which is typically bilateral.

Atheromatous renovascular disease

While ARVD is usually associated with progressive CKD it does increase the risk of AKI when renal perfusion is compromised:
- hypovolemic states;
- ACEIs or ARBs;
- NSAIDs;
- radiological contrast administration.

Prescription of ACEIs in the presence of renal artery stenosis (RAS, bilateral or in a single functioning kidney) can precipitate AKI. This process is generally but not always reversible. Patients with RAS are dependent upon angiotensin II to maintain the efferent arteriolar tone and therefore glomerular capillary pressure and filtration.

Patients with atheromatous renovascular disease are also at increased risk of contrast-induced AKI due to both contrast-induced vasoconstriction and direct tubular toxicity.

Clinical features

Clinical manifestations will differ between atheroembolism (cholesterol embolization), thromboembolism and thrombosis in situ.

Thromboembolism and thrombosis in situ more commonly result in complete arterial occlusion whereas atheroembolism more commonly leads to partial occlusion of distal vessels and more widespread extrarenal ischemia.

Renal manifestations of the disease are dependent upon whether the arterial occlusion is acute or occurs subacutely on the background of underlying atherosclerotic arterial disease.

Acute renal artery occlusion secondary to thromboembolism or thrombosis in situ in the absence of pre-existing renal artery stenosis is associated with:
- fever;
- loin or flank pain;
- low back pain or abdominal pain;
- nausea and vomiting;
- hypertension (secondary to renin release);
- AKI with oliguria/anuria (if bilateral occlusion or occlusion of single functioning kidney).

Atheroembolism (less common with thromboembolism) may be associated with the following extra-renal features:
- livedo reticularis;
- necrotic skin ulceration;
- Hollenhorst plaques (yellow deposits on fundoscopy);
- digital ischemia;
- gastrointestinal bleeding;
- hepatitis;

Table 10.8.1 Arterial causes of ischemic acute kidney injury

Embolic
Thromboembolic
  Cardiac source
  • atrial fibrillation
  • infective endocarditis
  • left ventricular mural thrombus
Atheroembolic
  Cholesterol embolus
Fat embolus
Tumor embolus

Thrombotic
Renal artery stenosis
Hypercoagulable states
  Nephrotic syndrome
  Protein S and C deficiency
  Factor V Leiden deficiency
  Antithrombin III deficiency
  Antiphospholipid syndrome
  Homocystinuria
Dissection of aorta or renal artery
  Marfan syndrome
  Ehlers–Danlos syndrome
  Traumatic
  Surgical intervention
  Radiological intervention
Vasculitis
  Polyarteritis nodosa
  Takayasu's disease
  Necrotizing vasculitis
Thrombotic microangiography
  Accelerated hypertension
  Hemolytic uremic syndrome
  Thrombotic thrombocytopenia purpura
  Scleroderma
  Polycythemia vera
  Hyperacute vascular allograft rejection

• angina;
• pulmonary edema;
• neurological dysfunction.

Digital ischemia may lead to gangrene or ulceration.

Livedo reticularis is the most common cutaneous manifestation, occurring in up to 50% of cases.

Cardiac failure and severe hypertension contribute to the high mortality.

The presence of pre-existing arterial disease results in chronic renal ischemia and promotes the development of a collateral renal blood supply.

Therefore subacute renal artery occlusion in the presence of pre-existing renal artery stenosis may present with very few signs and symptoms unless it occurs in a solitary functioning kidney. In this scenario clinical features will be secondary to AKI.

Additional signs and symptoms will depend upon the extrarenal extent of atheroembolism.

Differential diagnosis

Clinical features may closely resemble that of systemic vasculitis.

Atheroembolic AKI is favored by the presence of atherosclerotic disease elsewhere.

Atheroembolic AKI following surgery or a radiological procedure needs to be differentiated from postischemic acute tubular necrosis (ATN) and contrast nephropathy.

Unlike postischemic ATN and contrast nephropathy the renal dysfunction associated with atheroembolic AKI generally fails to recover.

Thromboembolic AKI needs to be differentiated from renal stone disease (renal colic) and acute pyelonephritis (loin pain).

Unlike thromboembolic AKI the latter two conditions are not associated with a rise in LDH.

Investigations

Blood tests

Full blood count, expect:
• anemia (normocytic);
• leukocytosis;
• eosinophilia (atheroembolism, 80%).

Clotting screen (perform if hypercoagulable state suspected):
• protein S and C deficiency;
• antithrombin III deficiency;
• factor V Leiden deficiency;
• lupus anticoagulant.

Urea and electrolytes, expect:
• elevated urea & creatinine;
• elevated CK (atheroembolism);
• elevated LDH (renal infarction);
• elevated amylase (atheroembolism);
• elevated CRP (atheroembolism, pyelonephritis).

Liver function tests, expect:
• elevated alkaline phosphatase.

Autoantibody screen:
• hypocomplementemia (atheroembolism);
• antiphospholipid antibody (spontaneous thrombosis);
• ANA, ANCA (to exclude vasculitis).

Urine

Urinalysis, expect:
• hematuria;
• proteinuria.

Urine microscopy, expect:
• hematuria;
• ± pyuria (pyelonephritis);
• ± eosinophiluria (atheroembolism).

Urine culture, expect:
• negative culture (exclude acute pyelonephritis).

Radiology

CXR:
• cardiomegaly/LV aneurysm (mural thrombus);
• pulmonary edema (may be present);
• tortuous aorta (may be present).

Ultrasound, expect:

- asymmetrical kidneys (if pre-existing ARVD);
- normal kidneys (if acute athero/thromboembolism);
- renal Doppler may demonstrate renal artery occlusion (less sensitive).

CT:

- spiral CT without contrast will exclude renal stone disease;
- enhanced CT will identify perfusion defects and areas of renal infarction.

MRA:

- will demonstrate renal artery occlusion.

Renal angiography:

- provides a definitive diagnosis;
- carries a risk of contrast nephropathy;
- increases the risk of further atheroembolism.

Radioisotope (DTPA) scan:

- will demonstrate segmental or generalized decreased renal perfusion.

Other
ECG:

- atrial fibrillation (thromboembolism).

Renal biopsy
Often not required when there are strong clinical and radiological grounds for diagnosis.

In atheroembolic AKI, birefringent, biconvex, elongated cholesterol crystals (frozen sections) will be seen on polarized light microscopy or cholesterol clefts (fixed sections) (Fig. 10.8.1). Cholesterol clefts represent areas of cholesterol embolization within vascular lumina. The cholesterol is dissolved during the processing of the histological specimen.

Eosinophilic infiltrates and surrounding tissue ischemia are often seen in association with cholesterol emboli.

Muscle biopsy
Lower limb muscle biopsy has a sensitivity of nearly 100%, but is rarely performed to diagnose atheroembolism.

Skin biopsy
Will be diagnostic in ~75% of atheroembolism.

Management
Identifying patients at risk of atheroembolism and thromboembolism is essential to allow prompt diagnosis and treatment.

In particular it is important to recognize that the majority of these patients will be at an increased risk of developing contrast-induced nephropathy if undergoing angiography.

The appropriate prophylactic measures to reduce the risk of radiocontrast induced nephropathy include:

- assessment to confirm that the investigation is appropriate;
- avoidance of nephrotoxic drugs, e.g. NSAIDs;
- adequate volume expansion prior to and following the procedure with 0.9% sodium chloride 1 mL/kg/h (volume administered will be dependent upon volume status);
- minimization of the volume of contrast media used;
- use of iso-osmolar contrast media.

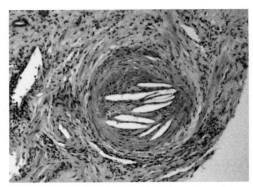

Fig. 10.8.1 Renal biopsy demonstrating cholesterol embolization within renal arterioles. The arteriolar lumen contains several cholesterol clefts. (Courtesy of Dr D. Leitch, St James's University Hospital, Leeds, UK.)

Thromboembolism and in situ thrombosis
Immediate management of thromboembolism and thrombosis *in situ* will be dictated by the clinical scenario and other organ systems affected.

The urgency of intervention depends upon whether there is a significant collateral blood supply to the kidney.

Anticoagulation is necessary if there is a hypercoagulable state or if the occlusion is secondary to an acute thromboembolic event (atrial fibrillation, mural thrombus).

Otherwise anticoagulation is not advisable in the acute setting if there is widespread atherosclerosis due to its destabilizing affect on atherosclerotic plaques.

Thrombolysis with intra-arterial recombinant tissue plasminogen activator is indicated if the occlusion has occurred to previously normal renal arteries or is related to recent renal artery instrumentation. The procedure is minimally invasive but there are no large series to support its efficacy.

Angioplasty may be successful following acute occlusion of an atherosclerotic renal artery. However, there are significant risks of precipitating atheroembolism related to the instrumentation.

Revascularization has been successfully performed following acute renal artery occlusion, up to several weeks after the event. Surgical intervention is not recommended if the occlusion is unilateral in the setting of two previously normal functioning kidneys due to the relatively high operative mortality.

Atheroembolism
There is no specific therapy for renal atheroembolism, but there are a number of general measures that can be considered.

ACEIs need to be stopped if implicated in the etiology. If not implicated they may be effective in managing the hypertension triggered by the atheroembolism.

Corticosteroids have been used in patients with an acute inflammatory response or those with gastrointestinal involvement. Their use is controversial and is based on small series and case reports.

Nutritional support should be considered as patients are often malnourished prior to the event.

Statins should be started or continued due to their anti-inflammatory properties and ability to stabilize plaques.

Hemodialysis is the preferred form of renal replacement therapy but should be performed with minimal anticoagulation if atherosclerotic disease is widespread.

Peritoneal dialysis is usually not practical due to previous abdominal surgery, gastrointestinal ischemia and nutritional compromise.

Prognosis

The overall prognosis of atheroembolic AKI is difficult to quantify and is dependent upon the associated comorbidities and extrarenal organ involvement.

Patients who develop cardiac failure and AKI following atheroembolism have a 1 year mortality of 50%.

Patients developing ESRD following atheroembolism have a 5 year mortality rate of 40%.

Indicators of a poor prognosis include:
* recurrent atheroembolism;
* gastrointestinal involvement.

One-third of patients with AKI due to atheroembolism remain dialysis dependent.

Renal vein thrombosis

Renal vein thrombosis (RVT) is a rare and often undiagnosed cause of AKI.

Epidemiology
This is poorly defined. There is a reported incidence of ~22% in patients with nephrotic syndrome.

Etiology
RVT may occur in patients who have a hypercoagulable state including:
* nephrotic syndrome;
* malignancy;
* pregnancy.

Patients with nephrotic syndrome secondary to membranous nephropathy and lupus nephritis are particularly at risk.

Extrinsic compression of the renal vein can occur secondary to retroperitoneal fibrosis and tumor.

Clinical features
* loin, testicular or flank pain;
* low grade fever;
* AKI with oliguria/anuria (bilateral or single functioning
* kidney);
* hematuria (microscopic);
* pulmonary embolus (as a consequence).

Investigations
Blood tests
Clotting screen if thrombophilia suspected.

Table 10.8.2 Causes of renal vein thrombosis

Nephrotic syndrome
Membranous nephropathy
Lupus nephritis
Amyloidosis
Malignancy
Renal cell carcinoma
Retroperitoneal tumor
Hypercoagulable states
Oral contraceptive
Pregnancy
Antiphospholipid syndrome
Protein S and C deficiency
Antithrombin III deficiency
Factor V Leiden mutation
Trauma
Surgical
Blunt
Renal transplantation
Acute pancreatitis
Thrombosis of inferior vena cava

Urine
Urinalysis, expect:
* hematuria;
* proteinuria.

Radiology
Ultrasound and Doppler:
* may demonstrate increased renal size and echogenicity;
* filling defect in renal vein;
* $\uparrow$ resistive indices.

MRA:
Can be used to make the diagnosis but is rarely necessary.

Renal biopsy
Not indicated.

Management
Management is dependent upon the underlying disease process.

Systemic anticoagulation to prevent thrombus extension and embolization.

Anticoagulation must be continued indefinitely if there is a hypercoagulable state.

Nephrectomy may be required for tumor-related RVT, capsular rupture or longer-term consequences of a non-functioning kidney such as hypertension or infection.

Catheter-directed thrombolysis with percutaneous thrombectomy has been reported to be successful in some cases.

Conservative therapy may be favored in the case of a left RVT because its extensive collateral venous supply may allow venous drainage and partial recovery of renal function.

Further reading

Harris R, Ismail N. Extrarenal complications of nephrotic syndrome. *Am J Kidney Dis* 1994; **23**: 477–497.

Modi KS, Rao VK. Atheroembolic renal disease. *J Am Soc Nephrol* 2001; **12**: 1781.

Paris B, Bobrie G, Rossignol P, et al. Blood pressure and renal outcomes in patients with kidney infarction and hypertension. *J Hypertens* 2006; **24**: 1649.

Scolari F, Tardanico R, Zani R, et al. Cholesterol crystal embolisation: a recognisable cause of renal disease. *Am J Kidney Dis* 2000; **36**: 1089.

Scolari F, Ravani P, Pola A, et al. Predictors of renal and patient outcomes in atheroembolic renal disease: a prospective study. *J Am Soc Nephrol* 2003; **14**: 1584–1590.

Internet resources

Acute Dialysis Quality Initiative:

http://www.ADQI.net

Acute Kidney Injury Network:

http://akinet.org/index.php

Renovascular Forum:

http://www.renovascularforum.org

Journal of Renovascular Disease:

http://www.journalrenovasculardisease.com/

See also

Clinical approach to acute kidney injury, p. 318

Renovascular disease, p. 292

Pigment-induced acute kidney injury

Introduction

AKI can occur secondary to the release of intracellular heme pigments. Muscle cell breakdown (rhabdomyolysis) results in the release of myoglobin and myoglobinuria whereas red blood cell breakdown (hemolysis) leads to the release of heme pigments and hemoglobinuria.

Epidemiology

There are wide variations in the reported incidence of AKI secondary to hemolysis and rhabdomyolysis, in many cases the discrepancy is due to the varying definitions of AKI used by investigators.

Rhabdomyolysis-related AKI is responsible for up to half of all cases of AKI requiring renal replacement therapy following earthquakes.

Etiology

Rhabdomyolysis

There are a number of causes of rhabdomyolysis (Table 10.9.1). The final common pathway involves striated muscle injury with the release of cellular contents including myoglobin.

In rhabdomyolysis there is sequestration of large volumes of fluid in damaged muscle (up to 15–20 L) which can result in volume depletion.

Myoglobin (17 kDa) is freely filtered by the glomerulus and in the setting of volume depletion and acidosis myoglobin binds more avidly to Tamm–Horsfall protein and sloughed tubular epithelial cells promoting the formation of casts.

Tubular degradation of reabsorbed myoglobin generates a highly toxic hydroxyl radical with subsequent free-radical-mediated cellular injury.

Hemolysis

Hemoglobinuria can occur following massive intravascular hemolysis (Table 10.9.2).

In this setting haptoglobin binding of free hemoglobin is overwhelmed.

Unbound hemoglobin dissociates into dimers (34 kDa) which are filtered by the glomerulus.

The filtered hemoglobin may cause tubular obstruction through cast formation or may be taken up by tubular epithelial cells and exert a toxic effect.

Clinical features

The clinical features of rhabdomyolysis can vary dependent upon the specific cause, but it should be suspected if oliguric AKI is associated with:

- fever;
- myalgia (50%);
- muscle weakness;
- compartment syndrome;
- crush injury.

Where the cause of AKI is hemolysis there will be features of anemia along with features of the precipitating cause (Table 10.9.2).

Differential diagnosis

The differential diagnosis will include other causes of oliguric AKI but the diagnosis is often readily apparent from a careful clinical evaluation and simple investigations.

An important distinguishing characteristic is that in the case of hemoglobinuria the plasma is dark (heme pigment), but it remains clear in rhabdomyolysis.

Investigations

Blood tests

Full blood count, expect:

- anemia (hemolysis);
- reduced platelet count (rhabdomyolysis);
- elevated reticulocyte count (hemolysis).

Blood film, expect:

- fragmented red blood cells (schistocytes);
- parasites (e.g. malaria), spherocytes (hemolysis).

Coagulation screen, expect:

- elevated D-dimers (rhabdomyolysis);
- reduced haptoglobin (hemolysis).

Red cell autoimmune screen, expect:

- positive direct Coombs test (some causes of hemolysis).

Serum biochemistry, expect:

- elevated urea and creatinine;
- elevated K^+ (rhabdomyolysis and hemolysis);
- elevated PO_4^{2-}, urate, lactate (rhabdomyolysis);
- reduced Ca^{2+} (rhabdomyolysis);
- elevated CK (usually >10 000 U/L in rhabdomyolysis);
- elevated LDH (rhabdomyolysis and hemolysis).

Liver function tests, expect:

- elevated bilirubin (hemolysis);
- elevated ALT/AST (rhabdomyolysis).

Thyroid function tests:

- elevated TSH (if hypothyroidism is the cause of rhabdomyolysis).

Autoantibodies:

- Anti-aminoacyl-tRNA synthetase antibodies, e.g. anti-Jo-1 (if polymyositis is the cause of rhabdomyolysis).

Toxicology screen:

- for evidence of causative drug ingestion (Tables 10.9.1 and 10.9.2).

Urine

Urinalysis, expect:

- strong positivity for blood (both myoglobinuria and hemoglobinuria);
- myoglobin (rhabdomyolysis).

Urine microscopy, expect:

- no red blood cells on microscopy;
- pigmented casts.

Microbiology

- Blood cultures.
- Serology (Tables 10.9.1 and 10.9.2).

Virology

- If a viral infection is suspected screen for suspected pathogens (Table 10.9.1).

Table 10.9.1 Causes of rhabdomyolysis and myoglobinuria

Muscle injury
Trauma
Compartment syndrome
Prolonged immobilization
Burns
Electric shock
Acute vascular occlusion
Seizures
Excessive exertion
Sickle cell disease
Polymyositis/dermatomyositis

Drugs
Statins
Fibrates
Antimalarials
Zidovudine
Heroin
Cocaine
Alcohol
Ecstasy
Amphetamines

Electrolyte abnormalities
Hypokalemia
Hypocalcemia
Hypophosphatemia
Hyponatremia
Hypernatremia

Toxins
Snake venom
Insect venom

Infections
Bacterial
• *Legionella* spp.
• *Streptococcus pneumoniae*
• *Salmonella* spp.
• *Staphylococcus aureus*
Viral
• influenza
• HIV
• EBV
• coxsackievirus

Familial
Malignant hyperthermia
Neuroleptic malignant syndrome
McArdle's disease
Carnitine palmitoyltransferase deficiency

Endocrine
Hypothyroidism
Diabetic ketoacidosis

Table 10.9.2 Causes of hemolysis and hemoglobinuria

Transfusion reactions
Falciparum malaria
Mycoplasma infection
Toxins
Snake bite
Insect bites
Poisoning
• copper sulfate
Autoimmune hemolytic anemia
Drug-induced hemolytic anemia
• aspirin
• chloroquine
Mechanical hemolysis
Bacterial endocarditis
Dysfunctional prosthetic heart valves

Radiology

Ultrasound, expect:
• normal renal tract;
• no specific abnormalities.

Intracompartment pressure measurement

If a compartment syndrome is suspected, measure intra-compartment pressure by tonometry.

Renal biopsy

A renal biopsy may be performed when a clinical diagnosis of AKI is not clearly secondary to rhabdomyolysis or hemoglobinuria.

Characteristic histopathological changes include features of acute tubular necrosis with granular tubular casts, which may stain positively for myoglobin in rhabdomyolysis (Fig. 10.9.1).

Muscle biopsy

This may be indicated if:
• there is no obvious precipitant for rhabdomyolysis;
• there is a history of myoglobinuria provoked by exercise;
• an underlying inflammatory disorder is suspected.

Electromyography

Polymyositis is associated with short polyphasic motor potentials, occasional spontaneous fibrillation and high frequency repetitive discharges.

Management

Prompt diagnosis and appropriate treatment may prevent the development of AKI following rhabdomyolysis.

Identification of the cause is important to allow more specific therapy.

Prophylactic fasciotomy in cases of rhabdomyolysis complicating a compartment syndrome may be required to save tissue/organ function.

Vigorous fluid resuscitation is essential.

Management should include:
• careful assessment of the volume status;
• central venous pressure monitoring;
• measurement of the urine output;
• IV 0.9% sodium chloride 10–15 mL/kg/h to achieve euvolemia;
• maintain urine output >200 mL/h.

Urinary alkalinization is controversial and is not routinely recommended. There is a risk of precipitating volume overload, hypernatremia and symptomatic hypocalcemia due to a fall in the ionized calcium concentration.

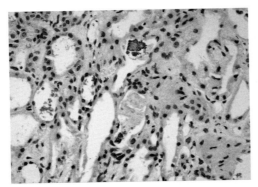

Fig. 10.9.1 AKI secondary to rhabdomyolysis. Immunoperoxidase staining demonstrates myoglobin within acutely injured dilated tubules with flattened epithelium. (Courtesy of Dr D. Leitch, St James's University Hospital, Leeds, UK.)

If urinary alkalinization is attempted, 1.26–1.4% sodium bicarbonate can be added to the IV fluid regimen to achieve a urinary pH >6.5.

There is little evidence to support a role for mannitol, which may precipitate a hyperosmolar state and worsen the degree of AKI.

Treat specific electrolyte abnormalities as required.

Hypocalcemia associated with rhabdomyolysis should not be routinely corrected unless there are complications such as tetany or arrhythmias.

Aggressive correction of hypocalcemia may cause metastatic calcification in the injured muscle.

Rebound hypercalcemia can occur during the recovery phase.

If attempts to prevent AKI are unsuccessful then renal replacement therapy will be necessary.

The management of hemoglobinuria involves treatment of the underlying disorder and vigorous fluid resuscitation.

Prognosis

Renal function generally returns to normal if the underlying cause is treated.

Further reading

Brown CV. Rhee P, Chan L, et al. Preventing renal failure in patients with rhabdomyolysis: do bicarbonate and mannitol make a difference? *J Trauma* 2004; **56**: 1191–1196.

Holt S, Moore K. Pathogenesis of renal failure in rhabdomyolysis: the role of myoglobin. *Exp Nephrol* 2000; **8**: 72–76.

Sever MS, Vanholder R, Lameire R. Medical progress; management of crush-related injuries after disasters. *New Engl J Med* 2006; **354**: 1052–1063.

Internet resources

Acute Dialysis Quality Initiative:

http://www.ADQI.net

Acute Kidney Injury Network:

http://www.akinet.org

See also

Clinical approach to acute kidney injury, p. 318

Renal replacement therapies in AKI 328

Acute kidney injury in tropical countries

Introduction
The causes and presentation of AKI in the tropics vary considerably from that seen in Western countries. There is also a varied spectrum of AKI even among tropical countries due to regional differences in bioecology, social behavior and socioeconomic development. In the larger cities, causes of AKI resemble those in the developed world, e.g. nephrotoxic drugs, prerenal AKI due to functional hypovolemia (cardiac failure) and AKI as a postoperative complication following complex cardiothoracic surgery.

Epidemiology
Reliable statistics regarding the true incidence of AKI in tropical countries are not available but it is estimated at an average annual incidence of 150 cases pmp.

Community-acquired AKI is more common, and patients are generally younger than in Western countries.

AKI associated with internal medicine practice
Medical causes of AKI predominate.
The overall incidence has remained unchanged for the last four decades (Table 10.10.1) but diarrheal disease, intravascular hemolysis due to glucose 6-phosphate dehydrogenase (G6PD) deficiency and self-poisoning have largely been replaced by sepsis, drugs and toxins as the main medical causes of AKI.

AKI associated with obstetric practice
AKI complicating childbirth is declining with improvements in prenatal care and obstetric practice.

Legalization of abortion in several developing countries has been followed by a substantial decline in the rate of AKI related to septic abortion.

AKI associated with surgical practice
Surgical AKI incidence is increasing.

This probably reflects the increasing complexity of surgery in addition to increasing age and comorbidity of patients in whom surgery is undertaken.

Infection-related AKI
There is a high prevalence of infection in the tropics due to bioecological factors:
- warm climate;
- abundant animal and insect vectors;
- poverty;
- overcrowding;
- poor hygiene;
- malnutrition.

Late/inadequate medical attention, particularly in remote areas, predisposes to complications such as AKI.

Infective causes of AKI include:
- diarrheal diseases;
- malaria;
- leptospirosis;
- hemolytic uremic syndrome;
- melioidosis.

Development of infection-related AKI is usually multifactorial (Table 10.10.2).

General management of infection-related AKI is supportive with close attendance to fluid balance and management of acute electrolyte disturbances and longer-term nutritional support.

Specific treatment recommendations will be discussed below.

Diarrhea-associated AKI
Diarrhea most commonly leads to prerenal AKI secondary to volume depletion with the development of ATN. Acute cortical necrosis may occasionally occur in pediatric cases with severe volume depletion.

Epidemiology
Children are more susceptible to the development of AKI following diarrhea than adults.

In India, diarrheal diseases account for 35–50% of pediatric AKI requiring dialysis.

The incidence is greatest in summer and peaks during the rainy season.

Common causative organisms
Viral:
- rotavirus and Norwalk agent.

Bacterial:
- *Escherichia coli*;
- *Campylobacter jejuni*;
- *Klebsiella pneumoniae*;
- *Shigella* spp.;
- *Salmonella enteritides*;
- *Vibrio cholerae*;
- *Pseudomonas aeruginosa*.

Clinical presentation
Dehydration, oliguric AKI ± severe metabolic acidosis and hypokalemia.

Investigations
Stool cultures ± stool hanging drop examination.

Treatment
Fluid replacement.

Correction of electrolyte abnormalities.

Antibiotics for specific infections.

Malaria-associated AKI
Malarial AKI results from a variable combination of ATN, interstitial nephritis and development of a mesangial proliferative glomerulonephritis.

Epidemiology
Malaria affects 300–500 million people annually, with 1–3 million deaths.

The overall prevalence of AKI in falciparum malaria is <1% but may reach 60% with severe infection.

Residents in endemic areas acquire various degrees of immunity to infection: their incidence of AKI is 2–5%.

Nonimmune visitors develop a more severe infection and are at higher risk of AKI (25–30%).

Table 10.10.1 Patterns and trends in AKI among tropical countries

Country	Time period	Authors	No. of cases	Proportion (%) of AKI cases associated with:		
				Internal medicine	Surgery	Obstetrics
Singapore	1964–73	Ku et al., 1975	143	60	24	16
Thailand	1960–70s	Sitprija et al., 1975	162	61	24	15
Ghana	1972–75	Adu et al., 1976	50	62	4	24
Nepal	1998–99	Khakurel et al., 2005	45	84	4	11
India	1965–74	Chugh et al., 1989	325	67	11	22
	1975–80	Chugh et al., 1989	510	55	24	21
	1981–86	Chugh et al., 1989	1027	61	30	9
Malaysia	1976–80	Suleiman, 1982	184	41	32	27
	1994	Chow et al., 2007	78	69	31	0
	2004	Chow et al., 2007	211	73	26	1

Causative organism
AKI is associated mainly with *Plasmodium falciparum*.

Very occasionally it complicates *Plasmodium vivax*.

Clinical presentation
AKI is usually oliguric, hypercatabolic and associated with other complications:

- jaundice (>75%);
- anemia (70%);
- thrombocytopenia (70%);
- hepatitis (20%);
- hypotension (20%);
- septic inflammatory response syndrome (5%).

Cerebral malaria is rarely associated with malarial AKI.

Investigations
Thin and thick blood film microscopy to diagnose and type the malarial parasite.

Proteinuria occurs in 60% but is usually <1 g/24 h.

Hyponatremia occurs in up to 55% due to internal dilution ± salt wasting.

Hyperkalemia may be striking due to hemolysis, rhabdomyolysis, acidosis and AKI.

Treatment
Once the diagnosis is suspected a rapid clinical assessment is required with transfer of the patient to the highest level of care available as soon as possible.

Supportive measures:

- intensive invasive/noninvasive monitoring of tissue oxygenation, fluid balance and conscious level;
- care is required with IV fluids, particularly in adults, due to the risk of noncardiogenic pulmonary edema. If CVP is available, target 0–5 cm water; if not, fluid therapy should be guided by physical findings/urine indices;
- regular assessment of FBC, clotting studies, serum biochemistry (U&Es, LFTs glucose and lactate levels), arterial blood gases and parasite counts are required.

Specific antimalarial chemotherapy:

In severe falciparum malaria, the drug of choice is either a parenteral cinchona alkaloid (quinine and quinidine) or artemisinin derivatives (artesunate, artemether and artemotil).

Quinine or quinidine dosage should be reduced by one-third after 48 h if there is no clinical improvement, if AKI persists or there is hepatic dysfunction.

No dose adjustment is necessary if the patient is on hemodialysis (HD) or hemofiltration (HF).

A switch to oral treatment can be made once the patient is able to tolerate oral medications. A 7 day treatment regimen should be completed.

In nonpregnant patients, doxycycline should be added for 7 days.

Indications for renal replacement therapy (RRT):

Initiate HD or HF early in established AKI or severe metabolic acidosis unresponsive to rehydration.

There are no comparative trials of HD versus HF.

HF is associated with more rapid correction of biochemical abnormalities and lower mortality compared with peritoneal dialysis.

Hyperparasitemia (>300 000/µL) may also be an indication for early RRT; this may reduce the number of organs failing by removing cytokines and toxic metabolites generated by the parasite and treatment.

Prognosis
Dialysis is required in up to 78% of cases.

Oliguria may last for a few days to several weeks.

The mortality ranges from 15 to 45%.

The prognosis depends on severity of AKI, associated extra-renal complications, early institution of antimalarial treatment and availability of RRT.

Leptospira-associated AKI (Weil's disease)
Renal failure may develop as a consequence of prerenal AKI and ATN due to hemodynamic instability or acute interstitial nephritis (AIN).

There may also be a direct nephrotoxic contribution from tubular hemoglobin and myoglobin casts.

Epidemiology
The peak incidence is between 11 and 40 years of age.

There is a male preponderance.

The incidence rises during or soon after the rainy season, especially post floods.

Table 10.10.2 Pathogenetic mechanisms of AKI in tropical infections.

Direct invasion of renal parenchyma	**Bacteria**
	Microabcesses (systemic melioidosis) or solitary abscesses (typhoid).
	Acute interstitial nephritis (leptospirosis, diphtheria, scrub typhus, tuberculosis and leprosy).
	Viruses
	Dengue fever.
	Hanta virus infection (hemorrhagic fever–renal failure syndrome).
	Protozoa
	Visceral leishmaniasis/kala-azar (acute interstitial nephritis).
Induction of an immune response leading to glomerular or tubulointerstitial damage	**Immune complex-mediated glomerulonephritis**
	Mesangial proliferative GN (acute typhoid fever, acute malaria).
	Diffuse proliferative GN (post-streptococcal GN, and GN associated with endocarditis or pneumococcal pneumonia).
	Vasculitis
	Severe streptococcal or falciparum malaria infection.
	Acute interstitial nephritis
	Postdysenteric hemolytic uremic syndrome
Hemodynamic disturbances ± other insults leading to acute tubular necrosis (ATN)	**Intravascular volume depletion**
	Dehydration from hyperpyrexia, excess sweating, vomiting and/or diarrhea.
	Compromise of renal microcirculation
	By sludging of red blood cells and platelets due to hemoconcentration.
	'Sticky' parasitized erythrocytes in falciparum malaria, which adhere to adjacent healthy erythrocytes, platelets and capillary endothelium to form rosettes and clumps, impede the microcirculation.
	Systemic inflammatory response syndrome
	Peripheral blood pooling and capillary leakage mediated by nitric oxide, TNF-α, prostaglandins, kinins and free oxygen radicals results in a reduced effective circulatory volume, renal ischemia and ATN.
	Pigment-related ATN
	Heme pigment, bilirubin, myoglobin.
	Increased mechanical fragility of parasitized erythrocytes in malaria causes intravascular hemolysis.
	Rhabdomyolysis may occur as a nonspecific effect of hyperpyrexia or due to specific viruses (influenza, HIV, coxsackie, Epstein–Barr virus) and bacteria (*Legionella* spp., *Francisella* spp., *Streptococcus pneumoniae*, *Salmonella* spp., *Staphylococcus aureus*).
Iatrogenic renal injury associated with treatment or prophylaxis against tropical infections	**Nephrotoxic drugs**
	For example, aminoglycosides, amphotericin, NSAIDs.
	G6PD deficiency
	Hemolysis induced by certain drugs, e.g. sulfur-based agents, primaquine.

Based on Barsoum (2004).

Causative organism
- *Leptospira interrogans* (a spirochaete which infects a wide range of mammals, and is shed in the urine).

Clinical presentation
The severity of illness ranges from mild constitutional symptoms to fulminant liver and renal failure (when known as Weil's disease).

Classically the clinical course is biphasic:

Initial phase:
- abrupt onset fever, myalgia, arthralgia, headache and conjunctival injection.

Second phase:
- jaundice with mild transaminitis, conjugated hyperbilirubinemia and subsequent development of AKI.

Investigations
Blood cultures (in first 10 days).

Urine cultures (up to 30 days).

Leptospira serology: a single titer >1:400 or a four-fold rise is considered significant.

Treatment
IV crystalline penicillin (1.5 million units every 6 h) or oral doxycycline (100 mg bd) for 7 days.

Aggressive nutritional support and daily dialysis may be required.

Prognosis
A poor prognosis is associated with:
- advanced age;
- pulmonary complications;
- hyperbilirubinemia;
- diarrhea;
- hyperkalemia;
- associated infection/underlying disease.

AKI usually recovers within 2 months.

Hemolytic uremic syndrome

This has been reported as one of the commonest causes of pediatric AKI in certain tropical countries, e.g. India.

Unlike Western countries where HUS is associated with verotoxin-producing E. coli (0157:H7), HUS in the tropics is linked with:

- Shigella dysenteriae serotype 1 (most commonly);
- Salmonella spp.;
- Klebsiella spp.;
- nonverotoxin producing strains of E.coli;
- Shigella flexneri;
- Proteus spp.;
- Pseudomonas spp.

Melioidosis

AKI commonly complicates acute septicemic melioidosis which may result in marked hemodynamic changes and prerenal AKI but also an acute interstitial nephritis and formation of multiple renal microabscesses.

Epidemiology
It is endemic in South East Asia and northern Australia.

Predisposing factors:
- diabetes;
- thalassemia;
- chronic kidney disease;
- alcoholic liver disease;
- occupation (rice paddy farmers).

Causative organism
Burkholderia pseudomallei (Gram-negative bacteria found in soil and water).

Clinical presentation
Fever, signs and symptoms of pneumonia, multiple cutaneous/visceral abscesses.

The infection exists in acute and chronic forms.

AKI occurs in up to 61% in acute septicemic melioidosis where mortality is >90% if untreated.

Investigations
A complete septic screen is required including cultures of blood, urine, sputum, throat swab, aspirated pus.

Serological tests may be of limited value in endemic areas.

Treatment
Intravenous antibiotics for 10–14 days:
- drug of choice: ceftazidime;
- alternatives: carbapenem/amoxicillin-clavulanate.

Maintenance treatment with oral cotrimoxazole and doxycycline is required for 12–20 weeks.

Other infections

Rarer causes of tropical infection-associated AKI:

Mucormycosis
Renal vascular invasion with renal infarction and necrosis.

Aspergillosis
Renal abscesses, infarcts, papillary necrosis and obstructive uropathy from fungal bezoars.

Kala-azar
Acute interstitial nephritis.

Typhoid
Intravascular hemolysis in G6PD-deficient patients, myoglobinuria, AIN from ciprofloxacin treatment and HUS.

Lepromatous leprosy
ATN, intravascular hemolysis, glomerulonephritis, and AIN secondary to rifampicin treatment.

AKI due to toxins and chemicals

Ingestion of traditional medicines/foods or accidental exposure to noxious local plants and animals contribute to toxin-related AKI. Chemical poisoning (e.g. copper sulfate, paraquat, etc.) is now relatively uncommon.

Snakebite nephropathy

Snake venom can lead to marked hemodynamic changes induced by release of cytokines and vasoactive mediators (± blood loss in severe hemorrhage).

Prerenal AKI is therefore a potential complication of various snakebites.

The development of prerenal AKI may be compounded by other contributory factors such as:
- hemolysis;
- rhabdomyolysis;
- intravascular coagulation;
- direct snake venom nephrotoxicity through metalloproteases and phospholipase.

The commonest findings in renal biopsy series are:
- ATN (70–80%);
- acute interstitial nephritis;
- acute cortical necrosis;
- mesangiolysis;
- glomerulonephritis;
- vasculitis.

Epidemiology
AKI following snakebites constitutes 1.2% of AKI in Thailand, 3% in India and up to 70% in Myanmar.

AKI is usually caused by snakebites from the Viperidae, Colubridae and Hydrophidae families, i.e. those with hemotoxic or myotoxic venom.

Clinical presentation
Pain, swelling ± tissue necrosis at the bite site

Systemic involvement:
- hypotension;
- disseminated intravascular coagulation;
- hemorrhage;
- intravascular hemolysis;
- rhabdomyolysis.

AKI is usually hypercatabolic and oligoanuric.

Apart from AKI, proteinuria and hematuria are commonly seen following snakebites.

Treatment
Early administration of antivenom, preferably monovalent.

Repeated doses may be required due to delayed absorption of venom from the bite.

Coagulation indices need to be tested for up to 3 days.

Replacement of blood loss with fresh blood.

Tetanus immune globulin administration.

Antibiotics may be required for pyogenic infection at site of bite wound.

Early institution of good fluid balance with maintenance of good urine flow and urinary alkalinization may reduce risk of AKI.

Dialysis should be instituted early if available.

Prognosis
AKI typically lasts 2–3 weeks.

With cortical necrosis there may be no recovery/delayed recovery with residual renal impairment.

Other animal toxins:
Scorpion and jellyfish stings, spider and centipede bites lead to AKI in 6–10% of incidents.

Oral ingestion of raw carp bile may be associated with gastrointestinal toxicity and lead to hematuria (77%), jaundice (62%) and AKI in up to 54% of cases.

Plant toxins and AKI
Mushrooms of the genera *Amanita*, *Galerina* and *Cortinarius* may produce gastrointestinal and hepatic toxicity, and AKI. Mortality can be >50% in severe cases.

Attractyloside, an alkaloid from tubers of *Callilepsis laureola* (commonly used in Southern and Central Africa as a traditional remedy) can cause AKI, hypoglycemia and liver dysfunction. The mortality rate is >50%.

Djenkolic acid in the djengkol bean from the *Pithecellobium jiringa/lobatum* tree in South East Asia can cause dysuria, hematuria, proteinuria, urolithiasis and AKI. The diagnosis can be confirmed by finding characteristic needle-shaped crystals of djenkolic acid on urine microscopy.

Other plant toxins:
- phenolic compounds (via skin exposure) in the sap of the marking-nut tree of India (*Semecarpus anacardium*);
- gaultherin in *Securidaca longipe dunculata*;
- divicine and isouramil in *Vicis favus* (broad bean) in G6PD deficient individuals.

For all the plant poisonings described above, treatment is mainly supportive.

With djenkol and *Vicis favus*, increasing fluid intake and alkalinizing urine may be helpful.

Glucose 6-phosphate dehydrogenase (G6PD) deficiency

This affects >400 million people worldwide, mainly in Africa, the Mediterranean, Middle and Far East.

It may confer a survival advantage in regions with malaria because infected erythrocytes are cleared more rapidly by the spleen.

It is associated with intravascular hemolysis on exposure to oxidative stress from infection, medication and certain foods.

AKI may occur after severe hemolysis due to heme pigment nephropathy.

Preventive measures include maintenance of a high urine output and urinary alkalinization.

Further reading

Adu D, Anim-Addo Y, Foli AK, Yeboah ED, Quartey JK, Ribeiro BF. Acute renal failure in tropical Africa. *Br Med J* 1976; **1**: 890.

Barsoum RS. Malarial acute renal failure. *J Am Soc Nephrol* 2000; **11**: 2147–2154.

Barsoum RS. Tropical acute renal failure. In: Ronco C, Bellomo R, Brendolan A (eds): *Sepsis, kidney and multiple organ dysfunction*. *Contrib Nephrol* 2004; **144**: 44–52.

Chow YW, Lim BB, Hooi LS. Acute renal failure in the same hospital ten years apart. *Med J Malaysia* 2007; **62**: 27–32.

Chugh KS, Sakhuja V, Malhotra HS, Pereira BJ. Changing trends in acute renal failure in third-world countries – Chandigarh study. *Q J Med* 1989; **73**: 1117–1123.

Chugh KS, Sitprija V, Jha V. Acute renal failure in the tropical countries. In: Davison AM, Cameron JS, Grunfeld J-P, et al. (eds), *Oxford Textbook of Clinical Nephrology*, 3rd edn. Oxford: Oxford University Press; 2005. Vol. 2, pp. 1614–1630.

Khakurel S, Satyal PR l, Agrawal RK, Chhetri PK, Hada R. Acute renal failure in a tertiary care center in Nepal. *J Nepal Med Assoc* 2005; **44**: 32–35.

Ku G, Lim CH, Pwee HS, Khoo OT. Review of acute renal failure in Singapore. *Ann Acad Med Singapore* 1975; **4** (Suppl):115–120.

Sitprija V. Snakebite nephropathy. *Nephrology* 2006; **11**: 442–448.

Sitprija V, Kashemsant U, Arthachinta S, Poshyachinda V. Pathogenesis of renal failure in tropical diseases. *Nippon Jinzo Gakkai Shi* 1975; **17**: 707–709.

Suleiman AB. Clinical review of acute renal failure: a 5-year experience at Kuala Lumpur. *Ann Acad Med* 1982; **11**: 32–35.

Vetter RS, Visscher PK. Bites and Stings of medically important venomous arthropods. *Int J Derm* 1998; **37**: 481–496.

Internet resources

WHO Global Malaria Programme:

http://www.who.int/malaria

Melioidosis Research Centre:

http://www.melioid.org/

G6PD Deficiency Association:

http://www.g6pd.org/favism/english/index.mv

Snake bites, a useful introduction to the subject:

http://www.usyd.edu.au/su/anaes/venom/snake-bite.html

See also

Clinical approach to acute kidney injury, p. 318

Renal replacement therapies in acute kidney injury, p. XXX

Dialysis and hemoperfusion treatment of acute poisoning, p. 336

Acute kidney injury in infants and children, p. 372

Acute tubulointerstitial nephritis, p. 344

Hemolytic uremic syndrome and thrombotic thrombocytopenic purpura, p. 348

Pigment-induced acute kidney injury, p. 362

Acute kidney injury in infants and children

Introduction

Acute kidney injury in children is defined as a rapid increase in blood concentrations of creatinine and urea and an inability to regulate fluid and electrolyte balances.

In a majority there is oliguria (urine output <0.5 mL/kg/h) or anuria but a proportion of children will experience normal urine output or polyuria. This is most common with tubular and interstitial diseases.

When a child presents with severe renal failure it is important to try to define if the child is suffering from AKI or acute on chronic renal failure.

Children with CKD can sometimes present acutely with ESRD, in which case AKI can initially be part of the differential diagnosis.

Epidemiology

In UK studies the incidence of AKI in children ranges between 6.4 and 8 per million population per year. AKI occurs more commonly in neonates and infants than in older children and it is also more common in hospitalized children.

Predisposing factors

Children with a lower initial nephron mass are more susceptible to injuries to the remaining nephrons.

Pre-existing CKD may have been unrecognized and children can present as AKI as a result of chronic disease.

Clinical features

Clinical features will depend on the cause of the AKI. The etiology of AKI varies with the age of the child.

It is useful to define the cause of the AKI as intrinsic, pre- or postrenal.

Pre-renal AKI

A major cause of AKI in children is decreased circulating blood volume (Table 10.11.1). This is mostly caused by dehydration or third spacing of fluids, as may occur in septicemia or the nephrotic syndrome, for example.

Blood loss in major surgery (for example in heart surgery) may also cause acute tubular necrosis with AKI.

Intrinsic renal AKI

The most common causes of intrinsic AKI in children are glomerular and some tubulointerstitial diseases.

These have a quite different diagnostic spectrum to that seen in adults.

Hemolytic uremic syndrome (HUS) is the commonest cause of intrinsic AKI (see below).

In neonates renal vein thrombosis is an important cause of AKI.

Post-renal AKI

In boys, posterior urethral valves are an important cause of AKI.

Unusually bilateral ureteral stenosis or obstruction in a single system can cause AKI.

Presentation of AKI

Presenting symptoms in children depend on the cause.

Generalized symptoms such as malaise, being unwell with sickness and vomiting are common.

Many children have edema and respiratory symptoms due to pulmonary edema.

Fever, rashes and other symptoms of infection or an inflammatory disease are common.

It is important to ask about urine output and whether there is hematuria.

It is also important to ask about symptoms such as polyuria and polydipsia which can help in distinguishing between an acute disease and a more longstanding cause for the renal failure.

Measurement of blood pressure: high blood pressure must be interpreted in conjunction with other clinical findings; with cool peripheries it suggests intravascular depletion and with warm peripheries it suggests volume overload.

Investigations

Initial investigations

Life-threatening symptoms must be addressed first.

Urgent analyses of serum creatinine, electrolytes and albumin should be performed.

Oxygen saturations and CXR should be undertaken in cases of suspected pulmonary edema.

Further investigations

All children need the work-up outlined below:
- blood and urine tests: see Tables 10.11.2 and 10.11.3;
- abdominal USS: looking for urinary obstruction, kidney size, echogenicity, cysts;
- CXR.

Additional investigations

These will depend on the clinical presentation:

Hemolytic uremic syndrome
- blood film (looking for fragmented red blood cells);
- blood grouping;
- stool culture;
- VTEC serology.

If nondiarrhea-associated HUS, test for alternative etiology:
- T-antigen *Streptococcus pneumoniae*;
- SLE;
- factor H deficiency.

Acute nephritic syndrome
- ESR;
- creatine kinase;
- complement (C3, C4, C3 nephritic factor);
- immunoglobulins (including IgA);
- throat swab;
- ASOT, anti-DNAse B;
- ANA, dsDNA, anti-GBM, ANCA, ENA, anticardiolipin antibodies.

Ongoing investigations
- Serum creatinine, urea, electrolytes and bicarbonate may be required up to every 6 h.
- Calcium, phosphate, albumin daily.
- Full blood count daily.
- Urine analysis daily.

Table 10.11.1 Causes of AKI in children

Prerenal AKI

Hypovolemia due to: dehydration, GI losses, renal losses or third-space losses as in sepsis and nephrotic syndrome

Circulatory failure

Bilateral renal artery or vein thrombosis

Intrinsic renal AKI

Acute tubular necrosis (ischemic–hypoxic injury, drug-induced or toxin-mediated)

Uric acid nephropathy/tumor lysis syndrome

Rhabdomyolysis

Glomerulonephritis (GN)

• postinfectious GN
• lupus nephritis
• membranoproliferative GN
• Henoch–Schönlein nephritis
• ANCA-positive nephritis
• nephritis of chronic infection
• GBM-positive GN
• idiopathic RPGN

Vascular lesions (HUS, renal venous or artery thromboses)

Interstitial nephritis

Postrenal AKI

Obstruction in a solitary kidney

Bilateral ureteral obstruction

Urethral obstruction

Table 10.11.2 Baseline blood and urine tests required for the evaluation of AKI

Urine examination

Urine analysis

Urine microscopy

Biochemistry

Electrolytes, creatinine, urea, calcium, bicarbonate, phosphate, PTH, liver function tests and CRP

Hematology

Full blood count and ESR

Coagulation screen

Microbiology

Blood culture

Urine microscopy and culture

The role of renal biopsy

A kidney biopsy should be done as soon as possible in all cases where the kidney function is deteriorating and the diagnosis from the above investigations is not clear.

Treatment

Supportive management

Fluid balance:

Determine if the child is dehydrated, euvolemic or overloaded and treat as outlined in Table 10.11.4.

Ongoing fluid management requires replacement of insensible losses (400 mL/m^2/day) and urinary output.

Monitor fluid balance on an hourly basis and weigh the child twice daily.

Table 10.11.3 Urinary findings evaluating the cause of AKI

Urine component	Prerenal AKI	Intrinsic renal AKI
Sediment	Normal	Cells and casts
Specific gravity	High >1.020	Fixed 1.010
Sodium	Low <10 mmol/L	High >40 mmol/L
	Neonates <20 mmol/L	
FE$_{Na}$	Low <1%	High >3%
	Neonates <2.5%	
Osmolality	High	Low

Adjust fluid replacement according to the child's fluid status. full replacement of insensible losses and urine output if euvolemic and restrict to 50–75% of this if overloaded.

Hyperkalemia:

Hyperkalemia is a potentially life-threatening situation that needs urgent treatment (Table 10.11.5).

Potassium >6.5 mmol/L is an indication for treatment until dialysis or urine output is established.

Hyponatremia

Mild hyponatremia is commonly seen and is often dilutional secondary to fluid overload.

If sodium >120 mmol/L, fluid restriction and fluid replacement with 0.9% saline will usually correct it.

If sodium <120 mmol/L there is a risk of seizures and treatment is required to return the sodium to ~125 mmol/L with hypertonic saline (3 %) according to formula:

Na dose (mmol) = (125 − measured Pl$_{Na}$ × weight × 0.6)

and given over 2 h. Pl$_{Na}$: plasma sodium concentration.

Severe hyponatremia with oliguria is an indication for dialysis.

Hypernatremia

This is much less common than hyponatremia

It may be caused by sodium retention or water depletion so careful assessment of fluid status is mandatory.

Mild hypernatremia:

• give IV furosemide 4 mg/kg;
• replace insensible losses with 0.45% saline.

Severe hypernatremia with oliguria is an indication for dialysis.

Hypocalcemia

Correct if severe: <1.9 mmol/L. Give IV 10% calcium gluconate 0.5 mL/kg over 30 min.

If less severe, treat with oral supplements and focus on treating the related hyperphosphatemia with calcium carbonate.

In acute on chronic renal failure consider starting 1α-calcidol.

Acidosis

Correct if serum bicarbonate <18 mmol/L.

The required dose is calculated as:

NaHCO$_3$ dose (mmol) = (18 − Pl$_{HCO_3}$) × 0.5 × weight

Administer half the dose over 1 h and re-evaluate. Give the rest if needed.

An oral dose is 1–2 mmol/kg/day in 2–4 divided doses.

Table 10.11.4 Assessment and management of fluid balance in the child with AKI

Hydration status	Clinical features	Initial management

Dehydrated	Tachycardic
	Cool peripheries:
	   >2 toe-core gap is significant
	   prolonged capillary refill time
	Dry mucous membranes
	Sunken eyes
	UNa <10 mmol/L (<20 mmol/L in neonates)
		Fluid resuscitation
		   10–20 ml/kg 0.9% saline over 1 h
		Then reassess

Euvolemic		Fluid challenge: 10–20 mL/kg normal saline over 1 h Consider furosemide up to 5 mg/kg if no urine response
Overloaded	Tachycardic Gallop rhythm Elevated jugular venous pressure Edema Hypertension	Furosemide 4 mg/kg if fluid overload is severe Dialysis if no response to furosemide

Table 10.11.5 Temporary treatment of hyperkalemia

Treatment	Dose	Comment
Salbutamol	Nebulized dose 2.5 mg If nebulized administration not possible, give 4–10 μg/kg over 10 min	Quick therapy, as it drives K into the cells but short-acting response
Calcium gluconate	10% solution 0.2–0.5 mL/kg IV over 30 min	Use if signs of cardiotoxicity stabilizes cardiac membrane
Calcium resonium	2(–4) g/kg orally or rectally	Should be given to provide a more sustained hypokalemic effect Give lactulose in addition
Sodium bicarbonate	1–2 mmol/kg as 4.2% solution	Use if acidotic (caution if hypocalcemic)
Insulin and dextrose	Give insulin 0.1 U/kg with 5 mL/kg of 10% dextrose	Can be used if other methods are ineffective Monitor for hypoglycemia

Hypertension

This is very often related to fluid overload. Diuretics (furosemide) should be given. Failure to respond is an indication for dialysis.

Oral nifedipine (1–2 mg/kg/day in 2–4 divided doses) is a good second-line drug.

In hypertensive emergencies labetalol IV is often effective in children. The starting dose is 500 μg/kg/h titrated up to maximum of 3 mg/kg/h.

Nutrition

AKI is often associated with a catabolic state and this might delay recovery. The aim is to provide sufficient calories. Dietetic advice is very important.

If possible use enteral feeding via a nasogastric tube if needed.

Parenteral nutrition should be used if enteral feeding is not possible.

Frequent dialysis may be required to allow adequate volumes of the nutrition to be given.

Adequate nutrition can help to prevent potassium and phosphate abnormalities

Drug treatment

It is important to adjust drug doses to the estimated renal function. In severe AKI assume GFR is <20 mL/min/m^2 until onset of improvement.

Doses of drugs will need to be changed when kidney function improves.

Avoid nephrotoxic drugs.

Dialysis

Indications for dialysis are given in Table 10.11.6.

Table 10.11.6 Indications for dialysis in children with AKI

Hyperkalemia >6.5 mmol/L
Severe fluid overload with pulmonary edema unresponsive to diuretics
Severe acidosis unresponsive to treatment
Severe hyperphosphatemia
Uremic symptoms
Anticipation of prolonged AKI, e.g. in HUS

The different modalities for dialysis in children are:
- peritoneal dialysis;
- hemodialysis;
- hemofiltration.

The choice of RRT depends on:
- the hemodynamic stability of the child (children in ITU are mostly managed with CVVH;
- the speed with which the abnormalities need to be corrected;
- the local expertise and availability of equipment.

Hemodialysis is the preferred option if plasma exchange is also needed.

Active intervention

This will depend on the cause of AKI (Table 10.11.1) and may include surgical intervention in cases of postrenal AKI or more specific medical therapies some of which are discussed below.

Hemolytic uremic syndrome (HUS)

This is the most important cause of severe AKI in children. HUS presents with the triad of renal failure, microangiopathic hemolytic anemia and thrombocytopenia.

There are many causes of HUS (Table 10.11.7) and they have traditionally been divided into:
- Diarrhea-positive (D$^+$, typical) HUS;
- Diarrhea-negative (D$^-$, atypical) HUS.

Diarrhea-positive HUS

This is most commonly caused by enteropathogenic E. coli of different serotypes, most commonly O157:H7, or sometimes by shigellosis. These strains produce an enterotoxin called VT (verocyte toxin).

Children present with severe, mostly bloody, diarrhea.

After a few days they develop generalized symptoms with hemolytic anemia and renal failure.

The incidence of VTEC (verocyte toxin E. coli) is variable but peaks during the warm season. The natural reservoir of VTEC is the intestinal tract of farm animals. The bacterium is often spread via milk and meat but can also spread via vegetables contaminated from farm animals.

Outbreaks have been described and as the infectious dose is very low person-to-person spread is also known to occur.

HUS is the tip of an iceberg as infections resulting in asymptomatic colonization of the GI tract can occur in some patients; others may just get bloody diarrhea. Only some 10% will develop the full-blown HUS.

Diarrhea-negative HUS

This can result from a range of different disorders (Table 10.11.7).

Over the last decade pneumococcal-related HUS has in the UK become the second most common cause of HUS accounting for 10–15% of all cases. The reason for this recent increase is not known.

In the UK atypical HUS from other causes comprises some 5% of all cases. Many of these cases never receive an etiological diagnosis. They are often familial and have a relapsing/remitting pattern.

The most commonly found diagnoses in this group are complement deficiencies, particularly mutation in the factor H gene with or without proven factor H deficiency.

Clinical features

The diagnosis is confirmed by the triad of:
- renal failure;
- hemolytic anemia;
- thrombocytopenia.

Many affected children will also develop symptoms in other organ systems, in particular cerebral involvement and pancreatitis. The cerebral symptoms can be severe including epileptic fits, confusion and frank psychotic symptoms.

Investigations

In D$^+$ cases the diagnosis needs to be confirmed by stool culture or by other means of establishing the infection such as detection of the toxin in feces or serology. In cases of atypical HUS there is a strong clinical benefit from establishing, if possible, the genetic diagnosis as this will inform the future clinical course and treatment.

Treatment

Treatment of children with HUS is mostly supportive with management of their fluid balance and, if needed, blood and platelet transfusions. More than 50% of the children will need acute dialysis.

Plasma exchange

This has been used in the group of children with worst prognostic markers: cerebral symptoms and high leukocyte counts (>17 $\times$ 10^9/L).

Antibiotics

Antibiotic treatment of hemorrhagic colitis has not been shown to be beneficial for children. On the contrary there are reports suggesting that antibiotics might make the HUS worse. Innovative treatments trying to bind the toxin within the gut have not been shown to be effective.

Prognosis and long-term outcome

During recent years the mortality from VTEC HUS has improved and is now <5% but up to 30% of survivors will be left with some CKD.

The other forms of HUS have significantly higher mortality and many have a significant chance of a relapsing course.

Acute glomerulonephritis

The spectrum of glomerulonephritides in children is different from that in adults and it is a relatively less important cause for renal failure than later in life.

Post-streptococcal GN (PSGN) is the most common diagnosis, which is made from the combination of a preceding streptococcal infection, mostly throat or skin infection, and the later development of clinical symptoms of nephritic syndrome including edema, pulmonary edema, high BP and hematuria and proteinuria.

Low serum levels of complement C3 and C4 together with raised streptococcal antibodies (ASOT) will support the diagnosis.

PSGN is normally a self-limiting disease but it can cause a rapidly progressive GN requiring dialysis.

Other forms of GN including Henoch–Schönlein nephritis, IgA nephropathy, SLE, ANCA-positive vasculitis, membranoproliferative GN and Goodpasture's syndrome can occasionally be seen in children.

Neonatal AKI

AKI is most commonly found in this age group. There are many causes related to the immature kidney function of

Table 10.11.7 Causes of hemolytic uremic syndrome (HUS) in children

| Diarrhea-associated HUS |
| E. coli |
| Shigella |
| Diarrhea-negative HUS |
| *Pneumococcus-associated HUS* |
| T-antigen-associated HUS |
| *'Atypical' HUS* |
| Complement abnormalities |
| • factor H, factor I, membrane cofactor protein |
| ADAMTS 13 deficiency |
| • von Willebrand factor-cleaving protease |
| *Secondary HUS* |
| Drugs (ciclosporin, cytotoxic drugs, etc.) |
| Bone marrow transplant |
| Autoimmune disorders (SLE) |
| Malignancy |

newborn babies and problems related to prematurity and neonatal intensive unit (NICU) care.

During the first few days of life serum creatinine values in neonates reflect those of the mother. Levels then decrease over the ensuing weeks but will, particularly in premature babies, continue to be higher than later in infancy, reflecting the lower GFR during the first year of life.

In infants, anuria is defined as a urine output <1 mL/kg/day. Eight percent of NICU babies develop AKI. The dominating causes are pre-renal AKI, often due to asphyxia or complications of NICU care. Hypoplastic or dysplastic kidneys with or without obstructing urinary disorders might manifest during infancy. Renal vein thrombosis is also a cause of AKI in neonates.

Post-renal AKI is another important cause of AKI in neonates and will lead to CKD if not adequately treated. The majority of cases are nowadays diagnosed prenatally, although this depends on local prenatal USS screening policies.

Ultrasound will normally confirm the diagnosis. The most common diagnosis is posterior urethral valves in boys. The urinary tract should be drained immediately the diagnosis is made. In most cases a per-urethral bladder catheter will suffice. The child should be sent to a pediatric urologist.

Renal vein thrombosis
Renal vein thrombosis occurs in neonates, especially in those with a thrombotic tendency, e.g. due to hemoconcentration, hypovolemia or a clotting problem such as protein C deficiency.

It is more common in neonates of diabetic mothers and more often seen after traumatic deliveries.

Thrombus normally develops within the kidney in the arcuate or interlobular vessels and then extends to the main renal veins and the vena cava.

The diagnosis should be suspected in infants with hematuria, often macroscopic, impaired kidney function and reduced urinary output. Anemia and thrombocytopenia will develop. The kidney enlarges and may become easily palpable.

Ultrasound and DMSA renogram can be useful in establishing the diagnosis.

Treatment of renal venous thrombosis is controversial. Some authors advocate an expectant approach while others use heparin or attempt to dissolve the clot with tissue plasminogen activator. Before considering such an aggressive approach the risks of an intracranial bleed need to be formally assessed.

The renal prognosis following renal vein thrombosis is highly variable and depends on the extent of venous thrombus formation.

Follow-up
All children recovering from AKI need follow-up, preferably by a pediatric nephrologist.

A formal GFR examination should be undertaken 1 year after the insult to establish the degree of remaining, if any, renal impairment. It is also important to evaluate whether any degree of proteinuria, hematuria or hypertension remain.

Most children who at the 1 year follow-up have normal GFR, BP and urine findings can be discharged from further follow up if the diagnosed illness has not been known to have a recurrent pattern, as in atypical HUS.

Nevertheless some authors advocate long-term follow-up of children with no signs of kidney damage or remaining disease, as there are reports suggesting an increased risk of CKD in this apparently healthy group of children.

Prognosis
The outcome in children who develop AKI depends on the cause of the illness. Children with ATN without other underlying disease have a much better long-term prognosis, whereas children developing AKI in the ITU reportedly suffer ≥50% mortality.

Further reading
Amirlak I, Amirlak B. Haemolytic uraemic syndrome: an overview. *Nephrology (Carlton)* 2006; **11**: 213–218.

Barletta GM, Bunchman TE. Acute renal failure in children and infants. *Curr Opin Crit Care* 2004; **10** 499–504.

Marks SM, Massicotte MP, Steele BT, *et al.* Neonatal renal venous thrombosis: clinical outcomes and prevalence of prothrombotic disorders. *J Pediatr* 2005; **146**: 811–816.

Strazdins V, Watson A, Harvey B, European Pediatric Peritoneal Dialysis working Group. Renal replacement therapy for acute renal failure in children: European guidelines. *Pediatr Nephrol* 2004; **19**: 199–207.

Internet resources
Patient Fact Sheet on hemolytic–uremic syndrome:

http://www.ich.ucl.ac.uk/factsheets/families/F060408/index.html

Treatment of adults and children with renal failure. UK Renal Association Standards and Audit Measures:

http://www.renal.org/Standards/RenalStandards_2002b.pdf

See also
Renal function in the newborn infant, p. 16

Hypertensive children, p. 304

Congenital abnormalities of the urinary tract, p. 658

Acute kidney injury in pregnancy

Introduction

There is no clear definition of AKI in pregnancy, therefore the reported incidence varies between studies. The severity of reported cases of AKI varies from uremia requiring immediate dialysis to a doubling of serum creatinine values, making comparisons across studies difficult.

Renal physiology in normal pregnancy

Early decreases in peripheral vascular resistance lead to lower BP in early pregnancy which then rises gradually to baseline at term.

Cardiac output increases (50% above nonpregnant at baseline).

Plasma volume increases (40% above nonpregnant baseline).

Red cell mass increases (proportionately less than increase in plasma volume, therefore a mild anemia results).

GFR increases by ~50% above baseline (Fig. 10.12.1) due to increased renal plasma flow (45% by 9 weeks and 70% in mid-pregnancy). This is due to dilatation of renal afferent and efferent arterioles and leads to a fall in serum creatinine which persists throughout normal pregnancy. There is no associated increase in intraglomerular pressure.

Plasma osmolality reduces in the 1st trimester and then remains constant during pregnancy.

Sodium reabsorption increases (increased GFR increases filtered sodium load).

A relative respiratory alkalosis develops (direct stimulus of respiratory center).

Glycosuria develops as the increased filtered load exceeds the maximum tubular transport capacity for glucose reabsorption (T_{max}).

Renal size increases with advancing gestation due to dilatation of the renal collecting system, especially on right side.

Epidemiology

Over the last 20 years the incidence of AKI has reduced in developed but less so in developing countries.

In the 1960s the incidence was reported as 1 in 3000 pregnancies but now the rate is almost ten times lower in Europe and North America.

AKI requiring dialysis now occurs in ~1 in 20 000 pregnancies in Europe and North America.

In the developed nations there has been little overall change in mortality which is reported to be 0–30%. In developing countries AKI in pregnancy continues to cause 20% of the total cases of AKI and mortality is as high as 50%.

Traditionally, early pregnancy AKI cases were mainly due to septic abortion and later cases due to obstetric complications including hemorrhage and pre-eclampsia (PeT).

The legalization of abortion and improvements in antenatal care with early detection of antenatal complications of pregnancy are the two main factors that have led to a reduction in AKI in pregnancy.

Hemorrhage and PeT remain the commonest causes of pregnancy-related AKI in developed countries whereas septic abortion and acute pyelonephritis are still common causes in developing countries.

60–90% women will fully recover kidney function following AKI in pregnancy.

Clinical features

Clinical features will depend on the cause of the AKI.

Pre-renal AKI

Volume contraction, hypotension and vasoconstriction can occur in numerous settings in pregnancy:
- persistent vomiting, diarrhea, or diuretic therapy;
- PeT is associated with profound vasoconstriction and volume depletion;
- ante-partum and postpartum hemorrhage.

Blood loss alone may cause hypovolemia but antepartum hemorrhage may also be associated with intravascular coagulation which also compromises intrarenal blood flow. In view of the pre-existing hypovolemic and increased vasoconstrictor response in women with PeT, they are at greater risk from the effects of hemorrhage.

Intrinsic renal AKI

Any of the possible causes of acute renal dysfunction can be encountered in pregnancy but the following are some of the more common causes:
- acute tubular necrosis;
- bilateral cortical necrosis;
- microangiopathy;
- acute interstitial nephritis;
- *de novo* glomerulonephritis.

Each will be discussed separately below.

Post-renal AKI

This is an uncommon cause of AKI in pregnancy. The urinary tract undergoes physiological dilatation in pregnancy especially on the right side in later pregnancy. However, pathological obstruction can occur.

Rarely women can develop an exaggeration of the normal physiological dilatation in the urinary tract in pregnancy. This is called 'the overdistention syndrome'.

Very rarely this syndrome may lead to rupture of the dilated urinary tract.

Urinary tract obstruction is difficult to assess in pregnancy. If the dilatation is gross or there are associated symptoms of flank pain, urinary tract infection or impaired renal function then further investigation and drainage may be required.

The pregnant uterus can rarely be the cause of obstruction. This may be more common in presence of extreme polyhydramnios or with twin pregnancies.

In later pregnancy obstruction is relieved by delivery, in earlier pregnancy stenting and amniotomy (for polyhydramnios) have been reported to delay delivery by 5–15 weeks.

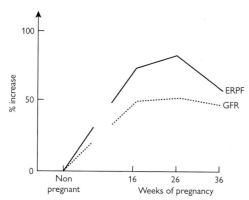

Fig. 10.12.1 Effect of pregnancy on glomerular filtration rate (GFR) and effective renal plasma flow (EFPF). (Redrawn from: Davison, 1987.)

Renal calculi
The incidence of renal stone disease is the same as non-pregnant women. Typical symptoms of loin pain, hematuria and urinary infection may occur but the diagnosis can be difficult in heavily pregnant women. Suspected cases should be referred to urologists for investigation and may require a ureteric stent or nephrostomy.

Clinical presentation
This will depend largely on the precipitating cause of AKI (Table 10.12.1).

It is important to establish the presence of:
• fever and other systemic symptoms of sepsis;
• symptoms of bleeding or other obstetric complications;
• specific disease associated symptoms e.g. rash in SLE, joint pains, vasculitic rash.

BP may be low in prerenal AKI or raised in the presence of glomerulonephritis or PeT.

Jugular venous pressure/volume status – may be low due to volume depletion or high when there is established renal impairment indicating hypervolemia and fluid overload, often associated with peripheral and pulmonary edema.

It is always important to ask the obstetrician to assess the fetal viability and growth and exclude antepartum hemorrhage and other intrauterine complications.

Acute tubular necrosis in pregnancy
This occurs most commonly due to prolonged volume depletion, hypotension and vasoconstriction. ATN can occur secondary to a number of underlying pathologies in pregnancy:

Pre-eclampsia, HELLP syndrome
PeT is accompanied by volume contraction and vasoconstriction and patients are more at risk of developing established ATN following any further volume depletion. PeT is often associated with intravascular coagulation and generalized 'endothelial activation', further compromising renal blood flow and leading to multiple organ dysfunction.

Acute fatty liver of pregnancy
This is part of the spectrum of the maternal systemic PeT disease process.

It is a rare but potentially fatal complication of the third trimester.

Incidence ranges from 1 in 10 000 to 1 in 15 000 deliveries.

It usually presents mid–late pregnancy (27–40 weeks), or occasionally postpartum.

Symptoms are usually of malaise, nausea, vomiting, neurological symptoms, upper abdominal pain and jaundice.

The clinical picture is similar to PeT and HELLP syndrome with hypertension, and with abnormalities in coagulation which are due to liver dysfunction rather than abnormal platelet consumption.

~40% of patients develop AKI.

Septicemia
This is a rare complication of pregnancy in developed countries.

It is one of the five leading causes of maternal death worldwide.

A decline in the number of cases of sepsis in pregnancy has been reported in the USA over last 25 years (from 0.6% to 0.3%).

Prevalence of bacteremia in pregnancy is 7.5 per 1000 admissions but most do not develop septicemia.

One in 8500 deliveries is complicated by septic shock.

Death from septic shock is uncommon in developed countries and outcome is good compared with nonobstetric patients.

Mortality rates vary widely – one recent study reported a mortality rate of 12.5%.

Mortality in developing (mainly African countries) was reported to be >1000 per 100 000 live births compared to < 20 per 100 000 live births in European countries.

Septicemia may arise from any cause in pregnancy, e.g. cholecystitis, ruptured appendix, etc. However, common causes in pregnancy are:

Septic abortion
This remains common in developing countries, but uncommon in developed countries following the introduction of antibiotics, oral contraception and legalized abortion.

It is usually caused by infection with *Clostridium* spp.

Patients present with systemic features of septicemic shock and may have evidence of gas formation in the uterus or abdomen.

Acute pyelonephritis
Patients may complain of fever, loin pain, lower urinary tract symptoms including dysuria, etc. In addition, if the infection is severe there may be symptoms and signs of systemic infection and septic shock, decline in renal function and multiple organ failure.

Other causes of ATN in pregnancy
Other complications of pregnancy that may result in prerenal AKI and established ATN include prolonged intrauterine death and amniotic fluid embolism.

Table 10.12.1 Causes of acute kidney injury in pregnancy

Prerenal causes of AKI

Volume contraction, hypotension and vasoconstriction due to:
water and electrolyte depletion
- persistent vomiting, diarrhea, or overdiuresis

edema-forming states
- pre-eclampsia, nephrotic syndrome

hemorrhage
- antepartum and postpartum hemorrhage

Pre-eclampsia

Renal causes of AKI

Acute tubular necrosis
Secondary to prolonged volume depletion, hypotension and vasoconstriction of any cause, e.g. pre-eclampsia, HELLP syndrome, hemorrhage

Septicemia
Bilateral cortical necrosis
Thrombotic thrombocytopenic purpura/hemolytic uremic syndrome
Acute interstitial nephritis
De novo glomerulonephritis
Amniotic fluid embolism

Postrenal causes of AKI

Physiological dilatation of pregnancy (hydronephrosis and/or hydroureter)
Renal calculi
Obstruction by gravid uterus
Tubular obstruction

Bilateral cortical necrosis

Any cause of sustained hypovolemia, hypotension or profound vasoconstriction can result in this condition. Pregnant women may be more susceptible than nonpregnant patients. The incidence is reported to be ~20% following septic abortion whereas the incidence is only 2% following other causes of AKI in pregnancy.

It most commonly occurs following severe PeT or antepartum hemorrhage.

Microangiopathic syndromes in pregnancy

These include:
- PeT/HELLP syndrome;
- thrombotic thrombocytopenic purpura;
- hemolytic uremic syndrome.

PeT/HELLP is discussed in detail in Chapter 9.5.

Thrombotic thrombocytopenic purpura

A rare complication of pregnancy.

Both acquired idiopathic TTP and familial TTP can occur in pregnancy.

Pregnancy is a predisposing factor for de novo disease or relapse of the condition.

It often occurs in the 2nd or 3rd trimester with mean onset at 23 weeks.

Clinical features
- thrombocytopenia;
- microangiopathic hemolytic anemia;
- fever;
- renal dysfunction;
- neurological symptoms;
- hypertension.

Laboratory investigations
- thrombocytopenia;
- anemia;
- schistocytes/fragmented red blood cells on blood film;
- elevated serum lactate dehydrogenase;
- reduced haptoglobin;
- impaired renal function.

Pathogenesis
In normal individuals, endothelial cell-derived von Willebrand factor multimers are cleaved by a metalloproteinase enzyme (ADAMTS13).

In patients with acquired TTP the ADAMTS13 activity is reduced, leading to aggregation and systemic circulation of excess von Willebrand factor multimers which cause endothelial cell damage, activation of the coagulation cascade and microangiopathy in the kidney and other organs.

Hemolytic uremic syndrome (HUS)

This is a very rare complication of pregnancy.

It may occur at any stage of pregnancy but most typically occurs postpartum (few hours to 8–10 weeks postpartum, but may be delayed several months).

The pregnancy and delivery in most cases have been unremarkable.

The resultant microangiopathy mainly affects the kidneys.

Clinical features
It frequently begins with flu-like symptoms, hypertension, edema and oligoanuria. Hypertension is present in half of cases. HUS can be very difficult to differentiate from PeT in the later stages of pregnancy. If renal failure is progressive a renal biopsy may be considered but is difficult if thrombocytopenia is present.

Laboratory investigations
These are similar to TTP.

Management of microangiopathy in pregnancy

This requires close liaison between hematologist, nephrologist and obstetric team.

Cryoprecipitate-poor fresh frozen plasma
Treatment is similar to nonpregnant cases. Cryoprecipitate-poor fresh frozen plasma is used to replace the deficient metalloproteinases. This treatment is often effective alone in nonoliguric patients (60%).

Plasma exchange
Oliguric or severely affected patients will require plasma exchange which also removes excess von Willebrand factor multimers and autoantibodies against the metalloproteinase ADAMTS13. Treatment is given daily and response to treatment is accompanied by reduced schistocytes on a blood film, increased platelet counts and reduction in LDH levels.

Platelet and blood transfusions
Platelet transfusions should be avoided given the potential risk of increased microvascular thrombosis unless there is risk of life-threatening bleeding.

Blood transfusion can be given if required.

Renal replacement therapy

Patients with significant renal dysfunction will require hemodialysis (see below).

Continuance of the pregnancy

Unlike severe PeT, HELLP syndrome or acute fatty liver of pregnancy – when the condition occurs in the early stages of gestation the pregnancy can be continued in patients with TTP/HUS. The mother may require ongoing treatment during pregnancy with plasma infusion/exchange and dialysis. In addition, the fetus needs to be closely monitored for signs of compromise to regularly determine whether the outcome of early delivery would be better than continuing pregnancy.

Outcome

HUS and TTP in pregnancy are associated with increased maternal morbidity and mortality. Recent case series report a reduction in maternal mortality with a rate of 0–10% (previously 40–50%). Similarly, fetal outcomes have improved with recent reports of 20% fetal loss (previous 80%). Most cases result in early delivery (average 26 weeks).

Acute interstitial nephritis

The pregnant patient may develop acute interstitial nephritis (AIN) which is often due to medication in pregnancy as in the nonpregnant patient.

In 1st and early 2nd trimesters a renal biopsy may be performed to establish the cause of sustained deterioration in renal function.

Drugs considered a potential cause of AIN should be discontinued and avoided. Steroid therapy can be administered in pregnancy if necessary.

Diagnosis is more difficult in mid/later pregnancy as it is technically difficult to perform a safe renal biopsy (see renal biopsy in pregnancy).

Associated clinical findings (rash, etc.) may indicate possible AIN and potentially nephrotoxic drugs should be discontinued. In later pregnancy it is again necessary to consider the relative merits and disadvantages to mother and fetus of continuing with the pregnancy *in utero* or considering an early delivery.

De novo glomerulonephritis

Any acute glomerulonephritis can present in pregnancy.

Hypertension and urinary abnormalities are often detected during routine antenatal care.

Glomerulonephritis can present at any stage of pregnancy and it may be difficult to distinguish a new presentation of glomerulonephritis in later pregnancy from PeT.

Clinical presentation of glomerulonephritis may be mild with hypertension, urinary abnormalities including microscopic hematuria and proteinuria with or without impaired renal function; or severe with renal failure, thrombocytopenia, edema and hypertension.

There may be associated clinical symptoms and signs which aid diagnosis as in the nonpregnant patient, e.g. symptoms and signs of other organ involvement: skin lesions and joint symptoms in systemic lupus erythematosis (SLE), purpuric rash in vasculitis.

Lupus nephritis in pregnancy

Pregnancy may exacerbate activity in SLE, especially if disease is active at the time of conception. In later pregnancy it can be difficult to distinguish between new onset of lupus nephritis and PeT.

It is important to consider the extrarenal manifestations of SLE and the effects on pregnancy.

30% patients with SLE have antiphospholipid antibodies.

Increased risk of thrombotic microangiopathy can result in hypertension, proteinuria and renal impairment which are difficult to distinguish from PeT.

For other manifestations of thromboembolic disease, anticoagulation needs to be considered with obstetric and hematology teams.

Some patients with SLE have anti-Ro/La antibodies which have been linked to neonatal cardiac problems with bradycardia and heart block. It is therefore important to discuss the need for fetal cardiac monitoring with the obstetricians.

In general, the outcome of SLE is good in pregnancy but depends on the severity and extent of organ involvement.

There is a high incidence of early-onset PeT. One series reported that PeT occurred in 15% of patients with SLE.

Complications are more severe in the presence of antiphospholipid antibodies.

Management of glomerulonephritis in pregnancy

This depends on the type of glomerulonephritis and the severity of the initial presentation.

In pregnancy, treatment for active SLE usually includes:

- corticosteroids;
- low dose aspirin;
- immunosuppressive medication (azathioprine or cyclophosphamide);
- hydroxychloroquine;
- antihypertensive medications (nifedipine, methyldopa and/or labetaolol);
- low molecular weight heparin (if antiphospholipid antibodies/significant proteinuria).

Mycophenolate mofetil is contraindicated in pregnancy.

The renal and obstetric teams need to liaise closely and determine issues regarding continuation of the pregnancy in consultation with the mother. The remainder of the management is as outlined below.

Investigations

These are essentially the same as for nonpregnant patients, but with particular emphasis on identification of specific causes related to pregnancy (Table 10.12.2).

Biochemistry

- urea and electrolytes;
- liver function tests;
- quantification of urinary protein excretion.

Blood film, LDH, haptoglobin and platelet count

- to exclude schistocytes and microangiopathic hemolytic anemia.

Urate

- raised in patients with diagnosis of PeT.

Immunology screen

- dsDNA antibodies;
- complement levels C3, C4;
- lupus anticoagulant and anticardiolipin antibodies;
- ANCA.

Renal ultrasound scan
- diagnosis of urinary tract obstruction may be difficult as dilatation of ureter and renal pelvis (especially on right) is a feature of normal pregnancy.

Renal biopsy
- Consider in certain cases if, for example, GN is suspected and results of a biopsy are likely to lead to specific therapy.

Renal biopsy in pregnancy

Rarely, when AKI of unknown cause or symptomatic *de novo* renal disease presents in a pregnant women, renal biopsy will need to be considered (Table 10.12.3). Recent studies have reported the complication rate to be the same as in nonpregnant patients.

In all cases USS should be performed to exclude obstruction and a urine culture to exclude infection before proceeding to a renal biopsy. In addition, platelet count, coagulation screen should be normal and BP well-controlled.

If possible a renal biopsy should be deferred until after pregnancy is completed. Although pregnancy confers no additional risk, the positioning of the patient may be more difficult and it may be uncomfortable for a woman to lie on her stomach, in which case the biopsy can be performed sitting. It is wise to liaise with the radiologists.

When a biopsy is performed in pregnancy there should be an expectation that the histological findings may lead to immediate treatment which would improve the outcome of pregnancy for the mother and fetus.

Investigation of newly identified urinary sediment abnormalities in pregnancy with normal renal function should be deferred until postpartum.

Treatment

The following are required:
- prompt identification and correction of volume depletion and electrolyte disturbances;
- prompt identification of sepsis with supportive treatment and commencement of broad spectrum and then specific antibiotics;
- prompt investigation and relief of urinary tract obstruction;
- discontinuation of medication likely to cause acute interstitial nephritis.
- specific therapy for some pathologies, e.g. SLE, may require immunosuppressive therapy; HUS may require fresh frozen plasma and plasma exchange;
- close monitoring of all biochemical parameters including urea and electrolytes, acidosis;
- when AKI occurs in pregnancy one of the most important treatment decisions is whether the outcome would be improved by immediate delivery.

Early delivery of the baby
The decision to deliver the baby depends upon:

1. Whether the cause of AKI is presumed to be PeT, HELLP or acute fatty liver of pregnancy where delivery is often the only way to stop the disease process or when the presence of an ongoing pregnancy prevents administration of adequate treatment to the mother.

2. The stage of pregnancy. Facilitating delivery is relatively easy in later pregnancy >28–32 weeks when the fetus is likely to be viable, but below this level of gestation the

Table 10.12.2 Investigation of AKI in pregnancy

Urine
- urine stick testing (blood, protein, leukocytes and nitrites)
- quantification of proteinuria (24 h urine collection or urine protein:creatinine ratio)
- urine culture
- microscopy/cytology

Biochemistry
- urea and electrolytes
- bone chemistry
- liver function tests
- lactate dehydrogenase and haptoglobin
- glucose
- urate
- C-reactive protein

Hematology
- full blood count
- blood film
- coagulation studies (include lupus anticoagulant in SLE)

Immunology
- autoantibodies (dsDNA, anticardiolipin antibodies and anti-Ro/La antibodies in SLE)
- complement

Microbiology
- blood cultures
- specific infections and virology as required

Radiology
- renal ultrasound (to exclude obstruction and assess renal size)

Renal biopsy
- see Table 10.12.3

Obstetric liaison
- arrange for obstetric monitoring of the fetus

---

pregnancy may be lost if immediate delivery takes place. In this situation if the maternal condition is stable and fetus is viable, a patient with AKI may be given dialysis during pregnancy. When renal impairment is present but not requiring dialysis then a decision may need to be taken regarding maximizing the viability of the fetus versus continuing the pregnancy and risking further deterioration in renal function. This requires close liaison between renal and obstetric teams.

Indications for dialysis in pregnancy
- volume overload;
- hyperkalemia;
- metabolic acidosis;
- uremia (urea >20 mmol/L).

There is no clear evidence to indicate the correct time to start dialysis in pregnancy; however, most nephrologists aim to keep the serum urea level <20 mmol/L in a pregnant patient.

Dialysis modality

Both peritoneal dialysis and hemodialysis have been successfully used in pregnancy. Hemodialysis is used most frequently and needs to be performed approximately daily to minimize uremia and intradialytic weight gain. Generally, 6 treatments per week (20 h) are recommended. Care needs to be taken to avoid hypokalemia and excessive fluid removal because hypotension and wide variations in volume status may affect placental perfusion.

Table 10.12.3 Indications for renal biopsy in pregnancy

Sudden deterioration in renal function before 28 weeks gestation of unknown cause

In this situation a biopsy may identify an important reversible pathology and lead to immediate treatment, e.g. SLE with lupus nephritis, renal vasculitis.

Symptomatic nephrotic syndrome before 28 weeks

Renal biopsy may identify a pathology which is treatable such as minimal change disease, SLE or a pathology for which you would not initiate further therapy during pregnancy, e.g. mesangiocapillary glomerulonephritis.

In this way a renal biopsy can also be useful to prevent initiation of potentially toxic empirical treatment with steroids during pregnancy.

All other situations

Generally, investigation by renal biopsy should be deferred until after delivery but may sometimes be considered in 1st trimester if the result would inform future management decisions:
- isolated proteinuria >3 g/24 h;
- previously diagnosed systemic disease associated with urinary abnormalities or renal impairment;
- unexplained chronic renal impairment.

Patients may also be anemic; hemoglobin should be maintained >10 g/dL units. Erythropoietin therapy appears safe in pregnancy.

Prognosis

Outcome depends on the cause of AKI.

When the cause of AKI is reversible, renal function often recovers in 3–4 weeks. Some patients will require dialysis and other intensive care measures. Unfortunately, bilateral cortical necrosis may also be a consequence and recovery of renal function may then be limited.

Full renal recovery is reported in 60–90% cases of AKI in pregnancy.

Follow-up

Postpartum follow-up of women with AKI in pregnancy is essential. The urgency and duration of follow-up depends on the nature of the AKI.

All women in the UK have a 6 week postnatal check but women with AKI may need early nephrological review to consider further investigation, i.e. renal biopsy and management of persisting problems.

Many medications are changed or omitted during pregnancy e.g. ACEIs. A full medication review is required postpartum to consider reintroduction of medications discontinued antenatally. It is important to consider the safety of medications in women who are breastfeeding and advice may be needed from a pharmacist.

Future prospects

The majority of the available data on renal disease and pregnancy dates from the 1970s and 1980s. There is a need for contemporary data to improve the advice we are able to give to pregnant mothers with renal disease.

It will be important that future collaborative studies are established and funded and that information regarding renal disease in pregnancy is accumulated by the National Obstetric and Renal registries – for example UK CORD (Collaboration in Renal disease in Pregnancy) and the UK Transplant Pregnancy Registry.

The Royal College of Obsterics and Gynecology and NICE are currently reviewing the evidence for treatment of hypertension in pregnancy and will publish their recommendations within the next 12 months.

Further reading

Davison JM. Overview: kidney function in pregnant women. *Am Kidney Dis* 1987; **9**: 248.

Dwyer PL, O'Reilly M. Recurrent urinary tract infection in the female. *Curr Opin Obstet Gynaecol* 2002; **14**: 537–543.

Evans R, Fernandez-Perez, Salman S, *et al*. Sepsis during pregnancy. *Crit Care Med* 2005; **33**(10, Suppl): S286–293.

Gammill HS, Jeyabalan A. Acute renal failure in pregnancy. *Crit Care Med* 2005; **33**(10, Suppl): S372–384.

Hou S, Firanek C. Management of the pregnant dialysis patient. *Adv Renal Replacement Therapy* 1998; **5**: 24–30.

Johnson RJ, Feehally J (eds). Renal Complications in the Normal Pregnancy. *Comprehensive clinical nephrology*, 2nd edn. London: Mosby; 2003. Chapter 44, pp. 567–581.

Karumanchi SA, Epstein FH. Renal complications in pregnancy. In: Feehally J, Floege J, Johnson RJ (eds) Comprehensive clinical nephrology, 3rd edn. Philadelphia, PA: Mosby; 2007; Chapter 41, pp 483–494.

Moroni G, Ponticelli C. The risk of pregnancy with lupus nephritis. *J Nephrol* 2003; **16**: 161–167.

Sturgiss SN, Dunlop W, Davison JM. Renal haemodynamics and tubular function in human pregnancy. *Ballières Clin Obstet Gynecol* 1994; **8**: 209–234.

Internet resources

SafeFoetus.com, useful site to assess safety of prescribing in pregnancy:

http://www.safefoetus.com/

Pregnancy as a test of renal function: a streamed lecture held on the RCP Edinburgh website:

http://rcpe.ac.uk/education/education/streamed_lectures/renal-med.php

Lupus UK, patient friendly information on planning pregnancy in patients with SLE:

http://www.lupusuk.com

Royal College of Obstetricians and Gynaecologists:

http://www.rcog.org.uk

National Collaborating Centre for Women's and Children's Health:

http://www.ncc-wch.org.uk/

See also

CKD in pregnancy, p. 476

Hypertensive disorders in pregnancy p. 310

Clinical approach to acute kidney injury, p. 318

Renal replacement therapies in acute kidney injury, p. 328

Acute kidney injury in the elderly

Introduction

Acute kidney injury (AKI) is more common in the elderly population resulting from a combination of physiological changes within the aging kidney, a higher frequency of associated comorbidities and differences in the etiological spectrum of AKI in the elderly population.

The 'biological age' of patients is likely to be of more relevance than chronological age, but is much more difficult to define. In studies of AKI, therefore, it is chronological age that is most widely used to define an elderly population. Despite this, there is considerable variation in the age used to define 'elderly' in the published literature.

The age demography of the developed world is that of an increasingly elderly population, a trend that is likely to continue as life expectancy rises. The age at which one is considered elderly also varies between countries with an average life expectancy in India of 62.5 years compared with 77.7 years in the UK (data from the US Census Bureau International Database 2000).

Epidemiology

The incidence of AKI in the elderly is difficult to quantify as the definitions of both 'elderly' and 'AKI' differ widely in the literature.

Studies also vary in their clinical setting (community, general hospital, ITU, etc.) making generalizations and comparisons between sets of data impossible.

The frequency of AKI increases with advancing age whichever definition is chosen.

A UK community-based study found that the incidence of AKI was:

- 17 pmp/year in <50-year-olds;
- 949 pmp/year in 80–89-year-olds.

From the same study: 72% cases of AKI occurred in patients aged >70 years.

More recently, another smaller UK study found the incidence of severe AKI to be:

- 68 pmp/year in <65-year-olds;
- 351 pmp/year in >65-year-olds.

In general, the incidence of AKI also appears to be increasing over time although some of this rise reflects the changing criteria for AKI and indications for treatment.

A Scottish study found the incidence of AKI requiring renal replacement therapy (RRT) to be 50 pmp/year in 1989–1990 and 297 pmp/year in 2002.

Predisposing factors

The elderly are at increased risk of developing AKI through a combination of physiological changes within the kidney and other demographic factors.

Structural and functional changes in the aging kidney

Under normal circumstances, the elderly kidney is capable of maintaining fluid and electrolyte balance and the physiological changes associated with age are clinically silent. However, the capacity to adapt is reduced and the response rate to change is slower, thus making the elderly kidney more susceptible to developing AKI.

Being less able to adapt to sudden changes in blood flow or salt and water balance leads to:

- blunted response to sodium depletion due to reduced tubular reabsorption capacity (salt wasting);
- blunted response to sodium loading, due to a reduced natriuretic response;
- reduced urinary concentrating ability;
- reduced urinary diluting ability;
- reduced sensation of thirst despite raised plasma osmolality;
- loss of renal blood flow autoregulation in response to a reduction in perfusion pressure (increased vascular tone and reduced vasodilatory response);

In addition to these functional changes, there is also an increased use of drugs interfering with autoregulation of blood flow (ACEIs, loop diuretics, NSAIDs, etc.).

As a consequence of these changes, the elderly patient is at increased risk of developing:

- dehydration and hypernatremia due to a reduction in maximal concentrating ability combined with reduced thirst perception;
- hyponatremia and fluid overload due to a reduction in maximal diluting ability combined with impaired ability to conserve sodium;
- hyperkalemic (type IV) renal tubular acidosis due to a reduction in basal renin and aldosterone activity. This increases the risk of hyperkalemia following a GI bleed and with drugs inhibiting the renin–angiotensin system (ACEIs, ARBs, heparin, tacrolimus, ciclosporin, NSAIDs) or those blocking sodium channels (trimethoprim, pentamidine, K^+-sparing diuretics).

Other factors

As well as physiological changes within the aging kidney, there are other factors which increase the risk of AKI amongst elderly populations:

Chronic comorbidity

Chronic conditions that lead to CKD, such as hypertension and diabetes mellitus, are more prevalent in the elderly.

Polypharmacy

The use of multiple medications is much greater among the elderly and often includes potentially nephrotoxic drugs (ACEIs, ARBs and NSAIDs).

Radiological tests and surgical interventions

More aggressive investigation and treatment has led to an increase in radiological tests and surgical interventions being performed on elderly patients with the attendant risk of contrast nephropathy and postoperative AKI.

Clinical features

As in other populations, AKI in the elderly is often multifactorial, making precise etiological classification difficult. Although the overall etiological spectrum in the elderly is similar to other populations, certain causes are more prevalent in older populations (Table 10.13.1).

The clinical features, investigation and management of specific causes are dealt with elsewhere in this book. The text below details specific features pertaining to the elderly.

Table 10.13.1 Causes of AKI occuring more frequently in the elderly

Prerenal AKI (all forms more common in the elderly)
True hypovolemia
Reduced intravascular volume (functional hypovolemia)
NSAID- or ACEI/ARB-induced hemodynamic changes
Renal artery thrombosis
Cholesterol embolization

Intrinsic renal AKI
Rapidly progressive glomerulonephritis
Focal segmental glomerulosclerosis
Ischemic ATN
Nephrotoxic ATN
Myeloma

Postrenal AKI
Benign prostatic hyperplasia or prostate cancer
Abdominal/pelvic malignancy

Prerenal AKI

Prerenal AKI is more common in the elderly and also more common in community-acquired AKI. It may result from a number of causes.

Hypovolemia

The elderly are more susceptible to true hypovolemia due to reduced maximal concentrating ability, reduced sodium reabsorption capacity, a reduced thirst impulse and an increased prevalence of diuretic usage.

Functional hypovolemia (interpreted by the kidney as a reduction in intravascular volume) from pre-existing conditions such as heart failure is also more common in the elderly.

Hemodynamic

Impaired renal blood flow autoregulation leaves the elderly kidney at increased risk from superadded hemodynamic effects from drug therapy.

Age alone, however, has not been shown to be a risk factor for AKI following either NSAIDs or ACEIs/ARBs.

Risk factors for NSAID-induced AKI include patient aged >60 years with concomitant cardiovascular disease, CKD and renal hypoperfusion.

Risk factors for ACEI/ARB-induced AKI include the presence of renal artery stenosis, severe chronic heart failure, polycystic kidney disease and intra-renal nephrosclerosis (often undiagnosed).

Renovascular disease

Both renal artery thrombosis and cholesterol embolism are more common in the elderly.

Cholesterol embolization is an important cause of AKI in the elderly. It most commonly occurs after vascular interventions with AKI, generally occuring up to 2–4 weeks after the procedure. It is thought to be responsible for a third of cases of AKI following AAA repair. Cholesterol embolization can also arise spontaneously in an individual with severe atherosclerotic disease, or following anticoagulation or thrombolysis.

Intrinsic renal AKI

Rapidly progressive glomerulonephritis, renovascular disease and myeloma are all seen more frequently in the elderly.

Glomerulonephritis

There is an increased incidence of rapidly progressive glomerulonephritis (RPGN) due to small vessel vasculitis in patients aged >60 years.

RPGN consistently accounts for approximately a third of cases in renal biopsy series in the elderly.

Lupus nephritis is very rarely found in renal biopsies in older populations.

Acute tubular necrosis

Acute tubular necrosis (ATN) is the commonest cause of AKI in both young and elderly populations, particularly for those patients who require ITU admission.

Although a distinction is frequently made between ischemic, nephrotoxic and septic ATN, in reality, ATN commonly results from a mixture of insults. The elderly also have an increased prevalence of comorbid conditions predisposing them to develop ATN (diabetes mellitus, hypertension, CKD and heart failure).

Ischemic ATN is more common in elderly populations where approximately one-third of cases are the consequence of surgical intervention. Raised serum creatinine or urea preoperatively strongly predict the likelihood of developing worsening renal function postoperatively. Cardiac and vascular surgery are most likely to result in postoperative AKI.

Septic ATN is common in younger adults as well as the elderly. Multiple organ failure in the elderly most frequently results from infection, and the development of AKI is a strong predictor of mortality in this age group.

The interaction of nephrotoxins and renal hypoperfusion is at least additive in the development of AKI and may be synergistic. Risk factors for the development of nephrotoxic ATN in the elderly are:

- radiocontrast use (prevalence increasing as more interventions carried out);
- an increased prevalence of polypharmacy;
- injudicious use of nephrotoxic drugs especially when dosage is not adjusted for the reduction in GFR. Aminoglycosides in particular are associated with an increased incidence of AKI amongst the elderly and should be avoided unless absolutely necessary whereupon monitoring of drug levels is essential.

Acute interstitial nephritis

The overall incidence of acute interstitial nephritis is not higher in the elderly, but theoretically they are more at risk due to the higher prevalence of polypharmacy. If diagnosis is suspected, renal biopsy should be performed promptly as early treatment with corticosteroids may improve renal recovery.

Intratubular obstruction

This is less common than urethral/ureteric obstruction. Intratubular obstruction due to myeloma (light chain precipitation) is more common in the elderly. Otherwise the causes of intratubular obstruction are similar to the general population.

Postrenal AKI

Obstructive renal failure is more common in the elderly than in younger adults.

The incidence in the general population is quoted as 1–10% but in elderly populations the incidence is increased to 9–22%.

AKI only develops where there is bilateral obstruction or obstruction to a single functioning kidney.

Urethral/ureteric obstruction

This is an important cause of AKI in the elderly and is often amenable to treatment. Important causes to consider in the elderly patient are:

- prostatic disease (benign prostatic hyperplasia and prostate cancer);
- intra-abdominal malignancy;
- retroperitoneal malignancy.

Presentation of AKI

The presentation of AKI in the elderly as in the general population is often nonspecific. However, the elderly are more likely to have an atypical presentation of AKI such as an acute confusional state.

Physical signs can also be misleading in the elderly.

In particular:

- loss of skin turgor is a common finding in the elderly and may be a reflection of aging rather than hydration status;
- orthostatic hypotension may occur in elderly patients without hypovolemia;
- edema may occur in the absence of fluid overload.

Investigations

In general, AKI occurring in an elderly patient should be investigated in the same way as in the general adult population.

The following pertain to issues specifically related to the elderly population.

Blood tests

The following should always be considered:

- serum immunoglobulins, serum protein electrophoresis and urine electrophoresis to exclude myeloma;
- ANCA and anti-GBM Ab (see below);
- LDH if renal infarction is suspected (raised in absence of LFT derangement).

Urinary electrolytes

The value of urinary indices in distinguishing types of AKI is controversial.

A high urine osmolality (>500 mosmol/kg) and a fractional excretion of sodium (FE_{Na}) <1% suggest pre-renal AKI.

Such parameters may be even less useful in elderly patients because FE_{Na} >1% and a urine osmolality <500 mosmol/kg can occur in pre-renal AKI in the elderly in the presence of:

- a decrease in the maximal concentrating ability of the kidney (with or without underlying CKD);
- an inability to maximize sodium reabsorption;
- diuretic use.

Conversely, FE_{Na} <1% may also be seen in intrinsic AKI in:

- early obstruction;
- acute glomerulonephritis;
- hepatorenal syndrome;
- following radiocontrast administration;
- sepsis.

Radiological investigations

Abdominal ultrasound

USS is imperative to diagnose or exclude obstructive AKI and should be performed without delay.

CT scan

An enhanced CT scan should be considered if renal artery occlusion is suspected.

Renal biopsy

There is no excess risk in performing a renal biopsy in the elderly patient and much potentially to be gained if a treatable condition is diagnosed. A biopsy should therefore be performed if clinically indicated. Interpretation of the biopsy can sometimes be more difficult due to the presence of age-related changes such as glomerulosclerosis. However, this should not be used as a reason for not performing a biopsy if it is otherwise indicated.

The most common diagnoses seen in renal biopsy series in elderly patients with AKI are:

- RPGN (one-third of all renal biopsies in the elderly);
- ATN;
- renovascular disease;
- acute interstitial nephritis.

One renal biopsy study in the elderly noted that the histological diagnosis was different from the clinical diagnosis in ~33% of cases, emphasizing the importance of biopsy in this population.

Treatment

There are currently no evidence-based guidelines for the management of AKI in the elderly. The following principles are based on expert opinion.

Fluid management

As the elderly are more prone to volume contraction, initial rehydration is an important first step when AKI is suspected (and there are no signs of fluid overload).

This should occur regardless of urinary indices.

Reversibility of renal impairment in response to fluid replacement is the most reliable indicator of prerenal AKI.

Whereas rehydration rapidly reverses prerenal AKI in the young, the elderly are likely to respond more slowly to a fluid challenge.

Furthermore, the cardiovascular system is frequently more rigid in older populations leading to an increased risk of fluid overload.

For these reasons, the assessment of fluid balance is often more difficult in elderly patients and generally CVP monitoring will be required to guide fluid resuscitation.

Care should be taken with fluid management in the elderly patient with obstructive AKI, being alert to the possibility of:

- Postobstructive diuresis (>4 L/day): fluid and electrolyte replacement needs to be carefully managed due to reduced urinary concentrating and diluting ability and blunted maximal response to alterations in sodium concentration.
- Hyperkalemic (type IV) renal tubular acidosis: the elderly are more susceptible (reduction in renin and aldosterone activity), and it may persist after correction of the obstruction.

Renal replacement therapy

Indications for dialysis are no different from the general population and individual patient characteristics and local service provision rather than age should determine the dialysis modality chosen.

There is currently no convincing evidence that elderly patients with AKI requiring RRT have a significantly worse outcome than their younger counterparts and dialysis should therefore not be withheld on the basis of age alone.

Crescentic (rapidly progressive) glomerulonephritis
Any form of RPGN has a much poorer prognosis in patients aged >60 years. However, the decision to treat patients aged >60 years with aggressive immunosuppression should be considered carefully as it is associated with a significantly increased relative risk of death compared with patients aged <60 years.

Prognosis
It is difficult to estimate immediate mortality risk or long-term prognosis for an individual patient due to the diversity of the different data series, reflecting the heterogeneity of both the underlying causes of AKI and population groups studied.

Whereas increasing age is associated with a worse outcome in the ITU population, there is no consensus as to whether mortality rates from AKI in the elderly are higher than the overall population. Mortality is lower in obstructive AKI and more common in elderly populations, which may have a bearing on mortality rates.

Mortality rates range from 40 to 65% but studies on AKI in the elderly are generally small.

Mortality is often not related to AKI *per se*.

The major causes of mortality in elderly patients with AKI published in the literature are:
- sepsis;
- multiple organ failure;
- GI bleeding;
- cardiac failure and arrhythmias.

Prognostic factors
Many studies have looked for factors which have prognostic significance for AKI in the elderly. Although no consensus exists, the following (in decreasing order) are those factors considered to have a negative prognostic significance, for which most agreement exists:
- primary diagnosis or underlying cause of AKI;
- increasing number of failing organ systems;
- requirement for dialysis;
- oliguria;
- hypotension;
- pre-existing cardiac disease.

Recovery of renal function
Renal tubular recovery is slower in the elderly and, although there is no firm evidence to suggest that the proportion of patients remaining dialysis dependent is different in young and elderly adults, studies suggest that full recovery of renal function occurs less often in elderly patients. Figure 10.13.1 combines the outcomes of 137 patients from two studies of AKI in elderly patients.

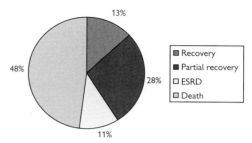

Fig. 10.13.1 Prognosis of AKI in patients aged >65 years. Renal function is taken from the time of discharge from hospital. Data are taken from two studies with 137 patients in total: Baraldi *et al.* (1998) and Klouche *et al.* (1995).

Further reading
Baraldi A, Ballestri M, Rapanà R, *et al.* Acute renal failure of medical type in an elderly population. *Nephrol Dial Transplant* 1998; **13**(Suppl 7): 25–29.

Feest TG, Round A, Hamad S. Incidence of severe acute renal failure in adults: results of a community based study. *Br Med J* 1993; **306**: 481–483.

Haas M, Spargo BH, Ernst-Jan C, *et al.* Etiologies and outcome of acute renal insufficiency in older adults: a renal biopsy study of 259 cases. *Am J Kidney Dis* 2000; **35**: 433–447.

Hegarty J, Middleton RJ, Krebs M, *et al.* Severe acute renal failure in adults: place of care, incidence and outcomes. *Q J Med* 2005; **8**: 661–666.

Klouche K, Cristol JP, Kaaki C, *et al.* Prognosis of acute renal failure in the elderly. *Nephrol Dial Transplant* 1995; **10**: 2240–2243.

Lameire N, Van der Noortgate N, Vanholder RC. The elderly. In: Davison AM, *et al.* (eds), *Oxford textbook of nephrology*, 3rd edn. Oxford: Oxford University Press; 2005.

Metcalfe W, Simpson M, Khan IH, *et al.* Scottish Renal Registry. Acute renal failure requiring renal replacement therapy: incidence and outcome. *Q J Med* 2002; **95**: 579–583.

Internet resources
Acute Dialysis Quality Initiative:
http://www.ADQI.net

See also
The aging kidney, p. 18
Clinical approach to acute kidney injury, p. 318
Renal replacement therapies in acute kidney injury, p. 328
Urinary tract obstruction, p. 652
Crescentic glomerulephritis, p. 120

Chronic kidney disease (CKD)

Chapter contents

Assessment of chronic kidney disease

Introduction

Chronic kidney disease (CKD) is a long-term condition which can arise from damage to the kidneys from a variety of diseases. When mild it results in few symptoms and may frequently go undetected. For such patients the major issue is the associated increased morbidity and mortality from cardiovascular disease (CVD).

In an important minority of people CKD is progressive and results in end-stage renal disease (ESRD). This is fatal unless treated by renal replacement therapy (RRT) – either dialysis or kidney transplantation. Such treatment is expensive, consuming a disproportionate amount of healthcare resource (in the UK >2% of the NHS budget is spent on the 0.1% of patients who receive RRT). The number of patients receiving RRT around the world is rising rapidly and is unlikely to reach steady state for many years.

Many healthcare economies are currently putting in place systems to allow the early detection of CKD. At the same time guidelines for CKD management are being implemented with the aim of either preventing or delaying the onset of associated cardiovascular complications as well as progression of CKD to a more advanced stage.

Definitions

In 2002 the K/DOQI Clinical Practice Guidelines provided a definition of CKD which is now widely used around the world.

To diagnose CKD there must be:
- Kidney damage for ≥3 months defined as either structural or functional abnormalities such as urinary sediment abnormalities or albuminuria. GFR may or may not be reduced.
- GFR ≤60 mL/min/1.73m² for ≥3 months with or without evidence of structural damage.

CKD is classified into five stages according to the level of GFR irrespective of the underlying diagnosis (Table 11.1.1).

It is essential to exclude causes of acute kidney injury (AKI) before classifying a patient as having CKD, or acute on chronic kidney before determining the stage of CKD.

Stage 5 CKD may be called established renal failure (ERF) or ESRD and reflects progression of CKD to a point where RRT may be required to maintain life. It is irreversible.

As understanding of the epidemiology of CKD has developed, modifications of the above classification have been suggested in order to allow improved risk stratification of patients with CKD. These include:

Subdivision of stage 3 into:
- stage 3A: a lower risk group with an eGFR of 45–59 mL/min/1.73 m²;
- stage 3B: a higher risk group with an eGFR of 30–44 mL/min/1.73 m².

Applying the suffix 'p' to all stages reflects the importance of proteinuria/albuminuria as an independent risk factor for adverse outcomes in CKD.

Epidemiology

CKD is increasingly recognized as a public health problem.

Mild-to-moderate CKD is very common in unselected populations; some surveys have suggested that as many as 16% of the adult population have CKD.

Generally, cross-sectional population studies in a number of countries suggest an overall prevalence of CKD 1–5 of >10%.

CKD stage 5 is relatively rare, but lesser degrees of CKD are frequently found in the community and are frequently asymptomatic.

Reported community prevalence of the various stages of CKD is typically of the order:
- CKD 5: 0.1%
- CKD 4: 0.2%
- CKD 3: 5%
- CKD 2: 3%
- CKD 1: 3%

However, in assessing the burden of disease it is important to understand the characteristics of the population since the prevalence of CKD is affected by:
- *Increasing age*: exponentially increasing so that 30–40% of population >75 years have CKD 3–5 (mostly CKD 3).
- *Ethnicity*: several-fold more common in Afro-Caribbean and South East Asian populations.
- *Presence of comorbidities*: higher prevalence in those with hypertension, diabetes, vascular disease, ischemic heart disease and heart failure.
- *Social deprivation*: increases with increasing deprivation.

First-degree relatives of a patient with ERF have a higher risk of developing CKD.

Data from the US (National Health and Nutrition Examination Surveys: NHANES) suggests that the prevalence of CKD has increased from 10% to 13% between 1988–1994 and 1999–2004. This may be partly explained by an increase in the risk factors for CKD including an aging population and increasing prevalence of diabetes and hypertension.

Typically in a cohort of patients with CKD 3–5:
- 60% will be aged >70 years;
- 25% will be known to have diabetes;
- 75% will have a history of hypertension.

CKD appears to be an independent and significant risk factor for progressive CVD.

CVD accounts for ~50% of the deaths in patients with CKD.

The relative risk of death from CVD increases with decreasing GFR even when adjusted for comorbidities such as known cardiovascular disease, hypertension and diabetes.

This relationship is maintained (although less pronounced) even into the 9th decade of life.

Etiology

There are many causes of CKD. These include:
- systemic diseases: diabetes, hypertension, immunological disease;
- glomerular diseases: resulting in so-called 'chronic glomerulonephritis';
- tubulointerstitial diseases;
- AKI, which does not recover.

The various causes of CKD are described in depth elsewhere in this book.

Table 11.1.1. Classification of CKD based on the NKF K/DOQI recommendations

CKD stage	Description	GFR (mL/min/1.73 m²)
1	Kidney damage with a normal or increased GFR There must be other evidence of kidney damage: • persistent microalbuminuria • persistent proteinuria • persistent hematuria • structural abnormalities of the kidneys demonstrated • on USS or other radiological tests • biopsy-proven chronic glomerulonephritis	>90
2	Kidney damage with mild reduction in GFR There must be other evidence of kidney damage (as above)	60–89
3	Moderate reduction in GFR	30–59
4	Severe reduction in GFR	15–29
5	Kidney failure	<15 (or dialysis)

There appears to be wide variation in the causes of CKD in different parts of the world. This may reflect geographical differences in the prevalence of the causative diseases which can lead to CKD or different racial susceptibilities to the adverse renal effects of those diseases.

However, the causes of CKD as listed within National Registries are frequently based on clinical assessment without histological examination of the kidney (the 'gold standard'). This can result in misclassification – for example most patients with CKD will be hypertensive, but it would be wrong to conclude that hypertension had caused the CKD without a thorough assessment.

Many patients present late in the course of their disease; a histological diagnosis is either not justified or not technically possible due to small, shrunken kidneys. In such cases the cause of CKD should be listed as 'cause unknown'.

The cause of CKD is unknown in 20–30% of patients starting RRT in the UK.

The increasing prevalence of diabetes means this is now the single commonest cause of CKD in the Western world. In the UK, 19–20% of patients start dialysis as a result of diabetes, and in the USA the rate is nearer 50%.

Pathophysiological changes within the kidney
Most forms of chronic injury to the kidney initiate a series of pathological events which result in the functional unit of the kidney (the nephron) being replaced by scar tissue.

This appears to be a nonspecific response to injury, but as a result renal function is lost resulting in CKD.

The pathological changes within the kidney are characterized by:

Glomerulosclerosis: this is considered the histological hallmark of CKD. It is characterized by expansion of the glomerular mesangium and deposition of extracellular matrix.

Tubulointerstitial fibrosis: there is tubular atrophy, an interstitial inflammatory cell infiltrate and deposition of extracellular matrix within the interstitium. A number of studies have demonstrated that tubulointerstitial disease correlates better with the level of renal function than glomerular disease.

Because of the nonspecific nature of the response the histological changes seen in the end-stage kidney are similar irrespective of the primary cause of the renal injury.

When the process is long-standing and the damage advanced it may be difficult to identify the primary renal disease with certainty.

At the same time the fibrotic process results in a loss of renal cortex and a contraction in the size of the kidneys (Fig. 11.1.1).

Thus in advanced CKD a renal biopsy is rarely indicated since it may be both technically difficult and unlikely to yield information that would be diagnostically or therapeutically useful.

Clinical features
Patients with CKD are frequently asymptomatic until the disease is advanced.

Symptoms related to progressive loss of tubular function may be seen in early CKD. The loss of urinary concentrating ability (lack of response to ADH) results in polyuria which may manifest itself as nocturia in adults or enuresis in children.

However, it is possible for the majority of the kidney's excretory function (GFR) to be lost without the patient experiencing any symptoms.

Symptoms are frequently not seen until CKD 4 and even at that stage they are often nonspecific. They may include:

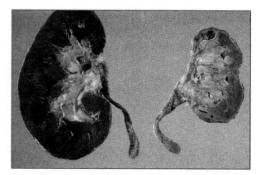

Fig. 11.1.1 Macroscopic section of a normal kidney (left) and a small, shrunken, end-stage kidney (right).

- lethargy and tiredness: at least in part related to renal anemia;
- pruritis: an ill-understood symptom but a cause of significant morbidity to the patient;
- skin pigmentation: a combination of deposition of melanin due to increased melanocyte-stimulating hormone and retained urochromes;
- easy bruising: due to platelet dysfunction;
- generalized aches and pains: a result of disturbed bone and mineral metabolism and secondary hyperparathyroidism;
- loss of appetite and nausea: often associated with a metallic taste;
- vomiting: unusual until CKD is advanced;
- sleep disturbance.

When the GFR is extremely low (<5 mL/min) the patient may develop:

- neurological disturbances (signs of neuropathy, altered conscious level, fitting and coma);
- 'uremic' pericarditis;
- a uremic 'frost' (deposits of urea and urate on the skin, especially around the mucous membranes).

With the routine availability of RRT, the symptoms and signs of preterminal uremia are now rarely seen except in patients being treated conservatively.

Frequently and especially in the early stages of CKD there may be little to find on examination other than hypertension (which is found in the majority of patients with CKD). Some patients will also have signs of salt and water retention (edema, pulmonary edema) or signs relating to any underlying systemic disease which has caused the CKD.

Early detection of CKD

Several types of intervention have been shown to reduce the risk of CVD, decrease the rate of progression of CKD and reduce mortality in CKD. Thus some countries have highlighted the early identification of CKD as a priority (including in the UK by the National Service Framework for Renal Services).

CKD may be detected by simple and readily available tests. These include:

- measurement of blood pressure;
- testing the urine;
- measuring the renal function.

Urine testing

Testing the urine for the presence of:

- protein;
- albumin;
- erythrocytes.

This can be conveniently undertaken on a spot urine sample using a commercially available reagent strip ('dipstick').

Persistent abnormalities provide evidence of kidney damage (although urological causes of hematuria need to be considered and excluded where appropriate).

In routine clinical practice, dipstick testing is a more reliable way of detecting hematuria than urine microscopy because of cell lysis during transport of the sample to the laboratory.

Dipsticks for proteinuria provide semiquantitative information and have limitations due to false-positive results.

Proteinuria is better quantified on a spot (ideally early morning) urine sample by measuring either:

- albumin:creatinine ratio (ACR);
- protein:creatinine ratio (PCR).

ACR and PCR results correlate well with those obtained from 'gold standard' 24 h urine samples.

As the latter are difficult to perform reliably in clinical practice they should not be routinely undertaken.

Table 11.1.2 Situations which may cause the eGFR to be unreliable

When the true GFR is normal	In particular values ≥60 mL/min/1.73 m² should be interpreted with caution
States of reduced muscle mass	Muscle wasting disease states
	Amputees
	Malnourished patients
Where there is an abnormal volume of distribution for creatinine	Edematous states
	Pregnancy (MDRD should not be used to estimate GFR in pregnancy)
At extremes of body size	
At extremes of age	Children require specific formulae (for example the Schwartz equation)
	MDRD underestimates GFR in the elderly
In particular ethnic groups	Formulae have not generally been validated in all ethnic groups
When there is a high or low dietary intake of creatinine or creatine	Ideally blood samples for GFR estimation should be obtained without the person having eaten any meat in the previous 12 h
Technical issues	Appropriate calibrated creatinine assays must be used and blood samples should be processed by the laboratory within 12 h

Measuring renal function

Measurement of GFR is considered the 'gold standard' assessment of kidney function but this is both expensive and complex to perform.

Traditionally, clinicians have relied on serum creatinine to assess renal function.

However, the serum creatinine level depends not only on renal function but also on muscle mass and, for a given level of renal function, serum creatinine will vary according to factors such as age, sex, body mass and ethnic origin since these are surrogate markers of an individual's muscle mass.

GFR may be estimated from the creatinine (eGFR) using a number of different formulae.

For adults the four-variable MDRD formula has been most widely adopted (see Appendix) since it relies only on:

- creatinine;
- age;
- sex.

This allows it to be reported automatically by laboratories when serum creatinine is requested. A correction for black race must be applied manually.

The widespread introduction of automated eGFR reporting has made the true prevalence of CKD readily apparent to clinicians.

It is important to remember that formulaic estimates of GFR do have limitations and may have wide confidence limits (Table 11.1.2). They must therefore be interpreted in the clinical context.

Formal measurement of GFR should only be required where a high degree of accuracy is needed such as for dosing of drugs with a narrow therapeutic window during chemotherapy or in the evaluation of renal function in potential living donors.

Who to screen for chronic kidney disease

Screening the general population for CKD is not justified.

However, targeted investigation of groups at high-risk of CKD does allow the majority of cases to be identified at an early stage and enables timely therapeutic intervention.

The following groups should be tested for CKD:
- patients with hypertension;
- patients with diabetes (types 1 and 2);
- patients with cardiovascular disease (ischemic heart disease, chronic heart failure, peripheral vascular disease and cerebral vascular disease);
- anyone found to have hematuria or proteinuria on an incidental medical examination;
- patients receiving drugs known to be potentially nephrotoxic (NSAIDs for example);
- patients known to have structural renal tract disease, renal calculi or prostatic hypertrophy;
- people with a family history of stage 5 CKD or hereditary kidney disease.

Further investigations

Further investigations should initially be directed at identifying the underlying cause of CKD.

This may require several different biochemical and immunological tests as well as some radiological interventions.

A renal USS is not justified in all patients with CKD but should be undertaken in anyone with:
- CKD stage 4 or 5;
- visible or invisible hematuria;
- symptoms of renal tract obstruction;
- rapidly declining GFR;
- family history of polycystic kidney disease;

In patients with unexplained CKD and a normal renal tract, renal biopsy may be required.

These investigations are discussed in detail elsewhere in this book in the relevant chapters.

Patients with CKD should also be investigated for complications of CKD, principally anemia and renal bone disease.

Epidemiological data suggest that the prevalence of CKD-associated complications increases sharply once GFR declines to <45 mL/min/1.73 m^2.

Therefore such patients should have the following measured:
- hemoglobin to identify anemia – other causes of non-CKD-related anemia should also be considered and excluded where necessary;
- calcium, phosphate and alkaline phosphatase;

- PTH should also be measured in people with CKD 4/5.

The frequency of testing of these parameters should be determined in the light of the initial values, the clinical circumstances and any treatments that are initiated.

Patients with CKD should be investigated for other end-organ damage related to hypertension. This may include an ECG and echocardiography looking for evidence of LV hypertrophy.

In addition, because of the high risk of death from CVD it is essential to fully assess cardiovascular risk factors (including lipids) in patients with CKD. However, it is important to recognize that cardiovascular risk tables significantly underestimate risk of death from CVD in people with CKD.

Other complications of CKD which may require further specific investigation include malnutrition and neuropathy.

Progression of CKD

CKD is a potentially progressive disease.

Experimental studies and observational data in humans suggest that CKD may progress as a result of both:
- ongoing injury from the primary renal insult;
- a maladaptive response that is initiated within the kidney following a renal injury.

Once a critical reduction in renal mass has occurred it appears that CKD progresses inexorably even if the initiating insult has resolved. This has led to the concept that a 'maladaptive' response occurs within the kidney which in turn leads to further damage (Fig. 11.1.2). There is a large body of experimental work which has examined potential maladaptive responses. Suggested mechanisms include:

Hemodynamic factors:
- systemic hypertension;
- intraglomerular hypertension.

Nonhemodynamic factors:
- proteinuria;
- hyperlipidemia;
- glomerular hypertrophy;
- mesangial cell activation and proliferation;
- biologically active infiltrating cells;
- production of prosclerotic cytokines and growth factors.

The extent to which any of these factors contributes to the progression of CKD in humans is unknown.

Observational studies suggest that whereas some patients with CKD experience a linear and predictable decline in renal function with time, others (possibly the majority) may have extended periods during which their renal function is completely stable but which are punctuated by sudden and stepwise decrements in renal function.

Longitudinal studies suggest that renal function declines with age. Whether this is part of the natural aging process (and therefore should be considered normal) or a pathological condition remains controversial. Such studies have generally included those at risk of CKD (diabetes, hypertension) and therefore the findings of an age-related decline in renal function may reflect unrecognized CKD in an aging population with comorbidity. Studies of people without comorbidities generally support the view that renal function declines only very slowly with age and that

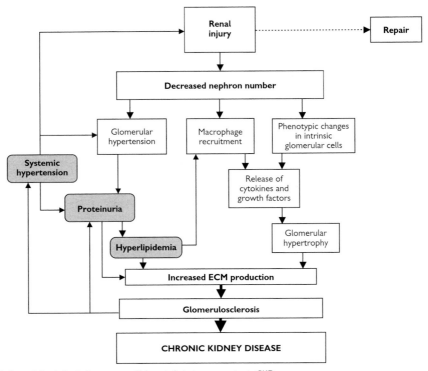

Fig. 11.1.2 Potential 'maladaptive' responses which contribute to progression in CKD.

GFR can remain normal into the 9th decade of life. Hence age alone is not a justification for dismissing the finding of CKD as unimportant.

The K/DOQI classification defines CKD at a given point in time. Clinically it is more useful to understand how CKD is progressing with time in order to focus efforts on those in whom a rate of decline of GFR would lead either to complications of CKD or to the need for RRT within their lifetimes This requires repeated measurement of renal function and for the results to be interpreted in the clinical context of the individual patient. For example, young patients with CKD 4 progressing at a slow rate may be at greater risk of requiring RRT within their lifetimes than elderly patients with CKD 2 progressing at the same or an even faster rate.

What constitutes progression of CKD is controversial.

NICE has recently suggested that progression of CKD should be defined as a decline in GFR of:

- >5 mL/min/1.73 m^2 within 1 year

or

- >10 mL/min/1.73 m^2 within 5 years in the absence of other causes of an alternative acute deterioration in renal function.

Progression of CKD is more likely when the following risk factors are present:

- cardiovascular disease;
- proteinuria;
- hypertension;
- diabetes;
- smoking;
- Afro-Caribbean or South East Asian.

Assessment of proteinuria
Either urinary protein or albumin excretion must be quantified in patients with CKD.

The level that constitutes 'significant proteinuria' and hence would trigger further intervention is debated but typically guidelines suggest a total protein excretion of 1 g/24 h (equivalent to a PCR of 100 mg/mmol or ACR of 70 mg/mmol) in non diabetic CKD, although NICE has recently proposed a lower protein excretion threshold of 0.5 g/24 h.

In diabetics, microalbuminuria (ACR ≥2.5 mg/mmol in men and ACR ≥3.5 mg/mmol in women) is an indication for the use of ACEIs or ARBs.

Treatment
The specific goals of treatment in CKD should be to:

- minimize the risk of any additional renal injury (in particular nephrotoxic drugs should be avoided);
- reduce the risk of death from CVD;
- reduce the rate of progression;
- manage the complications of CKD.

Cardiovascular disease
It is important to remember that at any stage of CKD the risk of premature cardiovascular death is far greater than the risk of progression.

For patients with CKD 3, the 5 year risk of progressing to require RRT has been estimated to be only 1% compared to a 25% risk of dying.

Many of the primary and secondary prevention studies in CVD excluded patients with CKD so the evidence base is generally poor.

However, the principles of prevention and management of CVD in people with early CKD should not be different from those employed in people without CKD and should include where appropriate:

- lifestyle measures;
- blood pressure control;
- lipid lowering;
- antiplatelet agents.

In more advanced CKD the underlying vascular pathology includes arterial medial calcification as well as atherosclerosis.

This may not respond to the modification of traditional risk factors (one prospective randomized trial in diabetic HD patients failed to show any survival benefit from statins).

In advanced CKD cardiovascular death is associated with abnormalities in markers of bone and mineral metabolism.

Although there is speculation of a potential benefit from treatments aimed at normalizng these abnormalities, there are no interventional studies available to demonstrate an improved clinical outcome from such intervention.

Reducing the rate of progression
Treatments which are important in preventing CVD have many similarities with those that should be used in preventing progression of CKD, and can be used to provide a straightforward health educational message to patients (Table 11.1.3).

In general there is also considerable overlap in management protocols for CKD, diabetes and CVD, and given that these commonly coexist in the same patient there is a strong argument for managing such patients as part of a chronic 'vascular risk' management program.

Treat the primary disease
Where possible, treatment aimed at the underlying primary disease should be instituted to minimize any subsequent or ongoing damage to the kidney.

Many renal diseases have no specific treatments, but examples include:

- optimal control of the blood sugar in diabetics has been shown to delay the onset of CKD and delay any subsequent progression that might otherwise have occurred;
- immunosuppression has been shown to delay progression of a small number of immunologically mediated renal diseases;
- prevention of urinary tract sepsis in children with reflux nephropathy.

Treat factors involved in any maladaptive renal response
Treatments aimed at minimizing ongoing renal damage from any maladaptive response that has occurred should be considered.

Such treatments are nonspecific but have proved highly effective in reducing the rate of progression in a number of controlled clinical trials.

Table 11.1.3 Key educational messages for patients and healthcare professionals for the management of CVD and CKD

Lifestyle advice	Stop smoking
	Exercise
	Weight management
	Healthy diet
Review medications	Avoid nephrotoxic agents (e.g. NSAIDs)
Treat diabetes (if present)	According to best practice guidelines
Treat hypertension	According to best practice guidelines Suggest patients buy their own BP meter Threshold for treatment is 140/90 mmHg Target BP is: 130/80 mmHg 125/75 mmHg if PCR >100 mg/mmol ACEIs or ARBs are first-line agents in proteinuric CKD
Treat hyperlipidemia	According to best practice guidelines for primary and secondary prevention
Antiplatelet agents (aspirin)	For secondary prevention
Vaccinations	According to local guidelines (for example annual influenza and pneumococcal vaccinations)

For patients these messages should be supported by information leaflets and there should ideally be a dedicated educational programme about CKD.

Treatments that may be effective in delaying progression include:

- treatment of hypertension;
- inhibition of the renin angiotensin system;
- dietary protein restriction;

Treatment of systemic hypertension in CKD can effectively reduce the rate of progression. The ideal target blood pressure is debated but suggested targets are:

- 130/80 mmHg for patients without proteinuria;
- 125/75 mmHg for those with proteinuria.

ACEIs and ARBs reduce the rate of progression of CKD in diabetic nephropathy and proteinuric CKD of any cause over and above what might have been expected from blood pressure control alone. Their mechanism of action may include reducing intraglomerular hypertension and proteinuria. ACEIs and ARBs are being used in combination in patients with proteinuric CKD to attempt to augment any antiproteinuric effect. There is some evidence to support this approach but the risk of side-effects (especially hyperkalemia) may be greater, requiring more intense monitoring.

The effect of low protein diets on the progression of CKD has been extensively studied with variable results. Such diets are difficult to maintain and if not properly monitored are associated with the risk of protein-calorie malnutrition which carries a poor prognosis in patients starting RRT. With the benefits obtained from lower BP targets and the use of ACEIs and ARBs, many nephrologists no longer routinely prescribe such diets for patients with CKD, although their use may be justified in a highly motivated patient with advanced CKD, as long as they are supervised by a dietician.

There is some evidence that statins can reduce the level of proteinuria in patients with proteinuric CKD, but their effect on progression is unknown.

Managing the complications of CKD

Treatments for specific CKD-associated complications (anemia, bone disease) are dealt with in other chapters of this book.

Follow-up

CKD is a potentially progressive disease associated with a number of significant complications and accelerated CVD. It is thus essential that any patient with CKD is monitored both for evidence of progression and for the development of complications.

The frequency with which monitoring is required and the type of monitoring needed is dependent on:

- stage of CKD;
- rate of progression;
- any risk factors for CVD or progression of CKD.

Thus it is important that patients receive an individualized plan for follow-up which is appropriate to their needs.

Patients at high risk of progression (those with proteinuria or difficult-to-control hypertension and those who have already demonstrated they are progressing) generally require more frequent monitoring than those without such risk factors.

Many health economies have devised guidelines to aid health professionals in their ongoing monitoring and assessment of patients with CKD. In order to improve their day-to-day utility, such guidelines have often been summarized into simple flow charts, e.g. Fig. 11.1.3.

However, it is important to stress that such guidelines provide an idealized overview of the optimal long-term management of a population with CKD. They were not designed to replace a careful clinical risk assessment of an individual patient, nor the development of an appropriate ongoing management plan for that patient.

Referral to specialist care

The majority of patients with CKD do not need follow-up by a renal specialist and can be appropriately managed by generalists in primary care according to locally agreed principles and guidelines (see Fig. 11.1.3 for a typical example).

Referral to a specialist may add value in the following settings.

To establish a diagnosis and agree a management plan in a patient with suspected CKD of any stage

This will include the identification and advice on control of risk factors for progression of CKD.

The majority of such patients do not need long-term specialist follow-up as the plan can frequently be implemented and the patient followed in primary care.

Any circumstances where by re-referral would be appropriate should be made explicit.

The treatment of complex kidney disease

Specialist expertise and the required monitoring will not be available in primary care.

For instance, this would include the treatment and ongoing monitoring of complex glomerular disease.

To allow timely planning for RRT

This will be necessary for all patients progressing to ESRD despite optimal treatment, since this has been shown to improve patient outcomes.

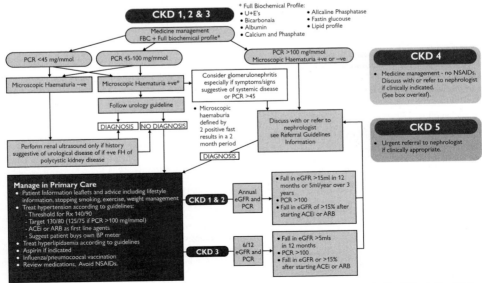

Fig. 11.1.3 Principles for the assessment, management and referral of adults with CKD. (Redrawn from the East Midlands Renal Network, http://www.emrn.org.uk/.)

In some cases specialist advice can appropriately be obtained using a 'virtual consultation' (letter or telephone discussion) without he need for the patient to visit the hospital.

Ideally specialist nephrology services should support primary care by providing 24 h telephone access to qualified advice.

Based on the principles outlined above, NICE has recently suggested that the following groups of patients may benefit from specialist advice.

Group 1

Those in whom it is likely to be useful to establish a diagnosis and in whom specialist treatment and monitoring may be required:

- proteinuria ≥1 g/24 h unless explained by diabetes (PCR ≥100 mg/mmol or ACR ≥70 mg/mmol);
- proteinuria ≥ 0.5 g/24 h and hematuria (PCR ≥50 mg/mmol or ACR ≥30 mg/mmol);
- suspected rare or genetic causes of CKD;
- suspected renal artery stenosis (suggested by a fall in GFR of >25% on initiating ACEI or ARB);
- hypertension that remains poorly controlled despite the use of at least four antihypertensive drugs at therapeutic doses.

Group2

Those at high risk of needing RRT in the near future:

- patients with CKD 4 and 5;
- patients with a rapidly declining eGFR
  - (>5 mL/min/1.73 m^2 in ≤1 year)
  - (>10 mL/min/1.73 m^2 over ≤5 years).

The importance of referral to allow timely planning and preparation for RRT (including pre-emptive transplantation) is well-accepted and was highlighted in the standards laid out in Part 1 of the National Service Framework for Renal Services.

Late referral of patients with advanced CKD is known to be associated with increased morbidity and mortality, increased length of hospital stay, and increased costs.

The lack of time to prepare patients referred late for dialysis, particularly the establishment of permanent vascular access for hemodialysis, appears to be the dominant factor in the adverse outcomes, but untreated anemia, bone disease, hypertension and acidosis may also contribute.

Palliative and supportive care

It is now recognized that not all patients with advanced CKD will necessarily benefit from RRT, especially when quality-of-life issues are considered.

Active conservative management of advanced CKD may allow the patient to maintain a good quality of life for several months, which may be preferable to multiple admissions to hospital as part of establishing RRT.

Some patients already on RRT but who develop intolerable symptoms from worsening comorbidities may also wish to withdraw from RRT.

End-of-life care is now recognized as part of the much wider area of (noncancer-related) palliative care and supportive care for people living, sometimes for years, with life-threatening conditions including CKD.

It is an active treatment option and requires multidisciplinary and multiagency input to be successful.

In the UK a Gold Standards Supportive Care Register has been developed on which a number of patients with CKD should be included in order to allow them to receive the most appropriate supportive care.

Inclusion on the register should be considered if any of the following apply:

- those with CKD 5 or frail individuals with CKD 4;
- those thought by the care team to be in the last year of life;
- those choosing conservative treatment (no RRT) or those discontinuing dialysis or opting not to restart dialysis if their transplant is failing;
- those with difficult physical symptoms (e.g. anorexia, nausea, pruritus, reduced function status, intractable fluid overload) or psychological symptoms despite optimal therapy.

Further reading

Royal College of Physicians and the Renal Association. Chronic Kidney Disease in Adults: UK Guidelines for Identification, Management and Referral. 2006 (http://www.renal.org/CKDguide/full/UKCKDfull.pdf).

NICE. Chronic Kidney Disease. National clinical guideline for the management of adults with chronic kidney disease in primary and secondary care (draft for consultation 2008). (http://www.nice.org.uk/guidance/index.jsp?action=folder&o=39905).

UK Department of Health. The National Service Framework for Renal Services. Part one: Dialysis and Transplantation; 2004. (http://www.dh.gov.uk/en/Publicationsandstatistics/Publications/PublicationsPolicyAndGuidance/DH_4070359).

UK Department of Health: The National Service Framework for Renal Services Part Two: Chronic Kidney Disease, Acute Renal Failure and End of Life Care; 2005. (http://www.dh.gov.uk/en/Publicationsandstatistics/Publications/PublicationsPolicyAndGuidance/DH_4101902).

Internet resources

East Midlands Renal Network:

http://www.emrn.org.uk

European Best Practice Group Guidelines of the ERA-EDTA:

http://www.ndt-educational.org/

National Kidney Foundation Kidney Disease Outcomes Quality Initiative (NKF KDOQI):

http://www.kidney.org/professionals/kdoqi/index.cfm

National Institute for Health and Clinical Excellence:

http://www.nice.org.uk

UK Renal Association:

http://www.renal.org/

UK Renal Registry:

http://www.renalreg.com/

See also

CKD in the elderly, p. 468

Dialysis strategies, p. 480

Hematological disorders in CKD, p. 426

Skeletal disorders in CKD, p. 432

Vascular access, p. 488

Endocrine disorders in chronic kidney disease

Introduction

Chronic kidney disease (CKD), including end-stage renal disease (ESRD), has major effects on the endocrine system. The failing kidney is associated with alterations of the production, transport, metabolism, elimination and protein binding of hormones. This may result in increased (most commonly seen in CKD), unchanged or decreased circulating hormone levels as summarized in Table 11.2.1. In addition, there may be decreased sensitivity to hormones, as a result of an altered target response (e.g. insulin). Therefore, the final effect of a particular hormone on its target may not necessarily reflect its circulating level.

Mechanisms of endocrine dysfunction in CKD

Increased circulating hormone levels

This may result from a number of processes.

Decreased GFR resulting in impaired renal clearance:

- prolactin;
- insulin;
- glucagons;
- calcitonin;
- leptin.

Increased secretion:

- parathyroid hormone (PTH).

Accumulation of inactive metabolites which may crossreact with a defined hormonal assay, thus artificially increasing the measured circulating level:

- PTH;
- calcitonin;
- prolactin.

Decreased sensitivity to hormones

Altered target response:

- insulin;
- growth hormone;
- PTH;
- erythropoietin;
- 1,25-$(OH)_2$ vitamin D3.

Decreased circulating hormone levels

Decreased secretion by the diseased kidney:

- 1,25-$(OH)_2$ vitamin D3;
- erythropoietin.

Decreased secretion by other endocrine glands:

- testosterone;
- estrogen;
- progesterone.

Thyroid hormones

A number of abnormalities in thyroid hormones have been described in CKD and ESRD.

Total and free thyroxine (T4) concentrations are either decreased or normal.

Total and free triiodothyronine (T3) concentrations are decreased.

There are subtle abnormalities in the hypothalamic–hypophyseal axis including:

- normal thyroid-stimulating hormone (TSH) despite low thyroid hormone levels (inappropriate TSH response to decreased levels due to a reset in the feedback loop to a lower TSH level for a given level of thyroid hormone);
- absence of the usual nocturnal TSH surge;
- blunted TSH response to thyrotropin-releasing hormone (TRH) administration (corrected by recombinant EPO);
- TSH administration results in an increase in T3, but in a blunted response in T4 (not corrected by recombinant EPO).

Significance of thyroid axis abnormalities in CKD

Despite these biochemical abnormalities, clinical thyroid disease is not common in CKD and ESRD.

Levels of T4 and T3 may be low without clinical hypothyroidism.

Despite the described biochemical abnormalities the TSH concentration in plasma remains a good indicator of hypo- and hyperthyroidism in CKD.

Abnormal thyroid function tests normalize after successful kidney transplantation.

Growth hormone

Plasma GH levels are increased because of:

- increased secretion;
- impaired clearance.

Sensitivity to GH is decreased.

Insulin-like growth factor-1 (IGF-1) levels are normal.

Significance of growth hormone abnormalities in CKD

Children

Growth retardation despite elevated GH and normal IGF-1.

Other factors may contribute to growth retardation in this setting including:

- protein wasting;
- metabolic acidosis;
- hyperparathyroidism;
- recurrent infections.

Recombinant human growth hormone (rHGH) can restore growth velocity and increases muscle mass without affecting epiphyseal closure and glucose tolerance.

Adults

The role of GH in general adult health remains unclear and therefore it has proved difficult to determine the clinical consequences of GH dysregulation in CKD and ESRD.

Preliminary results of small clinical trials have shown that rHGH may be useful in improving muscle wasting, a common feature in patients on hemodialysis. Further data are awaited from large randomized controlled clinical trials.

Prolactin

Basal levels of prolactin are increased up to six times normal in patients with CKD.

Increased prolactin in CKD is due to a decrease in prolactin inhibitory factor (PIF), which in turn is the consequence of a decrease in dopaminergic activity.

Significance of increased prolactin levels in CKD

Hyperprolactinemia may be associated with:

- amenorrhea;
- impotence;
- gynecomastia.

Table 11.2.1 Changes in hormone concentrations in CKD

Hormonal system	Changes in CKD
Hypothalamo-pituitary axis	Growth hormone ↑
	Prolactin ↑
Thyroid axis	Free T3 ↓
	Free T4 normal or ↓
	TSH normal
Gonads	Testosterone ↓
	Oestrogen normal or ↓
	Progesterone ↓
	LH normal or ↑
	FSH normal
Pancreas	Insulin ↑
	Glucagon ↑
Adrenal glands	Aldosterone normal or ↓ or ↑
	Cortisol normal or ↑
	ACTH normal or ↑
	Catecholamines normal or ↑
Kidneys	Erythropoietin ↓
	Renin ↓
	1,25-$(OH)_2$ vitamin D_3 ↓

Antidopaminergic medications may aggravate hyperprolactinemia in CKD, and should be avoided where possible. These include:

- α-methyldopa;
- neuroleptics;
- metoclopramide;
- cimetidine.

Treatment of hyperprolactinemia

Bromocriptine reduces prolactin levels but may not correct symptoms of hyperprolactinemia. Side-effects (nausea and vomiting) are common in CKD and limit its use.

Recombinant human EPO treatment may normalize prolactin levels and improve impotence in men and menstrual irregularities in women.

Adrenal hormones

Glucocorticoids

Adrenocorticotropic hormone (ACTH) is either normal or elevated.

Basal cortisol levels are normal.

The circadian rhythm of cortisol secretion is unaltered.

Responses of the glucocorticotropic axis in CKD:

- corticotropin-releasing hormone (CRH) induces a normal or blunted ACTH response;
- standard ACTH stimulation test for diagnosing hypoadrenalism is not affected;
- insulin-induced hypoglycemia fails to raise plasma cortisol;
- dexamethasone suppression test to assess hyperadrenalism is blunted;
- a high dose of oral (8 mg) or IV (1 mg) dexamethasone is necessary to suppress the gland because of an altered

set point of the axis and decreased oral absorption of dexamathasone.

Significance of glucocorticoid abnormalities in CKD

Despite these biochemical abnormalities, clinical abnormalities of glucocorticoid function are not common in CKD and ESRD.

The cortisol response to major stress such as surgery is preserved.

Mineralocorticoids

Renin production is low in CKD due to the loss of renal tissue and volume expansion.

Aldosterone levels may be low, normal or elevated.

Because of low renin levels, hyperkalemia may be the major stimulus for aldosterone secretion in CKD.

Significance of mineralocorticoid abnormalities in CKD

Elevated levels of aldosterone in CKD are associated with:

- stimulation of colonic loss of potassium;
- increase in blood pressure;
- stimulation of mesangial and vascular collagen synthesis.

Elevated levels of aldosterone in CKD may play a role in the progression of CKD.

Diagnosis of hyperaldosteronism in CKD is difficult because of the changes in renin and aldosterone that occur with renal failure. Adrenal vein blood sampling and adrenal imaging studies may be required to confirm a diagnosis.

Catecholamines

Catecholamine levels are increased due to:

- decreased degradation;
- decreased neuronal reuptake.

Significance of catecholamine abnormalities in CKD

Increased cathecholamine levels in CKD may contribute to the sympathetic overactivity seen in these patients.

The diagnosis of a pheochromocytoma should be made using total and free plasma metanephrines, as urinary excretion will be reduced or absent in CKD and ESRD.

Insulin and carbohydrate metabolism

Abnormalities of carbohydrate metabolism in CKD include:

- insulin resistance (IR);
- circulating inhibitors of insulin action;
- decreased islet cell insulin secretion.

Peripheral IR is the consequence of a blunted response to a normal insulin level in plasma.

Insulin resistance has been described in patients with preserved renal function and CKD.

As GFR decreases, IR is accompanied by an accumulation of circulating inhibitors of insulin action and a decrease in islet cell insulin release.

Mechanism of insulin resistance in CKD

This has not been fully elucidated.

It is thought to be due to postreceptor abnormalities induced by several factors:

- accumulation of uremic toxins;
- metabolic acidosis;
- lack of vitamin D;
- proinflammatory cytokines;

- other potential contributors such as uric acid, pseudou-ridine, advanced glycation end-products.

Significance of insulin resistance in CKD

Insulin resistance is associated with the development of endothelial dysfunction, an early step in the pathogenesis of atherosclerosis.

The presence of IR correlates with cardiovascular mortality in nondiabetic dialysis patients.

Insulin resistance contributes to muscle catabolism in dialysed patients.

Insulin resistance may also contribute to the progression of CKD via deleterious renal hemodynamic effects.

Assessment of insulin resistance

Insulin resistance is assessed by the HOMA-IR (homeostasis model assessment of insulin resistance).

HOMA-IR calculation:

$$\frac{\text{insulin concentration (}\mu\text{U/ml) } \times \text{ fasting glucose (mmol/L)}}{22.5}$$

Impact of dialysis technique on insulin resistance

Hemodialysis and peritoneal dialysis only partially correct the IR seen in patients with CKD.

PD is associated with higher insulinemia than HD and a more severe IR due to the result of the glucose load absorbed from glucose-based dialysis fluids.

The use of icodextrin and aminoacids as glucose-free peritoneal dialysis fluids reduces IR.

Drugs known to improve insulin resistance

- ACEIs.
- ARBs.
- 25-(OH) vitamin D3.
- Thiazolidinediones.

Adipokines

Adipokines are a group of hormones and cytokines secreted by adipocytes.

The most important adipokines identified to date are leptin and adiponectin.

The known biological actions of leptin include:

- anorexia;
- increased energy expenditure;
- proinflammatory effects;
- proatherogenic effects.

The known biological actions of adiponectin include:

- a potent insulin-sensitizing effect;
- antiatherogenic effects;
- anti-inflammatory effects.

Adipokines in CKD and ESRD

There is marked hyperleptinemia (5–7 times normal in ESRD: PD > HD).

There is moderate hyperadiponectinemia (~2-fold increase in ESRD).

Factors other than renal function modulate the hyperleptinemia and hyperadiponectinemia associated with CKD and include:

- fat mass;
- inflammation;
- hyperinsulinemia;
- acidosis.

The accumulation of adipokines in CKD may directly contribute to the development of CKD and associated complications:

- hyperleptinemia may contribute to protein-energy wasting observed in patients with ESRD;
- hyperleptinemia may worsen the sympathetic overactivity seen in CKD and ESRD;
- hyperleptinemia promotes hypertension.

The role of hyperadiponectinemia in CKD and its complications is unclear and is awaiting further investigation.

Further reading

Axelsson J, Stenvinkel P. Role of fat mass and adipokines in chronic kidney disease. *Curr Opin Nephrol Hypertens* 2008; **17**: 25–31.

Carrero JJ, Qureshi AR, Axelsson J, et al. Clinical and biochemical implications of low thyroid hormone levels (total and free forms) in euthyroid patients with chronic kidney disease. *J Intern Med* 2007; **262**: 690–701.

Feldt-Rasmussen B, Lange M, Sulowicz W, et al.; APCD Study Group. Growth hormone treatment during hemodialysis in a randomized trial improves nutrition, quality of life, and cardiovascular risk. *J Am Soc Nephrol* 2007; **18**: 2161–2171.

Ritz E. Metabolic syndrome and kidney disease. *Blood Purif* 2008; **26**: 59–62.

Seikaly MG, Salhab N, Warady BA, Stablein D. Use of rhGH in children with chronic kidney disease: lessons from NAPRTCS. *Pediatr Nephrol* 2007; **22**: 1195–204.

Internet resources

Insulin Resistance and Pre-Diabetes:

http://diabetes.niddk.nih.gov/dm/pubs/insulin-resistance/

International Committee for Insulin Resistance (ICIR):

http://www.insulinresistance.us/about.php

Growth hormone for children with chronic kidney disease (The Cochrane Collaboration):

http://www.cochrane.org/reviews/en/ab003264.html

Adipocytye.co.uk, a website devoted to the adipocyte and adipokines:

http://adipocyte.co.uk/Adiposetissuepeptides.htm

See also

Sexual disorders in CKD, p. 402

Hypertension in CKD, p. 406

Cardiovascular risk factors in CKD, p. 412

CKD in diabetic patients, p. 472

Sexual disorders in chronic kidney disease

Introduction

Sexual dysfunction is a common problem in patients with chronic kidney disease (CKD) both in males and in females. The pathophysiology of these disorders is primarily organic in origin. Many factors contribute including:

- hormone abnormalities;
- peripheral vascular disease;
- peripheral neuropathy;
- autonomic dysfunction;
- drug therapy;
- psychological factors associated with CKD and its treatment.

Sexual dysfunction in males

Clinical features include:

- loss of libido;
- impotence;
- testicular atrophy;
- gynecomastia;
- infertility.

Hormonal abnormalities

Testosterone is decreased, indicating peripheral testicular failure.

Luteinizing hormone (LH) is increased.

Follicle-stimulating hormone (FSH) is increased.

Response to LH-releasing hormone (LHRH) is unpredictable (blunted, normal or exaggerated), indicating central hypothalamic abnormalities.

Hyperprolactinemia and hyperparathyroidism may also contribute (see below).

Factors involved in the pathogenesis of impotence

Gonadal dysfunction:

- decreased production of testosterone;
- hypothalamic–pituitary function;
  - blunted increase in serum LH levels;
  - decreased amplitude of LH secretory burst;
  - variable increase in serum FSH levels;
  - increased prolactin levels.

Psychological factors related to CKD.

Zinc deficiency.

Medications.

Anemia.

Secondary hyperparathyroidism.

Impaired arterial inflow and venous drainage of the penis.

Autonomic neuropathy.

Treatment of impotence

Stop β-blockers.

Start sildenafil or analogues.

Consider an erythropoesis-stimulating agent: reduces hyperprolactinemia and hyperparathyroidism, but has no effect on plasma testosterone. May alleviate the impact of lack of energy and fatigue on impotence.

In some cases: cavernous injections may be tried; should be used with caution in hypertensive patients (vasoconstrictor effect).

In nonresponders, vacuum erector devices or penile implants may be used.

Psychological interventions may also be useful.

An approach to sexual dysfunction in the male patient is summarized in Fig. 11.3.1.

Sexual dysfunction in females

Clinical features include:

- loss of libido;
- irregularity of menstrual cycle;
- amenorrhea;
- anovulation;
- sterility.

<10% of women with ESRD on dialysis have regular menses.

Hormone abnormalities

Estradiol levels are normal to low.

Estrone levels are normal to low.

Progesterone levels are normal to low.

Testosterone levels are normal to low.

FSH is normal.

LH is mildly elevated.

Increased LH:FSH ratio similar to that seen in prepuberty.

Impaired positive hypothalamic feedback in response to estrogens.

No mid-cycle surge of LH and FSH, resulting in no ovulation.

Treatment of sexual dysfunction

Much less is known about the factors contributing to sexual dysfunction in women with CKD and therefore treatments are lacking.

There is some evidence in the non-CKD population that sildenafil may be useful for the treatment of female sexual dysfunction although there is no evidence in the CKD population.

There may be a role for psychological interventions in some women.

Pregnancy in CKD

Female patients with ESRD on dialysis may occasionally become pregnant.

Residual renal function may improve the likelihood of pregnancy.

Daily dialysis may improve both the likelihood of pregnancy and the maternal and fetal outcomes once pregnancy has occurred.

Impact of renal transplantation

Rapidly restores fertility in pre-menopausal women.

Ovulation usually starts within a month of transplantation.

Stable graft function, adequate control of blood pressure and minimal immunosuppression are advised before conception is considered, i.e. a waiting time of ~2 years after transplantation is usual.

Data on the effectiveness of contraceptive agents in this setting are lacking.

An approach to sexual dysfunction in the female patient is summarized in Fig. 11.3.2.

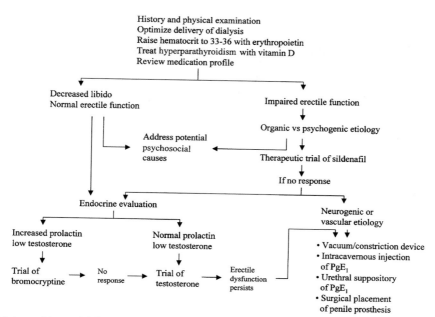

Fig. 11.3.1 Approach to sexual dysfunction in the male patient with CKD. (Reproduced with permission from Palmer, 1999.)

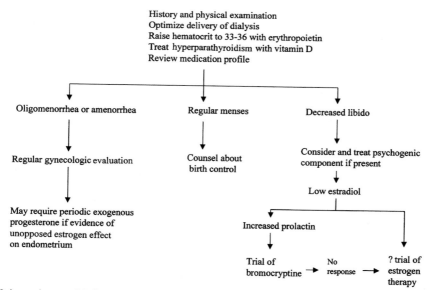

Fig. 11.3.2 Approach to sexual dysfunction in women with CKD. (Reproduced with permission from Palmer, 1999.)

Further reading

Bellinghieri G, Santoro D, Lo Forti B, *et al.* Erectile dysfunction in uremic dialysis patients: diagnostic evaluation in the sildenafil era. *Am J Kidney Dis* 2001; **38**(4 Suppl 1): S115–117.

Bellinghieri G, Savica V, Santoro D. Vascular erectile dysfunction in chronic renal failure. *Semin Nephrol* 2006; **26**: 42–45.

Finkelstein FO, Shirani S, Wuerth D, Finkelstein SH. Therapy insight: sexual dysfunction in patients with chronic kidney disease. *Nat Clin Pract Nephrol* 2007; **3**: 200–207.

Lai CF, Wang YT, Hung KY, *et al.* Sexual dysfunction in peritoneal dialysis patients. *Am J Nephrol* 2007; **27**: 615–621.

Palmer BF. Sexual dysfunction in uremia. *J Am Soc Nephrol* 1999; **10**: 1381–1388.

Internet resources

Clinical trials website listing trials in sexual dysfunction:

http://clinicaltrials.gov/

Erectile dysfunction:

http://kidney.niddk.nih.gov/kudiseases/pubs/impotence/index.htm

Sexuality and the renal patient:

http://aakp.org/newsletters/KB-The-Magazine/Feature-Story/Sexuality/

Sex problems with renal failure:

http://www.kidney.org.uk/Medical-Info/sex-problems/index.html

See also

Endocrine disorders in CKD, p. 398

Psychological aspects of treatment for renal failure, p. 538

Hypertension in chronic kidney disease

Introduction

Hypertension (HTN) is frequent in all types of primary kidney disease, and is nearly universally present in patients with advanced CKD. All types of HTN, even those due to 'nonrenal' causes such as endocrine HTN, involve alterations in the way the kidney handles salt and water.

Hypertension is a major risk factor for progression of most types of CKD, so untreated HTN leads to a 'vicious cycle' resulting in progressive worsening of excretory kidney function and rising blood pressure (BP). However, excretory kidney function is partly dependent on the pressure perfusing the glomeruli, so reduction of BP can also cause deterioration of kidney function.

Clinicians treating patients with kidney disease and HTN therefore need some understanding of the pathophysiology of these conditions.

Autoregulation of renal blood flow

The kidneys have extensive capacity to autoregulate in response to changes in systemic arterial pressure.

In healthy people GFR is independent of BP over a wide range.

This autoregulatory range is reduced in CKD and in severe congestive cardiac failure, so that GFR becomes pressure dependent (Fig. 11.4.1).

Diagnosis

The diagnosis of HTN depends on repeated, careful measurements of resting BP.

Blood pressure should be measured according to British Hypertension Society standards:
- patient seated for ≥5 min;
- free from caffeine and nicotine for the preceding 30 min;
- arm supported at heart level;
- appropriate-sized cuff;
- two measurements a few minutes apart;
- further measurements until two measurements within 5 mmHg of each other are obtained.

NICE recommends that HTN is diagnosed when:
- clinic or surgery systolic BP (SBP) >140 mmHg or diastolic BP (DBP) >90 mmHg;
- confirmed on two further occasions.

HTN should not be diagnosed on the basis of a single BP measurement.

Epidemiology

Hypertension is extremely common in patients with CKD.

83% of 1795 patients screened for the Modification of Diet in Renal Disease study were hypertensive, and the frequency of HTN increased with reducing glomerular filtration rate (GFR).

Hypertension is very common among patients on dialysis and frequently persists after kidney transplantation, partly due to the effects of calcineurin inhibitors on BP regulation.

Cause or effect?

Although HTN is a common consequence of renal injury, it is also a major risk factor for progressive kidney damage, and the kidney is therefore both 'villain and victim' in HTN.

Whether 'essential' HTN (defined as HTN in the absence of 'primary' kidney disease) can cause significant kidney damage has been controversial, largely because most large-scale long-term studies (with 20 year follow-up, at least, being necessary to answer this question) have not included exhaustive tests to exclude primary renal disease at baseline.

The histological entity of 'hypertensive nephroangiosclerosis' is well defined (having first been described in wedge biopsies of patients undergoing surgical lumbar sympathectomy as the only treatment then available for HTN) and is distinct from other forms of renal injury such as glomerulonephritis – although of course the two conditions can, and often do, coexist.

It is also probable that chronic atheromatous embolism (resulting from ulcerated atheromatous plaques in the renal arteries or upstream aorta) contributes to the parenchymal damage seen in patients with CKD and HTN.

The association of HTN with a higher risk of progressive loss of GFR among individuals with CKD does not, however, prove causality.

It is possible, for instance, that both HTN and progression are determined by the nature of the underlying kidney disease.

Proof that the association is causal comes from numerous studies demonstrating that antihypertensive treatment reduces the rate of progression of most types of kidney disease, with the possible exception of polycystic kidney disease.

Types of kidney disease causing hypertension

Hypertension is a frequent feature of all types of parenchymal kidney disease.

Normal BP in the presence of reduced GFR suggests coincident heart failure, but can occur in salt-wasting types of kidney disease (e.g. after relief of bilateral urinary tract obstruction).

Renal artery stenosis is an important treatable cause of HTN, and is not necessarily associated with a reduction of GFR.

A so-called 'Page kidney' is caused by encasement of a kidney by scar tissue, for instance after trauma; release of the scar tissue can cure the HTN.

Chronic high pressure retention of urine is also an important treatable cause of HTN.

Etiology

The major contributors to HTN in CKD are:
- increased activity of the renin–angiotensin system (RAS);
- increased peripheral sympathetic nervous system (SNS) activity;
- expansion of extracellular volume.

RAS overactivity is seen in renal artery stenosis, but also in many types of parenchymal kidney disease.

SNS overactivity has been demonstrated in ESRD, and appears to be caused by an afferent signal arising in

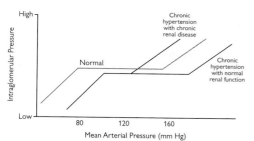

Fig. 11.4.1 Relationship between mean arterial pressure and intraglomerular pressure in health and chronic kidney disease.

diseased kidneys; no increased traffic is seen in patients who have undergone bilateral nephrectomy, and the activity is reduced by ACEIs.

Other endocrine effects

A number of changes in intrarenal and systemic vasoactive mediators have all been implicated in HTN in the presence of kidney disease:

• increased production of endothelin;
• reduced production of medullolipin (a vasodilator lipid produced in the renal medulla);
• reduced renal or systemic synthesis of nitric oxide (possibly due to accumulation of asymmetric dimethylarginine, an inhibitor of nitric oxide synthase);
• deficient production of renalase, a circulating monoamine oxidase that catabolizes circulating catecholamines.

Secondary hyperparathyroidism and sleep apnea (common in advanced CKD) may also contribute.

Salt sensitivity

Humans and experimental animals vary in their response to altered salt intake, with 'salt-sensitive' and 'salt-resistant' phenotypes.

By definition, higher salt intake causes more of a rise in BP in salt-sensitive than in salt-resistant individuals.

In general, salt-sensitive HTN is more common in people of Black race and in older people, but is also common in CKD.

Salt-sensitive HTN responds to restriction of dietary salt intake and to diuretic treatment, both of which are therefore important in the treatment of HTN in CKD.

Salt sensitivity is associated with renal microvascular changes causing local ischemic damage.

Risk factors for the development of salt-sensitive HTN include:

• low birth weight (associated with reduced nephron number);
• Black race;
• obesity;
• insulin resistance;
• hyperuricemia;
• low-level lead intoxication.

Crosstransplantation experiments and observations

Evidence that the kidneys themselves are major contributors to HTN comes from a variety of sources.

Transplantation of kidneys from hypertension-prone strains of rat causes the recipient to have higher BP than transplantation of kidneys from normotensive strains.

Similarly, transplantation of kidneys from human donors with a history of HTN is associated with higher post-transplant BP in the recipient than transplantation of kidneys from normotensive donors.

Hypertension complicating correction of anemia

Rapid correction of longstanding renal anemia can cause severe HTN (and hypertensive encephalopathy), particularly in patients with pre-existing HTN.

This may be caused by:

• increases in blood viscosity;
• extracellular volume expansion;
• persistence of raised cardiac output;
• direct effect of erythropoiesis-stimulating agents on peripheral vascular tone;

Glomerular hyperfiltration in proteinuric CKD

Intraglomerular pressure, and single nephron GFR, are both increased in many types of kidney disease, including diabetic nephropathy.

These changes, together with glomerular hypertrophy, are also seen after experimental reduction in nephron number, and are maladaptive, leading eventually to glomerulosclerosis and further loss of functioning nephrons.

The increased glomerular pressure causes an increase in proteinuria, which causes tubular damage and further contributes to nephron loss.

The degree of proteinuria is an accurate predictor of the risk of progression of CKD.

Reduction of urine protein excretion is an important therapeutic target in CKD.

Drugs that selectively decrease intraglomerular pressure, such as ACEIs and ARBs, also reduce proteinuria.

These drugs may also have other beneficial effects, for instance on glomerular hypertrophy and fibrosis.

Drugs that increase intraglomerular pressure, such as dihydropyridine calcium channel antagonists, often increase proteinuria.

Reduction of glomerular HTN also reduces glomerular hyperfiltration, and treatment with ACEIs and ARBs can be expected to cause a reduction in GFR of up to 30% in proteinuric patients.

Short-term treatment-induced reduction of GFR has been shown to be associated with long-term stability of GFR among proteinuric patients.

Arterial hypertension as a treatable risk factor for progressive kidney disease

Patients with kidney disease have more to gain from adequate treatment of HTN, both because they are at increased risk of cardiovascular disease and because of the risk of progressive loss of GFR.

Patients with proteinuria are more at risk of progression, and have more to gain (in terms of prevention of progression) from BP reduction.

Treatment thresholds and targets

Current UK guidelines state that the threshold for initiation of treatment, and the target BP, should be lower in the presence of proteinuria (defined as a random urine PCR of ≥100 mg/mmol/L).

No proteinuria:
- threshold ≥140/90 mmHg
- target <130/80 mmHg.

With proteinuria:
- threshold ≥130/80 mmHg
- target <125/75 mmHg.

These guidelines (along with all other guidelines on BP) can be difficult to implement because current antihypertensive therapy does not allow the clinician to manipulate SBP and DBP separately.

Pulse pressure (SBP minus DBP) rises as a consequence of reduced compliance of conduit vessels, which is common in kidney disease and aging.

For patients with high pulse pressures, it is reasonable to titrate treatment against mean arterial blood pressure (MAP), as was done in the trials on which these recommendations were based.

MAP = diastolic + 1/3 pulse pressure.

For example, the MAP is ~92 at 125/75 but also at 146/65, 156/60, 166/55, and 176/50.

Importance of salt restriction
Hypertension in the presence of established kidney disease is nearly always salt-sensitive, and restriction of dietary intake of sodium chloride is therefore important.

Sodium bicarbonate does not have the same effect on extracellular volume or BP as sodium chloride, and so can be used in the treatment of acidosis in CKD without compromising BP control.

Restriction of salt intake is particularly important in the presence of proteinuria: a high salt intake completely abrogates the antiproteinuric effect of ACEIs.

Salt intake can be assessed by measurement of 24 h urinary sodium excretion. Intakes of >300 mmol/24 h are common in the UK but intakes of <100 mmol/24 h can be achieved by dietary modification, although many find this very difficult to accomplish.

Choice of antihypertensive drug treatment
The choice of which drug to use is far less important than the BP reduction achieved.

A combination of drugs is nearly always required to achieve perfect BP control.

The effect of antihypertensive drugs on intraglomerular pressure (a measure of the extent to which systemic pressure is transmitted to the glomerulus) varies.

ACEIs and ARBs decrease intraglomerular pressure, whereas dihydropyridine calcium channel blockers increase it.

Reduction of proteinuria, and prevention of progressive kidney damage, is associated with reduction in intraglomerular pressure, so ACEIs and ARBs are the drugs of first choice, particularly if the systemic BP remains above target.

If compliance with dietary salt restriction is poor, diuretic therapy can also augment the antiproteinuric effect of RAS inhibition.

It is widely stated, without good evidence, that thiazide diuretics are ineffective in advanced CKD. These drugs have the advantage of promoting potassium excretion, which can be useful in advanced CKD, particularly when ACEIs or ARBs are used.

Renal artery stenosis
Reduction in renal perfusion caused by stenosis of the renal artery results in increased renin release from the underperfused kidney, which causes systemic HTN.

If the other kidney has a normal arterial supply, pressure-natriuresis occurs, causing volume contraction.

This can occasionally cause the 'hyponatremic hypertensive syndrome', a type of hyponatremia caused by hypovolemia-induced secretion of antidiuretic hormone.

If both kidneys are involved, volume expansion occurs, with a risk of recurrent 'flash' pulmonary edema, a form of hypertensive heart failure that can occur despite normal left ventricular systolic function.

Types of renal artery stenosis
Fibromuscular dysplasia (FMD) is a nonatherosclerotic, nonvasculitic, noninflammatory disease most commonly affecting the renal and cerebral arteries.

The main subtype, medial dysplasia, is characterized by variable thickness of the arterial media, causing a 'string of beads' appearance on angiography. It may be complicated by aneurysm formation or dissection. Intimal and adventitial fibroplasias are rarer.

FMD is said to be a disease of young women, but can occur in both genders and at any age.

Atherosclerotic renal artery stenosis (ARAS) is usually associated with widespread atherosclerotic disease and most commonly affects the ostium of the renal artery.

Kidney function in renal artery stenosis
Even in severe bilateral FMD, the GFR is seldom reduced.

Reduced GFR in ARAS is caused by parenchymal kidney disease, to which the diseased plaque may contribute by causing repeated showers of atheromatous ('cholesterol') emboli into the renal circulation.

Diagnosis of renal artery stenosis
In skilled hands and with slender patients, duplex USS has good diagnostic accuracy.

Isotope renography has largely been supplanted by CT or MR angiography.

Direct angiography is usually only undertaken when it is proposed to proceed to treatment by angioplasty.

Treatment of renal artery stenosis
Percutaneous balloon angioplasty is the standard of care for FMD of the renal arteries.

For treatment of ARAS, angioplasty is nearly always followed by stent placement.

Various surgical revascularization techniques including autotransplantation are available for patients in whom percutaneous treatment is impossible for technical reasons.

When to look for, and treat, renal artery stenosis
Investigating patients for 'treatable' causes of HTN requires an analysis of the costs and complications of investigation versus the likelihood of benefit from treatment.

Most guidelines suggest that investigation for RAS should be reserved for patients with atypical presenting features:
- young age;
- recurrent pulmonary edema with normal systolic function;

- rise in serum creatinine >20% from baseline during ACEI or ARB treatment;
- resistance to standard drug therapy.

The likelihood of finding ARAS is greater in:
- smokers;
- patients with known atherosclerotic disease;
- patients with abdominal bruits.

The effect of correction of RAS on BP is greater in FMD than in ARAS.

Whether treatment prevents progressive loss of GFR in ARAS is uncertain.

Two large clinical trials (ASTRAL, CORAL) are currently investigating the effect of angioplasty and stent placement on the outcome of ARAS.

Adverse effects of renin–angiotensin axis inhibition in the presence of reduced renal perfusion
Autoregulation of GFR is achieved, in part, by local activation of the RAS in response to decreased renal perfusion.

Locally produced angiotensin II causes preferential vasoconstriction of efferent glomerular arterioles, with less effect on afferent arterioles.

This mechanism maintains glomerular pressure and filtration in a number of settings, including:
- severe renal artery stenosis;
- severe hypovolemia (diarrhea, vomiting, or hemorrhage);
- effective hypovolemia caused by heart failure.

In these settings, use of ACEIs or ARBs can precipitate an acute fall in GFR.

This is more likely to be noticed (if using serum creatinine as a filtration marker), and the clinical consequences likely to be more severe, if the GFR is already low – and may go unrecognized if baseline renal function is near normal (e.g. in unilateral renal artery stenosis).

Among patients referred because of a clinical suspicion of ARAS, a rise in serum creatinine ≥20% is highly predictive of significant RAS on angiography.

The reduction in GFR is reversible if the ACEI or ARB is withdrawn promptly, but irreversible renal atrophy may be the consequence of continued use of ACEI or ARB in the presence of severe RAS.

The risk of this complication has to be weighed against the benefits of ACEI or ARB treatment in heart failure and atherosclerotic vascular disease.

Current recommendations for the use of ACEIs and ARBs require that serum creatinine is checked:
- prior to initiation;
- within 2 weeks after initiation;
- after each dose increase.

Repeated measurements are required to confirm a suspected deterioration of kidney function.

Referral is recommended if a rise in serum creatinine of >20% is detected.

These recommendations may appear to conflict with the recommendation that ACEIs or ARBs are used in parenchymal kidney diseases, and that a treatment-induced rise of serum creatinine of up to 30% is acceptable and may predict future stabilization of kidney function.

The recommendations are based on evidence collected in very different populations.

In patients with a high prior probability of ARAS, treatment-induced rise in serum creatinine probably indicates functionally significant ARAS, with GFR being preserved by intense angiotensin-II-mediated efferent arteriolar vasoconstriction; in patients with parenchymal kidney disease, the same phenomenon probably indicates a reduction in intraglomerular hypertension by efferent arteriolar vasodilatation.

Proteinuria is probably the best single discriminator between these two states.

In addition to these recommendations, it is also good practice to advise patients (and their GPs) that ACEIs and ARBs should be discontinued temporarily in the face of intercurrent illness, particularly if associated with hypovolemia or hypotension.

Hypertension in end-stage renal disease

Hypertension is common, and is probably a major contributor to the high cardiovascular mortality in patients receiving dialysis.

Short-term observational studies showing higher mortality with lower BP are a good example of 'reverse causation': systolic failure causes low BP and is associated with a high risk of death.

Systolic failure in dialysis patients may itself result from sustained poorly controlled HTN, and this would be an argument for aggressive treatment of HTN in these patients.

How to achieve this safely remains controversial.

Treatment of hypertension in patients on dialysis
An oversimplified but useful clinical approach is to regard all HTN in kidney failure as a combination of:
- volume overload and
- overactivity of the RAS,

with different contributions from each in individual patients.

It follows from this simplification that BP can usually be controlled in patients receiving conventional thrice weekly hemodialysis (HD) by the achievement of 'dry weight' combined with the use of ACEIs or ARBs.

β-Blockers should be used in the presence of ischemic heart disease or systolic dysfunction.

Vasodilator drugs increase the risk of intradialytic hypotension, which itself may contribute to progressive myocardial injury, and should be avoided if possible.

It is possible to obtain excellent drug-free BP control by volume control alone, using long slow dialysis, at the expense of frequent muscle cramps for the first 4–6 weeks of treatment and loss of residual urine output.

BP slowly normalizes during this 4–6 week period (the 'lag phase') and normotension is associated with a low systemic vascular resistance ('paradoxical vasodilatation') despite volume contraction, suggesting that salt depletion causes changes in resistance vessels during the 'lag' phase.

Patients treated with daily HD also often achieve drug-free normotension.

The following pragmatic rules are useful in the management of HTN in dialysis patients:
- In a dialysis patient with poor BP control, whose BP was previously well controlled on the same or less drug treatment, the patient has lost body weight, and the

HTN will respond to a progressive reduction in target weight.
- In patients with no kidneys (bilateral nephrectomy, no transplant kidneys *in situ*), HTN is always caused by fluid overload, and antihypertensive drug treatment is never necessary.
- Symptomatic hypotension during dialysis does not necessarily mean that the target weight is set too low; it might result from many other factors, including vasodilatation caused by drugs or heat transfer, the rate of fluid removal, rapid reduction in plasma urea concentration, etc.
- A rise in BP during HD is nearly always due to fluid overload, not fluid depletion; so-called 'paradoxical HTN' due to removal of too much fluid is very rare.
- Achieving sodium balance in PD patients can be difficult due to differential removal of sodium and water ('sodium sieving'); dietary restriction of sodium intake is important, particularly in those with low residual kidney function.

Future prospects
Both the ASTRAL trial and the CORAL trial may give further information on how to treat atherosclerotic renal artery stenosis. Preliminary reports from ASTRAL indicate no benefit from revascularisation over medical treatment, despite inclusion of many patients with bilateral stenoses.

Further reading
Guyton AC. Renal function curve – a key to understanding the pathogenesis of hypertension. *Hypertension* 1981; **10**; 1–5.

Johnson RJ. Subtle acquired renal injury as a mechanism of salt-sensitive hypertension. *N Engl J Med* 2002; **346**: 913–923.

Palmer BF. Renal dysfunction complicating the treatment of hypertension. *N Engl J Med* 2002; **347**: 1256–1261.

Internet resources
British Hypertension Society: guidelines on measurement of blood pressure and on treatment:

http://www.bhsoc.org/

NICE guideline on hypertension:

http://www.nice.org.uk/CG034

Fibromuscular Dysplasia Society of America:

www.fmdsa.org

ASTRAL trial website:

www.astral.bham.ac.uk

CORAL trial website:

www.coralclinicaltrial.org

UK CKD guidelines:

www.renal.org/CKDguide/ckd.html

KDOQI guidelines:

www.kidney.org/professionals/kdoqi/guidelines_bp/index.htm

Useful site for calculating Mean Arterial Pressure:

www.mdcalc.com/map

See also
Clinical approach to hypertension, p. 286

Renovascular disease, p. 292

Hypertensive children, p. 304

Hypertensive disorders in pregnancy, p. 310

Cardiovascular risk factors in CKD, p. 412

Cardiovascular risk factors in chronic kidney disease

Introduction

Cardiovascular disease is the single leading cause of morbidity and mortality in patients with CKD at all stages. The risk of a cardiovascular event (defined as hospitalization for coronary disease, heart failure, stroke, or peripheral arterial disease) increases inversely as the GFR falls (Fig. 11.5.1). It is increasingly recognized that even minor impairment of kidney function is a powerful risk factor for cardiovascular disease. Patients who reach ESRD are a minority who have survived. In all but young patients with CKD, the risk of death, primarily from cardiovascular causes, is higher than the risk of needing dialysis or transplantation.

Arterial disease in CKD is a combination of:
- atherosclerosis (characterized by focal lipid-laden intimal plaques);
- arteriosclerosis (characterized by diffuse medial thickening and reduplication of the internal elastic lamina).

Fundamental to each of these processes is endothelial dysfunction.

Myocardial damage may be the result of:
- ischemic damage following coronary artery occlusion;
- diffuse muscular hypertrophy and fibrosis.

In addition to conventional risk factors it is increasingly recognized that there are a number of factors peculiar to CKD that markedly increase the risk of cardiovascular disease.

Each of these is discussed below.

Albuminuria

The presence of albuminuria suggests an increase in glomerular permeability and it may be an easily measured marker of diffuse endothelial dysfunction.

Albuminuria is a potent risk factor for cardiovascular disease in individuals with and without diabetes, and has been associated with increased cardiovascular risk independently of GFR.

It is now increasingly recognized that cardiovascular risk begins to rise at levels of urinary albumin excretion within the currently defined normal range (albumin/creatinine ratio (ACR) as low as 0.5 mg/mmol) and that the risk increases along a continuum.

For every 0.4 mg/mmol increase in the ACR, the adjusted hazard of major CV events increases by 5.9%.

In the SAVE study cohort, albuminuria and reduced eGFR were independently and additively associated with increased mortality.

Whether these two risk factors influence outcomes by the same or separate mechanisms has not yet been established; endothelial dysfunction would be a potential common pathway.

Two large studies have demonstrated that reduction of albuminuria with an ARB in diabetic and nondiabetic subjects results in a reduction in cardiovascular risk.

Altered conduit artery function

Endothelial dysfunction, arteriosclerosis and vascular calcification all interfere with the cushioning effects of large arteries, causing increased pulse wave velocity and earlier reflection of the systolic pressure wave.

This results in a widened pulse pressure which in the heart results in:
- increased systolic pressures causing left ventricular hypertrophy;
- reduced subendocardial perfusion during diastole, exacerbating the effects of relatively minor coronary stenoses.

Pulse wave velocity is raised in:
- patients with CKD stage 3 or higher;
- patients with ≥1 g/24 h proteinuria.

Increased pulse wave velocity is correlated with the extent of cardiovascular disease in CKD and with poorer survival in dialysis patients.

Anemia

The prevalence of anemia increases with falling GFR and there is a strong association between anemia and cardiovascular disease.

In observational studies, anemia is associated with LVH independently of HTN and is also associated with the development of LV dilatation and death.

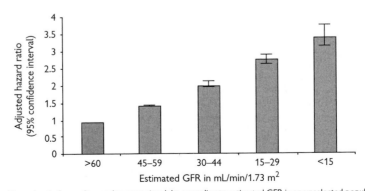

Fig. 11.5.1 Adjusted hazard ratio for cardiovascular events in adults according to estimated GFR in an unselected population of 1 120 295 adults.

Randomized controlled trials (RCTs) comparing different strategies for correcting anemia with erythropoiesis-stimulating agents (ESAs) have shown that partial correction of renal anemia:

- prevents the development of LVH;
- improves physical functioning;
- improves quality of life.

Several studies (the normal hematocrit study, CREATE, and CHOIR) comparing partial with full correction of anemia in CKD and in hemodialysis patients have both failed to show that full correction reduces cardiovascular risk, and in fact they suggest an increased risk.

Whether this increased risk is due to the higher hemoglobin (Hb) concentration achieved *per se,* or to the high doses of ESA (and iron) required in some (sicker) patients to achieve the higher target Hb, remains uncertain.

The TREAT study, a large double-blind, RCT of treatment with an ESA versus placebo in diabetics is still ongoing.

The NICE guidelines on correction of anemia state that ESA treatment should be initiated, after exclusion of other causes of anemia, in patients with CKD whose Hb <11 g/dL, and once on treatment, Hb concentration should be maintained between 10.5 and 12.5 g/dL.

Diabetes

Patients with CKD and diabetes have a greatly increased risk of cardiovascular disease.

Control of HTN and dyslipidemia is at least as important as good glycemic control in reducing this risk.

Dyslipidemia

Kidney disease is associated with alterations in lipoprotein structure and function, including:

- reduced high density lipoprotein (HDL) cholesterol;
- increased intermediate density lipoprotein;
- increased proatherogenic lipid particles.

In addition, a number of biochemical alterations in uremia contribute to increased oxidation of low density lipoprotein (LDL).

All of these changes promote atherogenesis.

The evidence that lipid-lowering drug treatment reduces cardiovascular event rates in patients with CKD is limited.

This is partly due to the exclusion of patients with advanced CKD from large statin trials, although *post hoc* analyses of these trials have suggested benefit in subgroups with low estimated GFR.

Competing cardiovascular risk from nonatherosclerotic vascular disease (e.g. arteriosclerosis, vascular calcification, hypertensive heart failure), may reduce the overall impact of lipid-lowering treatment on outcomes, particularly in advanced CKD.

The *Die Deutsche Diabetes Dialyse* (4D) study showed no benefit from lowering of cholesterol by atorvastatin in type II diabetic patients on dialysis.

The ALERT study compared fluvastatin against placebo in kidney transplant recipients. There was no significant reduction in the prespecified composite endpoint, but there were fewer cardiac deaths and fewer nonfatal myocardial infarctions.

Two large ongoing RCTs, SHARP and AURORA, will provide further evidence in the next few years.

SHARP will compare the combination of simvastatin and ezetimibe with placebo on the risk of major vascular events among 9000 patients with CKD who do not have established coronary heart disease on enrolment.

AURORA is examining the effect of rosuvastatin versus placebo on cardiovascular disease in >2750 patients on hemodialysis.

Pending the results of these trials, current UK guidelines suggest adoption of the guidelines for primary and secondary prevention of cardiovascular disease that apply to the general population:

- statin treatment for those with a 10 year risk of cardiovascular disease of ≥30%.

The calculation is based on the Joint British Societies' chart or the cardiovascular risk calculator (despite the fact that these have not been validated in patients with renal disease).

The dose of statin should be increased to achieve:

- total cholesterol of <5 mmol/L;
- 30% reduction from baseline; or
- fasting LDL-cholesterol of <3 mmol/L.

The aim is to achieve the target which represents the greatest reduction.

Endothelial dysfunction

Impairment of endothelial function is one of the initial steps in the pathological process leading to atherosclerosis.

Endothelial dysfunction is related to generic factors which can be present in patients without CKD:

- hypertension;
- smoking;
- diabetes;
- obesity;
- dyslipidemia.

In patients with CKD there are a number of additional factors including:

- retention of homocysteine and asymmetric dimethyl-arginine (ADMA);
- reduced intrarenal generation of nitric oxide;
- oxidative stress;
- reduced activation of vitamin D;
- reduced production of erythropoietin, renalase, and bone morphogenic protein 7;
- insulin resistance;
- low level persistent chronic inflammation;
- activation of the renin–angiotensin system.

Hyperhomocysteinemia

Raised plasma homocysteine levels are strongly associated with an increased risk of cardiovascular disease, both in the general population and in CKD, which is associated with marked hyperhomocysteinemia.

Hyperhomocystinemia in CKD is multifactorial, but can be partially corrected by B vitamin supplementation.

A recent large RCT of reduction of homocysteine with folic acid, pyridoxine and cyanocobalamin in patients with advanced CKD showed no reduction in the vascular event rate.

Nitric oxide and asymmetric dimethyl arginine

One of the main factors involved in endothelial dysfunction in CKD is the reduced bioavailability of nitric oxide.

Nitric oxide is produced and released in the vascular endothelium by endothelial nitric oxide synthase from L-arginine.

ADMA is a competitive inhibitor of nitric oxide synthase which is retained as GFR falls.

In CKD, ADMA levels in plasma are markedly elevated from an early stage, even when the GFR is still within the normal range.

Increased ADMA levels have been associated with progression to ESRD and increased mortality.

Whether L-arginine supplementation or administration of nitric oxide donors reduces cardiovascular events is unknown.

Oxidant stress

Oxidative stress occurs when there is an imbalance between the production of reactive oxygen species (ROS) and the body's ability to inactivate them or easily repair the resulting damage.

In CKD, levels of ROS are high, and levels of antioxidants such as vitamin E are often low.

While studies of vitamin E supplementation in high risk people in the general population (e.g. the Heart Outcomes Prevention Evaluation trial) have conclusively shown no evidence of reduced cardiovascular risk, some still argue that antioxidants, including vitamin E and acetylcysteine, may be of benefit in CKD.

The existing trials evidence suggests that the benefit from vitamin E and acetylcystine were too small to allow any definite conclusions.

Abnormalities of bone mineral metabolism

Hyperphosphatemia
Raised serum phosphate is associated with an increased risk of death in both early CKD and in patients receiving dialysis.

Serum phosphate can be reduced by a combination of dietary restriction of phosphate intake and ingestion with meals of phosphate binders to reduce phosphate absorption. Phosphate binders may contain:

- calcium carbonate;
- calcium acetate;
- sevelamer hydrochloride;
- lanthanum carbonate.

Sevelamer also reduces serum cholesterol.

It has been reported that sevelamer reduces the risk of progression of established coronary artery calcification in patients starting dialysis.

Direct comparison of sevelamer with calcium acetate in 1068 hemodialysis patients followed for a mean of 20 months (the DCOR study) showed no clear advantage of one or other on cardiovascular deaths.

Current recommendations in the UK are to achieve a serum phosphate of:

- 0.9–1.5 mmol/L in CKD 3 and 4;
- 1.1–1.8 mmol/L in dialysis patients.

The choice of phosphate binder is up to individuals.

Hyperparathyroidism
Parathyroid hormone has a number of adverse effects on cardiac myocytes *in vitro*, and in animal experiments may contribute to defective capillary supply to cardiac muscle.

In patients, it is difficult to distinguish the effects of hyperparathyroidism on the cardiovascular system from the conditions that contribute to it, including the duration of CKD, reduced 1,25-(OH) vitamin D concentrations, hyperphosphatemia, and hypocalcemia.

Correction of severe hyperparathyroidism is probably beneficial in calcific uremic arteriolopathy.

The effect of correction of hyperparathyroidism by cinacalcet on cardiovascular events is currently being studied in the EVOLVE trial.

Insulin resistance and hyperinsulinemia

Insulin resistance and consequent hyperinsulinemia play a central role in the development of atherosclerosis.

Insulin resistance and hyperinsulinemia are present very early in the course of kidney disease, even when GFR is still within the normal range.

Insulin resistance can be measured using the homeostatic model assessment (HOMA) technique, from fasting glucose and insulin concentrations. The HOMA index has been shown to predict survival in dialysis patients.

Insulin resistance and endothelial dysfunction are inextricably linked with vascular damage.

Diet, exercise and drugs may reduce insulin resistance by a number of mechanisms and may reduce endothelial dysfunction and reduce cardiovascular mortality.

It remains uncertain whether the 'glitazones' or other insulin-sensitizing drugs reduce cardiovascular events in CKD.

Low grade inflammation

Chronic inflammation is strongly associated with atherosclerosis both in the absence and presence of CKD.

In CKD, chronic inflammation is also associated with reduced levels of fetuin-A, a potent inhibitor of vascular calcification.

Whether any specific strategies to identify and treat the cause of chronic low-grade inflammation are of benefit remains uncertain.

Hypertension

Hypertension (HTN) is frequently found in patients with CKD and is a powerful risk factor for cardiovascular disease.

Although large short-term observational studies of patients on dialysis show that the highest risk of death is among those with the lowest blood pressure, this is almost certainly because low blood pressure is a marker for heart failure, which may often have been caused by poorly controlled HTN over the longer term.

Lack of exercise

Exercise is of proven benefit in reducing cardiovascular risk in the general population.

In CKD, aerobic exercise:

- decreases microalbuminuria;
- reduces oxidative stress;
- may increase GFR.

Aerobic exercise in hemodialysis patients has been reported to:

- enhance insulin sensitivity;
- improve lipid profile;

- increase hemoglobin;
- increase strength;
- decrease BP;
- improve quality of life;
- improve survival.

Left ventricular dilatation

Left ventricular dilatation may develop as an end result of:
- LVH;
- valvular disease;
- ischemic injury.

It carries a particularly poor prognosis.

Left ventricular hypertrophy

Left ventricular hypertrophy (LVH) is a strong predictor of mortality in patients on dialysis.

LVH is present from the early stages of CKD and the prevalence of LVH correlates with the degree of renal impairment.

In one series the prevalence of LVH was:
- 26.7% if the CrCl was >50 mL/min;
- 30.8% if the CrCl was 25–49 mL/min;
- 45.2% if the CrCl was <25 mL/min.

Causes of LVH in CKD include:
- hypertension;
- volume overload;
- anemia;
- decreased conduit artery compliance.

Aldosterone

Raised aldosterone levels in CKD may contribute to left ventricular fibrosis.

The role of aldosterone antagonists in the prevention of cardiovascular events in CKD remains uncertain.

Obesity

There is a strong association between body mass index, progression of CKD, and cardiovascular disease.

Obesity is associated with:
- insulin resistance;
- oxidative stress;
- endothelial dysfunction.

Adipose tissue secretes a number of adipokines, the serum levels of which are elevated in CKD, probably due to decreased renal excretion. These adipokines are implicated in endothelial dysfunction and insulin resistance.

Weight reduction has been shown to have beneficial effects on:
- hypertension;
- glomerular hyperfiltration;
- albuminuria;
- insulin resistance;
- progression of CKD.

There is no direct evidence that weight reduction (either through diet or bariatric surgery) is of benefit in patients with CKD.

For reasons that are highly debated, obesity appears to confer a survival advantage in dialysis patients.

Smoking

Smoking is an important risk factor for progression of CKD and a major risk factor for atherosclerotic vascular disease in diabetic and nondiabetic patients.

Cigarette smoking causes:
- endothelial dysfunction;
- reduced synthesis and bioavailability of nitric oxide;
- atherosclerosis and thrombosis;
- coronary artery disease;
- stroke.

All patients with CKD and a reasonable life expectancy should be strongly advised to stop smoking.

Valvular disease

Calcification of the mitral valve annulus and the aortic valve cusps is common with failing renal function.

Calcification may be associated with valvular regurgitation or (particularly with the aortic valve) with significant stenosis.

Vascular calcification

Vascular calcification may be the result of calcification of either atherosclerotic plaques or the media.

It is increasingly recognized as an actively regulated process and not just the result of passive precipitation of calcium and phosphorus crystals.

Vascular calcification is a multistep process similar to bone formation.

Vascular smooth muscle cells undergo a phenotypic switch into osteoblast-like cells and then express alkaline phosphatase, osteocalcin and osteopontin. Expression of these bone-associated proteins leads to mineralization of the extracellular matrix (ossification).

There is now abundant evidence that phosphate retention is a major factor in vascular calcification.

An increase in intracellular phosphate induces vascular smooth muscle cells to undergo the phenotypic changes described above.

Several regulatory factors that induce or inhibit vascular calcification have also been identified.

The five key inhibitors currently implicated in vascular calcification associated with CKD are:
- fetuin A (α2-Heremans-Schmid glycoprotein (AHSG);
- matrix-carboxyglutamic acid protein (MGP);
- bone morphogenic protein (BMP) 7;
- osteoprotegerin (OPG);
- pyrophosphate.

Of these, BMP-7 shows the most promise as a future therapeutic agent.

BMP-7 inhibits vascular calcification, maintains vascular smooth muscle cell differentiation and prevents osteoblastic transformation.

BMP-7 is mainly expressed by the kidney and its expression is decreased from the early stages of CKD resulting in a progressive loss of ability to inhibit vascular calcification.

In mice, treatment with BMP-7 has been shown to reduce vascular calcification.

Recombinant human BMP-7 in putty has been used in several human trials for osseous repair after bone fracture, and was shown to be safe and well-tolerated.

Calcific uremic arteriolopathy (CUA)

CUA (often referred to as 'calciphylaxis') is characterized by diffuse calcification of the media of small-to-medium arteries and arterioles.

Intimal proliferation and thrombosis occur resulting in painful skin ulceration and necrosis.

Parathyroidectomy may be of benefit if there is marked hyperparathyroidism.

Warfarin may precipitate the syndrome, probably by inhibition of factor VII-dependent anticoagulant proteins.

CUA carries a very poor prognosis, with a high mortality from cardiovascular disease.

Future prospects

A number of large RCTs will report in the next few years which may help in the stratification and management of cardiovascular risk in CKD. These include:

- SHARP;
- TREAT;
- AURORA;
- EVOLVE.

Bone morphogenic protein 7 (BMP-7) shows the most promise as a future therapeutic agent.

Further reading

Cozzolino M, et al. Vascular calcification and uremia: what do we know? Am J Nephrol 2008; 28: 339–346.

Go AS, et al. Chronic kidney disease and the risks of death, cardiovascular events, and hospitalization. N Engl J Med 2004: 351: 1296–305.

Kaysen GA, Eiserich JP. The role of oxidative stress-altered lipoprotein structure and function and microinflammation on cardiovascular risk in patients with minor renal dysfunction. J Am Soc Nephrol 2004; 15: 538–548.

Internet resources

NICE guideline on hypertension:

http://www.nice.org.uk/CG034

Joint British Societies' Guidelines on prevention of cardiovascular disease in clinical practice:

www.bcs.com/download/651/JBS2final.pdf

UK CKD guidelines:

www.renal.org/CKDguide/ckd.html

KDOQI guidelines:

www.kidney.org/professionals/kdoqi/guidelines_bp/index.htm

SHARP trial website:

http://www.sharpinfo.org/

See also

Clinical approach to hypertension, p. 286

Renovascular disease, p. 292

Hypertension in CKD, p. 406

Chronic kidney disease in diabetic patients, p. 472

Medical management of dialysis patients, p. 528

Gastrointestinal disorders in chronic kidney disease

Introduction
Three-quarters of patients with ESRD have gastrointestinal (GI) complaints. There is an increased prevalence of irritable bowel disease, bleeding from angiodysplasia, gastroparesis, gastritis and duodenitis in ESRD patients compared with the normal population. However, prevalences of dyspepsia, ulcer disease, and *Helicobacter pylori* gastritis are not significantly different from the general population. GI disorders are a leading cause of hospitalization in ESRD patients and account for 8–15% of admissions.

Upper GI tract
Pathogenetic factors of upper GI disorders
Serum levels of hormones involved in the modulation of GI motility and in the regulation of hunger and satiety (e.g. gastrin, cholecystokinin, neurotensin and glucagons) are significantly raised as a consequence of renal failure.

Humoral abnormalities (hypercalcemia, hypokalemia and acidosis) may play a role in GI dysmotility and acid secretion alteration.

Anorexia.
Loss of appetite is common, occurring in one-third of ESRD patients and associated with increased morbidity and mortality.

Pathogenesis is largely unknown.

Therapy options include:
- dietetic counseling and nutritional supplements;
- appetite stimulants;
- improvement of dialysis adequacy;
- renal transplantation.

Gastric emptying and gastroesophageal reflux
Patients with CKD have a high prevalence of:
- prolonged gastric emptying;
- GI dysmotility;
- anorexia;
- nausea and vomiting.

Patients on PD and those with dialysis-related amyloidosis have a greater incidence of gastroesophageal reflux.

Pathogenesis
Autonomic and enteric nervous system dysfunction due to uremia.

Increased levels of GI peptides (gastrin, cholecystokinin, neurotensin) due to impaired renal clearance.

PD patients show a higher prevalence of delayed gastric emptying compared with HD and predialysis patients.

Peptic ulcer disease
There is no evidence of a higher duodenal ulcer and *H. pylori* infection prevalence compared to the general population.

Biopsy proven chronic active gastritis is the most common histological diagnosis among with upper GI symptoms, patients and is closely associated with *H. pylori* infection.

The urea breath test remains a valid diagnostic tool for *H. pylori* infection in CKD and ESRD.

H. pylori eradication
14 days treatment with:
- omeprazole 20 mg bd, or lansoprazole 30 mg od;
- clarithromycin 500 mg bd and amoxicillin 1 g bd or metronidazole 500 mg tds.

Biliary tract disease and pancreatitis
There is no increase in the incidence of cholecystitis, cholelithiasis and pancreatitis in patients with ESRD.

Patients with CKD often have elevated serum amylase and lipase levels but they do not normally exceed three times the upper limit of normal.

Lower GI tract
Colonic perforation
Spontaneous colonic perforation may occur as a consequence of:
- diverticulitis;
- fecal impaction;
- dehydration;
- dialysis-related amyloidosis.

The incidence of diverticular disease is no different from the general population except in cases of autosomal dominant polycystic kidney disease where there is an increased incidence.

In patients who have been on dialysis long-term, there may be β2-microglobulin deposition in the GI tract causing dysmotility, perforation or necrosis.

Ischemic bowel disease
Symptoms include sudden onset of fever, vomiting and abdominal pain.

In patients on peritoneal dialysis this may mimic peritonitis.

Predisposing factors:
- atheromatosis;
- increased blood viscosity;
- constipation (high intraluminal pressure);
- digoxin (splachnic vasoconstrictor).

Precipitating factors:
- severe hypovolemia;
- congestive heart failure (decreased cardiac output);
- hypoxia;
- excessive ultrafiltration with intradialytic hypotension.

The diagnostic method of choice is mesenteric angiography.

Hemorrhoids and proctitis
There is a high prevalence in ESRD, due to diet and drugs (phosphate binders).

Fecal impaction
This may occur secondary to a number of medications commonly prescribed in CKD and ESRD including phosphate binders, analgesics and oral iron supplements.

Treatment includes:
- stool softeners (e.g. sodium docusate);
- osmotive laxatives (e.g. lactulose, disacodyl).

Idiopathic dialysis ascites
This is an exudative ascites.

The main cause is inadequate dialysis.

Incidence is declining due to improvements in nutrition and delivered dialysis dose.

It is a diagnosis of exclusion.

The differential diagnosis includes:
- constrictive pericarditis;
- cirrhosis;
- occult infection (e.g. tuberculosis);
- encapsulating peritoneal sclerosis
- neoplasia;
- granulomatous peritoneal disease;
- inferior vena cava stenosis.

Treatment includes:
- salt and fluid restriction;
- aggressive ultrafiltration;
- intermittent paracentesis;
- daily HD;
- switching from HD to PD;
- renal transplantation (best treatment).

The prognosis is poor: 35% mortality at 1 year.

Intestinal pseudo-obstruction

Chronic intestinal pseudo-obstruction
Symptoms are those of mechanical bowel obstruction but without an anatomical obstructing lesion.

Clinical manifestations include:
- abdominal pain;
- vomiting;
- constipation or diarrhea.

Several potential contributory factors can affect GI neuromuscular function:
- amyloidosis (including β2-microglobulin amyloidosis);
- diabetes mellitus;
- scleroderma;
- medications (e.g. calcium channel blockers and anti-cholinergic antidepressants).

Investigations:
- plain abdominal X-ray;
- gastric and small bowel transit tests using either scintigraphy or manometry.

There is no proven treatment other than supportive care:
- temporary parenteral nutrition can be used in severe cases;
- prokinetic agents (e.g. erythromycin).

Acute intestinal pseudo-obstruction
Predisposing factors:
- chronic constipation;
- diabetic autonomic neuropathy;
- medications (e.g. kayexalate, opioid analgesics).

The acute abdomen
All common causes of an acute abdomen are seen in patients with renal failure.

Common causes to consider include:
- small bowel or colon obstruction (particularly if previous PD and risk of intra-abdominal adhesions);
- visceral perforation;
- bowel ischemia or necrosis (high incidence of accelerated atherosclerosis in CKD and ESRD);
- intracyst infection and hemorrhage in patients with polycystic kidney disease;

- bacterial peritonitis or pseudoperitontis (due to icodextrin sensitivity) in patients on peritoneal dialysis.

Pneumoperitoneum and GI perforation in PD
Important points to note are:

Free subdiaphragmatic air on an erect CXR has a low specificity for the diagnosis of GI perforation in CAPD patients.

PD fluid may dilute the initial intraperitoneal contamination and, together with intraperitoneal antibiotics, mask clinical signs.

Perforation is suggested by the presence of mixed Gram-negative or anerobic organisms in PD fluid cultures.

The presence of feces, food or bile in the PD effluent indicates visceral perforation.

GI manifestations of polycystic kidney disease
The most common are:

Hepatic cysts which may be associated with:
- chronic abdominal pain;
- hemorrhage;
- infection;
- rupture;
- early satiety (stomach compression);
- lower limb edema (inferior vena cava compression).

Renal cyst infection will require antibiotics that concentrate inside the cysts (quinolones) and occasionally percutaneous drainage.

Colonic diverticulae which may be associated with:
- constipation;
- diverticulitis;
- hemorrhage;
- perforation.

Umbilical and inguinal hernias.

Gastrointestinal bleeding
There is an increased incidence of GI bleeding in patients with ESRD due to:
- a higher incidence of lesions producing bleeding (particularly a high incidence of erosive gastritis and angiodysplasia);
- impairment of hemostasis (anemia, uremia);
- intradialytic anticoagulation;
- drugs (e.g. antiplatelet agents and warfarin);
- coexistent GI tract disease (β2-microglobulin amyloidosis).

Practical points:
- high incidence of angiodysplasia in elderly patients;
- high incidence of amyloidosis in long-term dialysis patients;
- consider NSAID enteropathy in patients with rheumatoid arthritis;
- constipation due to phosphate binders or kayexalate exacerbating rectal bleeding;
- uremia-related coagulation abnormalities – often primary cause or exacerbating factor.

Upper GI tract bleeding
The incidence of upper GI bleeding has decreased due to improvements in dialysis practices and treatment with H_2 antagonists/proton pump inhibitors.

Nevertheless, upper GI bleeding accounts for 3–7% of all deaths in ESRD patients.

Common causative conditions are listed in Table 11.6.1.

Cardiovascular disease, current smoking and increasing debility are associated with a greater risk of upper GI bleeding in patients with ESRD.

Gastric antral vascular ectasia (watermelon stomach) is an angiodysplastic lesion confined to the gastric antrum. It is characterized by submucosal capillary dilatation and fibromuscular hyperplasia.

General therapy
- review need for antiplatelet agents and warfarin;
- maximize hematocrit (EPO and red cell transfusion);
- minimize effect of uremia with increased dialysis dose;
- DDAVP (desmopressin);
- antifibrinolytic agents (tranexamic acid);
- cryoprecipitate;
- recombinant activated factor VII.

Tranexamic acid is a potent inhibitor of the fibrinolytic system and can be used both orally and IV. One suggested protocol is 20 mg IV followed for the next 4 weeks by 10 mg/kg/48 h orally.

Specific therapy
Bleeding peptic ulcer: endoscopic laser therapy, topical injection of adrenaline, ethanol or polidocanol.

Esophageal varices: endoscopic sclerotherapy, endoscopic variceal band ligation, balloon tamponade, somatostatin or octreotide infusion.

Hemorrhagic gastritis: antacids, H_2 receptor antagonists, proton pump inhibitors, sucralfate.

Lower GI tract bleeding
Angiodysplasia is the commonest cause (Table 11.6.1).

Angiodysplasia is a vascular abnormality affecting the microcirculation of the GI mucosa and submucosa.

It commonly causes GI hemorrhage in the elderly.

The incidence is increased in HD patients and responsible for ~20% of all GI hemorrhages in HD population.

Investigations include:
- endoscopic procedures (colonoscopy, fine fibre enteroscopy);
- selective visceral angiography.

General therapy
- review need for antiplatelet agents and warfarin;
- maximize hematocrit (EPO and red cell transfusion);
- minimize effect of uremia with increased dialysis dose;
- DDAVP;
- antifibrinolytic agents (tranexamic acid);
- cryoprecipitate;
- recombinant activated factor VII.

Specific therapy
- estrogen/progesterone preparations;
- therapeutic endoscopy (electrocoagulation and laser therapy);
- surgical resection.

Diarrhea
Diarrhea is frequently seen in patients with advanced CKD and ESRD and its cause is often multifactorial:
- autonomic neuropathy;
- nonspecific antibiotic-induced diarrhea;

- effects on colonic motility of iron supplements, digoxin, phosphate binders and antihypertensive therapy.

Clostridium difficile-associated pseudomembranous colitis is more common, more severe and has a higher recurrence rate in patients with renal failure, due to a reduced threshold for use of antibiotics in relatively immunocompromised patients with ESRD, in older patients, and topical enteral factors (dysmotility, abnormal bile acid profiles).

Other pathogens such as CMV in HIV-positive patients and *Strongyloides stercoralis* may be the causative agents of severe enterocolitis in patients with renal failure.

GI complications in patients on PD
The most commonly seen are:
- gastroparesis;
- malabsorption;
- pancreatic dysfunction;
- protein-losing enteropathy.

Additionally, increased intra-abdominal pressure can result in hernia formation, delayed gastric emptying and gastroesophageal reflux.

A reduction in supine intraperitoneal fluid with adjustment of dialysis prescription to maintain adequate clearance may help gastroesophageal reflux.

Oral or intraperitoneal erythromycin may improve gastroparesis.

In women, pain on infusion of dialyzate and hemoperitoneum may be seen during menstruation and ovulation and can also be seen in endometriosis.

Pain during dialyzate infusion is not uncommon and may be due to:
- the acidic pH of lactate-buffered dialyzate;
- catheter malposition;
- hypertonic dialysis solutions.

Treatment options include:
- switching to bicarbonate-based PD solutions;
- catheter repositioning or replacement;
- slowing the infusion rate;
- injection of local anesthetic into the PD solution before infusion.

Scrotal or labial swelling may be seen due to a patent processus vaginalis or a dissection through the peritoneal

Table 11.6.1 Common causes of GI bleeding in patients with ESRD

Upper tract bleeding
Esophageal varices
Mallory–Weis tear
Gastritis/duodenitis
Peptic ulcer
Angiodysplasia
Gastric antral vascular ectasia
Dieulafoy malformation
β2-Microglobulin amyloidosis
Lower tract bleeding
Angiodysplasia
Diverticulae
β2-Microglobulin amyloidosis
Colorectal polyps
Hemorrhoids/anorectal tears
Stercoral ulcers

membrane. This usually requires surgical repair of the hernia or patent processus vaginalis.

Abdominal wall edema, due to dialyzate leak into the anterior abdominal wall, may resolve following a period of resting from PD or transfer onto automated PD. Surgical repositioning of the catheter may be required if conservative measures fail.

Encapsulating peritoneal sclerosis is a rare complication of PD and is associated with a number of GI complications, the most serious of which is malabsorption and consequent malnutrition.

GI complications in patients with diabetes

Diabetic gastroparesis

This is related to diabetic autonomic neuropathy of the GI tract.

Clinical signs include:
- abdominal bloating;
- early satiety;
- episodic vomiting.

It compromises glycemic control and impairs absorption of orally administered drugs.

There are no anatomic alterations of the upper GI tract on imaging studies.

Investigation:
- scintigraphic measurement of gastric emptying.

Treatment:
- low fat and low fiber diet with frequent small meals;
- if severe enteral (via jejunostomy) or parenteral nutrition;
- drug therapy with dopamine antagonists (metoclopramide, domperidone) and motilin receptor stimulants (erythromycin);
- gastric electric stimulation and pyloric botulinum toxin injection have been successfully used in a small number of cases.

Diabetic enteropathy

This presents with episodic watery and painless diarrhea due to:
- diabetic autonomic neuropathy (vagal, sympathetic and enteric nervous system damage); and
- bacterial overgrowth (resulting in bile acid deconjugation and fat malabsorption).

Treatment involves both supportive therapy with loperamide and octreotide and treatment of any contributing microbial cause of the diarrhea.

Further reading

Bossola M, Tazza L, Giungi S, Luciani G. Anorexia in hemodialysis patients: an update. *Kidney Int* 2006; **70**: 417–422.

Etemad B. Gastrointestinal complications of renal failure. *Gastroenterol Clin North Am* 1998; **27**: 875–892.

Strid H, Simrén M, Stotzer PO, Abrahamsson H, Björnsson ES. Delay in gastric emptying in patients with chronic renal failure. *Scand J Gastroenterol* 2004; **39**: 516–520.

Tsai CJ, Hwang JC. Investigation of upper gastrointestinal hemorrhage in chronic renal failure. *J Clin Gastroenterol* 1996; **22**: 2–5.

Internet resources

National Library of Guidelines Specialist Library:

http://www.library.nhs.uk/guidelinesFinder/

British Society of Gastroenterology:

http://www.bsg.org.uk/

American College of Gastroenterology:

http://www.acg.gi.org

See also

Liver disorders in chronic kidney disease

Hepatitis B

Hepatitis B virus (HBV) is a dsDNA hepadnavirus. It is relatively stable in the environment and can remain viable for at least 7 days on environmental surfaces. HBV is transmitted by percutaneous (i.e. puncture through the skin), permucosal (i.e. direct contact with mucous membranes) or perinatal exposure to infectious blood. Chronic hepatitis B virus (HBV) infection can be associated with the development of:

- cirrhosis;
- hepatocellular carcinoma (HCC);
- hepatic failure.

Patients with renal failure have an increased risk of acquiring the virus through blood transfusions and contact with contaminated bodily fluids during hemodialysis.

Epidemiology

While the prevalence of HBV hepatitis appears to have decreased in recent times in Europe and the USA, HBV infection still poses a significant public health burden in Asia and South America.

Hepatitis B surface antigen (HBsAg) positivity rates among dialysis patients tend to correlate with rates in the endemic population.

A lower prevalence of HBV infection has been reported in patients on PD compared with patients treated with HD.

Predisposing factors

The most common risk factors for HBV infection in dialysis patients are:

- multiple transfusions;
- local levels of hepatitis B carriage;
- duration of HD;
- presence of HBsAg$^+$ patients in the dialysis unit and non-separation of infected from noninfected patients;
- failing to follow standard infection practices, e.g. sharing multidose vials and IV solutions or equipment in contact with blood;
- not periodically screening patients for HBsAg;
- not vaccinating susceptible patients;
- staff members who simultaneously care for both HBV-infected and susceptible patients.

Clinical features

HBV causes both acute and chronic hepatitis.

The incubation period ranges from 45 to 160 days.

Acute HBV infection in dialysis patients is often mild or asymptomatic and many will become chronic carriers due to impaired uremia-related antiviral immune responses.

When present, clinical symptoms and signs might include:

- anorexia and malaise;
- nausea and vomiting;
- abdominal pain;
- jaundice.

Chronic HBV infection is defined as persistence of HBsAg for >6 months with histological changes on liver biopsy and/or persistently elevated alanine aminotransferase (ALT) levels.

In ESRD progression of chronic HBV infection to hepatic cirrhosis and HCC can occur with a less marked hepatic inflammatory response.

Investigations

Liver function tests

Aspartate aminotransferase (AST) and ALT levels may be elevated and reflect hepatocellular injury.

Total serum alkaline phosphatase may be elevated but alkaline phosphatase is also produced by the intestine, liver and bone and so may not correlate well with the extent of liver involvement.

Measurement of other enzymes, such as 5-nucleotidase and γ-glutamyltransferase, may provide some additional information on extent of liver injury.

Liver biopsy

This is the 'gold standard' for the assessment of the liver's functional reserves, the activity and chronicity of liver disease.

Serological assays

- HBsAg

A positive result indicates ongoing HBV infection and potential infectivity. It appears 30–60 days after exposure to HBV and persists for variable periods) (Fig 11.7.1 & Table 11.7.1).

- HBeAg

This is positive in acute and chronic HBV infection and correlates with viral replication and high infectivity.

HBeAg-negative patients:

1 these are quiescent and were previously known as the 'healthy' or 'inactive' carriers; or

2 are actively replicating 'pre-core' mutants.

'Pre-core' mutants have a mutation in the pre-core region of the HBV DNA. They have a worse prognosis and poorer response to therapy than HBeAg-positive patients.

- HBcAb

Antibodies against the HBV core antigen appear in the early stages of infection and persist long term.

IgM anti-HBcAb indicates recent infection and persists for ~6 months.

- HBsAb

Antibodies against the HBV surface antigen indicate immunity from HBV infection, either natural (anti-HBsAb$^+$ and anti-HBcAb$^+$) or after successful vaccination (only anti-HBsAb$^+$).

- HBeAb

Antibodies against the HBcAg envelope antigen correlate with nonreplicating virus and with lower levels of virus.

Nucleic acid detection

A quantitative test for HBV DNA copy number is available and measures hepatitis B viral load (expressed in copies/ml). It is used:

- in suspected cases when other tests are inconclusive (e.g. before the HBsAg becomes positive, in cases of occult HBV (with a negative HBsAg) or pre-core mutants);
- prior to initiation of antiviral therapy;
- to estimate the success of antiviral therapy.

Screening for hepatocellular cancer
- α-Fetoprotein (AFP):

In HBsAg$^+$ patients AFP should be measured every 6 months.

It is elevated in 60% of liver cancers.
- Liver ultrasound:

Should be performed every year in HBsAg$^+$ patients.

It is diagnostic in 80% of cases of liver cancer.

Treatment

The goals of therapy are (Fig 11.7.2):
- suppression of viral replication;
- prevention of hepatic fibrosis;
- seroconversion from HBsAg$^+$ to HBsAb$^+$ and from HBeAg$^+$ to HBeAb$^+$.
- Commonly used antiviral agents include (Table 11.7.2):

Interferon-α

This is an antiviral, antiproliferative and immunomodulatory agent.

Side-effects are common and include:
- flu-like symptoms;
- neutropenia;
- thrombocytopenia;
- neuropsychiatric symptoms;
- exacerbation of hepatitis.

Treatment duration for HBeAg$^+$ patients is 16 weeks and for HBeAg$^-$ patients is 12 months.

Pegylated interferon-α has improved pharmacokinetics and allows for a weekly dosing schedule. It is associated with a 30–35% HBeAg seroconversion rate, compared to 16–20% with standard interferon.

Lamivudine

A cytosine analogue that inhibits HBV reverse transcriptase. It is well-tolerated and safe.

Lamivudine-resistant HBV variants have emerged, with a mutation in the YMDD locus of the HBV DNA polymerase. The prevalence of resistance increases with the duration of treatment and HBeAg$^-$ disease.

Adefovir dipivoxil

This is a phosphonate nucleotide analogue of adenosine that binds competitively to HBV DNA polymerase.

It is safe and effective in patients with lamivudine-resistant HBV and renal disease.

It is cleared by the kidneys and patients with renal insufficiency should receive reduced doses.

Prophylaxis

General measures
- universal infection control precautions;
- routine serologic testing for markers of HBV infection and prompt review of results;
- isolation of HBsAg$^+$ patients with dedicated room, machine, other equipment, supplies and staff members;
- testing susceptible patients monthly for HBsAg, particularly those who have not yet received hepatitis B vaccine, are in the process of being vaccinated, or have not responded to vaccination;
- dialysis staff should be vaccinated and wear protective gloves that must be changed before proceeding from one patient to another;

- no reuse of dialyzers in HBsAg$^+$ patients.

When a seroconversion occurs
- review all patients' laboratory results to identify additional cases;
- investigate potential sources of HBV infection;
- in patients newly infected with HBV, repeat HBsAg and test for HBcAb (including IgM HBcAb) 1–2 months later;
- 6 months later, repeat HBsAg testing and test for HBsAb to determine clinical outcome;
- patients who become HBsAg$^-$ are no longer infectious and can be removed from isolation.

Immunization

There is no difference in effectiveness between plasma-derived and recombinant type of vaccines.

Success rates of vaccination in HD patients are lower compared to the general population due to immunosuppression related to uremia.

Vaccine success is inversely related to the degree of renal dysfunction, therefore early vaccination is recommended.

There is no evidence to support the use of alternative vaccination routes (e.g. intradermal) or coadministration with other agents (e.g. erythropoietin or IL-2).

A three or four dose recombinant vaccine schedule of 40 μg at 0, 1 and 6 months or 0, 1, 2, and 6 months respectively is recommended for patients with CKD and ESRD.

All vaccinated patients should be tested for HBsAb 1–2 months after the last primary vaccine dose, to determine response.

Adequate response:
- >10 sample ratio units (SRU);
- >10 mIU/mL (North America);
- > 100 IU/L (Europe).

Responders should be retested annually.

Revaccination of nonresponders with three additional doses is recommended.

No additional doses of vaccine should be given if there is still no response to the second series.

In responders whose HBsAb levels decline below protective levels a booster dose is recommended.

Patients as peritoneal dialysis should be similarly vaccinated.

Hepatitis C

Hepatitis C virus (HCV) was discovered in 1989 and causes the majority of cases previously labelled as non-A, non-B hepatitis.

HCV is a small RNA hepacivirus of the Flaviviridae family.

At least six different genotypes and >90 subtypes of HCV exist, with genotype 1 associated with more severe disease and worse clinical outcomes.

Unlike HBV virus, infection with one HCV genotype or subtype does not protect against reinfection or superinfection with other HCV strains.

There is no correlation between the severity of hepatic lesions and viral genotype or viral load.

HCV infection increases the risk of all cause death in ESRD patients.

HCV is transmitted via direct percutaneous exposure to infectious blood.

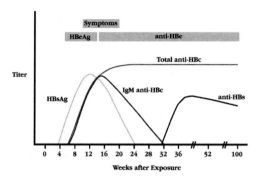

Fig. 11.7.1 Serologic course of hepatitis B virus infection.

Table 11.7.1 Interpretation of the hepatitis B panel

HBsAg	HBsAb	HBcAb	HBeAg	HBeAb	Interpretation
+	–	–	+	–	Incubation period.
+	–	IgM	+	–	Acute hepatitis B or persistent carrier state, high infectivity.
+	–	IgG	+	–	Chronic hepatitis B, high infectivity.
+	–	IgG	–	+	Chronic hepatitis B with low infectivity or 'pre-core mutant' hepatitis B.
–	±	IgG	–	+	Recovery from natural infection.
–	–	IgM	–	–	Infection with HBV without detectable HBsAg.
–	+	–	–	–	Post immunization or recovery from infection with loss of detectable anti-HBcAb.

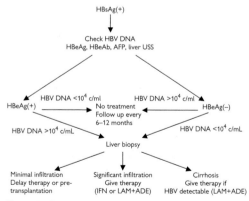

Fig. 11.7.2 Diagnostic and therapeutic algorithm for management of hepatitis B infection in patients with renal disease. IFN, interferon-α; LAM, lamivudine; ADE, adefovir; c/mL, copies/mL.

Table 11.7.2 Dosing recommendations in patients with ESRD

Drug	Dosage
IFN-α-2b	3 million units (MU) SC three times per week[a]
PEG-IFN-α-2a	135 µg SC once per week[a]
PEG-IFN-α-2b	0.5–1.0 µg/kg SC once per week[a]
Lamivudine	35 mg first dose, then 10 mg PO qds
Adefovir	10 mg PO every week

[a] These drugs should be administered post HD.

Epidemiology

The prevalence of HCV infection is 8–20% in HD patients in Europe and North America (10-fold greater than in the general population) and much higher in Asia and South America.

Risk factors

- multiple transfusions;
- local levels of hepatitis C carriage;
- duration of HD;
- prevalence of HCV-positive patients in the unit;
- failing to follow standard infection practices;
- not periodically screening patients for HCV;
- dialysis modality (greater incidence in in-centre than home hemodialysis or peritoneal dialysis);
- previous organ transplantation;
- IV drug abuse.

Clinical features

HCV causes both acute and chronic hepatitis. The incubation period ranges from 14 to 180 days (average: 6–7 weeks).

HCV-infected ESRD patients are usually either asymptomatic or have a mild clinical illness and rarely show biochemical evidence of active liver disease, i.e. fluctuating ALT levels.

ESRD patients with HCVAb are at risk of developing hepatic cirrhosis and HCC.

Investigations

Liver biopsy is the most accurate tool for assessing severity of HCV infection.

Serological assays

- HCVAb

There are three generations of tests for antibodies against HCV, with the newer tests having higher sensitivity and specificity.

They include the general screening enzyme immunoassays (EIAs) and the recombinant immunoblot assay (RIBA™) which is used to confirm the EIA or clarify inconclusive tests.

Nucleic acid detection

A quantitative test for HCV viral copy number is available and measures hepatitis C viral load (expressed in copies/mL).

Treatment

Interferon-α and pegylated interferon-α are the only available therapeutic agents for HCV infection in patients with ESRD.

HCV genotype is the strongest predictive factor of response to treatment.

Infection with genotypes 2 and 3 have a better response to therapy than patients with genotype 1.

Ribavirin is also used for treating HCV infection but is cleared by the kidneys and cannot be removed by dialysis.

It may cause a marked hemolytic anemia and because of this it is not used in patients with advanced CKD and ESRD.

Prophylaxis

General measures

- Segregation of HCV-infected patients from uninfected patients during dialysis.

- National and international recommendations do not include dedicated machines for patients with HCV.
- Despite this, some centers have separate HD machines in dedicated areas (not necessarily a single room) for HCV infected patients.
- Screening of all new patients and the HCV⁻ patient population for HCVAb every 3–6 months.
- Adherence to infection control precautions.

HCV-infected patients should be screened for the presence of hepatic cirrhosis and HCC.

Hepatitis D

Delta hepatitis is caused by the hepatitis delta virus (HDV), a defective virus that causes infection either as a coinfection with HBV or as a superinfection in a person with chronic HBV infection.

Infection carries a high risk of subsequent hepatic cirrhosis and hepatocellular cancer.

HDVAb measurement is only indicated in HBV-infected patients.

Prevention of HBV infection will prevent HDV infection.

Isolation of HDV-infected patients from other dialysis patients is recommended, especially those who are HBsAg positive.

Further reading

European Best Practice Guidelines on Hemodialysis. *Nephrol Dial Transplant* 2002; **7**(Suppl 7): 78–86.

Olsen SK, Brown RS. Hepatitis B treatment: lessons for the nephrologists. *Kidney Int* 2006; **70**: 1897–1904.

Russo MW, Goldsweig CD, Jacobson IM, Brown RS. Interferon monotherapy for dialysis patients with chronic hepatitis C: an analysis of the literature on efficacy and safety. *Am J Gastroenterol* 2003; **98**: 1610–1615.

Sweny PS, Rubin R, Tolkoff-Rubin N (eds). *The infectious complications of renal disease.* Oxford: Oxford University Press; 2003.

Wong P-N ,Fung T-T, Mak S-K, et al. Hepatitis B virus infection in dialysis patients. *J Gastroenterol Hepatol* 2005; **20**: 1641–1651.

Internet resources

MMWR Recommendations for Preventing Transmission of Infections Among Chronic Hemodialysis Patients:

http://www.cdc.gov

Clinical Practice Guidelines for the Care of Patients with Chronic Kidney Disease UK Renal Association. (Guideline CKD 3.3):

http://www.renal.org/guidelines/

European Best Practice Guidelines:

http://www.ndt-educational.org/guidelines.asp

Department of Health. Good practice guidelines for renal dialysis/transplantation units: prevention and control of bloodborne virus infection:

http://www.library.nhs.uk/guidelinesFinder/

European recommendations for the management of healthcare workers occupationally exposed to hepatitis B virus and hepatitis C virus:

http://www.eurosurveillance.org

See also

Medical management of dialysis patients, p. 528

Polycystic kidney disease in children, p. 586

Autosomal dominant polycystic kidney disease, p. 590

Hematological disorders in chronic kidney disease

The patient with failing renal function is susceptible to disorders of erythrocyte synthesis, platelet function and leukocyte function.

Anemia

Anemia may be defined as:

- hemoglobin <11.5 g/dL in females;
- hemoglobin <13.5 g/dL in males.

Relative erythropoietin (EPO) deficiency occurs in early CKD although overt anemia is unusual prior to CKD 4 (EPOETIN DARBOPOETIN ERYTHROPOETIN eDER eGFR <30 mL/min/1.73 m^2).

The cause of anemia in patients with renal disease extends beyond a relative deficiency of EPO and is frequently multifactorial.

Normal erythropoiesis

Red cell production in the bone marrow maintains a circulating population of >1 × 10^{14} erythrocytes.

Under the influence of EPO, burst-forming units—erythroid (BFU-E) multiply and differentiate into proerythrocytes and finally mature red cells.

EPO is predominantly secreted from peritubular fibroblasts within the renal cortex. In response to hypoxia, the number of EPO-secreting cells increases.

A small proportion of circulating EPO originates in the liver.

Anemia is the most prominent stimulus to EPO release.

Oxygen-sensing mechanisms
The rate of secretion of EPO from the renal cortex is determined by the number of functioning nephrons and the difference between parenchymal oxygen supply and demand.

EPO gene expression is regulated by the binding of hypoxia-inducible factor (HIF), a transcription factor, to the hypoxia response element (HRE) at the loci of the *EPO* gene on chromosome 7q22.

HIF is a heterodimer consisting of a constitutively expressed β-subunit and an α-subunit which, in the kidney, can be induced by hypoxia.

In conditions of normoxia HIF-α undergoes hydroxylation by oxygen-dependent hydroxylases. Hydroxylated HIF-α binds to von Hippel–Lindau ubiquitin ligase prompting subsequent proteosomal destruction.

In hypoxic conditions hydroxylation of HIF-α does not occur. Heterodimerization with the β-subunit forms the active transcription factor (Fig. 11.8.1).

Causes of anemia in CKD

Common causes of anemia in CKD are listed in Table 11.8.1.

Erythropoetin deficiency
As renal dysfunction worsens the number of functioning EPO-secreting cells decreases and an appropriate compensatory response to anemia is not possible.

The response of the remaining functioning cells to hypoxia is blunted as a consequence of decreased oxygen use by the damaged parenchyma and the effect of inflammatory cytokines.

Decreased red cell survival
Circulating erythrocytes have a lifespan of ~100 days in health. Uremia can induce chronic hemolysis, reducing red cell half-life by up to 50%.

Overt or occult blood loss
May occur as a result of platelet dysfunction, 'lost lines' during hemodialysis, uremic gastritis or gastric antral vascular ectasia.

Decreased bone marrow response
Absolute or functional iron deficiency is the commonest cause (see below).

Aluminium toxicity may contribute but is seen less commonly than in the past.

Numerous 'uremic inhibitors' of erythropoiesis have been postulated including parathyroid hormone and polyamines such as spermine.

Adequate dialysis and control of hyperparathyroidism lead to decreased EPO requirements but a pathogenic role for these compounds in impaired erythropoiesis has not been established.

Anemia related to underlying disease
Common secondary causes of renal disease may be associated with anemia such as systemic lupus erythematosus (SLE), multiple myeloma, sickle cell disease or amyloidosis.

Treatment of the underlying disease may ameliorate the anemia.

Anemia secondary to treatment of underlying disease
Immunosuppressant therapy for vasculitis or SLE leads to bone marrow suppression. Dose modification may be required or alternative treatment regimes prescribed.

Chemotherapy for multiple myeloma and other neoplastic disease is commonly associated with decreased erythropoiesis. Antiviral therapy for chronic hepatitis or the human immunodeficiency virus may lead to hemolysis or myelosuppression.

Anemia secondary to concurrent disease
Patients with failing renal function are just as likely as the general population to have common unrelated conditions which may lead to anemia such as pernicious anemia, hypothyroidism, celiac disease and primary hematological disease.

Treatment

There is marked variability in EPO levels between patients and the measurement of serum EPO levels is neither recommended nor useful in diagnosis (Fig. 11.8.2).

EPO replacement therapy for patients with CKD should be considered after investigation for alternative causes of anemia (Table 11.8.2).

Erythropoiesis-stimulating agents (ESAs)
Recombinant human EPO may be administered SC or IV.

Patients receiving hemodialysis may prefer the IV route.

SC administration offers higher bioavailability and ~20% lower dosing.

Dosing schedules are summarized in Table 11.8.3.

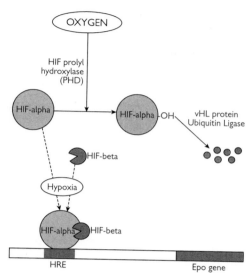

Fig. 11.8.1 Oxygen sensing and regulation of the erythropoietin gene.

Table 11.8.2 Investigation of anemia in CKD

Recommended initial investigations
- Hemoglobin concentration
- Mean corpuscular volume and hemoglobin
- Reticulocyte count
- Serum ferritin
- Serum transferrin saturation *or* reticulocyte hemoglobin content *or* percentage hypochromic red cells
- C-reactive protein

Further investigation in selected patients
- Serum vitamin B12 and folate concentration
- Parathyroid hormone concentration
- Haptoglobin, lactate dehydrogenase, bilirubin, direct Coombs test
- Serum and urine protein electrophoresis
- Hemoglobin electrophoresis
- Serum aluminium
- Faecal occult blood and/or GI endoscopy

Table 11.8.1 Causes of anemia in CKD

Erythropoietin deficiency

Decreased red cell survival
- Chronic uremic hemolysis
- Gastric antral vascular ectasia or other GI loss
- Hemodialysis

Decreased bone marrow response
- Absolute iron deficiency
- Functional iron deficiency
- 'Uremic inhibitors'
- Aluminium toxicity

Relating to underlying disease
- Myeloma
- SLE
- Amyloid
- Sickle cell

Relating to treatment
- Immunosuppressant therapy
- Idiosyncratic reactions

Concurrent unrelated disease
- Pernicious anemia
- Hemoglobinopathies
- Celiac disease
- Hypothyroidism

In practice, patients are usually started on a dose of ESA that corresponds as closely as possible to one of the available prefilled syringes.

Higher initial doses may be appropriate in severe anemia (hemoglobin <8.0 g/dL).

Darbepoetin-α has two additional glycosylation chains and eight additional sialic acid residues making it more resistant to metabolic degradation.

One microgram of darbepoetin-α is approximately bioequivalent to 200 U of epoetin-α, -β and -δ.

Mircera® (methoxy-polyethylene glycol–epoetin-β) is a continuous erythropoietin receptor activator which has a longer biological half-life allowing monthly dosing.

Newer ESAs in development include:
- biosimilars/generic ESAs (e.g. epoetin-γ);
- erythropoietin-mimetic peptides (hematide);
- oral agents which inhibit hydroxylation of HIF-α.

Clinical benefits of ESAs include:
- increased exercise tolerance;
- decreased angina episodes;
- decreased left ventricular hypertrophy;
- improved quality of life;
- improved cognitive function.

Inadequate correction of anemia limits these benefits.

Conversely, correction of anemia to 'normal values' may lead to increased cardiovascular morbidity.

Treatment guidelines
There is slight variation between the various national and international guidelines for the management of renal anemia and these are summarized in Table 11.8.4.

Assessment of response to treatment by hemoglobin concentration measurement is recommended every 2 weeks until target hemoglobin is reached with a stable ESA dose.

Hemoglobin concentration should not rise by >2 g/dL/month.

When hemoglobin is stable, hemoglobin concentration should be checked every 1–2 months and ESA dose adjusted accordingly (Fig. 11.8.3).

Iron
Erythropoiesis requires 30–40 mg of iron per day. In the steady state this is available from red cell destruction. During the correction phase of anemia supplemental iron is required.

Insufficient availability of iron is the most common cause of an inadequate response to ESA therapy.

Absolute iron deficiency occurs when iron loss, usually as a result of blood loss, exceeds the erythropoietic requirement.

Functional iron deficiency is a result of inadequate mobilization of iron from stores to bone marrow.

Target values for iron stores are higher in CKD than those regarded as normal in the non-CKD population (Table 11.8.4).

Measurement of iron stores is challenging (Fig. 11.8.4).

Iron staining of bone marrow is widely quoted as the 'gold standard' but is invasive.

Serum iron measurement is effectively obsolete as the amounts present are minute and quantities are markedly labile.

Serum ferritin offers an estimation of reticuloendothelial iron, the predominant source of stored iron. Ferritin may be elevated in infection, inflammation, malignancy or liver disease, independent of iron stores. A low ferritin is diagnostic of iron deficiency

Transferrin acts as a binding protein to transport iron to bone marrow. The percentage of transferrin saturated with iron (TSAT) reveals the balance between iron supply and demand.

The percentage of red cells which are hypochromic is more sensitive at confirming iron deficiency but is less available.

Reticulocyte hemoglobin concentration is a more accurate assessor of functional iron status but, again, this is not widely available.

Oral supplemental iron is rarely adequate to maintain erythropoiesis in CKD. Tolerability is limited by gastrointestinal side-effects. Interaction with phosphate binders in the gut limits iron bioavailability.

IV iron preparations are more effective in increasing measurements of iron store availability and attaining hemoglobin target. Newer preparations have a low incidence of side-effects.

ESA resistance
An inadequate response to ESA may be caused by:
- absolute or relative iron deficiency;
- inflammation;
- underdialysis;
- hyperparathyroidism;
- malignancy;
- other hematinic deficiencies;
- aluminium toxicity.

Acute illness in patients with advanced CKD frequently precipitates anemia. Increasing ESA dose is rarely effective and blood transfusion may be required.

Side-effects of ESA therapy
ESA therapy may be associated with:
- hypertension;
- vascular access thrombosis;
- encephalopathy;
- influenza-like symptoms;
- hyperkalemia.

Iatrogenic polycythemia should be avoided.

Pure red cell aplasia is a rare complication of ESA therapy characterized by:
- antibodies against EPO;
- absent erythropoiesis on bone marrow examination and very low reticulocyte count;
- ESA resistance;
- transfusion-dependent anemia.

Immunosuppressive regimes using corticosteroids and cyclophosphamide, ciclosporin and rituximab have led to the disappearance of anti-EPO antibodies in some patients. Reintroduction of ESA therapy may be successful in those without measurable antibody titers following treatment.

Table 11.8.3 Recommended dosing for ESA therapy

ESA	Initiation	Maintenance
Epoetin-α	50 U/kg 3 times per week	1–3 times/week
Epoetin-β	20 U/kg 3 times per week	1–3 times/week
Epoetin-δ	50 U/kg 3 times per week (IV) 2 times per week (SC)	1–3 times/week
Darbepoetin	450 ng/kg Once per week	Weekly or fortnightly (or monthly if predialysis)
Mircera®	0.6 µg/kg Once per 2 weeks	Monthly

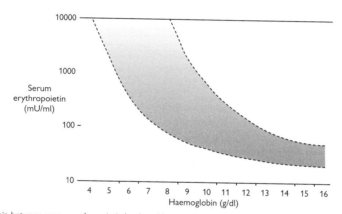

Fig. 11.8.2 Relationship between serum erythropoietin levels and hemoglobin in patients with normal renal function.

Table 11.8.4 Guidelines for target indices in managing renal anemia

European Best Practice Guidelines (2004)	Hb 11.0–12.0 g/dL[a]	Ferritin >100 ng/ml TSAT >20% or hypochromic red cells <10% or CHr >29 pg/cell
NICE (2006)	Hb 10.5–12.5 g/dL	Ferritin 200–500 ng/mL TSAT >20% or hypochromic red cells <6%
Renal Association (2007)	Hb 10.5–12.5 g/dL	Ferritin 200–500 ng/mL (HD) or 100–500 ng/mL (non-HD) TSAT >20% or hypochromic red cells <6%
NKF-K/DOQI (2007)	Hb 11.0–12.0 g/dL	Ferritin >200 ng/mL (HD) or >100 ng/mL (non-HD) TSAT >20% or CHr >29 pg/cell

[a]Target Hb up to 14.0 g/dL for patients with chronic obstructive pulmonary disease.

Hb, hemoglobin; TSAT, transferrin saturation; CHr, reticulocyte hemoglobin concentration; HD, hemodialysis.

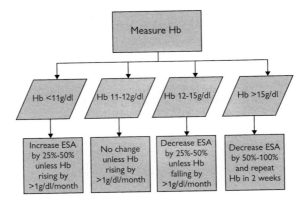

Fig. 11.8.3 Adjusting ESA dosage.

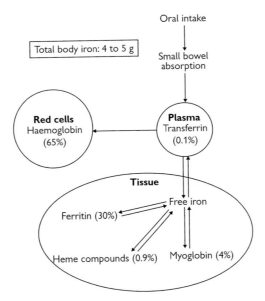

Fig. 11.8.4 Iron utilization.

ESA therapy and tumor progression

The use of ESAs in treating anemia associated with malignancy has shown an increase in the rate of tumor progression in some patients.

Increased rates of malignancy in patients with CKD treated with ESAs have not been identified.

Other therapies

Patients with profound symptomatic anemia or ESA resistance may benefit from blood transfusion. Repeated transfusions can be complicated by:

• iron overload;
• transmission of bloodborne infections;
• HLA sensitization.

Androgens stimulate endogenous EPO production and can decrease ESA requirements and blood transfusions. They have limited efficacy, however, and treatment can be complicated by hepatobiliary disease, virilization and muscle damage.

Polycythemia

Excess erythrocyte production is uncommon in patients with failing renal function.

Increased EPO secretion may be associated with:

• autosomal dominant polycystic kidney disease;
• hydronephrosis;
• renal cell carcinoma;
• simple renal cysts.

The etiology is unclear, although local tissue hypoxia secondary to structural changes has been implicated.

Post-transplant polycythemia

Up to a fifth of patients develop polycythemia following renal transplantation.

This can be secondary to increased bone marrow sensitivity, or to recovery of the hypoxic response of fibroblasts in the native kidney leading to excess EPO synthesis.

Treatment with ACEIs is effective at reducing the polycythemic response.

Venesection is recommended if the hematocrit remains >50%.

Platelet dysfunction

Impaired platelet function in renal impairment is characterized by:

• impaired von Willebrand factor-dependent platelet aggregation;
• impaired endothelial adhesion;
• reduced thrombopoiesis and decreased mean platelet half-life.

Thrombocytopenia is uncommon but may be associated with hepatitis C infection or following heparin exposure in hemodialysis.

By contrast, platelet dysfunction is common in patients with CKD and manifests as bruising, purpura and epistaxis. Platelet function is further impaired by aspirin, dipyridamole or heparin. Platelet count and coagulation cascade studies do not reveal abnormal platelet function.

Platelet function improves after:

• correction of anemia;
• adequate renal replacement therapy;
• desmopressin.

Desmopressin promotes the release of preformed von Willebrand factor and can improve platelet function for up to 4 h. Treatment is with 0.2–0.3 μg/kg of desmopressin IV prior to renal biopsy or surgery.

Leukocyte abnormalities

Functional defects of humoral and cellular immunity are common with uremia. Phagocytic activity of circulating neutrophils is decreased and rates of lymphocyte maturation and activation are reduced. Adequacy of dialysis does not correlate with recovery of leukocyte function.

Vaccination in patients with advanced renal insufficiency is often unsuccessful.

Lymphoid and myeloid suppression may also be associated with underlying disease and its treatment, including:

• SLE;
• rheumatoid arthritis;
• myeloma;
• human immunodeficiency virus;
• hepatitis C.

Further reading

Drüeke TB, Locatelli F, Clyne N, *et al.* Normalization of hemoglobin level in patients with chronic kidney disease and anaemia. *N Engl J Med* 2006; **355**; 2071–2084.

Mannucci PM, Remuzzi G, Pusineri F, *et al.* Deamino-8-D-arginine vasopressin shortens the bleeding time in uraemia. *N Engl J Med* 1983; **308**: 8–12.

Ratcliffe PJ. Understanding hypoxia signalling in cells – a new therapeutic opportunity? *Clin Med* 2006; **6**: 573–578.

Singh AK, Szczech L, Tang KL, *et al.* Correction of anaemia with epoetin alfa in chronic kidney disease. *N Engl J Med* 2006; **355**; 2085–2098.

Internet resources

Renal Association Clinical Practice Guidelines:

`http://www.renal.org/pages/pages/clinical-affairs/guidelines.php`

National Kidney Federation Dialysis Outcomes Quality Initiative (NKF-KDOQI):

`http://www.kidney.org/professionals/kdoqi/`

European Best Practice Guidelines:

`http://www.ndt-educational.org/guidelines.asp`

National Institute for Clinical Excellence:

`http://www.nice.org.uk/`

See also

Coagulation disorders in CKD, p. 444

Immune function in CKD, p. 440

Medical management of dialysis patients, p. 528

Skeletal disorders in chronic kidney disease

Introduction
Renal bone disease (osteodystrophy) has its origins early in the course of CKD, so that by the time GFR has fallen to 50% of normal (CKD 3), ~50% of patients have abnormal bone histology. This approaches 100% in patients by the time of starting dialysis (CKD 5). Disordered skeletal metabolism is associated with an increased risk of cardiovascular disease.

Bone as a tissue
The skeleton is continually remodeled in health, with a balance between synthesis, mineralization and resorption.

Bone is formed from parallel bundles of collagen, calcified by fixation of hydroxyapatite crystals.

There are three main cell types in bone:
- osteoblasts (build new bone) at bone surfaces;
- osteoclasts (cut into and resorb bone) releasing calcium and phosphate;
- osteocytes buried within calcified bone, connected to one another by microfilaments within canaliculi.

Classification of skeletal lesions
Little is known about skeletal lesions in CKD 3 and 4, but most patients have abnormal histology in CKD 5.

There are three main diagnostic groups:

High turnover lesions
Associated with high PTH, hyperactive bone cells and excess bone resorption.

Low turnover lesions
Associated with normal or low PTH and little or no bone cell activity (adynamic bone).

Mixed lesions
Features of high and low turnover, and no correlation with PTH levels.

In addition, elderly patients, or those exposed to steroids, may have superimposed osteoporosis.

Osteomalacia due to aluminium deposition or vitamin D deficiency is now rare except in certain ethnic groups.

Pathogenesis
Control of bone metabolism is incompletely understood, even in health, and therefore many aspects of renal bone disease remain controversial.

It is multifactorial, and dependent on complex interactions between:
- vitamin D metabolism;
- PTH & calcium;
- phosphate;
- magnesium;
- acid–base balance.

For simplicity each will be considered individually:

Vitamin D deficiency
Vitamin D3 (calciferol) circulates in the blood bound to vitamin D-binding protein, and is metabolized in the liver by vitamin-D-25-hydroxylase to form 25-(OH) vitamin D.

In the kidney 25-(OH) vitamin D is further metabolized by 1α-hydroxylase to form 1,25-(OH)$_2$ vitamin D3 (calcitriol), the biologically active form of vitamin D.

In CKD, deficiency of 1α-hydroxylase results in calcitriol deficiency. If not replaced this results in:
- reduced dietary calcium uptake;
- hypocalcemia and PTH stimulation;
- failure to directly suppress parathyroid cells.

Vitamin D also has immunoregulatory functions and may be involved in immune surveillance for tumor cells.

Parathyroid hormone and calcium
PTH is a single-chain protein of 84 amino acids, synthesized in the parathyroid chief cell.

Increased secretion increases both number and activity of osteoclasts and osteoblasts.

PTH secretion is:
- controlled by the concentration of ionized calcium, so hypocalcemia stimulates, and hypercalcemia suppresses, PTH levels;
- stimulated by hyperphosphatemia;
- suppressed by oral or IV vitamin D, via receptors on parathyroid cell nuclei, and by severe hypomagnesemia.

PTH is incompletely metabolized in CKD 4/5 so that PTH fragments accumulate and may give false readings with certain PTH assays.

Mild elevations of PTH are evident even at a GFR of 60 mL/min.

Phosphate
Hyperphosphatemia is associated with vascular and cardiac calcification and mortality.

Increased serum phosphate levels:
- suppress 1α-hydroxylase activity and therefore vitamin D production;
- directly stimulate PTH production;
- stimulate mineralization of vascular tissue *in vitro*.

Magnesium
Levels tend to be elevated in CKD, but overall importance unclear.

Low magnesium levels are uncommon in CKD, but:
- moderate hypomagnesemia stimulates PTH production;
- severe hypomagnesemia inhibits PTH production.

Acid–base balance
Acidosis tends to stimulate PTH production and osteoclast activity. Treatment with sodium bicarbonate can reduce PTH levels by up to 20%.

Clinical features
History
Important factors to consider include:
- gender;
- menopausal status;
- duration of renal impairment;
- chronic back pain;
- previous fractures with minimal trauma;
- drug history (steroids, ciclosporin, thyroid hormone, anticonvulsants, heparin);
- alcohol intake.

Symptoms and signs

Low turnover lesions are usually asymptomatic, but osteomalacia and advanced high turnover lesions with very high PTH cause nonspecific symptoms such as proximal muscle weakness and fatigue.

High PTH also causes:

- depression;
- limb and abdominal aches and pains;
- tendon ruptures.

Unless the patient has severe hyperparathyroidism it is unlikely that there will be signs on examination, but established osteoporosis may be evident, particularly in elderly females.

Investigations

Few CKD patients undergo formal skeletal assessment despite being high risk for a variety of skeletal problems including osteoporosis.

Parathyroid hormone

Measurement of circulating PTH is the most useful method of assessing bone turnover rate.

Measurement of PTH every 3 months is usual in dialysis patients.

Measurement of PTH should also be considered in earlier stages of CKD (CKD 4 and possibly CKD 3) although opinion varies about the required frequency and utility of this.

There is no indication to measure PTH in CKD 1 or 2 in the absence of a suspected disorder of bone and mineral metabolism.

Older assay methods detect PTH fragments as well as whole PTH molecules, but values still appear to reflect bone turnover.

Values between 0 and 2× upper limit of normal (ULN) suggest a low turnover lesion.

Values >8× ULN suggest a high turnover lesion.

Values between 2 and 8× ULN on a single measurement are unhelpful; the trend may help to guide treatment.

Calcium, phosphate and alkaline phosphatase

In high turnover bone lesions, serum calcium and phosphate may be elevated because of release from the skeleton by overactive osteoclasts, rather than dietary intake.

In low turnover adynamic lesions, hypercalcemia is common because excess calcium cannot be incorporated into bone by inactive osteoblasts.

Alkaline phosphatase is produced by intestine, liver and bone, so does not correlate well with bone turnover. The bone-specific isoenzyme gives a better correlation but is not used in routine practice.

Radiology, bone density and isotope studies

Skeletal surveys are not regularly used to monitor osteodystrophy, except when myeloma is suspected.

Plain radiographs will only detect advanced osteodystrophy, but will reveal vascular calcification.

DEXA measurement of bone density at the start of dialysis is useful if locally available, so that sequential studies enable meaningful monitoring of change.

Bone biopsy

Transiliac bone biopsy is the only way to accurately diagnose the type and severity of osteodystrophy.

It is relatively invasive, and requires two doses of tetracycline at 14 days and 4 days before the biopsy, which appear in the bone as discrete bands on fluorescent microscopy, enabling measurement of bone growth rates.

It can be helpful, but few laboratories have the expertise to process and analyse biopsies so it is only routinely used within research projects.

Treatment

By controlling serum values of various ions and molecules, mineral metabolism can be influenced.

Many guidelines exist but almost all are based on opinion.

Significant differences exist between UK and US practice.

Table 11.9.1 summarizes UK Renal Association guidelines.

In CKD 5, management is difficult unless dialysis adequacy is appropriate and basic dietary advice is being followed.

Currently only ~10% of dialysis patients achieve all targets simultaneously.

Once adequate dialysis and dietary management are in place almost all patients require pharmacological intervention too.

If phosphate remains very high with adequate doses of phosphate binder, severe high turnover bone lesions should be considered as a possible cause, not dietary intake.

Table 11.9.2 summarizes the assessment and treatment of the patient with CKD 5 and suspected disorder of bone and mineral metabolism.

Available agents include:

Oral sodium bicarbonate

Usually not required in PD patients, but may be required to maintain serum bicarbonate within the normal range in HD patients and CKD 4/5.

Oral phosphate binders

These must be in the stomach with food to bind phosphate and reduce serum levels.

As many patients only eat two main meals per day, twice daily dosing is common, divided 2/3 and 1/3 in proportion to meal size.

All binders cause GI side-effects in up to 20% of patients.

Aluminium hydroxide

Effective but significant toxicity limits usefulness.

Requires 3-monthly serum aluminium monitoring.

Avoid if possible.

Inexpensive.

Calcium carbonate/acetate

Effective binders but increasing (unproven) concern exists about calcium loading contributing to cardiovascular mortality.

Avoid if there is hypercalcemia.

Inexpensive.

Sevelamer hydrochloride

- Large doses and pill burden may be required.
- Expensive.

Lanthanum carbonate

- Effective with reduced pill burden.
- Expensive.

Table 11.9.1. UK Renal Association targets for calcium, phosphate, PTH and calcium phosphate product in CKD

Serum calcium	
CKD 1–4	Should be maintained within the local laboratory's normal range.
	Hypercalcemia will accelerate loss of renal function.
CKD 5	Should be maintained within the local laboratory's normal range (albumin-corrected, measured before a 'short gap' dialysis session in HD patients).
	Ideally keep <2.5 mmol/L.
	Higher values are associated with vascular calcification and (in retrospective studies only) increased mortality.
Serum phosphate	
CKD 1–4	Should be maintained between 0.9 and 1.5 mmol/L: dietary restriction initially.
CKD 5	Should be maintained between 1.1 and 1.8 mmol/L (measured before a 'short gap' dialysis session in HD patients).
	Ideally keep <1.4 mmol/L.
	Higher values are strongly associated with vascular calcification and (in retrospective studies only) increased mortality.
	Values <1.0 mmol/L suggest poor nutrition and should prompt dietetic review.
	Phosphate clearance can be improved by intensifying the dialysis regimen.
	Slow prolonged dialysis (>8h at night) or daily dialysis increases phosphate removal.
	However, these options may be feasible only for patients on home dialysis.
Calcium × phosphate product	Should be maintained <4.8 mmol^2/L^2 (with comment now in brackets underneath) (If the calcium and phosphate are within the desired ranges, then the product will be also, and calculating the product is probably unnecessary.– authors opinion)
Parathyroid hormone	UK target ranges for CKD, and post transplant, as follows:
CKD 1–3	Within the normal range.
CKD 4	Between the ULN and 2× ULN.
CKD 5	Between 2 and 4× ULN.

ULN, upper limit of normal.

Vitamin D analogues

Vitamin D therapy is used to reduce PTH levels.

A significant side-effect is increased intestinal absorption of calcium and phosphate which may aggravate skeletal problems.

Care must be taken not to oversuppress PTH and push the skeletal lesion towards adynamic bone.

Although newer expensive vitamin D analogues (e.g. paricalcitol) are said to have advantages over calcitriol or alfacalcidol, this remains to be proven. No prospective outcome studies have shown benefit.

CKD 3–4

Current UK recommendation is that if the PTH is above target range, 25-(OH) vitamin D levels should be measured and replacement therapy started if <75 nmol/L.

Many laboratories are unable to provide the 25-(OH) vitamin D assay so the recommendation is variably applied.

NICE is currently reviewing guidelines for the investigation and management of patients with CKD (available 2008).

CKD 5

Calcitriol or alfacalcidol therapy suppresses PTH in dialysis patients, and can be used in two ways.

If serum calcium <2.3 mmol/L:
- give daily oral dosages (250–500 ng) to raise calcium towards 2.5 mmol/L

If serum calcium >2.3 mmol/L:
- try twice weekly 'pulse therapy' (1.0–2.0 µg) either orally or IV and monitor effect on calcium and PTH.

Pulse therapy probably has a less hypercalcemic effect and achieves higher serum calcitriol levels.

Bisphosphonates

These can be used for osteoporosis if GFR >30 mL/min.

Bone biopsy recommended before use.

If GFR <30 mL/min, risks need to weighed against benefits, but remember that major fractures can be fatal.

Parathyroidectomy and calcimimetics

Surgical parathyroidectomy is indicated for treatment of symptomatic uncontrollable, tertiary hyperparathyroidism.

Features include:
- bone pain, anemia, malaise;
- PTH >10× ULN and rising;
- calcium and phosphate uncontrolled;
- calcific uremic arteriolopathy (calciphylaxis).

Surgery can be subtotal, total, or total with some tissue reimplanted in a limb.

Perioperative risk is greater in people with CKD, and there is the risk that any remaining parathyroid tissue may become hyperplastic and require repeat surgery.

Cinacalcet

Cinacalcet is a calcimimetic which increases the sensitivity of calcium-sensing receptors to extracellular calcium ions, inhibiting the release of PTH.

The starting dose is 30 mg daily, titrated every 2–4 weeks to maximum of 180 mg daily, to achieve the target level of intact PTH.

Table 11.9.2. Management of mineral metabolism in CKD stage 5

History

Review skeletal history: gender, age, fractures

Review previous drug history, especially steroid use if previously received renal transplant

Check for symptoms of skeletal disease, including non-specific aches/pains and depression

Examination

Vertebral collapse: 'Dowager's hump'

Proximal muscle weakness

Initial radiology

Plain radiographs of hands and pelvis

Look for vascular calcification

Consider DEXA bone density measurement

Biochemistry targets

Serum calcium within normal range, ideally <2.5 mmol/L

Serum phosphate 1.1–1.8 mmol/L

Serum PTH 2–4× ULN

General interventions

Arrange appropriate dietary modification

Ensure dialysis adequacy is optimal

Check dialyzate calcium concentration is appropriate

Pharmacological interventions

Oral sodium bicarbonate to correct venous serum bicarbonate

Oral phosphate binder taken with main meals

If PTH >4× ULN give alfacalcidol:

• 0.25 µg daily if serum calcium <2.3 mmol/L

• 2.0 µg twice weekly if serum calcium >2.3 mmol/L

Monitoring

Monthly biochemistry if on hemodialysis

1–3-monthly biochemistry if on PD

PTH check every 3 months, and look at trend

Education

Educate patient regarding significance of biochemistry results

Review adherence to diet, dialysis, drugs

Review latest results with patient

NICE guidelines (UK) on its use are:

Not recommended for the routine treatment of secondary hyperparathyroidism in patients with ESRD on maintenance dialysis therapy.

Recommended for the treatment of refractory secondary hyperparathyroidism in patients with ESRD (including those with calciphylaxis) only in those:

• with 'very uncontrolled' plasma levels of PTH (>85 pmol/ L (800 pg/mL)) and refractory to standard therapy, and a normal or high adjusted serum calcium level,

and

• in whom surgical parathyroidectomy is contraindicated, in that the risks of surgery are considered to outweigh the benefits

Treatment should be continued only if a reduction in PTH of ≥30% is seen within 4 months.

Tumoral calcification

This is often periarticular, and occasionally associated with acute periarticular inflammation.

It is usually associated with severe hyperphosphatemia in CKD 5.

Occasionally it may be mistaken for osteosarcoma.

It will regress if phosphate and calcium can be tightly controlled to <1.4 and <2.5 mmol/L respectively.

Calcific uremic arteriolopathy

This is a rare complication that can occur in people with CKD 5, usually with severe hyperparathryoidism.

It causes painful, purple/red cutaneous nodules (singular or numerous).

It progresses rapidly to ulceration, necrosis and sepsis of the skin and subcutaneous tissues.

Skin biopsy may make ulceration worse.

Mortality is high at ~50%, but it may respond to tight phosphate control and parathyroidectomy or cinacalcet treatment.

Future prospects

There is a pressing need for randomized prospective outcome studies in CKD to examine cost:benefit ratios of newer expensive pharmacological agents, as well as benefits of phosphate and PTH control (currently unproven).

Measurement of vascular calcification (with latest generation CT scanners or possibly plain X-ray) may identify patients who should avoid calcium-containing phosphate binders.

New oral noncalcium phosphate binders are in development including magnesium iron hydroxycarbonate and ferric citrate (both effective in phase II studies).

Prevention of intestinal phosphate absorption may be possible in the future by blockade of the ileal sodium-dependent phosphate cotransporter.

Further reading

Favus MJ (ed.). *Primer on the metabolic bone diseases and disorders of mineral metabolism*, 6th edn. American Society for Bone and Mineral Research; 2006.

Bushinsky D (ed). *Renal osteodystrophy*. Philadelphia: Lippincott–Raven Press; 1998.

Internet resources

UK Renal Association Mineral Bone Disease Guidelines:

http://www.renal.org/guidelines/module2.html

The National Kidney Federation Dialysis Outcomes Quality Initiative Bone and Mineral Metabolism Guidelines:

http://www.kidney.org/professionals/kdoqi/guidelines_bone/index.htm

European Best Practice Guidelines:

http://www.ndt-educational.org/guidelines.asp

National Institute for Health and Clinical Excellence (NICE):

http://www.nice.org.uk

See also

Medical management of dialysis patients, p. 528

Cardiovascular risk factors in CKD, p. 412

β2-Microglobulin amyloidosis in chronic kidney disease

β2-Microglobulin amyloidosis (Aβ2M) is a systemic disorder characteristically observed in individuals with chronic uremia.

The hallmark of the disease is the abnormal tissue deposition of amyloid fibrils of which the primary constituent is β2-microglobulin (β2M).

The underlying process is unaffected by mode of dialysis and potentially Aβ2M can be detected in predialysis patients.

Aβ2M carries with it a significant morbidity and mortality to patients with ESRD although changes in practice are aiming to reduce its burden.

Understanding the early pathological changes is crucial and makes this a fertile research field.

Pathogenesis

β2M is a nonglycosylated polypeptide of 11.8 kDa.

It is a component of the class I major histocompatibility complex and is present on the cell surface of virtually all nucleated cells.

Clearance occurs by glomerular filtration followed by proximal tubular cell (PTC) uptake and catabolism.

A raised serum level of β2M is a prerequisite for Aβ2M formation. This can result from increased production or decreased clearance of the molecule.

Causes of increased β2M production include:

- lymphoid cell activation (clonal B-cell disorders, various viral infections, rheumatoid arthritis, Crohn's disease and systemic lupus erythematosus);
- interferon-α therapy;
- metabolic acidosis;
- bioincompatibility of HD membranes.

Factors affecting clearance of β2M include:

- falling GFR;
- the mode of dialysis in ESRD.

A seemingly trivial residual GFR in ESRD can significantly increase renal clearance of β2M.

Although raised serum β2M levels are a prerequisite this alone is insufficient to initiate Aβ2M.

Generation of amyloid fibrils

Although it is well-documented that β2M can spontaneously assemble into amyloid fibrils *in vitro* there is discordance between the physicochemical conditions required for this and those that would occur pathophysiologically.

It is unclear how fibril seeds form *in vivo* although transient unfolding of the native protein under mildly acidic conditions has been suggested.

Once formed, fibril seeds can be stabilized by biologically relevant molecules (serum amyloid protein, apolipoprotein E, glycosaminoglycans, collagen and prostaglandins).

Such seeds then provide a focus for further elongation into fibrils using β2M. This process may be enhanced by the addition of uremic serum.

At a histological level these deposits will eventually disrupt tissue architecture and have a deleterious effect on function. There is also evidence that amyloid-derived fibrils are able to modify cell function at a much earlier point in the natural history, before clinical disease becomes apparent.

An interaction between advanced glycation end-products (AGE) and β2M has been reported resulting in activation of the receptor for AGE (RAGE) and a variety of intracellular signaling processes. This occurs prior to the histological detection of Aβ2M.

If pathophysiologically relevant processes are active before clinical disease becomes apparent, new therapies may be able to interrupt the long term effects of Aβ2M.

Epidemiology

This is markedly dependent upon the time spent on dialysis.

Post-mortem studies indicate a prevalence of ~20% after 1 year on dialysis rising to >90% after 9 years.

Clinical or radiological features are unlikely before 5 years on dialysis but then rise to ~50% at 15 years.

Histological detection is much greater than that found on clinical or radiological grounds.

Changes in practice would imply that greater clearances of β2M will result in a falling prevalence.

Clinical features

The major clinical features of Aβ2M relate to the musculoskeletal system.

Carpal tunnel syndrome (CTS)

This is one of most frequently encountered manifestations of Aβ2M.

On the basis of neurological involvement it is clinically indistinguishable from other causes of CTS.

It is, however, more likely to be exacerbated by dialysis sessions and at night.

A high index of suspicion should remain for other causes of CTS in renal patients (diabetes mellitus, myeloma and AL-amyloid).

Scapulohumeral periarthritis

The most commonly affected joint in Aβ2M is the shoulder.

Amyloid deposits are found in the synovial tissue and subacromial bursa.

Effusive arthropathy

This is commonly bilateral and affects the knees and shoulders.

It is characterized by restricted movement and pain.

It is exacerbated during dialysis and is worse at night.

Amyloid deposits may be found in the synovial fluid.

Bone cysts

These occur at the ends of long bones and contain amyloid deposits.

They may cause pathological fractures.

Spondyloarthropathy

This is radiologically characterized by cysts and narrowing of the intervertebral space.

Osteophytes are not a feature.

It can be compounded by coexistent hyperparathyroidism and aluminium overload.

It is associated with back pain of variable severity.

Rarely encroachment on the spinal cord may result in paralysis or a cauda equine syndrome.

Visceral involvement
Visceral involvement at postmortem is well-described though the functional consequences of such infiltration are less clear.

GI tract
Involvement is serosal rather than mucosal and at postmortem this gives a rippled appearance to the entire GI tract. It can cause bleeding, pseudo-obstruction, perforation, infarction and diarrhea.

Cardiovascular system
The literature is not extensive but the predominant sites of involvement are the walls of the small blood vessels supplying the myocardium. These changes have been reported at postmortem but there is no information on any functional correlation.

Risk factors for cardiac involvement are age at onset of dialysis and the duration of dialysis treatment.

Respiratory system
It is a rare cause of pulmonary hypertension but has been described as a cause of exudative pleural effusions in long-term hemodialysis patients.

Skin
Cutaneous involvement has been described although it is rare.

Investigations

Histology
The 'gold standard' remains the histological examination of affected tissue.

In common with other forms of amyloid, Aβ2M stains with Congo Red and there is apple-green birefringence under polarized light.

Joint aspiration may yield Aβ2M in synovial tissue fragments.

Biopsy of rectal mucosa is of low yield and may reflect the serosal rather than mucosal pattern of involvement.

Radiology

Plain radiography
Features include:
- swelling of the soft tissues around the joint;
- preserved or widened joint space with juxta-articular cystic bone lesions.

Typical joints affected are the wrist, shoulder and hip.

Over time the size and number of cysts increases ($\geq$30% per year).

For a diagnosis of Aβ2M changes must be present in at least two joints.

CT and MRI
Useful when lesions are too small to see with plain radiography.

Particularly useful for investigating potential involvement of the nonaxial skeleton.

MRI is useful for the diagnosis of Aβ2M spondyloarthropathy and spondylodiscitis.

Ultrasonography
May be of use in detecting synovial sheath thickening or rotator cuff enlargement.

Scintigraphy
Serum amyloid P (SAP) is a liver synthesized glycoprotein that binds noncovalently and in a calcium-dependent manner to virtually all forms of amyloid fibrils.

Use of radiolabelled SAP for the detection of Aβ2M has been limited largely by the poor sensitivity and specificity of the investigation.

Use of [131I]β2M has produced mixed results. Generally the sensitivity and specificity are better than the combined use of clinical and radiological evidence. The high cost of the investigation precludes its widespread use in clinical practice.

Treatment

Medical management
Simple analgesia

Intra-articular corticosteroid injections are useful when a single joint is affected. As with all joint injections their effect is transitory and carries a definite risk of septic arthritis.

Oral prednisolone (0.1 mg/kg/day) may be helpful.

Surgical management
The natural history is for nerve entrapment syndromes to be progressive and therefore early intervention is warranted to prevent permanent neurological deficit.

Arthroscopic or open surgery for affected shoulder joints and removal of affected synovium has a marked analgesic effect.

Curettage of cysts within the femoral head and subsequent bone grafting has been reported to reduce hip pain.

Prosthetic replacement of affected joints may be considered on an individual basis and may result in beneficial effects on pain and mobility.

Renal transplantation
Renal transplantation results in the most significant improvement in symptoms and may arrest disease progression.

β2M levels fall to the normal range.

Pain from affected joints is reduced. This has been attributed in the short term to the beneficial effects of steroids but the effect continues despite steroid dose reduction.

Regression of Aβ2M deposits following transplantation is difficult to assess.

Radiological lesions including bone cysts remain for 15 years post transplantation suggesting that pre-existing lesions may not regress.

Measures to reduce Aβ2M in patients with ESRD
Guidelines to reduce the risk of Aβ2M have been published (Table 11.10.1).

The use of high flux HD membranes reduces β2M levels probably by a combination of diffusion/convective mass transport and adsorption.

Hemodiafiltration also results in a substantially higher clearance of β2M as a result of convective removal.

Increased frequency and duration of dialysis will also reduce levels of β2M.

Whether lowering β2M levels equates to an improved clinical outcome has not been clearly established.

Trials of high flux dialysis, β2M and survival

A systematic review of 27 randomized trials comparing cellulose, modified cellulose and synthetic membranes showed a significant reduction in end-of-study β2M values when high flux synthetic membranes were used and one small study showed that dialysis-related amyloid occurred less frequently with this treatment.

The potential benefit of high flux membranes was examined prospectively in the HEMO study. No differences in overall mortality or secondary endpoints were observed between the groups that received high- or low-flux treatment. A 10-fold increase in β2M clearance was observed in the high flux group (β2M clearance of ≥20 mL/min) versus the low flux group. Secondary analysis of those that had been on dialysis for >3.7 years suggested that there may be an advantage to high flux dialysis on overall mortality.

The impact of high flux dialysis on outcome in HD is currently being assessed in the Membrane Permeability Outcome study (MPO) which has now finished recruitment.

Prognosis

Over time there is an inevitable increase in the deposition of β2M.

The rate of deposition is altered by reducing the production or clearance of β2M. Transplantation arrests disease progression. No other intervention achieves this effect.

There is no clear relationship between deposition of β2M and function of the affected organ.

Individual prognosis is difficult to assess. Genetic variability is important: polymorphisms in various cytokines, including transforming growth factor-β (TGF-β), are important in modifying disease progression.

Prognosis is affected by the clearance of other 'middle molecules' that have neutrophil inhibitory effects. This is thought to underly the susceptibility to infection of those with elevated serum β2M levels.

Future prospects

Extra- and intracorporeal techniques are being developed to facilitate removal of β2M although these are not currently in clinical use.

Immunoabsorbent technology using membrane-fixed antibodies against β2M has been developed and under laboratory conditions is capable of removing β2M.

In animal studies megalin-expressing cells implanted under the skin have been shown to bind and endocytose β2M. Megalin is a member of the low-density lipoprotein receptor superfamily that is expressed on a variety of secretory epithelia including the PTC and mediates uptake of a large number of ligands.

Further reading

Cheung AK, Rocco MV, Yan G, et al. for HEMO Study Group. Serum β-2 microglobulin levels predict mortality in dialysis patients: results of the HEMO Study. *J Am Soc Neph* 2006; **17**: 546–555.

Dember LM, Jaber BL. Dialysis-related amyloidosis: late finding or hidden epidemic? *Semin Dial* 2006; **19**: 105–109.

Grovender EA, Kellogg B, Singh J, et al. Single-chain antibody fragment-based adsorbent for the extracorporeal removal of β₂-microglobulin. *Kid Int* 2004; **65**: 310–322.

Jadoul M, van Ypersele C. β2M Amyloidosis. In: Davidson et al. (ed.), *Oxford Textbook of Nephrology*. Oxford: Oxford University Press; 2005. pp. 1861–1867.

Saito A, Geyjo F. Current clinical aspects of dialysis-related amyloidosis in chronic dialysis patients. *Ther Apheresis Dial* 2006; **10**: 316–320.

Winchester JF, Salsberg JA, Levin NW. Beta-2 microglobulin in ESRD: an in-depth review. *Adv Renal Replacement Therapy* 2003; **10**: 279–309.

Internet resources

Renal Association Clinical Practice Guidelines for Hemodialysis:

http://www.renal.org/guidelines/module3a.html

The Renal Registry:

http://www.renalreg.org

National Kidney Federation Dialysis Outcomes Quality Initiative:

http://www.kidney.org/professionals/kdoqi/

European Best Practice Guidelines:

http://www.ndt-educational.org/guidelines.asp

See also

Hemodialysis, hemofiltration and hemodiafiltration, p. 494

Adequacy of dialysis, p. 518

Medical management of dialysis patients, p. 528

Table 11.10.1 Guidelines for the management of β2-microglobulin amyloidosis (Aβ2M)

UK Renal Association (2007)

- Ultrapure water is easily available and should be regarded as standard.
- The use of high flux synthetic and modified cellulose dialysers can be justified on the basis of potentially beneficial biological effects and equivalent cost.
- The balance of evidence supports the use of a dialysis regimen that promotes the clearance of middle molecules in either incident patients predicted to stay on dialysis for several years (personal choice, age, HLA sensitization, risk of recurrent disease, rare tissue type or other contraindications), or prevalent patients that have been on dialysis for >3.7 years.
- At the current time there is no evidence to support the routine use of hemofiltration or hemodiafiltration in the management of ESRD.

K/DOQI (2003)

- Screening for Aβ2M, including measurement of serum levels of β2M, is not recommended.
- No currently available therapy (except kidney transplantation) can stop disease progression or provide symptomatic relief.
- Kidney transplantation should be considered to stop disease progression or provide symptomatic relief in patients with Aβ2M.
- In patients with or at risk for Aβ2M, noncuprophane, high flux dialysers should be used.

Immune function in chronic kidney disease

Introduction
The effect of failing renal function on the immune system is insidious and far reaching. Both innate and adaptive immune responses are affected and this leads to a number of clinically important consequences.

All patients with CKD stage 5, whether they are approaching ESRD or already on dialysis, share the common immunologic defects caused by the uremic milieu.

Epidemiological studies have consistently shown that infection is the second commonest cause of morbidity and mortality in patients on dialysis after cardiovascular disease.

Abnormalities of immune function
Abnormalities of immune function arise as a consequence of:
- direct effects of uremic toxins on immune cell function;
- underlying renal condition;
- treatment of the underlying renal condition;
- effects of proteinuria.

Effects of uremia
There is an increasing body of evidence supporting the role of uremia in abnormalities of the innate and adaptive immune systems in CKD and ESRD.

Uremia is associated with hypermethylation of a number of genes associated with inflammation, atherosclerosis and aging. Hypermethylation of gene promoter regions will result in changes in gene expression and ultimately cell function.

Adaptive immune system: T- and B-cell function
The exact mechanisms underlying lymphocyte dysfunction *in vivo* remain unknown.

Transfer of lymphocytes from a uremic to nonuremic environment *in vitro* results in a return to normal lymphocyte function implying that the effects of uremia are potentially reversible.

Uremia has been shown to affect:
- T-cell maturation;
- T-helper (CD4) cell function;
- T-cell activation through defective costimulatory signaling.

Innate immune system: neutrophil function
A number of peptides have been identified in both hemodialysis ultrafiltrate and peritoneal dialysis effluent that inhibit neutrophil function.

These include:
- granulocyte inhibitory proteins (GIP);
- degranulation inhibitory proteins (DIP).

These proteins inhibit all stages of the neutrophil response including:
- chemotaxis;
- phagocytosis;
- degranulation.

This inhibition of neutrophil function is believed partly to explain the increased susceptibility to bacterial infections in CKD and ESRD.

Innate immune system: monocyte/macrophage function
Uremia is associated with changes in cell surface expression of a number of costimulatory molecules necessary for effective antigen presentation and T-cell activation.

In parallel there are defects in phagocytosis further compounding antigen presentation.

Activation of monocytes by advanced glycation end-products is thought to be an important factor in the development of the syndrome of malnutrition, inflammation, and atherosclerosis (MIA).

Effects of the underlying renal condition
In the UK and other developed countries diabetes is the most common cause of ESRD requiring RRT.

The World Health Organization lists diabetes as a cause of secondary immunodeficiency.

Hyperglycemia has been shown to impair both the innate and adaptive immune systems with defects being reported in chemotaxis, phagocytosis and cidal activity of lymphocytes and neutrophils.

Other causes of CKD and ESRD associated with significant immune dysfunction include amyloidosis, multiple myeloma and the multisystem autoimmune diseases where many abnormalities have been described in T-cell and antibody function.

Effects of treatment of the underlying renal condition
Immunosuppression
Immunosuppression with steroids, cytotoxic agents, calcineurin inhibitors and biologics will invariably accentuate the immunosuppressive effect of the uremic syndrome.

Different immunosuppressive regimens will have variable effects on T-cell (calcineurin inhibitors) and/or B-cell (mycophenolate mofetil, rituximab) function.

It is clearly important when commencing immunosuppressive therapy in a patient with CKD or ESRD that the risks of further immunosuppression are discussed with the patient; that appropriate monitoring is in place to assess the leukocyte count; and that antibiotic prophylaxis is commenced when necessary.

Plasma exchange
There are theoretical concerns that the removal of immunoglobulin and complement during plasma exchange increases the risk of infection.

There are no data to support an increase in infection specifically due to the institution of plasma exchange although these patients invariably have AKI and will be receiving immunosuppression.

Effects of proteinuria
Proteins lost in the urine by the nephrotic patient with nonselective proteinuria include immunoglobulins (principally IgG) and complement components.

Nephrotic range proteinuria may therefore lead to impairment of both the innate (complement) and adaptive (IgG) immune systems.

In practice this increases the risks of infection, particularly with encapsulated bacteria such as *Pneumococcus* spp.

The risk of infection is further increased when there is a breakdown in skin integrity that may develop in patients with severe edema.

Vaccination

In an attempt to reduce the risk of infection most guidelines advocate the following vaccinations in patients with CKD and ESRD:

- hepatitis B;
- pneumococcus;
- influenza;
- tetanus;
- meningococcus (serogroup B).

As one might expect, however, patients with CKD and ESRD are less likely to respond to these vaccinations.

Hepatitis B

It is recommended that all patients approaching ESRD should be vaccinated against hepatitis B in order to avoid the potential for transmission among patients and between patients and staff.

Hepatitis B outbreaks continue to occur in hemodialysis centres and vaccination is the most effective measure to prevent infection.

The response to hepatitis B vaccination reduces as serum creatinine and age rise.

Vaccination is more likely to be successful in patients with mild–moderate CKD, and is successful in only ~37% of patients on hemodialysis.

Furthermore, patients with CKD require larger doses of vaccine than patients with normal renal function.

The immune defects leading to the reduction in response to hepatitis B vaccination has been the focus of much research.

Impaired T-helper cell function is thought to be important and arises due to abnormal cytokine signaling and reduced expression of HLA class II molecules by antigen-presenting cells in CKD and ESRD.

A typical hepatitis B vaccine schedule would be a 40 μg vaccination repeated at 1, 2 and 6 months.

Seroconversion is conventionally said to have occurred when the hepatitis B surface antibody is >10 IU three months after the last vaccination.

Other vaccinations

Each year influenza viruses cause significant morbidity and mortality, particularly in immunocompromised patients, including those with CKD.

In the UK as part of the national NHS Influenza Immunisation programme all patients with ESRD and CKD should be offered the influenza vaccine.

Influenza vaccination is associated with a significant reduction in hospitalization and death in patients with ESRD but uptake of the vaccination is variable.

Cancer

Immune surveillance is an important mechanism for the early detection and deletion of potentially cancerous cells.

Immune dysfunction in kidney disease may therefore increase the risk of cancer in a number of ways:

- direct effect of uremic toxins on immune cell function;
- underlying renal condition;
- treatment of the underlying renal condition.

Cancer and uremia

Despite the theoretical risk of an increased incidence of cancer in uremic patients this has not been confirmed in a number of retrospective studies.

A retrospective case note study of 834 patients with CKD failed to demonstrate an increased incidence of cancer.

A separate study of 28 000 patients on dialysis found no statistically significant increase in cancer incidence (excluding nonmelanoma skin cancer, multiple myeloma, kidney cancer, and uterine cervix cancer).

There is some evidence for a slight increase in cancer of the kidney and urinary tract in patients on dialysis and transplant recipients.

Cancer and primary renal disease

von Hippel–Lindau disease is a familial, autosomal dominant, multisystem cancer syndrome. Patients develop multiple benign and malignant tumors in many organs. The CNS, kidneys, adrenal glands and pancreas are most commonly affected.

An association between analgesic nephropathy and transitional cell carcinoma has been described; perhaps related to a common toxic insult.

Similarly, Balkan nephropathy may be associated with the development of transitional cell carcinoma.

There is no evidence for an increased risk of renal cell carcinoma in the ADPKD population. However, if renal cancer is present it is more likely to be bilateral, multicentric and sarcomatous.

Cancer and the treatment of renal disease

There is an increasing body of evidence that cytotoxic agents such as cyclophosphamide used in the treatment of a number of glomerulonephritides and vasculitides are associated with an increased incidence of neoplasia.

This increase may not become apparent until many years or decades after treatment, often making it difficult to directly link the two.

It is clearly important when commencing immunosuppression in a patient with CKD or ESRD that the risks of further immunosuppression, including neoplasia, are discussed with the patient

Cancer in renal transplant recipients

It is unclear whether the incidence of cancer is increased or decreased in transplant recipients when compared with uremic patients both on and off dialysis.

Certain cancers are more common in transplant recipients: nonmelanoma skin cancer, post-transplant lymphoproliferative disease.

The risk of neoplasia is linked to the immunosuppressive regimen used and there is some evidence that mTOR inhibitors such as rapamycin may in fact have an antiproliferative effect and reduce the risk of neoplasia.

Other factors influencing immune function

Parathyroid hormone

Parathyroid hormone (PTH) mobilizes calcium from bone and increases urinary phosphate excretion.

Uremic patients invariably develop secondary hyperparathyroidism with raised levels of circulating PTH.

PTH is also a potent modulator of immune function.

Lymphocytes bear PTH receptors and there is evidence that B-lymphocyte proliferation and T-lymphocyte activation are reduced in uremic patients with hyperparathyroidism.

Changes in polymorphonuclear cell function have also been reported.

Iron and erythropoiesis-stimulating agents
Patients with CKD stages 4 and 5 commonly develop anemia.

Erythropoiesis-stimulating agents (ESAs) are most effective when iron stores are replete, prompting the frequent prescription of IV iron to patients receiving ESA.

It has been recognized for some time that chronic iron overload (hemochromatosis and β-thalassemia) is associated with impaired immune function.

High circulating levels of iron in the uremic patient may interfere with normal immune function in a number of ways:

- reduction of macrophage cytotoxic effector function;
- impairment of the complement system;
- impairment of T-helper-1 cell function.

As a consequence of these effects there is a theoretical concern that high levels of iron could further increase susceptibility to infection and neoplasia.

The effects of ESAs on the immune system are uncertain with conflicting studies reporting:

- an antineoplastic effect;
- B-cell-stimulating properties;
- reduced cell-mediated immune responses;
- immunosuppression in patients on dialysis;
- enhanced tumor growth.

It remains unclear at present whether tumor cells express erythropoietin receptors that can be stimulated by ESAs.

Mood disorders
There is increasing evidence to support the theory that depression and mood disorders impact negatively on immune function.

These findings are most marked in the elderly and those who are hospitalized.

Depression may affect as many as one-third of all dialysis patients.

Recent studies suggest that chronic inflammation and immune activation may lead to mood disorders.

Recognition and treatment of psychiatric disorders in patients with failing renal function and those on dialysis may also have a positive impact on immune function.

Nutrition
Intake of essential nutrients is integral to maintaining a healthy immune system.

Patients with failing renal function may have a decreased appetite due to uremia, altered taste sensation, dyspepsia and other comorbid conditions.

Metabolic acidosis increases protein catabolism.

Malnutrition affects up to 50–70% of hemodialysis patients.

It has been shown in hemodialysis patients that peripheral blood lymphocyte counts correlate with serum albumin and cholesterol levels.

Skin integrity
Repeated breaches of the skin and mucosal surfaces predispose patients with CKD to the development of bacterial infection.

This includes the formation of hemodialysis and peritoneal access and its repeated use for dialysis.

In particular, vascular and peritoneal catheters (both tunneled and nontunneled) are a common portal of entry for micro-organisms.

Gram-positive organisms account for two-thirds of dialysis access-related infections.

Methicillin-sensitive (MSSA) and -resistant (MRSA) *Staphylococcus aureus* infections can be associated with serious metastatic complications including endocarditis, discitis and abscess formation.

UK Department of Health initiatives (High Impact Interventions) have been developed to reduce healthcare-associated infections (HCAIs). These have particularly focused on MRSA as a surrogate marker of all HCAIs. In the UK, renal departments typically account for 10% of all hospital-acquired MRSA infections.

Body temperature
In a significant proportion of hemodialysis patients intradialytic body temperature is ~1°C lower than normal.

This can make identification of infection more difficult due to the apparent absence of pyrexia.

Malnutrition inflammation and atherosclerosis (MIA)

Malnutrition, inflammation and atherosclerosis (MIA) syndrome describes wasting as part of an inflammatory state associated with cardiovascular disease. It is not responsive to increasing dietary nutrient intake.

MIA was proposed to explain the enormously increased risk of cardiovascular disease in those with failing renal function and those on dialysis.

The evolution of atherosclerosis is an inflammatory process, and there is increasing evidence that C-reactive protein (CRP) enhances this process.

Patients with CKD have raised circulating levels of CRP and a number of proinflammatory cytokines including IL-6.

The low serum albumin levels seen in MIA rather than reflecting poor nutritional intake instead reflect ongoing inflammation, as well as cytokine action on the GI tract.

Children with failing renal function

In contrast to adult patients with failing renal function, relatively few studies have investigated immune function in children with CKD.

Most studies have found that children with uremia are not overtly immunocompromised, but do have detectable abnormalities in many areas of immune function.

Further reading
Bush A, Gabriel R. Cancer in uremic patients. *Clin Nephrol* 1984; **22**: 77–81.

Fraser GM, Ochana N, Fenyves D, et al. Increasing serum creatinine and age reduce the response to hepatitis B vaccine in renal failure patients. *J Hepatol* 1994; **21**: 450–454.

Gilbertson DT, Unruh M, et al. Influenza vaccine delivery and effectiveness in end-stage renal disease. *Kidney Int* 2003; **63**: 738–743.

Kantor AF, Hoover RN, *et al.* Cancer in patients receiving long-term dialysis treatment. *Am J Epidemiol* 1987; **126**: 370–376.

Pecoits-Filho R, Lindholm B, Stenvinkel P. The malnutrition, inflammation, and atherosclerosis (MIA) syndrome – the heart of the matter. *Nephrol Dial Transplant* 2002; **17**(Suppl 11): 28–31.

Stenvinkel P, Karimi M, *et al.* Impact of inflammation on epigenetic DNA methylation – a novel risk factor for cardiovascular disease? *J Intern Med* 2007; **261**: 488–499.

Internet resources

European Best Practice Guidelines:

http://www.ndt-educational.org/guidelines.asp

Renal Association Clinical Practice Guidelines:

http://www.renal.org/guidelines/

UK Department of Health High Impact Interventions:

http://www.dh.gov.uk/en/Publichealth/
Healthprotection/Healthcareacquiredinfection/
Healthcareacquiredgeneralinformation/index.htm

See also

Hematological disorders in CKD, p. 426

Nephrotic syndrome, p. 80

Medical management of dialysis patients, p. 528

Coagulation disorders in chronic kidney diesase

Introduction

Disturbances in blood coagulation mechanisms are commonly seen in patients with failing renal function. The nature of these changes depends on the underlying cause of the renal disease but complex situations involving both hypo- and hypercoaguable states can arise, leading to a precarious balance of bleeding and thrombotic risk. In order to understand the effects of renal failure a basic appreciation of normal hemostasis is required.

Normal hemostasis

Hemostasis is the process of repair to damaged vessels. Highly developed coagulation and fibrinolytic systems coordinate to form a thrombus which is localized to the site of injury, whilst avoiding unwanted systemic changes and physiological disturbance at critical sites.

Three simultaneous mechanisms are triggered at the moment of vascular damage:

- platelet adhesion and activation;
- initiation and propagation of coagulation pathways, culminating in the formation of fibrin;
- vasoconstriction, to reduce blood flow to the damaged area and to bring circulating platelets and leukocytes in contact with the broken endothelium.

Primary hemostasis

Involves platelet adhesion, mediated by the binding of von Willebrand factor (vWF) to both exposed subendothelial collagen and platelets through their glycoprotein 1b (GP1b) receptor.

On activation platelets change shape from discs to tiny spheres with projections, to enhance surface area and bring platelet granules to the surface, where they release their contents, of pro- and anticoagulants, into the microenvironment.

Platelet aggregation accelerates.

Microparticles bleb from the activated platelet membrane, increasing phospholipid surfaces to which the activated clotting factors bind.

Secondary hemostasis

Involves a highly complicated network of clotting factor reactions taking place on cell surfaces.

Key reactions include:

- exposure of tissue factor (TF) which activates factor VII;
- TF–FVII complex activates factor X, both directly and indirectly through the intrinsic pathway;
- the tenase complex, involving activated factor X, activated factor V and prothrombin, generates thrombin;
- thrombin amplifies its own production in a powerful positive feedback loop, involving the activation of cofactors V and VIII, the intrinsic pathway via factor XI and further activation of platelets;
- the thrombin burst leads to the formation of fibrin from fibrinogen and the activation of factor XIII to crosslink the fibrin monomers and stabilize the clot.

Natural inhibitors to coagulation

There are three major anticoagulation mechanisms:

- tissue factor pathway inhibitor (TFPI);
- the protein C system;
- the antithrombin pathway.

Deficiencies in the latter two are associated with an increase in thrombotic risk, whereas the clinical significance of TFPI deficiency is not yet clear.

TFPI is responsible for the inactivation of FVIIa bound to tissue factor.

Antithrombin neutralizes several of the activated coagulation factors, including thrombin. Its action is catalyzed by heparin-like proteoglycans synthesized by the endothelial cell.

Protein C is activated by the binding of thrombin to thrombomodulin on the endothelial cell surface. The activated protein C, with protein S as a cofactor, inactivates Va and VIIIa.

Relationship between coagulation and inflammation

The coagulation system is strongly related to inflammation. In inflammatory states, prothrombotic potential is increased, with risk of disseminated intravascular coagulation or systemic thrombosis in extreme circumstances.

Inflammatory cytokines enhance platelet numbers and reactivity and stimulate monocytes to synthesize tissue factor.

The change in shape of platelets and monocytes and release of microparticles provide increased phospholipid surfaces to support hemostatic reactions.

Leukocyte adhesion molecules such as P-selectin and E-selectin, synthesized by the endothelial cell, enhance binding of activated platelets to circulating microparticles.

C-reactive protein facilitates endothelial cell–monocyte interactions and further promotes tissue factor expression. It also activates complement, thereby increasing platelet activation and available procoagulant membrane surfaces.

Anticoagulant function is downregulated by the disappearance of thrombomodulin from the endothelial cell surface, reducing the ability of thrombin to activate the protein C system. Antithrombin inhibitory activity is also reduced.

The fibrinolytic system is impaired and fibrinogen, being an acute phase reactant, is increased in inflammatory states.

Coagulation disorders secondary to renal disease

Uremic bleeding

Hemostatic mechanisms, particularly those of primary hemostasis, are impaired in patients with CKD.

Clinical bleeding, in the form of bruising, bleeding at venepuncture sites, menorrhagia and gastrointestinal blood loss, occurs in up to 50%.

Contributing factors include:

- reduced hematocrit;
- thrombocytopenia;
- platelet dysfunction (intrinsic platelet abnormalities and impaired platelet–vessel wall interaction).

Comorbidities and medications such as antiplatelet drugs or anticoagulants may compound the problem.

Hematocrit

There is an inverse correlation between bleeding time and hematocrit, with a prolonged bleeding time in patients with renal anemia.

Platelet adhesion to the subendothelium increases progressively as hematocrit rises. As red cells travel through the blood vessels in the fast stream at the center of the lumen, platelets diffuse radially, increasing the chance of adhesion to sites of injury. Decreases in hematocrit allow fast passage of platelets in the central luminal flow reducing platelet–endothelial cell interaction. Also, platelet aggregation is affected by lower production of ADP and thromboxane from red cells and reduced availability of hemoglobin to scavenge nitrous oxide.

Conversely, disproportionate increases in hematocrit and whole blood viscosity, aggravated by the use of diuretics, enhance thrombotic risk. Uremic erythrocytes can display increased procoagulant activity due to increased phosphatidylserine exposure on the surface membrane. Thus a steady hematocrit of ~30% should be maintained when managing patients with renal failure.

Platelet dysfunction
In the absence of dialysis, platelets are usually quantitatively normal (or slightly reduced) but function is often impaired, largely due to increases in urea and other retention solutes such as creatinine, phenolic acids and methylguanidine.

Ineffective adhesion to the subendothelium arises from reduced expression of Gp1b receptors and reduced affinity for vWF.

Conformational changes occur in platelet fibrinogen receptors, affecting platelet activation, and *in vitro* platelet aggregation responses to agonists, such as ADP, collagen and epinephrine, are impaired. This is variable and does not correlate with the severity of the renal disease.

Production of nitrous oxide, PGI_2, calcium and cAMP is increased, inhibiting platelet aggregation and causing vasodilatation.

Thrombocytopenia
Hemodialysis is often associated with thrombosis as a result of chronic platelet activation due to contact with artificial surfaces. However, this consumes platelets and the resulting thrombocytopenia along with the anticoagulants used in the hemodialysis process may in fact contribute to bleeding.

Investigations for uremic bleeding
Full blood count
A full blood count is essential to ensure adequate hemoglobin, hematocrit and platelet count.

Coagulation tests
These include the prothrombin time (PT) and activated partial thromboplastin time (aPTT), which measure the integrity of the extrinsic and intrinsic pathways respectively. They are usually normal in patients with uremic bleeding but, where they are abnormal, other conditions such as disseminated intravascular coagulation should be excluded.

Fibrinogen and D Dimers are acute phase reactants and are raised in inflammatory states. Being partially cleared by the kidneys, D Dimers accumulate in CKD.

Bleeding time
Using a disposable lancet device, two small longitudinal incisions are made in the volar aspect of the forearm, with a sphygmomanometer cuff above the elbow inflated to 40 mmHg. Blood is gently blotted at 15 s intervals and the time until bleeding ceases is recorded. The normal range is ~2–7 min but in-house normal ranges should always be determined.

The test is time-consuming, poorly standardized, subject to interobserver error and results do not correlate with the clinical incidence of bleeding. It has now been largely replaced by PFA-100.

The PFA-100 system
This is an *in vitro* system which attempts to reproduce the high shear circulation involving vWF binding and the platelet adhesion, activation and aggregation processes. It determines the time to platelet closure over a tiny aperture in a membrane coated with collagen and either ADP or epinephrine. It is sensitive to abnormalities of vWF and platelet adhesion but certain activation processes and granule secretion defects are not detected.

Closure times have been shown to shorten following DDAVP and dialysis; however, the role of the PFA-100 in therapeutic monitoring of platelet function in patients with renal failure remains to be established.

Management of uremic bleeding
The choice of agent used in the management of uremic bleeding depends on the clinical circumstances.

Agents used for the treatment of uremic bleeding or for emergency surgery:

DDAVP
DDAVP (arginine vasopressin) acts on endothelial vasopressin V_2 receptors and cAMP-mediated signaling, leading to exocytosis of vWF from Weibel–Palade bodies where it is stored.

Larger vWF factor VIII multimers are noted in the serum after an infusion of DDAVP and are associated with a shortening of the bleeding time.

It is the first-line agent in the management of uremic bleeding as onset of action is rapid. The half-life is ~10 h and the bleeding time tends to reverse to baseline within 24 h.

A single infusion of 0.3 µg/kg is usually sufficient to cover renal biopsy and does not appear to cause fluid overload or changes in serum electrolytes, although an increase of ~10% in urine osmolality lasts for 48 h.

It is contraindicated in cardiac insufficiency.

Cryoprecipitate
Transfusion of cryoprecipitate, rich in vWF, factor VIII and fibrinogen can partially or fully reverse the disturbances of primary hemostasis within minutes.

It should be given if DDAVP fails to control bleeding or in conjunction with DDAVP for urgent surgery, providing the increase in intravascular volume can be tolerated.

This is an old version of the submitted text and has missed out the following.

Platelet transfusion
Platelet transfusions can temporarily eliminate the bleeding tendency, with a haemostatic effect lasting for 4–5 hours and should be used if the above agents are ineffective or inappropriate. The incidence of alloimmunisation with subsequent platelet refractoriness has been reduced by the current practice of pre-storage leucodepletion.

Red cell transfusion
Red cell transfusion allows margination of platelets and has been shown to improve many markers of platelet activation, including platelet retention on glass beads, prothrombin consumption index and serum thromboxane levels.

Tranexamic acid

Tranexamic acid inhibits fibrinolysis by forming a reversible complex with plasminogen and preventing its conversion to plasmin.

Single doses can be a useful adjunct to treatment when DDAVP has been used which, in addition to the above effects, stimulates release of tissue-plasminogen activator from the Weibel–Palade bodies.

As excretion is via glomerular filtration, oral or IV doses should be reduced to 5 mg/kg every 24 h and prolonged treatment should not be given.

Recombinant activated factor VII

Recombinant activated factor VII, at a dose of 90 μg/kg, has been successfully used for emergency bleeding which has failed to respond to first-line therapy.

It is capable of binding directly to activated platelets and stimulating a thrombin burst.

It has a short half-life and repeat doses may be needed at 2-hourly intervals. For this reason it has not been used prophylactically in this setting.

Agents used for the prevention of uremic bleeding and preparation for elective surgery:

Erthyropoetin

Recombinant human erythropoetin induces erythropoiesis, increasing hematocrit and facilitating margination of platelets.

There is also evidence for enhanced platelet signaling through tyrosine phosphorylation, an increase in metabolically active reticulated platelets and improved hemoglobin availability for scavenging of nitrous oxide.

The effect on bleeding time takes several days and therefore there is little benefit in the acute setting but it is an important agent in the management of hemodynamically stable patients with uremic bleeding where hematocrit is <30%.

Adequate iron stores should be ensured and concomitant iron supplements are usually required.

The hematocrit should be maintained at 30% for optimal hemostasis as well as oxygen delivery.

Conjugated estrogens

Conjugated oestrogens increase synthesis of vWF and factor VIII and reduce protein S levels. They reduce bleeding time and improve clinical bleeding.

The required dose is 0.6 mg/kg IV over 30–40 min once daily for 5 days, although there is some evidence for positive effects with oral and transdermal estrogens.

Time to onset of action is 6 h with maximum effect at 5–7 days, lasting for 14–21 days.

They are ideally used in preparation for elective surgery and the short duration of therapy is also suitable for male patients.

Dialysis

Dialysis, particularly peritoneal dialysis, has been shown to improve the abnormalities of platelet function and is important in the prevention of uremic bleeding.

Renal biopsy in the uremic patient

The kidneys are highly vascular organs, receiving 20% of the cardiac output and therefore percutaneous biopsy carries a significant bleeding risk.

Clinically overt bleeding has been reported in 2–8% of patients. A much higher percentage has hidden bleeding and perirenal hematoma has been demonstrated by CT scan in up to 90%.

The risk of bleeding depends on the degree of renal insufficiency, being highest in patients with advanced uremia.

DDAVP at 0.3 μg/kg given 30–60 min before the biopsy reduces the potential for bleeding in these patients. However, the balance of risks for all cases must be carefully considered and contributing factors assessed and eliminated as far as possible.

Prebiopsy evaluation should assess:
- personal and family bleeding history;
- recent ingestion of aspirin or NSAIDs;
- platelet count;
- hematocrit;
- PT and aPTT.

Aspirin has been shown to produce a greater effect on platelets in uremic patients than in those with normal renal function and should, where possible, be discontinued 2 weeks prior to the procedure.

Warfarin should be stopped 5 days before biopsy, if necessary bridging with heparin, omitting the heparin on the day of the biopsy and ensuring normal antiXa levels or aPTT before biopsy.

The transjugular approach may be an option for patients with known bleeding risk, in whom renal biopsy is mandatory for diagnosis and management.

Only two-thirds of bleeding complications are evident in the first 8 h and a 24 h postoperative observation time is advised in uremic patients.

Thrombotic disorders

Despite the effect of uremia on platelet function, patients with CKD usually have a hypercoagulable state with:
- enhanced thrombin generation due to tissue factor pathway activation;
- platelet, monocyte and endothelial activation or injury;
- resistance to activated protein C;
- reduced antithrombin levels.

Increased hepatic synthesis of factors II, V, VII, VIII, X and XIII further augments thrombin formation and fibrinolytic activity is reduced.

Cellular activation is boosted by dialysis, advancing progression of atherosclerosis.

Thrombotic complications in uremic patients can occur at:
- sites of vascular access;
- in the deep venous system (DVT);
- in the coronary, cerebral, and retinal arteries.

Hyperhomocysteinemia

Homocysteine levels increase with failing renal function and hyperhomocysteinemia is universal in patients with ESRD.

It is an independent risk factor for arterial thrombosis and contributes to the high incidence of cardiovascular deaths in patients on dialysis.

It is also a risk factor for venous thrombosis and although levels can be reduced by vitamins B6, B12 and folic acid, there is no conclusive evidence that this treatment lowers the incidence of vascular events or improves survival.

Homocysteine also causes endothelial dysfunction through increased inactivation of nitrous oxide.

Treatment with folic acid has been shown to improve endothelial function, although this effect may be independent of the fall in homocysteine levels.

Thromboprophylaxis

Most hospitalized patients have one or more additional risk factors for venous thromboembolism (VTE) such as advanced age, obesity or immobility.

These risk factors are generally cumulative and without prophylaxis, the incidence of objectively confirmed, hospital-acquired DVT is ~10–40% among general medical patients.

One-quarter to one-third of these thrombi involve the proximal deep veins and are much more likely to produce symptoms and to result in pulmonary embolism.

Therefore the value of thromboprophylaxis is substantial and the need for this should be assessed in all patients.

They should be informed of the potential risk for thrombosis and encouraged to mobilize as much as possible.

Providing there are no bleeding manifestations or thrombocytopenia, pharmacological thromboprophylaxis should be considered for immobile patients.

Low molecular weight heparin (LMWH) at prophylactic doses can be used safely in patients with renal impairment. However, chronic LMWH administered at fixed-weight doses and without monitoring show unpredictable anticoagulant effects in patients with severe renal impairment, leading to serious and occasionally fatal adverse incidents. Thus the need for anti-Xa assays should be considered.

Where heparin is contraindicated due to thrombocytopenia and/or bleeding, thromboembolic deterrent stockings should be used, providing there is no overt evidence of peripheral vascular disease.

Investigation of suspected venous thromboembolism

The clinical probability of VTE should always be estimated before testing, so that objective diagnostic tests can be employed in an efficient, safe, and cost-effective manner.

A number of scoring systems have been proposed, the Wells score being most commonly used.

D Dimers are the breakdown products of crosslinked fibrin and are highly sensitive for acute thrombus formation. Thus, in patients with a low clinical probability score, negative D Dimers can reliably exclude acute thrombosis. However, their accumulation in renal failure makes them less likely to be helpful in this cohort of patients and imaging is required more often.

There have been reports of the use of raised D Dimers as a predictive tool for vascular access thrombosis but it may be that they are merely reflecting the degree of renal impairment.

Use of anticoagulants in patients with renal impairment

Kidney function should be evaluated in all patients commencing anticoagulants.

Heparin

In patients with normal renal function, LMWH is the preferred agent for initial treatment of VTE in view of the predictable bioavailability and long half-life, enabling once daily administration.

LMWHs, as well as other factor Xa inhibitors such as fondaparinux, are primarily eliminated by the kidneys and dose accumulation may occur in patients with renal impairment.

Dose reduction is therefore required, with close clinical observation for bleeding and/or thromboembolic complications and monitoring of anti-Xa activity levels.

Unfractionated heparin currently remains the preferred anticoagulant even though its use is associated with increased bleeding in this group of patients.

Anti-Xa assay

The concentration of LMWHs in the patient's plasma is determined by the amount of inhibition of a fixed quantity of factor Xa in the presence of calcium, platelet substitute and factor X-depleted plasma.

Anti-Xa assays are important to exclude heparin accumulation, but limitations of the assay must be realized – the therapeutic range has not been clearly validated, and a recent survey from the UK National External Quality Assurance Scheme (NEQAS) showed considerable interlaboratory variation of results.

Heparin-induced thrombocytopenia (HIT)

Around 5% of patients on unfractionated heparin, particularly bovine heparin, develop a severe immune-mediated reaction associated with increased platelet and endothelial cell activation and a significant risk of potentially fatal thrombosis.

HIT has been reported in 0–12% of hemodialysis patients, although a recent UK survey showed 0.26%.

The process results from the formation of antibodies to complexes of heparin and platelet factor 4, a heparin-neutralizer released from platelet α granules. The antibodies induce platelet activation via their Fc receptors, with formation of procoagulant microparticles, increasing the phospholipid surface area for hemostatic reactions.

Simultaneous endothelial cell activation results in overexpression of tissue factor and thrombin generation is enhanced, increasing the risk of arterial and venous thrombosis, with clinical manifestations in up to 50% of untreated patients, most commonly occurring at sites of existing pathology.

Clotting in the extracorporeal circuit or site of vascular access can occur or other clinical features including skin necrosis, cutaneous allergy and acute systemic reactions.

The immune-mediated etiology gives rise to the specific timing of the fall in platelet count, which occurs at day 5–10 of exposure.

Rapid onset HIT only occurs where there has been previous exposure to heparin, particularly within the last 3 months.

Delayed HIT is unusual but may occur when there is substantial platelet activation even after the heparin has been stopped.

The diagnosis is made on the basis of a clinical probability score, taking into consideration the timing of the drop in platelets, the likelihood of an alternative explanation and the presence of thrombosis (Table 11.12.1).

Serological confirmation can be obtained by a variety of HIT assays. Functional assays such as the serotonin release assay are the gold standard but these are time-consuming and not practical for most laboratories.

Table 11.12.1. Pretest probability score, described by Warkentin et al. as the 'four Ts', to assess the clinical likelihood of heparin-induced thrombocytopenia

	2 points	1 point	0 points
Thrombocytopenia	50% fall or platelet nadir 20–100 × 10⁹/L	30–50% fall or platelet nadir 10–19 × 10⁹/L	<30% fall or platelet nadir <10 × 10⁹/L
Timing of platelet count fall or other sequelae	Clear onset between days 5 and 10; or <1 day (if heparin exposure within past 100 days)	Onset of thrombocytopenia after day 10	Platelet count fall too early (without recent heparin exposure)
Thrombosis or other sequelae (e.g. skin lesions)	New thrombosis; skin necrosis; post-heparin bolus acute systemic reaction	Progressive or recurrent thrombosis; erythematous skin lesions; suspected thrombosis not yet proven	None
Other cause for thrombocytopenia not evident	No other cause for platelet count fall is evident	Possible other cause is evident	Definite other cause is present

Points: 0, 1, or 2 for each of four categories: maximum possible score = 8.
Pretest probability score: 6–8 = high; 4–5 = intermediate; 0–3 = low.

ELISA assays are more widely available but although they are highly sensitive to the presence of antibody, specificity for clinical HIT is limited.

Although HIT is most commonly seen with unfractionated heparin, it can occur with LMWH and even heparin line flushes. Therefore once the diagnosis is suspected all forms of heparin must be stopped and, in view of the significant risk of thrombosis, an alternative anticoagulant started.

Warfarin is contraindicated in the acute stages of the disease as initial therapy further enhances hypercoagulability by reduction in protein C and S levels.

In patients with renal failure the choice of anticoagulant can be difficult and commencement of hirudins or danaparoid must be decided on an individual basis.

Anticoagulation for hemodialysis
Unfractionated heparin has conventionally been used to prevent clot formation in the dialyser.

There is now evidence for the safety and efficacy of LMWH given as a single bolus in the arterial line at the beginning of dialysis.

The advantages include lower incidences of bleeding, HIT and osteoporosis and possible benefits in uremic dyslipidemia.

Pharmacokinetic and pharmacodynamic properties differ between the various LMWH but either weight-based regimens or fixed doses of all the different preparations have been used successfully.

Anti-Xa levels of ~0.4 IU/mL at 3 h post dialysis appear to be optimal. However, despite clinically effective anticoagulation, subclinical platelet and coagulation activation still occurs and dialysis time itself is an independent risk factor for clotting.

Warfarin
Warfarin is metabolized in the liver and does not accumulate in patients with renal disease.

It is associated with increased bleeding risk for patients on hemodialysis.

When monitoring the INR in patients on dialysis, care must be taken to avoid heparin contamination of the sample.

Use of antiplatelet drugs in patients with renal impairment

Aspirin
Aspirin affects platelet function by inducing an irreversible defect in thromboxane synthesis, through the modification of cyclo-oxygenase.

Additional effects of aspirin have also been postulated, including cyclo-oxygenase-independent platelet inhibition, anticoagulant and anti-inflammatory properties and enhanced fibrinolysis.

The use of aspirin in patients with CKD is controversial. However, these patients have an extremely high risk of death from cardiovascular disease and aspirin has an undoubted beneficial impact on the progression of this disorder.

Therefore, provided measures to prevent uremic bleeding are optimized, such as maintaining a steady hematocrit of 30%, the benefits should outweigh the risks in patients with cardiovascular disease and therapy should be recommended.

The pathogenesis of allograft rejection after kidney transplant has many features in common with atherosclerosis and aspirin has been shown to improve graft function and survival.

Clopidogrel
Clopidogrel blocks the ADP pathway, suppressing its amplifying effect on platelet activation. The effect on the platelet is permanent.

Where aspirin has been used in conjunction with clopidogrel, in an attempt to maintain patency of vascular access, this has resulted in a two-fold increased risk of bleeding including substantially more episodes that are life-threatening.

The risk/benefit balance of combined therapy should be considered in conjunction with the prescribing team.

Glycoprotein IIb/IIIa inhibitors
Glycoprotein (GP) IIb/IIIa inhibitors (GPIs) block the binding of fibrinogen to activated platelet GP IIb/IIIa receptors and prevent the formation of platelet thrombi.

They are important adjunctive therapies for patients with non-ST elevation acute coronary syndromes and are pivotal in the success of percutaneous coronary intervention (PCI) in these patients. Clinical trials confirm reduced periprocedural thrombotic complications but with an inevitable increased incidence of bleeding.

CKD is associated with heightened risk of both thrombotic complications in these clinical settings as well as bleeding with GPIs, and the benefit versus risk of therapy needs to be assessed on an individual basis.

Baseline PT and aPTT should be measured and patients should be monitored for bleeding complications or a fall in hemoglobin or platelet count in the 24 h following commencement of a GPI.

As GPIs are cleared by the kidneys, dose reductions are recommended.

Tirofiban should be reduced by 50% for patients with GFR <30 mL/min.

Clearance of eptifibatide, a small, highly selective heptapeptide, shows strong correlation with creatinine clearance and should be avoided if GFR <30 mL/min. In those with a GFR between 30 and 50 mL/min, the maintenance infusion dose should be reduced by half, but the bolus loading dose remains unchanged.

No dose reduction has been recommended for abciximab, although it is specifically contraindicated in patients with severe renal impairment or on dialysis.

Anticoagulation of the pregnant patient with renal disease

Pregnancy is associated with a 10-fold increase in relative risk for venous thrombosis, which increases to 25-fold after delivery, returning to baseline at ~6 weeks postpartum.

This is augmented in renal failure and particularly so in nephrotic syndrome, where there is a disproportionate loss of lower molecular weight anticoagulant factors.

Associated acquired antithrombin deficiency can result in a risk of venous thromboembolism as high as 40%.

Management requires close collaboration between the patient and the multidisciplinary team.

All patients should be considered for thromboprophylaxis, based on the degree of proteinuria, antithrombin levels and other contributing patient factors.

LMWH does not cross the placenta and can be used safely, both during pregnancy and breastfeeding, providing anti-Xa levels are measured to exclude drug accumulation.

Meticulous attention to anemia helps to prevent bleeding.

Further reading

Hetzel GR, Sucker C. The heparins: all a nephrologist should know. *Nephrol Dial Transplant* 2005; **20**: 2036–2042.

Hutchison CA, Dasgupta I. National survey of heparin-induced thrombocytopenia in the haemodialysis population of the UK. *Nephrol Dial Transplant* 2007; **22**: 1680–1684.

Geerts WH, Pineo GF, Heit JA. Prevention of venous thromboembolism: the Seventh ACCP Conference on Antithrombotic and Thrombolytic Therapy. *Chest* 2004; **126**(3 Suppl)**:** 338S–400S.

RCOG Guidelines. *Thromboprophylaxis during pregnancy, labour and after vaginal delivery.* London: RCOG; 2004.

Warkentin TE, Heddle NM. Laboratory diagnosis of immune heparin-induced thrombocytopenia. *Curr Hematol Rep* **2003; 2**: 148–157.

Warkentin TE, Greinacher A. *Heparin-induced thrombocytopenia*, 3rd edn. New York: Marcel Dekker; 2004.

Wells P, *et al.* Value of assessment of pretest probability of deep vein thrombosis in clinical management *Lancet* 1997; **350**: 1795–1798.

Internet resources

LifeBlood: The Thrombosis Charity:

http://www.thrombosis-charity.org.uk/old/index.htm

Heparin-induced thrombocytopenia information:

http://www.heparininducedthrombocytopenia.com/

Royal College of Obstetricians and Gynaecologists:

http://www.rcog.org.uk

See also

Renal replacement therapies in acute kidney injury, p. 328

Hemodialysis, hemofiltration, and hemodiafiltration, p. 494

CKD in pregnant women, p. 476

Dermatologic disorders in chronic kidney disease

Introduction
Cutaneous disorders are common in patients with ESRD, 50–100% of patients having at least one dermatologic condition. By contrast, skin changes are rare in acute kidney injury (AKI). Improvements in early diagnosis and treatment of renal disease mean that some dermatologic conditions such as uremic frost are now rarely seen.

Anemia
Pallor of the skin and conjunctivae is a common early cutaneous sign in ESRD.

Development of anemia in CKD is multifactorial:
- anemia of chronic disease;
- decreased erythropoiesis;
- increased hemolysis;
- significant reduction in cutaneous blood flow on dialysis.

Treatment involves the use of:
- erythropoetin;
- IV iron dextran.

Cutaneous hyperpigmentation
Occurs in 25–70% of patients on dialysis with incidence increasing with duration of renal disease.

It is seen equally in hemodialysis (HD) and peritoneal dialysis (PD) patients although a yellowish hue is more prevalent in patients on HD.

Patients have a distinctive grey-yellow hue with diffuse hyperpigmentation of sun-exposed skin.

Etiology
- Deposition of melanin (possibly due to impaired renal processing of melanocyte-stimulating hormone, MSH).
- Accumulation of carotenoid and nitrogenous pigments in dermis.

Dry skin (xerosis)
50–75% of dialysis population have excessively dry skin.

The incidence of xerosis in patients with CKD is unknown.

Patients will have dry roughened skin, sometimes with fine scaling.

Etiology
- Reduction in the size of eccrine sweat glands.
- High dose diuretic treatment.
- Fluid restriction.

Treatment
- Regular use of paraffin-based bland emollients.
- Urea-containing emollients.
- Emollient-based soap substitutes.

Pruritus
Clinically significant pruritus affects 50–90% of the dialysis population and is more prevalent in patients on HD.

Pruritus is unusual in AKI.

Etiology
Exact pathogenesis is unknown and likely to be multifactorial:
- patients receiving dialysis with less permeable membranes experience more severe pruritus;

- possible increase in tissue mast cells;
- dryness of skin is a contributing factor but not sole cause;
- correlation with predialysis blood urea levels not established; an increase in dialysis dose may not improve symptoms;
- possible correlation with hyperphosphatemia due to secondary hyperparathyroidism but symptoms may recur after subtotal parathyroidectomy.

Treatment
Difficult.

A long list of published treatment options bears witness to the lack of a consistently effective therapy.

General measures
- Removal of cause, where possible.
- Paraffin-based emollients.
- Topical steroids.
- Physical methods to cool the skin, including use of cotton clothing and avoidance of wool.

Specific measures
- Phototherapy (narrow band Ultraviolet B).
- Oral cholestyramine and activated charcoal.
- Thalidomide.
- Erythropoetin.
- Opioid antagonists: based on reports of elevated plasma levels of opioid peptides and serotonin (e.g. oral naltrexone, oral ondansetron).
- Lowering magnesium concentration of dialyzate may help.

Purpura
This is a common cutaneous finding in ESRD especially in those patients on HD.

Patients may have:
- petechiae or ecchymoses (bruising);
- mucosal bleeding;
- also reflected in poor wound healing in dialysis patients.

Etiology
- Mild thrombocytopenia and platelet dysfunction.
- Malnutrition.

Half-and-half nails
These will be present in up to 50% of patients with ESRD.

The incidence increases with duration of dialysis.

It is more prevalent in patients on HD.

Patients have whitish or normal-colored proximal portion of the nail plate, with abnormally brown/red distal portion. Latter comprises more than one-third of nail plate.

Etiology
An increased level of MSH causes increased melanin pigment within the nail plate.

Treatment
There is no specific treatment but it may disappear with successful renal transplantation.

Skin cancer
Squamous cell and basal cell carcinomas are the commonest types of skin cancers seen in CKD and ESRD.

The incidence rises with increased time on dialysis.

Lesions are distinct from the multiple dysplastic and frankly malignant skin lesions which can develop in the immuno-suppressed patient with a renal transplant.

Clinical features

Excessive wrinkling and yellowing of skin, especially over the neck.

Senile lentigines (liver spots, age spots).

Vascular dilatations (telangiectases).

Actinic keratoses:
- precancerous lesions;
- red spots with a rough surface (easier to feel (rough) than see);
- found on sun-exposed surfaces.

Nonhealing enlarging skin lesions suggest cancer.

Etiology

Acceleration of cutaneous aging is a function of time on dialysis.

Individuals at higher risk include:
- fair skin that burns easily;
- light-colored eyes;
- red hair;
- numerous freckles;
- past history of heavy sun exposure.

Treatment

Sun protection advice

Prevention is the best course of action:
- cover up with sun hat, long sleeves and trousers in sunny weather;
- stay in shade particularly between 11:00 and 15:00;
- apply sun-block of sun protection factor (SPF) ≥25 every 3 h;
- do not use sunbeds.

Active management

Excision of suspected skin tumors under local anesthetic.

Cryotherapy (freezing the lesion with liquid nitrogen).

Topical 5-fluorouracil or imiquimod cream.

Photodynamic therapy.

Reduce/stop immunosuppression in aggressive skin cancers.

Hypertrichosis lanuginosa

This is a common finding in patients with CKD and ESRD.

There is a uniform increase in growth of fine hair over the cheeks and thickening of the eyebrows.

The etiology is unknown.

Some cases are iatrogenic:
- corticosteroids;
- ciclosporin;
- penicillamine.

Uremic neuropathy and neuropathic skin ulcers

Up to 60% of patients with ESRD or on long-term HD develop some degree of peripheral neuropathy.

Neuropathy is mainly sensorimotor and can lead to pressure ulcers.

This will be compounded in patients with ESRD due to conditions independently associated with development of peripheral neuropathy, e.g. diabetes and amyloidosis.

Cutaneous calcification

Benign nodular calcification is not uncommon and develops in the setting of CKD complicated by prolonged secondary and tertiary hyperparathyroidism.

Large calcium deposits may be found in the skin and subcutaneous tissue, particularly periarticular sites.

The number and size correlate with severity of hyperphosphatemia.

It is usually asymptomatic except for the pressure they can place on surrounding structures.

Etiology

Disruption of normal calcium regulatory pathways can lead to 'metastatic' calcification and/or ossification of skin:
- impaired renal phosphate clearance;
- impaired synthesis of 1,25-(OH) vitamin D3;
- decreased absorption of calcium from intestine with resulting hypocalcemia;
- increased parathyroid hormone and mobilization of calcium and phosphate from bone;
- solubility product of calcium × phosphate exceeded.

Treatment

Phosphate binders.

Surgical excision of symptomatic lesions.

Calciphylaxis

Vascular calcification is a common incidental finding in ESRD.

Rarely vascular calcification may lead to cutaneous necrosis or gangrene as a result of thrombosed vessels, an entity known as calciphylaxis (calcific uremic syndrome).

In contrast to benign nodular calcification, this condition is a medical emergency and carries a poor prognosis.

1–4% of patients with ESRD develop calciphylaxis.

Incidence has increased over the last decade, possibly due to the increased use of parenteral vitamin D and iron dextran.

It is more common in:
- females (3:1);
- Caucasians;
- diabetics;
- obese;
- longstanding ESRD and renal replacement therapy.

Lesions develop suddenly and progress rapidly.

Early lesions appear as violaceous mottling, livedo reticularis or erythematous purpuric papules.

Later, lesions have a stellate purpuric configuration with central cutaneous ulceration and necrosis.

Less commonly, lesions present as blisters or subcutaneous erythematous nodules.

Intense pain is a constant finding.

90% of lesions occur on lower extremities.

More proximal lesions occur in 44–68% of cases, predominantly on thighs, buttocks and lower abdomen.

Multiple lesions of variable age may be present.

Visceral involvement is not uncommon.

Intact pulses help distinguish calciphylaxis from atherosclerotic peripheral vascular disease.

Etiology
Reported triggering factors include:

- recent and sudden weight loss;
- infusion of medications such as iron dextran, corticosteroids;
- concurrent use of warfarin.

Investigations
Parathyroid hormone is usually markedly elevated.

Serum calcium, phosphate and calcium × phosphate are likely to be high.

Skin biopsy shows nonspecific changes with calcium deposition in vessel walls. There is risk of subsequent ulceration at biopsy site.

Treatment
Analgesia.

Urgent normalization of serum calcium and phosphate, which may require daily dialysis.

Careful wound care and aggressive treatment of wound infection lowers risk of systemic sepsis.

Surgical debridement of necrotic painful lesions.

Parathyroidectomy.

Anecdotal success has been reported with hyperbaric oxygen and low calcium dialysis.

Secondary hyperuricemia (gout)

This may present as:

- acute monoarthritis;
- tophi in chronic gout.

Acute monoarthritis:

- most commonly in the great toe;
- affected joint; warm, swollen, erythematous and very painful.

Tophaceous gout:

- firm asymptomatic dermal or subcutaneous nodules or fusiform swelling;
- painful ulceration may occur;
- commonly affects helix or antihelix of ear, along ulnar surface of forearm and index fingers and olecranon bursa (other tissues in <10% cases).

There is male predominance.

Prevalence increases with obesity, diabetes mellitus and alcohol consumption.

Etiology
Decreased excretion of uric acid occurs secondary to diuretic therapy and CKD.

In some renal disorders, e.g. medullary cystic disease and chronic lead nephropathy, hyperuricemia may occur with minimal renal insufficiency.

Investigations
Serum uric acid levels are raised during an acute attack.

Joint aspiration may be diagnostic in acute gout; sodium urate crystals show positive birefringence under polarized light.

Joint X-ray: subcortical cysts, calcification in pseudogout.

Histological examination of tophi if diagnosis in doubt.

Treatment for chronic gout
Low purine diet: avoid meat, poultry, fish, seafood, alcohol, beans and peas.

Allopurinol: xanthine oxidase inhibitor.

Partial/complete resolution of tophi when serum uric acid normalized.

Cryotherapy, intralesional corticosteroids or surgical excision of individual symptomatic tophi.

Secondary oxalosis (hyperoxaluria)

Insoluble calcium oxalate may be deposited in the skin and other organs in CKD and ESRD, particularly in those patients on long-term HD.

Tiny millet seed-like (miliary) deposits can be found on fingers and palmar surfaces.

Livedo reticularis with peripheral cyanosis is rare.

Investigations
Serum oxalate levels.

Skin biopsy shows birefringent crystals in vessel walls.

Treatment
Where possible improvements in hydration and urine alkalinization may be beneficial.

Arteriovenous fistula

Cutaneous complications affecting the limb in which the hemodialysis AV fistula is situated include:

- infection;
- phlebitis;
- hematoma;
- irritant and contact allergic dermatitis.

Venous hypertension syndrome, with or without ulceration, together with pseudo-Kaposi's sarcoma is rare.

Acquired perforating dermatoses

This can occur in up to 10% of patients on HD.

It is more common in African-Americans.

Patients develop hyperkeratotic papules or nodules 1–10 mm diameter, often umbilicated with central crust-filled crater.

There is a linear or serpiginous distribution on trunk and extensor surfaces.

The face and scalp are rarely affected.

Spontaneous resolution can occur along with development of new lesions.

Etiology
It is associated with ESRD and diabetes mellitus.

Proposed mechanisms include:

- diabetic microangiopathy;
- dysregulation of vitamin A or D metabolism;
- abnormality of collagen or elastic fibers;
- inflammation and connective tissue degradation caused by dermal deposition of substances such as uric acid and calcium pyrophosphate.

Investigations
Skin biopsy shows transepidermal elimination of both collagen and elastic fibers.

Treatment
Potent topical or intralesional steroids.

Cryotherapy.

Phototherapy.

Systemic retinoids.

Nephrogenic fibrosing dermopathy (NFD)

This is a progressive fibrosing condition associated with the use of gadolinium-containing contrast used in MRI.

It is rare.

It has mainly been described in patients with ESRD, mostly on long-term HD, but has been reported in AKI.

Red indurated plaques develop over weeks leading to extensive thickened skin with a 'woody texture'.

It starts at extremities with progressive involvement of the trunk.

The face and neck are usually spared.

Flexion of adjacent joints is inhibited.

Pruritus is common.

Systemic involvement of lung, myocardium, striated muscle have been reported.

Etiology
This is unknown.

Recombinant erythropoetin has fibrogenic properties and it has been suggested may play a role.

Investigations
Skin biopsy shows:
• proliferation of fibroblasts in dermis and subcutaneous septae;
• increased dermal and septal collagen and mucin detected by Alcian Blue stain;
• absence of inflammatory cell infiltrate.

Treatment
Improvements have been reported with correction of renal failure following renal transplantation.

Decreasing erythropoetin dose may ameliorate (but not cure) the condition.

Phototherapy and plasma exchange have been reported in the literature but there is insufficient evidence to recommend these at present.

Bullous disease of HD (pseudoporphyria)

This resembles porphyria cutanea tarda (PCT) with mechanical skin fragility and crops of delicate blisters or crusted erosions on sun-exposed areas (hands and face).

Incidental trauma may precede lesions.

Atrophic scarring, milia and hyperpigmentation may also be seen.

It may be seen in patients with advanced CKD not on dialysis.

The reported prevalence is 1–18% in patients on HD.

Etiology
This is unclear.

Possible mechanisms include:
• phototoxic reaction or inadequate excretion of porphyrins;
• HD patients may produce or be exposed to compounds altering normal heme synthesis;
• drugs including tetracyclines, nabumetone, nalidixic acid, naproxen, frusemide and phenytoin.

Investigations
Serum, urine and stool porphyrins normal (unlike PCT).

Skin biopsy shows subepidermal separation.

Treatment
Sun-protection advice.

Phlebotomy and IV erythropoetin (patients likely to have concurrent anemia and may not tolerate phlebotomy).

Renal transplantation leads to complete resolution.

Further reading

Abdelbaqi-Salhab M, et al. A current review of cutaneous manifestations of renal disease. *J Cutan Pathol* 2003; **30**: 527–538.

Avermaete A, et al. Skin changes in dialysis patients: a review. *Nephrol Dial Transplant* 2001; **16**: 2293–2296.

Johnston GA, Graham-Brown RAC. The skin and disorders of the alimentary tract, the hepatobiliary, kidney and cardiopulmonary systems. In: Wolff K, Goldsmith L, Katz S, Gilchrest B, Paller A, Leffel D (eds), *Fitzpatrick's dermatology in general medicine*, 7th edn. New York: McGraw-Hill. pp. 1445–1460.

Internet resources

British Association of Dermatologists has a number of useful patient information leaflets:

www.bad.org.uk

International Center for Nephrogenic Fibrosing Dermopathy Research (ICNFDR):

http://www.pathmax.com/dermweb/

See also

Medical management of dialysis patients, p. 528

Neuropsychiatric disorders in chronic kidney disease

In this chapter the common neuropsychiatric manifestations of renal failure, and related issues, are discussed.

Peripheral neuropathy

Renal failure results in neurological dysfunction due to uremia.

Peripheral neuropathy is a common complication of ESRD and is usually a uremic neuropathy, although other causes of neuropathy such as ethanol-related neuropathy, chronic inflammatory demyelinating polyradiculoneuropathy, and diabetic neuropathy should be borne in mind.

Epidemiology

There is a widely variable prevalence ranging from 10 to 100% (commonly accepted figure of 60–65%).

It is more common in females.

It can occur at any age but is uncommon in children.

It usually develops below GFR of 12 mL/min, and the severity is moderately correlated with the severity of renal insufficiency.

Pathogenesis

Uremia is the common denominator and pathological changes are similar to other neuropathies. The exact mechanism is unknown although there are many theories.

The search for a specific uremic neurotoxin remains elusive. Urea, creatinine, guanidine, methylguanidine, guanidinosuccinic acid, uric acid, oxalic acid and a host of other substances have been proposed.

The 'middle molecule hypothesis' postulates that there may be accumulation of slowly dialyzable neurotoxic molecules of molecular weight 300–2000 Da.

Newer research attributes an important role to K^+ (chronic hyperkalemic depolarization) necessitating the need to maintain the serum K^+ within normal limits.

Clinical features

Uremic neuropathy presents as a symmetric distal sensorimotor polyneuropathy with greater lower limb involvement.

It is usually of insidious onset, with progression over months.

Clinical features include:

- tingling and prickling in the lower limbs;
- paresthesia (commonest and earliest symptom);
- weakness, muscle wasting;
- impaired vibration sense;
- pain that is partly relieved by movement.

The clinical features reflect large fiber involvement.

Mononeuropathies can occur at compression points: median nerve (carpal tunnel syndrome), ulnar nerve or peroneal nerve. A positive Tinel sign may be present.

The vestibulocochlear nerve is the most common cranial nerve affected and can manifest with variable loss of hearing that tends to improve with dialysis.

Investigations

These mainly focus on ruling out other causes of neuropathy.

Use of imaging has not been shown to be beneficial.

Electrophysiology studies show reduced conduction velocities.

Histology reveals axonal degeneration in distal nerve trunks. Myelin sheaths may appear normal on transverse electron microscopy but splitting of myelin lamella may be noted.

Management

Management is essentially focused on ensuring adequate dialysis.

Vitamin supplements have been used but have not been shown to be consistently beneficial.

Tricyclic antidepressants (amitryptiline, nortriptyline) and anticonvulsants such as gabapentin can be used for symptomatic relief of neuropathic pain. Care must be taken if prescribing high doses due to the underlying renal insufficiency as well as cardiac adverse effects of the medications themselves.

Local anesthetics such as lidocaine may be beneficial by stabilizing neuronal membranes and thus decreasing pain intensity.

The use of high flux dialyser membranes and alteration of hemodialysis schedules have been studied but have not been shown to be consistently beneficial.

Renal transplantation, especially if performed early in the course of the neuropathy, has been shown to be effective. All but the most severe cases are usually reversed.

Myopathy

Most patients with ESRD have muscle weakness and fatigue.

Uremic myopathy refers to the cluster of functional and occasionally structural muscle abnormalities in patients with CKD that may be attributed to the uremic state itself.

Epidemiology

The incidence of myopathy in CKD is unknown due to the lack of well-conducted studies.

Increasing age and female sex are risk factors.

The estimated prevalence is 50%.

Pathogenesis

The pathogenesis is inadequately understood.

The 'middle molecule hypothesis' (toxins incompletely dialysed and harmful to muscle) has been postulated.

In many cases uremic myopathy is related to secondary hyperparathyroidism and is superimposed on osteomalacia-associated myopathy.

Clinical features

Proximal limb weakness and wasting.

Easy fatiguability and poor endurance.

Functioning is worsened by bone pain and tenderness.

Reflexes may be impaired due to concomitant neuropathy.

Muscle strength is usually impaired (<50% of normal).

Investigations

Electromyography (EMG) and serum creatine kinase are normal.

Muscle biopsy findings are often nonspecific but can show fiber necrosis.

Management

High doses of vitamin D3 have been recommended but have not been shown to be consistently effective.

The condition is less common among well-dialysed patients, suggesting a role for optimization of dialysis adequacy.

Successful renal transplantation has been associated with improvement although may not restore full physical working capacity.

Autonomic dysfunction

Autonomic dysfunction may present as postural hypotension, sweating and diarrhea.

Epidemiology

It is more commonly seen in diabetic and elderly patients.

It is found in ~50% of patients with advanced CKD.

Investigations

Sympathetic skin responses (SSR) can be assessed with routine EMG equipment. They reveal a delayed or absent sympathetic skin response.

Other tests include:

- plasma noradrenaline levels in response to posture;
- Thermoregulatory Sweat Test (TST);
- Quantitative Sensory Testing (QST).

Esophageal manometry can also be useful in patients with possible autonomic neuropathy and dysphagia.

Management

Supportive management includes advice regarding reducing sudden changes in posture and recumbent dialysis.

Anemia should be avoided.

Pharmacologic treatment is attempted when conservative treatment is unsuccessful although results are variable:

- fludrocortisone;
- SSRIs (serotonin reuptake inhibitors);
- NSAIDs.

Midodrine, a selective α1-adrenoreceptor agonist which is metabolized to desglymidodrine, may be used. It acts by arterioconstriction and venoconstriction.

Erythropoetin therapy will not only correct renal anemia but may also increase norepinephrine levels and can be effective.

Psychological dysfunction

There is a higher prevalence of psychiatric illnesses in people suffering from physical disorders when compared to the general population.

Studies have consistently shown higher rates for admission in patients with comorbid depression, anxiety disorders, dementia, substance misuse psychoses and personality disorders.

One has also to be mindful of the stigma that mental illnesses continue to have in society. This may result in patients hiding their diagnoses or symptoms, resulting in inadequate psychological treatment, which may in turn influence the treatment of the physical disorder.

Affective disorders

Depression

Depression is the commonest of the affective disorders associated with CKD.

Symptoms include:

- low mood;
- easy fatiguability;
- inability to derive pleasure from activities that were previously enjoyed;
- decreased sleep and early morning awakening;
- decreased appetite and weight loss;
- diurnal variation of mood;
- decreased motivation, concentration and self-esteem;
- ideas of helplessness, hopelessness and worthlessness and suicidal ideations.

Sometimes the symptoms may be 'understandable' in the context of the physical illness but they still deserve assessment and treatment.

Use of screening questionnaires such as the Beck's Depression Inventory or General Hospital Questionnaire may be helpful but there is no better screening tool than a good clinical enquiry of symptoms.

Depression may worsen at certain stages of the illness, such as at times of diagnosis, clinical worsening of the condition, awareness of poor prognosis or transplant failure. It is important to be more vigilant at these times.

Management includes use of antidepressants and psychological therapies such as cognitive behavior therapy (CBT). There is no evidence for the use of 'counseling' and unfocussed therapies have the potential for harm.

SSRIs are the drugs of choice although dose adjustments may be necessary.

Tricyclic antidepressants usually do not require dosage adjustments in renal dysfunction but they have other adverse effects (anticholinergic, sedation) and are not drugs of first choice.

CBT focusses on the 'here and now' and uses techniques such as Socratic questioning and behavioral exercises to bring about change.

Bipolar disorder

This disorder is characterized by episodes of depression and/or mania.

The main issue is usually the safe and effective management of bipolar illness considering that patients may be prescribed lithium and this has the potential to worsen uremia.

The dose of lithium is difficult to manage in CKD and therefore other mood stabilizers such as sodium valproate may be used.

Close liaison with the treating psychiatrist is essential.

Case reports of mania being associated with uremia and improved with dialysis have been published.

Anxiety disorders

Anxiety may be related to diagnosis, prognosis or treatments such as dialysis and renal transplantation.

Patients may also suffer anxiety due to the intimidating environment of a sophisticated renal unit and the complexity of treatments required for progressive CKD.

Some patients may develop a phobia for the unit or the treatment. Others may have pre-existing specific phobic disorders such as needle phobias which may interfere with treatment.

Post-traumatic stress disorder may pre-exist or may develop with the stress of the illness.

Clinical features include physical symptoms such as:

- palpitations;
- dizziness;
- sweating;
- tremulousness.

Psychological symptoms include a sense of impending doom.

A careful enquiry must be made of these symptoms as it is easy to subsume them (especially the physical symptoms) under the symptoms of renal failure.

Treatment includes both pharmacological measures (such as SSRIs) and psychological measures (such as CBT).

Psychoses

These are unlikely to be caused by uremia.

The important issue is to distinguish 'functional' psychotic symptoms from the symptoms of encephalopathy.

It is useful to recognize that visual hallucinations and disorientation usually indicate an 'organic' cause.

Auditory hallucinations and persistent delusions in clear consciousness are indicative of primary psychotic illnesses.

It is also important to be aware that schizoaffective disorder may be treated by lithium.

Antipsychotics such as sulpiride and amisulpiride are excreted by the kidneys and their dose must be adjusted or they must be discontinued altogether depending on the renal function.

Cognitive dysfunction

Cognitive functioning can be affected by many medical conditions including encephalopathy and cerebrovascular disease.

Aluminium accumulation may be a contributing factor and other factors suggested include trace metal ions found in the dialyzate including manganese, cadmium, boron and tin.

Uremia can also depress cognitive function and this is partly improved with dialysis. Rapid dialysis may also contribute to cognitive dysfunction.

The Mini-Mental State Examination is a good tool to screen for cognitive problems. Bedside examination of cortical lobes is also useful. Specialized psychometric tests are indicated for prolonged or severe difficulties.

EEG shows bursts of high voltage slowing and frontal spiking in relation to excess aluminium. In dementia, the EEG shows slow waves.

Treatment depends upon the etiology. Commencing dialysis or increasing the dialysis dose has been suggested and there is evidence that correction of anemia with erythropoietin therapy may improve cognitive dysfunction.

Uremic encephalopathy

Uremic encephalopathy is an organic brain syndrome seen in advanced CKD. The symptoms are nonspecific and are seen in a wide range of encephalopathies.

Cognitive symptoms include difficulty with attention and memory. Patients find it difficult to perform tasks that require mentation or those that require multiple ideas at once. Frontal lobe signs and myoclonic jerks may be present.

Hallucinosis, paranoid ideations, emotional lability can be seen.

Autonomic (e.g. dizziness) and neuromuscular disturbances (e.g. fatigue) are also present.

The sleep–wake cycle is disrupted in the later stages.

The course is fluctuating and can change over days or even hours. In the later stages delirium may be prominent with disorientation, perceptual abnormalities and agitation leading to difficulty in management on the ward. The final stages are marked by torpor, a semicomatose state and generalized tonic–clonic seizures.

Neurological examination reveals increased tone and hyperreflexia with tremors (leading to asterixis), ankle clonus and an extensor plantar response.

Deterioration in renal function is associated with increased severity. Other contributing factors include electrolyte imbalance and drug toxicity.

The pathophysiology is not well-defined although electrolyte imbalances are a postulated cause. Most changes are nonspecific. Abnormalities of sodium, calcium and magnesium levels are common.

There seems to be little correlation between the level of uraemia and the clinical presentation.

Imaging is not usually helpful except to rule out other suspected causes of an acute confusional state.

Lumbar puncture may reveal aseptic meningitis.

EEG shows a generalized slowing, most prominent in the frontal region. Spike and wave discharges may be present.

Treatment is with the careful institution of dialysis to avoid dialysis disequilibrium syndrome.

Symptoms such as sluggishness and sleep–wake cycle abnormalities may persist.

Dialysis disequilibrium syndrome

This was first described when patients were dialysed infrequently and rapidly, and refers to the development of acute neurological symptoms occurring during or after intermittent dialysis.

The incidence is unknown. Risk factors include:

- severe uremia;
- first dialysis;
- young or old age;
- pre-existing neurological disease (head injury, stroke, malignant hypertension).

Symptoms usually occur at the end of or after dialysis.

Mild symptoms include:

- nausea;
- severe headaches;
- restlessness;
- muscle cramps.

These can rarely progress to:

- confusion and delirium;
- myoclonus;
- generalized tonic clonic seizures;
- cardiac arrhythmias;
- blurring of vision (due to papilloedema and raised intraocular pressure).

Disequilibrium syndrome is linked to:

Rapid changes in the osmotic gradient between the plasma and the brain. This is especially so with rapid dialysis or in people with severe uremia. Removal of urea during dialysis occurs slower across the blood–brain barrier than from plasma. This generates a 'reverse osmotic gradient' causing water movement into the brain leading to cerebral edema.

A decrease in cerebral intracellular pH by mechanisms that are not completely understood has been proposed as an alternative hypothesis: intracellular acidosis is associated with an increase in unmeasured organic acids which increase cerebral osmolality thus leading to cerebral edema.

Management is mainly focussed on prevention. Frequent dialysis (every 1–2 days) of short duration (2 h) using a smaller dialyser will facilitate slow removal of urea.

Dialysis dementia

Dialysis dementia, also known as dialysis encephalopathy, is a progressive, often diffuse encephalopathy which occurs in some patients on chronic HD.

Prevalence is estimated to be ~1%. It is equally prevalent among the sexes and different age groups.

Communication difficulties are often the presenting feature with dysarthria, dysphasia and slurred, stuttering speech.

This may initially be present only during or after dialysis.

Other cognitive signs such as dyslexia, dyspraxia and dyscalculia may be seen.

Impairment of memory, depression and paranoid ideation may occur.

Progression to myoclonus, asterixis, seizures and personality change may be seen.

In the later stages the patient may become mute.

Death usually occurs within 15 months.

EEG abnormalities of bilateral spike and wave complexes and frontal slow waves are seen, usually about 6 months prior to the onset of symptoms. There is a marked slowing of background rhythm.

Neuroimaging has not been shown to be diagnostically helpful.

Histopathological changes at postmortem are nonspecific.

Histochemically there is significant elevation of brain aluminium content especially in those cases that are geographically clustered.

Cerebrospinal fluid aluminium concentrations are of no diagnostic benefit, the disorder occurring at widely varying concentrations.

Management must focus on prevention by use of aluminium-free dialyzates, purification of water, and avoiding dietary intake of aluminium.

Benzodiazepines such as clonazepam and diazepam are effective in controlling myoclonus.

Desferroxamine can be used to chelate aluminium and is used in the treatment of established cases. The chelated complex is removed by dialysis. Improvement is slow and treatment may need to be continued for a year. Chelation can lead to an initial deterioration that may be progressive and occasionally fatal.

Sporadic dementia not related to aluminium excess is not amenable to chelation treatment.

Other disorders

Subdural hematomas, either due to an intrinsic coagulopathy in uremia (or due to administration of heparin when the patient starts dialysis) may occur. Clinical manifestations are not specific and can fluctuate. Cognitive impairment can be present.

Wernicke's encephalopathy resulting from thiamine deficiency (which may be made worse when the patient starts dialysis due to thiamine egress during dialysis) can occur. An underlying genetic predisposition, chronic malnutrition with anorexia, and the administration of glucose containing IV fluids are contributory factors. The classic triad (ophthalmoplegia, ataxia and confusion) is rarely present. Treatment is by thiamine replacement. Early treatment prevents progression to Korsakoff's psychosis which is not amenable to thiamine replacement.

Sleep disorders. The commonest sleep problems reported with CKD are insomnia, restless leg syndrome and excessive daytime sleepiness. Other reported syndromes include obstructive sleep apnea syndrome, sleepwalking and narcolepsy. Uremia is postulated as the common denominator and commencement of dialysis may improve symptoms but rarely results in complete resolution.

Psychotropic drug use in the patient with failing renal function

The common drugs and the implications for prescribing in patients with CKD and ESRD are reviewed in Table 11.14.1.

Issues of capacity and consent

The law (in England and Wales) assumes that all adults have the capacity to make decisions unless otherwise proven.

Different laws may apply in other countries and the following are only general principles.

Difficulties and ethical dilemmas arise when issues regarding extent of capacity arise. Some important concepts to note are:

- Capacity is specific to the planned treatment.
- Different suggested treatments may require different levels of capacity. Generally more invasive treatments require a greater understanding of risks and benefits.
- Capacity may be present to consent for one treatment but not for another even at the same time.

Informed consent is the heart of clinical ethics and it is the duty of the treating physician to satisfy the criteria required and to make an assessment of capacity.

The principles of assessment of capacity can be summarized in the following questions:

- Does my patient understand the information provided regarding the treatment in question?
- Does my patient believe the information provided?
- Does my patient understand the pros and cons of having this treatment versus any other treatment or even no treatment at all?
- Can my patient retain the information provided long enough for him/her to make a decision?
- Can my patient communicate (not necessarily by verbal means) the decision made?

If the answer to any of the above questions is 'No', it usually signifies a lack of capacity.

Common law has supported the principles of Best Interests, Necessity and Duty of Care in managing patients without capacity.

The above principles hold true for any individual aged >18 years. For those aged <18 years, the law (in England and Wales) is different. Some important principles are:

Young people (<18 years) CAN CONSENT to treatment if they satisfy the requirements of capacity assessment. However, in practice an adult with parental responsibility is usually involved in the decision-making process.

Young people (<18 years) CANNOT REFUSE to have any treatment if an adult with parental responsibility consents, even if the young person fulfills the criteria for capacity assessment. The decision of the adult with parental responsibility usually overrides any decision made by the young person. If in doubt, it is appropriate to consult with persons with experience in the legal aspects as they apply to young persons.

If the patient is deemed not to have capacity, The Mental Capacity Act (2005) (in England and Wales) provides a legal framework for decision-making. The Act also allows adults with capacity to make decisions in the event of future incapacity in some areas (including refusal of specific treatments).

When a patient is unable to make an autonomous choice, the health professional must act in the best interests of the patient. Second opinions are usually appropriate. The Act lays down some principles for acting in the patient's best interests:

• To ensure that if the decision can be clinically delayed in the likely event of regaining capacity, it is.
• To encourage and optimize the participation of the patient as far as is possible.
• To thoroughly investigate any past or present wishes or values of the patient or any other relevant factors.
• To consider the views of other relevant people who may be carers or people interested in their welfare.

The Court of Protection is the final arbiter (in England and Wales) in case of dispute.

Finally, it is important to realize that people have the right to make unwise decisions and this does not necessarily indicate lack of capacity. In complex cases it would be reasonable to ask for expert advice.

Further reading

Brown T, Brown R. Neuropsychiatric consequences of renal failure. *Psychosomatics* 1995; **36**: 244–253.

Cohen LM, Tessier EG, Germain MJ, Levy NB. Update on psychotropic medication in renal disease. *Psychosomatics* 2004; **45**: 34–46.

Phipps A, Turkington D. Psychiatry in the renal unit. *Adv Psychiat Treatment* 2001; **7**: 426–432.

Table 11.14.1 Common drugs used for the treatment of neuropsychiatric disorders with specific consideration of changes in CKD and ESRD

Drug group	Notes on prescribing in renal impairment
Antipsychotics	<1% of haloperidol is excreted by the kidneys (recommended dose in ESRD is 1–2 mg bd or tds).
	<1% of aripiprazole is excreted by the kidneys but there are reports of drug interactions with other drugs; not much is known in terms of safety in renal impairment. No dose reduction is recommended in ESRD.
	No dose adjustments recommended for olanzapine or quetiapine by their respective manufacturers.
	Clozapine excreted in only trace amounts in urine but the anticholinergic side-effects, especially urinary retention, may be a problem.
	Sulpiride and amisulpiride are excreted by the kidneys and risperidone clearance is reduced in ESRD.
Antimanic agents	Lithium is a common source of concern.
	Avoid altogether if possible. If not, reduce dose.
	It can be removed by dialysis, hence best to administer as a single, reduced dose post dialysis.
	Contraindicated in severe renal impairment.
	Other mood stabilizers such as sodium valproate, carbamazepine and lamotrigine are not significantly excreted in urine.
	There is a risk of increased free levels of valproate in ESRD, hence the need to monitor 'free' drug levels in severe renal impairment. Safest principle is to 'start low and go slow'.
Antidepressants	SSRIs are generally drugs of first choice.
	If using paroxetine, reduce dose. No change recommended with other SSRIs.
	Tricyclic antidepressants are not significantly excreted by the kidneys; however, their use is to be balanced with potential for adverse effects (especially anticholinergic) and risk of mortality in overdose.
	Nefazodone is not excreted by the kidneys but risk of hepatotoxicity is high, hence use with caution.
Anxiolytics	Benzodiazepines are primarily excreted via the liver.
	Adjust dose only in severe renal impairment and monitor for excessive sedation.
	Zolpidem and zopiclone may be used but it is prudent to start with a low dose.

Internet resources

National Institute of Mental Health:

http://www.nimh.nih.gov

National Phobics Society:

http://www.phobics-society.org.uk

Royal College of Psychiatrists:

http://www.rcpsych.ac.uk/mentalhealthinforma-
tion.aspx

British Association for Behavioural and Cognitive Psychotherapies (BABCP):

http://www.babcp.org.uk

See also

Psychological aspects of treatment for renal failure, p. 538

β2M amyloidosis, p. 436

Drug-induced nephropathies, p. 698

Special problems in chronic kidney disease

Chapter contents

Chronic kidney disease in children

Introduction
Children need to grow and develop into adults. Chronic kidney disease (CKD) can have a major impact upon physical growth as well as psychological, social and scholastic development.

Organization of facilities
It is appropriate to treat and follow such children in specialized units which provide access to multidisciplinary teams including:
- pediatric nephrologists;
- specialist nurses;
- pediatric urologists;
- dieticians;
- social workers;
- psychologists;
- play specialists;
- hospital teaching staff;
- youth workers.

Pediatric units are likely to use the transplantation expertise of local adult units.

Pediatric and adult care is a continuum and young people with CKD should be prepared for transition to adult units.

This should take place when they are mature and have completed growth and development.

The same categories of chronic kidney disease (CKD 1–5) are used for children as with adults.

Dialysis should be seen only as a temporary option in children before transplantation becomes available.

A good functioning transplant offers the best opportunity for growth and long-term rehabilitation.

Epidemiology
Incidence of CKD 5 is low compared to adults with an annual take on rate for dialysis of ~2–3 pmp (8 pmp aged <15 years).

Prevalence of mild–severe CKD (stages 2–5) is 35–40 pmp.

Prevalence of CKD 5 in South Asian children is ~3× that of Caucasian population due to high incidence of inherited disease.

Prevalence of CKD is higher in male patients (ratio of 1.54:1) due to predominance of renal dysplasia and obstructive uropathy in males.

Etiology
The majority of patients in childhood have an identifiable cause for CKD.

Congenital abnormalities (55%)
- Renal dysplasia/hypoplasia
- Obstructive uropathies
- Reflux nephropathy

Hereditary conditions (17%)
- Nephronophthisis
- Alport's syndrome
- Congenital nephrotic syndrome
- Cystinosis
- Autosomal recessive polycystic kidney disease
- Oxalosis

Glomerulonephritis (10%)
- Focal and segmental glomerulosclerosis
- Other chronic glomerulonephritides

Multisystem disorders (6%)
- Hemolytic uremic syndrome
- Henoch–Schönlein purpura
- Lupus erythematosus

Miscellaneous (9%)
- Renal vascular disease
- Kidney tumour (usually bilateral Wilms')
- Denys–Drash syndrome

Cause unknown
- 3%

Clinical presentation
Children are often asymptomatic until CKD is very advanced.

There may be nonspecific symptoms including:
- lethargy;
- tiredness after school and poor concentration;
- poor appetite;
- urinary symptoms including polyuria or enuresis (bed-wetting).

The use of antenatal USS has enabled the detection of renal tract malformations before symptoms develop or superimposed problems occur such as urinary tract sepsis with posterior urethral valves.

Modes of presentation include:
- incidental on antenatal USS;
- urinary tract infection with underlying dysplasia and/or reflux nephropathy;
- polyuria and enuresis (renal concentrating defect with nephronophthisis);
- failure to thrive and short stature related to poor nutritional intake or tubulopathy;
- bone abnormalities or rickets due to tubulopathy (cystinosis or CKD);
- hematuria or proteinuria;
- hypertension and congestive cardiac failure;
- failure to recover from AKI;
- seizures and hypertensive encephalopathy;
- investigation of a child with lethargy or pallor;
- investigation of siblings with familial condition;
- investigation of child with syndrome known to have an associated renal abnormality.

Investigations
General investigations
Urine
- Urinalysis (pH, blood, protein, glucose, nitrites, leukocytes);
- Urine culture if urinalysis positive, especially if any symptoms;
- Proteinuria quantified by early morning urine protein: creatinine ratio (PCR, normal <20 mg of protein/mmol of creatinine).

Blood
- Full blood count, ferritin and transferrin saturation (TSAT)
- Urea and electrolytes, creatinine, bicarbonate, calcium, phosphate, alkaline phosphatase and albumin
- Parathyroid hormone (PTH)
- Estimated GFR (Schwartz formula should be used for children between 2 and 14 years of age [mL/min/1.73 m^2 = 40 × height cm/creatinine μmol/l])

Radiology
- Renal tract USS – invaluable to have expert pediatric radiology advice as USS is informative and noninvasive. Size of kidneys related to patient's height to define hypoplasia/dysplasia.
- Hand and wrist X-ray for bone age and signs of renal osteodystrophy.

Cardiac review
- ECG/echocardiography: for signs of left ventricular hypertrophy, especially if hypertensive.

Special investigations
The choice will be guided by history (including detailed family history), examination and general investigations especially urinalysis and USS.

GFR can be formally measured by [^{51}Cr]EDTA method or inulin or iohexol clearance.

Further radiological investigations are best discussed at nephrouroradiology conferences. Further imaging could include micturating cystourethrography, radionuclide imaging (DMSA or MAG3), CT or MRI studies.

Children presenting with nephritic or nephrotic syndrome require complement levels, autoantibody screen and ANCA levels ('nephritic screen').

Children with urinary calculi should be investigated with a 'stone-former protocol' looking for conditions such as hyperoxaluria and disorders of purine metabolism.

Suspected cystinosis can be confirmed by white cell cystine levels and slit lamp examination for corneal crystals.

Liaison with the genetics department is important as a large number of hereditary/familial conditions can now be recognized by mutations:
- oxalosis;
- congenital nephrotic syndrome;
- cystinosis;
- Denys–Drash syndrome;
- nephronophthisis;
- Alports.

Renal biopsy is generally undertaken when chronic glomerulonephritis is suspected, the etiology of CKD unexplained and genetic testing not possible.

Management
Patients with CKD 1 and 2 can be seen infrequently (12- or 6-monthly respectively) and can attend shared care regional clinics to reduce travel time to the nephrology centre.

Disturbances in phosphate metabolism and rises in PTH have been documented in CKD 3 patients and so dietary evaluation should be undertaken.

CKD 4 and 5 patients require more frequent monitoring with access to the center's multidisciplinary team.

Treatment has to be individualized for each child.

For the child born with major urinary tract abnormalities the testing time is whether the child has sufficient renal reserve to grow adequately in the first 2 years of life.

Renal function often declines slowly in mid-childhood. The greatest challenge is whether the child has sufficient renal reserve to get through the pubertal growth spurt.

The diagnosis of CKD in a child in any family can cause great anxiety, especially with the uncertainty of deterioration.

Information and support need to be available to the family throughout the childhood period and are cornerstones of good practice.

Prevention of progression of CKD
Monitoring of all children with CKD should include measurement of an early morning urine for PCR or albumin: creatinine ratio (ACR).

Urine taken at a morning clinic is acceptable but beware orthostatic proteinuria, especially in adolescents.

There is currently no agreement at what level of proteinuria treatment should be started (normal PCR <20 mg/mmol).

For increasing proteinuria an ACEI is first choice (usually enalapril) starting at 2.5 mg and gradually increasing to maximally tolerated dose.

Monitor blood pressure and plasma potassium and creatinine at clinic visits.

Aim to maximally reduce proteinuria but without hypotension or hyperkalemia.

Concordance remains problematical in adolescents.

Teenage girls need to be informed of the risk from ACEIs of fetal malformations in pregnancy.

Evidence is emerging that children with CKD due to congenital abnormalities of the urinary tract (the major group) do not respond to ACEIs as well as those with chronic glomerulonephritis.

There is very limited experience of adding ARBs (e.g. losartan) to ACEI treatment and there are no recommendations for this in children.

Nutrition
The involvement of a renal dietician trained in pediatrics is essential.

In mild renal failure healthy eating diet advice should be provided including advice on 'no added salt' (children love salty snack foods!).

In CKD 3–5, phosphate restriction may be required.

Low protein diets are not advocated.

Patients with CKD 4 and 5 require regular dietary assessments with comparisons to Reference Nutrient Intakes (RNIs) to optimize nutritional status.

Supplements may be required to achieve RNI.

Dialysis patients often require nasogastric or gastrostomy feeds.

The required protein intakes depend upon stage of CKD and the age of the patient.

Vitamin supplements including B-complex, iron, zinc and copper should be given to dialysis patients and CKD 4 patients after assessment. Vitamin A needs to be avoided and a suitable vitamin and micronutrient is Pediatric Renal Dialyvit.

Fluid and electrolyte balance

Avoid potassium-containing foods, e.g. certain fruits, chocolate.

If hypertensive and fluid overloaded, sodium restriction and diuretics are required.

In children with congenital abnormalities of the urinary tract and polyuria, salt wasting may be prominent and sodium supplements may be required (also in infants also on peritoneal dialysis).

Acid base balance

Acidosis has an adverse effect on growth and sodium bicarbonate supplements should be prescribed to maintain plasma bicarbonate in normal range.

Renal osteodystrophy

This is particularly important in children because the lesions of hyperparathyroidism are superimposed on the growth zone lesions – hence the old term 'renal rickets'.

Such bones can deform easily and result in the need for orthopedic intervention.

Treatment primarily involves control of plasma phosphate by dietary intake along with phosphate binders which are usually calcium carbonate compounds. Patients should be involved in choice of medication which might improve compliance. Sevelamer is not licensed for children but increasingly used.

Vitamin D analogues such as 1α-hydroxycholecalciferol or 1,25-dihydroxycholecalciferol are prescribed aiming to keep the PTH level within the normal range.

Three-monthly monitoring of PTH should be undertaken or monthly in young infants on dialysis.

Annual X-ray to assess bone age.

Anemia

Assess iron status by hemoglobin, ferritin and TSAT.

Oral iron supplements, e.g. Sytron liquid in younger children or ferrous sulphate tablets in older children. Poor compliance is again a problem and clear instructions regarding time of taking tablets is important.

IV iron may be required in hemodialysis patients and can safely be administered on an outpatient basis to patients on PD and before dialysis.

SC erythropoetin to maintain hemoglobin at target levels of ≥11 g/dL in older children and ≤10 g/dL if aged <2 years.

Hypertension

Defined by reference to published centile charts for sex and height.

Blood pressure should be at least <90th centile.

Appropriate sized cuff should be used for each child.

Automated oscillometric measurements are commonly used but cause discomfort in some children.

Check blood pressure with aneroid sphygmomanometer and Doppler device for systolic pressure in small infants.

If doubt about 'white-coat hypertension' then blood pressure can be assessed using 24 h ambulatory blood pressure monitoring.

Address salt intake which is invariably high in children.

Calcium channel blockers such as nifedipine (twice a day modified release) or once daily slow release preparations are favored as initial treatment.

In renin-dependent hypertension use ACEI (captopril and then enalapril). Cautionary use in teenage girls who may become pregnant.

Many drugs have not been fully evaluated in children but should be prescribed as advised in the British National Formulary for Children.

Infection

When children have congenital abnormalities of the urinary tract recurrent infection is common.

Parents/carers should be properly informed about obtaining appropriate urine samples (clean-catch urine preferable to bag urine) in primary care.

Prophylactic antibiotics

Trimethoprim 2 mg/kg or nitrofurantoin 1 mg/kg are generally employed for those with grade 3–5 vesicoureteric reflux for at least the first 2 years of life.

Surgical intervention

Close liaison is required with pediatric urologists for those with recurrent infections and consideration given to procedures such as establishing bladder drainage, ureteric reimplantation or endoscopic correction (STING procedure) or, ultimately, nephrectomy in a kidney with <10% function.

Growth

Many of the above factors impact upon growth which is a good indicator of adequacy of CKD treatment.

There may also be psychosocial factors affecting the child's well-being which require careful exploration by a team member, such as a social worker and/or psychologist.

Height and weight should be measured at each clinic visit and charted on the appropriate growth charts (with corrections made for prematurity in the first 2 years).

Head circumference should be measured regularly in children <2 years of age and also plotted on appropriate centile charts.

Growth hormone is licensed for use in children with CKD who fail to grow adequately when all other aspects of management have been optimized. Child qualify for growth hormone if their height standard deviation score (SDS) is below −2 or if their height velocity SDS is below the mean, but only if adequate nutrition and metabolic abnormalities have been corrected.

Growth hormone is administered subcutaneously on a daily basis. Information on its use is provided by the relevant manufacturers.

Preparation for dialysis and transplantation

Children who have a slowly progressive deterioration of renal function should be given information about future dialysis and transplant options which can be discussed with the family over a long period.

Some patients may present needing urgent chronic dialysis ('crash-landers'). This invariably occurs when patients present with AKI such as a crescentic glomerulonephritis which then progresses rapidly to a chronic state. Sometimes CKD is undetected and the child suddenly presents in teenage years with persistent anorexia and anemia. Such acute patients and their families can have major difficulties adjusting to the 'double-hit' of both acute and chronic renal failure.

Transplantation is the ultimate goal for children with CKD 5 and there has been increasing focus on pre-emptive transplantation which is regarded as the treatment of choice.

Information needs of children and families can be addressed by multimedia methods which should involve the whole family.

Home visits by members of the team, including social worker and experienced nurse, are very beneficial in assessing family set-ups, facilities for possible home dialysis and allowing the family to ask questions in their own home environments.

Families may benefit from being linked either to other families with the same condition or to a child of similar age or same sex.

If children have been seen only in a regional referral clinic, investigations that are needed before dialysis or transplantation can be co-ordinated on dedicated renal assessment days. Families should also have the opportunity to visit the dialysis unit and meet other members of the multiprofessional team. Some children are very apprehensive about needles (needle phobia) and it is essential that the unit has play therapists who can help relieve anxiety often in discussion or supervision with the clinical psychologist.

A child may be depressed or have major behavioral disturbance and may require assessment by a child psychiatrist.

A number of children entering the dialysis/transplant program have disabilities. If severe, the ethical imperative is to act in the best interests of the child and maximizing conservative treatment without dialysis is a treatment option. This will require discussions with a number of agencies and possibly a clinical ethics committee to help formulate the best plan.

Immunizations

All children must complete routine childhood vaccinations including:
- haemophilis influenzae Type B conjugate (HIB);
- pneumococcal vaccine;
- meningococcal group C conjugate.

Infants with CKD should be considered for vaccination against rotavirus.

Children approaching dialysis and transplantation require vaccination for:
- hepatitis B;
- varicella;
- BCG.

Hepatitis B vaccine can be given at any age at intervals of 0, 1 and 6 months. Check anti-HBS antigen antibodies 2–3 months after the 3rd dose.

BCG may be given to some newborns routinely.

Over the age of 6 years BCG should only be given if tuberculin skin test negative.

Transplantation should be delayed for 3 months after BCG.

Annual immunization with influenza vaccine is recommended.

Dialysis and transplant options

Transplantation

For all children dialysis should be seen only as a temporary measure before transplantation.

Restoration of good kidney function after transplantation offers the best opportunity for improved growth, school attendance and long-term psychosocial rehabilitation.

For many children with congenital or familial conditions causing their CKD, deterioration in renal function (particularly around puberty) can be anticipated and pre-emptive transplantation considered.

Living–related donor transplantation (LRD) is strongly favored, especially with laparoscopic donor nephrectomy. With decreasing numbers of deceased donor offers, living donation is now being extended from the parents to other family members or emotionally related donors.

Altruistic donation and paired donor schemes are exceptional at present.

Evaluation for transplantation is similar to that of adult patients with a urology opinion essential for children with suspected abnormal bladders. It is essential to ensure that the bladder is of adequate capacity, empties adequately and does not generate high pressures before transplantation.

Most pediatric centers use the transplantation expertise of local adult units with postoperative medical management being in a pediatric facility.

Standard immunosuppressive regimes at present typically consist of:
- tacrolimus (calcineurin inhibitor of choice based on randomized trials and fewer side-effects than ciclosporin);
- prednisolone (minimization or steroid-avoidance regimes are being trialled);
- azathioprine.

The latter may be substituted by mycophenolate mofetil after rejection episodes and increasingly mycophenolate is used de novo.

Concordance with therapy is a major problem in the long term, especially in the adolescent age group. Enquiries about who supervises medications as well as ongoing education and support from team members such as youth workers may assist.

Excellent patient survival rates (96% at 5 years) with 5 year graft survival rates of 78% for deceased donors and 83% for living related donors.

Peritoneal dialysis therapy

Automated peritoneal dialysis (APD) is preferred. It can be performed overnight in the patient's home with hopefully minimal impact upon schooling and social life.

APD machines are mobile and hence family holidays are possible.

Two parents or carers should be trained – there is a very heavy burden of care on mothers with infants receiving APD as well as enteral feeds and medications.

Home support and respite care need careful consideration.

Peritonitis is the main risk. The Renal Association standard is one episode in 18 patient-months (3 year average).

Adequacy of dialysis should be assessed using both clinical and biochemical parameters.

Hemodialysis

Jugular venous catheters are the commonest form of vascular access as there is usually only a short period of hemodialysis before transplantation. There are inherent difficulties of creating arteriovenous fistulas in small children.

Logistical problems occur transporting patients from long distances to central specialized pediatric hemodialysis units.

Hemodialysis is therefore chosen for mainly social reasons or when peritoneal dialysis access is not possible, i.e. peritonitis or abdominal problems.

Bicarbonate dialysis should be standard and machines should be capable of ultrafiltration control.

Hemodiafiltration may have advantages over hemodialysis but requires ultrapure water.

Hemodialysis regimes are usually 4 h three times per week.

Daily dialysis may result in better growth, improved bone disease and less anemia.

Home hemodialysis is feasible but should only be attempted in those predicted to need long-term dialysis and who have good vascular access and a dedicated carer.

Psychosocial support

This is an essential component of pediatric care.

Every child should be seen in the context of the family and stress upon the patient, parents and siblings recognized.

A social worker should assess each family at home to assess needs and any entitlement to state support, e.g. disability allowance.

A psychologist can help with the impact of illness upon the child, i.e. needle phobias, behavior disturbance, nightmares.

Educational support is mandatory for children on hemodialysis but it is also important to liaise with schools if the child is on peritoneal dialysis and post transplantation.

Most specialist units have a holiday strategy which can include support for families, holidays for a patient group to build self-esteem and give families a break, and sport-oriented camps to increase participation and socialization.

Youth workers can help support young people (aged 12–20 years) having major adjustment issues.

Children and families should be discussed at regular psychosocial team meetings in order to share knowledge and anticipate problems.

Follow-up

The survival rate of children with CKD is good and the majority will transfer to adult care.

In patients with CKD 1–3 this may be the primary care physician with instructions to refer back to adult services if increasing proteinuria or creatinine develop.

Patients with CKD 4 or 5 need an organized transfer to adult units when they have followed a transition process with adequate information and preparation. Transition issues need to be addressed in both the pediatric and adult units and processes agreed so that follow-up and hopefully patient compliance is assured.

Further reading

Batte S, Watson AR, Amess K. The effects of chronic renal failure on siblings. *Pediatr Nephrol* 2006; **21**: 246–250.

Dixon P, Iurilli J, Watson AR, Neill E, Foy J, Martin M. Acceptability of a reformulated renal-specific micronutrient supplement. *Pediatr Nephrol* 2004; **19**: 1433–1443.

Fischbach M, Edefonti A, Schroder C, Watson A, The European Pediatric Dialysis Working Group. Hemodialysis in children: general practical guidelines. *Pediatr Nephrol* 2005; **20**: 1054–1066.

Klaus G, Watson A, Edefonti A, et al. Prevention and treatment of renal osteodystrophy in children on chronic renal failure: European guidelines. *Pediatr Nephrol* 2006; **21**: 151–159.

Lewis M, et al. Demography and management of childhood established renal failure in the UK. In: Ansell D, Feest TG, Tomson C, Williams AJ, Warwick G (eds), *UK Renal Registry Report*. Bristol: UK Renal Registry; 2006. Chapter 13.

Smith GC, Inward C. How and when to measure blood pressure. In: Webb N, Postlethwaite R (eds), *Clinical paediatric nephrology*. Oxford: Oxford University Press; 2003. pp. 135–150.

Watson AR. Strategies to support the families of children with end stage renal failure. *Pediatr Nephrol* 1995; **9**: 628–631.

Watson AR. Meeting the information needs of children and their families. In: Postlethwaite R, Webb N (eds), *Clinical paediatric nephrology*, 3rd ed. Oxford University Press, Oxford; 2003. pp. 465–474.

Watson AR. Hospital youth work and adolescent support. *Arch Dis Child* 2004; **89**: 440–442.

Watson AR. Problems and pitfalls of transition from paediatric to adult renal care. *Pediatr Nephrol* 2005; **20**: 113–117.

Internet resources

British National Formulary for Children:

http://www.bnfc.org

NKF K/DOQI Guidelines. Clinical Practice Guidelines and Clinical Practice Recommendations. 2006 Updates. Peritoneal Dialysis Adequacy:

http://www.kidney.org/professionals/kdoqi/guideline_upHD_PD_VA/pd_wg.htm

Child and carer information on kidney disease:

http://www.nuh.nhs.uk/ext/ckn/information.htm

http://www.ich.ucl.ac.uk/factsheets/index.html

NICE Clinical Guidance CG39. Anaemia management in people with chronic kidney disease. Sept 2006:

http://guidance.nice.org.uk/CG39

See also

Urinary tract infections in infancy and childhood, p. 252

Hypertensive children, p. 304

Acute kidney injury in infants and children, p. 372

Congenital abnormalities of the urinary tract, p. 658

Vesicoureteric reflux and reflux nephropathy, p. 648

Chronic kidney disease in the elderly

Introduction

Life expectancy in most developed countries has increased substantially in recent years. Around 20% of the total population are aged >65 years and 6% are >75 years; these figures are likely to increase further. The greater life expectancy of females means that they increase as a proportion of the population in older cohorts and among those with CKD.

The presence of ESRD requiring dialysis increases the risk of death three-fold at the age of 75 years compared to the healthy population. However, it should be noted that the increase in risk and years of life lost are substantially less than for the middle-aged dialysis patient.

The incidence of newly diagnosed CKD increases significantly with age and the mean age for new referrals in developed countries is now 60–65 years. The median age of patients starting dialysis in the UK in 2006 was 65 years, which has changed little over the previous 6 years.

Elderly patients with ESRD have been significantly disadvantaged in terms of referral for RRT and transplantation.

This has been because of a combination of reluctance to use scarce facilities for those with less to gain and a perception that the elderly will tolerate the process less well.

Late referral of elderly patients has been a particular problem with its attendant increased mortality and morbidity, increased time of hospitalization, and disadvantage with regard to choice of therapy and access to transplantation.

The introduction of reporting of eGFR in the UK in 2006 was primarily to reduce late referral by highlighting that relatively low levels of creatinine in elderly patients may represent advanced renal impairment.

The marked aging of the dialysis population in recent years can be attributed to:
- an expansion in the number of places;
- increased referral rates (supported by concerns about agism);
- technical advances that have made dialysis more tolerable;
- improved survival on dialysis.

Elderly patients with CKD have increasing numbers of comorbidities including dementia although these vary greatly. These factors have to be taken into account when discussing treatment options with patients and selecting appropriate candidates for dialysis.

It is clear, however, that chronological age alone is not a reason to exclude patients from RRT. Some physicians evoke the concept of biological age although this is, in reality, a subjective judgement.

The presence of severe vascular disease and diabetes carries a particularly poor prognosis.

Social and psychological factors may also be crucial factors determining the success or otherwise of dialysis.

The elderly have greater challenges in adjusting to dialysis regimens:
- they find learning techniques more difficult;
- they spend more time in hospital;
- they are more vulnerable to complications;
- they have a greater mortality from infection and cardiovascular disease;
- they survive for shorter periods;

Treatment costs are higher for elderly patients compared to younger patients.

There are inevitable difficulties in making selection decisions over life-prolonging treatment in elderly patients who develop ESRD. However, it is widely accepted that some frail elderly patients are unsuitable for dialysis.

Some units will offer a 'trial of dialysis' in more marginal cases with the agreement of clinicians, family and patient that the decision will be reviewed at an interval and the explicit possibility that it may subsequently be appropriate to withdraw treatment.

Causes of chronic kidney disease in the elderly

The causes of renal failure among elderly patients differ substantially when compared to younger cohorts (Table 12.2.1).

The most common diseases leading to renal failure are:
- vascular disease including hypertension;
- diabetes;
- obstructive uropathy;

Although there is no identifiable cause in a significant minority.

Glomerulonephritis accounts for a smaller proportion of cases than in younger groups.

Cardiovascular disease is highly prevalent in the elderly in developed countries.

Vascular disease of the main renal arteries should be suspected as a cause in patients with asymmetrical kidneys, cardiac or peripheral vascular disease, and diabetes mellitus.

Renal artery stenosis is present in 15–20% of many series of patients with ESRD and is more common with increasing age.

The benefit of renal artery angioplasty ± stenting remains under study, but is probably indicated in patients with deteriorating function and 'flash pulmonary edema'.

Prostatic obstruction is a potential cause that should always be considered in elderly males. Relief of the obstruction may lead to significant recovery of renal function.

Amyloidosis is also increasingly common with age, being a significant cause of nephrotic syndrome in the elderly. Periorbital hemorrhage is a classic sign. The prognosis is often poor because cardiac amyloid may lead to terminal cardiac failure.

Renal replacement therapy in the elderly

The main treatment options available for elderly patients with ESRD are:
- home-based peritoneal dialysis (CAPD or APD);
- hospital-based hemodialysis;
- renal transplantation.

The proportion receiving each will depend on the availability of hospital-supervised dialysis spaces and of donor organs.

Table 12.2.1 Causes of chronic kidney disease in the elderly

Cause	Approximate frequency
Atherosclerotic disease	17–38%
Diabetes	10–28%
Unknown cause	12–29%
Glomerulonephritis	6–28%
Infective/obstructive	1–17%
Neoplastic	2–4%
Hereditary	2–6%
Toxic	1–18%
Congenital	<1%
Miscellaneous	1–2%

Historically in the UK as many as 70% of patients aged >65 were allocated to peritoneal dialysis.

The choice between home- or center-based treatments should be made with consultation between the patient and renal team.

An assessment by trained members of the multidisciplinary dialysis team, performed in the patient's home, is invaluable in determining the suitability of individuals for peritoneal dialysis.

All patients should have an optimal hemoglobin concentration.

Those with poor cardiac function or myocardial ischemia (likely causes of mortality) should be assessed and treated.

Transplantation should be considered in fit patients up to the age of 70 years and is increasingly an option in selected patients over that age. Patients should be screened for cardiac (including coronary angiography if appropriate), respiratory and urological disease. All diabetic patients should have full cardiovascular assessment including coronary angiography.

Peritoneal dialysis

Peritoneal dialysis has some important potential advantages for older patients, although only ~15% of elderly patients in Europe and 8% in the USA are treated by this method.

Advantages include:
- independence from the dialysis unit;
- more physiological removal of fluid and electrolytes;
- reduced cardiovascular instability;
- preservation of native renal function.

There are also some limitations particularly relevant to older patients.

PD requires:
- manual dexterity;
- personal hygiene;
- visual acuity;
- strength to lift bags of fluid;
- motivation;
- preserved cognitive function;
- the ability to learn new skills.

The demands on the patient can be reduced by automation but are still considerable for many elderly patients.

There are moves in the UK to assist patients with automated PD (APD) by daily carers visiting to help with machine set-up and emptying waste bags (assisted APD). This is likely to help elderly patients wishing to receive therapy at home and has increasingly become standard practice in a number of countries over the past few years.

There are a number of relative contraindications to PD that are relevant in older patients including:
- previous abdominal surgery;
- severe chronic obstructive airways disease;
- diverticulitis;
- untreatable hernias.

In contrast to hemodialysis, where technique-related dropout occurs early, dropout from PD is continuous.

Most renal registries suggest that the survival of elderly uremic patients is broadly equivalent whether PD or hemodialysis is used.

Infection (peritonitis, exit site and tunnel infections) is no more common in the elderly than in younger patients.

Some quality of life studies suggest that patients managing PD in their own home fair better than those undergoing hospital-based hemodialysis.

Hemodialysis

Given the complexity of managing PD, a greater proportion of elderly compared to younger patients are on unit-based hemodialysis.

Establishing vascular access can pose significant difficulties because peripheral arterial disease and small, fragile veins make good fistula formation difficult.

However, the increased risk of bacteremias with tunneled lines (internal jugular and subclavian) means that fistula formation should be attempted if at all feasible and can be aided by Doppler and arteriographical imaging.

The increased maturation times of fistulae in the elderly and increased surgical failure rates mean that access surgery should be planned early.

Older patients are more vulnerable to the recognized adverse effects of hemodialysis including:
- hypotension;
- arrythmias;
- chronic malnutrition;
- increased incidence of infection;
- depression.

Outcomes of dialysis

Both quality and quantity of life are important.

However, both are difficult to measure because of:
- variable referral patterns;
- differing take-on rates;
- unequal access of elderly patients to transplantation.

Various tools have been used to measure quality of life, e.g. Karnofsky scores and Short Form (SF)-36. As with survival, there is likely to be an effect of selection for acceptance for dialysis.

Studies suggest that the patient's support and environment, as well as selection for treatment, may determine the degree of rehabilitation.

Erythropoetin has a clear role in improving quality of life in both dialysed and nondialysed patients.

Overall survival of the elderly on dialysis improved considerably during the 1980s; this continued but at a reduced rate into the 1990s.

There is still a significant actuarial shortfall in life expectancy, but the shortfall is much less than in younger populations.

Cause of death, as in younger populations, is led by cardiovascular disease and infection.

The issue of withdrawal from dialysis is increasingly important as older and frailer patients embark on RRT.

Decision-making may be complicated by the deterioration of mental capacity due to a variety of causes.

Discontinuation of dialysis is the second most common cause of death after cardiovascular disease in many countries.

Significant factors associated with discontinuation are the emergence of dementia or malignancy.

Withdrawal of RRT is likely to increase in the future if more 'marginal' cases are given a 'trial of dialysis'.

Transplantation

Transplantation in elderly patients remains an area of debate in spite of the widespread acceptance that this is the optimal approach to the treatment of ESRD in most patients.

A very small proportion of elderly patients receive a transplant (<1% in those aged >70 years).

This restriction could be justified in former years when allograft survival was poor amongst older patients.

There is now an increasing number of grafts allocated to patients aged >65 years: in 1999, 8.4% of cadaver grafts in the USA were placed in patients aged 65–75 years.

The shortage of donor organs is now the main factor limiting transplantation in older patients.

The principal cause of graft loss in the elderly is death with a functioning graft.

Selection of potential recipients who are likely to have the best survival is therefore important in maximizing the use of scarce cadaver kidneys.

This usually takes into account an assessment of cardiovascular health (looking for evidence of cardiac, cerebrovascular and peripheral disease), the presence of prostate disease and other general factors such as physical incapacity and dementia.

Healthy elderly subjects are subject to some reduction in activity of both humoral and cellular immune responses to antigens. Uremia itself is associated with generalized immunosuppression. Perhaps as a consequence, it is well-recognized that older graft recipients have fewer and milder episodes of early acute rejection.

However, they are also more vulnerable to bacterial and viral infections and have a much higher death rate from infection.

These factors have persuaded most clinicians of the need to reduce the doses of immunosuppressive drugs in the elderly, especially corticosteroids.

Furthermore, the metabolism of both prednisolone and ciclosporin in the microsomal P450 system is less active.

Mycophenolate mofetil has been associated with increased rates of serious infection when compared to azathioprine in patients aged >60 years.

Survival of older transplant recipients (65–69 years) at 5 years seems relatively good at 70% although 10 year survival is ~33%, which is less than half the rate in younger patients.

In a single series examining the outcome in recipients aged >70 years, the patient and graft survival at 5 years were both just over 50%.

Interestingly, if graft survival figures are adjusted to take into account death with a functioning graft (i.e. discounting grafts lost due to death of the recipient) then graft survival in most series equates to that in younger cohorts. This indicates the impact of recipient death on graft survival.

While rejection stands out as the major cause of graft loss in the younger recipient, 'death with a functioning graft' is the major cause of loss in the elderly and accounts for ~50% of graft losses.

The majority of deaths are from cardiovascular disease followed by infection.

It should also be noted that malignancy is substantially increased as a cause of death compared with the age-matched general population, with skin cancers and lymphoma standing out.

Given the scarcity of donor organs an important question is whether there are significant benefits to transplantation compared to dialysis in older patients?

Analysis is complicated by the bias towards selection of fitter patients for transplantation but comparisons can be made between recipients and waiting list patients.

The data suggest that graft recipients have about half the rate of death compared to those who remain on dialysis. The only cause of death increased in recipients is malignancy.

Studies of quality of life suggest significant improvements in those who are transplanted compared to those remaining on dialysis.

It has been suggested that, given the scarcity of donor organs, elderly patients should have 'age-matched' donor organs that might be considered 'marginal' for younger recipients.

Few units have an overt policy in place but series suggest that such matching probably occurs.

While overall patient survival may not be compromised, older more marginal kidneys are associated with:

- delayed graft function;
- reduced graft survival;
- worse renal function.

Conservative management in the elderly

There is increasing interest in conservative care of patients with ESRD, largely in those with extensive comorbidities. Many, but not all, are elderly patients.

One study, comparing dialysis with conservative therapy, concluded that dialysis did not confer a significant survival benefit (judged by the putative start date for dialysis) in a cohort of patients recommended for palliative care by a multidisciplinary team. These patients tended to be older, diabetic and were more functionally impaired.

Many units have developed links with palliative care services and/or have appointed specialist palliative care renal nurses to manage the increasing numbers of elderly, debilitated patients being referred to renal services.

There is also a growing appreciation of the range of debilitating symptoms experienced, especially by the elderly receiving dialysis. These specialist palliative–renal nurses may facilitate management of some of these symptoms such as pain, nausea, tiredness and constipation.

The increasing emphasis on palliative care is likely to improve communication about end-of-life issues between the multidisciplinary team, patients and their carers.

Specific problems in the elderly with renal disease

Cardiovascular disease

Cardiovascular disease is the major cause of morbidity and mortality in patients with ESRD and is even more marked in older patients.

Hypertension is a major cardiovascular risk factor, develops with progressive renal impairment and is associated with left ventricular hypertrophy, ischemic heart disease, arrhythmias and sudden death.

Anemia is another very important precipitant of left ventricular hypertrophy, and treatment of hemoglobin to a concentration of 10–12 g/dL with erythropoetin is considered optimal.

An important cause of dialysis failure in the elderly is poor cardiac output often in association with a dilated ischemic cardiomyopathy. This possibility should be carefully assessed and may demand revascularization procedures in selected cases.

Peripheral vascular disease is frequent in elderly patients with ESRD.

Malnutrition

The healthy elderly have some reduction in the absorption of nutrients and tend to have diets that are higher in carbohydrates.

They may also be somewhat limited financially which may reduce the intake of foods rich in protein and essential nutrients.

Older patients may also become depressed and stop eating.

Malnutrition may become evident as nonfluid weight loss, low serum albumin and a reduction in creatinine due to loss of muscle mass.

Patients should be encouraged to take ≥1 g/kg of protein per day and should also be given water-soluble vitamins that might be lost during dialysis (folate, pyridoxine) and alphacalcidol.

Neuropsychiatric issues

Older dialysis patients are predisposed to developing neurological complications due to:
- intradialytic hypotension;
- reduced cerebral blood flow;
- carotid disease;
- malnourishment.

Cerebral atrophy is known to be commoner among even younger dialysis patients.

Bone disease

The elderly are predisposed to bone disease even in the absence of renal disease.

Osteopenia and reduction in bone trabecular volume are found in 'normal' elderly.

A balanced diet, exercise and sunlight are all of importance.

Conclusions

Renal failure is predominantly a disease of the elderly; the underlying conditions vary from younger patients.

Dialysis should not be withheld on the grounds of age alone.

Significant numbers of the very elderly may opt not to receive dialysis or be thought to be unsuitable for treatment because of extensive comorbidities.

Ideally, patients should make an informed choice as to their modality of renal replacement therapy; in reality there are often economical and logistical factors pressuring the decision.

Transplantation is an excellent treatment for fit elderly patients but the scarcity of cadaver kidneys means some selection occurs.

Further reading

Cameron JS, Macías-Núñez JF. Chronic renal failure in the elderly. *Oxford textbook of clinical nephrology*, 3rd edn. Chapter 14.2: pp. 2165–2191.

Lamping DL, Constantinovici N, Roderick P, et al. Clinical outcomes, quality of life, and costs in the North Thames Dialysis Study of elderly people on dialysis: a prospective cohort study. *Lancet* 2000; **356**(9241): 1543–1550.

Ouseph R, Hendricks P, Hollon JA, Bhimani BD, Lederer ED. Under-recognition of chronic kidney disease in elderly outpatients. *Clin Nephrol* 2007; **68**: 373–378.

Smith C, Da Silva-Gane M, Chandna S, Warwicker P, Greenwood R, Farrington K. Choosing not to dialyse: evaluation of planned non-dialytic management in a cohort of patients with end-stage renal failure. *Nephron Clin Pract* 2003; **95**: c40–46.

Wong CF, McCarthy M, Howse ML, Williams PS. Factors affecting survival in advanced chronic kidney disease patients who choose not to receive dialysis. *Ren Fail* 2007; **29**: 653–659.

Internet resources

British Geriatrics Society:

http://www.bgs.org.uk/

Chronic kidney disease and older people—implications of the publication of the Part 2 of the National Service Framework for Renal Services:

http://ageing.oxfordjournals.org/cgi/content/full/34/6/546

Geriatrics and Ageing: CME Portal to Clinical Issues Specific to the Care of Ageing Adults:

http://www.geriatricsandaging.ca/

See also

Acute kidney injury in the elderly, p. 384

Dialysis strategies, p. 480

Medical management of dialysis patients, p. 528

Selection and preparation of recipients, p. 544

Chronic kidney disease in diabetic patients

Introduction

The coexistence of diabetes and chronic kidney disease (CKD) is associated with a high burden of complications resulting from synergistic effects on cardiovascular and metabolic-related morbidity and mortality.

The complexity of treatments used in patients with diabetes and CKD requires a co-ordinated multi-disciplinary approach with particular emphasis on involvement of patients themselves in their ongoing management.

Preservation of renal function

Preservation of renal function in diabetics is based on achievement of therapeutic goals.

It is important to realize that these goals are continually under review as more evidence emerges.

Blood pressure

Aim for a target blood pressure of ≤130/80 mmHg.

Avoid systolic BP of <110 mmHg.

Where possible ACEIs and/or ARBs should be used as the antihypertensive drugs of choice in view of their antiproteinuric effect.

Proteinuria

Aim for the greatest decrease in microalbuminuria possible with ACEI and/or ARB.

Aim for the greatest possible reduction in overt proteinuria with ACEI and/or ARB.

Moderate salt restriction (4–6 g/24 h (Na$^+$<100 mmol/day)) increases the antiproteinuric effect of ACEI and ARB.

Glycemic control

Aim for an HbA$_{1C}$ ≤6.5%.

Prevention of AKI

It is important to be aware of the potential risks to renal function in diabetic patients and to try to avoid or minimize their impact.

Dehydration

Loss of sodium and extracellular water (e.g. from diarrhea) may lead to worsening kidney function, particularly in patients taking ACEIs, ARBs and diuretics.

Patients should provisionally stop diuretics if there is a risk of dehydration.

Drugs

Avoid drugs that can worsen renal function:

- NSAIDs;
- aminoglycosides.

Diagnostic imaging

When iodinated contrast agents must be used (e.g. for a CT scan or angiography) the following preventative measures should be considered:

- stop NSAIDs, aminoglycosides and metformin;
- give IV hydration with 0.9% saline or 1.4% sodium bicarbonate (1 mL/kg/h for 6–12 h before and after);
- use a low osmolal contrast agent;
- use the smallest volume of contrast agent possible;
- consider the use of oral or IV acetylcysteine (efficacy is not established).

Cardiovascular risk

Most patients with diabetes and CKD will not reach CKD 5, because they die earlier from cardiovascular causes.

All measures aimed at preserving renal function also reduce cardiovascular risk, particularly the reduction of blood pressure and proteinuria.

Lifestyle and nutrition

Patients should be advised to perform aerobic exercise on a regular basis (aim for ≥30 min each day).

Smoking cessation should be encouraged.

Weight loss to a target body mass index within the normal range (18.5–24.9 kg/m^2) should be encouraged.

Protein

Protein intake restriction should be considered and discussed with the patient.

Protein restriction may slow progression of CKD but may also lead to protein-calorie malnutrition.

Protein restriction to 0.6–0.8 g/kg/day should therefore only be undertaken with appropriate education, detailed dietary assessment and supervision to ensure that malnutrition is prevented.

In patients with CKD 5 treated by dialysis, intake should be ≥1.2 g/kg/day.

Carbohydrates and fat (unsaturated fats and ω-3-enriched)

These should be increased to reach an appropriate caloric intake (≥35 kcal/kg/day in patients <60 years if no weight loss is needed).

Salt

Salt intake should be restricted to 4–6 g/day (for better blood pressure control).

Dyslipidemia

Aim for an LDL-cholesterol concentration of ≤3 mmol/L (100 mg/dL).

Dietary advice is necessary.

Statins need to be used in many patients to reach the target LDL-cholesterol.

In patients on chronic hemodialysis, treatment with statins should be restricted to those with a specific indication (e.g. after myocardial infarction), since no clinical benefit has been proven, even in patients with high LDL-cholesterol.

Pharmacological treatment of diabetes

Patients with CKD 3–5 are at risk of hypoglycemia because of:

- decreased renal clearance of insulin and sulfonylureas;
- impaired renal gluconeogenesis.

Type 1 diabetes

Insulin needs may change with decreasing renal function, since CKD is associated with insulin resistance and there is decreased renal clearance with advancing CKD.

Type 2 diabetes

A number of different oral hypoglycemic drugs are available (Table 12.3.1).

The benefits of intensive therapy are independent of the type of treatment administered.

Table 12.3.1 Modifications of antidiabetic drugs in patients with type 2 diabetes (adapted from the K/DOQI guidelines)

Class	Drug	Dosing recommendation CKD stages 3, 4, or kidney transplant	Dosing recommendation dialysis
First-generation sulfonylureas	Acetohexamide, tolazamide, tolbutamide	Avoid	Avoid
	Chlorpropamide	Avoid when GFR <50 mL/min/1.73 m^2	Avoid
Second-generation sulfonylureas	Glipizide, gliclazide	Preferred sulfonylurea. No dose adjustment necessary.	Preferred sulfonylurea. No dose adjustment necessary.
	Glyburide	Avoid	Avoid
	Glimepiride	Initiate at low dose, 1 mg daily	Avoid
α-Glucosidase inhibitors	Acarbose, miglitol	Not recommended if SCr >180 µmol/l	Avoid
Biguanides	Metformin	See text	Avoid
Meglitinides	Repaglinide	No dose adjustment necessary	No dose adjustment necessary
	Nateglinide	Initiate at low dose, 60 mg before each meal	Avoid
Thiazolidinediones	Pioglitazone, rosiglitazone	No dose adjustment necessary	No dose adjustment necessary
Incretin mimetic	Exenatide	No dose adjustment necessary	No dose adjustment necessary
Amylin analog	Pramlintide	No dose adjustment necessary for GFR 20–50 mL/min/1.73 m^2	No data available
DPP-4 inhibitor	Sitagliptin	Reduce dose by 50% (50 mg/day) when GFR <50 and ≥30 mL/min/1.73 m^2 and by 75% (25 mg/day) when GFR <30 mL/min/1.73 m^2	Reduce dose by 75% (25 mg/day)

DPP-4, dipeptidyl peptidase-4.

Metformin

This should be used with caution in patients with CKD.

The use of metformin in CKD carries a risk of severe lactic acidosis; the risk increases with decreasing GFR.

Various thresholds have been proposed to withdraw metformin based on serum creatinine:

• 140 µmol/L in men;
• 130 µmol/L in women;

or GFR:

• 40–50 mL/min/1.73 m^2.

The use of metformin should be reviewed when the patient reaches CKD 3 and is contraindicated in CKD 4 and 5.

Sulfonylureas

First-generation sulfonylureas should be avoided.

Second-generation sulfonylureas may be used in patients who have learnt to prevent hypoglycemic episodes, as long as diabetes is controlled and nutritional status is satisfactory.

Thiazolidinediones

These may be used in patients without heart failure.

Caution is advised in patients with ischemic heart disease.

Higher rates of fractures have been reported in patients treated by thiazolidinediones.

Insulin

When insulin therapy is used care should be taken to avoid hypoglycemic episodes as the renal clearance of insulin falls with advancing renal impairment.

Consequences of decreased kidney function

Patients with diabetes and CKD should be referred early to a nephrologist for management of the complications of progressive CKD.

Referral criteria vary, but all diabetic patients should be reviewed when they reach CKD 3.

Anemia

Anemia increases the risk of cardiovascular events in diabetics with CKD.

Anemia should be treated by erythropoetin-stimulating agents (ESAs) when Hb <11 g/dL, and after excluding:

• iron deficiency (transferrin saturation >20% and ferritin >100 µg/L);
• chronic or acute inflammation (C-reactive protein <5 mg/L);
• folate or vitamin B12 deficiency.

The target Hb is between 11 and 12 g/dL, with a rate of increase of ≤1 g/dL over 2 weeks.

ESAs should not be used in the presence of uncontrolled hypertension.

Mineral metabolism

Disturbances in mineral metabolism increase cardiovascular risk, and are associated with renal osteodystrophy in diabetics with CKD.

Targets for calcium, phosphate and PTH are identical to those defined for patients with CKD from other causes.

Electrolyte disturbances

Metabolic acidosis should be corrected by bicarbonate supplementation.

Hyperkalemia may result from diet, adverse effects of renin–angiotensin inhibitors, or acidosis at CKD stages 3 and higher.

Fluid retention

Fluid retention is frequent in diabetic CKD.

Salt restriction and diuretic therapy are the basis of fluid control in these patients.

Malnutrition

Malnutrition is common in diabetics with CKD.

Inappropriate dietary counselling may lead to malnutrition through excessive dietary restriction.

End-stage renal disease

Therapeutic strategies

All techniques of renal replacement therapy (RRT) may be used in patients with diabetes.

A decision should be made early (when the GFR falls to <30 mL/min/1.73 m^2) with the patient on the type of RRT to be used.

Vaccination against hepatitis B should be performed early in all patients with progressive CKD (stage 3).

It is important to avoid venous punctures in the nondominant arm to preserve the veins for creation of an arteriovenous fistula (AVF) for hemodialysis.

Kidney transplantation

RRT by renal transplantation is associated with a lower morbidity and mortality, and should be encouraged wherever possible.

Cardiovascular morbidity is the main limitation for transplantation in diabetic patients.

Kidney transplantation may be performed in patients with type 1 or type 2 diabetes.

The threshold for kidney transplantation will vary between centres but is usually <20–10 mL/min/1.73 m^2.

Kidney transplantation may be performed either from a living or a cadaveric donor.

Combined kidney and pancreas transplantation

Combined kidney and pancreas transplantation should be considered in patients with type 1 diabetes.

It is inappropriate in patients with type 2 diabetes.

The criteria for acceptance onto the combined list and the threshold for kidney and pancreas transplantation will vary between centers (combined transplantation usually considered below 20 mL/min/1.73 m^2).

Various techniques may be used for pancreas transplantation, including islets transplantation.

In some centers peritoneal dialysis is contraindicated in patients in whom pancreas transplantation is planned.

Peritoneal dialysis

Peritoneal dialysis may be performed in patients with type 1 or type 2 diabetes.

The technique is well-suited to patients who are waiting for a cadaveric transplant.

The glucose load associated with peritoneal dialysis might be as high as 100–200 g/day (i.e. 400–800 kcal/day).

In patients treated with the starch-containing solution icodextrin, a glucose-specific monitor and test strips should be used, as metabolites of icodextrin interfere with many glucometers.

Hemodialysis

Hemodialysis may be performed in patients with type 1 or type 2 diabetes.

If the patient chooses hemodialysis, vascular access should be planned and undertaken early (typically when the patient reaches CKD 4).

The best form of vascular access is a native AVF.

Prosthetic grafts should only be used when it is not possible to form a native AVF.

Vascular catheters should only be used in emergency circumstances or if no other type of vascular access can be made.

Catheter use is associated with more frequent infective complications and increased mortality.

Other complications of diabetes

Cardiovascular disease

Coronary artery disease

Asymptomatic patients should be screened every 2 years using a noninvasive method (exercise test, echocardiography with dobutamine).

Coronary angiography is frequently needed as part of the pretransplant evaluation.

Diabetic patients with CKD and coronary artery disease should be treated aggressively with β-blockers, statins, and aspirin or clopidogrel.

Peripheral vascular disease

Peripheral vascular disease is a frequent complication in patients with diabetes and CKD.

Patients should be regularly assessed by clinical examination with appropriate investigations as needed.

Erectile dysfunction

This is a frequent complication often resulting from a combination of vasculopathy and the side-effects of drugs used to treat hypertension and ischemic heart disease.

Phosphodiesterase type 5 inhibitors (sildenafil, tadalafil, vardenafil) may be used unless the patient has uncontrolled ischemic heart disease or uses nitrates.

Diabetic retinopathy

Annual screening for diabetic retinopathy should be undertaken.

Diabetic foot

Diabetic patients with CKD have a high risk of diabetic foot lesions.

High risk patients (previous ulcer or peripheral neuropathy) require specific advice about the use of appropriate footware and recognizing the early signs of infection.

Close liaison with local podiatry services is important.

Feet should be examined periodically and should form part of the regular assessment of the diabetic patient in both nephrology and dialysis clinics.

Pregnancy

Women with diabetes and CKD are at increased risk of preterm birth, pre-eclampsia, and worsening of renal function.

Preconception counseling should be offered to all women wishing to start a family so that medical care can be optimized and the risks of pregnancy discussed.

Insulin should be used to control blood sugars during pregnancy.

ACEIs and ARBs should be discontinued as soon as pregnancy is confirmed if they have not been stopped preconception, because of the risk of teratogenicity.

Patients' involvement in their own care

Patients should be educated to be proactive in their own treatment, particularly with regard to:
- glycemic control;
- blood pressure;
- nutrition;
- exercise.

Further reading

Genuth S, Eastman R, et al. Implications of the United kingdom prospective diabetes study. *Diabetes Care* 2003; **26**(Suppl 1): S28–32.

K/DOQI Clinical Practice Guidelines and Clinical Practice Recommendations for Diabetes and Chronic Kidney Disease. *Am J Kidney Dis* 2007; **49**: S1–S179.

Lewis EJ, Hunsicker LG, et al. The effect of angiotensin-converting-enzyme inhibition on diabetic nephropathy. The Collaborative Study Group. *N Engl J Med* 1993; **329**: 1456–1462.

Nathan DM, Cleary PA, et al. Intensive diabetes treatment and cardiovascular disease in patients with type 1 diabetes. *N Engl J Med* 2005; **353**: 2643–2653.

Internet resources

National Diabetes Support Team, UK guidelines:

`http://www.diabetes.nhs.uk/downloads/NICE_and_Diabetes.pdf`

UK Renal Association guidelines for diabetic patients with CKD:

`http://www.renal.org/CKDguide/full/CKDprintedfullguide.pdf`

US National Kidney Foundation KDOQI guidelines:

`http://www.kidney.org/professionals/kdoqi/guideline_diabetes/`

See also

Diabetes mellitus, p. 144

CKD in pregnancy, p. 476

Selection and preparation of recipients, p. 544

Chronic kidney disease in pregnancy

Introduction

Chronic kidney disease in pregnancy provides a clinical challenge for nephrologists and obstetricians tasked with managing the reciprocal effects of pregnancy on renal disease, and of underlying pre-existing renal disease on pregnancy outcomes.

In order to assess these women it is necessary to appreciate the changes in renal physiology and function that occur in normal pregnancy:

Changes in renal physiology and function in normal pregnancy

Kidney length and volume increase, and the collecting system dilates – more markedly on the right side.

Renal plasma flow increases by 80%.

Gestational vasodilatation results in decreased maternal blood pressure in the first and second trimesters.

Glomerular filtration rate (GFR) increases by 50% in the first trimester.

Serum creatinine concentration falls by 10% in the first trimester and 30% by the last trimester.

In the third trimester maternal plasma volume is increased by 40% over prepregnancy values.

There is a concurrent fall in serum albumin concentration to 30–35 g/L.

Many of these functional changes are attenuated or absent when renal disease is present.

Therefore blood tests and other clinical investigations must be interpreted in the light of these functional changes.

For example in pregnant women:
- 'normal' serum creatinine may represent significantly impaired renal function;
- formulaic estimations of glomerular filtration rate (eGFR) are not valid in pregnancy;
- a dilated collecting system does not generally reflect underlying obstruction to urinary flow;
- a depressed serum albumin concentration in a proteinuric patient does not necessarily indicate nephrotic syndrome.

Effect of renal disease on obstetric outcomes

In general, pregnancies of women with renal disease are associated with increased risks of adverse obstetric outcomes, including an increased incidence of:
- pre-eclampsia;
- babies born prematurely;
- babies born small for gestational age;
- reduced fetal survival.

The key determinants of adverse obstetric outcomes are:
- the presence of hypertension;
- the degree of underlying renal impairment.

Poorly controlled blood pressure (MAP >105 mmHg) is associated with an ~10-fold increase in the risk of fetal death.

With respect to degree of renal impairment, it is conventional to stratify women as follows:

1. Mild: serum creatinine ≤124 μmol/L.
2. Moderate: serum creatinine 124–220 μmol/L.
3. Severe: serum creatinine >220 μmol/L.

Pregnant women in the mild category have a rate of live outcomes similar to that of the pregnant population as a whole, despite an increase in prematurity.

Results are less certain in the moderate and severe categories. Premature delivery is very common, and reports of fetal loss cluster in those women with worse renal function.

Nonetheless with modern neonatal surveillance and intensive care most women can anticipate a successful obstetric outcome.

The underlying renal disease seems to be of little importance as a determinant of outcome, although pregnancies in women with renal involvement in some systemic diseases such as vasculitis and lupus nephritis may be associated with a poorer prognosis.

Effect of pregnancy on underlying renal disease

As with obstetric outcomes the probability that pregnancy will adversely affect maternal renal function is largely dependent on remaining renal function and blood pressure control.

The identity of the underlying renal disease *per se* appears to have little influence.

Women with mild renal impairment demonstrate a gestational increase in GFR, and renal function is usually maintained.

However, those with severe renal impairment may suffer significant loss of renal function in pregnancy, with a steeper trajectory of decline compared to that observed before conception.

In some this may recover after delivery but in others functional deterioration accelerates after delivery.

Those with a serum creatinine >180 μmol/L have a 33% chance of ESRD by 12 months postpartum.

The presence of >1 g proteinuria/24 h is an aggravating factor.

Prepregnancy risk stratification for women with renal disease based on renal function may change with the advent of new CKD classifications and eGFR reporting.

More women with identified pre-existing renal impairment identified by eGFR may be encountered by renal/obstetric services in the future.

Preconception counseling and preparation of women with CKD for pregnancy

Ideally all women with CKD should be offered preconception counseling to discuss the risks of pregnancy to the mother and foetus, and the potential impact on maternal renal function.

In addition it is often necessary to discontinue unsafe medications in pregnancy with the substitution of more 'pregnancy-friendly' agents.

The following antihypertensives are safe and commonly used in pregnancy:
- methyldopa;
- labetalol;
- hydralazine;
- nifedipine.

Other antihypertensives should be avoided.

If a woman with treated hypertension is planning a pregnancy, sufficient time must be allocated to ensure adequacy of blood pressure control following transition from usual medication onto 'pregnancy-friendly' antihypertensives.

The following commonly prescribed drugs in CKD should be discontinued, preferably before pregnancy:
- ACEIs;
- ARBs;
- statins;
- bisphosphonates;
- cytotoxic agents.

Renal biopsy in pregnancy

Experience suggests that renal biopsy in pregnancy is no more hazardous than in the nonpregnant situation.

Some caution is required because the published experience of renal biopsy in pregnancy amounts to only a few hundred cases compared to several thousand in nonpregnant subjects.

The standard cautions and contraindications used to guide the performance of renal biopsy in nonpregnant patients apply equally in pregnancy.

After 24 weeks gestation it may be difficult or uncomfortable for women to assume the prone position for biopsy. In this case potential operators should avoid the performance of renal biopsy in an unfamiliar manner or with the patient in an unusual position as this may increase the risk of complications.

Renal biopsy in pregnancy may be indicated to assist in the management of:
- acute kidney injury;
- nephrotic syndrome;
- altered activity of a pre-existing systemic disease such as lupus nephritis.

However, renal biopsy in pregnancy is not recommended for the investigation of:
- stable CKD;
- non-nephrotic proteinuria;
- pre-eclampsia.

If a maternal indication for renal biopsy develops at a stage of pregnancy when fetal survival is likely to be good (certainly after 32 weeks, and possibly after 28 weeks gestation) the pregnancy should be brought to an end and biopsy performed thereafter.

Pregnancy in the dialysis patient

Fertility is severely curtailed in women receiving dialysis. Nonetheless studies show that pregnancy occurs in 1–7% of women of childbearing age on dialysis.

Regular menstrual periods are now more common in premenopausal dialysed women, and improved dialytic techniques and anemia management may have increased fertility and the incidence of conception on dialysis.

The incidence of pregnancy is better in those with residual renal function and is 2–3× greater in hemodialysis patients compared to those treated by peritoneal dialysis.

Appropriate contraceptive advice should therefore be provided to female dialysis patients who may conceive.

Fetal survival is of the order of 30–50% with an average gestation of 32 weeks.

Maternal BP control may be problematic and should be rigorously managed, but deaths are rare.

Increasing dialysis dose improves fetal outcomes.

Prescribing hemodialysis to pregnant patients
More frequent/daily dialysis.

16–24 h dialysis per week.

Aim for predialysis urea <20 mmol/L.

Establishing target weights may be difficult.

Aim for lowest ultrafiltration possible per treatment.

Adjustment of dialyzate composition may be required to avoid alkalosis, hypocalcemia and hypokalemia.

Minimize heparin.

Prescribing peritoneal dialysis to pregnant patients
Increasing abdominal girth in pregnancy may necessitate lower dialyzate dwell volumes.

Frequency of exchanges should be increased.

Difficulty may be encountered in achieving adequate dialysis.

Other considerations in dialysis management
Erythropoetin is safe and a 50% increase in dose may be required.

IV iron sucrose preparations can be used in pregnancy.

Modify dietary advice to ensure adequate nutrition.

Vitamin D dosages may require adjustment.

Pregnancy in the renal transplant patient

Successful renal transplantation often restores fertility in women with ESRD.

More than 14 000 pregnancies have been documented in renal allograft recipients and registry data indicate a live birth rate of ~80%.

Nonetheless these are high risk pregnancies requiring frequent monitoring due to obstetric problems:
- 30% worsening hypertension/pre-eclampsia;
- ~50% preterm delivery;
- 20% intrauterine growth retardation.

As in pregnant women with native kidney CKD, the risk of adverse obstetric outcomes is dependent largely on:
- the degree of graft (dys)function;
- adequacy of BP control.

The pelvic location of the transplanted kidney does not hinder vaginal delivery and cesarean section is reserved for obstetric reasons only.

Guidelines for considering pregnancy in renal transplant recipients
Stable graft function with serum creatinine <180 µmol/L.

No ongoing or recent acute rejection.

Normal or well-controlled BP.

Minimal or absent proteinuria.

Low risk of opportunistic infection.

If these criteria are met then pregnancy can be considered from 1 year after transplantation.

Effect of pregnancy on renal graft survival
Pregnancy exerts minimal effects on both short- and long-term survival of stable, well-functioning grafts.

A harmful effect on renal function is more likely if the pre-pregnancy serum creatinine is >180 µmol/L.

Transplant immunosuppresive drugs in pregnancy

Prednisolone <15 mg/day.

Azathioprine is safe and should continue at prepregnancy levels.

Ciclosporin and tacrolimus can be continued according to levels; dosage may need to be increased.

Mycophenolate mofetil and rapamycin are contraindicated in pregnancy. These agents should be discontinued at least 6 weeks before conception.

Methylprednisolone is the drug of choice for the treatment of acute rejection in pregnancy.

Further reading

Davison JM. Renal disorders in pregnancy. *Curr Opin Obstet Gynecol* 2001; **13**: 109–114.

Holley JL, Reddy SS. Pregnancy in dialysis patients: a review of outcomes, complications, and management. *Semin Dial* 2003; **16**: 384-387.

Jones DC, Hayslett JP. Outcome of pregnancy in women with moderate or severe renal insufficiency. *N Engl J Med* 1996; **335**: 226–232.

Krane NK, Hamrahian M. Pregnancy: Kidney diseases and hypertension. *Am J Kidney Dis* 2007; **49**: 336–345.

McKay DB, Josephson MA. Reproduction and transplantation: report on the AST consensus conference on reproductive issues and transplantation. *Am J Transplant* 2005; **5**: 1592–1599.

Sibanda N, Briggs JD, Davison JM, Johnson RJ, Rudge CJ. Pregnancy after organ transplantation: a report from the UK transplant pregnancy registry. *Transplantation* 2007; **83**: 1301–1307.

Internet resources

SafeFetus.com, useful site to assess safety of prescribing in pregnancy:

http://www.safefetus.com/

Pregnancy as a test of renal function: a streamed lecture held on the RCP Edinburgh website:

http://rcpe.ac.uk/education/education/streamed_lectures/renal-med.php

Lupus UK, patient friendly information on planning pregnancy in patients with SLE:

http://www.lupusuk.com

British Transplantation Society:

http://www.bts.org

American Society of Transplantation:

http://www.a-s-t.org/

See also

Renal biopsy, p. 32

Acute kidney injury in pregnancy, p. 378

Hypertensive disorders in pregnancy, p. 310

Dialysis

Chapter contents

Dialysis strategies

Introduction

Many kidney diseases cause a slowly progressive decline in renal function over 10–20 years. There are few curative treatments and, even where the primary disease is inactive (e.g. vasculitis), renal function often continues to decline once a critical nephron mass has been lost. Intensive treatments aimed at tight BP control, blockage of the renin–angiotensin system and control of other cardiovascular risk factors may reduce the rate of renal function loss. However, this may only delay the time before replacement of renal function is required.

Epidemiology of end-stage renal disease

The incidence of CKD requiring replacement of renal function is expressed as new patients per million of the population (pmp) per year starting renal replacement therapy (the 'take-on' rate).

There is considerable variation in this rate between countries (Fig. 13.1.1). Lack of resources and the cost of dialysis therapy account for the low rate in many underdeveloped countries. In these countries, the dialysis 'take-on' rate underestimates the incidence of CKD requiring renal replacement.

However, even among developed countries there is considerable variation. For instance, the rates of >300 per million of the population per year in Taiwan and the USA are three times the rates in the UK, The Netherlands, Australia, New Zealand and Nordic countries.

Some of these differences may be due to real differences in the incidence of advanced CKD which increases dramatically with:

- increasing age;
- ethnicity (particularly South East Asian, Polynesian, Native American);
- social deprivation.

However, this variation probably also reflects attitudes of nephrologists and other healthcare workers as to which patients will benefit from dialysis and variation in the level of renal function at start of dialysis.

The prevalence of CKD is also highly variable between countries (Fig. 13.1.2).

In the UK in 2005, there were 706 patients pmp receiving treatment by dialysis or transplantation. The prevalence rate in Japan, Taiwan and USA is more than twice that in the UK.

The pool of patients continues to expand with an increase in the UK of 5% per year since 2000.

Modeling suggests that the pool of patients will continue to grow for at least another 20 years.

Clinical features of progressive CKD

In most patients:

- symptoms of CKD will only develop once GFR <30 mL/min/1.73 m^2 (CKD stage 4);
- severe symptoms will generally only appear when GFR <15 mL/min/1.73 m^2 (CKD stage 5).

As the GFR falls to <15 mL/min/1.73 m^2 the typical symptoms of uremia occur and virtually any organ system may be affected (Table 13.1.1).

Ideally patients with progressive kidney disease should be referred for nephrology assessment well before this point.

This will allow:

- identification and treatment of reversible causes of CKD;
- slowing of progression of renal disease;
- management of complications of CKD (e.g. bone disease, anemia, salt and water imbalance, acidosis, increased cardiovascular risk);
- preparation of patients for renal replacement therapy.

Preparing patients for renal replacement therapy

When it is clear that renal function is progressively declining and that eGFR will fall to <10–15 mL/min/1.73 m^2, preparations should be made to inform patients about treatment choices so that renal replacement therapy (RRT) may start in a planned and programmed manner.

The options to consider are:

- RRT by dialysis:
  hemodialysis (HD);
  peritoneal dialysis (PD).
- RRT by renal transplantation;
- Supportive treatment without dialysis.

A particular advantage of this approach is that vascular or peritoneal access can be established well in advance of the time when treatment will be required.

The optimal time to start preparation is unknown but may be as long as a year before dialysis is required.

Potential problems are:

- estimating accurately when dialysis will be required (see optimal time to start dialysis);
- the rate of decline of renal function is not always predictable;
- the level of function at which patients develop symptoms or signs attributable to uremia is also variable.

The low clearance/predialysis clinic

There is good evidence that patients with progressive CKD are best managed in dedicated clinics often termed low clearance or predialysis clinics. These clinics are run with a multidisciplinary team which may include:

- experienced renal nurses;
- specialist renal dieticians;
- social workers;
- clinical psychologists;
- renal pharmacists;
- trained counselors;
- nephrologists.

An important objective of these clinics is to educate and inform the patients and family/carers about the progressive nature of the renal failure and the importance of making a plan for treatment.

Clinic visits are often supplemented by other support which may include:

- home visits;
- support group meetings;

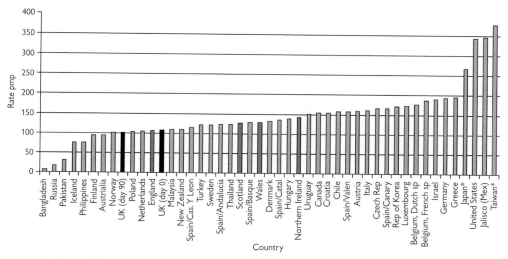

Fig. 13.1.1 Incidence of CKD 5 requiring renal replacement therapy in different countries. pmp, per million population.

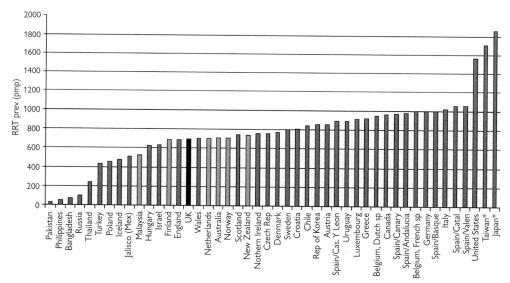

Fig. 13.1.2 Prevalence of renal replacement therapy (RRT) in different countries. pmp, per million population.

- patient information days;
- visits to HD units;
- visits to PD training centers;
- meetings with established patients.

Written and visual material is used to supplement these visits and demonstrations. This allows patients to select the modality of RRT which is most suitable taking into account medical problems, social issues, lifestyle and other factors. It requires time, patience and persistence.

Issues regarding choice of RRT modality

It is important to emphasize that many patients with established kidney failure often require more than one modality of treatment.

The options of HD, PD, renal transplantation and supportive care should be viewed as an integrated package of care for patients with established kidney disease.

Over time, patients may move between different forms of dialysis at different sites (home versus hospital), to renal transplantation and back to dialysis.

Table 13.1.1 Symptoms and signs of uremia

System	Symptoms	Signs
Gastrointestinal	Weight loss Anorexia Nausea/vomiting Diarrhea	
Cardiorespiratory	Breathlessness	Edema Signs of volume overload
Neurological	Paresthesia Restless legs Insomnia Seizures Coma	Peripheral neuropathy
Endocrine	Impotence Menstrual irregularity	
Hematological	Tiredness, lethargy Bruising Increased bleeding	Pallor
Dermatological	Pruritus	Dry skin Excoriation

Different treatments may be appropriate at different times in an individual's treatment 'career'.

Equally it is important to give a realistic picture of life on RRT.

Even those who do well are likely to have temporary periods where they experience intercurrent illness or problems related to dialysis treatment.

Psychosocial aspects of predialysis care

Many patients may feel well with no symptoms despite significant reductions in GFR.

In some societies and cultures, there may be difficulties in accepting advice about preparation for a future illness.

There may be complex psychological and social issues regarding acceptance/denial of the diagnosis and prognosis; adherence to treatment regimens; participation in predialysis counseling/ education.

There are several other aspects which should be considered in predialysis clinics:

Employment

An important part of planning for RRT should be to minimize disruption for patients who are in employment.

Social interactions

Involvement of family, carers and often professional social workers is helpful to maintain normal social function and to assist with access to support at home and other benefits.

Sexual health

Advice is often sought about sexual activity. There is a high prevalence of erectile dysfunction and low libido. Although pregnancy is rare in patients with advanced CKD, patients of childbearing age should be advised about contraception.

Hepatitis B vaccination

This should be performed using a high dose regimen as soon as it is clear that patients will progress to RRT; earlier vaccination leads to a greater rate of seroconversion.

Table 13.1.2 Guidelines for initiating renal replacement therapy

Source	Year	Indicative eGFR (mL/min/1.73 m^2)	Other criteria/descriptors
US NKF K/DOQI	2006	<15	If evidence of characteristic complications of uremia.
European Best Practice	2002	8–10	Dialysis may be started at any time if GFR <15 and symptoms or signs attributable to uremia; in all patients dialysis should be started before GFR <6 irrespective of symptoms.
CARI	2005	6–10	Commence dialysis if GFR <10 or if there is evidence of uremia or its complications such as malnutrition; if there is no evidence of uremia or its complications, commence dialysis when GFR falls to <6.
UK Renal Association	2002	<14	Where there is evidence of malnutrition; symptoms interfere with quality of life; or there is predictable decline in GFR.

K/DOQI, Kidney Disease Outcomes Quality Initiative; CARI, Caring for Australians with Renal Impairment.

Choosing the time to start dialysis treatment

There is no universal agreement on the optimal time for starting dialysis.

Dialysis imposes considerable physical, social and economic costs for patients. These have to be balanced against the benefits of control of uremia and salt and water balance in terms of symptom improvement, quality of life and prolongation of survival.

Absolute indications for starting dialysis

These are all the consequences of advanced renal failure and are usually accompanied by a severe biochemical disturbance:

- uncontrolled uremic symptoms (e.g. nausea, vomiting, itching, insomnia, neuropathy);
- salt and water overload;
- persistent hyperkalemia;
- progressive malnutrition;
- pericarditis;
- severe acidosis.

Guidelines for commencement of dialysis

Exactly when dialysis should be started for individual patients is not clear.

Patients known to a nephrologist should be started on dialysis before the onset of life-threatening complications.

The inability to reliably predict when an individual patient will become symptomatic has led many experts and guidelines to recommend starting dialysis electively based on measurements of GFR.

Guidelines from different authorities regarding the level of renal function to start dialysis are shown in Table 13.1.2. However, all of these still leave room for clinical judgement.

GFR at commencement of dialysis

Over the last 20 years the level of renal function (as estimated by derived GFR) at which dialysis has started has tended to increase.

Data from the United States Renal Data System (USRDS) show that the mean eGFR at start of dialysis has increased progressively since 1995 and was 9.8 mL/min/1.73 m^2 in 2004.

In the UK the mean eGFR of patients starting RRT was:
- 6.0 mL/min/1.73 m^2 in 1997;
- 7.9 mL/min/1.73 m^2 in 2005.

The starting eGFR seems to be stable over more recent years.

Predicting rate of decline in GFR

Even with the use of eGFR-vs-time plots to extrapolate when a certain eGFR value (e.g. 10 mL/min/1.73 m^2) will be reached, many patients develop symptoms earlier than anticipated or conversely kidney function may stabilize for many years.

Commencing dialysis with a higher GFR: 'early start'

Some experts have suggested that starting dialysis earlier will lead to improved survival. However, there are no controlled studies proving this and there are conflicting data from observational and cohort studies.

An important confounding factor is adjustment for lead time bias. Survival must be counted from the point where dialysis may have been started and therefore will include a period of nondialysis treatment for patients starting later.

A randomized study to investigate this is difficult due to issues with funding earlier dialysis treatment and patient consent/recruitment. Despite these problems, one such trial is underway in Australia and New Zealand (The IDEAL study: Initiation of Dialysis Early and Late) in which patients are being randomized to start RRT at estimated GFRs of 5–7 versus 10–14 mL/min/1.73 m^2 (Cockcroft–Gault formula). The study is due to report in 2010 and potentially will give important information on this difficult question.

Choosing an initial mode of renal replacement therapy

The choice of initial treatment for patients with progressive renal failure is influenced by a whole range of factors – medical, social and psychological.

Absolute and relative contraindications to both PD and HD are listed in Table 13.1.3.

Although many centers claim to offer a free choice of treatments, this is influenced by the views and opinions of health professionals and often by the availability and local experience of different forms of therapy.

The initial mode of RRT varies considerably between centers and countries, probably reflecting available facilities, geography and physician opinion/prejudice:
- worldwide, 90% of patients starting dialysis start on HD.
- In the UK in 2005, 23.7% of all incident patients were on some form of PD at 90 days from start of RRT. This figure varied from 4.6 to 58.3% among units offering PD.

Hemodialysis

Hemodialysis (HD) therapy is often the default for many patients, especially those presenting late as uremic emergencies without established vascular or peritoneal access or after PD has failed.

Home HD

Home HD is a successful treatment with excellent outcomes in terms of survival and quality of life.

This form of treatment was pioneered in the late 1960s when chronic dialysis started and is still the treatment of choice in some centers around the world.

Home HD was endorsed by the UK National Institute for Clinical Excellence in 2002 although this was not a surprise to experienced nephrologists.

Over the years, both the percentage and absolute numbers of patients carrying out HD at home has declined. This reflects the aging dialysis population and the increased availability of center or satellite unit based dialysis nearer patients' homes.

Nevertheless, it is important to identify suitable candidates for home HD in the predialysis phase based on local facilities/resources, patient preference and the availability of a suitable helper and home premises.

These patients can then be fast-tracked to an independent treatment at home.

Unit-based HD

Many patients choose HD at a main center or satellite unit when offered choice.

In the UK, the percentage of patients starting HD (versus PD or pre-emptive transplantation) as initial therapy has increased from 58% in 1998 to 76% in 2005.

Some of this reflects the previous overreliance on PD due to a lack of HD facilities.

Contraindications for HD

Patients with extremely poor peripheral veins or severe cardiac disease which might cause hemodynamic instability are often considered to do badly on HD. However, neither of these are absolute contraindications.

Vascular access can nearly always be obtained in the short term using a tunneled dialysis catheter and the hemodynamic response to dialysis is quite variable.

Recent studies have shown better outcomes from HD for patients with impaired cardiac function compared to PD.

Vascular access planning

Planning for vascular access is an essential and important part of the predialysis process.

Patients should be advised to preserve the forearm veins in their nondominant arm by restricting venepuncture and avoiding the use of intravenous lines.

For patients planned to have HD, an arteriovenous fistula (AVF) should be constructed >6 months before the predicted time when dialysis will be required. This gives time for the fistula to develop adequately.

Once formed, the AVF should be carefully monitored and assessed. When adequate vessel enlargement does not develop, revision by surgery or percutaneous angioplasty may be required or a second fistula may be created.

Although it may be argued that all patients should have an AVF formed even if their initial mode of therapy will be PD (due to the limited longevity of this form of treatment), studies have shown that only a small proportion of such AVFs are ever used for HD.

Peritoneal dialysis

Peritoneal dialysis (PD) was first described as a chronic form of treatment for renal failure in 1976. Its potential was not fully accepted initially but, in the 1980s, PD programmes expanded rapidly in certain countries, notably the UK and Mexico. This reflected inadequate investment in HD facilities at a time when dialysis programmes were expanding rapidly.

Patients who are informed about the options for RRT may choose PD because of:
- its relative simplicity and ease of learning;
- desire for independence;
- geography (distance from a HD unit);
- home circumstances.

Overnight automated PD has made this a more attractive option for those with responsibilities during the day (e.g. work, childcare).

There are few absolute contraindications to PD (Table 13.1.3). However, there are many relative contraindications but even major disabilities such as blindness and severe arthritis of the hands can be overcome by use of a variety of ingenious devices to permit patients to carry out exchanges.

During the predialysis phase it is important to clarify that PD is unlikely to be a long-term option. As residual renal function declines, patients may not obtain adequate control of solute balance or salt and water overload, necessitating transfer to HD.

Table 13.1.3 Contraindications to different forms of dialysis

Modality	Absolute	Relative
Hemodialysis		Severe cardiac disease
		Extensive vascular disease (e.g. absent pulses in arms)
		Poor venous access
		Geographical isolation
		Body image (concern regarding appearance of arteriovenous fistula)
		Needle phobia
Peritoneal dialysis	Gastrointestinal or urinary stoma	Multiple abdominal operations
	Known peritoneal sclerosis	Ascites
	Diaphragmatic fluid leak	Morbid obesity/large muscle bulk
		Hernia
		Severe organomegaly (e.g. massive polycystic kidneys)
		Severe respiratory disease
		Ongoing nephrotic syndrome
		Suppurative or broken abdominal skin wound
		Severe back pain
		Lack of manual dexterity
		Unsuitable home environment
		Body image
		Cognitive problems

The timing of catheter insertion for PD is crucial. Ideally the catheter should be inserted at least 2 weeks before required to allow wound healing and to reduce the risk of leaks along the catheter track. This requires careful planning which may be easier if there is easy access to day-case insertion by nephrologists.

An interesting development over recent years has been the early insertion of PD catheters with subcutaneous placement of the external part of the catheter. This can then be quickly exteriorized when required to permit dialysis to start.

Supportive nondialysis treatment

Over 40 years of RRT the average age of patients starting dialysis has gradually increased. Many patients with comorbid conditions which would previously have excluded them from treatment are now accepted onto dialysis programmes and there is general agreement that age by itself is not a contraindication to treatment. Previous policies restricting access to dialysis on the basis of age were often driven by resource issues or physician prejudice.

However, increasingly the benefit in terms of long-term survival and quality of life in frail elderly patients with multiple comorbidities has been questioned. Many physicians believe that for some patients in this category, a conservative and supportive approach is justified. This approach focuses on dealing with medical problems which can be treated without dialysis (e.g. anemia, fluid overload, acidosis, disturbances of bone mineral metabolism) and careful attention to symptom control. In addition, patients' psychological and social needs are addressed and, as patients become more symptomatic, a clear plan for end-of-life care including symptom control and place of death can be agreed by the patient, their family and carers and the multidisciplinary team.

There is evidence from observational studies that elderly patients with multiple comorbid conditions and poor functional status treated in this way have similar or even improved survival compared to those starting dialysis programs. However, this has not been tested in a randomized trial and probably never will be. Thus nephrologists and multidisciplinary teams have to discuss with such patients and their families the advantages and disadvantages of dialysis and promote supportive care as a valid choice for many patients.

Where there is uncertainty about the benefits of RRT, one option is to initiate a time-limited trial of dialysis. A specific date can be set, often 30–60 days after starting dialysis, to review with patients and their families whether quality of life has improved sufficiently to justify continuing treatment.

Pre-emptive transplantation

Where patients with CKD are known to have progressively declining renal function, pre-emptive (i.e. before dialysis is required) transplantation is an attractive option.

Many studies have shown that patients transplanted pre-emptively have better outcomes in terms of transplant and patient survival.

Pre-emptive transplants may be carried out by:
- living related or living unrelated transplantation;
- cadaveric transplantation with a kidney obtained through a national or regional waiting list.

In recent years, living related and living unrelated transplantation has increased in many countries. Where this service is available, every effort should be made to identify a living donor as part of the predialysis education process. This allows a programmed, elective transplant to be performed when the recipient's condition is stable.

Different rules and regulations govern the placement of predialysis patients on cadaveric kidney transplant lists. In the UK, patients may be added to the national cadaveric transplant list if it is estimated that they will need dialysis within 6 months – although as discussed elsewhere in this chapter this is notoriously hard to predict.

One group of patients who may particularly benefit from the pre-emptive approach is those with type I diabetes mellitus and advanced CKD who may be worked up for simultaneous pancreas and kidney (SPK) transplantation from a cadaveric donor. These patients have a predictable decline in renal function and often have unstable diabetes mellitus and benefit doubly from successful SPK transplants.

Late referral

Many patients with CKD and diabetes mellitus, hypertension and vascular disease are known to primary care or to general physicians. Despite this, late referral to nephrologists continues to handicap the care of patients who will require dialysis or transplantation. These patients are sometimes referred to as 'crash-landers'.

There is no universally agreed definition of late referral.

Most studies have included patients referred within 3 or 4 months of the need to start dialysis. However, recent studies in this area suggest that it may take up to a year to prepare a patient for dialysis or transplantation.

Implications of late referral

Numerous studies over the years have shown that patients referred for nephrology care late have poorer outcomes compared to patients known to nephrology services for longer. These include:

- increased mortality;
- reduced treatment choices with more patients receiving HD;
- reduced access to transplantation;
- increased morbidity and hospitalization.

This reflects the complexity of the process regarding choice of RRT.

Late-referred patients have to cope with the implications of the diagnosis, undergo educational programs and quickly make a decision about modality of dialysis and transplantation.

Local facilities and resources may dictate the speed with which vascular or peritoneal access can be established.

For many patients, late referral restricts choice and patients are often established on HD via a tunneled HD catheter. Peritoneal dialysis is less likely to be the initial mode of therapy and the opportunity to perform pre-emptive transplantation is lost.

More importantly, for elderly and frail patients and their families, the opportunity to have information and a careful consideration of the benefits of dialysis compared to supportive treatment is lost. Some patients may start dialysis inappropriately when they present as uremic emergencies.

There is an association between late referral and poorer outcomes but this may not be causal. Although late referral may be associated with increased complications associated with acute hospitalization and temporary vascular access,

these patients may be predetermined to have poorer outcomes as a result of comorbid conditions which may have delayed their referral in the first place.

Reasons for late referral

The reasons why patients are referred late is not clear. Studies have shown that up to 50% of patients were already known to have renal impairment and opportunities to refer were missed by both primary and secondary care physicians. This may be because the severity or progression of the renal disease is missed or because the patient is not considered to be a candidate for RRT until the last moment.

Outcomes of different modes of RRT

An important question for patients starting RRT is which modality will improve survival.

There is unequivocal evidence that renal transplantation provides the best chance of survival and improves quality of life.

Earlier studies which compared survival post transplant with patients on dialysis were flawed by the selection bias of those who had been transplanted. However, studies comparing outcomes only with patients listed for transplantation clearly show the survival benefit of transplantation over those who remain on the waiting list even in higher risk patients with diabetes mellitus or older age.

Controversy exists about the survival advantage of PD versus HD. Over the years there have been conflicting reports favoring each modality. However, all the studies are retrospective or observational and it is difficult to control for other factors, particularly comorbidity, which have a major influence on survival.

There are no controlled trials randomizing patients to these treatments. One such study was attempted in The Netherlands but recruitment was difficult and the study was abandoned.

The best source of comparative data is probably from large registries (Table 13.1.4 and Fig. 13.1.3).

USRDS survival data

The 5 year survival adjusted for age, gender, race and primary renal diagnosis is:

- 34.1% for PD;
- 34.7% for HD.

European registry data

Data for survival on PD and HD are shown in Fig. 13.1.3 and again there is no difference although there is improved

Table 13.1.4 United States Renal Data Systems survival of incident patients by modality of first RRT adjusted for age, gender, race and primary renal diagnosis

Dialysis modality	No. of years survival	Year of incident cohort	% survival unadjusted	% survival adjusted
Peritoneal dialysis	3	2000	59.3	55.7
	5	1998	37.0	34.1
	10	1993	12.2	11.1
Hemodialysis	3	2000	50.2	53.2
	5	1998	31.4	34.7
	10	1993	9.7	11.9

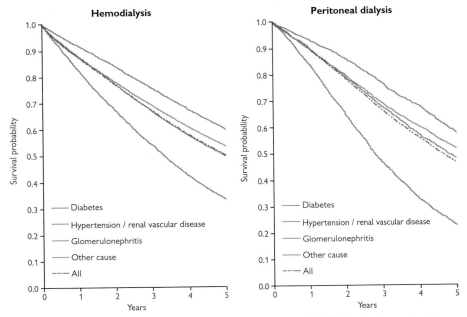

Fig. 13.1.3 Adjusted survival from day 91 for incident patients 1995–1999 from European Renal Registry by primary diagnosis.

survival compared to USRDS data. This is a consistent finding comparing USRDS data to European and Japanese data.

Within the limitations of these data, there appears to be no clear survival advantage of one form of dialysis treatment.

The importance of residual renal function

Replacement of renal function by dialysis, although life-sustaining, is a very crude, empiric and inadequate therapy.

Peritoneal dialysis will deliver an average clearance of small molecules of ~5-8 mL/min and although the efficiency of HD is much greater the time-averaged value will be similar for conventional thrice weekly sessions.

Therefore, when a patient starts dialysis with an eGFR of 5–10 mL/min/1.73 m^2, solute clearance will often be greater through native kidney function than by dialysis.

Those patients who retain this residual renal function often remain healthier on dialysis with better appetite, improved solute and phosphate control, better BP and salt and water balance and less anemia.

Unfortunately, over time for many kidney diseases, the GFR continues to decline once dialysis is started.

Most studies suggest that this happens more quickly on HD but this is not a universal finding.

Some have advocated the continued use of renin–angiotensin blockage once dialysis has started to preserve residual function but the evidence for this strategy is weak.

Diuretic therapy has not been shown to preserve GFR.

The loss of residual renal function is particularly important for patients on PD where the scope for increasing dialysis dose is limited. When residual renal function declines, total

clearance may be inadequate especially for larger patients. This is a major cause of technique failure and transfer to HD.

Withdrawal of dialysis

The increasing age and comorbidity of the prevalent dialysis population means that patients and nephrologists are frequently faced with choices about continuing dialysis treatment.

Data from North America suggest that stopping dialysis accounts for ~20% of all deaths of patients on RRT. This outcome is less often reported in Europe.

Death usually follows within 7–14 days of stopping RRT although some patients may survive much longer especially if they retain some residual renal function.

Withdrawal of dialysis occurs more frequently in association with:

- increasing age;
- diabetes mellitus;
- widespread vascular disease;
- race (Caucasians > Blacks in USA);
- female sex;
- greater educational attainment;
- poor functional and physical status.

This decision may be initiated by the patient, family/carer or nephrologist.

Often the decision is made after a progressive decline in physical and mental capacity due to comorbid illness or sometimes after a severe acute illness.

Some patients judge that their quality of life has declined to the point where the difficulties associated with dialysis are no longer acceptable.

Most societies accept the autonomy of the competent patient to make this decision. Difficulties may arise where the patient is no longer competent and differences of opinion arise between the family and the physician.

In the USA, the Renal Physicians Association and the American Society of Nephrology have produced useful clinical practice guidelines on these issues (see 'Further reading').

Increasingly patients may draw up an advanced directive about their treatment should their mental capacity change.

When patients choose to stop dialysis, it is important to control symptoms including pain, vomiting and pruritus and to prevent pulmonary edema by judicious fluid management and use of opiate drugs.

Further reading

Ansell D, Feest TG, Tomson C, *et al.* UK Renal Registry Report. Bristol: UK Renal Registry; 2006.

Galla JH. Clinical practice guideline on shared decision-making in the appropriate initiation of and withdrawal from dialysis. *Am Soc Nephrol* 2000; **11**: 1340–1342.

Horl WH, Koch KM, Lindsay RM, Ronco C, Winchester JF (eds), *Replacement of renal function by dialysis.* Dordrecht: Kluwer; 2004.

UK Department of Health. The National Service Framework for Renal Services Part One: Dialysis and Transplantation, January 2004.

US Renal Data System. USRDS 2006 Annual Data Report: Atlas of End-Stage Renal Disease in the United States. Bethesda, MD: NIH, NIDDKD; 2006.

Sources of information for patients and carers

Stein A, Wild J. *Kidney failure explained.* London: Class Health; 2006.

Walser M, Thorpe B. *12-Step treatment program to help you avoid dialysis.* Hoboken, NJ: Wiley; 2004.

Internet resources

The Renal Association:

`http://www.renal.org/`

The Renal Registry:

`http://www.renalreg.org`

National Kidney Federation Dialysis Outcomes Quality Initiative:

`http://www.kidney.org/professionals/kdoqi/`

UK National Kidney Federation:

`http://www.kidney.org.uk/`

Care for Australians with Renal Impairment:

`http://www.cari.org.au/`

European Best Practice Guidelines:

`http://www.ndt-educational.org/guidelines.asp`

See also

Clinical assessment of renal function, p. 12

Selection and preparation of recipients, p. 544

Vascular access, p. 488

Hemodialysis, hemofiltration, and hemodiafiltration, p. 494

Peritoneal dialysis, p. 506

Vascular access

Introduction

Vascular access is currently the rate-limiting component for hemodialysis. Despite major advances in dialysis technology, without satisfactory access to the circulation, dialysis adequacy will remain poor. Blood needs to be taken from the patient, pumped through the dialysis machine and returned back to the patient. The conduit from which blood is taken and through which it is returned is defined as the vascular access.

Types of vascular access

Autogenous arteriovenous fistula (AVF).

Prosthetic graft fistula.

Biological graft fistula.

Central venous catheter.

Requirement for dialysis

Blood flow should be sufficient to enable adequate hemodialysis.

Generally blood flows of >400 mL/min through fistulas are preferable although flows less than this are usual for dialysis central venous catheters.

Autogenous fistula blood flow can range from <250 mL to several litres per minute, the former being inadequate and the latter excessive with risk of cardiac failure.

Graft fistula blood flow needs to be >600 mL/min to avoid thrombosis but again can reach several litres per minute.

Acceptable fistula blood flow rates range between 500 mL/min and 1.5 L/min.

Guiding principles in vascular access surgery

Use upper limb before lower limb (less risk of infection).

Use distal fistula sites (wrist) before proximal sites (allows proximal sites to be preserved for later use).

Use autogenous vein before prosthetic graft (for reasons given below).

Use nondominant arm before dominant arm (allows the patient to use dominant arm for eating, writing, etc., while on dialysis).

Whilst creating the current fistula, the surgeon needs to plan ahead to the next procedure.

Assessment of patients for vascular access

Clinical examination of the upper limbs with a tourniquet in place in a warm room.

Inspection of veins in both forearms and arms and checking the radial and brachial pulses.

Duplex scan to map veins and flow in arteries may be undertaken routinely if available but is always required when there is clinical doubt, particularly in a diabetic, elderly or complex patient.

Venography or MR angiography is required when there is concern about central vein or arterial stenosis.

Types of autogenous AVF

Upper limb fistulae

Radio-cephalic

This is eponymously known as the Cimino–Brescia AVF.

The cephalic vein is joined to the radial artery at the wrist (Fig. 13.2.1).

It is the commonest vascular access fistula.

Distal ulnar-basilic or radio-basilic

This involves mobilizing the forearm basilic vein and either directly anastomosing to the ulnar artery or transposing to join the radial artery at the wrist.

Brachio-cephalic

The median cephalic vein is joined to the brachial artery in the antecubital fossa.

It is the second commonest form of fistula in Europe.

Brachio-basilic transposition

The basilic vein is anastomosed to the brachial artery after being transposed superficially and laterally from its deep lying medial position.

Saphenous vein transposition to the arm

Lower limb fistulae

Saphenous vein thigh loop

This involves mobilizing the saphenous vein and tunneling it in a U-shape bend to join the femoral artery.

Superficial femoral vein transposition

This is a rare fistula which mobilizes the superficial femoral vein and transposes it superficially and laterally, anastomosing it to the superficial femoral artery

Prosthetic and biological grafts

These can be:

- Expanded polytetrafluoroethylene (ePTFE).
- Polyurethane.
- Dacron (rarely used).
- Bovine mesenteric vein.
- Bovine ureter.
- Bovine carotid artery.

Prosthetic grafts

ePTFE (the coating used in nonstick frying pans) has been used for the past 30 years.

Despite lack of compliance, PTFE grafts are resilient due to hydrophobic properties making blood less likely to stick to it.

The holes created by dialysis needles do not heal and are sealed by a pseudointimal lining and platelet plugs.

The polyurethane graft does have self-sealing properties but has a greater risk of thrombosis.

Biological grafts

The bovine biological grafts are essentially acellular collagen tubes.

They are similar to vein, easier to implant but are more expensive than prosthetic grafts.

Outcomes are similar to grafts.

Types of graft fistula

Upper limb

Forearm straight graft

Run from radial artery to antecubital vein.

Forearm loop graft

Run from brachial artery to antecubital vein in a U-shaped loop.

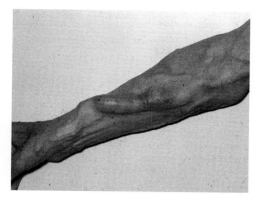

Fig. 13.2.1 A mature radio-cephalic AVF used for hemodialysis.

Arm graft
Run from brachial artery to axillary vein.

Lower limb

Thigh loop graft
Run from femoral artery to saphenous or femoral vein in the groin.

Thigh straight graft
Run from the distal superficial femoral artery to the saphenous or femoral vein in the groin.

Advantages of autogenous AVF

Biological tissues generally handle better than prosthetic.

The long-term patency is better (Figs 13.1.3 and 13.1.4).

There is resilience to thrombosis in hemodynamically unstable patients.

There are low rates of septic complications which generally respond to antibiotic therapy.

There is ease of needling for dialysis except in obese patients

Low cost.

Disadvantages of autogenous AVF

There is an early failure rate of up to 30% for radio-cephalic AVFs, but less for others.

Often suitable veins are not available due to prior usage for IV infusions.

They need a maturation time of several weeks before usage.

Fistula vein may need transposition to a superficial position in obese patients.

Cosmetically less satisfactory, especially if they develop aneurysmal dilatation.

Advantages of prosthetic or biological grafts

Good quality grafts are easily available 'off the shelf' in appropriate lengths.

They allow earlier needling for dialysis, particularly the prosthetic grafts. In an emergency, the graft can be needled almost immediately although there is greater risk of infection and bleeding at this early stage.

Biological grafts are easy to handle and anastomose compared to prosthetic grafts.

They are cosmetically more acceptable.

Disadvantages of prosthetic or biological grafts

There is a lower long-term patency (Figs 13.2.3 and 13.2.4).

The risk of thrombosis due to the development of neointimal hyperplasia at the venous anastomosis is significantly greater.

There is a greater risk of infection requiring excision of the graft.

Biological grafts are susceptible to aneurysm formation.

The cost is high.

Complications of fistulas

Thrombosis

This is the greatest risk, requiring radiological or surgical intervention to re-establish the fistula.

Infection

This is less with autogenous fistulas and usually responds to appropriate antibiotic therapy but grafts frequently have to be removed when infection develops.

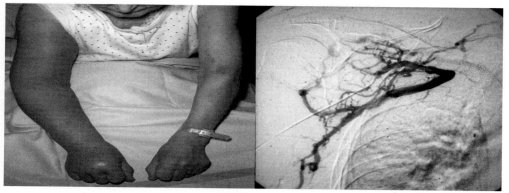

Fig. 13.2.2 Complications of AVF formation: central venous occlusion following previous central venous catheter insertion. Right arm swelling following brachio-cephalic AVF formation due to a right subclavian vein occlusion following a previous right subclavian vein catheter. Note the occluded subclavian stent previously inserted to open up the vein. The AVF had to be ligated eventually.

Steal syndrome
See below.

Aneurysm formation
The risk is greatest with biological and autogenous fistulas.

High output cardiac failure
This occurs when fistula blood flow becomes excessive.

One extraordinary case report revealed a blood flow of >30 L/min before the surgeon banded the fistula down to a flow of 600 mL/min.

Venous hypertension
This may develop in the fistula limb and be exacerbated by central vein stenoses from previous central venous catheters (Fig. 13.2.2).

If it fails to settle as venous collaterals open, options include central vein angioplasty with or without stent insertion or ligation of the AVF.

Seroma
This may occur with prosthetic fistulas.

Physiological changes after fistula surgery
Creation of an AVF or graft produces a new low pressure circuit through which blood flows preferentially.

The limb with a fistula attracts increased blood flow compared to the other limb.

The fistula vein dilates rapidly over the first 2–3 weeks after surgery and then at a slower rate subsequently. The artery also remodels and dilates although less than the vein. However, in some patients the artery can become huge over time.

Major hemodynamic changes take place at the fistula anastomosis due to changes in flow patterns.

The normal laminar blood flow becomes turbulent with changes in wall shear stress, leading to variable degrees of intimal hyperplasia and fistula vein stenosis.

Percutaneous angioplasty or surgical revision of the fistula will be necessary in severe cases.

Failure of AVF maturation
The radio-cephalic AVF has a high incidence of nonmaturation (up to 30%) but when successful can survive >20 years without thrombosis.

The causes of nonmaturation can be related to:
• small size and quality of vein or artery;
• raised blood viscosity;
• intimal hyperplasia in the segment just distal to the anastomosis.

More proximal fistulas using the brachial artery as inflow have less risk of failure and a higher blood flow. However, there is a potential for development of a 'steal syndrome'.

Steal syndrome
A steal syndrome typically presents with:
• a cool/cold hand;
• paresthesia;
• numbness in the fingers;
• loss of the radial pulse;
• cyanosis of finger tips.

If the patient starts to wear a glove on the fistula hand then suspect steal syndrome.

It may present even more dramatically as complete anesthesia of the fingers, pain in the hand or forearm, loss of movement, and eventually with ulceration and gangrene.

This presentation is a surgical emergency and is due to ischemia of the hand and forearm, with loss of sensory and motor nerve function. Unless the fistula is taken down or revised rapidly, it will lead to long-term loss of hand/forearm function.

No patient should develop pain in the hand after proximal fistula surgery and so the operating surgeon should be notified to assess the possibility of a steal syndrome.

Physiological changes after graft surgery
Usually 6 mm PTFE grafts are implanted and the grafts should not change in size with time.

The principle problem with grafts is neointimal hyperplasia which causes a gradual narrowing of the venous anastomosis leading to fistula thrombosis.

Flow monitoring has been suggested as a means of detecting risk of graft thrombosis although evidence from the literature is mixed.

Percutaneous thrombectomy and angioplasty of the venous stenosis is the procedure of choice to re-establish patency with surgery as an alternative.

Revision of the venous anastomosis may be required.

Vascular access in special groups
Diabetics
Pose problems due to poor vessels.

Often veins have already been used and arteries are calcified.

Are more likely to need a proximal fistula hence greater risk of steal syndrome.

Similar principles for vascular access planning apply in diabetics but there is a greater necessity for preoperative vessel imaging.

Elderly patients
Need to be evaluated more carefully before access performed.

If survival prospects are poor then a long-term tunneled catheter may be appropriate, but if the prognosis is good then an AVF/graft should be considered.

Children
PD is the preferred treatment but an AVF remains an option.

When to needle a fistula
AVFs can be needled mostly between 4 and 6 weeks (occasionally earlier if well-developed).

Needling is too often delayed in the UK compared to other European countries.

Grafts can be needled within 2 weeks after the pain of the tunneling has settled and a pseudointima allowed to develop.

Central venous catheters
Types of catheters
Catheters are generally made of polyurethane and may be single lumen, double lumen or two separate single catheters inserted for drawing and returning blood.

Temporary catheters
Used for emergency dialysis and short-term access.

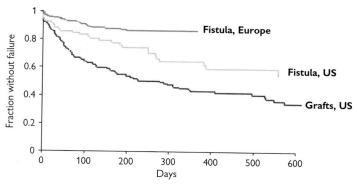

Fig. 13.2.3 Fistula versus graft survival in patients starting hemodialysis with permanent vascular access. Data kindly provided by DOPPS 2005; adjusted for differences in age, gender, diabetes, peripheral vascular disease and body mass index.

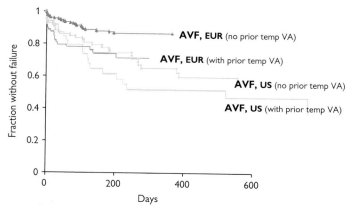

Fig. 13.2.4 Survival of first AVF in incident patients with or without prior temporary vascular access (VA). Data kindly provided by DOPPS 2002; adjusted for differences in age, gender, diabetes, peripheral vascular disease and body mass index.

Tunneled or 'permanent' catheters
Used for long-term dialysis.

They have a subcutaneous Dacron cuff into which tissue grows, fixing the catheter in position and reducing passage of organisms up around the catheter.

They are generally of larger bore than temporary catheters.

Insertion of catheters
Catheter placement is usually performed under local anesthetic, in a clean area, using strict aseptic technique, preferably with radiological screening.

Catheter tip placement ideally should be in the right atrium for maximum blood flow.

Sites of insertion:
• internal jugular vein;
• femoral vein;
• subclavian vein.

The subclavian vein should be avoided unless there is absolutely no other option since subsequent stenosis of the vein will cause severe arm swelling if an ipsilateral fistula is created (Fig. 13.2.2).

The inferior vena cava may be used *in extremis* when there is no other access site.

Benefits of central dialysis catheters
They can be inserted quickly for emergency dialysis, as in late presenters.

They offer painless dialysis once catheter inserted, hence are popular with patients.

They are useful as permanent dialysis for patients with poor cardiac output and poor prognosis.

Disadvantages of central dialysis catheters
There is a much greater infection risk compared to AVFs (5–8× that of a fistula according to DOPPS data), including a high rate of MRSA infection.

There is a risk of central vein stenosis, especially with subclavian vein catheters.

Vein thrombosis can occur, especially the iliac veins when using femoral catheters.

Catheter use is associated with:

- higher rate of hospitalization: 50% greater in centers where >20% of patients dialyze through catheters compared to AVFs;
- higher mortality rate: 20% higher in centers with >28% catheter use versus centres with <7% catheter use.

Data from the DOPPS study suggest prior central vein catheters reduce the long-term patency of subsequent autogenous and graft fistulas.

Complications of central venous catheterization

- Carotid artery/femoral artery injury.
- Hemo-/pneumothorax.
- Lymphatic injury.
- Cardiac tamponade.
- Nerve injury.

Current problems in vascular access

Vascular access is fundamental to enable good dialysis and sustain the quality of life of patients.

More effort needs to be made to preserve the veins in renal patients to facilitate autogenous fistula formation. Venepuncture can be performed using veins on the dorsum of the hand. Use of the cephalic vein in the nondominant hand should be avoided since this potentially is the best resource for long-term dialysis.

Early placement of vascular access (≥6 months before dialysis is necessary) is recommended by the UK National Service Framework. Patients are frequently not referred early enough to surgeons for timely fistula creation.

There is frequently a long delay from referral to preoperative investigations and surgery. Hence too many patients start hemodialysis with central venous dialysis catheters, with all their known complications.

Increasing the number of patients dialysing through an autogenous AVF or graft, and reducing the number dialyzing through tunneled or nontunneled dialysis central venous catheters, will improve morbidity and mortality of patients on hemodialysis.

Further reading

Bakran A, Mickley V, Passlick-Deetjen J (eds). *Management of the renal patient: clinical algorithms on vascular access for haemodialysis*. Berlin: Pabst Science Publishers; 2003.

Davies AH, Gibbons CP (eds). *Vascular access simplified*, 2nd edn. Shrewsbury: TFM Publishing; 2007.

Fluck R, Rao R, van Schalkwyk D, Ansell D, Feest T. The 9th Renal Registry Report, 2005. Southmead Hospital, Bristol: UK Renal Association Renal Registry.

Pisoni RL, Young EW, Dykstra DM, et al. Vascular access use in Europe and the United States: results from the DOPPS. *Kidney Int* 2002;**61**:305–316.

Pisoni RL, Albert JM, Elder SE, et al. Lower mortality risk associated with native arteriovenous fistula (AVF) vs graft (AVG) use in patient and facility-level analyses: results from the DOPPS. *J Am Soc Nephrol* 2005;**16**:259A.

Internet resources

Vascular Access Society:

www.vascularaccesssociety.com

The Renal Registry:

http://www.renalreg.org

National Kidney Federation Dialysis Outcomes Quality Initiative:

http://www.kidney.org/professionals/kdoqi/

European Best Practice Guidelines:

http://www.ndt-educational.org/guidelines.asp

Dialysis Outcomes and Practice Patterns Study (DOPPS):

http://www.dopps.org/Dopps_Default.aspx

See also

Dialysis strategies, p. 480

Hemodialysis, hemofiltration, and hemodiafiltration, p. 494

Psychological aspects of treatment for renal failure, p. 538

Hemodialysis, hemofiltration and hemodiafiltration

Principles of hemodialysis

Hemodialysis (HD) is the default therapy for all forms of renal replacement therapy (RRT).

HD requires an integrated machine with the following essential components:

- a pump to deliver blood from the vascular access to the dialyzer;
- a dialyzate concentrate proportionating system to prepare dialysis fluid from treated water and then deliver the dialysis fluid to the dialyzer;
- a volumetric control system for fluid removal (ultrafiltration);
- a range of patient safety monitors and alarms.

HD employs the use of countercurrent flow of the blood and dialyzate pathways in the dialyzer to maximize the concentration gradient for diffusive transport.

Diffusive transport is greater for smaller and uncharged solutes.

HD also employs the use of a hydrostatic gradient across the dialyzer membrane to induce ultrafiltration (UF) of water and convective transport of solutes by solvent drag.

The permeability of the membrane to larger solutes, such as vitamin B12 or β2-microglobulin, is used to categorize dialyzer membranes into low, mid or high flux.

Dialyzer membranes have widely different capacities to permit flow of water across the membrane and the ultrafiltration coefficient (Kuf) of dialyzers ranges from 3 to >60 mL/min/h per mmHg transmembrane hydrostatic pressure.

Prescription of hemodialysis

Small solute clearance rates

The urea clearance rate (K) will depend on whichever of the following prescription variables is the lowest:

- blood flow rate (200–500 mL/min)
- dialyzer urea mass transfer coefficient (>300 mL/min)
- dialyzate flow rate (500–800 mL/min)

There has been a trend to prescribe higher blood flow rates (300–450 mL/min) and use dialyzers with higher urea mass transfer coefficients to provide higher efficiency HD than in the past.

The commonest rate-limiting factor for urea clearance is the blood flow rate that can be achieved from the patient's vascular access.

Increasing the dialyzate flow rate results in a relatively small increase in urea clearance rates, e.g. a 60% rise in dialyzate flow rates from 500 to 800 mL/min increases the rate of urea clearance by only 5–10% when a high efficiency dialyzer is used and the blood flow rate is 350 mL/min.

Ultrafiltration

The interdialytic fluid (weight) gain is removed under volumetric control by the HD machine which adjusts the transmembrane pressure to achieve the prescribed UF rate.

Choice of dialyzer

Biocompatible dialysis membranes

Synthetic and modified cellulose membranes have been shown to be more biocompatible than unmodified cellulose membranes.

The reported beneficial biological effects of the more biocompatible membranes include:

- lower activation of complement and leukocytes;
- greater adsorption of cytokines;
- greater adsorption of β2-microglobulin;
- higher flux and removal of middle molecules e.g. β2-microglobulin.

A systematic Cochrane review showed no evidence of benefit either in reduced mortality or reduction in dialysis-related adverse symptoms when synthetic membranes were compared with cellulose/modified cellulose membranes. A comparison of unmodified cellulose and modified cellulose membranes was not performed.

Despite the lack of evidence of improved patient outcomes the use of more biocompatible dialyzers instead of unmodified cellulose seems justifiable on the basis of the evidence for their biological benefits and equivalent costs.

High or low flux biocompatible dialyzers

Most of the currently used dialyzers are manufactured from modified cellulose or synthetic materials which are more biocompatible than unmodified cellulose membranes.

The key decision when using these more biocompatible membranes is whether to prescribe a low, mid or high flux dialyzer.

Removal of middle molecules

The proven benefits of high flux synthetic membranes in randomized trials are limited to advantages arising from improved biocompatibility and enhanced removal of middle molecules, such as β2-microglobulin, rather than better patient survival rates.

A systematic review of 27 randomized trials comparing cellulose, modified cellulose and synthetic membranes showed a significant reduction in end-of-study β2-microglobulin values when high flux synthetic membranes were used and one small study showed that dialysis-related amyloid occurred less frequently with this treatment.

The HEMO study

This is the only large prospective randomized trial to study the effect of dialyzer membrane flux on patient outcomes (Table 13.3.1).

The study was designed to detect a 25% reduction in the predicted baseline all-cause mortality rate. The limited benefit observed with high flux membranes has been attributed to several factors in its design:

- enrolment of prevalent rather than incident patients;
- exclusion of patients with major comorbidity;
- failure to use ultrapure water whilst using dialyzer reuse;
- the high and low flux groups may have been separated inadequately since pre-dialysis β2-microglobulin levels were only 19% lower in the high flux group;

The MPO study

Most of the confounding factors listed above have been addressed in the Membrane Permeability Outcome (MPO) study.

This study is a randomized, multicenter European study of high flux membranes in incident HD patients who have few

Table 13.3.1 Summary of the HEMO study findings

Study design	Prospective randomized controlled trial of 1846 prevalent HD patients.
	Patients were on dialysis for a median of 3.7 years at the time of recruitment to the study.
	2 × 2 factorial study design: high and low flux; high and standard dialysis dose.
Outcomes	871 of the 1846 randomized patients died during the study after a mean follow-up period of 2.8 years.
	Ten-fold increase in β2-microglobulin clearances in the high flux group (β2-microglobulin clearances of ≥20 mL/min) versus low flux group.
	No difference in:
	primary outcome of all cause mortality;
	first cardiac hospitalization or all cause mortality;
	first infectious hospitalization or all cause mortality;
	first 15% decrease in serum albumin or all cause mortality;
	all nonvascular access-related hospitalizations.
Secondary analysis	For the patient subgroup which had been on HD for median of >3.7 years before enrolment:
	use of high flux dialysis membranes was associated with a 32% reduction in all cause mortality;
	use of high flux dialysis membranes was associated with a 37% reduction in cardiac death.
	When the number of prevalent years on HD was analysed as a continuous variable, the interaction of flux and years of dialysis on patient survival was not significant.

exclusion criteria and do not reuse dialyzers. This study has now finished recruitment.

Report of the French Group for Nutrition in Dialysis
A multivariate Cox proportional hazards analysis of a prospective nonrandomized study of 1610 prevalent HD patients from 20 centers in France showed that the following were associated with poorer survival:

- increasing age;
- diabetes;
- lower serum albumin;
- use of low flux dialyzer membranes.

Patients on high flux dialyzers had a 38% lower risk of death ($P = 0.01$) than patients on low flux membranes.

Effect of high flux dialysis on control of anemia
A multicenter, randomized controlled trial has failed to show a beneficial effect on anemia in stable HD patients treated over a 12 week study period with high flux biocompatible membranes instead of conventional cellulose membranes.

Effect of high flux dialysis on residual renal function
One small prospective study has shown better preservation of residual renal function when using high flux membranes combined with ultrapure water.

Preservation of residual renal function is desirable as residual renal function is a predictor of survival in HD patients, decreases β2-microglobulin levels and lessens the need for ultrafiltration.

Conclusions
The French study and *post hoc* analysis of the HEMO study provide some evidence that long-term HD patients may have better survival from the use of high flux dialyzers but this observation needs to be confirmed in a large prospective randomized study, such as the MPO study.

As long as high flux membranes cost significantly more than low flux synthetic and modified cellulose membranes, the use of high flux membranes should be a higher priority in patients who are:

- likely to remain/have been on HD for ≥3.7 years;
- have no residual renal function at the start of dialysis.

These patients are at the greatest risk of developing dialysis-related amyloidosis.

Treatment time on hemodialysis per week
Weekly solute removal rates may be increased by either increasing the frequency and/or duration of HD sessions.

Frequency of hemodialysis
HD frequency is a more powerful determinant of weekly solute removal than the duration of each session.

HD twice per week is not regarded as an adequate long-term form of chronic RRT and should be avoided.

The frequency of twice-weekly HD has decreased worldwide, including in the USA where it fell from 12.9% to 3.6% of incident patients between 1990 and 1996.

Twice-weekly HD may be acceptable provided that:

- the patient has a significant level of residual renal function (e.g. mean of combined urinary urea and creatinine clearance >5 mL/min/1.73 m^2);
- the patient's residual renal function is monitored at least every 3 months;
- the frequency of dialysis is increased when renal function decreases.

A thrice-weekly HD schedule evolved from the belief that it reconciled adequate treatment with adequate breaks between treatments to provide the patient with a reasonable quality of life within a 7 day treatment cycle.

It is common practice to prescribe daily HD in the short term when patients with ESRD develop an acute intecurrent illness or pericarditis.

Daily dialysis strategies
Two forms of more frequent, long-term HD have been advocated recently:

Short daily HD

- usually prescribed as 6 'daily' sessions of dialysis of 2–3 h with one rest day per week.

Nocturnal daily HD

- usually prescribed as slow overnight treatment for 5–7 nights per week while the patient is sleeping.

Both forms of daily HD have been shown to provide a number of medical advantages compared with standard duration, thrice-weekly HD:

- improved well-being and better quality of life;
- regression of left ventricular hypertrophy;
- improved fluid balance and BP control;
- reduced need for erythropoetin;
- lower hospital admission rate;
- higher dietary protein intake and better nutritional status.

Short daily HD offers the additional benefit of:

- higher weekly removal of small and large molecular weight solutes (e.g. potassium, phosphate, urea, β2-microglobulin) for the same total time on HD per week.

Daily nocturnal HD provides:

- very large doses of dialysis (weekly Kt/V of almost 6 and much greater removal of middle molecules);
- greatly reduced need for phosphate binders;
- reduction in sleep disturbance and sleep apnea.

Based on the above medical advantages the NHS in the UK has included daily HD as a treatment option in planning future renal services.

During the past few years a small number of patients have commenced daily home HD, and these patients and their helpers continue on daily HD in spite of the potential inconvenience arising from the long-term need for set-up, treatment, and disconnect time on a daily basis.

Clinical trials evaluating impact of frequency of HD
Randomized prospective trials thus far have compared outcome data only in patients receiving thrice-weekly HD. On the basis of observational studies of the clinical benefits of short daily and nocturnal daily HD the National Institutes of Health (NIH) has commenced two prospective randomized studies (Frequent Haemodialysis Network Studies) of 250 patients comparing each form of frequent HD with standard thrice-weekly HD.

Duration of hemodialysis

It is difficult to separate the influence of dialysis duration and dose on patient outcomes.

The National Co-operative Dialysis Study (NCDS), a historical US randomized trial where cellulose membranes and acetate dialyzate were used, is the only randomized study so far to address the issue of optimal dialysis time. This 2×2 factorial design study randomized nondiabetic patients into one of four dialysis regimens:

- two with short (2.5–3.5 h) dialysis times;
- two with longer (4.5–5.0 h) dialysis times;
- two with different time-averaged urea concentrations.

Longer dialysis gave a better but statistically insignificant outcome.

A crossover study of standard and higher efficiency HD prescriptions delivering equal dialysis dose (urea removal) measured by direct dialyzate quantification has shown that shorter duration, higher efficiency dialysis is associated with:

- lower phosphate and β2-microglobulin removal;
- less bicarbonate absorption.

Improved clearance of iohexol has also been observed on longer duration HD with similar Kt/V.

Thus, when short and standard duration HD provide equal urea clearances, delivered dialysis therapy should not be regarded as equivalent.

Clinical impact of dialysis duration
There has been a gradual reduction in the average length of HD sessions in many areas of the world during the last two decades.

This trend was most likely due to better patient tolerance of higher efficiency HD arising from the routine use of bicarbonate dialyzate, more biocompatible dialyzers and machine improvements, such as volumetric control of UF, combined with patient preference for shorter times and economic constraints.

However, several observational studies have shown an association between risk of death and shorter dialysis duration:

- very low mortality rates were observed in patients treated with long duration thrice-weekly HD with mean spKt/V of 1.67 + 0.41 in Tassin, France;
- increments in dialysis duration up to 5.5 h were associated with improved patient survival rates in a large Japanese population after adjusting for dialysis dose;
- patients in the USA who received dialysis for <3.5 h per session three times per week had approximately twice the risk of death of patients on HD for >4 h three times per week;
- data from the Dialysis Outcomes and Practice Patterns Study (DOPPS) have shown that patient survival, independent of dialysis dose, was greater in patients with treatment times >4 h;
- data from the Australian and New Zealand Dialysis and Transplant Registry have shown that patient survival, independent of dialysis dose, was greater in patients with treatment times >4.5 h.

These observations suggest that the duration of thrice-weekly HD should not be reduced to <4 h unless the patient has significant residual renal function and indicate that a randomized controlled study of longer dialysis sessions in thrice-weekly HD is needed.

Ultrafiltration on hemodialysis

Ultrafiltration of fluid is required to maintain the patient at estimated dry body weight. Treatment time and UF rates are related inversely in HD. Patients with excessive interdialysis weight gain or hemodynamic instability may require isolated ultrafiltration.

Long-term observational data from Tassin, France have demonstrated that target 'dry' body weight and good control of BP without antihypertensive medication are more likely to be achieved with long duration HD sessions and lower rates of UF.

Higher rates of UF may be poorly tolerated and associated with a greater risk of death.

The Dialysis Outcomes and Practice Patterns Study

This was an international observational study of the risk of death in 22 000 HD patients. It adjusted for demographics, comorbidity, dialysis dose (including RRF) and body size and showed that:

- UF rate >10 mL/h/kg was associated with a higher risk of intradialytic hypotension;
- UF rate >10 mL/h/kg was associated with a higher risk of death.

Factors affecting patient safety on HD

Hemodialysis machine monitors and alarms

HD machines must be serviced and maintained in full working order at all times to ensure that all of the safety monitors and alarms are functional:

- blood pump speed (nominal dialyzer blood flow rate);
- ultrafiltration rate and volume;
- heparin infusion pump;
- dialyzate conductivity monitor and alarm;
- dialyzate temperature monitor and alarm;
- arterial pressure monitor and alarm;
- venous air detect alarm and air trap;
- venous pressure monitor and alarm;
- dialyzate blood leak detector and alarm;
- BP monitor (optional);
- ionic dialysance or online urea clearance for dialysis dose (optional).

Vascular access

Integrity of the extracorporeal blood circuit is paramount for patient safety on HD. Dislodgement of vascular access needles or catheters and disconnection of the HD lines should be very uncommon complications of HD and should be detected promptly if they do occur.

Patients are at greater risk of exsanguination following dislodgement of the venous needle or line as the patient will continue to lose blood at the rate of the blood pump speed unless the HD venous pressure alarm is activated.

The venous alarm may only activate after venous line disconnection when the venous pressure alarm is set close to the prevailing venous pressure of the HD circuit.

Anticoagulation during hemodialysis

Extracorporeal anticoagulation is usually required to prevent thrombosis of the dialyzer and extracorporeal circuit.

Unfractionated heparin

This may be used as the standard anticoagulant in view of its proven efficacy, ease of use and safety record.

It is best administered as a loading dose followed by a continuous infusion of 500–1500 units/h that is discontinued ~30 min before the end of the dialysis session in patients using an arteriovenous fistula or graft (mean half-life 1.5 h).

The dosage of heparin may need to be increased if there has been a substantive rise in the hematocrit after correction of renal anemia or reduced if the patient is on warfarin or antiplatelet drugs.

Low molecular weight heparin

This is an alternative agent that has been associated with a lower risk of bleeding, less frequent episodes of hyperkalemia, and an improved lipid profile than standard heparin.

A systematic review of 11 trials comparing the use of low molecular weight heparin and unfractionated heparin in HD patients concluded that there was no difference in the incidence of bleeding complications, bleeding from the vascular access after HD or thrombosis of the extracorporeal circuit.

For patients with heparin-induced thrombocytopenia either heparinoids (danaparoid) or hirudin should be used instead of heparin.

Reuse of dialyzers

Dialyzers are generally marked for 'single use only' although some are now designed for multiple use in an individual patient.

Reprocessing of dialyzers for reuse requires a combination of cleaning, disinfection and sterilization processes.

It is standard practice to discard the dialyzer whenever the hollow fiber volume (total cell volume) is <80% of the initial measured value but this method may not always be reliable in detecting dialyzer dysfunction.

Changing from multiple to single use of dialyzers has been reported recently to result in a reduction in the mortality rate in a large population in the USA.

The cost of high flux dialyzers has fallen gradually and the use of high flux biocompatible dialyzers is now cost-effective without reuse.

Water quality for hemodialysis

Quality assurance of the water used in the preparation of dialysis fluid is of paramount importance.

HD exposes the blood of the patient to >300 L of water per week through a nonselective dialyzer membrane in contrast to an average of 12 L per week through a highly selective membrane (intestinal tract) in healthy individuals.

Intact dialyzer membranes are permeable to bacterial contaminants, and permit back-diffusion and filtration of chemical contaminants from the dialyzate.

A subset of contaminants that should always be included in routine testing are listed in Table 13.3.2. This is because they occur in relatively high levels and are not restricted in drinking water (chlorine, calcium, magnesium and potassium), or where the drinking water limit is more than five times the recommended limit for water for dialysis.

Sodium is included in the 'mandatory' group because, although the drinking water limit is 200 mg/L, additional sodium is introduced by softening.

In water treated by reverse osmosis, these contaminants will only exceed the limits in Table 13.3.3 if they occur at relatively high levels in the water supplied to the unit. These contaminants can be omitted from routine tests if data are available to show that the levels in the water supplied to the unit rarely exceed the limit in the table. These data should be obtained from the municipal water supplier or from tests on the raw water if it is obtained from a private source.

Routine testing is not required for other contaminants (barium, beryllium, silver, thallium, tin and zinc) for which limits are defined for the water used for dialysis as these trace elements are not considered to occur in levels that give cause for concern and, if low levels are present, they are removed effectively by reverse osmosis. Testing is only required if there is evidence of high levels in the local water supply (zinc, for example, can be introduced in the pipework).

The tests used for monitoring microbial contamination of water for dialysis should be appropriate to the type of organisms found in water. A low nutrient agar, such as Tryptone Glucose Extract Agar or Reasoner's 2A, should be used and samples should be incubated for ≥7 days at 20–22°C.

Table 13.3.2 Maximum recommended concentration of chemical and microbial contaminants in water for dialysis for which routine testing is mandatory

Contaminant	Maximum recommended concentration (mg/L = ppm)	Standards on which limit is based	Initial test frequency
Aluminium	0.01	EP, AAMI, ISO	3-monthly
Calcium	2 (0.05 mmol/L)	EP, AAMI, ISO	3-monthly
Total chlorine	0.1	EP	Not less than weekly
Copper	0.1	AAMI, ISO	3-monthly
Fluoride	0.2	EP, AAMI, ISO	3-monthly
Magnesium	2 (0.08 mmol/L)	EP	3-monthly
Nitrate (as N)	2 (equates to 9 mg/L NO3)	AAMI, ISO	3-monthly
Potassium	2 (0.05 mmol/L)	EP	3-monthly
Sodium	50 (2.2 mmol/L)	EP	3-monthly
Bacteria (total viable count)	100 cfu/mL	EP, ISO	Not less than monthly
Endotoxin	0.25 IU/mL	EP	Not less than monthly

Table 13.3.3 Chemical contaminants in water for dialysis which only require routine testing if the concentration in the water supply exceeds the maximum recommended concentration for treated water

Contaminant	Maximum recommended concentration (mg/l = ppm)	Standards on which limit is based	Initial test frequency
Ammonium	0.2	EP	3-monthly
Arsenic	0.005	AAMI, ISO	3-monthly
Cadmium	0.001	AAMI, ISO	3-monthly
Chloride	50	EP	3-monthly
Chromium	0.014	AAMI, ISO	3-monthly
Lead	0.005	AAMI, ISO	3-monthly
Mercury	0.0002	AAMI, ISO	3-monthly
Sulphate	50	EP	3-monthly

EP, European Pharmacopoeia; AAMI, Association for the Advancement of Medical Instrumentation; ISO, International Organization for Standardization.

The water quality standards in Tables 13.3.2 and 13.3.3 have been endorsed by the Association of Renal Technologists and UK Renal Association Clinical Practice Guidelines on HD (Table 13.3.4).

Clinical impact of water quality

The use of ultrapure water in a randomized study of 30 incident HD patients was associated with a reduction in both CRP levels and the rate of loss of residual renal function.

Impure dialysis fluid has also been implicated in the pathogenesis of dialysis-related amyloidosis. While this hypothesis has not been tested in clinical practice it would seem prudent to ensure that water is as pure as reasonably possible.

Ultrapure water

Ultrapure water (defined as <0.1 cfu/mL and bacterial endotoxins <0.03 IU/mL) is readily achievable using modern water treatment techniques and should be regarded as the standard for all newly installed water treatment plants. The European Best Practice Guidelines recommend the use of ultrapure water for conventional as well as high flux HD.

Table 13.3.4 Summary of water standards adopted by the UK Renal Association

Limits for chemical contaminants derived from:
    Association for the Advancement of Medical Instrumentation
    International Organization for Standardization
    European Pharmacopoeia
Limits for bacterial counts (100 cfu/mL) and endotoxin (0.25 IU/mL) based on:
    European Pharmacopoeia
    European Renal Association Best Practice Guidelines
With exception of nitrate, where standards differ in their recommendations, the most stringent limit has been adopted.

Achieving this standard of purity usually requires:
- softening
- carbon filtration
- reverse osmosis
- effective disinfection programme for pipework between the treatment plant and dialysis machines

Water quality limits should not be difficult to meet with a correctly specified and maintained water plant.

If routine monitoring of treated water demonstrates contamination in excess of the desired levels a programme to improve this should start immediately.

Hemofiltration and hemodiafiltration

Reinfusion fluid, used in hemofiltration and hemodiafiltration, must be sterile (<1 cfu/1000 L) and, particularly where large exchange volumes are required, have an endotoxin level of <0.03 IU/mL.

Even with ultrapure water, this standard of purity can only be achieved with 'online' fluid production with multiple filtration of the dialysis fluid.

Machines designed to produce reinfusion fluid usually require a water supply which can produce ultrapure water.

Modifiable factors affecting clinical outcomes on hemodialysis

Mode of vascular access

A native arteriovenous fistula is the preferred access in the great majority of HD patients as it provides the highest

Table 13.5.5 Biochemical and hematological factors predictive of improved survival in patients on hemodialysis

Pre-dialysis serum:

- bicarbonate: 20–26 mmol/L
  (measured with minimum delay after venepuncture)
- potassium: <6.5 mmol/L
- phosphate: 1.1–1.8 mmol/L
- calcium: within normal range for local laboratory (adjusted for serum albumin)
- Ca × P: ≤4.8 mmol^2/L^2 (serum albumin-corrected)

Pre-dialysis:

- hemoglobin <12.5 g/dL (in patients receiving erythropoietin-stimulating agents)

blood flow rates, minimizes the risk of sepsis and has the greatest longevity.

The rate of vascular access-related infection has been reported as:

- 2.5 per 1000 dialysis sessions with native fistulae or grafts;
- 13.6 per 1000 dialysis sessions for tunneled central venous catheters;
- 18.4 per 1000 dialysis sessions with temporary central venous catheters.

The CHOICE study of 616 incident patients showed that the adjusted relative risk of death compared with a reference group with an arteriovenous fistula was:

- 1.2 for an arteriovenous graft;
- 1.5 for a central venous catheter.

Adequacy of dialysis

A global assessment of the adequacy of the delivered rather than the prescribed HD treatment is required to optimize patient outcomes.

The assessment of dialysis adequacy should include:

- Clinical assessment of patients, including:
  general well-being;
  nutritional status;
  quality of life;
  BP;
  fluid status.
- Measures of clearance of putative uremic toxins by the dialysis process.
- Monitoring of biochemical and hematological parameters.

Dialysis dose

Prospective randomized controlled trials of thrice-weekly HD have indicated that the minimum 'dose of dialysis' should be:

- urea reduction ratio (URR) of 65%; or
- eKt/V of 1.2.

A target URR >70% or eKt/V >1.4 is required if this 'dose of dialysis' is to be achieved consistently (see Chapter 13.5).

Large observational studies have shown that survival in patients on thrice-weekly HD is highest when predialysis biochemical and hematological measurements are within set target ranges (Table 13.3.5).

Blood sampling for biochemical and hematological measurements in HD patients needs to be standardized and should be performed before a mid-week HD session using a dry needle or syringe.

Interdialytic weight gain and blood pressure

The impact of BP control and interdialytic weight gain on HD patient survival is uncertain.

Observational studies have shown an association between excessive interdialytic fluid gains and reduced survival rates whereas patients with hypotension rather than uncontrolled hypertension have the lowest life expectancy.

In particular the frequency of dialysis-related hypotension, defined as an acute symptomatic fall in BP during dialysis requiring immediate intervention to prevent syncope, is an indicator of poor prognosis for survival in HD patients. This may reflect underlying overt or occult cardiac disease in patients with dialysis-related hypotension.

Dialyzate composition

Recognition of the adverse effects of acetate intolerance led to the introduction of bicarbonate in the early 1980s as the standard dialysis fluid buffer.

A systematic review of 18 randomized trials indicated a reduction in the number of treatments complicated by headaches, nausea, vomiting and symptomatic hypotension when bicarbonate was used.

It should be noted, however, that 'bicarbonate' dialyzate still contains moderate amounts of acetate.

There are no set standards for the other components of the dialyzate.

HD treatment in nondiabetic patients using glucose-free dialyzate may result in asymptomatic hypoglycemia without inducing an associated counterregulatory response.

The potential for adverse long-term effects from repeat episodes of dialysis-induced hypoglycemia can be avoided if the dialyzate contains glucose.

Individualization of dialyzate potassium concentrations may be required in patients with hypokalemia, and adjustment of dialyzate sodium concentrations during HD (sodium profiling) may be beneficial in patients with hemodynamic instability.

Relative importance of modifiable factors on hemodialysis patient survival

Data from DOPPS have evaluated the relative risk of death of HD patients who fail to meet clinical practice guidelines for five modifiable clinical variables.

This observational data suggests that the use of central venous catheters for vascular access and nutrition/inflammation are at least as important as adequate dialysis dose or control of hyperphosphatemia in influencing patient survival rates (Table 13.3.6).

Hemofiltration

Hemofiltration (HF) is an alternative form of extracorporeal dialysis which removes solutes by convection rather than diffusion as in HD.

The highly permeable membrane in the hemofilter allows UF of large volumes of fluid which is measured gravimetrically and replaced by infusion of the substitute fluid either into the arterial line (predilutional HF) or the venous line (postdilutional HF).

HF is not commonly used as a mode of chronic RRT because adequate intermittent HF requires:

- large exchange volumes (40% of body weight three times per week);
- high blood flow rates (350–450 mL/min);
- additional costs.

Continuous or daily HF is often performed instead of daily HD for management of AKI in many critical care settings since continuous HF can maintain fluid balance and may promote cardiovascular stability.

The introduction of online production of substitution fluid in the new range of HF machines has obviated much of the extra cost of this form of therapy.

Hemodiafiltration

Hemodiafiltration (HDF) is a hybrid of HD and HF and can be used to increase middle molecule clearances without the need for an increase in treatment time.

HDF superimposes convective removal of middle molecules onto the diffusive removal of the HD technique.

As well as removal of 'unwanted' larger solutes, such as β2-microglobulin, HDF removes other 'wanted' solutes, such as amino acids and small proteins. Vitamin B12 supplements are often required in patients receiving long-term HDF.

Usually ~20 L of 'extra' fluid, over and above the patients' interdialytic fluid gain, is removed through the hemodiafilter and an equal volume of physiological 'replacement' fluid is returned to the blood before (predilutional) or after (postdilutional) the hemodiafilter.

Outcomes with HD, HF and HDF

A recent systematic review of 18 small, randomized trials showed no difference between HD, HDF and HF on the outcomes of patients on long-term RRT.

Hemodynamic stability was found to be similar in a study comparing HDF and low flux HD with equivalent dialysis dose, UF volume and core temperature.

A large retrospective observational study has shown a survival advantage for patients treated with high efficiency HDF (Table 13.3.7). In view of the potential influence of selection bias and other confounding factors the authors of this study concluded that evidence of the benefits of HDF from a controlled clinical trial was required before HDF could be recommended instead of low flux HD in the management of ESRD.

The Dutch CONvective TRAnsport STudy (CONTRAST) is a 3 year randomized study in progress that addresses whether all-cause mortality and/or fatal and nonfatal cardiovascular events differ between HDF and low flux HD in almost 800 HD patients.

Renal replacement therapy for AKI

Modality of renal replacement therapy

At present there is no evidence to show whether continuous or intermittent renal replacement therapies, or HF or HD provide better survival in patients with AKI.

In a randomized, risk stratified, dose equivalent prospective comparison of continuous venovenous HD (CVVHD) versus intermittent HD in 80 intensive care unit patients with AKI, the CVVHD group had greater daily fluid volume removal but no improvement in patient survival, preservation of urinary output or recovery of renal function.

A randomized study of extended daily HD and continuous HD in intensive care patients with AKI showed no difference in hemodynamic stability.

The ongoing prospective, multicenter, Veterans study in the USA may clarify which modality of RRT should be used in AKI.

Frequency of HD in AKI

There is evidence that survival in patients with AKI is better with daily than alternate day RRT. In a randomized prospective study of 160 critically ill patients with AKI the mortality rate using an intention-to-treat analysis was 28% with daily HD and 46% with alternate day HD ($P < 0.01$).

Choice of dialyzer

Initial randomized studies showed that the use of high flux biocompatible membranes was associated with improved patient survival rates in AKI but this has not been confirmed in follow-up studies. In one study 58% of the 90 patients randomly assigned to bioincompatible Cuprophan dialyzers survived compared with 60% of the 90 patients assigned to polymethylmethacrylate membranes.

Dialysis dose

A randomized study of continuous venovenous HF in AKI has shown improved patient survival in patients prescribed an UF rate of ≥35 mL/h/kg body weight.

Conclusions

Both daily treatment and dialysis dose have been shown to improve patient survival.

Extended daily HD and postdilutional CVVHD are widely utilized in the management of AKI and both provide long duration therapy to help maintain adequate fluid balance whilst keeping adverse hemodynamic effects to a minimum in this critically ill patient group.

Center HD versus home HD

The National Institute for Clinical Excellence (NICE) has recommended that all suitable patients should be offered the opportunity to perform HD at home.

This statement is based on observations that patients on home HD have better survival than center HD patients after adjustment for comorbidity and that annual treatment costs are significantly less on home than center HD.

These comparisons are based on patients receiving three sessions of HD per week.

Home HD vs peritoneal dialysis

In most countries, patient choice of dialysis modality is limited to patients who are able to perform dialysis at home.

Observational studies have shown that short-term survival rates of patients on home HD and peritoneal dialysis are similar but technique survival is much poorer on peritoneal dialysis, mainly because of catheter-related infections and inadequate dialysis.

The relative advantages and disadvantages of home HD are summarized in Table 13.3.8.

Home HD may be considered more suitable for patients with:

- large body weight or body mass index;
- low residual renal function;
- heavy proteinuria and/or hypoalbumemia;
- previous major abdominal surgery.

Table 13.3.6 Adjusted relative risk of mortality of patients who fail to achieve clinical practice guidelines (DOPPS I and DOPPS II) and percentage of British patients outside each guideline or practice pattern

Modifiable practice pattern	Level at which clinical practice guideline parameter was achieved	Relative risk of mortality[a]	P-value	% British patients outside each parameter[b]
Dialysis dose	Single pool Kt/V <1.2	1.13	0.0023	17.8%
Anemia management	Hemoglobin <10 g/dL	1.21	<0.0001	21.5%
Mineral metabolism	PO_4 >1.8 mmol/L	1.11	0.001	41.6%
Nutrition/inflammation	Albumin <35 g/L	1.48	<0.0001	36.6%
Vascular access	Facility catheter use >10%	1.20	<0.0001	76.8%

[a]DOPPS I and DOPPS II.
[b]UK DOPPS II data only.

Table 13.3.7 Mortality risk for patients receiving HDF versus HD: European results from the DOPPS

Multicenter study of 2165 patients from 1998–2001 in five European countries patients stratified into four groups:
- low flux HD
- high flux HD
- low efficiency HDF
- high efficiency HDF

High efficiency HDF group had a 35% lower mortality risk than patients on low flux HD (after adjusting for the dialysis dose and comorbidity).

No significant differences observed between high flux HD and HDF.

Table 13.1.8 Comparison of home hemodialysis (HD) with peritoneal dialysis

Advantages of home HD	Disadvantages of home HD
• Higher doses of therapy per unit time	• Need for vascular access
• Ability to prescribe ultrafiltration volume	• Need for anticoagulation and risk of bleeding
• No need for peritoneal access	• Need for a designated treatment room or portacabin at home
• Quality control of the dialyser membrane as well as the dialysis fluid and so no loss of dialysis efficiency with time	• Most home HD training centers require that the patient has a helper at home
	• Training of the patient is more difficult and requires more time
• Lower daily protein losses	• Unphysiological unless performed daily

Complications of hemodialysis, hemofiltration and hemodiafiltration

Access-related infections

The relative risk of bacteremia in a large prospective cohort of incident HD patients compared to patients with an arteriovenous fistula was:
- 1.95 for HD with tunneled catheters;
- 1.05 for HD with grafts.

Infection-related hospitalization in the HEMO study was also shown to be more frequent in patients relying on central venous catheters for vascular access but was not reduced by the use of high flux dialyzers or a higher dialysis dose.

Patients with central venous dialysis catheters and a consequent risk of catheter-related infection have been shown to require higher doses of erythropoiesis-stimulating agents (ESAs) to maintain similar or slightly lower mean hemoglobin values.

Vascular access using central venous dialysis catheters is also associated with a higher risk of central venous stenoses and lower blood flow rates.

Loss of patency of central venous catheters is common.

Nontunneled versus tunneled central venous catheters
The incidence of bacteremia in a prospective study of non-tunneled HD catheters was 5% after 3 weeks of placement in the internal jugular vein.

Cuffed, tunneled rather than nontunneled central venous catheters are preferred if vascular access is likely to be required for >3 weeks since tunneled catheters are associated with a lower rate of infections and can provide higher blood flow rates.

Acute hemolysis
This uncommon complication should be suspected if:
- the patient develops backache, chest tightness or breathlessness;
- the blood in the venous line has a port-wine appearance;
- there is pink plasma in the venous chamber.

This complication may be due to:
- excessive dialyzate temperature;
- kinking of the venous line;
- water contamination with chloramines, nitrates or copper.

Air embolism
This life-threatening complication should be prevented by the machine alarms if a disconnection of the arterial line or arterial access occurs.

Foam is often seen in the dialysis lines and the commonest symptoms are chest tightness if the patient is recumbent, and impaired conscious level or seizures if the patient is sitting upright.

If suspected the blood pump should be stopped, the venous line clamped immediately and the patient placed in the recumbent position on their left side and with their head tilted downwards.

Dialyzer reactions
Chemical sterilization of dialyzers and tubing with ethylene oxide has been associated with anaphylactoid reactions.

This can be avoided by routinely using either steam- or γ-radiation-sterilized dialyzers.

The concurrent use of AN 69 dialyzer membranes in patients on ACEIs has been reported to cause hemodynamic instability attributable to bradykinin. This interaction is preventable by changing the ACEI to an ARB or changing to a different dialysis membrane.

Dialysis dysequilibrium

Nausea, vomiting, restlessness, headache, confusion, somnolence and, more rarely, seizures may occur during or shortly after dialysis when patients with advanced ESRD receive high intensity dialysis.

As the symptoms result from cerebral edema, presumed due to disequilibrium between cerebral water and blood water solute or H^+ concentrations, this syndrome can be avoided by increasing the dialysis dose gradually in patients starting RRT, e.g. 2 h, 3 h and then 4 h treatment for the first three dialysis sessions.

Dialysis-related amyloidosis

Dialysis-related amyloidosis is a disabling, progressive condition caused by the polymerization of β2-microglobulin within tendons, synovium, and other tissues.

β2-Microglobulin is a large molecular weight molecule (MW 11 600), which is released into the circulation as a result of normal cell turnover but is not excreted in renal failure and is not removed by cellulose membranes.

Exposure to bioincompatible membranes may increase β2-microglobulin generation.

Symptoms are typically first reported 7–10 years after commencing HD although tissue accumulation of dialysis-related amyloid in the joints and bone can be demonstrated much earlier.

The most common clinical presentations of dialysis-related amyloid are:
- carpal tunnel syndrome (usually after ≥7 years of HD);
- joint pains and stiffness especially in hands, arms and shoulders (usually after ≥10 years of HD);
- tenosynovitis of tendons in the hands;
- pathological fractures due to amyloid bone cysts;
- destructive spondylarthropathy.

Symptoms from dialysis-related amyloidosis may occur earlier if patients have no significant residual renal function or are elderly at the onset of dialysis.

High flux HD membranes remove β2-microglobulin by a combination of diffusive clearance and adsorption; HDF removes substantially more as a result of additional convective clearance. Both treatments are thought to reduce the risk of developing dialysis-related amyloid and have been recommended for use in patients who are predicted to remain on dialysis for at least 3.7 years.

Renal transplantation usually results in improvement in amyloid-related symptoms.

Dialysis-related hemorrhage

Bleeding from an arteriovenous fistula, graft or the GI tract is not uncommon in HD patients and should be treated as an emergency.

Great care is required with the use of anticoagulants during HD and heparin-locking solutions in patients with central venous catheters.

For patients with an increased risk of bleeding, anticoagulation should be avoided or kept to a minimum by using a high blood flow rate and regular flushing of the extracorporeal circuit with saline every 15–30 min.

Alternatively heparin may be replaced by a prostacyclin infusion or regional citrate anticoagulation. The former may induce hypotension and is expensive whereas the latter requires careful replacement of calcium, monitoring of serum calcium levels during HD and is too complex for routine use.

Dialysis-related symptomatic hypotension

Hypotension is the most frequent complication of HD and can shorten treatment times, thus reducing the delivered dialysis dose. It is important to exclude a range of uncommon alternative causes when a patient develops hypotension on dialysis:
- cardiac disease (arrthymias, myocardial infarction, pericardial tamponade);
- autonomic neuropathy;
- occult hemorrhage;
- septicemia;
- dialyzer reactions;
- air embolism;
- acute hemolysis.

Dialysis-related hypotension is an independent predictor of poor patient survival and patients experiencing frequent dialysis-related hypotension are at higher risk of death probably because dialysis-related hypotension is a marker of severe cardiac disease.

The frequency of dialysis-related hypotension is, therefore, an important indicator of the quality of dialysis.

The risk of dialysis-related symptomatic hypotension can be reduced by:
- increase in postdialysis target weight if the patient is assessed as below 'dry' weight;
- reduction in interdialytic weight gain;
- decrease in the rate of fluid removal;
- reduction in dialysate temperature during dialysis;
- increase in dialysate sodium concentration;
- avoiding the administration of BP-lowering medication before dialysis;
- reduction in food intake during dialysis.

Dialyzate sodium modelling or 'ramping' can reduce intradialytic cramps and hypotension but may increase thirst, weight gain and hypertension between dialysis sessions.

A recent randomized trial of intradialytic blood volume monitoring demonstrated no difference in weight, BP or frequency of dialysis-related complications although hospitalization and mortality rates were lower in the control group assigned to conventional monitoring.

A recent systematic review of 22 studies has concluded that a reduction in dialyzate temperature is effective in decreasing the incidence of intradialytic hypotension without affecting dialysis adequacy.

An increase in the dialysis treatment time combined with a reduction in the fluid UF rate or a decrease in the dialyzate fluid temperature are the most reliable methods of reducing intradialytic hypotension without causing adverse sequelae.

Hyperkalemia

Hyperkalemia is a common indication for emergency dialysis among patients already on HD and hyperkalemia is the probable cause of death in 3–5% of HD patients.

Nonconcordance with the dialysis prescription and diet are the commonest contributory factors but medications such as ACEIs, ARBs, NSAIDs, β-blockers and potassium supplements may be implicated.

Performing an urgent electrocardiogram is of proven use in guiding management of patients with serum potassium concentrations >6 mmol/L and can be used to dictate which patients should receive emergency administration of intravenous calcium chloride.

HD is the most appropriate emergency treatment for hyperkalemia in the dialysis patient. Serum potassium levels usually fall by 1 mmol/L during the first hour of treatment and by a further 1 mmol/L during the next 2 h. The rate of potassium removal is increased by using a higher dialyzer blood flow rate, higher dialyzate bicarbonate concentration or lower dialyzate potassium concentration.

Incidence and prevalence of comorbid medical conditions

The incidence and prevalence of a wide range of comorbid medical conditions is higher in chronic HD patients:

- myocardial infarction;
- cerebrovascular disease;
- peripheral vascular disease;
- falls and fractures;
- infective endocarditis;
- metastatic staphylococcal infections.

The management of these medical complications is akin to standard clinical practice but needs to take account of a reduction in the dosage of drugs excreted by the kidneys and the patient's ongoing dialysis therapy.

Further reading

Astor BC, Eustace JA, Powe NR, *et al.* Type of vascular access and survival among incident hemodialysis patients: the Choices for Healthy Outcomes in Caring for ESRD (CHOICE) Study. *J Am Soc Nephrol* 2005; **16**: 1449–1455.

Canaud B, Bragg-Gresham JL, Marshall MR, *et al.* Mortality risk for patients receiving haemodiafiltration versus hemodialysis: European results from the DOPPS. *Kidney Int* 2006; **69**: 2087–2093.

Charra B, Calemard E, Ruffet M, *et al.* Survival as an index of adequacy of dialysis. *Kidney Int* 1992; **41**: 1286–1291.

Chauveau P, Nguyen H, Combe C, *et al.* Dialyser membrane permeability and survival in hemodialysis patients. *Am J Kidney Dis* 2005; **45**: 564–571.

Cheung AK, Levin NW, Greene T, *et al.* Effects of high-flux hemodialysis on clinical outcomes: results of the HEMO study. *J Am Soc Nephrol* 2003; **14**: 3251–3263.

Eknoyan G, Beck GJ, Cheung AK, *et al.* Effect of dialysis dose and flux on mortality and morbidity in maintenance hemodialysis patients: primary results of the HEMO study. *N Engl J Med* 2002; **347**: 2010–2019.

Goldfarb-Rumyantzev AS, Leypoldt JK, Nelson N, *et al.* A crossover study of short daily haemodialysis. *Nephrol Dial Transplant* 2005; **21**: 166–175.

Grooteman MPC, Nube MJ. Impact of the type of dialyser on clinical outcome in chronic haemodialysis patients: does it really matter? *Nephrol Dial Transplant* 2004; **19**: 2965–29701.

Held PJ, Levin NW, Bovbjerg RR, *et al.* Mortality and duration of hemodialysis treatment. *J Am Med Assoc* 1991; **265**: 871–875.

Ishani A, Collins AJ, Herzog CA, Foley RN. Septicaemia, access and cardiovascular disease in dialysis patients: the USRDS Wave 2 study. *Kidney Int* 2005; **68**: 311–318.

Karamperis N, Sloth E, Jensen JD. Predilution hemofiltration displays no hemodynamic advantage over low-flux hemodialysis under matched conditions. *Kidney Int* 2005; **67**: 1601–1608.

Lim W, Cook DJ, Crowther MA. Safety and efficacy of low molecular weight heparins for hemodialysis in patients with end-stage renal failure: a meta-analysis of randomised trials. *J Am Soc Nephrol* 2004; **15**: 3192–3206.

Locatelli F, Andrulli S, Pecchini F, *et al.* Effect of high-flux dialysis on the anaemia of haemodialysis patients. *Nephrol Dial Transplant* 2000; **15**: 1399–1409.

Locatelli F, Pozzoni P, Di Filippo S. What are we expecting to learn from the MPO study? *Contrib Nephrol* 2005; **149**: 83–89.

Lowrie EG, Parker TF, Parker TF, Sargent JA. Effect of the hemodialysis prescription on patient morbidity: report from the National Cooperative Dialysis Study. *N Engl J Med* 1981; **305**: 1176–1181.

Macleod AM, Campbell M, Cody JD, *et al.* Cellulose, modified cellulose and synthetic membranes in the haemodialysis of patients with end-stage renal disease. *Cochrane Database Syst Rev* 2005(3).

Mactier RA, Madi AM, Allam BF. Comparison of high-efficiency and standard haemodialysis providing equal urea clearances by partial and total dialysate quantification. *Nephrol Dial Transplant* 1997; **12**: 1182–1186.

Marshall MR, Byrne BG, Kerr PG, McDonald SP. Associations of hemodialysis dose and session length with mortality risk in Australian and New Zealand patients. *Kidney Int* 2006; **69**: 1229–1236.

Owen WF, Lew NL, Lowrie EG, *et al.* The urea reduction ratio and serum albumin concentration as predictors of mortality in patients undergoing haemodialysis. *N Eng J Med* 1993; **329**: 1001–1006.

Penne EL, Blankestijn PJ, Bots ML, *et al.* Effect of increased convective clearance by on-line hemodiafiltration on all cause mortality in chronic hemodialysis patients – the Dutch CONvective TRAnsport STudy (CONTRAST): rationale and design of a randomised controlled trial. *Curr Control Trail Cardiovasc Med* 2005; **6**: 8.

Pierratos A. Nocturnal home haemodialysis: an update on a 5-year experience. *Nephrol Dial Transplant* 1999; **14**: 2835–2840.

Rabindranath KS, Strippoli GF, Roderick P, *et al.* Comparison of hemodialysis, hemofiltration, and acetate free biofiltration for ESRD:systematic review. *Am J Kidney Dis* 2005; **45**: 437–447.

Reddan DN, Szczech LA, Hasseblad V, *et al.* Intradialytic blood volume monitoring in ambulatory hemodialysis patients:a randomised trial. *J Am Soc Nephrol* 2005; **16**: 2162–2169.

Roberts TL, Obrador GT, St Peter WL, *et al.* Relationship among catheter insertions, vascular access infections and anaemia management in hemodialysis patients. *Kidney Int* 2004; **66**: 2429–2436.

Saran R, Bragg-Gresham JL, Levin NW, *et al.* Longer treatment time and slower ultrafiltration in hemodialysis: associations with lower mortality in the DOPPS. *Kidney Int* 2006;**69**:1222–1228.

Schiffl H, Lang SM, Fischer R. Ultrapure dialysis fluid slows loss of residual renal function in new dialysis patients. *Nephrol Dial Transplant* 2002; **17**: 1814–1818.

Selby NM, McIntyre CW. A systematic review of the clinical effects of reducing dialysate fluid temperature. *Nephrol Dial Transplant* 2006; **21**: 1883–1898.

Shinzato T, Nikai S, Akiba T, *et al.* Survival in long-term haemodialysis patients: results from the annual survey of the Japanese Society of Dialysis Therapy. *Nephrol Dial Transplant* 1997; **12**: 884–814.

Stevenson KB, Adcox MJ, Mallea MC, *et al.* Standardized surveillance of hemodialysis vascular access infections: 18-month experience at an outpatient, multi-facility, hemodialysis centre. *Infect Control Hosp Epidemiol* 2000; **21**: 200–203.

Termorshuizen F, Dekker FW, van Manen JG, *et al.* Relative contribution of residual renal function and different measures of adequacy to survival in hemodialysis patients: an analysis of the Netherlands Cooperative Study on the Adequacy of Dialysis (NECOSAD)-2. *J Am Soc Nephrol* 2004; **15**: 1061–1070.

Internet resources

Renal Association Clinical Practice Guidelines for HD:

http://www.renal.org/pages/pages/clinical-affairs/guidelines.php

The Renal Registry:

http://www.renalreg.org

National Kidney Federation Dialysis Outcomes Quality Initiative:

http://www.kidney.org/professionals/kdoqi/

European Best Practice Guidelines:

http://www.ndt-educational.org/guidelines.asp

Frequent hemodialysis clinical trials:

www.niddk.nih.gov/patient/hemodialysis/hemodialysis.htm

Cochrane Renal Group:

http://www.cochrane-renal.org/

International Organization for Standardization (standards for concentrates and water for HD):

www.iso.org

European Pharmacopoeia:

http://online.pheur.org/entry.htm

Association for the Advancement of Medical Instrumentation:

http://www.aami.org/

International Society for Haemodialysis:

http://www.hdintl.org/

Australia and New Zealand Dialysis and Transplant Registry:

http://www.anzdata.org.au/

National Institute for Clinical Excellence:

http://www.nice.org.uk/

Association of Renal Technologists:

http://www.artery.org.uk/site/ART/home

See also

Renal replacement therapies in acute kidney injury, p. 328

Dialysis and hemoperfusion treatment of acute poisoning, p. 336

Dialysis strategies, p. 480

Vascular access, p. 488

Adequacy of dialysis, p. 518

Medical management of dialysis patients, p. 528

Peritoneal dialysis

Introduction

Since the initial description of continuous ambulatory peritoneal dialysis (CAPD) to treat ESRD in the 1970s, peritoneal dialysis (PD) has become established as a major option for long-term renal replacement therapy. PD now offers a variety of modalities to allow treatment to be tailored to the individual patient's requirements.

The place of PD in the integrated care of the patient with ESRD

The relative merits of different dialysis modalities have been debated but no evidence clearly shows one to be superior.

Rather than debating whether any mode of dialysis is superior, it is better to consider that most patients will receive a variety of renal replacement modalities (including transplantation) and these should be used in combination over the patient's life to achieve the optimal patient outcomes and quality of life.

It may be advantageous to use PD as the initial mode of dialysis therapy as part of an integrated care concept:

- PD may be associated with better preservation of residual renal function and this may account for superior early outcomes on PD compared to HD.
- Initial PD use preserves possible sites for vascular access, which will be available later if a transfer to HD is required.
- Some evidence suggests that initial treatment with PD and subsequent transfer to HD has a superior outcome than treatment with a single dialysis modality.

In most cases there are no contraindications to either dialysis mode, leaving patients to choose according to personal preference and social/lifestyle factors.

Contraindications to PD include:

- psychosocial factors preventing patient or carer performing PD;
- abdominal stomas;
- morbid obesity.

Previous abdominal surgery is not usually a contraindication, although in some cases intra-abdominal adhesions may limit its success.

PD may be specifically indicated in patients where HD is difficult due to limited options for vascular access or hemodynamic instability.

Anatomy and physiology of the peritoneal cavity

PD involves infusion of dialysis fluid into the peritoneal cavity, with movement of solutes between the patient's blood and dialysis fluid across the semipermeable peritoneal membrane.

The peritoneal cavity represents the space between the abdominal viscera and abdominal wall. It is lined by the peritoneal membrane which comprises the parietal peritoneal membrane lining the abdominal wall, and visceral peritoneal membrane covering the intra-abdominal viscera.

The anatomical surface area of the peritoneal membrane in adults is typically 1.7–2 m^2 but effective surface area varies with anatomical factors and peritoneal blood flow.

The membrane is lined by mesothelial cells which are attached to a submesothelial connective tissue layer containing the peritoneal capillaries and lymphatics.

The peritoneal vasculature is central to the physiology of PD. The peritoneal capillary endothelium provides the major barrier to solute and fluid removal between patient and dialysis fluid.

Factors affecting peritoneal capillary blood flow alter peritoneal membrane function.

Peritoneal lymphatics contribute to fluid removal from the peritoneal cavity.

The three-pore theory of movement of solutes and water

This theory describes movement of solutes and water between patient and peritoneal dialyzate.

It describes the barrier between capillary blood and dialyzate according to three different sizes of pores in the capillary endothelium:

Large pores:
- possibly interendothelial cell clefts;
- are few in number;
- allow passage of macromolecules such as proteins into the dialyzate.

Small pores:
- the gaps between endothelial cells;
- represent the majority of the total pore area;
- allow small solute diffusion between blood and dialyzate (removal of urea and creatinine, and absorption of solutes from dialyzate such as glucose);
- account for part of fluid removal by ultrafiltration.

Ultra-small pores:
- transcellular aquaporin water channels;
- allow passage of water;
- impermeable to solutes;
- account for ~50% of water removal by the osmotic effect of dialyzate glucose.

PD catheters and exit site care

Permanent peritoneal access is crucial to successful PD. Catheter-related problems are a major cause of treatment interruption and transfer to HD. PD catheters should provide fast, reliable flow of dialysis fluid in and out of the peritoneal cavity, and avoid leaks and infection.

Catheter types

Most catheters are made from silicone or polyurethane. They have either one or two subcutaneous cuffs which anchor the catheter in position.

There is some evidence that single-cuffed catheters have a shorter time to the first episode of peritonitis and more exit site complications. However, they may produce equivalent outcomes to double-cuffed catheters, if the cuff is placed in a deep rather than superficial position.

There are various designs for the intraperitoneal portion of the catheter.

The commonest is the straight Tenckhoff design.

A coiled catheter design provides increased size of catheter tubing to separate catheter tip from the peritoneum and may provide better dialyzate flow, less inflow pain and less risk of migration or omental obstruction, though evidence for this is inconclusive.

The Toronto–Western Hospital catheter has two discs near the catheter tip, perpendicular to the catheter, which separate drainage holes from the peritoneum and viscera.

A T-fluted catheter has a T-shaped terminal portion with grooves designed to improve dialyzate flow.

A presternal catheter has a long subcutaneous tunnel, with the exit site on the chest wall in the presternal region. This may be used for patients with:

• abdominal stomas;
• fecal incontinence;
• no suitable abdominal site for an exit site;
• severely obese subjects.

The subcutaneous portion of the catheter may be straight or have a preformed bend (e.g. Swan-necked catheter) designed to ensure a downward-pointing exit site. This can also be achieved by appropriate tunneling of a straight catheter.

Exit site infection rates are significantly lower when the exit site is formed in a downwards direction.

Catheter insertion techniques

• surgical dissection and placement under direct vision;
• blind placement by Tenckhoff trocar or Seldinger technique;
• peritoneoscopic placement;
• laparoscopic placement.

There are various potential advantages and disadvantages to the different techniques, often with benefits at the expense of greater complexity.

Laparoscopy allows visualization of the catheter tip position, and other procedures can be performed at the same time (e.g. suturing the catheter tip in position, division of adhesions, omentectomy and hernia repair) but may be accompanied by greater surgical complications.

There is no clear evidence favoring any of the options. The experience and skill of the operator inserting the catheter and procedures for planning and preparing for the procedure are the most important factors affecting catheter insertion outcome.

Preinsertion preparation

Preparation before catheter insertion is important.

The presence of hernias and abdominal wall weakness should be sought, with defects being repaired either before or at the time of catheter insertion.

The position of the exit site should be determined and marked prior to surgery. Areas of pressure should be avoided (e.g. it should be above or below the patient's beltline).

Preoperative skin preparation includes washing with soap or detergent on the morning of surgery, and if necessary, clipping of abdominal wall hair.

Bowel preparation and avoidance of constipation is important. Patients should be started on laxatives prior to catheter insertion, and these should continue postoperatively.

An enema on the day prior to surgery is sometimes administered.

The bladder should be emptied prior to surgery to reduce the risk of accidental perforation during the procedure.

Antibiotic prophylaxis prior to catheter insertion may reduce the risk of developing exit site or wound infections postoperatively. Antibiotic choice depends on local patterns of infection. There is some evidence supporting the use of vancomycin, but this needs to be balanced against risk of development of antibiotic resistance.

Postinsertion care

Postinsertion management aims to allow healing and minimizing any risks of infection or leakage.

Dressings should be gauze or similar to avoid pooling of discharge around the exit site.

Dressing changes should be minimized in the initial period after insertion, with the initial dressing left unchanged for a week unless there is suspicion of infection.

The catheter should be immobilized with tape or dressings to reduce trauma due to movement.

It is desirable to delay commencing PD for 1–3 weeks after catheter insertion to promote healing, although there is increasing evidence that it is safe to use low volume APD immediately after insertion when the catheter has been placed using a percutaneous technique.

If early dialysis is required, this should be done with small dialyzate volumes (1–1.5 L) in a recumbent position, to reduce intra-abdominal pressure and the risk of leaking.

A 1 year catheter survival of 80% has been suggested as a desirable catheter outcome target.

Exit site care

Chronic exit site care involves regular assessment and cleaning.

There are no trials showing superiority of any particular cleansing agent or dressings.

Frequent cleaning is necessary to prevent the build-up of bacteria at the exit site, and most units recommend that this is done daily.

Cleaning should also be performed if the exit site becomes dirty or wet.

Patients should be taught to undertake hand washing and appropriate sterile technique, to assess their exit site and to detect the presence of infection or other problems.

Various cleansing agents are used, including povidone iodine, chlorhexidine solution and antibacterial liquid soap products.

There is no evidence in adults for superiority of any particular dressing and many types are used.

Some patients and centers may not use a dressing, and again there is no evidence of any adverse effect on outcomes.

Antibiotic or antibacterial preparations such as mupirocin cream may be used at the exit site (mupirocin ointment should be avoided with polyurethane catheters due to reports of resulting damage to the catheter).

Different modalities of peritoneal dialysis
CAPD

CAPD was the original modality allowing widespread uptake of PD for the treatment of ESRD. It consists of manual exchanges of dialyzate, with spent dialyzate drained by gravity from the peritoneal cavity and replaced by fresh fluid for a dwell period until the next exchange.

Typical CAPD regimes involve four exchanges per day. Some patients may perform fewer exchanges where clearances allow, and occasional patients perform five exchanges per day.

Automated peritoneal dialysis (APD)

An automated dialyzate cycling machine performs a number of dialysis cycles overnight while the patient is asleep.

A number of variants of APD have been developed.

Continuous cycling peritoneal dialysis (CCPD)

This comprises a series of automated dialysis exchanges performed overnight, with a long fluid dwell remaining in the peritoneal cavity during the day, which drains out at the start of next overnight session.

Variations include having a shorter daytime dwell – either by drainage of the day exchange before the night, with a subsequent dry period, or by leaving the peritoneum dry after the night cycles and draining in a day dwell later in the day.

Optimized cycling peritoneal dialysis (OCPD)

This involves two daytime dwells, with fluid left in the peritoneal cavity after the night-time cycles and an additional exchange performed at some time during the day.

It is used particularly to enhance solute clearances, or to improve daytime ultrafiltration.

Nocturnal intermittent PD (NIPD)

This involves overnight automated cycles, with subsequent dry peritoneal cavity during the day. It avoids peritoneal fluid during the day which may help patients with problems due to intra-abdominal pressure, but clearances are inferior to other APD regimes.

Tidal APD

The cycler is programmed to leave a percentage of the preceding dwell in the peritoneal cavity before the next fluid instillation during night-time cycles, so that the peritoneal cavity never completely empties.

It is useful for patients with abdominal pain between cycles and those with frequent 'low drain' alarms overnight, but generally does not improve clearances, which was the original aim of its development.

Choice of PD modality

A number of features determine choice of PD modality. Social and lifestyle reasons are important. CAPD is simpler, not requiring a cycling machine or connection to it overnight. However, APD, with few or no exchanges during the day, suits many patients, including individuals where employment would make CAPD difficult, or where a carer performs the dialysis, since it allows freedom from undertaking dialysis exchanges during the day.

Lower intraperitoneal pressure in the supine position means that APD is useful where problems arise from raised intra-abdominal pressure such as hernias and fluid leaks. It allows larger dwell volumes to be instilled at night, which may help to obtain target small solute clearances. Shorter dwell periods overnight on APD enhance ultrafiltration in higher peritoneal membrane transport status patients, due to reduced time for loss of osmotic agent during the dwell.

PD equipment design

A variety of designs of PD equipment have been developed, with the aims of reducing peritonitis rates and increasing the ease of performing dialysis (e.g. for patients with reduced manual dexterity or visual impairment).

A major development in CAPD was the introduction of disconnect Y-systems which resulted in a major reduction of peritonitis.

Mechanical devices exist which aid connection, including those incorporating a UV light sterilization component to the connection procedure.

Peritoneal dialysis solutions

Peritoneal dialysis fluids consist of solutions of electrolytes, a buffer to correct metabolic acidosis and an osmotic agent to achieve net fluid removal (Table 13.4.1).

Electrolytes

Sodium

Dialyzate sodium concentration is slightly below the normal plasma range. This prevents sodium diffusion into patients with hyponatremia, but achieves minimal sodium removal by diffusion.

Some studies have investigated the use of lower sodium concentrations in dialyzate to enhance sodium removal and improve BP control.

Potassium

Potassium is absent from dialyzate, facilitating removal from the patient.

Calcium

Solutions are available with varying calcium concentrations.

Previously, standard solutions had a calcium concentration of 1.75 mmol/L (greater than the ionized calcium concentration in blood).

This allowed correction of hypocalcemia but frequently resulted in hypercalcemia when used in conjunction with calcium-containing phosphate binders or vitamin D analogues to control hyperparathyroidism.

The majority of patients now receive lower calcium concentration dialyzate (e.g. 1.25 mmol/L), with choice of solution according to individual biochemistry parameters.

Correction of acidosis by dialyzate buffer content

Correction of acidosis in PD is achieved by absorption of buffer contained within the dialyzate.

Standard solutions contain lactate which is absorbed by the patient and undergoes hepatic conversion to bicarbonate, thereby correcting the acidosis.

Solutions with differing buffer content are available which may result in differing degrees of correction of acidosis or even development of alkalosis.

Use of bicarbonate as a buffer had been precluded due to instability and reaction with metal ions such as calcium and magnesium during storage.

Newer twin-chamber design bags for dialyzate have overcome this problem, with bicarbonate separated from divalent metal ions during storage, being mixed shortly prior to infusion.

To achieve serum bicarbonate levels in the normal physiological range, higher concentrations of buffer need to be present in the dialysis fluid, typically 35–40 mmol/L.

Osmotic agents

Glucose

Glucose has been the standard osmotic agent in PD solutions, but has several limitations.

Table 13.4.1 Typical composition of peritoneal fluid

Solute	Concentration
Electrolyte	
Sodium	132–3 mmol/L
Potassium	0 (–2) mmol/L
Calcium	1.0–1.75 mmol/L
Magnesium	0.25–0.75 mmol/L
Chloride	95–102 mmol/L
Buffer	
Lactate	35–40 mmol/L
or	
Lactate/bicarbonate	25/10–15 mmol/L
or	
Bicarbonate	34–39 mmol/L
Osmotic agent	
Glucose (anhydrous)	1.36–3.86 g/dL
or	
Amino acids	1.1 g/dL
or	
Icodextrin	7.5 g/dL

It is absorbed from the peritoneum relatively quickly (especially with higher peritoneal membrane transport status). This leads to loss of its osmotic effectiveness and reduced or negative ultrafiltration on longer dwell times.

Absorbed glucose results in metabolic complications such as hyperglycemia, hyperinsulinemia, hyperlipidemia and weight gain.

Exposure of the peritoneal membrane to high concentrations of dialyzate glucose adversely affects peritoneal membrane structure and function.

Amino acids
Amino acid dialyzate solutions contain amino acids instead of glucose as the osmotic agent.

An exchange of 1.1% amino acid solution achieves equivalent ultrafiltration to 1.36% glucose solution and typically provides ~20–25% of the patient's daily nitrogen requirements by absorption of amino acids from the dialyzate.

Usually only one exchange is used per day as more can result in the development of uremia and acidosis.

Icodextrin
Icodextrin is a large glucose polymer and acts as a colloid osmotic agent (similar to large molecules such as albumin).

It acts at the small intercellular pores and is only slowly lost from the peritoneal cavity.

Unlike glucose, it produces gradual and sustained ultrafiltration over long dwell periods and may be more effective in achieving ultrafiltration in higher transporters.

It is used for a single long dwell daily–overnight in CAPD or the day dwell in APD.

Being glucose free, it may avoid the adverse peritoneal membrane and metabolic effects of glucose.

Some icodextrin metabolites are absorbed. This leads to a small fall in serum sodium and increase in osmolality or osmolar gap in plasma, which is not of clinical significance. These absorbed metabolites can cause overestimation of blood glucose by some patient glucometers (with risk of undiagnosed hypoglycemia).

Biocompatibility of PD fluid
Biocompatibility of PD fluid can be defined as the ability to perform its role without inducing adverse effects in the patient – particularly change in peritoneal membrane, and also immune cell dysfunction.

Bioincompatibility of PD fluids is due to the toxicity of:
• high glucose concentrations;
• high osmolality;
• acid pH;
• lactate buffer;
• glucose degradation products (GDPs) produced from heat sterilization of glucose solutions.

Solutions have been developed to try to overcome these factors.

Icodextrin and amino acid fluids have some biocompatible features.

A variety of newer glucose-containing solutions are available which are low in GDPs, have neutral pH and use bicarbonate or a mixture of bicarbonate and lactate as a buffer.

Neutral pH reduces symptoms of infusion pain.

Long-term clinical benefits of these fluids are currently under investigation.

Peritoneal membrane function testing
Peritoneal membrane function differs between individuals. Variability occurs in the rate of movement of small solutes between the patient and the dialyzate. More rapid movement equates to the presence of a greater number of small pores, or effective vascular surface area (higher transporters).

Peritoneal equilibration test (PET)
This is the common test of peritoneal membrane function.

Two litres of 2.27% glucose dialyzate is infused into the peritoneal cavity for a 4 h period.

Dialyzate samples are taken after infusion, and at 2 and 4 h and analysed for creatinine and glucose.

A blood sample is taken at 2 h.

Graphs are plotted of the ratio of dialyzate to plasma (D:P) creatinine concentrations and the ratio of dialyzate glucose concentrations at sample time to that at time zero.

Comparison with standard curves derived from population studies allows classification of the patient's solute transporter status as:
• low;
• low average;
• high average;
• high.

Increasing transport state is associated with more rapid rise in dialyzate creatinine and fall in dialyzate glucose concentrations over time.

The net ultrafiltration at 4 h is also useful, with a value <100 mL suggesting ultrafiltration failure.

Standardized permeability analysis (SPA)
The test is similar to the PET, but:
• uses 3.86% glucose dialyzate;
• has an additional sample of dialyzate extracted at 1 h;
• dialyzate samples also analysed for sodium.

SPA classifies transport status in the same way as PET.

The fall in dialyzate sodium at 1 h (sodium dipping) reflects aquaporin function.

Net UF <400 mL at 4 h with 3.86% glucose is a more robust definition of ultrafiltration failure than that with PET.

Fluid balance management

Maintaining normal fluid balance is a primary role of PD.

Hydration depends on a balance of intake and input.

Determining correct dry weight is a difficult and imprecise process.

Clinical assessment can be insensitive to significant fluid imbalance.

Fluid overload is associated with adverse cardiovascular effects such as hypertension, and development of left ventricular hypertrophy and dysfunction.

Hypertension in the absence of other evidence of fluid overload may be due to fluid excess and respond to fluid removal, but care is necessary to avoid dehydration and loss of residual renal function in patients who still pass urine.

Appropriate individualized instructions should be given to patients with regard to their fluid and sodium intake allowances.

Water and sodium loss occur through dialysis and also residual renal function.

Urine volume (but not clearance) may be enhanced by prescription of high doses of loop diuretics.

Ultrafiltration with PD

Dialyzate fluid removal is dependent on:

- the osmotic agent;
- duration of dwell;
- peritoneal membrane transport status.

Ultrafiltration may be increased by:

- using more hypertonic glucose dialyzate;
- shorter dwell times (and thus less time for loss of glucose and its osmotic effect).

It is essential to avoid dwells with negative ultrafiltration. This is most likely to occur in the long day dwell of APD or the overnight dwell of CAPD and can be managed by:

- adding additional exchanges to shorten dwell times;
- using more hypertonic glucose;
- use of solutions containing icodextrin (whose sustained ultrafiltration profile is better-suited to long dwell periods than glucose).

There is clear evidence that for the long dwell, icodextrin can improve fluid balance compared with glucose.

Ultrafiltration failure

Ultrafiltration failure is an important cause of PD technique failure that may require transfer to HD.

It may be specifically defined as net fluid removal below a defined value during peritoneal membrane function testing:

- < 100 mL/4 h in PET test with 2.27% glucose;
- < 400 mL/4 h in SPA test with 3.86% glucose.

Sodium removal

During the course of a dwell, sodium concentrations between dialyzate and plasma will tend to equilibrate by diffusion.

Peritoneal sodium removal is however largely achieved by sodium accompanying water removal by ultrafiltration, with little sodium loss occurring by diffusion.

Thus patients with low ultrafiltration will develop sodium overload and hypertension.

Sodium sieving

Part of the ultrafiltration induced by glucose is water passage without accompanying solutes, through the ultra-small pores.

This water transport without sodium is termed sodium sieving.

The measured fall in dialyzate sodium at 1 h in the SPA reflects sodium sieving and aquaporin function.

Over a 4 h dwell, sodium concentrations will equilibrate between dialyzate and plasma by diffusion.

With hypertonic glucose exchanges and very short dwell times (e.g. in APD), sodium removal may be low relative to ultrafiltration volume (i.e. sodium sieving greater), as there is less time for dialyzate sodium concentration to equilibrate with plasma by diffusion.

Assessment of fluid overload in PD

Fluid overload has many potential causes and careful systematic assessment is essential to make the correct diagnosis and institute correct treatment. The majority of cases are not due to primary peritoneal membrane failure.

Excessive fluid intake

Fluid overload from excess fluid intake can result from:

- thirst due to high sodium intake or hyperglycemia in poorly controlled diabetes;
- inadequate education or instruction about intake;
- nonconcordance.

It is important to recognize these as they are reversible.

Loss of residual renal function

Loss of residual urine output may cause fluid retention in otherwise stable subjects. It should be recognized and treated by:

- reduction of fluid intake allowance;
- altered dialysis prescription to increase fluid removal;
- high dose loop diuretics to increase urinary water and sodium excretion.

Catheter dysfunction and other mechanical problems

Mechanical problems such as catheter malfunction and peritoneal fluid leaks also lead to inadequate fluid removal despite a healthy peritoneal membrane.

PD prescription errors

PD prescription errors commonly result in inadequate fluid removal and fluid retention. Problems include inadequate strength glucose dwells or too long cycles. The long dwell is a particular problem (overnight in CAPD or day in APD) as the long time period allows greatest loss of osmotic agent.

Ultrafiltration failure

Where initial assessment fails to reveal a reversible cause, assessment of peritoneal membrane function can aid in confirming and classifying ultrafiltration failure.

If fluid removal in the peritoneal function test is satisfactory, this suggests that the patient does not have ultrafiltration failure and further search for other reversible causes should be made.

Where achieved ultrafiltration is low, this suggests ultrafiltration failure and the transport characteristics determined by the test can suggest the mechanism.

Higher transporter status

The commonest cause of ultrafiltration failure is a high peritoneal membrane transport state, which results in rapid loss of osmotic agent from the peritoneal cavity for small solutes such as glucose and amino acids. This commonly develops after time on PD and episodes of peritonitis. Improvement of ultrafiltration requires PD with:

• greater glucose concentrations;
• shorter exchanges.

Higher transport patients may have most effective ultrafiltration with the short dwell times of APD regimes.

Icodextrin achieves its ultrafiltration effect at the small pores, which are relatively impermeable to it, and therefore in contrast to glucose it may actually be more effective in patients with higher transport status.

Low transport status

Ultrafiltration failure with a low transport state is rare and a serious situation, resulting in both poor fluid management and solute clearance.

It implies major damage or disruption to the intraperitoneal space.

This pattern can, however, also result from the coexistence of a low transport status with a reversible mechanical problem and this combination should be excluded.

High average and low average transporters

Ultrafiltration failure with high average or low average transport state may result in situations where there is enhanced fluid absorption from the peritoneal cavity (increased lymphatic or abdominal wall fluid absorption) aquaporin deficiency or the presence of a mechanical complication.

Management of UF failure:

Where the primary problem is reduced ultrafiltration capacity of the membrane, strategies include:

• Use of hypertonic glucose exchanges.
• Shortened dwell time:
  overnight APD cycles;
  additional daytime CAPD dwells;
  shortening long dwell times by additional overnight exchange in CAPD (by automated exchange device); manual exchange during day in APD.
• Use of icodextrin for long dwell of CAPD or APD.

Nutrition

Malnutrition occurs when there is inadequate nutrient intake or nutrient imbalance leading to adverse consequences for health.

There is a high prevalence of malnutrition in patients on PD (as also occurs in hemodialysis).

Malnutrition is a potent adverse prognostic marker for patient survival.

Many factors lead to malnutrition and wasting in patients on PD. Some are common to all patients with advanced renal failure, whereas others are specific to PD.

Causes of malnutrition in renal failure

Reduced nutrient intake due to uremic anorexia.

Coexistent acute and chronic medical conditions.

Metabolic factors:

• acidosis;
• insulin resistance;
• abnormalities of growth hormone metabolism.

Protein catabolism due to an inflammatory state in uremia.

Malnutrition, inflammation and atherosclerosis (MIA) syndrome describes wasting as part of an inflammatory state associated with cardiovascular disease, and is not responsive to increasing dietary nutrient intake and may be seen in patients on PD.

Causes of malnutrition specific to PD

In PD, glucose absorption and abdominal fullness may lead to appetite suppression.

Delayed gastric emptying may occur (especially in patients with diabetic autonomic neuropathy).

Protein and amino acids are lost in dialyzate, varying between 5 and 15 g/day (increased in peritonitis).

Dietary protein requirements are up to 1.2 g/kg body weight in PD (higher than healthy individuals in part to balance dialyzate losses).

Many patients have an intake as low as 0.8 g/kg but maintain stable state in the absence of additional nutritional stresses (but are at risk of decompensation with any added insult).

An energy intake of 35 kcal/kg is recommended.

Management of malnutrition

Optimizing dialytic clearances.

Correcting reversible factors.

Dietetic supervision of intake.

Nutritional supplementation.

PD catheter-related infections

Exit-site infection

An acute exit-site infection is defined as the presence of purulent discharge from the exit site which may be associated with:

• erythema;
• edema;
• granulation tissue;
• tenderness.

Exit-site infections can lead to development of peritonitis.

They may be resistant or relapsing and may require catheter removal for cure.

A variety of organisms may cause exit site infections. *Staphylococcus aureus* and *Pseudomonas spp* are common and most likely to lead to peritonitis or catheter loss.

A chronic exit-site infection may develop from an untreated or inadequately treated exit site infection.

Investigations

The responsible organism should be identified by culture of the exit site.

A positive culture without clinical features of infection is due to bacterial colonization and does not require antibiotic treatment.

Management

Management of the infected exit site includes local measures including regular cleaning of the exit site and removal of exuberant granulation tissue.

Hypertonic saline cleaning has also been suggested for aggressive infections.

Antibiotic treatment is essential for exit-site infections.

Antibiotic treatment should be guided by microbiological results, but empirical treatment is often initiated before they are available.

Initial treatment should be active against *Staphylococcus aureus*. *Pseudomonas* spp. should also be covered if the patient has had previous exit-site infections with this organism.

Duration of therapy should be for a minimum of 2 weeks, with further extension if resolution is slow or incomplete.

Catheter removal is required for persistent exit-site infection, or where there is an associated peritonitis.

Revision of the catheter tunnel and shaving of the external cuff of a two-cuff catheter have been advocated for persistent exit-site infections in an attempt to preserve the catheter.

Simultaneous removal of the infected catheter and insertion of a new catheter on the other side of the abdomen can be performed, with ongoing antibiotic treatment, in the absence of peritonitis.

Tunnel infection
A tunnel infection is defined by the presence of signs of inflammation along the track of the subcutaneous portion of the catheter and may be associated with purulent discharge from the exit site.

Investigations are the same as those for an exit-site infection and USS may be used to confirm the presence of a localized collection associated with the catheter.

Antibiotic treatment is essential for tunnel infections and empirical treatment is the same as for exit-site infections.

Tunnel infections are more likely to fail to respond to antibiotic treatment and there is a high chance that the PD catheter will need to be removed.

PD peritonitis
Peritonitis is one of the most important complications of PD.

Despite improvements in 'connectology', dialysis procedures and prophylaxis, peritonitis is an important cause of acute and long-term PD technique failure, morbidity, hospitalization and occasionally death.

Route of infection
Peritonitis can arise through varying routes of infection into the peritoneal cavity.

Passage of organisms may occur via the catheter lumen after contamination at the connection procedure. Coagulase-negative staphylococcal peritonitis commonly occurs via this route. The incidence of this infection may be particularly affected by improvements in 'connectology' and the performance of dialysis procedures by the patient.

Pericatheter passage of bacteria from the skin along the catheter tunnel may also occur, often associated with a catheter tunnel infection. Organisms commonly causing peritonitis via this route include *Staphylococcus aureus* and *Pseudomonas aeruginosa*.

Enteric organisms may cause peritonitis by passage from the bowel lumen into the peritoneal cavity. This may be associated with the presence of diverticular disease of the large bowel, or through transmural migration of organisms. Rarely PD peritonitis results from acute surgical abdominal conditions such as visceral perforation.

Other rarer routes of infection leading to PD peritonitis include bloodborne infection and ascending infection from the female genital tract.

Prevention of peritonitis
Intensive training of patients by specialist PD nurses in performing dialysis procedures and aseptic technique significantly reduces the risk of peritonitis.

Regular follow-up assessment of the patient and reassessment in those suffering infections are advised.

PD systems may also influence the rate of peritonitis. There is some evidence suggesting a lower rate of peritonitis in patients on APD compared to CAPD. However, the evidence is inconsistent and APD systems involving 'spiking' of the dialyzate bags may be associated with an increased peritonitis risk.

The introduction of CAPD systems incorporating a 'double-bag' design with flushing of the connection and drainage of dialyzate before filling with fresh dialyzate had a major effect on reducing PD peritonitis rates. These should be systems of choice for patients receiving CAPD.

Guidelines suggest that a peritonitis rate of <1 episode of peritonitis per 18 patient-months of PD treatment should be obtained.

Diagnosis of PD peritonitis
Clinical presentation of peritonitis is most commonly with cloudy dialysis fluid associated with abdominal pain.

Rarely PD peritonitis presents as abdominal pain with initially clear dialyzate which subsequently becomes cloudy.

Peritonitis should not therefore be excluded in the PD patient with abdominal pain if the initial dialysis fluid sample is clear, though alternative causes for abdominal pain should be sought.

Dialysis fluid samples are obtained to determine fluid white cell count and for microbiological testing.

A dialyzate sample with >100 white cells/μL (of which $\geq$50% are neutrophils) indicates peritoneal inflammation, with PD peritonitis being the most likely cause.

There are concerns that fluid from short dwells may provide a false-negative result in the presence of infection due to a low white cell count.

If in doubt, dialyzate can be instilled for a period of 1–2 h and the resulting fluid white cell count is reliable in confirming or excluding the presence of peritonitis.

The Gram stain is often negative, but may be useful in demonstrating the presence of a fungal infection.

Fluid should ideally be sent for culture before commencing antibiotic therapy. Correct culture techniques are essential to maximize the chance of obtaining a positive bacterial culture.

Centrifugation of 50 mL of dialyzate for 15 min, with resuspension of the sediment in 3–5 mL of saline and subsequent inoculation onto culture medium has been advocated as the most effective method.

Alternatively 5–10 mL of dialyzate can be inoculated directly into blood culture bottles.

It is recommended that microbiological investigations of peritonitis should have a culture-negative rate of <20%.

Management of PD peritonitis
Antibiotic therapy should be initiated as soon as peritonitis is suspected and after collecting samples for culture.

Initial treatment is commenced before culture results become available and should cover both Gram-positive and Gram-negative organisms (including *Pseudomonas aeruginosa*).

Debate has raged over the most appropriate initial antibiotic regime, particularly regarding the relative benefits (convenience and efficacy) and risks (antibiotic resistance) of empirical use of vancomycin.

The 2005 International Society of Peritoneal Dialysis (ISPD) guidelines suggest center-specific protocols based on the pattern of organisms and sensitivities observed in individual practices.

Gram-positive organisms should be covered by vancomycin or a cephalosporin. Gram-negative organisms should be covered by an aminoglycoside, third-generation cephalosporin (or quinolone if there is a high proportion of sensitive organisms in local results).

Antibiotics are commonly given intraperitoneally either by:

- continuous dosing with the antibiotic present in all infused dialysis fluid;
- intermittent dosing where the antibiotic is only administered for the long dwell period.

It is important to confirm the stability of the antibiotic in the dialysis fluid being used.

Increasing data are becoming available for intraperitoneal antibiotic dosing regimes.

Antibiotics may also be administered orally or intravenously.

Treatment of peritonitis is more complicated on APD due to the intermittent nature of the treatment. However, infections can be effectively treated while maintaining patients on their usual APD dialysis regime without swapping to CAPD.

Intermittent dosing regimes are available for a number of antibiotics, where they may be administered once daily into the long day dwell of APD patients or overnight in CAPD. Vancomycin is slowly cleared and may be administered less frequently, with doses given once every 3–7 days as determined by blood vancomycin levels.

Many episodes of peritonitis are accompanied by only mild symptoms and the patient may be treated as an outpatient. In more severe cases treatment may require hospitalization.

The minimum recommended duration of antibiotic treatment for PD peritonitis is 2 weeks, extended to 3 weeks for more serious or slowly responding infections.

Heparin may be added to dialyzate when large amounts of fibrin are present, to maintain flow and prevent catheter occlusion.

Specific infections

Once culture and sensitivity results become available, subsequent antibiotic therapy should be adjusted appropriately according to advice from microbiology (local practice may vary).

Coagulase-negative Staphylococcus aureus

This infection is often clinically mild, but may lead to relapsing infection due to catheter biofilm formation.

The organism commonly exhibits methicillin resistance and antibiotic choice is between vancomycin and first-generation cephalosporins.

Some units advocate the use of a urokinase flush of the PD catheter if there is recurrent peritonitis in an attempt to strip the catheter of biofilm.

Staphylococcus aureus

This organism often causes severe infection and arises from catheter infection or touch contamination of the dialysis procedure.

Catheter-related infection may require catheter removal to allow resolution.

Streptococcal and enterococcal infections

These are treated with intraperitoneal ampicilllin.

An aminoglycoside may be added for synergistic effect in enterococcal infections.

Vancomycin-resistant infections have been reported.

Pseudomonas infection

This is typically severe and often associated with catheter infection.

Treatment with a combination of two antipseudomonal antibiotics is recommended.

Other Gram-negative infections are also often serious, with worse outcomes than Gram-positive infections.

Treatment is with an appropriate antibiotic chosen on the basis of sensitivities (typically a cephalosporin or aminoglycoside).

Culture-negative peritonitis

This results from:

- fastidious organisms;
- previous antibacterial therapy;
- limitations of culture techniques.

If clinical improvement is occurring, initial antibiotic therapy can be continued, though continuation of Gram-negative cover may not be necessary.

If not responding, culture for unusual organisms may be performed, but catheter removal is usually required.

Polymicrobial infection

Polymicrobial infection with multiple Gram-negative bacteria, especially when with anerobic organisms, is often associated with underlying intra-abdominal pathology.

Surgical and radiological assessment is essential.

Antibiotic therapy should include appropriate Gram-negative cover and metronidazole.

Infection with multiple Gram-positive organisms carries a better prognosis and frequently responds to antibiotic therapy.

Fungal peritonitis

Fungal peritonitis carries a significant risk of mortality.

Catheter removal is considered mandatory.

Initial treatment may be with a combination of amphotericin B and flucytosine until identification of the organism and sensitivities.

Mycobacterial peritonitis

Mycobacterial peritonitis, due to *Mycobacterium tuberculosis* or nontuberculosis mycobacterium, is a rare cause of PD peritonitis.

Diagnosis may be made on repeated fluid culture in suspected cases.

Laparotomy and peritoneal biopsy may be needed.

Treatment is as for extrapulmonary mycobacterial disease with adjustment of regime as appropriate for the use and safety of drugs in renal failure.

The necessity for catheter removal is uncertain.

Complicated infections

Refractory peritonitis:
• an infection failing to clear after 5 days of appropriate antibiotics.

Relapsing peritonitis:
• an infection within 4 weeks of completing antibiotics with the same organism or sterile culture.

Recurrent peritonitis:
• an infection within 4 weeks of completing antibiotics with a different organism.

Repeat peritonitis:
• an infection after 4 weeks of completing antibiotics but with the same organism.

Catheter removal is required for:
• refractory and relapsing peritonitis;
• fungal peritonitis;
• nonresponding mycobacterial infection.

In relapsing infection the catheter may be removed and simultaneously replaced after resolution of the second infection and with appropriate ongoing antibiotic cover.

Surgical causes of peritonitis in PD

It is important to consider the possibility that an underlying surgical pathology may present with apparent PD peritonitis.

Causes include:
• acute appendicitis;
• diverticulitis;
• perforated viscus (peptic ulcer or diverticular disease);
• acute pancreatitis.

Surgical disease should be considered particularly when:
• the patient is disproportionately unwell;
• systemic signs of sepsis;
• suggestive clinical history;
• multiple enteric/anerobic agents on PD fluid culture.

When investigating suspected acute pancreatitis, serum amylase may be misleadingly low in patients receiving icodextrin dialyzate due to interference of icodextrin metabolites with the amylase assay.

Malignancy may also present as cloudy dialyzate and may be identified by radiological imaging or presence of malignant cells on cytology of spent dialyzate.

Complications of PD peritonitis

PD peritonitis may result in malnutrition due to:
• increased peritoneal protein loss;
• reduced nutrient intake;
• acute catabolism.

There may be a temporary reduction in ultrafiltration during peritonitis due to increased peritoneal vascularity increasing the transport status of the membrane as a result of peritoneal inflammation. This may be managed by:
• shortening dialysis exchanges;
• hypertonic fluids;
• use of icodextrin for long dwells.

Episodes of infection are also associated with long-term changes in peritoneal membrane function leading to increased transport state and eventual ultrafiltration failure.

Peritonitis may contribute to the development of encapsulating peritoneal sclerosis.

Adhesion formation after infection may prevent the further use of the peritoneum for dialysis.

Severe sepsis can occasionally be fatal.

PD infections and antibiotic prophylaxis

Some antibacterial prophylactic regimes reduce the incidence of exit-site infections.

Mupirocin daily at the exit site or nasally for 5–7 days per month (either in all patients, or those carrying S. aureus on screening nasal swabs) has been shown to reduce the risk of exit-site infections, but there is concern about the risk of development of mupirocin resistance.

If applied to the exit site, mupirocin cream rather than ointment should be used, as the latter may damage some catheters.

Exit-site application of gentamicin cream has also been demonstrated to reduce exit-site infection rates.

Antibiotic prophylaxis may be indicated to prevent development of peritonitis in the PD patient undergoing invasive procedures.

Dialysis fluid should be drained out before any procedures involving the abdomen or pelvis.

Noninfective causes of cloudy dialyzate

Eosinophilic peritonitis

Eosinophilic peritonitis is characterized by cloudy dialyzate with a high proportion of eosinophils on differential white cell count in dialyzate.

This is most commonly seen early after commencing PD and may reflect an allergic reaction to components of dialysis fluid, bags or tubing or PD catheter.

It often settles spontaneously on continuing dialysis but rarely corticosteroids or antihistamines have been used.

Other causes include exposure to intraperitoneal antibiotics.

Chylous ascites

Chylous ascites produces creamy white dialyzate with a very high triglyceride content.

Arises from blockage or damage to intra-abdominal lymphatics.

Can be associated with malignancy involving the lymphatics, including lymphoma.

May occur intermittently, related to fat-containing meals.

Icodextrin

Cases of sterile peritonitis have occurred in patients treated with batches of icodextrin fluid, attributed to contamination with high peptidoglycan concentrations.

Mechanical complications of PD

Catheter drainage problems

Drainage problems may occur because of:
• constipation;
• malposition/migration of the catheter;
• abdominal adhesions;
• catheter occlusion (e.g. fibrin, and omental wrapping).

Clinical features include slow drainage, which may be predominantly slow drainage out, or alternatively slow inflow (accompanied by slow outflow if fluid infusion is possible).

Investigations:

- plain abdominal X-ray (which will show catheter position and presence of constipation);
- injection of radiocontrast down catheter with screening (to show flow of dialyzate and presence of adhesions);
- CT peritoneography.

Management

Laxatives improve slow drainage due to constipation and sometimes reverse catheter migration.

Heparin is instilled if catheter blockage results from fibrin or blood, and urokinase may be used if heparin is ineffective.

Catheter repositioning may be attempted:

- radiologically (by passage of guidewire and attempts to move the catheter tip under X-ray screening);
- open surgically;
- laparoscopically.

If surgical intervention is required, partial omentectomy may be performed and the catheter can be sutured into the pelvis.

Alternatively, the catheter may be removed and replaced.

If catheter change is required, temporary HD may be avoided by resting from dialysis for the usual catheter healing time if residual renal function is sufficient, or by earlier commencement of PD post surgery using small volume exchanges in supine position (e.g. APD with dry day).

Fluid leaks

Pericatheter leaks

Pericatheter leaks may occur early or late after tube insertion and may be precipitated by coughing, straining or heavy lifting.

Presentation is with fluid leaking externally with wetness of the exit site or dressing.

Abdominal wall leaks

Abdominal wall edema may also arise by leaking through the catheter site or previous abdominal incisions. There may be induration or a spongy feeling of the abdominal wall skin and *peau d'orange* appearance.

Patients may experience a loss of ultrafiltration without change in transport characteristics.

Abdominal wall leaks may be demonstrated by CT peritoneography or MRI.

Genital edema

Genital edema is an uncommon but distressing complication of PD.

Mechanisms include tracking of fluid leaking around the catheter or an incision site via the subcutaneous tissues or leak via a hernia or patent processus vaginalis.

Investigations

Diagnosis of any leak and identification of the cause may include:

- CT peritoneogram with intraperitonal contrast;
- MRI with dialyzate *in situ*;
- USS (may identify the presence of herniae containing dialsate);
- abdominal scintigraphy (dialyzate containing radiolabeled tracer).

Management

Management of fluid leaks is a period of rest from PD to allow the leak to heal.

PD should be recommenced initially with lower volume exchanges with or without omission of the ambulant day dwell if the patient is on APD and clearances allow.

Persistent leaks require catheter change or surgical repair.

Hernias in PD

Hernias are a relatively common complication of PD.

Pre-existing hernias should be repaired before commencing PD. This may be combined with catheter insertion.

They may also develop after starting PD as a complication of the increase in intra-abdominal pressure. Sites include:

- inguinal;
- para-umbilical/umbilical;
- catheter insertion site;
- other incision sites;
- ventral hernias.

Problems include:

- pain;
- risk of bowel incarceration and strangulation.

In cases of Gram-negative peritonitis one should always consider the possibility of bowel strangulation as the hernial orifice may not always be obvious.

Management

Management is by surgical repair.

This may require a period of discontinuation of PD and temporary HD.

Some PD patients may have adequate residual function to allow a period without dialysis.

It is also possible to recommence PD very soon after a hernia repair, especially when a mesh repair has been performed, with initial use of low dialyzate volumes in the supine position.

Hydrothorax

Pleural effusions may occur for a number of reasons on PD.

Pulmonary and pleural disease may occur as in other subjects and it is also important to consider fluid overload and cardiac failure as causes in PD patients.

Diaphragmatic leak

Effusions may also occur due to peritoneo-pleural leakage of dialyzate when dialyzate passes through areas of deficiency in the diaphragm. This most commonly occurs on the right side.

The presence of an effusion may be identified clinically and confirmed on chest X-ray. Effusion size varies but may be large enough to cause respiratory difficulties.

Thoracocentesis should be performed with fluid undergoing standard biochemical, microbiological and cytological tests. The presence of low protein in keeping with a transudate and high glucose content (greater than in blood) suggests the diagnosis.

Management may include therapeutic pleural aspiration of pleural fluid and temporary discontinuation of PD.

Occasionally a period of rest and recommencement of PD with initially smaller volumes may be successful.

If the effusion recurs, pleurodesis may allow ongoing treatment with PD.

Other complications of PD

Pain with PD exchanges

Inflow pain

Inflow pain is the most common problem.

It may occur soon after commencing PD and disappear with time whilst continuing PD.

Persistent inflow pain may relate to the low pH of standard PD fluids and may improve with use of neutral pH solutions.

An alternative is the use of tidal PD for patients on APD.

Pain may relate to movement of the PD catheter out of its correct position which can be diagnosed on AXR.

Outflow pain

Outflow pain is less common.

It may be due to peritonitis or be a temporary phenomenon after commencing PD.

Back pain

Back pain may occur or be exacerbated by the presence of PD fluid which alters normal posture.

Other treatable or serious causes of back pain should be excluded by investigation.

Reducing volumes of fluid in the abdomen during the day, which may involve transfer to APD with reduced daytime dwell volume, or NIPD with a dry daytime period may help.

Hemoperitoneum

The presence of blood-stained dialyzate may be alarming for patients.

Commonly it is a transient self-limiting event of unknown cause, possibly related to catheter trauma of the peritoneal membrane.

It occurs in women in relation to the menstrual cycle, at times of menstruation and ovulation.

Occasionally it is a feature of peritonitis, which should be excluded by microbiological evaluation of a dialyzate sample.

Rare causes may include:
- abdominal malignancy;
- pancreatitis;
- hepatobiliary disease;
- bleeding from a polycystic kidney;
- liver disease;
- encapsulating peritoneal sclerosis.

Flushing with heparin-containing dialyzate may help to prevent catheter blockage.

Constipation

Constipation is common in PD due to:
- older average age of patients on PD;
- effect of dialyzate on bowel motility;
- low fiber content of diet;
- constipating medication;
- electrolyte imbalance.

Adverse effects include:
- reduced fluid drainage and ultrafiltration;
- catheter migration;
- possible increased risk of peritonitis due to enteric organisms.

Management includes:
- regular use of laxatives;
- patient education about the importance of avoiding constipation;
- dietary fibre supplements.

Encapsulating peritoneal sclerosis (EPS)

This is a rare but serious complication of long-term PD.

The incidence increases with time on PD.

Patients develop marked fibrotic thickening of the peritoneal membrane forming a cocoon surrounding and binding the intestine.

It may be preceded by a progressive increase in membrane transport state.

Although typically presenting in patients whilst on PD, it may still occur after the patient has been transplanted or transfered to HD.

Risk factors
- long-term exposure to bioincompatible dialysis fluid;
- previous episodes of bacterial peritonitis;
- use of acetate as a buffer in dialysis fluid;
- chlorhexidine contamination (used during sterilization of the exchange procedure);
- previous surgery;
- malignancy;
- β-blockers;
- autoimmune disease.

Clinical features
- bowel obstruction;
- abdominal pain;
- hemoperitoneum;
- weight loss;
- diarrhea;
- malnutrition.

Malnutrition is common, may be severe and is associated with a high mortality.

Clinical features and high index of suspicion are important in making the diagnosis.

Investigations

Radiological investigations include:
- plain AXR;
- ultrasound;
- CT scanning is the modality of greatest diagnostic value..

Radiological features include:
- peritoneal calcification;
- features of bowel obstruction;
- thickening of peritoneal membrane.

EPS may also be diagnosed by appearance of the peritoneum at laparotomy.

Patients may have elevated inflammatory markers and ongoing sepsis must be excluded where EPS develops soon after an episode of bacterial peritonitis.

Management

Management of nutrition is crucial. In patients with obstructive symptoms or malabsorption TPN is often required.

It is generally thought that stopping PD is mandatory, though discontinuation of PD may also be a triggering factor for developing EPS in some cases.

Immunosuppression:
- lacks significant evidence base;
- corticosteroids are most commonly used;
- other immunosuppressant drugs anecdotally reported to be useful;
- development of postrenal transplant EPS in patients heavily immunosuppressed casts doubt on role of these drugs;

Some reports suggest that tamoxifen may have a beneficial antifibrotic effect in EPS, but this is unconfirmed.

Surgery:
- may be indicated for persisting bowel obstruction;
- earlier studies described high associated mortality;
- more recent experience suggests that excellent surgical outcomes can be achieved by experienced operators.

Prognosis
High mortality in severe cases due to malnutrition and sepsis.

Optimal medical and nutritional management and timely surgical intervention where obstructive symptoms persist despite conservative measures may be the best current approach and lead to improved survival rates.

Lipid abnormalities in PD
Lipid abnormalities are common in renal disease and differ between dialysis modalities. PD is associated with increases in cholesterol and triglyceride concentrations.

VLDL and LDL lipoproteins and lipoprotein (a) increase on PD.

Treatment of elevated serum cholesterol is most commonly with statins. Fibrates are also effective but require dose reduction and carry increased risk of myopathy in PD patients.

The effectiveness of lipid-lowering therapy in reducing cardiovascular disease in PD is currently unknown.

Further reading
European Best Practice Guidelines for Peritoneal Dialysis. *Nephrol Dial Transplant* 2005; **20**(Suppl 9).

Flanigan M, Gokal R. Peritoneal catheters and exit-site practices towards optimum peritoneal access: a review of current developments. *Peritoneal Dial Int* 2005; **25**: 132–139.

Mujais S, Nolph K, Gokal R, *et al.* Evaluation and management of ultrafiltration problems in peritoneal dialysis. International Society for Peritoneal Dialysis Ad Hoc Committee on Ultrafiltration Management in Peritoneal Dialysis. *Peritoneal Dialysis Int* 2000; **20**(Suppl 4): S5–S21.

Piraino B, Bailie GR, Bernadini J, *et al.* Peritoneal dialysis-related infections recommendations: 2005 update. *Peritoneal Dial Int* 2005; **25**: 107–131.

Internet resources
International Society of Peritoneal Dialysis:

http://www.ispd.org

Peritoneal Dialysis International:

http://www.pdiconnect.com

Renal Association Clinical Practice Guidelines for PD:

http://www.renal.org/guidelines/module3b.html

The Renal Registry:

http://www.renalreg.org

National Kidney Federation Dialysis Outcomes Quality Initiative:

http://www.kidney.org/professionals/kdoqi/

European Best Practice Guidelines:

http://www.ndt-educational.org/guidelines.asp

National Institute for Clinical Excellence:

http://www.nice.org.uk/

See also
Renal replacement therapies in acute kidney injury, p. 328

Dialysis strategies, p. 480

Adequacy of dialysis, p. 518

Medical management of dialysis patients, p. 528

Adequacy of dialysis

Introduction

Adequacy of dialysis can be defined as the ability to correct the clinical features of uremia, promote rehabilitation and prolong survival of patients with ESRD.

Dialysis may prevent death in patients with terminal renal failure, and increases in dialysis may improve the clinical status of patients with symptoms of uremia. However, with current techniques for renal replacement, morbidity and mortality remain high. This has led to interest in objective measures of treatment to quantify and improve outcomes. For many years 'adequacy' has focused on dialytic solute clearances, though more recently has expanded to include a broader assessment of outcomes and well-being.

Therefore, in addition to a measurement of the clearance of putative uremic toxins by the dialysis process the assessment of dialysis adequacy should also include a global assessment of the patient's general well-being, nutrition, hemoglobin concentration, blood pressure and fluid status.

Uremic toxicity

Solutes of widely varying molecular size accumulate in patients with renal failure.

These substances are believed to be toxic and to result in many of the features of uremia.

Most of these substances increase in parallel in uremia, so it is difficult to determine which are the most important causes of clinical disease.

Retained solutes include:
- inorganic substances such as electrolytes;
- small organic molecules (<300 Da) such as urea and creatinine;
- medium molecular weight organic substances, 'middle molecules' of size 300–2000 Da;
- larger substances (up to 50 000 Da) such as β2-microglobulin (β2M).

The assessment of adequacy has primarily focused on small solute clearances.

Blood concentrations of urea and creatinine increase with deteriorating renal function and are reduced by removal during dialysis.

Outcomes do not, however, directly relate to blood concentrations of serum urea and creatinine and, paradoxically, lower values also carry an adverse prognosis.

The serum creatinine concentration depends on both clearance and generation. Creatinine is generated from muscle metabolism and the rate of generation depends on muscle mass. Low levels may be an adverse prognostic marker, reflecting reduced muscle mass due to malnutrition and wasting. Similarly, serum urea is also dependent on generation rates, reflecting protein intake and catabolism, as well as clearance.

Adequacy of hemodialysis

The molecular weights of solutes to be cleared by dialysis range over three orders of magnitude, from small (water, urea) to large (β2M).

Adequate clearance of the whole range of molecules by dialysis is important and monitoring of β2M levels may be used in the future to assess dialysis adequacy.

For practical reasons HD adequacy thus far has been measured using small, easily measured solutes such as urea.

The two commonly used measures of HD adequacy are:
- urea reduction ratio;
- Kt/V_{urea}.

Urea reduction ratio (URR)

This is the simplest method and is the percentage fall in blood urea achieved by a dialysis session.

It is measured as follows:
- $(Urea_{post}/Urea_{pre}) \times 100\%$.

The URR is easy to perform and is the index of dialysis dose which is most widely used in the UK.

URR does not take into account:
- solute removal via ultrafiltration;
- residual renal function;
- urea generation during dialysis.

Adjustment of dialysis dose to achieve a particular target URR will therefore result in higher overall urea removal than predicted from the percentage reduction in blood urea.

These theoretical drawbacks are not important if the main aim of measuring small solute removal by HD is to ensure that a minimum target dialysis dose is delivered consistently.

Kt/V_{urea}

This can be calculated in a number of different ways with mathematical formulae of increasing complexity.
- K: dialyzer clearance of urea;
- t: dialysis time;
- V: patients total body water.

Depending on the mathematical method used it is possible to calculate:
- a single-pool Kt/V (spKt/V);
- an equilibrated Kt/V (eKt/V);
- a standardized Kt/V (stdKt/V).

Each can be calculated using different formulae (see Appendix).

These formulae give different results for Kt/V.

If Kt/V is being used for comparative audit it is important that the raw data are collected to allow calculation of URR and Kt/V using a single formula.

The second-generation formula for estimating spKt/V, which was reported and validated by Daugirdas, is recommended.

Single-pool Kt/V

This assumes that urea is removed from a single compartment during dialysis and is the easiest to calculate, requiring:
- pre- and postdialysis urea concentrations;
- duration of dialysis;
- weight loss during dialysis.

Equilibrated (or double-pool) Kt/V

This attempts to take into account the amount of rebound in blood urea concentration at the end of dialysis due to redistribution of urea from the multiple body compartments.

Standardized Kt/V
This takes into account more variables including residual renal function but is correspondingly more complex to calculate.

Urea kinetic modeling (formal UKM)
Urea kinetic modeling is the most complex measure and involves analysis of:
- the fall in blood urea concentration during HD;
- the rise in blood urea and urea clearance by residual renal function in the next interdialytic period;
- the total clearance predicted from the dialyzer urea mass transfer area coefficient;
- blood and dialyzate flow;
- time on dialysis;
- fluid removal during dialysis.

Therefore UKM requires collection of additional data on dialyzer clearance, an interdialytic urine collection for measurement of urea concentration and volume, and measurement of predialysis urea concentration in the subsequent dialysis.

These data are fed into a computer program which, assuming steady state, calculates Kt/V_{urea} and normalized protein catabolic rate.

Kt/V measured by formal UKM allows accurate prediction of the effects of changing one particular component of the dialysis prescription (e.g. dialyzer size, dialysis duration, blood flow rate) on the delivered dialysis dose although this benefit has been overstated given the limited number of practical options for changing the dialysis prescription.

UKM may also give information on the urea generation rate and protein catabolic rate. If the patient is in a steady state nutritionally, this gives information on current protein intake, and may be a useful adjunct to other methods of assessment of nutritional status.

Disadvantages of Kt/V
Doubts have been raised as to whether Kt/V is a good index of dialysis dose since survival rates on HD are higher in patients with larger body size and better nutrition even though this patient group tends to have lower Kt/V values.

Non-normalized dialysis dose (Kt) has been proposed as an alternative and better index of dialysis dose adequacy to Kt/V since the former index obviates the tendency to accord a higher dialysis dose in smaller and poorly nourished patients.

In a large cross-sectional analysis using Kt as the index of dialysis dose, mortality risk was observed to fall if the delivered dialysis dose was a minimum Kt of 42 L in women and 48 L in men.

A further difficulty with the use of the Kt/V index for other than thrice-weekly HD is that the significance of any weekly Kt/V value depends on the frequency of dialysis since more frequent dialysis therapies, such as daily HD, will deliver greater small solute removal at the same weekly Kt/V.

Most HD units only measure pre- and postdialysis urea concentrations and a minority undertake formal UKM routinely. Therefore, to allow comparative audit, the choice is between calculation of URR and estimation of Kt/V urea.

Methods of postdialysis blood sampling
All measures of urea removal are derived from the ratio of postdialysis/predialysis blood urea concentrations and so the method of postdialysis blood sampling should be standardized.

The true venous blood urea concentration rises rapidly in the first few minutes after dialysis as the effects of access and cardiopulmonary recirculation dissipate. It continues to rise at a rate higher than that expected from urea generation for up to 30 min as a consequence of continued transfer of urea from peripheral body compartments into the bloodstream.

Falsely low measurements of the postdialysis blood urea concentration can occur due to a combination of:
- the dilutional effect of blood returning from the dialyzer (access recirculation);
- the dilutional effect of blood returning via the heart and lungs directly to the fistula or other access device (cardiopulmonary recirculation);
- contamination of the postdialysis blood sample by recently administered saline or other intravenous fluid.

For these reasons the earlier the sample is drawn the higher the apparent delivered dialysis dose.

Small variations in the timing and technique of postdialysis blood sampling can, therefore, result in clinically important errors in the estimated dose of dialysis. Such variation has been shown to be common in the past in the USA and UK.

The reinfusion method of postdialysis blood sampling should not be performed because of the dilutional effects of the saline washback. Three other methods of postdialysis blood sampling are still used:

Stop dialyzate flow method
At the end of the dialysis time, stop dialyzate flow but keep the blood pump running.

After 5 min with no dialyzate flow take a blood sample from anywhere in the blood circuit (i.e. the arterial or venous port).

Slow-flow method
At the end of the dialysis time turn the blood pump speed down to 100 mL/min.

Override alarms to keep the blood pump operating.

Wait 15–30 s and take samples from the 'arterial' line sampling port.

If more than one blood sample is required, the sample for urea should be the first one taken.

Simplified stop-flow method
When you are ready to take the sample turn the blood pump speed slowly down to 50 mL/min.

Start counting to five; if the venous pressure alarm has not already stopped the blood pump when you get to five, stop the pump manually.

Table 13.5.1. The effect of urea rebound on URR and Kt/V urea measurements in 70 hemodialysis patients

	Time of blood urea sampling after HD		
	0 min	5 min	30 min
Mean urea (mmol/L)	4.1 ± 1.7	4.6 ± 1.8	5.1 ± 1.9
% urea rebound	–	14.9 %	27.3 %
URR	76.9 ± 5.9	74.1 ± 5.9	71.4 ± 6.0
Kt/V urea	1.55 ± 0.30	1.42 ± 0.24	1.32 ± 0.22

Disconnect the arterial line and take a sample from the needle tubing (or the arterial connector of the catheter) within 20 s of slowing the blood pump speed to 50 mL/min.

If more than one blood sample is required, the urea sample should be the first one taken.

The slow-flow and stop-flow methods were devised to give early postdialysis measurements which avoid the effects of access recirculation but do not allow for cardiopulmonary recirculation which continues for the first 2 min after the end of HD using a fistula or graft.

The stop- and slow-flow methods will underestimate postdialysis 'equilibrated' blood urea concentrations more than the stop dialyzate flow method and consequently overestimate urea removal by HD.

The stop dialyzate flow method has several advantages:
- it avoids the dilutional effects of both access and cardiopulmonary recirculation;
- it is a simple two-step process;
- It is easily reproducible as accurate timing of blood sampling is less critical;
- blood sampling can be performed from either the arterial or venous line;
- it is suitable for all forms of vascular access;
- it is validated in hemodiafiltration as well as HD;
- it has been used by all of the HD units in Scotland since 1999 and is the most widely used method in the UK.

Equilibrated postdialysis urea concentration
Postdialysis rebound in venous blood urea concentration results from continued return of blood from poorly dialysed body 'compartments', and is particularly marked after high efficiency dialysis.

Accurate comparison of delivered dialysis dose therefore requires estimation of the equilibrated blood urea concentration and calculation of 'equilibrated' Kt/V.

Full re-equilibration takes ~30 min but it is impractical to ask patients to wait this long for postdialysis blood sampling on a routine basis.

The amount of rebound is determined by several factors including the efficiency of dialysis and the size of the patient. Table 13.5.1 demonstrates the degree of overestimation of dialysis dose if blood sampling does not allow for urea rebound during the first 5 min (as measured by the stop dialyzate flow method) and first 30 min after the end of dialysis.

Formulae have been validated for predicting 30 min postdialysis or 'equilibrated' blood urea from blood samples using either the stop dialyzate flow method or similar sampling methods to the slow-flow and stop-flow methods (Appendix).

The stop dialyzate flow and slow-flow methods are the two methods included in both Guideline 3.4 of the latest update of the K/DOQI Clinical Practice Guidelines on Haemodialysis Adequacy and the UK Renal Association Clinical Practice Guidelines on HD.

Minimum and target dialysis dose in HD
The optimal dialysis dose has not been well-defined but minimum targets of delivered dose measured by URR and Kt/V have been established.

A retrospective analysis of the National Co-operative Dialysis Study suggested that a Kt/V of 1.0 was the watershed between 'good' dialysis (Kt/V >1.0) and inadequate dialysis (Kt/V <1.0).

A large observational study of HD patients showed that variations in URR were associated with significant differences in mortality and this study led to the recommendation that the URR should be ≥65%.

Subsequent observational studies have generated conflicting results and suggest either a reduction in mortality rates with further increments in dialysis dose or no further reduction in mortality rates with a Kt/V >1.3 or URR >70%. These studies led to the setting up of the HEMO study (Table 13.5.2).

An association between higher dose and lower mortality rates in women but not in men was confirmed using the average URR of incident HD patients in the USA, and eKt/V of HD patients in the DOPPS data from seven countries.

Based upon this evidence the minimum dialysis dose delivered thrice weekly should be:
- URR of 65%;
- eKt/V of 1.2;
- spKt/V of >1.3 (calculated from pre- and postdialysis urea concentrations, duration of dialysis and weight loss during dialysis).

To achieve a URR >65% or eKt/V >1.2 consistently in the vast majority of the HD population, clinicians should aim for a minimum target URR of 70% or minimum eKt/V of 1.4 in individual patients.

Table 13.5.2 Summary of the HEMO study findings

Study design	Prospective randomized controlled trial of 1846 prevalent HD patients.
	Patients were on dialysis for a median of 3.7 years at the time of recruitment to the study.
	2 × 2 factorial study design: high and low flux; high and standard dialysis dose; • standard dose goal of an equilibrated Kt/V of 1.05 (URR ~65%); or • high dose goal of an equilibrated Kt/V of 1.45 (URR ~75%).
Outcomes	871 of the 1846 randomized patients died during the study after a mean follow-up period of 2.8 years.
	Even though dialysis doses were well-separated no difference was observed in: • primary outcome of all-cause mortality; • first cardiac hospitalization or all-cause mortality; • first infectious hospitalization or all-cause mortality; • first 15% decrease in serum albumin or all-cause mortality; • all non-vascular access-related hospitalizations.
Subgroup analysis	Differences in dialysis dose and membrane flux had no effect on the proportion of infection-related deaths.
	Survival rates in women randomized to the higher dose group were higher than in women in the lower dose group after adjusting for different indices of body size.

Aiming for these target doses also addresses the concerns raised by recent data suggesting that women and patients of low body weight may have improved survival rates if the URR is maintained at >70% or the eKt/V is ≥1.4.

The achievement of these clinical practice guidelines is dependent on patients' concordance with treatment.

This includes the agreement of the patient to increase treatment duration if the delivered dialysis dose is inadequate after the dialyzer blood flow rate, dialyzate flow rate and dialyzer performance have been increased to the maximum that can be achieved.

Increased understanding among patients of the benefits of an adequate dialysis dose should help to improve outcomes.

The use of β2M to assess adequacy of HD

Time-dependent Cox regression analysis of the HEMO study provides support for the use of β2M to assess adequacy of HD:

- mean predialysis serum β2M levels but not dialyzer β2M clearances were associated with all cause mortality
- the relative risk of death was 1.11 per 10 mg/L rise in the β2M concentration above a reference value of 27 mg/L after adjusting for residual renal function and prestudy years on dialysis.

The apparent disparity between the prognostic effects of serum β2M levels and β2M dialyzer clearances is most likely due to the limited mass removal of β2M in high efficiency dialysis.

This is due to intercompartmental transfer resistance of high molecular weight solutes within the patient during HD which results in rebound of serum β2M levels at the end of therapy.

In future, β2M levels may also be used to assess the adequacy of dialysis by serving as an indicator of patient outcome and as a surrogate marker of middle molecule removal.

Adequacy of peritoneal dialysis

Small solute clearances

As already alluded to, blood levels of retained solutes are unreliable measures of the efficiency of dialysis, and the clearance of small solutes is determined instead.

In PD, clearances of urea and creatinine are routinely measured. In HD the intermittent nature of the treatment allows calculation of clearance from the change in blood levels of urea before and after dialysis. This is not possible in PD due to the continuous nature of the therapy, so PD clearances are determined by collection of drained dialyzate over a 24 h period, and a simultaneous 24 h urine collection in subjects who are not anuric.

A blood sample is also taken, which should be midway through the dialyzate and urine collection period, especially for fluctuating therapies, i.e. APD.

To calculate clearances, it is necessary to know the amount of solute removed in 24 h periods by dialysis and by residual renal function. This requires knowledge of fluid volumes and their solute concentrations.

For dialyzate, the drained volume of dialyzate in a 24 h period is determined and the concentrations of urea, creatinine and glucose in the dialyzate are measured.

For APD, the drained volume may be determined from the measurements derived from cycler machines. For CAPD, the fluid from all bags may be pooled, the total volume

measured, and an aliquot extracted for biochemical analysis.

Alternatively, individual bags may be measured and aliquots taken in volumes proportional to the drained volumes (e.g. 1%) and combined in a final sample sent for biochemical analysis.

24 h urine samples are collected according to standard procedures. Incomplete collection may occur due to inaccuracy of timing of the collection and incomplete collection. Additional error may arise in patients where urine volumes are small and voiding infrequent, and in patients with conditions leading to incomplete bladder emptying.

Methods of assessing small solute removal on PD

Dialytic Kt/V urea

Since urea clearance is the basis of assessment of HD adequacy, there was interest in providing a comparable measurement for PD.

In HD urea clearance is expressed as the Kt/V for urea per dialysis session. For PD, urea clearance is also expressed as Kt/V, but with values quoted as Kt/V per week.

Kt is the clearance of solute removed in time t, and is determined from 24 h dialyzate collections.

In the expression Kt/V, clearance, Kt, is normalized for body size by division by V, the volume of total body water, which is the volume of distribution of urea.

Unlike in HD, in PD the volume V is estimated separately from Kt and biochemical measurements. In clinical practice, V is calculated from equations estimating V from anthropometric and demographic variables (Appendix). These equations have been developed by regression against total body water measured by dilution techniques. The most commonly used equation is that of Watson and Watson.

One limitation of anthropometric equations is that there is a degree of inaccuracy in the estimation of total body water in individuals. Also, obesity results in overestimation of V as fat is largely anhydrous, but increasing the weight term of the equations will increase estimated V. This leads to underestimation of Kt/V in obese individuals.

A further limitation of normalization of clearances to V is that patients with low body weight resulting from wasting and malnutrition will have lower values for V and thus higher Kt/V. For these patients the optimum clearance required will be greater than that suggested from these calculations.

It has been suggested that V should be calculated from ideal weight in malnourished patients.

Dialytic creatinine clearance

The other standard measure of dialytic clearance in PD is creatinine clearance.

This is determined by measurement of the quantity of creatinine removed in a 24 h dialyzate collection and is calculated in an analogous fashion to urinary creatinine clearance for measurement of the GFR.

It is usually expressed in liters per week and normalized to 1.73 m^2 body surface area (L/1.73 m^2/week).

Body surface area is determined by anthropometric equations (the formula of DuBois is commonly used).

Glucose interferes with some assays for creatinine estimation. High dialyzate glucose concentrations may result in spuriously high dialyzate concentrations of creatinine and overestimation of creatinine clearance.

It is important to determine the effect of dialyzate glucose in your local laboratory, and to measure glucose concentration in the collected dialyzate so that an appropriate correction to dialyzate creatinine concentration can be made.

Residual renal function urea and creatinine clearance
Residual renal function can make a significant contribution to small solute clearances in PD.

Renal clearances of urea and creatinine are measured from 24 h urine collections and values may be added to dialytic clearances to give total clearances.

Renal urea clearances are measured from 24 h urine urea and blood urea concentrations and expressed as residual renal Kt/V urea using similar calculations to dialytic Kt/V.

Creatinine is an imperfect measure of renal function due to tubular secretion. This leads to overestimation of renal function, which is proportionally greater with lower clearances and especially so for residual renal clearance in patients on dialysis.

To correct for this, 'residual renal creatinine clearance' is calculated as the mean of creatinine and urea clearances, as urea is passively reabsorbed in the tubules leading to underestimation of actual renal clearance.

Total small solute clearances
Total small solute clearances are calculated by adding dialytic and residual renal clearances together. However, they are not truly interchangeable.

Residual renal function is an important determinant of survival, whereas dialytic clearances beyond a minimum target are not.

There is also a proportionally different contribution of residual renal function and dialysis to urea and creatinine clearances.

Even with correction of renal creatinine clearance by calculation as a mean of creatinine and urea clearances, residual renal function contributes a greater proportion of total creatinine clearance than total Kt/V urea.

Patients with significant residual renal function have a relatively greater creatinine clearance than Kt/V urea.

Table 13.5.3 Recommended small solute clearance targets in PD

Organization	Recommendations
ISPD guidelines for solute and fluid removal in adults (2006)	Minimum total Kt/V urea of 1.7 and minimum target creatinine clearance of 45 L/1.73 m²/week(required only for APD and not CAPD)
NKF K/DOQI Guidelines (2006)	Minimum total Kt/V urea of 1.7
Renal Association (UK) Guidelines (2007)	Minimum total Kt/V urea of 1.7 or minimum target creatinine clearance of 50 L/1.73 m²/week
European Best Practice Guidelines for PD (2005)	Minimum total Kt/V urea of 1.7 and minimum target creatinine clearance of 45 L/1.73 m²/week(required only for APD and not CAPD)

Conversely, in anuric patients, it is more difficult to achieve clearance targets for creatinine clearance than Kt/V urea by increasing dialysis dose.

Kt/V urea or creatinine clearance?
The relative merits of urea and creatinine clearances have been debated and are unclear.

Neither is superior in performance in reflecting other features of uremia or predicting outcomes.

The two measures may vary discordantly in different clinical situations.

Important factors leading to differences between urea and creatinine clearances include PD modality and prescription, membrane transport type and presence of residual renal function.

Minimum and target dialysis dose in PD
There has been huge interest in defining optimal measures of dialysis, to allow objective determination of ideal dialysis prescription, with the aim of reducing the high morbidity and mortality of patients on dialysis, while avoiding unnecessarily intrusive dialysis regimes that would reduce patient quality of life without any clinical benefit.

Various guidelines have been produced by national and international organizations over time and have been rewritten as advances in the evidence base relating to aspects of clearance and patient outcomes have been made.

Initial guidelines focused exclusively on small solute clearance measurements and were based on the flawed assumption that control of uremic toxicity is related to total small solute clearance, and that clearance of molecules such as urea and creatinine has equivalent impact on outcome, whether by dialysis or residual renal function.

1997 NKF DOQI guidelines and the CANUSA study
These early guidelines were based on outcomes of observational studies. The largest and most influential was the CANUSA study.

This was a large observational study of PD patients in Canada and USA.

The original publication of this study showed that decreases in total Kt/V urea and total creatinine clearance were associated with a decline in nutrition and increased mortality.

This was the basis of the influential 1997 NKF DOQI guidelines for minimum small solute clearances in PD. These were a minimum weekly Kt/V of 2.0 and creatinine clearance of 60 L/1.73 m²/week for CAPD.

Because of the intermittent nature of APD, it was decided on the basis of opinion that targets should be even higher for APD than CAPD to counter theoretical increased toxicity from higher peak solute concentrations.

These targets were often challenging to achieve, especially in larger or anuric patients, raising concerns as to whether PD could provide adequate treatment for such patients.

Paradoxically, data (including some from the CANUSA study) showed that patients with lower peritoneal membrane transport status, in whom it was most difficult to achieve the highest clearance values, actually had a better survival than higher transporters.

In other words, patients whose transport status conferred a survival benefit on PD were most likely to fail PD due to inadequate clearances.

This led to revisions of some guidelines to account for transport status, with lower clearance targets required by lower transporters.

Reanalysis of the CANUSA study data showed that the effect of clearance on outcomes was explained by variation in residual renal function, with no effect of dialytic clearance alone.

More recent trial evidence for target dialysis dose in PD

Two large randomized controlled trials from Mexico (ADEMEX trial) and from Hong Kong have compared outcomes in patients randomized to PD regimes achieving different small solute clearances.

Both studies demonstrated that prescribing dialysis regimes prospectively to achieve clearances greater than the lower clearance groups did not improve survival and that survival was again dependent on residual renal function.

Based on these data, more modest minimum small solute clearance targets have been produced, on the basis that there is no benefit in routinely increasing dialysis to achieve higher clearances than those achieved in the low clearance groups in these two trials (Table 13.5.3).

It is important to appreciate that these are minimum clearance targets.

It is still acknowledged that lower clearances are likely to result in a significant risk of complications.

It is appropriate to increase the dialysis prescription in subjects who demonstrate features of uremia such as anorexia or malnutrition despite achieving the minimum small solute targets.

Dialysis prescriptions should not routinely be reduced in those with clearances greater than these targets.

Most guidelines now routinely state that adequacy of treatment extends beyond small solute clearances to include:

- fluid balance control;
- other electrolyte control (e.g. acidosis and bone biochemistry);
- nutrition;
- anemia;
- patient symptoms;
- quality of life and rehabilitation.

All of these should be considered and not neglected by focusing simply on solute clearances.

PD prescription and small solute clearances

Every dialysis prescription needs to be written and adjusted on an individual patient basis.

Factors that determine small solute clearance include:

- volume of dialysis fluid;
- length of dialysis dwell times;
- peritoneal membrane transport status;
- eventual drained dialyzate volume.

A higher transport state is associated with more rapid diffusion of solutes and often makes it easier to achieve clearance targets. However, a higher transport state is also associated with less good ultrafiltration and when this results in lower eventual drained volume this can adversely affect clearances. A higher transport state is associated with poorer fluid removal and, despite higher small solute clearances, in many studies it is associated with greater mortality than a lower transport state.

CAPD

Increasing clearance on CAPD is often achieved by increasing exchange volumes.

The use of large volumes does increase the risk of hernias and fluid leaks and because of the increase in intra-abdominal pressure may even have an adverse effect on ultrafiltration.

It is important to ensure that adequate ultrafiltration is achieved to ensure fluid balance is maintained and because clearance depends on the volume of dialyzate that is drained.

Clearances on CAPD may also be increased by increasing the number of exchanges per day.

CAPD is well-suited to lower transport status patients as longer dwell times allow greater equilibration of solutes between blood and dialyzate.

APD

APD presents more permutations for treatment modification in individual patients.

Nightly cycles can be altered in number, duration and volume of exchange over a wide range, which impacts on both clearance and ultrafiltration.

Increasing cycle volumes increases clearance and larger volumes are tolerated by the patient in the supine position in bed at night.

The number of exchanges may also be increased to increase total dialyzate volume, which often means reducing individual cycle duration if the overnight treatment time is constant.

However, increasing the number of cycles also increases the number of gaps between cycles during which the fluid volume in the peritoneum is reduced or absent and less dialysis occurs. Thus increasing the cycle number and thereby the total dialyzate volume may not always increase clearance, and may even reduce it, especially with lower transporter status.

Overnight APD regimes are adjusted according to membrane transport status.

With higher transport status, more rapid equilibration of solutes between the blood and dialyzate results in greater benefit of increasing the cycle number to increase the total drained volume. This will also aid ultrafiltration.

In lower transporters, time of dialysis, and thus the effect of lost time between cycles, becomes more important. In lower transport state patients it is preferable to prescribe fewer, longer dwells. With nightly dialysis, clearance is best optimized by maximizing dwell volumes rather than number.

Daytime exchange(s) are very important in APD. As the long duration allows full equilibration of small solutes, they make a proportionally greater contribution to clearance per liter of dialyzate than nightly cycles.

Most patients will have at least a single daytime dwell. Clearances may be significantly increased by adding an additional second daytime dwell (optimized cycling peritoneal dialysis (OCPD)).

Due to the slower diffusion of larger creatinine molecules than the smaller urea molecule, creatinine is less easily removed by short nightly APD cycles. Thus dialytic clearances of creatinine may be proportionally lower than urea for patients on APD compared with those on CAPD.

Changes in PD prescription can be guided by prescription-modeling computer programmes that predict the effect of a change in dialysis prescription in a patient where data such as transport status are known. It is important to repeat clearance measurements in patients soon after any prescription changes to determine their actual effect.

PD prescription and larger solute clearances

Although the focus of blood tests and dialytic clearance measurements has been on small molecules, it is likely that many manifestations and adverse effects of renal failure are due to the retention of larger solutes.

The diffusion of these substances is slower than urea and creatinine and increasingly so with increasing molecular size.

Thus clearance of these molecules does not change in proportion with smaller solutes on changing the dialysis prescription.

When equilibration is very slow, measures that increase small solute clearance such as increasing exchange number and volumes will have a much lesser effect on the clearance of large molecules.

For large molecules clearance is more dependent on the duration of dialysis.

This is important since some regimens, such as NIPD which has a long 'dry' period without dialyzate present in the peritoneal cavity, may produce small solute clearances equivalent to CCPD, but have inferior removal of important larger molecules due to the lesser time of dialysis.

Importance of preservation of residual renal function

There is strong evidence to support the relationship of residual renal function to outcome in PD.

Residual renal function may be better preserved on PD than HD. There are a number of possible explanations for this including:
- stable fluid status without the periods of hypotension and hypovolemia that occur in HD;
- the absence of the systemic inflammatory changes that occur in HD due to exposure of blood to bioincompatible dialysis membranes.

There are several possible explanations why an equivalent amount of renal small solute clearance appears to have greater 'value' than the same clearance achieved by PD:
- Renal function may provide better clearance of larger molecules than dialysis.
- Remaining kidney function may also be a marker for ongoing beneficial metabolic and endocrine activity of the kidney that is not provided by dialysis.
- Residual renal function may lead to better preservation of fluid status, with evidence that later loss of residual renal function on PD may be associated with fluid overload and hypertension.

Given the great clinical and prognostic importance of residual renal function, efforts should be made to preserve it for as long as possible.

Where possible, nephrotoxic insults, such as NSAID prescription and radiocontrast media administration, should be avoided.

The effect of aminoglycosides, used in the management of peritonitis, on residual renal function is unclear. Evidence from studies is conflicting.

Episodes of dehydration have been observed to be associated with loss of residual function and so whilst overhydration is a serious problem, dehydration resulting from overaggressive fluid removal should also be avoided.

Preservation of residual renal function has been shown with ACEIs and ARBs and these agents should be considered in patients who still have residual renal function.

Other aspects of adequacy in PD

A philosophy of optimizing care in PD has developed to encompass not only optimizing small solute clearances but also to consider multiple aspects of treatment and patient well-being.

Nutrition

Reduced appetite and nutrient intake may result from inadequate dialysis and be an important reflection of uremic toxicity. This may contribute to malnutrition which is associated with an increased risk of morbidity and mortality.

The nutritional state may be assessed by dietary history and physical examination.

Urea is the major breakdown product of protein metabolism. If a patient is in neutral protein balance, excreted nitrogen in the form of urea is equal to the nitrogen of protein intake.

Urea values from dialysate and urine collections can be used not only to assess small solute clearance but also to calculate protein intake.

This is called the protein equivalent of total nitrogen appearance (PNA). It is normalized to body weight as nPNA.

Normalization in malnourished patients with low body weight may lead to relatively high nPNA values. This may result in a failure to diagnose inadequate protein intake in malnourished patients.

There is debate as to whether PNA should be normalized to ideal body weight or the subject's premorbid body weight.

Care should be taken in interpreting nPNA in patients with weight loss.

Another limitation of nPNA is the underlying assumption of neutral nitrogen balance.

In catabolic patients protein breakdown will result in increased nitrogen excretion that is in excess of intake, giving a misleadingly high estimate of protein intake in patients at risk of wasting and malnutrition. Conversely, nPNA will underestimate protein intake in anabolic patients.

Salt and water balance

Fluid balance is a fundamental role of dialysis.

Fluid excess causes hypertension, cardiac dysfunction and left ventricular hypertrophy and is likely to be a major factor in mortality of dialysis patients.

Reduced sodium and water removal have been associated with poorer survival in a number of observational studies.

European Best Practice Guidelines for PD have set a minimal ultrafiltration target of 1 L though other organizations have stated that the evidence does not provide a rationale for such a target.

Whilst fluid overload is to be avoided there is no evidence for a beneficial effect of achieving 1 L ultrafiltration in all patients on PD.

Patients with low volume ultrafiltration should be assessed for the presence of fluid overload, deteriorating peritoneal membrane function, and poor nutritional intake before increasing fluid removal.

Fluid management and small solute clearances need to be considered jointly when adjusting PD dialysis prescriptions.

Acidosis

Correction of acidosis is important as acidosis both contributes to malnutrition by promoting protein catabolism, and causes bone demineralization.

Serum bicarbonate should be maintained within the normal range, with some evidence that the nutritional state may benefit if the serum bicarbonate is maintained in the higher part of this range.

Calcium, phosphate and parathyroid hormone

Abnormal bone biochemistry has been increasingly recognized to be important in dialysis, not just with respect to skeletal complications, but also in the development of cardiovascular disease.

Adverse cardiovascular effects include development of vascular calcification with cardiac, cerebral and peripheral vascular disease, cardiac valvular calcification, and cardiac dysfunction.

The key aims of treatment are to avoid hypercalcemia, control serum phosphate and to avoid an excessively high calcium × phosphate product. Control of serum PTH is also necessary.

Quality of life

Achieving optimum quality of life for patients on PD is as important as maximizing survival and achieving biochemical and other medical targets.

Questionnaire assessment tools have been developed which allow standardized determination of various physical and psychosocial aspects of the patient's well-being.

Important goals of PD are to achieve optimal rehabilitation of patients with minimal intrusion of their illness and treatment in their lives. Being able to continue normal social activities and employment are crucial outcomes of treatment.

When to start PD?

Debate continues as to whether an 'early' start of PD on biochemical grounds will help to delay the complications of renal failure, or whether this simply exposes the patient to the inconvenience and potential hazards of PD unnecessarily early.

On the basis of older interpretations of adequacy studies it has been proposed that patients should start PD when renal clearance declines to the equivalent of target clearances for PD.

This would equate to a renal creatinine clearance of ~10 mL/min to match a weekly Kt/V target of 2.

This is partly based on the assumption of equivalence of renal and dialytic clearances which, as discussed, is not necessarily the case.

It seems reasonable therefore to start PD at significantly lower levels of renal function, provided that there are no features of uremia and, in particular, no features of malnutrition or an inability to achieve target nutritional intake that may be attributable to renal failure.

Further reading

Hemodialysis adequacy

Allon M. Depner TA, Radeva M, et al. Impact of dialysis dose and membrane on infection-related hospitalisation and death: Results of the HEMO study. *J Am Soc Nephrol* 2003; **14**: 1863–1870.

Beto JA, Bansal VK, Ing TS, et al. Variation in blood sample collection for determination of haemodialysis adequacy. *Am J Kidney Dis* 1998; **31**: 135–141.

Canaud B, Morena M, Cristal JP, Krieter D. Beta-2-microglobulin, a uraemic toxin with a double meaning. *Kidney Int* 2006; **9**; 1297–1299

Cheung AK, Rocco MV, Yan G, et al. Serum beta-2-microglobulin levels predict mortality in dialysis patients: results of the HEMO study. *J Am Soc Nephrol* 2006; **17**: 546–555.

Daugirdas JT, Schneditz D. Overestimation of hemodialysis dose depends on dialysis efficiency by regional blood flow but not by conventional two pool kinetic analysis. *ASAIO J* 1995; **41**: M719–M724.

Daugirdas JT. Second generation logarithmic estimates of single-pool variable volume Kt/V; an analysis of error. *J Am Soc Nephrol* 1993; **4**: 1205–1213.

Depner T, Daugirdas J, Greene T, et al. Dialysis dose and the effect of gender and body size on outcome in the HEMO study. *Kidney Int* 2004; **65**: 1386–1394.

Eknoyan G, Beck GJ, Cheung AK, et al. Effect of dialysis dose and flux on mortality and morbidity in maintenance hemodialysis patients: Primary results of the HEMO study. *N Engl J Med* 2002; **347**: 2010–2019.

Geddes CC, Traynor JP, Walbaum D, et al. A new method of post-dialysis blood urea sampling: the 'stop dialysate flow' method. *Nephrol Dial Transplant* 2000; **15**: 517–523.

Gotch FA, Sargent JA. A mechanistic analysis of the National Cooperative Dialysis Study (NCDS). *Kidney Int* 1985; **28**: 526–534.

Lai YH, Guh JY, Chen HC, Tsai JH. Effects of different sampling methods for measurement of post dialysis blood urea nitrogen on urea kinetic modeling derived parameters in patients undergoing long-term hemodialysis. *ASAIO J* 1995; **41**: 211–215.

Li Z, Lew NL, Lazarus JM, Lowrie EG. Comparing the urea reduction ratio and urea product as outcome-based measures of hemodialysis dose. *Am J Kidney Dis* 2000; **35**: 598–605.

Lowrie EG, Li Z, Ofsthun N, Lazarus JM. Measurement of dialyser clearance, dialysis time, and body size: death risk relationships among patients. *Kidney Int* 2004; **66**: 2077–2084.

Owen WF, Lew NL, Lowrie EG, et al. The urea reduction ratio and serum albumin concentration as predictors of mortality in patients undergoing haemodialysis. *N Eng J Med* 1993; **329**: 1001–1006.

Port FK, Wolfe RA, Hulbert-Shearon TE, et al. High dialysis dose is associated with lower mortality among women but not among men. *Am J Kidney Dis* 2004; **43**: 1014–1023.

Priester-Coary A, Daugirdas JT. A recommended technique for obtaining the post dialysis BUN. *Semin Dial* 1997; **10**: 23–25.

Schneditz D, Kaufman AM, Polaschegg HD, et al. Cardiopulmonary recirculation during hemodialysis. *Kidney Int* 1992; **42**: 1450–1456.

Traynor JP, Geddes CC, Ferguson C, Mactier RA. Predicting 30-minute postdialysis rebound blood urea concentrations using the stop dialysate flow method. *Am J Kidney Dis* 2002; **39**: 308–314.

Traynor JP, Oun HA, McKenzie P, et al. Assessing the utility of the stop dialysate flow method in patients receiving haemodiafiltration. *Nephrol Dial Transplant* 2005; **20**: 2479–2484.

Peritoneal dialysis adequacy

Bargman JM, Thorpe KE, Churchill DN. Relative contribution of residual renal function and peritoneal clearance to adequacy of dialysis: a reanalysis of the CANUSA Study. *J Am Soc Nephrol* 2001; **12**: 2158–2162.

Churchill DN, Taylor DW, Keshaviah PR for the CANUSA Peritoneal Dialysis Study Group: Adequacy of dialysis and nutrition in continuous peritoneal dialysis: association with clinical outcomes. *J Am Soc Nephrol* 1996; **7**: 198–207.

European Best Practice Guidelines for Peritoneal Dialysis. *Nephrol Dialysis Transplant* 2005; **20**(Suppl 9).

Paniagua R, Amato D, Vonesh E, *et al.* Effects of in-creased peritoneal clearances on mortality rates in peritoneal dialysis: ADEMEX, a prospective, randomized, controlled trial. *J Am Soc Nephrol* 2002; **13**: 1307–1320.

Lo WK, Ho YW, Li CS, *et al.* Effect of Kt/V on survival and clinical outcome in CAPD patients in a randomized prospective study. *Kidney Int* 2003; **64**: 649–656.

Lo WK, Bargman JM, Burkart J, Krediet RT, Pollock C, Kawanishi H, Blake PG for the ISPD Adequacy of Peritoneal Dialysis Working Group. Guideline on targets for solute and fluid removal in adult patients on chronic peritoneal dialysis. *Peritoneal Dialysis Int* 2006; **26**: 520–522.

Internet resources

Renal Association Clinical Practice Guidelines:

`http://www.renal.org/guidelines/index.html`

The Renal Registry:

`http://www.renalreg.org`

National Kidney Federation Dialysis Outcomes Quality Initiative:

`http://www.kidney.org/professionals/kdoqi/`

European Best Practice Guidelines:

`http://www.ndt-educational.org/guidelines.asp`

Cochrane Renal Group:

`http://www.cochrane-renal.org/`

Australia and New Zealand Dialysis and Transplant Registry:

`http://www.anzdata.org.au/`

National Institute for Clinical Excellence:

`http://www.nice.org.uk/`

International Society of Peritoneal Dialysis:

`http://www.ispd.org`

See also

Hemodialysis, hemofiltration and hemodiafiltration, p. 494

Peritoneal dialysis, p. 506

Dialysis strategies, p. 480

Medical management of dialysis patients, p. 528

Medical management of the dialysis patient

Introduction

Caring for the patient with end-stage renal disease (ESRD) encompasses care related to both renal and nonrenal disease. As well as renal-specific issues such as anemia, bone disease, nutrition, pruritis and hypertension, the nephrologist will also be called upon to optimize the medical management of comorbid conditions such as cardiac disease and diabetes, as well as focusing on primary prevention. Close co-ordination with other services is required.

Management of renal anemia

Many of the symptoms associated with ESRD such as fatigue, depression, reduced exercise tolerance and dyspnea are attributable to anemia. The treatment of anemia was revolutionized by the introduction of recombinant human erythropoietin (EPO).

Management of anemia in ESRD should also include:

- prevention of blood loss;
- ensuring adequate iron stores;
- provision of adequate dialysis;
- control of hyperparathyroidism;
- avoidance of aluminium overload.

Most anemia guidelines recommend a target hemoglobin level of >11 g/dL in ESRD. However, therapy does carry side-effects (Table 13.6.1) and there is increasing evidence that there is little benefit and possibly some risk in maintaining hemoglobin levels >13 g/dL.

Iron management

There is a synergistic relationship between iron and EPO therapy: EPO increases iron requirements by stimulating red blood cell formation while adequate iron increases red blood cell production and reduces EPO requirements.

This is especially important during initial therapy when EPO is being used to correct rather than maintain hemoglobin. ESRD patients will typically require iron supplementation.

Historically, iron stores have been assessed using ferritin and transferrin saturation, but it is now recognized that ESRD patients with values in the normal range may still have both an absolute and functional iron deficiency. Several other tests have been introduced to determine iron stores (Table 13.6.2). Typically these are assessed monthly in ESRD patients.

Some PD patients will maintain hemoglobin level within the target range without EPO or supplemental iron therapy. Typically a proportion of PD patients will require oral iron supplementation, whereas most HD patients will require intravenous iron supplementation.

Intravenous iron is available in several forms and is generally safe. Rarely anaphylaxis may occur and careful monitoring is recommended during administration.

Treatment with erythropoiesis stimulating agents

Several erythropoiesis stimulating agents (ESAs) are commercially available although this varies from country to country.

Available ESAs include:

- epoetin alpha;
- epoetin beta;
- epoetin delta;
- epoetin zeta;
- darbepoetin alpha;
- Mircera®.

The latter two ESAs have a longer half-life and may be administered monthly.

The response to all ESAs is dose dependent but the dose required to achieve the target hemoglobin varies from patient to patient. The route and frequency of administration will also influence response.

The choice of ESA, route and frequency of administration should be based on the physician's choice and discussion with the patient. Usually for ESAs with a short half-life twice- or thrice-weekly administration is required and for those with a long half-life weekly to monthly treatment is required.

Subcutaneous administration is associated with a reduced EPO requirement but may carry an increased risk of pure red cell aplasia. However, this side-effect is rare.

In the initiation phase of treatment both iron stores and hemoglobin levels should be assessed fortnightly. Once in the maintenance phase of therapy iron and hemoglobin levels should be monitored monthly.

Iron supplementation and ESA dosing should be tailored to the individual patient's response.

Resistant anemia

Some ESRD patients are relatively resistant to therapy with ESAs. This should be investigated in patients who fail to attain the target hemoglobin while receiving doses of EPO >300–450 IU/kg/week.

A variety a conditions may produce resistance (Table 13.6.3); this is most often due to an absolute, relative or functional iron deficiency.

A further escalation in the EPO dose will result in achievement of the target hemoglobin in up to 10% of patients with resistant anemia, in whom these conditions have been excluded or treated.

Management of renal bone disease

Changes in bone and mineral metabolism appear early in CKD. Several types of lesions may be present in the ESRD patient. Typically these are thought of as disorders of high or low bone turnover (Table 13.6.4).

Clinical manifestations

The clinical symptoms of renal bone disease are often nonspecific and include:

- acute and chronic bone pain;
- pain around individual joints;
- muscle weakness;
- skeletal deformities;
- pruritis;
- extraskeletal calcifications including calciphylaxis.

Diagnosis

Double tetracycline labeling followed by bone biopsy remains the gold standard for the diagnosis of renal osteodystrophy but is not routinely performed in clinical practice.

Conventional X-rays are frequently performed but are an insensitive test.

Table 13.6.1 Potential benefits and risks of partial or complete correction of anemia with erythropoetin

Improvements in:	Increased risk of:
Cardiac function	Hypertension
Quality of life	Graft thrombosis
Exercise capacity	Pure red cell aplasia
Cognition	Seizures/encephalopathy
Sexual function/menses	Cardiovascular disease
Nutrition	(if Hb >13.5 g/dL)
Sleep	
Immune function	
Coagulopathy	

Table 13.6.2 Laboratory tests used to assess iron stores in ESR

Ferritin
Transferrin
Transferrin saturation
Serum iron
Protoporphyrin
Percent hypochromic red cells
Reticulocyte hemoglobin
Serum transferrin receptor

Table 13.6.3 Conditions associated with erythropoietin resistance in ESRD patients

Absolute, relative or functional iron deficiency
Inflammation/infection
Hyperparathyroidism
Aluminium overload
Vitamin deficiency (B12, folate)
Myeloma/myelofibrosis/other hematological disorders
Malignancy
Malnutrition
Patient concordance with treatment

Table 13.6.4 Bone lesions in ESRD

Osteitis fibrosis cystica
  Characterized by very high bone turnover with marrow fibrosis
Mild bone disease
  Less severe disease characterized by an increase in the osteoid surface and high/normal bone formation
Osteomalacia
  Characterized by an excess of unmineralized osteoid
Adynamic bone disease
  Characterized by low bone formation
Mixed renal osteodystrophy
  There is both an increase in marrow fibrosis and unmineralized osteoid
Other, e.g. β2-microglobulin amyloidosis

Serum biochemical markers are routinely used as surrogate markers of renal bone disease and include:
● calcium;
● phosphate;
● parathyroid hormone;
● alkaline phosphatase.

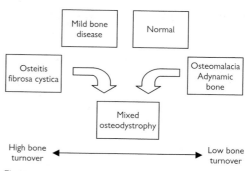

Fig.13.6.1. The spectrum of renal bone disease.

These are routinely measured in patients with CKD and ESRD and can be used to guide treatment.

Management
Treatment should begin early in the course of CKD in order to prevent skeletal changes developing.

In ESRD patients serum calcium, serum phosphate and calcium phosphate product should be assessed monthly and PTH concentration should be assessed 3-monthly.

These parameters should be considered together when determining the appropriate management.

Achieving ideal targets is challenging with conventional dialysis and currently available therapies.

Control of serum phosphate
Control of phosphate is the key to effective therapy and the serum concentration of phosphate should be maintained between 1.1 and 1.78 mmol/L.

Initially a renal dietician should provide education and counseling about restriction of dietary intake of phosphate.

If this is ineffective the next step is use of a phosphate binder. Various agents have been used including:
● aluminium hydroxide;
● magnesium salts;
● calcium salts;
● sevelemar;
● lanthanum carbonate.

Calcium salts are currently first-line therapy, although daily doses may need to be limited due to the risk of hypercalcemia and the potential to worsen vascular calcification.

Control of serum calcium
The serum calcium should be maintained in the range of 2.1–2.4 mmol/L.

This should be assessed using a predialysis sample in HD patients and ideally should be maintained at the lower range of normal unless this worsens hyperparathyroidism.

This may be achieved by oral calcium supplementation, use of calcitriol, which will increase both calcium and phosphate concentrations, and by manipulating the dialyzate calcium.

The ideal calcium dialyzate concentration is unclear.

The calcium phosphate product

The calcium phosphate product (serum calcium mulitplied by serum phosphate) has been regarded as a risk factor for extraskeletal calcification.

A calcium phosphate product of <4.0 mmol^2/L^2 is ideal.

Control of serum PTH

In ESRD patients concentrations of intact PTH in the normal range suggest low bone turnover whereas concentrations >3× normal are suggestive of high bone turnover.

An iPTH level of 2–3× normal (16.5–33 pmol/L) is thought to be optimal.

This may be achieved by manipulation of serum phosphate, calcium and use of calcitriol.

Surgical parathyroidectomy may be indicated in certain patients (Table 13.6.5).

Calcimimetic agents increase the sensitivity of the calcium-sensing receptors in the parathyroid glands, which is the dominant regulator of PTH secretion and parathyroid gland hyperplasia. The exact role of these agents is as yet unclear but they are likely to prove important in the treatment of hyperparathyroidism and reduce the need for surgical parathyroidectomy.

β2-Microglobulin amyloidosis

ESRD patients typically have serum concentrations of β2-microglobulin (β2M) 30–50-fold greater than normal and are at risk of developing amyloidosis (Aβ2M) affecting the skeletal system.

Risk factors for development of Aβ2M include:

- older patients;
- duration on dialysis;
- loss of residual renal function.

Other factors potentially involved include:

- type of HD membrane;
- high bone turnover renal osteodystrophy;
- use of impure dialyzate;
- skeletal accumulation of iron and aluminium.

Several clinical manifestations occur (Table 13.6.6). The initial presentation of Aβ2M is often subtle and only becomes apparent with time. Often more than one clinical syndrome may occur.

Conventional X-ray is an inexpensive, readily available screening test but will usually underestimate disease.

Ultrasonography, radionuclide scanning and CT scanning have all been used; if available, MRI is the best radiological test.

Histological examination of affected tissue will confirm the clinical and radiological diagnosis.

Successful renal transplantation will restore β2M concentrations to the normal range but it is unclear whether this will cause established lesions to regress.

Table 13.6.5 Indications for parathyroidectomy

Severe hyperparathyroism and:
- uncontrollable hyperphosphatemia;
- unresponsive to calcium and calcitriol;
- metastatic calcification;
- a potential renal transplant recipient.

Hyperparathroidisim and calciphylaxis

Table 13.6.6 Clinical syndromes of β2-microglobin amyloidosis

Carpal tunnel syndrome
Peripheral arthropathy
Tendon rupture/contracture
Spondyloarthropathy
Osseous involvement
Subcutaneous masses
Renal calculi

Although of unproven benefit it is reasonable to consider the use of biocompatible HD membranes, hemofiltration or hemodiafiltration at high blood flow rates with ultrapure dialyzate.

Patients with Aβ2M require symptomatic treatment and can require prompt surgical measures from orthopedic, neurosurgical or urological services.

Nutrition

Part of the routine care of the dialysis patient will include an initial and then regular review of their nutritional status, typically performed in conjunction with a renal dietician.

Malnutrition is common in dialysis patients and associated with worse morbidity and mortality.

The effect of dialysis on nutritional requirements

Dialysis itself carries specific nutritional demands for the patient.

HD is associated with protein loss into the dialyzate and an increase in protein catabolism. Thus when starting HD an increase in the protein and caloric intake is required to maintain a neutral nitrogen balance. Water-soluble vitamins are removed in the dialyzate and should be supplemented.

Recommended daily vitamin supplements in patients on HD are:

- vitamin C, 100 mg daily;
- folic acid, 1 mg daily;
- vitamin B6, 10 mg daily.

Patients on PD absorb, on average, 70% of the glucose infused from the dialyzate. Patients will often reduce their oral carbohydrate intake to compensate for the glucose load from the dialyzate. Typically 5–15 g of protein, mainly in the form of albumin, is lost each day in the dialyzate. This loss increases, during episodes of PD peritonitis, and remains increased for weeks after resolution of the episode.

Other factors affecting nutrition in dialysis patients

A number of other factors may contribute to malnutrition in dialysis patients (Table 13.6.7).

Progressive uremia is associated with a decline in appetite and inadequate dialysis may contribute to a reduced intake in ESRD patients.

Other factors which need to be considered include slowed gastric emptying and depression.

Metabolic acidosis stimulates protein catabolism and may contribute to a reduction in the level of the anabolic steroid IGF-1. Correction of metabolic acidosis will limit this catabolic state.

Endocrine abnormalities may also contribute to malnutition. Observational data have shown elevated levels of leptin in ESRD patients associated with reduced dietary intake.

Table 13.6.7 Causes of malnutrition in patients with ESRD

Reduced intake
Inadequate dialysis
Poor dentition
Cultural food preferences
Inability to obtain or prepare food
Slowed gastric emptying
Depression
Metabolic abnormalities
Metabolic acidosis
Altered amino acid metabolism
Insulin resistance
Endocrine abnormalities
Hyperleptinemia
Insulin resistance
Catabolism from PTH
IGF-1 resistance
Systemic inflammation
Intercurrent illness

Elevated PTH is also associated with increased protein degradation.

Inflammatory processes are common in ESRD patients and may contribute to malnutrition. This may be related to increased frequency of infections, uremia, proinflammatory cytokines and atherosclerosis. The malnutrition, inflammation and atherosclerosis (MIA) syndrome describes wasting as part of an inflammatory state associated with cardiovascular disease, and is commonly seen in patients with ESRD on dialysis.

Assessment of nutritional status
Typically the nutritional status of the ESRD patients is assessed using several methods (Table 13.6.8).

Symptoms such as anorexia, vomiting or weight loss should be elicited by direct questioning.

Regular assessments of the target weight should be performed – typically monthly in the stable HD patient and 3-monthly in the stable PD patient. This should be compared with the recommended ideal weight and previous target weight assessments.

Assessment of the food intake over a short period of time should be performed, and the 3 day food diary is typically used.

Body fat and muscle mass may be estimated using anthropometry which is rapid, noninvasive, and can be performed

Table 13.6.8 Assessment of nutrition in patients with ESRD

Presence of GI symptoms, e.g. anorexia, nausea, vomiting
Changes in the target weight
Assessment of food intake (food diary)
Protein catabolic ratio (PCR) and normalized protein equivalent of nitrogen appearance (nPNA)
Anthropometry
Plasma proteins, e.g. albumin, transferrin
Blood urea nitrogen/creatinine
Dual-energy X-ray absorbimetry (DEXA)
Bioimpedance analysis (BIA)

by the renal dietician. If repeated by the same person then interobserver error is small.

More sophisticated measures such as dual-energy X-ray absorbimetry (DEXA) and bioimpedance analysis (BIA) are not commonly performed in routine clinical practice.

Laboratory tests will also alert the clinician as to the nutritional state of the patient: serum potassium, phosphate, albumin, prealbumin, transferrin, urea and creatinine may all decline in the malnourished patient.

The protein catabolic ratio (PCR), also known as the normalized protein equivalent of nitrogen appearance (nPNA), may be used to assess nutrition in ESRD patients in a steady state.

In HD patients it is determined by measuring the interdialytic appearance of urea in body fluids as well as any urea excreted in the urine, where there is residual renal function.

In PD since the removal and generation of urea is relatively constant, urea generation is estimated from measurement of dialyzate and urinary urea losses.

A target of 1.0–1.2 g/kg per day or higher is recommended.

Treatment of the malnourished ESRD patient.
Often the etiology of malnutrition is multifactorial. Identifying any reversible causes of malnourishment by careful assessment is vital, with therapy then targeted to the underlying cause.

Determining the adequacy of the dose of dialysis should be done at regular intervals and this may need to be increased as part of the treatment of malnutrition.

Inflammation resulting from a specific source should receive targeted therapy.

Metabolic acidosis should be corrected.

Conflicting data exist as to the effectiveness of nutritional support but this should be considered in all patients with malnutrition (Table 13.6.9).

Initially, counseling, by a renal dietician, to increase dietary protein and energy intake should be undertaken. If this is ineffective then various renal-specific oral products are available for the malnourished dialysis patient.

If problems persist then nasogastric or nasojejunal feeding should be considered. Percutaneous endoscopic gastrostomy (PEG) feeding is generally avoided in adult PD patients, due to the increased risk of peritonitis, but may be considered in HD patients.

Using the gastrointestinal tract to support nutrition remains the most physiologic way of providing nutrition and when possible this should be used.

Table 13.6.9 Options for nutritional intervention

Oral supplements
Nasogastric/nasojejunal/PEG feeding
Intradialytic parenteral nutrition (HD patients)
Amino acid dialyzate (PD patients)
Total parental nutrition
Growth hormone
Anabolic steroids
Appetite stimulants

PEG, percutaneous endoscopic gastrostomy.

Table 13.6.10 Factors contributing to uremic pruritis

Inadequate dialysis
Hyperparathyroidism
Hyperphosphatemia
Increased calcium and phosphate product
Elevated aluminium
Increased β2-microglobulin
Anemia/erythropoietin deficiency
Immune dysfunction
Dry skin
Peripheral neuropathy

Table 13.6.11 Factors contributing to hypertension in ESRD

Sodium loading
Hypervolemia
Activation of the RAS system
Activation of the sympathetic nervous system
Activation of baroreceptors
Use of erythropoietin
Essential hypertension
Atrial naturetic peptides
Endothelium-derived vasoactive factors
Calcification of the arterial tree

Total parenteral nutrition should be considered for the malnourished patient in whom enteral feeding is ineffective. Typically this is in hospitalized patients with intercurrent illness, and in whom more frequent dialysis can be provided to allow protein and fluid load to be optimized.

Parenteral nutrition, delivered during HD, has been used to provide additional nutritional support and compensate for loss of amino acids into the dialyzate. Only a few studies evaluating its long-term effects show benefit, and these benefits have generally been modest.

Amino acid peritoneal dialyzate is a novel form of nutritional supplementation available for the PD patient that avoids glucose loading and allows absorption of infused amino acids. Most studies assessing effectiveness have been short-term, with small numbers of patients and variable benefits. Consistent long-term benefits have yet to be demonstrated.

Growth hormone, anabolic steroids and appetite stimulants have all been used in small short-term trials, with no clear indications established for their use.

Uremic pruritis

Uremic pruritis remains one of the most common and disabling symptoms in ESRD patients.

There is increased release of histamines from skin mast cells. A number of other factors may also contribute (Table 13.6.10) but no specific etiology has been identified.

It is important to note that ongoing scratching may lead to secondary skin conditions, which may be treated by targeted therapy.

The treatment of uremic pruritis remains challenging. It is important to ensure that the patient is adequately dialysed and that calcium, phosphate and PTH are normalized.

Other therapies that may be used include oral antihistamines, EPO, ultraviolet B light, opioid antagonists, topical capsaicin, oral evening primrose oil and gabapentin.

Hypertension

Hypertension occurs in up to 85% of patients with ESRD and is multifactorial (Table 13.6.11) with retention of sodium, water and activation of the sympathetic nervous system key factors.

In dialysis patients the relationship between blood pressure and cardiovascular events does not follow a linear relationship.

Low systolic BP (<110 mmHg) and high systolic BP (>180 mmHg) are associated with reduced survival.

Controlled studies showing an improvement in survival with better BP control have not been performed in ESRD patients. Nevertheless hypertension is recognized as an important predictor of cardiovascular disease and control of BP is widely agreed to be of great importance in improving long-term survival.

The ideal target BP for dialysis patients is uncertain.

JNC-VII recommendations are to achieve a target BP of <130/80 mmHg.

K/DOQI recommend pre- and postdialysis BP goals of 140/90 and 130/80 mmHg respectively.

Treatment of hypertension
Management of hypertension in the dialysis patient typically requires a combination of:
- lifestyle modification;
- optimization of fluid and volume status with dialysis;
- optimization of the dialysis prescription;
- antihypertensive therapy.

Lifestyle modification
This should include:
- dietary sodium restriction;
- encouragement of physical activity;
- restriction of ethanol intake;
- elimination of cocaine and amphetamine use.

Achieving a 'dry weight'
The 'dry weight' is typically defined as the body weight at the end of dialysis below which further reduction results in hypotension.

When a patient is started on dialysis the optimal dry weight should be aimed for by reducing the target weight by 1–2 kg per week over the course of several weeks.

Overzealous ultrafiltration and concurrent use of antihypertensive agents may result in symptomatic hypotension and thus frequent review of the dry weight and cautious withdrawal of antihypertensive agents are usually required.

High dose loop diuretics are a useful in patients who have a degree of residual function.

Excessive ultrafiltration during a single HD session may also result in symptomatic hypotension.

Patients should be advised to limit salt and fluid intake so that any ultrafiltration required to achieve the dry weight is modest.

Optimization of dialysis
For patients on HD the dialysis prescription may be altered to achieve better BP control.

A fixed low dialyzate sodium (e.g. 135 mmol/L) may help to control hypertension but is often associated with more muscle cramps and symptomatic hypotension.

Programmed variable dialyzate sodium is another strategy which may be employed for hypertension with, for example, a programmed exponential decrease of dialyzate sodium from 155 to 135 mmol/L. This strategy aims to limit hypotensive side-effects and postdialysis thirst and serum sodium rises.

Observational data suggest that increasing the duration, frequency or the duration and frequency of HD is the most effective method of controlling BP.

Antihypertensive therapy
If hypertension persists then antihypertensive agents may be required.

The presence of comorbidities may influence the choice of agents, i.e. β-blockers, may be avoided in patients with asthma, but used preferentially in patients with ischemic heart disease.

The pharmacokinetic profile of the agent should be considered, including the effect of renal failure and dialysis on the half-life of the drug and its active metabolites.

Water-soluble drugs are more readily removed by dialysis than lipid-soluble drugs and this may contribute to post dialysis hypertension.

Typically, agents inhibiting the renin–angiotensin system are recommended as first line antihypertensive agents.

β-Blockers are particularly indicated in patients who have underlying cardiac dysfunction.

Calcium channel blockers do not require additional postdialysis dosing, are usually well-tolerated and may be useful in patients with cardiac disease unable to tolerate other agents.

Resistant hypertension
If patients have predialysis BP of >140/90 mmHg despite three drugs, after achieving their target weight, then they are labeled as having resistant hypertension.

Several factors may need to be considered in this setting (Table 13.6.12).

For nonconcordant patients and those patients unable to take medications at home, administration of long-acting oral antihypertensive medications in the dialysis unit or long-acting transdermal clonidine patches may be useful.

In the rare patient with significant hypertension, unable to be otherwise controlled, bilateral nephrectomy should be considered.

Atherosclerotic vascular disease
Artherosclerotic vascular disease is common in incident patients on dialysis, and accelerates in prevalent patients.

Table 13.6.12 Causes of resistant hypertension in dialysis patients

Incorrect dry weight
Inadequate sodium restriction
Excessive fluid gain
Unrecognized secondary hypertension (e.g. pheochromocytoma, Conn's syndrome)
Erythropoietin
Inadequate drug regimen
Patient concordance with medications
Drug–drug interactions (e.g. NSAIDs, oral contraceptive pill)

Cardiovascular disease accounts for just under half of the deaths in patients with ESRD.

Risk factors
Patients with ESRD have a high prevalence of other disorders independently associated with cardiovascular disease including hypertension and diabetes mellitus (Table 13.6.13).

ESRD is also associated with a lower prevalence of some other traditional cardiovascular risk factors such as obesity, use of tobacco, and LDL-cholesterol.

Several factors related to uremia are likely to contribute to accelerated artherosclerosis (Table 13.6.13).

Hyperhomocysteinemia
Hyperhomocysteinemia is common in the dialysis population due to reduced renal clearance, low serum concentrations of vitamin cofactors and possible impaired metabolism.

Studies using folic acid and vitamin B supplementation to lower homocystine concentrations have not demonstrated a lower cardiovascular event rate.

Arterial calcification
Arterial calcification is common in patients with ESRD and is associated with:
● time on dialysis;
● increased calcium intake;
● elevated serum calcium and phosphate concentrations.

Deposition of calcium may occur in both the intima and media of arteries and appears to be an active process with inhibitors of vascular calcification, such as fetuin-A, normally being produced by vascular smooth muscle cells.

In the largest observational cohort study of dialysis patients mortality was independently predicted by:
● phosphate concentration >1.62 mmol/L;
● higher adjusted serum calcium concentrations;
● moderate–severe hyperparathyroidism (PTH>66 pmol/L).

Calcium, phosphate and PTH are potentially modifiable cardiovascular risk factors in CKD and ESRD.

The target for phosphate is 1.1–1.78 mmol/L and the target for PTH is 16.5–33 pmol/L.

Oxidative stress
Oxidative stress is increased in ESRD. Asymmetric dimethylarginine and other markers of oxidative stress

Table 13.6.13 Risk factors for atherosclerotic vascular disease in ESRD

Traditional risk factors
Hypertension
Left ventricular hypertrophy
Diabetes mellitus
Reduced physical activity
Low HDL-cholesterol
Uremia-related risk factors
Hyperhomocysteinemia
Arterial calcification
Oxidative stress
Elevated lipoprotein (a)
Malnutrition
Anemia

accumulate. Antioxidant therapy, with N-acetylcysteine and vitamin E, has been trialled in dialysis patients with some promise.

Serum lipids

Dialysis patients will often have lower than ideal HDL-cholesterol levels but also have low LDL-cholesterol.

Lipoprotein(a), a cholesterol ester-rich lipoprotein, is thought to be atherogenic in patients without kidney disease and is typically elevated in dialysis patients.

No clinical trials of prevention of coronary heart disease have evaluated the effects of specific lipoprotein-(a)-lowering therapies.

The 4D study (Die Deutsche Diabetes Dialyse Studie) is the only published randomized control trial of cholesterol lowering therapy in dialysis patients and did not show a benefit in reducing cardiovascular events.

Other large randomized control trials evaluating the effect of lipid-lowering agents are currently underway.

Clinical presentation of ischemic heart disease

Atypical presentations of ischemic heart disease are more common in ESRD than in the general population. Ischemic heart disease should be considered in dialysis patients with episodic hypotension, breathlessness or recurrent arrhythmias.

Management of stable coronary artery disease

Aspirin

There are no randomized controlled trials of therapy with aspirin in ESRD. However it is commonly prescribed for secondary prevention and any increased risk of bleeding due to uremic platelet dysfunction appears minor.

Treatment of anemia

Partial correction of anemia to a target of 11–13 g/dL is generally recommended.

Treatment of hypertension

Hypertension should be controlled by removal of excess fluid. β-Blockers should be considered in patients with ischemic heart disease. Antianginal agents may reduce BP which may necessitate night-time dosing.

Management of acute coronary syndromes

Patients with ESRD and unstable angina or acute myocardial infarction should be managed with standard therapy.

Aspirin, β-blockers and nitroglycerin should be used if no contraindications exist.

Thrombolysis

Although it is unclear if ESRD patients obtain the same benefits from thrombolytic agents (most studies have excluded patients with significant renal dysfunction) this should be used as per standard criteria.

Heparin

Heparin should be considered in patients with unstable angina. Unfractionated heparin is usually preferred for dialysis patients.

Although the low molecular weight heparin enoxaparin is considered as effective as unfractionated heparin for the treatment of acute coronary syndrome there are no clear dosing recommendations for patients with ESRD. A meta-analysis of patients not on dialysis, with creatinine clearance <30 mL/min, concluded that standard therapy with enoxaparin results in elevated concentrations of anti-Xa and an increased risk of major bleeding.

Glycoprotein IIb/IIIa inhibitors

Few data exist on the use of glycoprotein IIb/IIIa inhibitors, as patients with renal dysfunction were excluded from published trials.

Abciximab is not thought to require dose alteration for dialysis patients and should be the preferred agent.

Invasive management of coronary artery disease

Patients on dialysis with ischemic heart disease have poor long-term survival.

Invasive intervention, with percutaneous coronary intervention (PCI), or coronary artery bypass grafting (CABG) is associated with better survival than standard medical therapy in patients with ESRD. However, the mortality and morbidity after both PCI and CABG is increased in patients with ESRD compared with nonuremic patients.

CABG surgery is associated with a better long-term prognosis when compared against PCI without stenting. Small studies suggest that PCI both with and without stenting is associated with significant rates of restenosis or recurrence of angina although some suggest that this may be overcome by using drug eluting stents.

When possible, CABG is the favored invasive treatment of severe coronary artery disease in ESRD.

Left ventricular dysfunction

Left ventricular dysfunction is common in incident and prevalent ESRD patients. Typically there is impairment of both systolic and diastolic function.

Observational data suggest that the prevalence of heart failure in dialysis patients is ≥10-fold that of the nonuremic population.

Risk factors for left ventricular dysfunction at the inception of dialysis include:

- hypertension;
- older age;
- anemia;
- ischemic heart disease;
- baseline systolic dysfunction.

These risk factors do not explain the progression of left ventricular dysfunction for patients who remain on dialysis.

As with coronary artery disease, nontraditional risk factors may play a role in the development of cardiac fibrosis, with inflammation, increased oxidative stress, calcium and phosphate abnormalities and a direct effect of uremia all likely to play a role.

As in nonuremic patients, the presence of left ventricular dysfunction independently predicts early mortality in ESRD. In a cohort of almost 2000 ESRD patients with diagnosed congestive heart failure mortality at 3 years was 83%.

Treatment

Strategies to reduce left ventricular mass index and left ventricular dysfunction should include correction of anemia and correction of hypertension.

Correction of volume overload and limiting interdialytic weight gain are also important. For some patients on HD this may require instituting a more intensive dialysis regime with longer hours, greater frequency of dialysis or a combination of both.

For patients on PD, manipulation of the dialysis prescription may be required, and consideration given to the use of icodextrin or automated PD.

First-line pharmacological therapy should be with carvedilol, the only agent that has been shown to be effective at lowering all-cause mortality, cardiovascular mortality and hospitalization in HD patients with symptomatic left ventricular dysfunction.

Consideration should also be given to the use of ACEIs and digoxin as second- and third-line therapies.

The K/DOQI guidelines recommend that, at initiation of dialysis, all patients should undergo baseline echocardiography and electrocardiography. This should generally be deferred until the hemoglobin and the goal dry weight is achieved.

Diabetic ESRD patients

The nephrologist will commonly have to deal with ESRD patients with diabetes and manage their multisystem complications.

The glycated hemoglobin (HbA1$_C$) is typically used to monitor glycemic control in ESRD patients. However the target HbA1$_C$ to achieve optimal outcomes is uncertain in ESRD patients and controversy exists as to whether tight control affects survival.

Most nephrologists will aim to achieve an HbA1$_C$ of 6–7%.

Hypoglycemic agents

Biguanides are generally avoided in ESRD patients due to the risk of lactic acidosis and drug accumulation.

α-Glucosidase inhibitors are also avoided due to concerns about their pharmacokinetic profile.

Shorter-acting sulphonylureas, which lack active metabolites, such as glipizide and gliclazide, are usually preferred.

The thiazolidinedones are hepatically metabolized and active metabolites do not appear to accumulate in ESRD, although concerns as to the effects of rosiglitazone on cardiovascular events and mortality have been raised.

The dose of insulin needs to be reduced in ESRD patients due to decreased renal excretion. There is no consensus as to the choice of insulin regimen and type of insulin and treatment should be individualized to the patient.

If patients are established on PD then their insulin requirements will change due to absorption of glucose from the dialyzate. Patients treated with PD can theoretically be treated with intraperitoneal insulin although there are no proven advantages and the practice is now rare.

Multisystem effects

Regular screening for other diabetic complications is essential with treatment by ophthalmology and podiatry services as required.

Peripheral vascular disease is common and will often require input from interventional radiology or vascular surgical services.

Peripheral neuropathy is also common as a result of both diabetes and uremia. This may respond to increasing the dose of dialysis as well as standard medical treatment.

ESRD patients undergoing surgery

Patients with ESRD, compared to patients without kidney disease, are at increased risk of prolonged hospital stay, morbidity and mortality associated with surgery.

A number of issues should be addressed in the ESRD patient (Table 13.6.14).

Table 13.6.14 Surgery for ESRD: issues to be addressed

Evaluation of hematological and biochemical parameters
Fluid balance
Nutritional state
Cardiac state
Coagulation
Vascular access
Anesthetic considerations
Antibiotics
Analgesia

Issues for patients on PD

PD patients should continue performing exchanges until the time of surgery and should be drained out just prior to surgery.

If undergoing an abdominal procedure, which may disrupt the peritoneal membrane, then placement of a HD catheter under anesthetic is useful.

If the patient is diabetic, stopping PD may alter any requirement for hypoglycemic drugs.

Hematological and biochemical parameters

A full blood count should be performed and anemia should be corrected to the target range where possible. A baseline set of electrolytes including serum glucose, urea, creatinine, potassium, bicarbonate calcium, phosphorus, magnesium and albumin should be evaluated and monitored closely in the immediate postoperative period.

Nutritional state

Malnutrition increases the risk of surgical complications and results in a prolonged length of stay due to infection, wound breakdown and multiple organ dysfunction.

Where possible elective surgery should be delayed to optimize nutrition.

Postoperatively the dose of dialysis should be optimized and may need to be increased as surgery will induce a catabolic state.

Drugs which impair appetite should be avoided. Gastroparesis should be treated aggressively and early, aggressive nutritional supplementation should be considered.

Fluid balance

An assessment of the volume state of the patient should always be performed preoperatively.

HD may be required prior to emergent surgery and should be performed prior to elective surgery to optimize fluid and electrolyte balance.

Dialyzate concentrations should be adjusted to normalize serum potassium and calcium concentrations.

Perioperative fluid requirements should be determined, after discussion with the surgeon and anesthetist.

In patients without kidney disease, solutions such as Plasmalyte and Lactated Ringer's solution, which contain potassium, are frequently used peri- and intraoperatively. The acid–base and electrolyte state of the ESRD patient will often require other solutions to be used.

Close monitoring of fluid balance in the immediate postoperative period is essential.

Cardiac state

Cardiovascular complications are common in ESRD patients. Where possible preoperative cardiac risk assessment will help determine the potential risks of surgery for the patient and may guide perioperative management.

Several clinical risk indices, validated in non-ESRD patients, are available including the Revised Cardiac Risk Index and the Eagle Criteria.

Usually patients at low clinical risk do not need further evaluation. Patients at high risk should be considered for coronary angiography prior to elective surgery. In patients at intermediate risk, noninvasive testing should be considered.

A number of noninvasive tests are available. Exercise tolerance testing with electrocardiography alone or with thallium imaging is often inadequate or impractical in dialysis patients.

[^{201}Tl]Dipyridamole imaging and dobutamine stress echocardiography tend to be more accurate in identifying ESRD patients who should proceed to coronary angiography.

The indications for coronary revascularization of the ESRD patient are unaltered, irrespective of whether the patient is being considered for surgery.

If percutaneous intervention is performed then elective surgery should be delayed until antiplatelet therapy can be safely stopped.

β-Blockers should not be halted perioperatively, due to the risk of rebound and it is reasonable to consider prescribing β-blockers in at-risk patients to minimize the risk of myocardial ischemia or arrhythmias.

Coagulation

Adequate dialysis will generally correct uremic coagulopathy.

If HD is being provided prior to emergency surgery then it is important to avoid prolonging anticoagulation. Where possible heparin-free dialysis should be performed.

If dialysis cannot be performed preoperatively then desmopressin and/or cryoprecipitate may be required to correct the uremic coagulopathy.

For elective procedures, the effects of unfractionated heparin on coagulation will wear off 4 h after heparin is halted.

Vascular access

Vascular access should be discussed with the anesthetist and junior staff.

Patients with ESRD may have complex vascular anatomy and this may influence where the anesthetist elects to place central venous access.

Where possible, subclavian veins or central lines on the same side as an arteriovenous fistula should be avoided.

Patients should be reminded to ask staff to avoid, where possible, blood taking, intravenous cannulas and BP measurements on areas being used for current or future vascular access.

A sign at the patient's bedside or even temporary marking of the access arm may be required.

Anesthetic management

Premedications, induction and perioperative agents, will need to be modified in patients with ESRD as metabolism of anesthetic medications is altered in renal failure.

Antibiotics

ESRD patients who are undergoing access procedures should receive prophylactic antibiotics.

Peri- and postoperative antibiotics, for other surgical procedures, should be administered as normal but will usually require dose adjustment.

Analgesia

Paracetamol can be used in ESRD patients without dose modification.

The effects of many opioid analgesics are prolonged in ESRD. Sufentanil and fentanyl have a short redistribution phase, lack active metabolites and appear to have an unchanged free fraction in ESRD, so are the drugs of choice.

Oxycodone and methadone may be used cautiously when converting to oral opiate analgesia.

Primary prevention

General healthcare issues should be addressed in ESRD patients. This will include immunizations and screening for malignancies.

Although dialysis patients have reduced response rates to immunization compared with the general population and controversy exists as to cost-effectiveness and overall benefits, most guidelines advocate the following vaccinations:

- hepatitis B;
- pneumococcal;
- influenza;
- tetanus;
- meningococcal B.

Patients should be reminded to undergo routine screening for malignancies such as breast, cervix and bowel as per local guidelines.

Palliative care of the dialysis patient

Withdrawal from dialysis is common, and is recorded as the cause of death in >20% of dialysis patients.

This may be when the patient faces imminent death from other causes, incurable malignancy, or other reasons including the burden of dialysis outweighing its potential benefit. In the latter scenario, understanding why the patient feels that therapy is too much of a burden may identify areas where treatment may be modified.

The survival of patients with significant residual renal function may be months but in anuric patients is typically <1 week.

Many dialysis patients who withdraw from therapy will die in hospital. However, the option of care at home with community support or hospice care should be considered.

Although often described as painless and associated with progressive somnolence, uremic death is often associated with weakness, fatigue, myoclonic jerks, twitching, agitation, dyspnea, pain and nausea.

General care should be instituted including withdrawal of unnecessary medication, removal of fluid and dietary restrictions and elimination of blood testing. Pain, nausea, constipation and other symptoms should be treated with medications at doses adjusted for the level of renal dysfunction.

Further reading

Chobanian AV, *et al.* Seventh Report of the Joint National Committee on Prevention, Detection, Evaluation, and Treatment of High Blood Pressure: the JNC 7 report. *J Am Med Assoc* 2003; **289**: 2560–2572.

Cice G, *et al.* Carvedilol increases two-year survival in dialysis patients with dilated cardiomyopathy: a prospective, placebo-controlled trial. *J Am Coll Cardiol* 2003; **41**: 1438–1444.

K/DOQI clinical practice guidelines for cardiovascular disease in dialysis patients. K/DOQI Workgroup. *Am J Kidney Dis* 2005; **45**(4 Suppl 3): S1–153.

Lim W, *et al.* Meta-analysis: low molecular weight heparin and bleeding in patients with severe renal insufficiency. *Ann Intern Med* 2006; **144**: 673–684.

Trespalacios FC, *et al.* Heart failure as a cause of hospitalization in chronic dialysis patients. *Am J Kidney Dis* 2003; **41**: 1267–1277.

Wanner C, *et al.* Atorvastatin in patients with type 2 diabetes mellitus undergoing hemodialysis. *N Eng J Med* 2005; **353**: 238–248.

Internet resources

The Renal Association:

http://www.renal.org/

The Renal Registry:

http://www.renalreg.org

National Kidney Federation Dialysis Outcomes Quality Initiative:

http://www.kidney.org/professionals/kdoqi/

UK National Kidney Federation:

http://www.kidney.org.uk/

Care for Australians with Renal Impairment:

http://www.cari.org.au/

European Best Practice Guidelines:

http://www.ndt-educational.org/guidelines.asp

See also

Endocrine disorders in CKD, p. 398

Hypertension in CKD, p. 406

Cardiovascular risk factors in CKD, p. 412

Hematological disorders in CKD, p. 426

Skeletal disorders in CKD, p. 432

β2M amyloidosis in CKD, p. 436

Dermatological disorders in CKD, p. 450

Psychological aspects of treatment for renal failure

Introduction

The diagnosis and treatment of renal failure can have a significant impact on patients' psychosocial functioning and their ability to cope with the inevitable changes to their lifestyle. For patients approaching ESRD, early referral to renal services is preferred with patients having time to prepare and adjust to their condition and treatment. Sudden onset may be traumatic and the identification of trauma-related symptoms can go unrecognized.

Diagnosis of end-stage renal disease

Common reactions

Following a diagnosis of ESRD, patients may experience a range of emotions similar to the stages of grief typically seen following a significant loss or bereavement:

Shock:
- 'This is not really happening to me.'

Uncertainty, worry, anxiety:
- 'How long will I need these treatments?'

Low mood/depression:
- 'What did I do to cause this?'

Anger:
- 'Why is this happening to me?'

Denial:
- 'My kidneys are going to start working again soon.'
- 'The doctors have made a mistake.'

Relief:
- 'Now I know why I was feeling unwell.'

Acceptance:
- 'I feel I can look to the future now.'

Management

Allow time for the patient to express how they are feeling and any concerns or worries they might have.

Communicate to the patient that they might expect to feel a variety of emotions in response to their illness.

Acknowledge that their reaction is a normal response to diagnosis of a chronic medical condition.

Provide an appropriate level of information and keep the atient informed in relation to their condition and treatment.

Refer for psychological intervention if the patient continues to have difficulty in adjusting.

Adjustment

Adjustment and ability to cope with the diagnosis and long-term implications of ESRD can be affected by a number of other demographic and psychosocial variables:
- comorbidity with other chronic health conditions;
- illness-related factors;
- medication;
- impact on current lifestyle;
- age at diagnosis;
- personality;
- social and cultural factors;
- support networks available.

The impact on family and carers also needs to be considered both from an emotional and practical perspective.

Decision-making

Involvement in decision-making and treatment choices has been associated with a reduction in anxiety and depression and surveys have indicated that many patients prefer to be involved in their own healthcare.

For patients diagnosed with renal failure, treatment choice (e.g. dialysis, transplantation, or conservative management) may be influenced by a number of factors including:
- physiological factors;
- involvement of others, e.g. health professionals and family/carers;
- degree of autonomy, control and independence;
- change in treatment modality;
- predialysis patient education;
- quality of life;
- capacity to make informed choice, e.g. advanced dementia or severe learning disability.

Commencement of dialysis

Anxiety and depressive disorders are frequently seen in hemodialysis patients and may affect how they perceive their health status.

Furthermore, these affective disorders may not be recognized or viewed as a normal reaction to the patient's illness.

A number of factors are important to consider from a psychological perspective in patients who are commencing dialysis:
- treatment complications, e.g. catheters blocking; access difficulties; infections;
- change in treatment modality;
- fear that treatment may not be successful;
- transport issues;
- financial concerns;
- impact on family and other lifestyle factors;
- anxiety about treatment procedures;
- body image concerns.

Hospitalization

Admission to hospital can be a stressful experience for patients, with challenges related both directly and indirectly to illness and treatment.

Loss of independence and uncertainty have been described as the two most stressful challenges faced during hospitalization. Other key issues include:

Loss of control

Over body:
- loss of privacy and independence;
- the need to be highly dependent on others;
- undergoing distressing or invasive procedures.

Over lifestyle:
- unable to perform typical activities;
- unable to fulfill their usual family, social and work roles.

Over ability to predict what will happen:
- not knowing what to expect;
- confusion and disorientation;
- unable to plan for the future.

Lack of information

Patients need to understand what is happening to them for a number of reasons:

- to inform their treatment decisions;
- to make sense of their symptoms and illness;
- to reduce anxiety (about outcome and procedures).

Management

It is important for staff to be aware of the types of emotional responses and coping strategies used by hospitalized patients.

Patients can be helped to cope with psychological distress in a number of ways:

- keep patients informed of their condition, diagnosis and treatment;
- help patients use problem-focused coping;
- provide patients with appropriate social support.

Depression

Depression is frequently seen in renal patients both as a reaction to diagnosis and treatment, as well as the losses experienced in terms of health, lifestyle, status, etc.

It is commonly seen in the early stages of renal failure and/ or as a response to setbacks with treatment or physical health (e.g. transplant failure).

The type of depression seen in renal patients is often reactive and usually transient in nature.

Epidemiology

Depression and anxiety are twice as common in medical patients as in the general population.

In relation to ESRD, it is estimated that up to 30% of hemodialysis patients have a depressive disorder. However, prevalence rates vary according to diagnostic criteria and measures used.

Recognition of an anxiety or depressive disorder can be difficult in a medical setting particularly as typical symptoms can be confused with those of a physical illness, e.g. uremia, fatigue, loss of appetite, sleep disturbance.

Clinical features

- persistent sadness or low mood;
- loss of interest or pleasure;
- fatigue or low energy;
- sleep disturbance (either difficulty falling asleep or early morning wakening);
- appetite disturbance (either loss or increase in appetite);
- poor concentration or indecisiveness;
- agitation or slowing of movement;
- decreased libido;
- low self-confidence;
- suicidal thoughts or acts;
- guilt or self-blame.

Assessing suicide risk

Questions should determine:

- the presence or absence of suicidal ideas;
- the persistence of these ideas;
- the likelihood of them being acted upon;
- the risk to others.

The National Institute for Mental Health in England (NIMHE) provides useful advice and guidance including assessing the severity of depression and suicide risk.

Topics to be included in risk assessment include:

- level of hopelessness;
- thoughts of ending life (if so, how persistent);
- thoughts about a specific, available method of suicide;
- ever acted on such thoughts in the past;
- feel able to resist them, make them disappear;
- ability to give reassurance about safety, e.g. until next appointment;
- circumstances likely to make things worse;
- willingness to turn for help if crisis occurs;
- risk to others.

Treatment/interventions

Recognize that depression can be a normal response to diagnosis and hospitalization.

Referral for further specialist intervention may be necessary (see guidelines at end of chapter).

A number of psychological approaches/models have proven effectiveness in the treatment of depression.

Recent guidelines recommend cognitive behavior therapy (CBT) as an effective psychological treatment for mild and moderate depression.

A combination of antidepressants and individual CBT should be considered for severe depression and treatment-resistant depression.

However, more research is needed regarding the effectiveness of CBT with chronically ill patients.

Key components of CBT for depression include:

- identifying, monitoring, and altering negative thinking patterns, beliefs and interpretations related to targets symptoms/problems;
- learning new coping skills: activity scheduling, problem-solving, and goal-setting.

Anxiety

Anxiety may be experienced in relation to:

- dialysis and treatment;
- understanding of renal failure;
- specific phobias such as needles and medical/invasive procedures;
- relationships;
- quality of life and the future;
- employment and financial status;
- impact on overall lifestyle and other family members.

Epidemiology

Anxiety disorders can cause considerable distress, are often chronic in nature, and often unrecognized and untreated in the general population.

Anxiety can be manifested in terms of physiological, cognitive, and behavioral responses.

A medical history is particularly important in recognizing physical symptoms that might be due to anxiety as opposed to physical illness or the side-effects of medication.

Clinical features

- frequent worrying thoughts;
- feeling tense;
- fearing the worst (e.g. that their condition will deteriorate or they might die);
- palpitations;
- sweating;
- hyperventilating;

- inability to be at ease or relax;
- restlessness;
- sudden feelings of panic;
- feeling dizzy or faint;
- indigestion or diarrhea.

Treatment/interventions

A range of effective interventions is available including medication, psychological therapies, and self-help.

Furthermore, it has been demonstrated that anxiety disorders with marked symptomatic anxiety are likely to benefit from CBT.

CBT for anxiety includes:
- identifying and altering negative thinking patterns and associated behaviors;
- learning new cognitive skills, e.g. distraction (useful for immediate symptom management), positive self-talk;
- affective education (provide information about anxiety), monitoring and management;
- relaxation and breathing techniques;
- exposure-based therapy to manage avoidance of feared situation.

Needle phobia

A phobia is a persistent and excessive fear of an object or situation that is not dangerous and is characterized by avoidance behavior.

Epidemiology

Fear of needles and medical/invasive procedures is frequently seen in renal patients, with estimated prevalence rates of 10% in the general population. However, more severe cases are probably not identified due to avoidance of medical settings.

Clinical features

A typical phobic response includes:
- vasovagal syncope or fainting in response to fall in blood pressure;
- fear and avoidance in absence of vasovagal response.

Key features can include:
- anxiety;
- avoidance;
- fear of pain;
- loss of control.

Treatment/interventions

Behavioral therapy in the form of *in vivo* exposure (i.e. graded and prolonged exposure to feared stimuli) is the treatment of choice for specific, uncomplicated phobias.

Applied tension can be taught to counter vasovagal response.

Cognitive behavioral techniques taught alongside gradual exposure to feared situation include:
- relaxation;
- breathing retraining;
- cognitive restructuring and distraction.

Body image

Changes in appearance as a result of certain procedures and dialysis treatment can have an impact on a patient's psychosocial functioning and relationships with other people.

Body image can influence psychosocial recovery, adaptation to illness and quality of life as well as the degree of psychological morbidity in a range of chronic illnesses.

Patients may view dialysis access as a form of 'mutilation' or feel disfigured:

Hemodialysis
- appearance of fistula, e.g. scarring, size;
- appearance of vascular access catheter.

Peritoneal dialysis
- appearance of abdomen;
- PD catheter and associated fears including concerns about sexual intimacy.

Treatment/interventions

Be aware of the potential impact of treatment procedures on appearance.

Acknowledge that patients might have a very different view of their fistula or catheter, i.e. perceive in terms of appearance as opposed to functional status.

Refer for further psychological intervention if body image disturbance is having a significant impact on treatment and overall psychosocial functioning.

Sexual difficulties

Sexual difficulties can arise at an early stage of renal failure, although may not be experienced by all patients.

Distorted body image and sexual difficulties can also be a psychological response to dialysis treatment.

Sexual difficulties may be influenced by vascular or hormonal changes arising from renal failure; side-effects of medication and/or as a psychological response.

Psychological factors include:
- adjustment to condition and treatment;
- anxiety and depression;
- change in body image;
- relationship difficulties.

Loss of physical health and vitality is also a factor, as is body image.

The most common sexual difficulties in renal patients are:

Men:
- erectile dysfunction;
- loss of libido;
- ejaculatory difficulties.

Women:
- dyspareunia (pain during sexual intercourse);
- change in libido;
- fears related to fertility and pregnancy.

Treatment/interventions

Psychosexual counselling (individual or couple).

Provision of information about common sexual difficulties experienced.

Involvement of partner is preferable.

Nonconcordance

Epidemiology

Reported medication nonconcordance rates in patients with ESRD are high. Nonconcordance rates of 50% or higher have been reported for different aspects of the HD patient's treatment regime. Psychosocial factors underlying nonconcordance in PD patients are less well understood.

Main areas of nonconcordance:
- fluid restriction;
- medication;

- dietary advice;
- continuing/withdrawing from treatment.

Key issues

Self-efficacy, i.e. patients' understanding of the treatment plan and ability to carry it out.

Patients' health-related beliefs and expectations regarding outcome.

Patient choice and involvement in decision-making.

Psychological factors, e.g. depression; impact of past or current psychological trauma; anxiety.

Concerns over long-term effects and dependence on medication.

Unpleasant side-effects of medication or other aspects of treatment.

Nonintentional, e.g. practical difficulties in daily living; forgetting aspects of treatment regime or information provided.

Management

Agree on treatment goals.

Ensure that the patient has an adequate understanding of their condition and treatment regime.

Identify any potential barriers to concordance.

Ensure good communication and patient involvement.

Refer for further specialist help if underlying psychological factors have been identified and are contributing to non-concordant behaviors.

Trauma/post-traumatic stress disorder (PTSD)

Traumatic experiences (e.g. severe life-threatening complications, emergency treatments) may give rise to symptoms of PTSD.

Past psychological trauma may be recalled and impact on a patient's ability to cope with treatment.

Typical reactions to trauma include:
Re-experiencing the traumatic event:
- flashbacks;
- intrusive memories;
- distressing dreams and nightmares.

Arousal reactions:
- sleep disturbance;
- irritability and/or anger;
- impaired concentration and memory;
- hyperalertness;
- exaggerated startle response;
- physiological response such as anxiety and panic attacks.

Avoidance (e.g. of situations connected with trauma) and emotional numbing.

Treatment/interventions

It is recommended that the following treatments should be provided to people who have been diagnosed with PTSD:
- trauma-focused CBT;
- eye movement desensitization and reprocessing (EMDR) therapy.

Sleep disorders

Research has demonstrated that many hemodialysis patients experience a sleep disorder, including delayed sleep onset and/or night-time waking.

Restless leg symptoms have also been described in patients experiencing insomnia.

Psychological interventions which specifically focus on the management of reported sleep difficulties are therefore important to consider.

Eating disorders

Eating disorders have not been widely reported among patients with ESRD, but may be more common than previously thought.

It is recommended that patients who present with low body weight and vomiting in a renal setting should be carefully assessed to exclude an underlying or coexisting eating disorder, such as anorexia or bulimia.

Referral to more specialist services

Referral to a clinical psychologist

May be necessary when the patient:
- responds to illness/hospitalization in a way that is unusual or unexpected;
- refuses to adhere to treatment or health advice;
- has a phobic response to illness/treatment;
- has difficulty coping with the demands of the illness/treatment;
- holds unusually negative beliefs about illness/treatment;
- has a level of distress that exceeds capacity of support available through the team and threatens to interfere with treatment or would have a negative impact on health status.

Referral to liaison psychiatry

May be necessary:
- if the patient is psychotic, severely depressed, is at a significant risk of self-harm, or has suicidal ideation;
- if level of distress is sufficient to require medication (e.g. antidepressants or anxiolytics – see Royal College of Psychiatrists guidelines).

Further reading

Stein A, Wild J. *Kidney failure explained*. London: Class Publishing; 2007.

White CA. *Cognitive behaviour therapy for chronic medical problems: a guide to assessment and treatment in practice*. Chichester: Wiley; 2001.

Internet resources

British Association for Behavioural and Cognitive Psychotherapies (BABCP):

http://www.babcp.org.uk

National Institute for Health and Clinical Excellence (NICE):

http://www.nice.org.uk

National Institute of Mental Health:

http://www.nimh.nih.gov

National Phobics Society:

http://www.phobics-society.org.uk

Royal College of Psychiatrists:

http://www.rcpsych.ac.uk/mentalhealthinformation.aspx

See also

Neuropyschiatric disorders in CKD, p. 454

Sexual disorders in CKD, p. 402

Dialysis strategies, p. 480

Renal transplantation

Chapter contents

Selection and preparation of the recipient

Introduction

Overall renal transplantation both increases survival and greatly improves the quality of life of recipients. Most benefit is seen when the patient is transplanted either just before or shortly after initiating dialysis.

Because of the imbalance between the numbers of those who could benefit from renal transplantation and the supply of organs it is sensible to exclude potential recipients who can be predicted to have a poor outcome.

Recommendations in this chapter are based on guidelines published by the American Society of Transplantation and the American Society of Transplant Surgeons as well as the European Best Practice Guidelines for Renal Transplantation published on behalf of the European Renal Association – European Dialysis and Transplant Association.

Cardiovascular disease

Cardiovascular disease is the major contributor to premature death in renal transplant recipients. An algorithm for the workup of cardiovascular disease in potential recipients is shown in Fig. 14.1.1.

Ischemic heart disease

Criteria to select asymptomatic patients for further investigation may include:

- age >50 years;
- diabetes;
- smoked cigarettes in the past 5 years;
- resting ECG shows a rhythm disturbance or ST segment abnormalities.

Exercise tests have the most discriminating power but may not be practical due to poor exercise tolerance. Pharmacologically driven cardiac stress testing is commonly used as an alternative.

If there is significant reversible ischemia, coronary angiography should be undertaken.

If left ventricular function is adequate and symptoms are controlled then transplant listing can be recommended.

Cerebrovascular disease

Screening asymptomatic potential renal transplant recipients for cerebrovascular disease is not recommended.

Patients with a completed stroke or a transient ischemic attack within the past 6 months should be referred for neurological assessment. Transplantation should be reconsidered after medical and surgical management has been optimized and the patient free of recurrent transient ischemic attacks for 6 months.

Carotid ultrasound screening after the discovery of an asymptomatic bruit is routine but the results of this and further investigations rarely alter the clinical decision.

Peripheral vascular disease

If patients are asymptomatic with good femoral pulses then only a plain X-ray is recommended to rule out extensive vascular calcification.

Patients with symptoms or lack of palpable femoral pulses require vascular imaging and a surgical assessment of whether it is technically possible to implant the graft and if the transplant would be predicted to lead to steal and critical ischemia in the ipsilateral distal leg.

Cancer

How long to delay transplantation in a potential recipient who has been previously treated for cancer and potentially cured is a common clinical issue. The key consideration is to minimize the risk of relapse of occult metastatic disease which may be accelerated by immunosuppression.

Transplant registries have demonstrated that in general recurrence rates of cancer are less the longer the waiting time, with:

- 53% recurring within 2 years;
- 34% between 2 and 5 years;
- remaining 13% recurring after 5 years.

Because of the survival advantage of transplantation compared to dialysis, a reasonable compromise is to wait 2 years after successful treatment for most cancers prior to transplant listing.

Current guidelines are summarized in Table 14.1.1.

Breast cancer

It is difficult to know how best to manage patients with treated cancer of the breast as the majority of relapses occur after 3 years.

Many cancers are heterogeneous conditions, with the prognosis depending on staging. Therefore, it is important to adopt an individualized approach to this problem with close consultation with the oncology team.

Breast cancer is twice as common in renal transplant recipients compared to the general population.

Screening for cancer

The issue of screening for occult de novo cancer in potential renal transplant recipients is contentious. It is reasonable to adopt an individualized approach with cancer screening based on symptoms, signs or in the presence of conditions known to particularly predispose to cancer.

Gastrointestinal disease

The rate of colonic perforation post renal transplantation is ~1% and most commonly associated with diverticular disease.

Screening of asymptomatic patients is not justified, as one study found that none of the patients with significant diverticular disease had symptomatic disease post transplantation.

Patients with symptomatic disease should undergo imaging and consideration given to resection of extensive disease.

Screening of asymptomatic individuals for peptic ulcer disease is not recommended because of the low morbidity rate even in patients with past peptic ulcer disease.

How best to manage incidentally noted cholelithiasis is not straightforward, although a detailed decision analysis recommended expectant management as the preferred strategy for kidney transplant recipients with asymptomatic cholelithiasis.

Genitourinary disease

Routine urological screening of potential transplant candidates is generally unnecessary.

Investigations by urologists should be carried out in the pediatric population when congenital obstructive uropathy

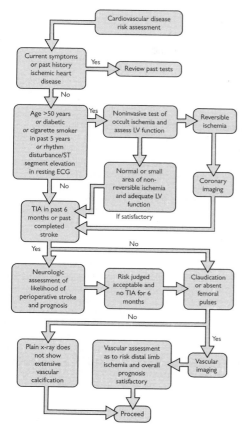

Fig 14.1.1 Algorithm for the work-up of cardiovascular disease in the transplant recipient. ECG, electrocardiogram; LV, left ventricular; TIA, transient ischemic attack. Reproduced with permission from Newstead and Davis (2007).

Table 14.1.1 Outline guidelines for recommended delay to transplant listing following diagnosis of cancer

No waiting time
Basal cell skin cancer
Low-grade bladder cancer
Asymptomatic renal cell carcinoma
In situ carcinoma
Focal neoplasm, with known very low rate of metastasis
2 years
Most cancers
>2 years (5 years advised)
Colorectal cancer
Breast cancer
Uterine cancer
Malignant melanoma

Modified from Penn (1993) with permission.

is suspected or in adult practice where bladder outlet obstruction or a neurogenic bladder resulting in high intravesical pressures is suggested by clinical history and examination.

Native nephrectomy is rarely indicated prior to listing for transplantation. Removal of both kidneys may be indicated for persistent sepsis especially in the presence of nephrolithiasis and/or pronounced reflux.

Uninephrectomy of a large polycystic kidney is occasionally required to make space for the allograft or if it is infected; there is no compelling evidence supporting whether the surgery should be pre-emptive or at the time of transplant.

The removal of a failed allograft may be required prior to listing if it is the source of sepsis or causing systemic inflammation from rejection or to allow space for a new allograft.

Histocompatibility

Blood group typing

ABO typing is routine as an incompatible transplant can result in immediate graft failure from hyperacute rejection.

HLA typing

Recipients also undergo HLA typing in which, as a minimum, the HLA-A, HLA-B and HLA-DR antigens of the major histocompatibility complex (MHC) are determined.

The degree of HLA mismatching may help to identify recipient and donor combinations that would be expected to result in poor graft survival, as well as influence immunosuppressive strategies.

In cadaveric graft allocation the level of HLA mismatching between donor and recipient influences the allocation protocol.

In live donor transplantation the degree of mismatching has much less influence on outcome.

Anti-HLA antibodies

Subjects undergoing transplantation are also tested for the presence of antibodies to HLA antigens.

Antibodies may develop following:
• previous transplantation of (mismatched) organs;
• pregnancy;
• blood transfusions.

On occasions there are no known risk factors.

These HLA antibodies may lead to immediate graft rejection or accelerated humoral rejection.

The presence of antibodies is detected by 'crossmatch' tests.

Current recommendations for detection and characterization of clinically relevant antibodies in solid organ transplantation have been summarized by the British Society of Histocompatibility and British Transplantation Society (BTS).

Assessment of histocompatibility

Formerly the presence of ABO incompatibility or of a positive crossmatch due to donor relevant HLA antibody would have precluded transplantation.

In recent years several groups have published reports of successful transplants in this situation using combinations of intravenous immunoglobulin, plasma exchange and immunoabsorption columns as well as augmented immunosuppressive treatment.

Reviews of the largest experience of HLA antibody desensitization have been published from the USA and Japan, particularly related to ABO 'incompatible' live donor renal transplantation.

Summary guidelines relating to 'Antibody Incompatible Transplants' are available from the BTS.

Infectious complications

The principal tests required for screening are shown in Table 14.1.2.

Geographic location determines screening requirements for some rare occult infections.

Epstein–Barr virus (EBV) and cytomegalovirus

Recipients with *negative EBV antibody titers* who receive EBV antibody-positive renal transplants have an increased risk of developing post-transplant lymphoproliferative disorder.

Recipient viral serology may therefore influence postgraft immunosuppressive strategies.

CMV serology at the time of grafting guides antiviral prophylactic strategies.

Human immunodeficiency virus

HIV infection is not an absolute exclusion for transplantation, with reports of graft and patient survival that are comparable to non-HIV infected recipients, but the work-up and postprocedure management are complex.

Guidelines have been produced in conjunction with the British HIV Association and are available on the BTS website.

Hepatitis B

Carriers of hepatitis B surface antigen may receive a renal transplant provided there is neither evidence of active viral replication nor evidence of chronic active hepatitis or cirrhosis.

Patients with active viral replication are recommended to undergo liver biopsy to stage the disease and to receive antiviral treatment prior to transplantation.

Patients with cirrhosis and active viral replication have a poor prognosis, and immunosuppressive therapy in these subjects can lead to worsening of the liver disease.

Patients should be monitored for the increased risk of hepatocellular carcinoma with yearly serum α-fetoprotein estimations and/or liver USS.

Hepatitis C

Candidates who have antibodies to hepatitis C virus (HCV) should be tested for HCV RNA and also undergo liver biopsy, since there is only a weak relationship between viral RNA load, conventional liver function tests and liver histology.

Subjects with mild liver disease and active infection should be treated with pegylated interferon while still on dialysis.

In the event that infection is not cleared, subjects may undergo renal transplantation, for even though viremia may increase with the immunosuppression, the survival of transplanted HCV-positive patients are improved compared to those remaining on dialysis.

For subjects with advanced liver disease on biopsy a simultaneous liver-kidney transplant may be considered.

Tuberculosis

Tuberculosis may reactivate following transplantation.

Practice with regard to screening for asymptomatic infection varies. CXR to look for inactive disease and a tuberculin skin (PPD) test is recommended in the USA.

While a positive PPD correlates with past infection, a negative skin test in the uremic patient may represent a false-negative result.

In one study the PPD was positive in only 20–25% of patients before transplant who developed active tuberculosis post transplant and many units chose not to screen.

Obesity

Obese subjects have an increased risk for wound infections and perioperative complications.

From an analysis of the USRDS data base, an advantage for transplantation for obese subjects could be shown for live donors, whereas for deceased donors the survival benefit was only shown if the recipient had a BMI <40 kg/m^2.

Transplantation of deceased donor kidneys into recipients with a BMI >40 kg/m^2 is not recommended.

Psychosocial issues

A number of psychosocial variables can influence the transplant work-up. If an adult has impaired capacity for consent, proxy arrangements need to be put in place.

Another concern relates to issues around treatment adherence and concordance, or the use of illicit drugs.

Some individuals can be identified prior to listing in whom additional support post procedure can minimize the risk of premature graft failure due to inability to comply with management.

Other individuals may demonstrate such poor adherence to medical management advice that placing them on the transplant waiting list would be inappropriate.

It is usual in these circumstances to seek views from several of the health professionals involved in the patient's care as well as from the patient and immediate family members.

Pulmonary disease

Pulmonary function tests should be performed if the history or examination suggest chronic lung disease.

All patients who smoke cigarettes should be advised to stop since smokers have a five-fold increased risk of pulmonary complications compared with those who do not smoke.

Patients with bronchiectasis require careful assessment as they carry significant risk of serious septic complications post transplantation.

Re-evaluation of patients on the waiting list

Following placement on the list, some patients wait years before receiving the offer of a transplant.

It is logical that a re-evaluation of suitability is undertaken at intervals, but there are no data to help decide how often this should be.

In Canada guidelines have been proposed which are significantly more rigorous than those recommended for initial evaluation in this Chapter and would, if followed, have very significant resource implications.

Regular assessment of hepatitis and HIV viral status should be undertaken and will generally occur as a part of routine dialysis care.

Table 14.1.2 Screening tests for occult infection.

Routine Serology	Where Indicated, Tests for	Other Routine Investigations
Hepatitis B virus	Human herpesvirus 8	Urine culture
Hepatitis C virus	HTLV	Chest radiograph
HIV	*Strongyloides stercoralis*	
Cytomegalovirus	Malaria	
Epstein-Barr virus	*Trypanosoma cruzi*	
	Schistosomiasis	

HIV, human immunodeficiency virus; HTLV, human T cell lymphotropic virus

Re-evaluation for progression of asymptomatic ischemic heart disease and atherosclerotic disease is the area most likely to be of benefit. However, no benefit of cardiac surveillance following wait-listing was shown in one observational study.

Nevertheless, in the absence of symptoms it seems reasonable that cardiac re-evaluation be performed every 4 years in nondiabetics and every 2 years in diabetic transplant wait-listed candidates using similar work-ups as in the initial evaluation.

Further reading

Berthoux F, Abramowicz D, Bradley B, *et al.* European best practice guidelines for renal transplantation (Part 1). *Nephrol Dial Transplant* 2000; **15**(Suppl 7).

Kasiske BL, Cangro CB, Hariharan S, *et al.* The evaluation of renal transplant candidates: clinical practice guidelines. *Am J Transplant* 2001; **1**(Suppl 2).

Newstead CG, Davis CL. Evaluation and preoperative management of kidney transplant recipient and donor. In: Feehally J, Floege J, Johnson RJ. *Comprehensive Clinical Nephrology*, 3rd edn. Amsterdam: Elsevier; 2007. p. 1056.

Penn I. The effect of immunosuppression on pre-existing cancers. *Transplantation* 1993; **55**: 742–747.

Internet resources

British Society of Histocompatibility:

http://www.bshi.org.uk/

British Transplantation Society:

http://www.bts.org.uk/

American Society of Transplantation:

http://www.a-s-t.org/

American Society of Transplant Surgeons:

http://www.asts.org/

Index of clinical trials including those in transplantation:

http://www.clinicaltrials.gov/

See also

Assessment of live renal donors 548

Medical management of dialysis patients 528

Psychological aspects of treatment for renal failure 538

Assessment of live renal donors

Introduction

Recipients who receive a kidney from a live donor have on average better graft function and survival than those receiving a kidney from a cadaveric donor.

In some countries receiving a live donor renal transplant is the only practical way of providing long-term treatment for ESRD.

Live donor surgery is elective and easier to organize prior to starting dialysis than when the renal donor is a cadaver.

Exchange schemes and strategies to overcome recipient antibodies to allow previously 'incompatible' transplants mean that there are increased opportunities for individuals to donate to assist their relative.

The advent of laparoscopic live donor nephrectomy has contributed to the acceptance of the procedure as it is seen as less traumatic for the donor.

The advantages to the recipient as well as the imbalance between the size of the waiting list and number of grafts performed have all contributed to a significant increase in live donor retrieval.

Living donors may be:
- 'blood relatives';
- not related (e.g. spouses);
- altruistic;
- part of an exchange scheme.

Practices vary from country to country.

Following successful donation there is usually an improved relationship with the recipient and self-image.

Risks of living donation

The undoubted advantage for the recipient of receiving a kidney from a live donor is balanced by the morbidity of the procedure for the donor.

The perioperative mortality risk is estimated at 1 in 3000.

Most deaths are related to occult ischemic heart disease or pulmonary thromboembolism.

Data from Scandinavia show an improved life expectancy for individuals who have been live renal donors with less risk than the general population of ESRD, but it is possible that this is falsely reassuring.

Acceptance of donors with medical morbidity that in the past would have precluded donation, or donors from certain ethnic groups, may result in unexpected late morbidity that only long-term follow-up will reveal.

The medical assessment of the donor

Medical evaluation of the living donor has been discussed at large consensus conferences with comprehensive guidelines available from several sources including the British Transplant Society (BTS) and UK Renal Association. An outline scheme for donor evaluation is shown in Table 14.2.1.

Cardiac disease

If the history, physical examination or a resting ECG suggests cardiac ischemia or valvular disease then an exercise or pharmacologic stress test and/or echocardiogram should be performed.

An individual with known or occult myocardial dysfunction or coronary ischemia should not donate.

Absolute contraindications to donation also include symptomatic valvular disease and severe valvular disease even if this asymptomatic.

Donor hypertension

If elevated blood pressure is detected the following should be performed looking for end-organ damage:
- CXR;
- ECG;
- echocardiogram;
- ophthalmic examination.

Donation from hypertensive individuals may be acceptable if:
- there is no evidence of end-organ damage;
- BP is subsequently controlled;
- GFR is normal;
- no proteinuria.

Pulmonary disease

Pulmonary function testing, echocardiogram and/or sleep studies should be performed, if indicated by the history and examination.

Contraindications to donation include chronic lung diseases that significantly increase the anesthetic risk.

In all cases, donors should cease smoking for ≥4–8 weeks before surgery to minimize the risk of pneumonia.

Donor obesity

Obesity increases the risk of:
- perioperative complications;
- nephrolithiasis;
- renal cell cancer;
- ESRD.

An arbitrary limit beyond which donation is absolutely contraindicated is difficult to define.

In practice, other significant comorbidity in the presence of marked obesity usually rules out donation.

Diabetes mellitus

The following should undergo an oral glucose tolerance test:
- obese prospective donors;
- nonobese subjects with a first-degree relative with diabetes;
- donors with a history of gestational diabetes.

An abnormal glucose tolerance is a contraindication to donation.

Renal function

Use of an age-related threshold GFR is sensible so that a prospective donor's predicted GFR post nephrectomy at age 80 years should be ≥50 mL/min/1.73 m^2.

This age-related threshold has been adopted in BTS/Renal Association guidelines and is shown in Fig. 14.2.1.

Nephrolithiasis

Patients with a history of bilateral or recurrent stones and those with systemic conditions associated with recurrent stone disease should not donate.

Table 14.2.1 Live donor evaluation checklist. CMV, cytomegalovirus; HBV, hepatitis B virus; HCV, hepatitis C virus; HIV, human immunodeficiency virus; HSV, herpes simples virus.

Live donor evaluation checklist
History (look for/ask about)
Hypertension
Diabetes
Nonsteroidal anti-inflammatory inhibitors/medications/herbs
Family history
Intravenus drug abuse
Infections
Vascular
Vocation/avocation
Willingness to donate
Physical Exam (evaluate/look for)
Blood pressure
Weight/height
Arthritis
Autoimmunity
Cancer
Prostate
Breast
Colorectal
Lymph node
Skin
Cardiovascular disease
Laboratory
Urinalysis
Electrolytes, liver panel
Fasting blood glucose and lipid profile
Complete blood count with platelets, coagulation screen
24-hour urine, creatinine clearance, protein excretion or glomerular filtration rate measurement (iothalamate clearance), and protein determination
Antiviral screening: HCV, HBV, HIV, EBV, CMV, HSV
Purified protein derivative test (PPD; controversial in nonendemic areas), rapid plasmin reagin tests
Electrocardiogram, chest radiograph
PAP smear, prostate examination
Age/family history determined
Exercise tolerance test, echocardiography
Colonoscopy, ultrasonography
Mammography/prostate-specific antigen
Anatomic Evaluation per the Local Expertise
Computed tomography angiography
Magnetic resonance imaging angiography
Arteriography

Reproduced with permission from: Newstead and Davis (2007).

The work-up for a prospective donor with a prior episode of nephrolithiasis should include:
- serum calcium;
- serum creatinine;
- serum albumin;
- serum parathyroid hormone;
- urinalysis;
- urine culture;
- spot urine for cystine;
- 24 h urine for oxalate and creatinine;

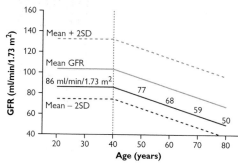

Fig. 14.2.1 Minimum acceptable age-associated GFR in living donor candidates. Black solid line shows the variation with age of mean GFR. The outer dashed lines show the ±2 population standard deviation limits. GFR is constant up to the age of 40 years and then declines at the rate of 9 mL/min/1.73 m^2 per decade. The grey line shows the safety limit of 86 mL/min/1.73 m^2 for young adults declining to 50 mL/min/1.73 m^2 at age 80 years. For transplant donors with preoperative GFR values above the grey line the GFR of the remaining kidney will still be >37.5 mL/min/1.73 m^2 at age 80 years.

- chemical analysis of the stone if available;
- a helical CT scan of the kidneys.

Malignancy

A past history of the following malignancies precludes live kidney donation:
- bronchial cancer;
- testicular cancer;
- renal cell carcinoma;
- choriocarcinoma;
- hematological malignancy;
- breast cancer;
- melanoma;
- monoclonal gammopathy.

A previous history of malignancy may not always preclude donation if the specific cancer is curable and the risk of transmission of the cancer thought to be acceptably low.

A donor with a successfully treated malignancy should only be accepted for donation if prior treatment did not decrease renal reserve or place the donor at increased risk for ESRD nor increase the risk of nephrectomy.

Uncontrolled Infections

A living donor should not be accepted when:
- there is a transmissible untreatable active infection;
- nephrotoxic treatment is required;
- the donor is at risk of developing renal disease from either the infection or the treatment.

Venous thromboembolism

Previous thromboembolism is a relative contraindication to live donation, and requires an assessment of the likelihood of recurrence.

Oral contraceptives and hormone replacement therapy increase the risk for postoperative venous thrombosis and should be withheld for at least 1 month prior to surgery.

Renovascular disease

Fibromuscular dysplasia where severe and diffuse precludes donation.

If present the donor must be normotensive, have normal renal function and have only unilateral disease.

Atherosclerotic renal vascular disease is a strong relative contraindication for living donation.

Careful investigation for occult coronary disease and peripheral vascular disease should be undertaken given their association with renal vascular disease.

Isolated hematuria

Isolated hematuria in a prospective donor is a relatively common problem.

The differential diagnosis includes:
- thin basement membrane nephropathy;
- IgA nephropathy;
- other glomerulonephritis;
- urinary tract infection;
- malignancy;
- nephrolithiasis.

A diagnosis needs to be established in the usual way.

Prospective donors with hematuria and thin basement membrane disease should only be considered when aged >50 years with a normal GFR.

IgA nephropathy is a contraindication to live donation. Isolated mesangial IgA deposition without proteinuria or impaired GFR may be not be a contraindication to donation. Any decision should be decided upon in the context of family history, GFR, the presence of interstitial disease, and age.

In a small numbers of caes despite full investigation no cause for isolated haematuria is found. Most units would accept such individuals for donation.

Further reading

Delmonico FL. A report of the Amsterdam forum on the care of the live kidney donor: data and medical guidelines. *Transplantation* 2005; **79**: S53–66.

Fehrman-Ekholm I, Elinder CG, Stenbeck M, Tyden G, Groth CG. Kidney donors live longer. *Transplantation* 1997; **64**: 976–978.

Jordan JC, Sann U, Janton A, et al. Living kidney donors' long-term psychological status and health behavior after nephrectomy – a retrospective study. *J Nephrol* 2004; **17**: 728–735.

Koushik R, Garvey C, Manivel JC, Matas AJ, Kasiske BL. Persistent, asymptomatic, microscopic hematuria in prospective kidney donors. *Transplantation* 2005; **80**: 1425–1429.

Newstead CG, Davis CL. Evaluation and preoperative management of kidney transplant recipient and donor. In: Feehally J, Floege J, Johnson RJ (eds), *Comprehensive clinical nephrology*, 3rd edn. Amsterdam: Elsevier; 2007. p. 1056.

Internet resources

British Transplantation Society:

`http://www.bts.org`

American Society of Transplantation:

`http://www.a-s-t.org/`

American Society of Transplant Surgeons:

`http://www.asts.org/`

See also

Selection and preparation of recipients, p. 544

Transplant surgery and surgical complications

Introduction

Renal transplantation is well-established as the best treatment for restoring quality and quantity of life to patients with ESRD. Although essentially comprising three anastomoses, the surgery can be challenging, particularly in the case of obese patients and complex graft anatomy. The inherently poor premorbid state of the recipients and the need for postoperative immunosuppression increases the risk of infection and bleeding. Although mostly rare, clinicians should be aware of the potential immediate complications of renal transplant surgery. A number require a high index of suspicion to identify and may result in graft loss if the diagnosis is delayed or missed.

Living donor nephrectomy

Over recent years, living donor renal transplantation has increasingly been used to offset the shortage of cadaveric kidneys. The safety of the procedure has been confirmed, and the improved outcome for the recipient over cadaveric grafts proven. However, controversy still remains about the optimal technique for removing the kidney. The options are as follows:

- Total laparoscopic donor nephrectomy (LDN);
- Hand-assisted laparoscopic donor nephrectomy (HALDN);
- Retroperitoneoscopic donor nephrectomy (RDN);
- Mini-incision open donor nephrectomy (MODN);
- Open donor nephrectomy (ODN).

Total laparoscopic donor nephrectomy

This involves dissection via 4–5 laparoscopic ports and removal of the kidney through a 6 cm Pfannansteil or lower midline incision.

Advantages

- Reduced post-operative pain and analgesia requirements compared to MODN and ODN.
- Quicker resumption of normal activities compared to MODN and ODN.
- Better cosmesis compared to MODN and ODN (Fig. 14.3.1).
- Better post-operative respiratory function compared to MODN and ODN.

Disadvantages

- Technically challenging procedure with a steep learning curve.
- Increased warm ischemic time compared to MODN and ODN.
- Increased operating time compared to MODN and ODN.
- Potentially increased risk of bowel injury and intra-abdominal adhesions compared to retroperitoneal approaches.

Hand-assisted laparoscopic donor nephrectomy

This is similar to LDN, but one port is a hand port, allowing placement of a hand within the peritoneal cavity. This allows tactile feedback and manual assistance with retraction and control of bleeding.

Advantages

- As for LDN.
- Shorter learning curve than LDN.

- Easier control of major bleeding than LDN.

Disadvantages

- As for LDN.
- Increased cost of consumables compared to LDN.

Retroperitoneoscopic donor nephrectomy

This technique involves approaching the kidney via the retroperitoneal space. The dissection is performed via laparoscopic ports and the kidney removed through a small flank incision. It can also be performed using a hand-assisted technique.

Advantages

- As for LDN.
- Shorter operating times than LDN.
- The peritoneal cavity is not entered, reducing the risk of bowel injury and adhesion formation compared to LDN.

Disadvantages

- Technically challenging procedure with a steep learning curve.
- Increased warm ischemic time compared to MODN and ODN.
- Increased operating time compared to MODN and ODN.
- Smaller working space than LDN.

Mini-incision open donor nephrectomy

This is similar to the traditional open procedure, but is performed through a smaller flank incision without rib resection.

Advantages

- Less painful than ODN.
- Better cosmesis than ODN.
- Shorter warm ischemic times than LDH, HALDN and RDN.

Disadvantages

- More painful and slower recovery than LDN, HALDN and RDN.
- Difficult access compared to ODN.
- May not be feasible in patients with higher BMI.

Open donor nephrectomy

This is performed through a flank incision, with or without resection of the 12th rib. The dissection is performed in the retroperitoneal space.

Advantages

- Least technically demanding of the various approaches.
- Allows easier control of major bleeding.
- No breach of the peritoneal cavity.
- Shortest warm ischemic time.

Disadvantages

- More post-operative pain and analgesia requirements than other techniques.
- Slower return to normal activities than other techniques.
- Risk of significant wound bulge due to paralysis of flank muscles.

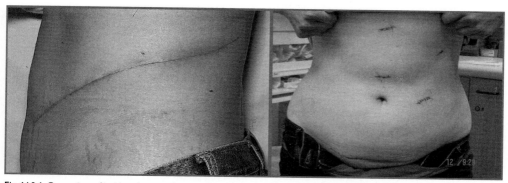

Fig. 14.3.1 Comparison of incisions for open donor nephrectomy and total laparoscopic donor nephrectomy.

Complications

Regardless of the surgical approach there are a number of potential complications of donor nephrectomy that clinicians should be aware of. These include:

- major post-operative bleeding, usually from the renal vessel stumps;
- deep vein thrombosis and/or pulmonary embolism;
- renal impairment;
- atelectasis and/or pneumonia.

Post-operative management is tailored to reduce the risk of these complications and includes:

- low molecular weight heparin;
- IV fluid to maintain urine output >50 mL/h;
- close monitoring of FBC and renal function;
- early mobilization.

Follow-up

Donors should be seen 4–6 weeks post-surgery for wound review and assessment of blood pressure and proteinuria.

Some centres also repeat an isotope GFR at this stage, but this is not mandatory.

All being well, follow-up should then be on a yearly basis. This should include measurement of blood pressure, renal function and urine dipstick, particularly looking for proteinuria.

Long-term sequelae

Following the initial decline in GFR, the rate of loss of renal function in kidney donors is no faster than expected with normal aging.

Overall, the risk of ESRD is ~0.2–0.5%.

Kidney donation does result in a small increase in urinary protein excretion secondary to hyperfiltration in the remaining kidney.

There is an increased risk of hypertension, with a mean increase of 5 mmHg compared with control groups.

The overall risk of long-term mortality among kidney donors is infact lower than the predicted age- and sex-matched mortality.

The transplant operation

Pre-operative preparation

The need for pre-operative dialysis is determined by the patient's fluid status and serum electrolytes, particularly potassium.

If fluid is removed, the patient should be maintained above their target weight to facilitate adequate postoperative fluid filling.

Consideration should be made of the likelihood of primary graft function, as this may affect the decision to dialyse.

Immunosuppression is commonly commenced preoperatively, usually in the form of an IL-2 receptor antibody.

Incision

An oblique or curvilinear incision is made from above the symphysis pubis towards the anterior superior iliac spine.

The decision concerning which groin is used varies between transplant centres. Arguments for the choice of groin are:

- a left kidney is placed in the right groin and vice versa as this places the renal pelvis and ureter anteriorly and facilitates the ureteric anastomosis;
- all kidneys are placed in the right groin as the right iliac vessels are more accessible and convenient for anastomosis than the left.

In the patient with a previous failed transplant in situ, the kidney is placed in the contralateral groin.

The muscles of the anterior abdominal wall are divided and the retroperitoneal space developed to expose the iliac vessels.

Vascular anastomoses

Renal vein

The renal vein is anastomosed end-to-side to the external iliac vein. If the renal vein is short this anastomosis may be facilitated by dividing the internal iliac vein, increasing the mobility of the external iliac vein

Renal artery

The renal artery is anastomosed to either the internal or external iliac artery.

Cadaveric kidneys with an aortic patch are conventionally anastomosed end-to-side to the external iliac artery (Fig. 14.3.2).

Live-donor kidneys, which do not have an aortic patch, are conventionally anastomosed end-to-end to the internal iliac artery (Fig. 14.3.3). However, an aortic punch may be used to create a circular arteriotomy in the external iliac artery, and an end-to-side anastomosis created.

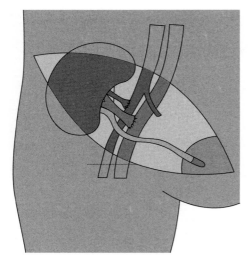

Fig. 14.3.2 End-to-side anastomosis between the renal artery and external iliac artery.

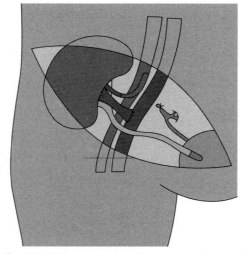

Fig. 14.3.3 End-to-end anastomosis between the renal artery and internal iliac artery.

Ureteric anastomoses

The transplant ureter is usually anastomosed directly onto the recipient's bladder.

A JJ stent may be placed in the transplant ureter to protect the anastomosis and prevent hydronephrosis; this is usually removed cystoscopically after 4 weeks.

A urethral catheter remains *in situ* for ≥5 days postoperatively.

If the transplant ureter is too short to anastomose to the bladder without tension, it may be anastomosed to the donor's ipsilateral native ureter. This is termed an uretero-ureterostomy.

Intra-operative fluid and drugs

Central venous pressure should be maintained >10 mmHg.

Mean arterial pressure should be maintained >90 mmHg.

Methylprednisolone and prophylactic antibiotics (e.g. co-amoxiclav or a cephalosporin) are given at induction of anesthesia.

Mannitol may be given immediately before clamp release to protect against renal cortical ischemia, and has been shown to reduce postoperative dialysis requirements.

Loop diuretics and dopamine are commonly used, but have not been shown to have any benefit on post-operative renal function.

Surgical complications

Bleeding

Early postoperative bleeding usually occurs in the first 24–48 h after surgery.

It is rarely due to bleeding from the vascular anastomoses, but may be from small hilar vessels damaged during the preparation of the graft.

Clinical features include a fall in hemoglobin, increased drain output, swelling at the operative site and blood seepage from the wound.

Ultrasound or CT examination may reveal a hematoma around the graft.

Treatment includes correction of any clotting abnormalities, blood transfusion and, if necessary, surgical exploration.

Wound infection

The use of prophylactic antibiotics has reduced the incidence of wound infection post-renal transplant to <1%.

If a wound infection does occur, treatment is with antibiotics and drainage of any collections as required.

Vascular thrombosis

This usually occurs within the first 48–72 h post-transplant.

Incidence is between 0.5 and 10%.

The risk of vascular thrombosis is reduced by the administration of post-operative aspirin, continued for 6–12 weeks post-surgery.

Renal transplant arterial thrombosis

Renal transplant arterial thrombosis is usually due to a technical error during procurement or transplantation, such as an intimal injury to either the renal or iliac arteries.

It is heralded by a sudden fall in urine output to zero.

Obviously, the diagnosis is harder to make in patients with good urine output from their native kidneys, or those with nonfunctioning grafts.

For this reason patients with delayed graft function should undergo regular USS examination with Doppler studies.

The treatment of arterial thrombosis is prompt surgery, and the advantage of diagnostic USS should be weighed against the risk of delaying treatment. Unfortunately the majority of grafts with arterial thrombosis are lost.

Renal transplant venous thrombosis
Renal transplant venous thrombosis is marked by:
- a fall in urine output;
- gross hematuria;
- graft swelling associated with pain.

Ultrasound examination shows:
- absent flow in the renal vein;
- reversal of arterial blood flow in diastole;
- peri-transplant hematoma due to capsular rupture.

Treatment is surgical and usually involves removal of the kidney and revision of the venous anastomosis.

Ureteric leak
This usually occurs due to necrosis of the distal transplant ureter or a technical problem with the ureteric anastomosis.

Clinical features of a urine leak from the ureteric anastomosis include:
- a fall in urine output;
- a rise or plateau in serum creatinine;
- pain and swelling at the operative site;
- increased drain output.

If a drain is *in situ* the diagnosis can be aided by sending drain fluid and urine for comparative biochemical analysis.

Ultrasound may show a peritransplant collection, which can be aspirated and sent for biochemical analysis.

If there is doubt about the diagnosis, a cystogram may demonstrate the site of the leak.

Treatment is prompt surgical repair of the leak.

Urinary tract obstruction
This diagnosis should be considered in grafts that initially produce urine and then urine output reduces or stops.

A common cause is blockage of the urethral catheter with clots, which can be solved by gentle irrigation of the catheter.

Obstruction of the transplant ureter is diagnosed by hydronephrosis on USS.

Early post-transplant this may be caused by blood or oedema, but this is rare with a JJ stent *in situ*.

Once the JJ stent has been removed, obstruction is usually due to an anastomotic stricture.

Initial treatment of ureteric obstruction is percutaneous insertion of a nephrostomy tube. This is followed by a nephrostogram to identify the site of the obstruction.

Ureteric anastomotic strictures may be treated radiologically, but long strictures often require surgery.

Lymphocele
A lymphocele is a collection of lymph at the operative site.

The incidence is 1–10% and may be reduced by the use of silk ligatures when dividing the lymphatics overlying the iliac vessels.

Presentation may be with:
- ureteric obstruction;
- deep vein thrombosis or leg swelling due to obstruction;
- swelling at the operative site.

Diagnosis is by USS examination, aspiration will reveal clear fluid with a high protein content.

Treatment depends on the size and presence of compressive complications and includes:
- aspiration;
- percutaneous drainage;
- drainage into the peritoneal cavity (can be done laparoscopically).

Further reading
Allen R, Chapman J. *A manual of renal transplantation.* London: Hodder Arnold; 1994.

Danovitch GM (ed.), *Handbook of kidney transplantation.* Philadelphia: Lippincott Williams & Wilkins, 2004.

Kahan BD, Ponticelli C (eds), *Principles and practice of renal transplantation.* London: Taylor & Francis; 2000.

Kuo PC, Bollinger RR, Dafoe DC, Davis RD (eds), *Comprehensive atlas of transplantation.* Philadelphia: Lippincott Williams & Wilkins; 2004.

Morris PJ. *Kidney transplantation.* Philadelphia: WB Saunders; 2001.

Tan HP, Marcos A, Shapiro R (eds), *Living donor transplantation.* New York: Informa Healthcare; 2007.

Internet resources
British Transplantation Society:

www.bts.org.uk

The Kidney Patient Guide:

www.kidneypatientguide.org.uk/site/transplants.php

American Society of Transplantation:

http://www.a-s-t.org/

American Society of Transplant Surgeons:

http://www.asts.org/

Laparoscopic live donor nephrectomy at the John Hopkins Medical Institute:

http://urology.jhu.edu/surgical_techniques/nephrectomy/index.html

See also
Early management of transplant recipients, p. 556

Recurrent disease and *de novo* disease post renal transplantation, p. 566

Drug-induced nephropathies, p. 698

Early management of transplant recipients

The first 48 hours

In the early period post surgery, frequent monitoring is critical in order to maintain appropriate fluid balance.

There is a small risk of hemorrhage that is common to all surgery.

Massive diuresis resulting in hypovolemia is a risk particular to renal transplant surgery.

As in any patient with ESRD there is also the significant risk that overaggressive fluid replacement can result in pulmonary edema and/or severe hypertension when the patient is oligo- or anuric.

Monitoring and prophylaxis

Frequent CVP monitoring, FBC, U+Es and monitoring of fluid balance is part of standard care.

Routine antibiotic prophylaxis should be prescribed for 48 h.

Routine heparin prophylaxis against deep vein thrombosis should be started.

In the immediate postoperative period some centers also routinely use:
- dopamine;
- mannitol;
- IV furosemide.

The intention is to reduce the rate of delayed graft function (DGF); there is no evidence base to justify the practice.

Blood transfusion

Well-compensated patients with ESRD without access to erythropoetin will often have tolerated a hemoglobin <7.5 g/dL for many months.

Transfusion may be appropriate if there is a fall in hemoglobin of >2.0 g/dL.

Patients with known or high risk of ischemic heart disease should be transfused to maintain a hemoglobin of ~10.0 g/dL.

Dialysis

Dialysis support is required for ~1/3 of patients in the post-transplant period.

Hyperkalemia that cannot be controlled by medical therapy is the most common indication.

If the patient is oligoanuric medical therapy will only achieve temporary control of hyperkalemia.

Peritoneal dialysis conventionally using low volume exchanges may be used post surgery although sometimes wound leakage of PD fluid due to surgical transgression of the peritoneum makes this impractical.

If urgent control of blood chemistry is required, as is often the case, then hemodialysis is the best treatment.

Complications in the first 48 hours

Oligoanuria

The majority of patients pass urine post surgery and this greatly simplifies management. However, some patients are oligoanuric from the outset. A third subgroup passes dilute urine with no or very little evidence of clearance of urea or creatinine and this group often becomes anuric between 10 and 20 h post procedure.

Where the patient is oliguric it is important to establish the cause of graft dysfunction.

A renal USS should be performed. This can usually reliably rule out significant urinary tract obstruction and confirm renal perfusion.

If the graft is obstructed then either re-exploration, further investigation with an isotope renogram or the placement of a nephrostomy is necessary.

Arterial thrombosis, which is usually asymptomatic, is almost never retrievable. Venous thrombosis, which is often associated with more periwound pain than is usual, can on occasion be treated with thrombectomy resulting in salvage of the graft.

If the USS confidently confirms absence or greatly compromised perfusion, urgent surgical exploration is preferred to further imaging such as an MRI, as any delay will have a serious negative impact on graft survival.

Urine leak

An early urinary leak is a rare complication. There will be a high volume of fluid in wound drains or an obvious wound leak of urine.

It may be necessary to measure the potassium and urea concentration in fluid to establish the diagnosis.

It is even rarer for a urinary leak to pass into the peritoneal cavity. The urine is then absorbed, making it very difficult to diagnose early, as usually the USS is normal. If this is suspected then an isotope scan should be performed with late films to show urine passage into the peritoneal cavity.

Rejection

When there is early graft dysfunction with unremarkable USS appearances the diagnosis of rejection needs to be considered. To make this diagnosis securely requires a biopsy and then prompt analysis of the histology.

Acute cellular rejection takes several days to cause graft dysfunction. Humoral rejection due to donor-directed antibodies that develop post grafting takes a similar interval to develop.

Only humoral rejection due to donor-directed antibodies that were present prior to implantation can cause rejection in the first 48 h.

At the inception of transplantation and before identification of these antibodies was possible, they were the cause of the hyperacute graft rejection that occurred very soon after reperfusion.

With modern crossmatch techniques and molecular HLA typing to ensure that patients are not transplanted with a kidney to which they have a known preformed antibody, the likelihood of humoral rejection is very small.

The important exception to this rule is when the transplant is performed in the presence of a known donor relevant antibody.

This is an increasingly common practice in the live donor setting when recipient preconditioning with plasma exchange usually in tandem with other strategies can achieve a situation that avoids hyperacute rejection but leaves the patient at risk of early accelerated humoral rejection.

Prophylactic plasma exchange is part of the routine management but it is almost never used before the third day post transplant.

In practice clinicians make a judgement of the likelihood that early graft dysfunction is due either to acute rejection or to acute tubular necrosis (ATN) based on the risk factors for the two scenarios.

The risk of delayed graft function due to ATN is more common where there is prolonged cold ischemia, a kidney from a nonheart-beating donor, or where there was donor renal impairment.

Ileus
Prolonged ileus is unusual but more common in patients with diabetes and if present IV medication is necessary.

Two to ten days post transplant

Monitoring and prophylaxis
During this interval the need for intensive monitoring of fluid balance is greatly decreased and CVP, peripheral lines, urinary catheter and wound drains are removed. Daily weighing to assess changes in fluid status is necessary.

In common with all abdominal surgical procedures there is a risk of pulmonary embolism, as well as wound and chest infections. In patients who have been treated with peritoneal dialysis there is also a small risk of peritonitis.

During this interval the majority of patients with delayed graft function due to presumed ATN will have a steadily increasing urine volume but a useful clearance of ~5 mL/min is rare until urinary volume >1 L in 24 h.

During this period, antimicrobial prophylaxis against *Pneumocysitis jiroveci* as well as cytomegalovirus should be started (if not already in place).

Immunosuppressants
During this time immunosuppressive dose adjustment is usually required, typically guided by thrice-weekly measurement of calcineurin levels.

Dose adjustment of antimetabolites and antilymphocyte preparations may be necessary, principally dictated by the leukocyte count, and sometimes anemia or thrombocytopenia.

Measurement of therapeutic drug levels apart from tacrolimus, ciclosporin and sirolimus is not routine but used principally in the research setting, in some units.

Complications

Delayed graft function
If the patient has protracted DGF it is important not to miss:

- occult acute rejection;
- urinary obstruction;
- urinary leak;
- renal arterial or venous compromise.

Although there are factors which predict ATN it is important to appreciate that acute cellular rejection is more common in grafts with ATN than in those with primary function.

A graft biopsy is the only way to make a confident diagnosis of rejection and to discriminate between the types of rejection.

When there is DGF, renal transplant biopsies at 5–7 day intervals are usual practice in order to ensure that acute cellular rejection is not missed.

Some units advocate 'protocol' biopsies even in patients with good graft function at, say, day 7 and at other intervals post surgery in the hope that treatment of clinically asymptomatic acute cellular rejection will improve long-term outcome.

Patient education
Patient education should be a major focus of care during this interval. The patient needs to understand completely new rules about fluid management as well as relaxation of any dietary restrictions.

It is often difficult for patients to absorb the changes in advice. A particularly critical issue is to ensure that patients understand and are capable of adhering to the complex medication regimens. The importance of medication concordance on graft survival should be emphasized.

Patients also need to be educated about the side-effect profile of drugs as well as symptoms of urinary tract infection and graft dysfunction.

Education about lifestyle choices that influence cardiovascular disease as well as the risk of cutaneous squamous cell carcinomas (common) and other malignancies can be conveniently made part of the predischarge education 'package'.

Two weeks to six months post transplantation

Monitoring
Outpatient follow-up during the early postdischarge period should be frequent because of the need to promptly diagnose acute graft dysfunction.

It is rare for acute graft dysfunction to be symptomatic so there is no substitute for regular measurement of serum creatinine and immunosuppressive drug levels.

Figure 14.4.1 shows the risk of acute rejection and how that changes with time. It is notable that:

- rejection is almost never diagnosed before 5 days post transplantation;
- virtually all episodes of acute rejection occur within the first 3 months;
- 93% of episodes of acute rejection occur within 1 month.

Therefore follow-up for the purpose of diagnosing occult acute rejection needs to be frequent in the first month (thrice weekly in many units) but can be much less frequent once the recipient is >3 months post surgery.

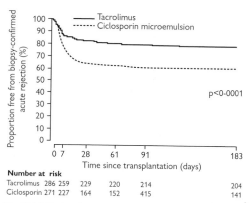

Number at risk						
Tacrolimus	286	259	229	220	214	204
Ciclosporin	271	227	164	152	415	141

Fig. 14.4.1 Timing of acute rejection post renal transplantation. (From: Margreiter et al., 2002.)

Immunosuppressants

Frequent follow-up also allows adjustment of immunosuppressive medication which is often necessary in the early period.

During this period there is usually adjustment to reduce the level of immunosuppressive therapy, in part because the risk of acute rejection decreases markedly with time but also to reduce that component of the risk of premature cardiovascular and late malignant disease that is attributable to drug therapy.

Complications

Acute graft dysfunction

Acute graft dysfunction should be investigated first by measurement of immunosuppressive drug levels as these drugs can be nephrotoxic.

A renal USS should be performed to rule out urinary obstruction. This can be secondary to the development of a significant perirenal lymphocele.

Further radiology such as as nephrostomy, isotope scans or arterial imaging for suspected renal artery stenosis may be directed by the USS appearances.

Most commonly, however, a renal biopsy needs to be performed.

In some cases staining for Simian BK virus/CMV or C4d antibodies will be indicated.

In the relatively rare situation where early recurrent glomerulonephritis is in the differential diagnosis then immunohistochemistry and electron microscopy need to be performed.

Infectious complications

Infectious complications of renal transplantation approximately follow the timetable as shown in Table 14.4.1. This information allows the initial diagnostic tests to be directed towards the most likely pathogens.

When managing an immunosuppressed patient who is unwell with what is probably an infection it is standard practice to take all appropriate specimens but then instigate treatment directed at the most likely pathogens while awaiting the results of the investigations.

Patient education

As well as lifestyle advice, especially smoking cessation and control of hyperlipidemia, the most important cardiovascular risk factor to control is hypertension.

Hypertension also significantly influences renal transplant survival.

Further reading

Amend WJC, Vincenti F, Tomlanovich. The first three posttransplant months. In: Danovitch G.M (ed.), *Handbook of kidney transplantation*, 4th edn. Philadelphia: Lippincott Willliams & Wilkins; 2005. pp. 212–233.

Kauffmann HM. Post-transplant de novo malignancies in renal transplant recipients: the past and present. *Transplant Int* 2006; **19**: 607–620.

Kotton CN, Fishman JA. Viral infection in the renal transplant recipient. *J Am Soc Nephrol* 2005; **16**: 1758–1774.

Margreiter R; European Tacrolimus vs Ciclosporin Microemulsion Renal Transplantation Study Group. Efficacy and safety of tacrolimus compared with ciclosporin microemulsion in renal transplantation: a randomized multicentre study. *Lancet* 2002; **359**(9308): 741–746.

Singer J, Gritsh HA, Rosenthal KR. The transplant operation and its surgical complications. In: Danovitch G.M (ed.), *Handbook of kidney transplantation*, 4th edn. Philadelphia: Lippincott Willliams & Wilkins; 2005. pp. 193–211.

Table 14.4.1 Approximate timetable of infections after renal transplantation

Time scale	Site of infection and common organisms
0–7 days	Chest infection
	Wound infection
	Line-associated sepsis
7–30 days	Urinary tract Infection
	Peritoneal dialysis peritonitis
	Herpes simplex (cutaneous and encephalitis)
	Clostridium difficile
	Candidiasis
30–180 days	Cytomegalovirus
	Primary CMV:
	• in absence of prophylaxis: 6 weeks
	• 2–8 weeks after completion of prophylaxis
	CMV reinfection/reactivation: 12 weeks
	Legionella pneumoniae
	Mycobacterium tuberculosis
	Pneumocystis jiroveci
	Nocardia spp.[a]
	Cryptococcus spp.[a]
	Toxoplasma spp.[a]
	Strongyloides spp.[a]
	Listeria spp.[a]
>180 days	Influenza/pneumococcus and other community-acquired viral and bacterial infections
	Varicella zoster virus reactivation
	Pneumocystis jiroveci
	Psitticosis spp.
	Listeria spp.
	Mycobacterium tuberculosis

[a] Less common or geographically limited infections.

Thaunat O, *et al.* To biopsy or not to biopsy? Should we screen the histology of stable renal grafts? *Transplantation* 2007; **84**: 671–676.

Internet resources

British Transplantation Society:

http://www.bts.org

American Society of Transplantation:

http://www.a-s-t.org/

American Society of Transplant Surgeons:

http://www.asts.org/

See also

Transplant surgery and surgical complications, p. 552

Immunosuppression for renal transplantation, p. 560

Recurrent disease and *de novo* disease post renal transplantation, p. 566

Drug-induced nephropathies, p. XXX

Clinical approach to acute kidney injury, p. 318

Renal replacement therapies in acute kidney injury, p. 328

Immunosuppression for renal transplantation

Introduction

The number of immunosuppressive agents available for use in renal transplantation has increased in the last 20 years.

In September 2004, the National Institute for Health and Clinical Excellence (NICE) published its guidance on the use of immunosuppressive therapy in adults following renal transplantation (NICE Technology Appraisal 85).

Randomized controlled trials (RCTs) comparing different agents have nearly all been funded by pharmaceutical companies with commercial interests and have had a number of shortcomings.

These have included:

- use of licensed rather than real-life dosing regimens;
- short-term follow-up only;
- inadequate power to detect statistical differences in patient and graft survival;
- until recently the use of acute rejection rates as the primary endpoint rather than allograft function.

Immunosuppressive regimens therefore have evolved within transplant centers based on local experience and need.

Although there is no consensus on the best regimen to use, the general principles are:

- to match the amount of immunosuppression with the perceived immunological risk;
- to use high doses in the early part of transplantation (induction) with phased reduction and even withdrawal of some agents thereafter (maintenance);
- to 'tailor' the type of agent with the patient's specific needs, e.g. cosmetic considerations.

All regimens are still based around the use of calcineurin inhibitors.

Individual drugs can be considered under two broad headings:

- 'Biological' agents: monoclonal or polyclonal antibodies used as induction therapy or to treat severe acute rejection.
- Agents used for maintenance immunosuppression:
  - calcineurin inhibitors (CNIs);
  - anti-proliferative agents;
  - corticosteroids.

Biological agents

Antithymocyte globulin (ATG)

A polyclonal antibody derived from rabbits with activity against human lymphocytes, particularly a number of T-cell markers.

Administration results in depletion of peripheral blood lymphocytes that are either lysed or cleared by the reticuloendothelial system.

In most UK centres its use is reserved for the treatment of steroid-resistant acute rejection although in the USA it is also used as induction therapy at the time of transplantation to prevent rejection.

It should be administered into a central vein (or fast-flowing vein such as an AVF) to avoid thrombophlebitis.

Side-effects relate largely to allergic reactions including chills, fevers, arthralgia and rarely anaphylaxis. These can be minimized by giving IV methylprednisolone and an antihistamine 30 min before use.

Thrombocytopenia and leukopenia are common.

Although fixed daily dosing regimens may be used, many clinicians dose according to total lymphocyte or CD3 count to avoid over-immunosuppression.

CMV and *Pneumocystis jiroveci (carinii)* prophylaxis should be considered mandatory, because of the increased risk of infections.

The use of ATG is associated with an increased incidence of post-transplant lymphoproliferative disease (PTLD).

OKT3 (Muromonab–CD3)

OKT3 is a mouse monoclonal IgG2a antibody that reacts with the T-cell receptor–CD3 complex chain of the T-lymphocyte on the surface of circulating human T-cells.

Deactivation of the CD3 complex causes the T-cell receptor to undergo endocytosis and the ineffectual T-cell is cleared by the reticuloendothelial system.

In the UK, OKT3 use tends to be restricted to the treatment of steroid-resistant rejection when ATG has failed or is contraindicated.

In the USA it has been used as induction therapy.

Potentially life-threatening side-effects including noncardiogenic pulmonary edema may occur during the first few days of treatment due to release of T-cell-derived cytokines (cytokine release syndrome). Its use therefore, is contraindicated in volume-overloaded patients. A sensible precaution is to dialyze/ultrafilter all patients to their target weight (or below) before its use.

Intravenous methylprednisolone, an antihistamine and oral paracetamol are given 15–60 min before the first and second doses.

Nearly all patients develop fever and rigors which usually abate after the third dose and can be treated with oral paracetamol.

Neurological side-effects are also common and self-limiting and range in severity from a mild headache to aseptic meningitis and encephalopathy.

Once again, CMV and *Pneumocystis jiroveci (carinii)* prophylaxis should be considered mandatory.

The use of OKT3 is associated with an increased incidence of post-transplant lymphoproliferative disease (PTLD).

With repeated use, antimouse antibodies may develop. For this reason, when a second course of OKT3 is used, monitoring of CD3⁺ cells is recommended to ensure that adequate depletion is being achieved.

Humanized anti-CD25 monoclonal antibodies

Basiliximab (Simulect)

Daclizumab (Zenapax)

These monoclonal antibodies are directed against the α chain (CD25) of the IL-2 receptor on activated T-cells.

As such they are used together with CNIs to prevent (but not treat) acute rejection.

Although derived from mouse, both monoclonal antibodies have been genetically engineered such that a large proportion of the antibody is replaced by human IgG.

Strictly speaking, basiliximab is a chimeric (xi) antibody (75% human, 25% mouse) whereas baclizumab is a humanized (zu) antibody (90% human, 10% mouse).

Both are of low immunogenicity and do not induce a significant human antimouse antibody response when administered.

Therefore first-dose reactions are rare and both have long half-lives.

Because basiliximab has a greater affinity for the IL-2 receptor, a less intense dosing regimen is required compared with daclizumab.

Despite increasing the early immunosuppressive burden, an increased incidence of opportunistic infections or PTLD over the control groups was not observed in the phase 3 studies which led to their clinical introduction.

Campath-1H (Alemtuzumab)

Campath-1H is an anti-CD52 humanized monoclonal antibody developed in the Cambridge Pathology Laboratories and licensed as a treatment for chronic lymphocytic leukemia.

When used off-label in transplantation, it results in profound and long-lasting lymphocyte depletion that may take many months to return to pretransplant levels.

It is used most commonly as induction therapy as part of a steroid-free low-dose maintenance immunosuppression regimen.

However, few long-term RCTs have been performed and its exact place as an immunosuppressive agent has yet to be determined.

Rituximab

Rituximab is a chimeric (mouse/human) monoclonal antibody directed against the CD20 antigen expressed on B lymphocytes.

Its use results in rapid and sustained depletion of both circulating and tissue-based B-cells.

Originally developed for the treatment of non-Hodgkin lymphoma, its use has been extended to a number of presumed B-cell-mediated autoimmune conditions.

In transplantation it has been used in a variety of ways, most notably in plasma exchange/immunoadsorption regimens to remove and prevent resynthesis of preformed antibodies in HLA- or ABO-incompatible living donor transplantation.

It has also been used to treat antibody-associated acute rejection as well as PTLD when CD20 is expressed.

Belatacept (LEA29Y or CTLA-4-Ig)

For an optimal and sustained T-cell response both antigen recognition by the T-cell receptor (signal 1) and costimulatory signals (signal 2) delivered through accessory T-cell surface molecules are required.

Experimental studies have suggested that interruption of costimulatory signals may lead to donor-specific graft tolerance.

Belatacept is a selective costimulation blocker that binds surface costimulatory ligands (CD80 and CD86) of antigen-presenting cells.

It is a cytotoxic T-lymphocyte antigen (CTLA)-4-Ig fusion protein homolog of CD28 which binds CD80 and CD86 with high affinity and blocks the interaction with CD28, thereby preventing full T-cell activation.

Short-term phase 2 studies have shown that belatacept when used in combination with basiliximab, mycophenolate mofetil (MMF) and corticosteroids, allows CNI avoidance with improved renal function when compared with ciclosporin-treated patients, although the incidence of acute rejection, graft and patient survival was similar between groups. Histological features of chronic allograft nephropathy were less common.

Agents used for maintenance immunosuppression

Calcineurin inhibitors

Ciclosporin A (CsA) and tacrolimus are the two major CNIs that have provided the cornerstone of maintenance immunosuppressive regimens in the modern era of solid organ transplantation.

Engagement of the T-cell receptor results in activation of calcineurin, a phosphatase that dephosphorylates a number of nuclear regulatory proteins including NFAT (nuclear factor of activated T-cells) thereby facilitating their movement into the nucleus where they upregulate the transcription of a number of important cytokines genes including IL-2, IL-4, interferon-γ (IFN-γ) and tumor necrosis factor-α.

The CNIs bind to their cytoplasmic receptor proteins (cyclophilin for CsA and FK-binding protein for tacrolimus).

The resulting complex binds to calcineurin, inhibiting its action thereby preventing T-cell activation and proliferation.

CsA is a small cyclic polypeptide (MW 1203) consisting of 11 amino acids derived from the fungus *Tolypocladium inflatum*. The most widely used preparation is a microemulsion formulation known as Neoral.

Tacrolimus is a macrolide antibiotic compound isolated from *Streptomyces tsukubaensis* (Tsukuba macrolide immunosuppressant).

Both drugs have a narrow therapeutic index; too little results in under-immunosuppression and too much in side-effects the most important of which is nephrotoxicity.

Furthermore, there is large inter- and intrapatient variation in drug metabolism and for these reasons therapeutic drug monitoring (TDM) is required with measurement of 12 h trough levels.

For Neoral, there is evidence that its 2 h postdose peak concentration (C2 level) correlates better with drug exposure than the C12 level and is used in preference in some centers.

Both agents are metabolized in the gut and liver by the cytochrome P450 IIIA system (CYP3A) found in the gastrointestinal tract and liver as well as by p-glycoprotein in gut.

The heterogeneity in intestinal CYP3A gene expression may account for some of the wide interpatient variability in drug metabolism.

Any drug that influences the CYP3A system in the gut or liver has a potential interaction with the CNIs and constant awareness is required.

Well-recognized interactions that increase CNI levels result from:

- calcium channel blockers, particularly diltiazem;
- antifungal agents such as fluconazole;
- macrolide antibiotics such as erythromycin or clarithromycin (but not azithromycin).

Interactions that reduce CNI concentration result from the use of:

- rifampicin;
- phenytoin;
- carbamazepine.

The CNIs may inhibit the metabolism of other drugs and important interactions occur with certain statins when used in full dose which may result in rhabdomyolysis.

Nephrotoxicity is the most important side-effect of both CNIs and appears to have two components.

The first is a reversible functional decrease in renal blood flow and GFR mediated by vasoconstriction of the afferent arteriole.

Long-term use is associated with chronic interstitial fibrosis which is a universal finding in longitudinal biopsy studies. Although fibrosis may be 'striped' and associated with hyaline arteriolar lesions, these are not specific features and similar findings may arise in response to a number of renal insults.

A thrombotic microangiopathy similar to HUS/TTP may rarely be observed.

Electrolyte abnormalities include hyperkalemia often associated with a hyperchloremic acidosis as in type IV RTA.

Hyperphosphaturia, hypermagnesuria and hypercalciura may all occur.

Hypertension is common, as are hyperuricemia and gout.

Cosmetic changes such as hypertrichosis and gum hyperplasia may be observed with CsA, whereas hair loss may occur with tacrolimus.

Glucose intolerance and new-onset diabetes after transplantation (NODAT) is observed with both agents, although these are commoner with tacrolimus as are neurological complications such as tremor.

By contrast, hyperlipidemia is commoner with CsA.

Corticosteroids

Corticosteroids inhibit the transcription of a number of cytokine genes including IL-1, IL-2, IL-3, IL-6, TNF-α and IFN-γ.

They act by inhibiting the translocation to the nucleus of nuclear factor-κ B (NF-κ B), an important transcription factor that regulates the expression of a large number of cytokine genes.

In addition, corticosteroids themselves translocate to the nucleus via a steroid–receptor complex which binds to glucocorticoid response elements (GREs) in the promoter region of several cytokine genes, preventing their transcription.

Corticosteroids also have nonspecific immunosuppressant and anti-inflammatory actions including inhibition of chemokines, vasodilators and blocking monocyte migration to sites of inflammation.

Although they have been part of most immunosuppressive regimens since the beginning of transplantation, their side-effects have led to new regimens that withdraw, minimize or avoid the use of these agents.

The most troublesome side-effects include:

- cosmetic changes and growth impairment, particularly in children and young adults;
- osteoporosis;

- delayed would healing and thin skin;
- glucose intolerance/NODAT;
- weight gain;
- cataracts;
- nontargeted immunosuppression resulting in increased susceptibility to infection.

Antiproliferative drugs

Azathioprine

Azathioprine is a purine analog which inhibits the synthesis of nucleotides for both DNA and RNA.

It prevents cell replication and inhibits T-cell proliferation.

Although used for many years as combination therapy with CNIs and corticosteroids, it has been largely superseded by MMF.

Its most important side-effect is generalized marrow suppression and regular monitoring of the FBC is mandatory in the first few months of therapy.

Patients with an inherited deficiency of the enzyme thiopurine methyltransferase (TPMT) metabolize azathioprine slowly. This results in rapid drug accumulation and pronounced marrow suppression with standard azathioprine doses.

Measurement of TPMT levels is recommended with dose reduction in patients with low enzyme levels.

Azathioprine is also metabolized by xanthine oxidase which is inhibited by concomitant use of allopurinol. This drug combination should therefore be avoided or used with great caution, i.e. azathioprine dose reduction to 25% of standard dose.

Other side-effects include hepatitis and cholestasis.

Mycophenolate mofetil (MMF) and mycophenolate sodium (MPS)

These are respectively the ester and sodium salt prodrugs of the active compound mycophenolic acid (MPA), a product of several *Penicillium* spp.

MPA is a reversible inhibitor of the enzyme inosine monophosphate dehydrogenase (IMPDH), a critical, rate-limiting enzyme in the *de novo* synthesis of purines.

Because lymphocytes lack the salvage pathway for purine synthesis that is present in other cell types, they are dependent on the *de novo* pathway and are therefore susceptible to its inhibition.

The antiproliferative effect of MPA is thus relatively selective for activated lymphocytes.

MPA blocks the proliferation of T- and B-lymphocytes, inhibits antibody formation and the generation of cytotoxic T-cells.

Mycophenolate mofetil and mycophenolate sodium are usually used in combination with CNIs and corticosteroids.

Mycophenolate mofetil has been shown to be more effective than azathioprine at preventing acute rejection when used in a triple therapy regimen.

Gastrointestinal side-effects are the most troublesome adverse effects, with diarrhea occurring in ~30% of patients and esophagitis and gastritis in 20%. Upper gastrointestinal hemorrhage has been observed.

Bone marrow suppression also occurs commonly and may necessitate a dose reduction.

The increased immunosuppression provided by MPA is associated with a slightly increased incidence of opportunistic infections and PTLD.

Therapeutic drug monitoring is not usually necessary.

There are few important drug interactions but MPA may increase aciclovir/ganciclovir levels by inhibiting renal tubular secretion.

Unlike azathioprine it can be used safely with allopurinol and no dose reduction is necessary.

mTOR inhibitors; sirolimus and everolimus
Sirolimus and everolimus are both inhibitors of the mammalian target of rapamycin, a key regulatory kinase that controls cell division.

Only sirolimus is licensed for use in the UK.

It is derived from a macrolide antibiotic first identified on Rapa Nui (Easter Island) and was originally called rapamycin.

Like tacrolimus, sirolimus binds to FKBP but the resultant complex inhibits mTOR blocking cytokine (IL-2)-dependent cellular (lymphocyte) proliferation at the G1–S phase of the cell cycle.

It was originally developed as combination therapy with ciclosporin and corticosteroids but was shown to potentiate the nephrotoxicity of ciclosporin.

This, together with other side-effects including delayed wound healing and lymphocele formation, has largely precluded its use as initial immunosuppression after transplantation.

Instead it has been used as switch therapy in place of a CNI after the first 3 months of transplantation.

It has also been used in regimens of CNI withdrawal.

It is metabolized mainly by the liver via both CYP3A and p-glycoprotein and therefore has a large number of drug interactions.

Therapeutic drug monitoring using a 24 h trough level is required.

In addition to lymphocele formation and delayed graft function it has a number of other side-effects that have limited its use.

These include:
- prolongation of delayed graft function;
- painful mouth ulcers;
- hyperlipidemia;
- bone marrow suppression;
- thrombotic microangiopathy;
- pneumonitis;
- rash.

It also has antiangiogenic effects (inhibits VEGF) and has been used successfully in the management of Kaposi's sarcoma when substituted for a CNI.

It may also inhibit other tumours.

Clinical use of immunosuppressant agents
Immunosuppressive regimens
Conventional regimens
These consist of:
- calcineurin inhibitor;
- corticosteroids;
- ± antiproliferative agent.

The antiproliferative agent is usually MMF in place of azathioprine.

Anti-CD25 antibody induction therapy may be included as a routine or reserved for patients at increased risk of acute rejection or delayed graft function.

Regimens that avoid, minimise or withdraw corticosteroids are becoming increasingly popular but carry risks.

Calcineurin inhibitor avoidance regimens
These are based around anti-CD25 induction, MMF and sirolimus, and have been associated with a high incidence of acute rejection and side-effects as well as worse graft function at 1 year.

CNI avoidance regimens based around belatacept use are currently more promising.

Acute cellular rejection
This is usually treated with high dose IV methylprednisolone on 3 consecutive days.

Background immunosuppression may be increased, i.e. addition of MMF if not already part of the regimen.

Steroid-resistant acute rejection
This is usually treated with ATG (occasionally OKT3).

Antibody-mediated acute rejection
This may be treated by plasma exchange ± IV immunoglobulin.

Rationale for antibody-based induction therapy
It provides rapid and profound early immunosuppression when acute rejection is most common.

In kidneys with a high risk of delayed graft function (long cold ischemia time, nonheart-beating donors etc.) it allows a delay to the introduction of CNIs (or use of reduced dose) when avoiding nephrotoxicity is particularly desirable.

Campath-1H may provide sufficient additional immunosuppression to permit corticosteroid minimization or avoidance.

ATG induction or anti-CD25 induction?
ATG induction has not been routinely adopted in UK compared with extensive use in the USA.

ATG use is associated with an increased incidence of opportunistic infections and PTLD.

Licensing studies of anti-CD25 induction showed a significant reduction in acute rejection rates with no increase in opportunistic infections or apparent adverse events compared with placebo.

A RCT of ATG (*n* = 141) versus basiliximab (*n* = 137) induction in patients at high risk of acute rejection or delayed graft function treated with CsA, MMF and prednisolone, showed a lower incidence of acute rejection in the ATG group (15.6% vs 25.5% *P* = 0.02). There was a similar incidence of delayed graft function as well as graft loss and death at 1 year. The incidence of serious adverse effects was similar between groups (3 PTLD in ATG vs 0 in basiliximab); there was a greater incidence of infection with ATG but a lower incidence of CMV disease.

Which calcineurin inhibitor?
Trials of head-to-head comparisons have been confounded by inadequate power and variable dosing regimens.

A large meta-analysis of 30 trials demonstrated a significant reduction in graft loss at 6 months in tacrolimus-treated recipients that persisted up to 3 years.

At 1 year, tacrolimus treated patients had:
- less acute rejection (RR 0.69);
- less steroid-resistant rejection (RR 0.49);
- more insulin-dependent diabetes mellitus (RR 1.86), tremor and headaches.

Ciclosporin-treated patients had more cosmetic side-effects and constipation.

There was no difference in incidence of infection or malignancy.

In a recent large RCT (ELITE–Symphony Study n = 1645), low risk patients were randomized to one of four immunosuppressive regimens. Patients receiving a low dose tacrolimus regimen (daclizumab induction, MMF and corticosteroids) had a significantly better 12 month calculated GFR than regimens based on CsA (standard dose CsA, MMF and corticosteroids or daclizumab induction, low dose CsA, MMF and corticosteroids).

Choice of CNI should also be influenced by patient characteristics:
- use tacrolimus in a dark-haired young female (avoid hypertrichosis and gum hyperplasia);
- use CsA in overweight patients with glucose intolerance (attempt to prevent development of NODAT).

Corticosteroid withdrawal, minimization and avoidance
The side-effects and morbidity associated with corticosteroid use has led to adoption of regimens that have avoided, minimized or withdrawn their use.

In 2004, 23% of US patients were discharged on steroid-free maintenance regimens.

Double-blind RCTs of corticosteroid withdrawal at 3 and 4 months in low risk patients maintained on CsA and MMF were discontinued because of an increased incidence of acute rejection in the withdrawal group (30.8 vs 9.8% and 20% vs 5% respectively).

An RCT of steroid avoidance, early steroid withdrawal (after day 7) or standard steroid therapy with basiliximab induction, CsA and MPS failed to demonstrate noninferiority in GFR at 12 months in the steroid avoidance or withdrawal groups compared with standard therapy. The incidence of acute rejection at 12 months was 36%, 29.6% and 19.3% in the avoidance, withdrawal and standard groups respectively.

Uncontrolled single center studies have demonstrated that steroid minimization regimens (used for first 7 days only) with tacrolimus and MMF are associated with excellent outcomes.

However, in an ongoing unpublished double-blind study by the Astellas Steroid Withdrawal Group, steroid minimization (used for first 7 days only) was associated with more clinical rejection and a significantly increased incidence of chronic allograft nephropathy at 4 years compared with maintenance therapy. Baseline immunosuppression was with ATG/anti-CD25 induction, tacrolimus and MMF.

In a 5 year follow-up study, low dose CsA monotherapy following Campath-1H induction demonstrated similar patient and graft survival and acute rejection rates as a retrospective contemporaneous group treated with CsA, azathioprine and prednisolone. More patients experienced late rejection (>1 year post transplant) in the Campath-1H group.

Further reading
Ahsan N, Hricik D, et al. Prednisone withdrawal in kidney transplant recipients on cyclosporine and mycophenolate mofetil – a prospective randomized study. Steroid Withdrawal Study Group. Transplantation 1999; **68**: 1865–1874.

Borrows R, Loucaidou M, et al. Steroid sparing with tacrolimus and mycophenolate mofetil in renal transplantation. Am J Transplant 2004; **4**: 1845–1851.

Brennan DC, Daller JA, et al. Rabbit antithymocyte globulin versus Basiliximab in renal transplantation. N Engl J Med 2006; **355**: 1967–1977.

Ekberg HE, Tedesco-Siva H, et al. Reduced exposure to calcineurin inhibitors in renal transplantation. N Engl J Med 2007; **357**: 2562–2575.

Vanrenterghem Y, Lebranchu Y, et al. Double-blind comparison of two corticosteroid regimens plus mycophenolate mofetil and cyclosporine for prevention of acute renal allograft rejection. Transplantation 2000; **70**: 1352–1359.

Vincenti F, Larsen C, et al. Costimulation blockade with belatacept in renal transplantation. N Engl J Med 2005; **353**: 770–781.

Vincenti F, Schena FP, et al. A randomized multicenter study of steroid avoidance, early steroid withdrawal, or standard steroid therapy in kidney transplant recipients. Am J Transplant 2008; **8**: 307–316.

Watson CJ, Bradley JA, et al. Alemtuzumab (CAMPATH 1H) induction therapy in cadaveric kidney transplantation – efficacy and safety at five years. Am J Transplant 2005; **5**: 1347–1353.

Webster AC, Woodroffe RC, et al. Tacrolimus versus ciclosporin as primary imunnosuppression for kidney transplant recipients; meta-analysis and meta-regression of randomised trial data. Br Med J 2005; **331**: 810–820.

Internet resources
Renal transplantation – immunosuppressive regimens (adults). NICE Technology Appraisal 85:

http://www.nice.org.uk/guidance/index.jsp?action=byID&o=11544

Renal transplantation – immunosuppressive regimens for children and adolescents. NICE Technology Appraisal 99:

http://www.nice.org.uk/guidance/index.jsp?action=byID&o=11576

British Transplantation Society Guidelines:

http://www.bts.org.uk/standards.htm

Eurotransplant:

http://www.transplant.org/

ANZDATA Australia and New Zealand Dialysis and Transplant Registry:

http://www.anzdata.org.au/ANZOD

United States Transplant Registry:

http://www.ustransplant.org

See also
Selection and preparation of recipients, p. 544

Long-term medical complications of renal transplantation, p. 566

Drug-induced nephropathies, p. 698

Long-term medical complications of renal transplantation

Introduction

For most patients, renal transplantation is the best form of renal replacement therapy. However, it does not provide a cure and is itself associated with a number of medical complications. In this section, long-term medical complications are those developing more than one year after transplantation.

Long-term medical complications arise as a result of:

Chronic drug therapy:

- e.g. osteoporosis associated with corticosteroid use.

Nonspecific consequences of immunosuppression:

- opportunistic infections;
- conventional infections;
- malignancy.

Chronic kidney disease:

- all renal transplant patients should be considered to have chronic kidney disease;
- the suffix T should be appended to the CKD classification (e.g. CKD stage 3T);
- CKD may be stable but associated with all the complications of CKD (e.g. anemia, renal bone disease);
- CKD can be progressive – chronic allograft dysfunction (CAD).

Accelerated cardiovascular disease.

It is most convenient to consider long-term medical complications under the following headings:

- Infection
- Malignancy
- Chronic allograft dysfunction
- Cardiovascular disease
- Chronic kidney disease
- Bone disease.

Infection

This is an important cause of death in kidney transplant recipients (18% in the Assessment of Lescol in Renal Transplant [ALERT] study, 2005).

It is an inevitable consequence of nonspecific immunosuppression.

Specific infections occur at different time-points after transplantation.

Opportunistic infections are more likely in the early post-transplant period because this is the time of greatest immunosuppression and the infection may be transmitted by the donor.

Most patients in the late post-transplant period have stable graft function and are maintained on minimal immunosuppressive therapy. The infections experienced by these patients are similar to those in the general population. However, some opportunistic infections may persist into the late transplant period or arise at any time that immunosuppression is increased, particularly in the absence of the chemoprophylaxis used in the early post-transplant period (e.g. trimethoprim-sulfamethoxazole, antiviral agents).

Viral infections

Human herpes virus (HHV)
HHV 1, herpes simplex virus 1
- cold sores.

HHV 2, herpes simplex virus 2
- genital herpes.

HHV 3, varicella zoster virus
- chicken pox;
- shingles.

HHV 4, Epstein–Barr virus (EBV)
- post-transplant lymphoproliferative disease (PTLD).

HHV 5, cytomegalovirus (CMV)
- retinitis or colitis (late infections).

HHV 8, Kaposi's sarcoma virus
- Kaposi's sarcoma.

Polyoma viruses
BK virus
- BK virus (BKV) nephropathy.

JC virus
- progressive multifocal leukoencephalopathy.

Human papilloma virus (HPV)
Squamous cell carcinoma of the:
- skin;
- vulva;
- anus
- cervix.

Parvovirus B19
Anemia.

HTLV 1
Tropical spastic paraparesis.

T-cell leukemia/lymphoma.

Other viruses
- Adenovirus.
- Hepatitis C.
- Hepatitis B.
- HIV.

Bacterial infections
These account for 80% of all infections.

Urinary tract infections
This is the most common primary site of infection associated with secondary bacteremia.

Patients with anatomically or functionally abnormal bladders or diabetes are particularly at risk.

A poor outcome is associated with:
- Gram-negative bacteria;
- multiresistant organisms;
- *Candida* spp.

Infection with *Corynebacterium urealyticum* is associated with encrustation and urinary tract obstruction and can be difficult to isolate with routine culture methods.

Problem bacteria
These may present as pneumonia, meningitis, cellulitis, osteomyelitis or generalized sepsis and include:
- *Listeria monocytogenes* (from unpasteurized dairy products);
- *Legionella* spp.;
- *Nocardia* spp.;
- *Mycobacterium tuberculosis* (especially in high risk patients from developing countries);
- Nontuberculous mycobacteria;
- Vancomycin-resistant *enterococcus* (VRE);
- Methicillin-resistant *Staphylococcus aureus* (MRSA).

Fungal infections
Pneumocystis jiroveci infection usually occurs in the first 6 months of transplantation but may occasionally occur later, particularly during periods of increased immunosuppression.

Cryptococcus neoformans can cause pneumonia and meningoencephalitis.

Aspergillus spp.

Histoplasmosis, coccidioidomycosis, and rarely blastomycosis (geographic or endemic fungal infections).

Parasitic infections
Strongyloides – there is a risk of hyperinfection syndrome in patients from endemic regions.

Toxoplasma gondi is associated with CNS disease and chorioretinitis.

Malignancy
This is a major cause of death in kidney transplant recipients (26% in the ALERT study).

There is an increased risk of most malignancies compared with:
- an age-matched general population;
- patients with ESRD on the transplant waiting list.

Risk factors include:
- age;
- immunosuppression;
- chronic viral infections;
- smoking.

The relative risk of malignancy ranges from a 2–3-fold increase for common malignancies (lung, prostate, breast, colon) to a 100-fold increase for nonmelanomatous skin cancers, PTLD and Kaposi's sarcoma.

An annual surveillance examination, especially of the skin, should be performed.

Otherwise age-appropriate screening as for the general population is indicated (e.g. mammography, cervical smears).

Reduction or modification of the immunosuppressive regimen should be considered when a malignancy occurs and the potential for graft loss balanced against the natural history and staging of the malignancy.

Sirolimus use has been associated with a reduced incidence of cancer (including skin cancer) in the first 2 years post transplantation but the benefit of switching to this form of immunosuppression in patients who develop malignancy has yet to be proved.

The Israel Penn Transplant Tumor Registry is a worldwide tumor database that has information on 8191 organ allograft recipients who developed 8724 de novo cancers. The great majority (6821) are kidney allograft recipients and there is a facility for nephrologists from around the world to enter their own data into the registry.

Post-transplant lymphoproliferative disease
Incidence: 1–2%.

Immunophenotypically it is a CD20$^+$ B-cell lymphoma.

Associated with EBV infection.

Seronegative recipients of an organ from a seropositive donor are at highest risk.

EBV transforms B-lymphocytes when immune surveillance is inadequate and may promote uncontrolled polyclonal/monoclonal proliferation.

There is an increased risk with the use of lymphocyte-depleting antibodies (ATG, OKT3, Campath-1H).

PTLD usually presents with lymphadenopathy but extranodal involvement is common (CNS, kidney, GI tract, liver, lungs) and multiple sites are often involved.

Renal transplant involvement may mimic severe rejection.

May respond to:
- significant reduction or withdrawal of immunosuppression (especially polyclonal disease);
- anti-CD20 humanized monoclonal antibody (rituximab);
- or may require conventional chemo- and radiotherapy

Antiviral agents are of no value.

PTLD carries a high mortality.

Poor prognostic factors include:
- increasing age;
- raised LDH levels;
- multiple organ involvement;
- constitutional symptoms.

Skin cancer
5–22% prevalence in UK.

Squamous cell carcinoma
More common than basal cell carcinoma (BCC) in transplant recipients, in contrast to the general population where BCC is more common.

Occur early, grow rapidly and are often multiple and metastasize.

Causative factors in the transplant recipient include:
- immunosuppression;
- UV light exposure;
- HPV (human papilloma viruses);
- genetic predisposition.

Risk factors include:
- presence of actinic keratosis;
- age at transplantation;
- male gender;
- history of smoking;
- increased UV light exposure;
- duration of immunosuppression.

Treatment depends on the size, site and number of lesions but includes:
- cryotherapy or surgical excision;
- radiotherapy;
- 5-fluorouracil;

- photodynamic therapy;
- immunosuppressive dose reduction.

Prevention includes photoprotection (avoid sun exposure, sun block creams).

Retinoids have been used as secondary prevention in patients with multiple recurrent lesions.

Kaposi's sarcoma
Uncommon.
- 60% are cutaneous;
- 40% are disseminated (GI, pulmonary, lymph nodes).

Associated with HHV 8 infection.

Immunosuppression dose reduction, retinoids and conventional chemotherapy have been used.

Regression with switching immunosuppression to sirolimus has been reported.

Chronic allograft dysfunction

Causes of chronic allograft dysfunction (CAD) include:
- chronic allograft nephropathy (CAN);
- BK virus nephropathy;
- transplant renal artery stenosis or pseudorenal artery stenosis;
- recurrent glomerular disease;
- *de novo* glomerular disease.

Chronic allograft nephropathy

CAN is the commonest cause of late allograft loss together with death with a functioning graft.

It is a histological diagnosis characterized by:
- tubulointerstitial fibrosis and tubular atrophy;
- fibrointimal proliferation and thickening of arteries with luminal narrowing;
- glomerular sclerosis.

It reflects cumulative and incremental damage from time-dependent immunological and nonimmunological causes.

It has been suggested by histopathologists that in most cases they are able to identify histologically the predominant lesion causing CAD.

Therefore they have proposed that the term CAN should be replaced by 'chronic allograft injury'.

However, because of the cumulative and multifactorial elements that result in chronic allograft damage, this claim seems exaggerated.

Immunological causes of CAN (alloantigen-dependent risk factors):
- clinical and subclinical acute rejection;
- degree of HLA mismatch;
- prior sensitization;
- suboptimal immunosuppression and medication non-concordance;
- chronic antibody-associated rejection (peritubular C4d deposition and demonstration of donor-specific antibodies).

Nonimmunological causes of CAN (alloantigen-independent risk factors):
- donor factors (age, donor type);
- prolonged cold ischemic time;
- calcineurin inhibitor (CNI) nephrotoxicity;
- hypertension;
- hyperlipidemia;
- infection (e.g. CMV);
- smoking.

Chronic calcineurin inhibitor nephrotoxicity
A paradox of modern transplantation is that CNIs, the agents that provide the cornerstone to most immunosuppressive regimes, are nephrotoxic.

This may account for the fact that despite a dramatic reduction in the rate of early acute rejection with a concomitant significant improvement in 1 year renal allograft survival after the introduction of ciclosporin (CsA) in the 1980s, there has been little improvement in graft half-life.

Long-term studies of protocol biopsies have demonstrated the natural history of CAN and emphasized that 90% of patients have evidence of chronic CNI nephrotoxicity 5 years after renal (mostly SPK) transplantation.

This is also emphasized by registry data documenting a CKD incidence of 16.5% in recipients 36 months after nonrenal solid organ transplantation.

In patients with a progressive decline in allograft function due to CAN, substitution of CNI with mycophenolate mofetil (MMF) may be effective in improving allograft function without risking acute rejection.

Substitution of CNI with sirolimus may also be effective in patients with suboptimal graft function.

CNI dose minimization with MMF introduction may also be an effective strategy.

BK virus nephropathy

BKV is a ubiquitous polyoma virus (60–80% of adults are seropositive).

BKV causes latent infection of the kidney with reactivation during immunosuppression.

Rates of infection range from 10 to 60%.

BKV infection was originally described as causing ureteral stenosis or stricture, but now is more commonly associated with a tubulointerstitial nephritis with associated allograft dysfunction.

The incidence of allograft failure in affected patients ranges from 15 to 50%.

The diagnosis requires a renal biopsy demonstrating:
- viral inclusion bodies in renal tubular cells;
- positive immunostains for SV40 T antigen.

Polymerase chain reaction (PCR) of serum for BKV DNA and viral load may be useful as a diagnostic and monitoring test.

Identification of characteristic cytological changes in tubular cells shed in the urine ('decoy cells') may be used for screening.

Specific antiviral therapy for BKV nephropathy does not exist.

Management involves a reduction in immunosuppression with close monitoring for rejection.

Low dose cidofovir or leflunomide may be effective in some patients.

Transplant artery stenosis or pseudoartery stenosis
Incidence: 1–3%.

Typically occurs 2 months to 2 years after transplantation either from atherosclerosis of the donor vessels, clamp/cannulation injury or poor surgical technique.

Immunological injury has also been proposed but is unproven.

May present as:
- graft dysfunction (especially with ACEI/ARB use);
- difficult-to-control hypertension;
- diuretic-resistant salt and water retention (peripheral edema);
- erythrocytosis.

There may be an associated bruit over the transplanted kidney.

Diagnosis may be confirmed by:
- color flow Doppler examination (but this is operator dependent and interpretation may be difficult);
- CT angiography;
- conventional angiography.

Given concerns over gadolinium-associated nephrogenic fibrosing dermopathy, MR angiography is no longer a favored method of investigation.

Treatment is with angioplasty and endovascular stenting or in recurrent cases operative revascularization.

Pseudorenal artery stenosis occurs if an atherosclerotic plaque in the recipient's iliac vessels impairs blood flow to the transplant renal artery. An iliac artery stenosis may also arise from intraoperative clamp damage.

Cardiovascular disease

This is the commonest cause of death after renal transplantation (34% of all deaths in the ALERT study).

The incidence of cardiovascular disease (CVD) is increased compared with a matched general population but it is not as high as in dialysis patients.

Both traditional and nontraditional risk factors contribute to CVD mortality and morbidity.

Nontraditional factors include CKD-associated LVH and myocardial fibrosis leading to arrhythmias and death. An association with CMV infection (in heart transplant recipients) has been observed but causality remains unproven.

Modifiable risk factors should be treated including:
- diabetes;
- hypertension;
- hypercholesterolemia;
- smoking.

The American Society of Transplantation and European Best Practice Guidelines (EBPG) recommend a target BP of:
- <135/85 mmHg;
- <125/75 in high risk patients or with proteinuria >1 g/day.

The metabolism of some statins (those metabolized via CYP3A) may be inhibited by CNIs and when used in high dose may rarely cause rhabdomyolysis. Hydrophilic statins such as pravastatin may be preferred.

New-onset diabetes mellitus after transplantation (NODAT)

A US registry study reported a cumulative incidence of 24% for developing NODAT at 3 years post transplantation.

NODAT significantly reduces patient and graft survival.

Risk factors for NODAT include:
- use of CNIs (tacrolimus greater risk than CsA);
- use of corticosteroids;
- age;

- hepatitis C infection;
- rejection episodes;
- Black race;
- high BMI.

Treatment is aimed at weight loss, diet and exercise, oral hypoglycemics as monotherapy or in combination with insulin to achieve tight glycemic control.

Post-transplant erythrocytosis

Occurs in up to 20% of patients, most commonly during the first 2 years after transplantation.

The mechanism responsible is uncertain but it may result from either overproduction of erythropoetin or of insulin-like growth factor-1 (IGF-1).

IGF-1 may increase the sensitivity of erythroid precursors to erythropoetin.

It requires treatment if the hematocrit is >52% to avoid the risk of increased viscosity and thrombosis (cardiovascular event).

ACEIs or ARBs are effective in most patients.

Theophylline may be used as an alternative.

Phlebotomy may be required in resistant cases.

Chronic kidney disease

The prevalence of CKD in renal transplant recipients from a UK registry study in 2007 showed that:
- 21.6% had CKD stage 2T;
- 57.5% had CKD stage 3T;
- 15.7% had CKD stage 4T;
- 3.1% had CKD stage 5T.

Complications of CKD are frequently observed and are either inadequately treated or resistant to treatment.

Many patients in stage 4T–5T have CKD-related complications but registry data would suggest that these complications are often less well-managed than in nontransplanted CKD stage 4–5 patients.

Anemia

The prevalence of anemia (Hb <11 g/dL) increases across CKD stages, reaching 51.5% in stage 5T.

Contributing factors in addition to CKD include:
- drugs (azathioprine, MMF, sirolimus, ACEI/ARB);
- chronic inflammatory state;
- infections (e.g. parvovirus).

Intravenous/oral iron and erythropoiesis-stimulating agents (ESA) should be used according to the same criteria applied to nontransplant patients.

Bone disease and metabolic acidosis

Hypocalcemia, hyperphosphatemia, hyperparathyroidism and metabolic acidosis should be managed as in nontransplant patients with CKD using phosphate-binders, calcitriol and sodium bicarbonate.

Preparation for dialysis

Patients need to be prepared for a return to dialysis or retransplantation in a timely manner when appropriate (e.g. AVF formation, relisting).

Bone disease

Renal bone disease

Almost all transplant recipients have some degree of renal osteodystrophy that persists after kidney transplantation.

EBPG recommend that patients with tertiary hyperparathyroidism (HPTH) should be observed for 1 year after transplantation to allow for spontaneous involution.

After the first year, tertiary HPTH may be treated by surgical parathyroidectomy although the procedure may be associated with a decline in renal allograft function through poorly defined mechanisms.

The calcimimetic agent cinacalcet may provide an alternative to surgical parathyroidectomy but its safety and cost-effectiveness needs to be established in transplantation.

Serum levels of calcium, phosphate and intact PTH (iPTH) should be maintained within the range for nontransplant CKD patients.

Osteoporosis

Osteoporosis (bone mineral density 2.5 SD below the young adult mean value or T-score) is common after transplantation.

There is a fracture rate of 7–11% (higher in diabetic patients receiving combined kidney pancreas transplants).

Maximum bone loss occurs during the first 6–12 months of transplantation and continues at a lower rate or stabilizes thereafter.

Risk factors include:
- corticosteroid use;
- CNI use;
- previous renal bone disease;
- persistent HPTH;
- hypogonadism;
- metabolic acidosis;
- smoking.

Treatment strategies to prevent osteoporosis include:
- corticosteroid minimization or avoidance;
- oral calcium and vitamin D supplementation;
- testosterone/estrogen replacement if appropriate;
- correction of metabolic acidosis;
- use of oral or IV biphosphonates.

However, effect of treatment on fracture rate is unproven.

There is concern over the use of biphosphonates in patients with low bone turnover.

Assessment of bone density with dual energy X-ray absorptiometry (DEXA) scan at intervals may be indicated in patients in whom it will change practice.

Avascular necrosis or osteonecrosis

This is associated with corticosteroid use although the pathogenesis is poorly understood.

The femoral head is affected in 90% of cases.

Avascular necrosis typically presents as hip or groin pain exacerbated by weight bearing.

MRI is the most sensitive imaging method for diagnosis.

Core decompression before the femoral head collapses may relieve pain but 60% of cases require total hip replacement.

Further reading

Ansell DA, Udayaraj UP, et al. Chronic renal failure in kidney transplant recipients. Do they receive optimum care?: Data from the UK Renal Registry. Am J Transplant 2007;**7**:1167–1176.

Bostom AD, Brown RS, et al. Prevention of post-transplant cardiovascular disease – report and recommendations of an ad hoc group. Am J Transplant 2002;**2**:491–500.

Davidson J, Wilkinson A, et al. New-onset diabetes after transplantation: International consensus guidelines. Transplantation 2003;**75**:SS3–24.

Dudley C, Pohanka E, et al. Mycophenolate mofetil substitution for cyclosporine a in renal transplant recipients with chronic progressive allograft dysfunction: the "creeping creatinine" study. Transplantation 2005; **79**: 466–475.

European Best Practice Guidelines for Renal Transplantation (Part 2). Nephrol Dial Transplant 2000; **17**(Suppl 4): 1–67.

Frimat L, Cassuto-Viguier E, et al. Impact of cyclosporine reduction with MMF: a randomized trial in chronic allograft dysfunction. The 'reference' study. Am J Transplant 2006; **6**: 2725–2734.

Holdaas H, Fellström B, et al. Assessment of LEscol in Renal Transplantation (ALERT) Study Investigators. Long-term cardiac outcomes in renal transplant recipients receiving fluvastatin: the ALERT extension study. Am J Transplant 2005; **5**: 2929–2936.

Kasiske BL, Snyder JJ, Gilbertson DT, Wang C. Cancer after kidney transplantation in the United States. Am J Transplant 2004; **4**: 905–913.

Nankivell BJ, Borrows RJ, et al. The natural history of chronic allograft nephropathy. N Engl J Med 2003; **349**: 2326–2333.

Ojo AO, Hold PJ, et al. Chronic renal failure after transplantation of a nonrenal organ. N Engl J Med 2003; **349**: 931–940.

Solez K, Colvin RB, et al. Banff '05 Meeting Report: differential diagnosis of chronic allograft injury and elimination of chronic allograft nephropathy ('CAN'). Am J Transplant 2007; **7**: 518–526.

Watson CJ, Firth J, et al. A randomized controlled trial of late conversion from CNI-based to sirolimus-based immunosuppression following renal transplantation. Am J Transplant 2005; **5**: 2496–2503.

Internet resources

British Transplantation Society Guidelines:
http://www.bts.org.uk/standards.htm

CTS – Collaborative Transplant Study:
www.ctstransplant.org/

European Best Practice Guidelines:
http://www.ndt-educational.org/

Eurotransplant:
http://www.transplant.org/

Australia and New Zealand Dialysis and Transplant Registry:
www.anzdata.org.au/

Israel Penn Transplant Tumor Registry:
http://www.ipittr.uc.edu/Home.cfm

United States Renal Data System (USRDS):
www.usrds.org/

UK Renal Registry:
www.renalreg.com/

United States Transplant Registry:
http://www.ustransplant.org

See also

Early management of transplant recipients, p. 556

Cardiovascular risk factors in CKD, p. 412

Hypertension in CKD, p. 406

Immunosuppression for renal transplantation, p. 560

Outcome of renal transplantation, p. 576

Recurrent and *de novo* disease post renal transplantation

Introduction

The most common cause of post-transplantation proteinuria is chronic allograft nephropathy (60%), followed by recurrent (15%) and *de novo* (10%) glomerulonephritis. The most common diseases associated with allograft glomerulonephritis and their recurrence rates post transplantation are:

- idiopathic focal glomerular sclerosis (25%);
- IgA nephropathy (25%);
- mesangiocapillary glomerulonephritis (type I, 25%, type II, 80%);
- membranous nephropathy (30%);
- hemolytic uremic syndrome (classic 1%, atypical, 20% familial 80%).

Clinical features of recurrent disease

In general, recurrence of disease affecting the renal transplant mimics the features of the original disease.

The discrimination between allograft dysfunction due to recurrent disease and that due to acute or chronic rejection, drug nephrotoxicity or pyelonephritis usually involves urine culture, measurement of proteinuria, measurement of immunosuppressive drug concentrations and ultrasound imaging. If recurrent renal disease is a likely diagnosis then a renal biopsy with full electron microscopy and immunohistological processing of a renal biopsy will be necessary.

Antiglomerular basement membrane disease

In patients with ESRD due to anti-GBM disease standard practice is to measure circulating anti-GBM antibodies periodically and most would advise waiting 12 months from when antibodies were negative before offering transplantation, whether from a cadaveric or a live donor source. Clinical disease is significantly less common than histological recurrence and rarely leads to graft loss.

De novo anti-GBM nephritis

Approximately 15% of patients with Alport's syndrome develop anti-GBM antibodies in response to what is for them the neoantigen of the α chain of type IV collagen. A small fraction of this subgroup develops severe crescentic glomerulonephritis with a poor outlook. However, given its rarity most authorities advise transplantation, whether from a live donor or a cadaveric source in Alport's syndrome.

ANCA-associated vasculitis

Patients are not listed for transplantation until they are in clinical remission. The duration of pretransplant dialysis does not appear, albeit based on small numbers, to have any significant influence on the risk of relapse. The presence of a positive ANCA at the time of transplantation does not preclude transplantation and subsequent serological monitoring would seem to be relatively unhelpful for predicting outcome.

Diabetic nephropathy

Histological recurrence of diabetic renal disease is seen in 100% of patients within 4 years of transplantation. Although histological recurrence rate is very high the frequency with which diabetic nephropathy is ascribed as a cause of graft loss is much smaller and was only 1.8% in the largest series.

In isolated renal transplantation the majority would argue for strict glycemic control with the early use of ACEIs, often in conjunction with ARBs to slow progression of glomerular renal disease.

De novo diabetic nephropathy

Renal transplant recipients are at risk of new-onset diabetes, particularly because of treatment with corticosteroids, tacrolimus and ciclosporin.

There is good evidence that the disorder has a significant impact on patient and graft survival.

It is therefore appropriate to aim for good glycemic control and to use ACEIs liberally if necessary in conjunction with ARBs for renal protection, irrespective of any favorable impact this management would be expected to have on cardiovascular disease. Attention to other modifiable risk factors such as physical activity, smoking and weight reduction are important.

Idiopathic focal segmental glomerulosclerosis

Focal segmental glomerulosclerosis (FSGS) is an especially important problem in pediatric practice. The absolute recurrence rate post transplantation in children varies with different series; but is between 20% and 30%. Data from the North American Pediatric Renal Transplant Co-operative Study show that patients with FSGS have the highest overall graft failure rate.

Risk of relapse is increased with:

- age <15 years;
- aggressive clinical course of original disease with the interval from diagnosis to ESRD less than ~3 years;
- diffuse mesangial proliferation on native biopsy.

Given the high frequency of recurrent disease it is important to advise patients and families about the relative merits of living verses cadaveric transplant donor sources.

Despite the high rate of graft loss, overall recipients of a living donor kidney have a better graft survival than recipients of cadaveric renal transplants at 50 months.

Many clinicians would avoid a living donor organ source as a primary transplant if the clinical course of the original disease was <3 years or if the patient was aged <15 years, especially if the FSGS was accompanied with diffuse mesangial proliferation.

If a primary transplant is lost to recurrent disease, a living related transplant should be avoided for subsequent grafting as the recurrence rate is in the order of 80%.

If the first graft was lost from rejection or another complication with no evidence of recurrence there is much less risk of recurrence in a subsequent graft.

It is important to emphasize that patients, often adults, with the histology of focal and segmental sclerosis where that is secondary to low renal mass, and who typically are not nephrotic, are not at risk of recurrent glomerulonephritis.

Treatment of recurrent FSGS

Treatment remains suboptimal with multiple case series of different strategies.

Treatments have included:

- ACEIs;
- indomethacin;

- immunoabsorption with protein A columns;
- IV immunoglobulin;
- high dose ciclosporin;
- cyclophosphamide;
- plasmapheresis;
- double filtration plasmapheresis.

Plasmapheresis is the most widely used technique in the treatment of recurrent nephrotic syndrome post transplantation.

This is usually in combination with other immunosuppressive treatments.

It is important to decide whether treatment with plasma exchange needs to be augmented with cyclophosphamide, especially in children.

The literature generally supports the early use of both plasma exchange and cyclophosphamide.

Familial FSGS

It is important to recognize familial FSGS, although rare, as it is a different syndrome from idiopathic FSGS.

Patients generally present in their 3rd or 4th decade and post-transplantation recurrent disease is rare with an overall 10 year graft survival of 62%.

Mutations in genes coding for podocyte proteins have now been reasonably well-characterized in hereditary FSGS.

In patients with two pathogenic *NPHS2* mutations there is a very low risk of recurrent disease; in other situations the prognostic value of genotyping is less clear.

Genetic testing is now available and can improve counseling before transplant.

De novo FSGS in renal transplants

This histological appearance is most commonly reported associated with other pathology, particularly chronic allograft nephropathy, or transplant glomerulopathy and occasionally ciclosporin toxicity or IgA disease.

In contrast to FSGS affecting native kidneys, only 24% of those with biopsy-proven glomerular disease have nephrotic syndrome.

This histological finding is associated with poor graft survival. The pathogenesis and whether this entity is separate from a chronic rejection process are unclear.

Hepatitis-B-associated glomerulonephritis

Concomitant hepatitis B infection has an important impact on survival of renal transplant patients.

Glomerulonephritis secondary to hepatitis B post renal transplantation is rarely an important clinical problem.

Membranous glomerulonephritis is the most common form of glomerular disease associated with hepatitis B. This has a far from benign prognosis, and a similar prognosis would be expected in renal transplant recipients who develop nephrotic syndrome.

Antiviral treatment is the mainstay of management.

Hepatitis-C-associated glomerulonephritis

Cryoglobulinemic nephritis with mesangiocapillary glomerulonephritis has been described after transplantation in patients infected with hepatitis C virus.

Although this has a poor prognosis in general it is liver failure that is responsible for most of the inferior graft and patient survival.

Hemolytic uremic syndrome (HUS)

It is critical to discriminate between:
- diarrhea-associated HUS;
- familial HUS;
- *de novo* HUS.

In the more common diarrhea-associated HUS recurrence rate with graft loss is of the order of 1%.

By contrast in the group with HUS with no diarrhea ~20% subsequently lose grafts due to recurrence.

In the subgroup with HUS associated with factor H deficiency, graft loss rates of the order of 80% are seen.

Family history is particularly important and molecular investigation of complement regulators as well as von Willebrand protease activity is advised; guidelines are available from the European Society of Paediatric Nephrology (ESPN).

Live related donation should only occur after a careful prediction of the risks of premature graft loss.

The clinical presentation may be gradual or relatively abrupt with marked thrombocytopenia, and hemolysis associated with progressive renal dysfunction.

Therapeutic options are limited with little evidence that altering calcineurin inhibitors changes prognosis.

In severe thrombocytopenia most practitioners would adopt treatment strategies similar to that used in classic HUS with plasma fraction infusions and plasma exchange.

In the event of life-threatening thrombocytopenia or hemolysis, particularly in the presence of severe allograft dysfunction, transplant nephrectomy may be required to restore stability.

De novo HUS

De novo HUS has been attributed to OKT3, tacrolimus, vascular rejection as well as ciclosporin post renal transplantation.

This syndrome occurs most frequently within a month of transplantation and is associated with graft loss in ~60% and patient death in 20% of cases.

Calcineurin dose minimization is usual as well as a treatment strategy similar to that used in diarrhea-associated HUS.

Henoch–Schönlein purpura

Because of the very small numbers of patients reported it is very difficult to predict accurately recurrence of this condition.

Overall the actuarial risk for renal recurrence and graft loss due to recurrence has been reported to be between 11% and 35% at 5 years after transplantation.

Importantly, recurrence may occur despite a >12 month delay between disappearance of purpura and transplantation.

The common advice to delay for a year between disappearance of purpura and transplantation may therefore not protect from recurrent disease.

IgA nephropathy

At a mean follow-up of 5 years ~13% of patients will have some recurrence-related renal graft dysfunction and 5% will lose the graft as a result of recurrence.

In the only series in which all patients were biopsied recurrence was found in 58%.

Younger patients are at greater risk of recurrence, as are those with a shorter duration of disease in the native kidneys.

At least one group has demonstrated clinically significant poorer graft survival in patients presenting with native cresentic glomerulonephritis.

Overall, graft survival at 5 and 10 years appears to be the same as average.

There is no established treatment for preventing or treating recurrent IgA nephropathy, but one group has reported a trend towards improved 5 and 10 year graft survival in those prescribed ACEI/ARB therapy.

The use of living related donors for recipients with IgA nephropathy has been the subject of some controversy. A large registry series found an increased rate of IgA nephropathy-related graft loss among zero HLA-mismatched recipients of kidneys from a live donor source. This offset the advantage normally seen among zero HLA-mismatched recipients. These authors argued that as overall survival was similar there was no reason to avoid live donor-recipient pairs with zero HLA mismatches.

Membranous nephropathy

In adults the rate of recurrence is ~30%.

No specific risk factor for recurrence has been clearly identified.

The outcome for graft survival is poor with a 52% graft loss at 10 years.

The clinical syndrome seems to be similar to the disease in native kidneys with progressively more severe nephrotic syndrome.

The management is usually based on extrapolation of data from management of native kidney disease and, similar to that situation, spontaneous remission, failures of immunosuppressive treatment as well as clinical response coincident with change of treatment have all been reported.

A recent case report of successful use of rituximab requires more experience and longer follow-up.

De novo membranous nephropathy

De novo membranous nephropathy is second only to transplant glomerulopathy as a cause of nephrotic syndrome after renal transplantation.

The mean time of diagnosis is at ~5 years post transplantation.

The addition of pulsed steroid therapy to the baseline immunosuppression in heavily nephrotic patients makes no obvious impact on outcome.

Mesangiocapillary glomerulonephritis (MCGN)

There are marked histological similarities between transplant glomerulopathy and MCGN, but immunofluorescence and electron microscopy can usually discriminate between the two diagnoses.

A recent report analysing the experience of a single country (Ireland) concluded that younger age at initial diagnosis and the severity of the native glomerular histology independently predicted the risk of recurrence, and not the classification of MCGN type, with the poorer reputation of type II disease explained by the more aggressive glomerular changes seen in that condition.

Mesangiocapillary glomerulonephritis type I

Where the renal disease is thought to be mediated by glomerular deposition of immune complexes generated after exposure, for example to native DNA (SLE) or hepatitis antigens, recurrence would be expected after transplantation as these antigens would be predicted to persist in the circulation post transplant.

Published experience suggests that type I MCGN recurs after renal transplantation in half the patients and that this frequency may be even greater in recipients of identical living related donor grafts.

Recurrence in a second transplant after recurrence in the first graft is extremely common and once diagnosed has an important detrimental impact on graft survival.

The risk of recurrence may be considerably less in Japanese patients with a rate of only 3% in one published series.

It is not possible to give any evidence-based advice with regard to treatment. Antiviral therapy would be logical in patients with persistent hepatitis B antigenemia.

Mesangiocapillary glomerulonephritis type II

The most comprehensive recent analysis is from the North American Pediatric database. Recurrent disease was seen in 67% and 5 year graft survival was 50%, compared to 74% on average. There was no correlation between severity of pre-transplantation presentation, pre- or post-transplantation C3 levels and prognosis.

No treatments are known to be effective: there are case reports describing successful use of plasma exchange and immunosuppression.

Systemic lupus erythematosus

The rate of recurrent lupus nephritis is ~1% at 5 years.

Pre-transplantation serological parameters are unreliable predictors of the likelihood of recurrence and also may not accurately reflect disease activity in the post-transplantation interval.

As would be expected given the small number of cases, there are no formal studies of the management of recurrent lupus nephritis.

Most clinicians would opt for management that mirrored that of native disease.

Anticoagulation during the early perioperative and early post-transplantation phase should be considered for patients with a history of thrombosis or those with the presence of lupus anticoagulant.

Systemic sclerosis

The evidence base in this condition is extremely small.

Most clinicians would manage patients with systemic sclerosis in a similar way to patients with SLE and recommend renal transplantation as a treatment option.

The majority would use ACEIs for antihypertensive control from the outset in patients who had ESRD secondary to scleroderma renal crisis.

Further reading

Bresin E, et al. Outcome of renal transplantation in patients with non-Shiga toxin-associated haemolytic uremic syndrome: prognostic significance of genetic background. Clin J Am Soc Nephrol 2006; **1**: 88–99.

Couser W. Recurrent glomerulonephritis in the renal allograft: an update of selected areas. Exp Clin Transplant 2005;**3**:283–288.

Floege J. Recurrent IgA nephropathy after renal transplantation. *Semin Neprol* 2004; **24**: 287–291.

Gera M, *et al.* Recurrence of ANCA-associated vasculitis following renal transplantation in the modern era of immunosuppression. *Kidney Int* 2007; **71**: 1296–1301.

Little MA, Dupont P, Campbell E, Dorman A, Walshe JJ. Severity of primary MPGN, rather than MPGN type, determines renal survival and post-transplantation recurrence risk. *Kidney Int* 2006; **69**: 504–511.

McDonald SP, Russ GR. Recurrence of IgA nephropathy among renal allograft recipients from living donors is greater among those with zero HLA mismatches. *Transplantation* 2006; **82**: 759–762.

Weber S. Tonshoff B. Recurrence of focal-segmental glomerulosclerosis in children after renal transplantation: clinical and genetic aspects. *Transplantation* 2005; **80**: S128–S134.

Internet resources

British Transplantation Society:

http://www.bts.org

American Society of Transplantation:

http://www.a-s-t.org/

American Society of Transplant Surgeons:

http://www.asts.org/

European Society of Paediatric Nephrology (ESPN):

http://.espn.cardiff.ac.uk

North American Pediatric Renal Trials and Collaborative Studies (NAPRTCS):

https://web.emmes.com/study/ped/

See also

Outcome of renal transplantation, p. 576

Early management of transplant recipients, p. 556

Long-term medical complications of renal transplantation, p. 566

Outcome of renal transplantation

Renal transplant outcome can be measured in a number of different ways including:

- graft survival;
- patient survival;
- graft function (serum creatinine);
- number of acute rejection episodes;
- days of hospitalization;
- quality of life.

Data about transplant outcome usually come from the large registries (for example, the US Renal Database System (USRDS), the Collaborative Transplant Study, and the Australia and New Zealand Dialysis and Transplant registry (ANZDATA)).

Patient and graft survival after renal transplantation have improved significantly over the last 25 years although the rate of improvement is now slowing.

Graft outcome is traditionally examined in two phases:

- early (the first 12 months post transplant);
- late (any time after the first 12 months).

Short-term outcomes of renal transplantation

Graft outcome

Currently the 1 year survival rate for deceased donor allografts is 90%, and 96% for living donor allografts.

The 1 year survival has steadily improved over the last 20 years from 74% and 89% for deceased donor and living donor allografts respectively in 1987.

Early graft loss is usually due to:

- acute rejection;
- renal artery thrombosis;
- patient death;
- primary nonfunction.

Patient outcome

The 1 year patient survival rate following a deceased or living donor allograft is 95% and 98% respectively.

The principal causes of death in the first 12 months are infection and cardiovascular events.

Long-term outcomes of renal transplantation

Graft outcome

Currently the 5 and 10 year graft survival for deceased donor allografts is 68 and 42% respectively. For living donor allografts 5 and 10 year graft survival is 80 and 55% respectively.

The longer-term outcome has also improved over the last 20 years (Fig. 14.8.1).

After the first year post transplant the major causes of graft loss are:

- patient death;
- chronic allograft nephropathy.

Less commonly late acute rejection and recurrent disease can develop.

Patient outcome

The 5 and 10 year patient survival is 80 and 61% respectively for recipients of deceased donor allografts, and 89 and 75% for recipients of living donor kidneys.

Over the past 20 years there has been a 5% and 8% improvement in 5 and 10 year patient survival following a deceased donor transplant, but a negligible improvement following a living donor transplant.

The principal causes of death beyond 1 year post transplant are:

- cardiovascular disease;
- infection;
- malignancy.

These three diagnoses account for 67% of deaths in the 45–64 year age group.

Survival benefit of renal transplantation

Numerous studies have demonstrated that transplanted patients have a better long-term outcome than those who remain on dialysis.

These studies have often been flawed by the inappropriate selection of the comparator group since nontransplanted patients may have more significant comorbidity that may prevent them from being transplanted in the first place.

A more appropriate comparison would be between transplanted patients and those who are on the transplant waiting list but remain untransplanted.

The best study of such a comparison indicated that before 106 days post transplant the relative risk of death was higher for transplanted patients, mainly because of the risks of the transplantation process (relative risk of death was 2.8 in the first 2 weeks post transplant). Thereafter transplantation conferred a survival benefit but the overall likelihood of survival did not become equal until day 244.

By 3–4 years post transplant, the relative risk of death was 68% lower in the transplanted group compared to those who remained on the transplant list (Fig. 14.8.2). Improved survival was seen in all groups but was particularly high in patients with diabetes mellitus.

Factors affecting renal allograft survival

Factors involving both donor and recipient

Delayed graft function

Delayed graft function is defined as the failure to function immediately post transplantation with the need for one or more dialysis sessions within a specified period (usually one week).

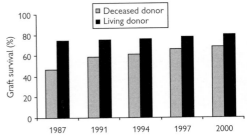

Fig. 14.8.1 Five-year renal survival probabilities (all transplants that survive beyond 1 year) adjusted by age, gender, race and primary diagnosis. (Data from USRDS 2007 Annual Data Report: www.usrds.org/2007/ref/F_tx_outcomes_07.pdf.)

Delayed graft function is associated with:
• worse graft survival;
• worse graft function;
• higher risk of recipient death;
• higher rate of acute rejection.

The increased risk of acute rejection may be because ischemia-reperfusion injury enhances the immunogenicity of the graft.

The rates of delayed graft function remain ~20% for deceased donor allografts and 3% for living donor allografts.

The risk of delayed graft function increases with:
• increasing donor age;
• longer cold ischemia time;
• Black recipients;
• presence of >50% panel reactive antibodies.

HLA matching
For deceased donor allografts better HLA matching is associated with improved survival.

For six antigen-matched kidneys this benefit outweighs the detrimental effect of prolonged cold ischemia. The foremost organ-sharing systems will sanction the transport of fully matched organs over long distances.

For mismatched grafts however, there is a progressive fall in graft survival with increasing cold ischemia time (1–2% per 12 h increase in cold ischemia time).

There is a progressive fall in graft survival with increasing mismatch.

For living donor allografts the effect of HLA matching is much less pronounced (although there is still a benefit seen in two haplotype-matched grafts). This is possibly due to the absence of significant ischemic injury.

Cytomegalovirus status of the donor and recipient
There is a small but demonstrable effect of CMV status on allograft outcome. CMV⁻ donor/CMV⁻ recipient combinations have better outcomes than CMV⁺ donor/CMV⁻ recipient combinations.

This difference is likely mediated by overt CMV infection/disease, but subtle effects of CMV on the immune system may be involved.

CMV prophylaxis has been shown to substantially reduce the incidence of acute rejection.

Timing of transplantation
Pre-emptive transplantation provides a survival benefit for both allografts and recipients.

The relative risk of graft loss and patient death have been shown to be reduced by 27% and 31% respectively following pre-emptive living donor transplantation. Similar benefit has been described in deceased donor transplantation.

The length of time on dialysis before transplantation also impacts on outcome. For example it has been demonstrated that 10 year allograft survival in living donor recipients transplanted pre-emptively was 75%.

10 year graft survival for those dialysed for:
• 0–6 months was 62%;
• 6–12 months was 56%;
• 12–24 months was 54%;
• >24 months was 49%.

The same effect was observed in recipients of deceased donor kidneys.

The beneficial effect of pre-emptive transplantation may be due to the:
• avoidance of the adverse consequences of dialysis (predominantly the development of cardiovascular disease and malnutrition);
• reduced incidence of delayed graft function;
• reduced incidence of acute rejection in the first 6 months post-transplantation;
• effect of socioeconomic factors. Pre-emptive transplantation tends to be undertaken in younger, Caucasian, and educated patients with fewer HLA mismatches.

Donor factors
Donor age
Increasing age of the donor reduces long-term allograft survival. The optimal donor age is 18–34 years.

The 5 year survival of an allograft from a donor aged 18–34 years is 78% compared to 55% for a kidney from a donor aged >65 years.

This is an increasingly important issue because all registries have reported that the average age of donors is increasing, presumably due to the general shortage of kidneys for donation and the acceptance of more marginal kidneys to increase the size of the donor pool.

Type of kidney
Living donor vs deceased donor. Living donor grafts are superior to deceased donor grafts. This is likely to be because of:
• the absence of significant cold ischemia;
• the absence of brain death;
• the better general health of the donor;
• higher nephron mass;
• possibly the shorter wait before transplantation.

Recipient concordance with immunosuppressive medication may also be better in the living donor setting.

Heart-beating vs nonheart-beating deceased donors. Allografts from a nonheart-beating deceased donor source do less well than those from a heart-beating donor.

The comparative 1 year graft survival is 72% and 84% for nonheart-beating and heart-beating sources respectively.

Longer-term survival appears to be very similar to that seen with heart-beating donors.

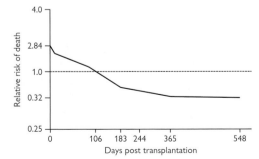

Fig. 14.8.2 Adjusted relative risk of death among 23 275 recipients of a first cadaveric transplant. (Reproduced with permission from Wolfe *et al.*, 1999.)

Extended criteria donors. Due to the mismatch between the supply of and demand for kidneys for transplantation, extended criteria donor kidneys are being used increasingly to expand the donor pool.

The extended criteria include kidneys from:
- donors aged >60 years;

or
- donors aged >50 years with two of the following features: a history of hypertension; death by CVA; terminal creatinine levels >133 μmol/L.

The use of extended criteria donor kidneys is associated with worse graft outcome with graft survival inversely correlating with the quality of the kidney (although the quality of a kidney can be hard to determine in practice).

It is estimated that the relative risk of graft failure with extended criteria grafts compared to those from an 'ideal' source is 1.7.

Donor gender
There is some evidence that grafts from deceased female donors have shorter survival, particularly when transplanted into male recipients. This is likely due to the relatively smaller size of the kidneys and nephron underdosing (see below).

Ischemia reperfusion injury
Longer cold ischemia increases the risk of delayed graft function and reduces long-term graft survival.

This risk is particularly high when cold ischemia exceeds 18 h and when kidneys are sourced from donors aged >60 years.

There is some evidence that pulsatile perfusion of harvested kidneys may improve long-term survival compared to simple cold storage (10% graft survival benefit at 2 years post transplantation).

Nephron mass
The transplantation of a kidney that contains an inadequate number of nephrons (nephron underdosing), may reduce long-term allograft survival.

This may occur when kidneys from old or very young donors are used, or when a normal kidney is transplanted into a large (>100 kg) recipient. The worse outcome of female-to-male transplantation may also be partially explained on this basis.

Recipient factors
Recipient age
Graft survival is less good at the extremes of age.

In young patients grafts are more likely to be lost due to technical issues such as vessel thrombosis, and acute rejection.

In older patients (>65 years) the commonest cause of graft loss is death with a functioning kidney.

There is also evidence that acute rejection is less common in elderly patients and therefore less aggressive immunosuppression may be appropriate in such patients.

Recipient race
In the USA, Black recipients have poorer deceased donor allograft survival than Caucasian recipients.

Potential explanations for this observation include:
- a higher incidence of delayed graft function;
- a higher incidence of acute rejection;

- enhanced immune responsiveness;
- poorer HLA-matching (with a predominantly Caucasian donor pool);
- a higher prevalence of hypertension;
- altered immunosuppressive pharmacokinetics and pharmacodynamics;
- socioeconomic factors may also play a role.

By contrast, Asian and Hispanic recipients in the USA have better graft outcomes than Caucasians.

Recipient gender
There are conflicting data about the influence of gender on renal allograft outcomes, with studies demonstrating both better outcomes in females who receive deceased donor kidneys, and in males who receive living donor kidneys.

Of relevance to transplantation, females are often sensitized to HLA and non-HLA antigens through pregnancy.

Acute rejection
In both living and deceased donor transplants, a single episode of acute rejection reduces the 5 year graft survival by ~10%.

The effect of acute rejection is cumulative: The 10 year graft survival following more than one episode of acute rejection was 54% compared to 88% and 96% following one or no episode of acute rejection respectively.

HLA antibodies
Anti-HLA antibodies are present in 20% of renal transplant recipients.

The presence of anti-HLA antibodies doubles the risk of graft failure by 1 year, and the *de novo* formation of anti-HLA antibodies trebles this risk.

Highly sensitized patients are less likely to be transplanted because of a positive pretransplant crossmatch. Nonetheless the presence of panel-reactive antibodies (PRA) increases the risk of acute rejection and graft loss. Thus the 5 year deceased donor allograft survival rates were shown to be:
- 70% for 0–10% PRA;
- 65% for 10–79% PRA;
- 63% for >80% PRA.

There is evidence from a variety of sources that non-HLA immunity is important in determining the outcome of patients with high level PRA.

Body mass index
Obesity is associated with:
- more transplantation-related surgical complications;
- more delayed graft function;
- higher mortality;
- poorer graft survival.

It has been suggested that, where possible, obese potential recipients should lose weight to achieve a BMI <30 kg/m^2 prior to transplantation. Nonetheless, transplanted obese patients derive a survival benefit when compared to those who remain on dialysis.

There is also evidence for increased mortality and graft loss in those with a low BMI (<18 kg/m^2).

Recipient hypertension
Hypertension adversely affects long-term allograft and patient survival.

It has been estimated that for every 10 mmHg rise in BP the relative risk of allograft failure is 1.3.

Recipient dyslipidemia

Some studies have suggested that hyperlipidemia and/or hypertriglyceridemia are associated with poorer allograft outcomes.

There are preliminary data indicating that lipid-lowering treatment with HMG-CoA reductase inhibitors may improve allograft outcome.

Recurrent or de novo glomerular disease

In patients with ESRD due to glomerulonephritis the 10 year incidence of graft loss due to recurrent glomerulonephritis is 8.4%. It is the third most common cause of graft failure behind chronic rejection and death.

It is likely that as overall allograft survival improves, graft loss due to recurrent or *de novo* glomerular disease will become a more significant problem.

Immune response gene polymorphisms

Genetic variations in the ability of the immune system to mount an immune response to an allograft may affect renal transplant outcome.

Candidate polymorphic genes would include those encoding cytokines, chemokines, adhesion molecules and their respective receptors.

It has been suggested for instance that recipients who harbour homozygous inactivating mutations of the CCR5 gene have a 20 year graft survival of 90% compared to 25% for other allografts.

These studies are inconclusive since they are often retrospective and do not account for other factors that may influence graft outcome.

Proteinuria

The degree of proteinuria correlates with renal allograft outcome. Proteinuria is undoubtedly a reflection of the severity of the underlying renal injury (chronic allograft nephropathy or recurrent/*de novo* glomerular disease), but there is also evidence that proteinuria *per se* can promote further renal injury.

There is a large body of evidence that RAS blockade in native kidneys slows renal disease progression although such data are lacking in the renal transplant setting.

Nonetheless RAS blockade with ACEI and/or ARB should be used in proteinuric renal allograft recipients.

Renal function should be monitored closely after introducing such agents since catastrophic renal failure can occur when there is undiagnosed transplant renal artery stenosis.

Strategies to improve renal transplant outcome

Measures that are likely to improve renal transplant outcome include:
- increased use of living donor kidney allografts;
- pre-emptive transplantation;
- use of younger, generally healthier donors;
- zero HLA mismatching;
- improved organ preservation;
- reduced cold ischemic time;
- nephron dosing;
- matching of donor/recipient with regard to nephron 'dose';
- minimized used of calcineurin inhibitors;
- RAS blockade;
- improved general medical care (including aggressive lipid-lowering and blood pressure control).

Further reading

Meier-Kriesche HU, Schold JD, Kaplan B. Long-term renal allograft survival: have we made significant progress or is it time to rethink our analytic and therapeutic strategies? *Am J Transplant* 2004; **4**: 1662–1668.

Pascual M, Theruvath T, Kawai T, Tolkoff-Rubin N, Cosimi AB. Strategies to improve long-term outcomes after renal transplantation. *N Engl J Med* 2002; **346**: 580–590.

Tang IY, Meier-Kriesche HU, Kaplan B. Immunosuppressive strategies to improve outcomes of kidney transplantation. *Semin Nephrol* 2007; **27**: 377–392.

Wolfe RA, Ashby VB, Milford EL, *et al.* Comparison of mortality in all patients on dialysis, patients on dialysis awaiting transplantation, and recipients of a first cadaveric transplant. *N Engl J Med* 1999; **341**: 1725–1730.

Internet resources

United States Renal Data System (USRDS):

www.usrds.org/

CTS – Collaborative Transplant Study:

www.ctstransplant.org/

Australia and New Zealand Dialysis and Transplant Registry:

www.anzdata.org.au/

UK Renal Registry:

www.renalreg.com/

See also

Inherited renal disease

Chapter contents

Investigation of inherited renal disease

Gene–protein–phenotype

The flow of genetic information

In every cell of the human body the nucleus contains ~35 000 structural genes that represent the entirety of genetic information. Tissue specificity, external stimuli, developmental stage and the current functional state of a cell determine which of these genes are actively expressed, i.e. a gene is transcribed into messenger RNA (mRNA), which is translated into a protein, which through its function, determines a phenotype of a cell (Fig. 15.1.1).

Monogenic diseases

Monogenic diseases are caused in any one patient by mutations in one gene only. In **recessive** diseases a mutation is on both parental chromosomes, whereas in **dominant** disorders a defect on one parental chromosome is pathogenic. Several hundred renal diseases are 'monogenic diseases'. Monogenic diseases are usually rare disorders in the range of 1:1 000 to 1:1 000 000 individuals.

Polygenic diseases

In polygenic diseases, for a given patient, only the actions of different gene defects together lead to the disease phenotype through interaction of the encoded proteins. Polygenic disorders are usually frequent diseases occurring in the range of up to 1:5 (e.g. essential hypertension) to 1:1000 individuals.

Genes

Positional cloning of disease genes

Family studies and haplotype analysis

The set of 46 human chromosomes consists of two sex chromosomes and a double set of 22 autosomes, one set of which is inherited from the father and one from the mother. Crossovers between parental homologous chromosomes can occur in meioses of the gametes that lead to a newborn child. In family studies these crossovers can be observed by examination of genomic DNA from affected individuals. This method is called haplotype analysis (Fig. 15.1.2). This critical region is narrowed down by identifying more crossovers in additional families, until only a few genes can be accommodated in this region. The exons of these genes will have to be examined by direct sequencing of DNA in affected individuals. Identification of mutations in a specific gene will then identify this gene as responsible for the disease.

Single nucleotide polymorphisms

There are ~3–5 million nucleotide positions in the human genome at which individuals may differ (single nucleotide polymorphisms SNPs) from each other (~0.1% of the genome). These SNPs can be detected by DNA microarray analysis. They are used for linkage analysis and are replacing microsatellite markers. This approach has already been very helpful for studies into polygenic diseases.

Known monogenic causes of renal disease

In the past few years the genes responsible for many monogenic renal disorders have been identified by positional cloning. There are renal cystic diseases, such as autosomal dominant polycystic kidney disease (ADPKD), autosomal recessive polycystic kidney disease (ARPKD), and nephronophthisis. There are monogenic glomerular diseases, e.g. mutations in the podocin gene in steroid-resistant nephrotic syndrome, and mutations in specific genes have been identified that are responsible for renal tumours, renal tubular disorders and nephrolithiasis.

Molecular genetic diagnostics

In a monogenic disease the specific gene defect represents the primary cause of this disorder. Gene identification allows for unequivocal molecular genetic diagnosis. In molecular genetic diagnostics two approaches are discerned:

Direct genetic testing: which can be applied if the disease-causing gene is known.

Indirect genetic testing: which is employed if the causative gene is unknown but has been localized to a specific chromosomal region by linkage analysis.

Direct genetic testing

Direct sequencing

In diseases in which the responsible gene is known, relevant mutations may be detected directly in affected individuals following amplification of exons by polymerase chain reaction and consecutive direct sequencing. Conditions that need to be met to allow for direct molecular genetic diagnostics are:

1. The disease gene must have been identified.
2. The functional relevance of mutations detected must be proven by absence from 100 healthy controls, or by a functional test.
3. The mutation may have been shown to be responsible for the disease phenotype in the literature.
4. If there are multiple affected individuals, the mutation must segregate within the pedigree.

For molecular genetic testing prior genetic counselling is mandatory, and ethical guidelines should be observed.

The GeneTests database provides help in finding laboratories all over the world that offer molecular genetic diagnostics for inherited renal diseases.

Indirect genetic testing

If the causative gene for a monogenic disorder is unknown, but a gene locus has been localized to a chromosomal region by positional cloning, indirect genetic testing by haplotype analysis at this gene locus can be performed for diagnostics (see also Fig. 15.1.2).

Electronic databases

Valuable resources are available from electronic databases on the Internet regarding genomic, proteomic and disease-related information. www.ncbi.nlm.nih.gov is a useful place to start.

Animal models of genetic renal disease

Transgenic mouse models are very helpful for the studies of human genetic disorders, and are greatly facilitated by the mouse genome sequence. Mouse models of renal disease have become available through identification of disease phenotypes that are based on spontaneously arisen mutations. In addition, mouse models of human renal genetic disease have been generated by targeted disruption of specific disease-causing genes.

Zebrafish

As a lower vertebrate the zebrafish (*Danio rerio*) has been a very useful model for the study of kidney organogenesis and human renal cystic diseases.

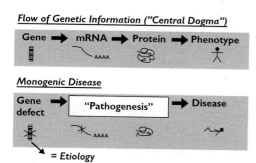

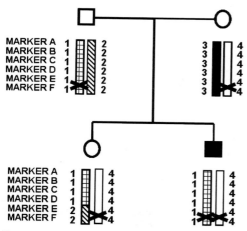

Flow of Genetic Information ("Central Dogma")

Gene → mRNA → Protein → Phenotype

Monogenic Disease

Gene defect → "Pathogenesis" → Disease

= Etiology

Fig. 15.1.1 Central dogma of molecular biology and its relation to monogenic disease mechanisms.

MARKER A	1	2	3	4	
MARKER B	1	2	3	4	
MARKER C	1	2	3	4	
MARKER D	1	2	3	4	
MARKER E	1	2	3	4	
MARKER F	1	2	3	4	

MARKER A	1	4	1	4	
MARKER B	1	4	1	4	
MARKER C	1	4	1	4	
MARKER D	1	4	1	4	
MARKER E	2	4	1	4	
MARKER F	2	4	1	4	

Fig. 15.1.2 The principle of haplotype analysis.

Caenorhabditis elegans

Many genes which cause renal cystic disease (*PKD1*, *PKD2*, *BBS*, *NPHP*) show conservation of sequence homology and of function in the nematode *Caenorhabditis elegans* (*C. elegans*). The genome has been fully sequenced and the cell lineage of every cell in development of *C. elegans* can be followed under a microscope using Nomarski optics. Therefore, *C. elegans* is a very useful model for the study for physiologic and pathophysiologic mechanisms.

Proteins

Generation and use of antibodies as molecular probes

Western blotting

In Western blotting proteins are first size-separated by sodium dodecyl sulphate–polyacrylamide gel electrophoresis (SDS–PAGE), then electroblotted onto a suitable membrane to yield a spatial representation of the result from size separation. This representation can then be visualized by staining with amido black or Ponceau S. The membrane is overlaid with 'primary' antibody directed against the protein of interest. Unbound antibody is then washed away, and secondary antibodies recognizing the Fc fragments of the primary antibody are added. The secondary

antibody has been coupled to a color detection tool, e.g. by using horseradish peroxidase or enhanced luminescence, which allows detection of the secondary antibody in its bound state to the primary antibody, and thereby detection of the band representing the protein of interest. If a suitable antibody is available, Western blotting thus allows detection of a protein of interest out of a complex protein mixture, such as total cell lysates from cell culture. As an example, Western blotting can be employed for detection of proteins from co-immunoprecipitation experiments (Fig 15.1.3). In very complex protein mixtures, size separation by SDS–PAGE alone may not yield sufficient resolution. Under these circumstances 2-dimensional gel electrophoresis may be used. In this method proteins are first separated by their characteristic isoelectric point through isoelectric focusing in a tube gel. Thereafter the linear tube gel is loaded onto an SDS–PAGE gel and proteins are size-separated in a direction perpendicular to the direction for isoelectric focusing. Thereby 2-dimensional size separation is achieved according to two independent characteristics: isoelectric point and molecular weight.

Protein–protein interaction

Co-immunoprecipitation

Protein–protein interactions can be demonstrated by co-immunoprecipitation experiments. Both proteins or fragments thereof are coexpressed in a suitable cell line through transfection of this cell line with expression-plasmids containing inserts encoding these proteins. If no cognate antibody is available for these proteins, they can be expressed as fusion proteins containing a peptide tag for which antibodies are available, such as myc-tags or FLAG-tags. After transfection and cell lysis the lysates are incubated with the antibody directed against one protein or its tag, antibodies with bound protein are precipitated and the precipitate isolated. The precipitate is then size-separated by SDS–PAGE, and protein–protein interaction partners are detected by Western blot analysis of the precipitate (Fig. 15.1.3A). The results usually have to be corroborated in the reciprocal form, i.e. if protein 'A' precipitated with protein 'B', protein 'B' should also co-precipitate with protein 'A' (Fig. 15.1.3B).

Pull-down assays (in vitro assays)

In so-called 'pull-down assays', *in vitro* protein interaction is examined by adsorption of one protein-binding partner as fusion protein to a solid phase, e.g. in a column of this solid phase material. The column is then equilibrated with a lysate that contains the binding partner under high salt conditions, allowing the binding partner to interact. Other nonbinding proteins from the lysate are washed out at high salt. Finally the binding partner is eluted under low salt conditions and detected, e.g. by Western blot analysis. In this way interaction of the proteins polycystin 1 and 2, the genes of which cause autosomal polycystic kidney disease types 1 and 2, respectively, has been demonstrated.

Mapping of protein–protein interaction domains

In vitro protein–protein interaction assays from *in vitro* interaction assays or from co-immunoprecipitation can be used to map protein–protein interaction domains. For this purpose specific constructs containing the full length of the protein and others that contain only fragments of the protein are tested for interaction. Depending on the result, regions necessary for interaction can be delineated.

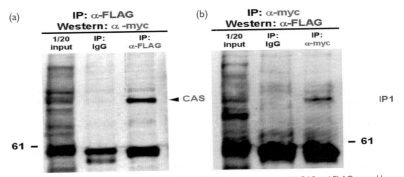

Fig. 15.1.3 Co-immunoprecipitation of nephrocystin-1 and p130CAS. (a) Myc-tagged murine p130CAS and FLAG-tagged human nephrocystin were co-expressed in baby hamster kidney cells. When nephrocystin was precipitated (IP) with the anti-FLAG-antibody, p130CAS was shown in a Western blot to co-precipitate using an anti-myc-ab (right lane; CAS). Also shown is 1/20 of the cell lysate input as positive control (left lane), and IP with an irrelevant antibody (middle lane). Strong bands at 60 kDa are immunoglobulin heavy chains. (b) Vice versa, if p130CAS was precipitated, nephrocystin-1 (NPHP1) co-precipitated, as detected by Western blot using an anti-FLAG-tag antibody.

Identification of new protein–protein interaction partners

In order to identify novel binding partners to a protein or peptide the yeast-2-hybrid system can be employed. In this way the protein p130CAS has been identified as a binding partner to nephrocystin, the product of the *NPHP1* gene, which if defective gives rise to juvenile nephronophthisis type 1 (Fig. 15.1.3).

Proteomics

The term 'proteomics' has been coined to represent the science of studying the entirety of proteins translated within a certain cell type or organism. The proteome of an organism is more complex than the genome, since each gene may be transcribed into alternative splice forms, leading to distinct translation products. Furthermore, post-translational modification, such as cleavage of a signal peptide or glycosylation, leads to additional protein products derived from the same gene. Modern techniques of protein biochemistry, such as high resolution 2-dimensional electrophoresis and mass spectrometry, allow rapid access to comparison of very complex protein expression patterns from whole cell extracts in a 2-dimensional pattern of protein 'spots'. The high sensitivity of mass spectrometry enables sequence-based identification of these spots. Together with sequence comparisons to genetic and protein databases, this provides a very strong approach to studying differential protein expression. As an example the total protein expression pattern of primary cilia from human trachea has been resolved by mass spectrometry.

This data set is very valuable for the study of renal cystic disease. Virtually all proteins involved in the pathogenesis of renal cystic disease in humans and mice are expressed in primary cilia or basal bodies of renal epithelial cells. High-throughput protein analysis can also be performed with the help of microarray techniques.

Phenotyping

Cell biological phenotyping

Immunofluorescence studies

Studies on subcellular localization of proteins can be very helpful to answer questions of the physiological and pathophysiological roles of newly discovered proteins. This is exemplified by subcellular localization studies of nephrocystin-1 and inversin which are mutated in nephronophthisis type 1 and 2 respectively.

Clinical phenotyping

Correct definition of the clinical disease phenotype is of paramount importance for studies of positional cloning. Data on co-segregation of the affected status with polymorphic markers can only be correctly interpreted if there is an *a priori* definition of which member of a pedigree is affected.

Genotype–phenotype correlation

Some genotype–phenotype correlations are emerging in monogenic renal diseases. They can be based on genetic locus heterogeneity, i.e. different genes cause a similar phenotype (as in polycystic kidney disease types 1 and 2), allelic differences of the same gene, i.e. different mutations of the same gene decide on phenotypic differences (as in Alport syndrome) or on the effect of modifier genes.

There are many more genes to be found for renal diseases. The rate-limiting step for disease gene identification is the availability of clinically well-characterized familial cases. Therefore, the three most important actions for nephrologists to partake in the process of gene identification of renal diseases are:

1. Take a family history and sketch a pedigree.
2. Check on the internet:
   - is the gene for the disorder in question known? (http://www.ncbi.nlm.nih.gov/sites/entrez?db=OMIM); and
   - are molecular genetic diagnostics available? (www.Genetests.org).
3. If the gene has not been identified and if a pedigree is informative:
   - autosomal recessive: ≥3 affected individuals of consanguineous parents;
   - autosomal dominant: ≥10 affected individuals.

Contact a molecular genetics laboratory to initiate the process of gene identification of novel genes causing renal disease and its subsequent functional evaluation.

Further reading

Burghes AH, Vessin HE, De La Chapelle A. Genetics. The land between Mendelian and multifactorial inheritance. *Science* 2001; **293**(5538): 2213–2214.

Gabriel SB, Schaffner SF, Nguyen H, *et al.* The structure of haplotype blocks in the human genome. *Science* 2002; **296**(5576): 2225–2229.

Glazier AM, Nadeau JH, Aitman TJ. Finding genes that underlie complex traits. *Science* 2002; **298**(5602): 2345–2349.

Hildebrandt F. Positional cloning and linkage analysis. In: Hildebrandt F, Igarashi P (eds), *Techniques in molecular medicine*. Berlin: Springer; 1999. pp. 352–366.

Ostrowski LE, Blackburn K, Radde KM, *et al.* A proteomic analysis of human cilia: identification of novel components. *Mol Cell Proteomics* 2002; **1**: 451–465.

Otto EA, Schermer S, Obara T, *et al.* Inversin mutations cause nephronophthisis type 2, linking renal cystic disease to the function of primary cilia and left–right axis determination. *Nature Genet* 2003; **34**: 413–420.

Sayer JA, Otto EA, O'Toole JF, *et al.* The centrosomal protein nephrocystin-6 is mutated in Joubert syndrome and activates transcription factor ATF4. *Nat Genet* 2006; **38**: 674-681.

Wolf MTF, Lee J, Panther F, *et al.* Expression and phenotype analysis of the nephrocystin-1 and nephrocystin-4 homologs in *C. elegans*. *J Am Soc Nephrol* 2005; **16**: 676–687.

Internet resources

National Center for Biotechnology Information:

`http://www.ncbi.nlm.nih.gov`

Online Medelian Inheritance in Man (OMIM):

`http://www.ncbi.nlm.nih.gov/sites/entrez?db=OMIM`

Ethical debates and advice on genetic testing:

`http://www.faseb.org/genetics/ashg/policy/pol-00.htm`

Resource for available genetic diagnostic testing:

`http://www.GeneTests.org`

Mouse genome informatics & GeneTrap project:

`http://www.jax.org/resources/index.html`

`http://tikus.gsf.de`

Genomic based drug discovery:

`http://www.lexgen.com`

Caenorhabditis elegans genome informatics:

`http://www.wormbase.org`

See also

History and clinical examination of patients with renal disease, p. 2

Polycystic kidney disease in children

Introduction

Cystic disease in childhood is common and encompasses both genetic and nongenetic causes. This chapter concentrates on autosomal recessive polycystic kidney disease (ARPKD), autosomal dominant polycystic kidney disease (ADPKD) and glomerulocystic disease.

Other common causes of childhood cystic disease (cystic dysplasia, juvenile nephronopthisis, medullary sponge kidney and rare malformation syndromes) will be discussed in later sections.

In ARPKD renal cysts originate from the renal collecting ducts while in ADPKD cysts arise from any segment of the nephron. ADPKD generally presents in adult life while ARPKD presents in childhood. Glomerulocystic disease is typically associated with minimal tubular involvement and can result from several different causes.

Autosomal recessive polycystic kidney disease

Epidemiology

ARPKD is a rare condition with an incidence of 1:20 000 live births and a carrier rate of 1:70. It is the most common inherited renal cystic disease in infancy and childhood.

Genetics

Inheritance of ARPKD is autosomal recessive with a 25% risk of each offspring inheriting the disease. All typical cases of ARPKD are linked to the polycystic kidney disease and hepatic disease 1 (PKHD1) locus on chromosome 6p21. PKHD1 has a complicated transcription profile that results in multiple variants of the integral membrane protein fibrocystin. The role of various splice forms is incompletely understood. Fibrocystin is found in the primary cilium and centrosome. PKHD1 gene products appear to be involved with regulation of cell proliferation, cellular adhesion and repulsion.

Allelic heterogeneity of a single gene is thought to account for differences in phenotypic concordance within and between families. Both genetic and environmental modifying factors may be present. Patients with two truncating mutations have the lethal phenotype. Missense mutations are more common in those with a moderate phenotype.

Previously ARPKD was classified into four groups according to age of onset and was thought to be caused by different mutant genes (Blyth and Ockenden, 1971). The four groups were perinatal, neonatal, infantile and juvenile. Earlier age of onset correlated with increased severity of renal disease and higher mortality. This classification has fallen out of favor recently and ARPKD is thought to be a spectrum of disease with a single gene defect.

Clinical features

The majority of patients are diagnosed in utero or at birth. There can be marked intra-familial phenotypic variability. All patients have renal and hepatic involvement to differing degrees. Renal disease usually begins in utero and hepatic fibrosis is evident by the time they reach adolescence. A distinction can be made between two groups of patients. The first group that presents in utero/perinatal with severe renal disease and high mortality and those that present later who have milder renal disease but more significant hepatic abnormalities.

Severe renal disease in the fetus causes a reduction in fetal urine output leading to oligohydramnios. Thoracic cage compression by the enlarged kidneys leads to severe pulmonary hypoplasia resulting in respiratory distress. The majority of these patients die shortly after birth secondary to respiratory failure. Pneumomediastinum and recurrent pneumothorax are common problems.

In milder renal disease, there is less reduction in amniotic fluid levels and perinatal respiratory compromise is less. Kidney enlargement tends to be mild with variable degrees of renal impairment. This results in better survival in the perinatal period. These patients tend to present later with splenomegaly and hepatic complications. Periportal fibrosis often leads to portal hypertension.

Investigations

The main differential diagnoses are:

- early onset ADPKD;
- glomerulocystic disease.

Screening of the parents to determine the pattern of inheritance is useful to distinguish between the two diseases- in ADPKD one would expect renal cysts in one of the parents.

However, a negative USS in the parents does not exclude ADPKD due to spontaneous mutation, nonpaternity, or a false negative result (in a parent <30 years of age).

The demonstration (usually by USS) of polycystic kidneys and portal hypertension is diagnostic of ARPKD, when parental USS would be expected to be normal.

Prenatal diagnosis

Typical features on USS include bilateral symmetrically enlarged hyperechoic kidneys, oligohydramnios and absence of urine in the fetal bladder. These changes may not be seen until the third trimester so early prenatal USS cannot accurately exclude ARPKD.

Fetal USS cannot reliably differentiate between ARPKD, ADPKD, glomerulocystic disease or Meckel syndrome. A thorough family history and parental screening should provide the diagnosis.

Severely affected fetuses as a result of oligohydramnios may demonstrate Potter's phenotype: low set flattened ears, deep eye creases, snubbed nose, micrognathia, pulmonary insufficiency, deformity of spine and limbs.

High risk pregnancies can now be screened as early as 13 weeks by chorionic villous sampling for haplotype based genetic testing. This requires a comparison with affected sibling(s) DNA, parental DNA and the assumption that the diagnosis is accurate in the index case. An alternative approach is mutational analysis of the PKHD1 gene.

Plain radiography

In the neonate, chest X-ray may show a small thorax with pulmonary hypoplasia. Pneumothorax and pneumomediastinum are often present. Abdominal X-ray may demonstrate bilateral flank masses with centrally displaced bowel.

Ultrasound

This is the modality of choice for diagnosis. In the neonate with significant renal disease, USS shows symmetrically enlarged, diffusely hyperechoic kidneys maintaining their reniform shape.

In children presenting later with mild renal disease, kidneys may appear normal or show changes similar to the neonate. Renal size usually peaks at 1–2 years of age, then declines and stabilizes by 4–5 years. Focal dilatation of the collecting tubules may produce discrete cysts. Appearances of macrocysts and renal fibrosis may mimic the appearances of ADPKD.

Ultrasound of the liver may show biliary ectasia or increased liver echogenicity in the periportal region from bile duct proliferation and fibrosis. In the older child there may be hepatosplenomegaly and evidence of portal hypertension depending on the severity of congenital hepatic fibrosis. Doppler studies may show reversal of portal blood flow. Prominent intrahepatic bile duct dilatation signifies the presence of Caroli's disease

CT and MRI
On unenhanced CT, the kidneys are smooth and enlarged with low attenuation reflecting the large fluid volume in the dilated ducts. Nephrocalcinosis is a common feature. With intravenous contrast, a striated pattern is seen. If renal function is impaired there may be poor opacification and excretion giving poor images of the kidneys. Other CT findings include focal liver cysts, and enlarged portal and splenic veins in portal hypertension.

MRI will show dilated ducts in a typical radial pattern. MRI is useful in the evaluation of liver disease.

Pathology
The cardinal features of this disease are renal collecting duct dilatation and biliary duct ectasia. Ectasia and dilatation are present in 10–90% of renal collecting tubules. Cysts are the result of circumferential epithelial proliferation leading to tubular lengthening and fusiform dilatation of collecting ducts extending from the medulla to the cortex. This cystic epithelium also has abnormal function by paradoxically becoming secretory in nature. Glomeruli are normal as is the collecting system with no component of obstruction. The kidneys are enlarged but smooth and reniform.

There is evidence of proliferation and ectasia of bile ducts which is a ductal plate malformation with periportal fibrosis. The hepatic parenchyma is normal. Significant fibrosis is termed congenital hepatic fibrosis (CHF) which can be found in other diseases and is not pathognomonic for ARPKD.

Widespread intrahepatic dilatation of bile ducts is referred to as Caroli's disease. This is present in 6–12% of patients. Congenital anomalies of other organs are rare.

Treatment
Treatment is centred on symptom and complication management. There is no curative treatment.

Hypertension
Hypertension is present in 61–70% of patients. It is often severe and associated with poor renal survival. If not managed adequately, it may result in cardiac hypertrophy, congestive cardiac failure and even death in infants. The exact mechanism is unknown but, activation of the renin–angiotensin axis and expansion of the intravascular volume has been demonstrated. Treatment with angiotensin converting enzyme inhibitors is recommended. Careful consideration and monitoring will be required in the context of existing renal impairment.

Hyponatremia
This is a common feature of ARPKD in infants. It is a consequence of a defect in free water excretion. Hyponatremia is augmented by the low sodium content of breast milk and formula. Due to the concentrating defect, ARPKD patients are at risk of significant dehydration with intercurrent illness. Careful fluid management is of great importance during these episodes. Thiazide diuretics have been used in severely polyuric patients to reduce distal nephron solute and water delivery. Hyponatremia spontaneously improves and is not seen in older children.

Infection, hematuria and proteinuria
Urinary tract infections occur in 30–43% of patients. Pyuria is a common finding but does not always signify infection. Microscopic and gross hematuria have been reported but is uncommon. Proteinuria is frequently found but nephrotic range proteinuria is rare.

Kidney
Bilateral or unilateral nephrectomy is performed especially in neonates where there is significant respiratory compromise or failure to thrive from malnutrition as a result of pressure effects.

The severity of renal disease is variable. Severe renal disease tends to present early in life with significant mortality and morbidity. Renal replacement therapy is indicated when patients are symptomatic or growth is compromised and refractory to medical management. Peritoneal dialysis is preferred in infants but in older children both peritoneal dialysis and hemodialysis can be used.

Transplantation is the treatment of choice. To enable transplantation, patients may require splenectomy for significant hypersplenism and nephrectomy especially in the neonate to provide surgical space or to reduce the risk of respiratory compromise.

Liver
The liver disease is referred to as congenital hepatic fibrosis (CHF). Hepatic involvement is variable in severity but is progressive and all patients develop hepatic fibrosis eventually. Liver synthetic function is usually normal as the liver parenchyma is preserved. Hepatic encephalopathy is rare. However CHF is not exclusive to ARPKD and can be associated with other kidney diseases (including ADPKD) or systemic disorders.

Portal hypertension is the main complication. The underlying mechanism to its development is not clear. When portal hypertension increases in severity, patients present with splenomegaly, variceal bleeding and hypersplenism. The age of onset is variable but tends to be in older children.

Variceal bleeding can be treated with sclerotherapy or banding. To reduce bleeding and formation of new varices consider transjugular intrahepatic portosystemic shunt placement. In a minority of cases surgical portocaval or splenorenal shunt insertion may be necessary. In anephric patients, portosystemic shunts have been noted to cause hyperammoniemia with fatal hepatic encephalopathy. In these patients, combined liver kidney transplantation should be considered. Hypersplenism may require splenectomy.

CHF may cause ascending cholangitis. Patients present with abdominal pain, fever and elevated liver enzymes. Patients have a higher risk if there are macroscopically dilated bile ducts. Cholangitis can lead to abscess formation, sepsis, fulminant hepatic failure and death. In severe cases surgical drainage or lobectomy may be required.

In a small minority of cases, liver transplantation is considered when severe hepatic dysfunction or chronic severe cholangitis is present.

Respiratory

Pulmonary hypoplasia is common in the affected fetus with corresponding respiratory failure. Bilateral nephrectomy and implementation of renal replacement therapy or continuous arteriovenous hemofiltration to reduce fluid overload have been advocated to improve pulmonary prognosis.

Growth

Growth retardation is correlated with the severity of renal impairment and is observed in ~25% of patients. It is important to ensure good nutrition. Where required, patients should have supplements, and nasogastric or gastrotomy feeding to improve nutritional status. Good management of electrolyte imbalance, fluid status and acid–base balance also play an important role. The use of recombinant growth hormone to improve growth should be considered.

Psycho-social

In addition to the medical problems one must not underestimate the psychosocial stress on the patient and family of the diagnosis and its complications. Reassurance, support and counselling will be required for both the family and the patient.

Follow-up

Frequency of follow-up will depend on the degree of renal impairment but should occur in specialist pediatric and adult renal units.

Prognosis

Within the first decade of life 50% of patients will require dialysis. Neonatal mortality is high at 25–35%. The most common cause of death at this stage is pulmonary insufficiency. The need for neonatal ventilation is a strong predictor of subsequent development of renal failure and death. The majority of patients who survive the neonatal period survive to adulthood with survival rates reported at 67–79% at 15 years of age of these 86% of patients are alive and 72% have adequate renal function at 40 years of age.

Genetic counseling

Parents of a child with ARPKD will both be carriers of the defective gene. Each offspring will have a 25% chance of inheriting the disease and 50% risk of being a carrier. The offspring of an ARPKD patient with a nonaffected partner will have <1% risk of inheritance but all children will be carriers.

Genetic counselling and preconception advise should be given to parents regarding subsequent pregnancies and to patients where appropriate.

Future prospects

Vasopressin receptor-2 antagonists are effective in a rat model of ARPKD, the Pck rat. It is possible that these compounds may be similarly beneficial in ARPKD.

Autosomal dominant polycystic kidney disease

Epidemiology

With advances in imaging and genetic testing, ADPKD is increasingly diagnosed in utero and in asymptomatic children.

Genetics

Inheritance is autosomal dominant. All early onset ADPKD is associated with PKD1. Recurrence rate of early onset ADPKD is 45% in affected siblings of early onset ADPKD patients. Bilateral enlarged kidneys are a common presentation. Glomerular cysts are prominent in very early onset ADPKD. Extrarenal cysts and intracranial aneurysms are rare in childhood.

Pathology

ADPKD is characterized by cystic dilatation of all parts of the nephron and generally presents in adulthood.

Clinical features

ADPKD is an uncommon cause of renal failure in childhood but is often symptomatic. The clinical spectrum is bimodal depending on the age of presentation – it can range from asymptomatic patients (in childhood) to severe nephronomegaly, renal failure, hypertension and pulmonary hypoplasia (at birth). The latter patients are phenotypically similar to ARPKD. Children with ADPKD diagnosed in utero or within the first year of life have higher perinatal mortality, more severe renal disease and reduced renal survival. Children presenting after this period generally have normal renal function.

Risk factors for increased renal volume growth include:

- early renal enlargement;
- >10 cysts by age 12 years;
- hypertension.

However these are not associated with a decline in renal function up to the age of 25 years. The impact on long term prognosis is unknown.

Gross hematuria is found in 10% of children and proteinuria in 28%.

Extrarenal cysts

These features are very rare in pediatric patients. There are rare reports of hepatic and pancreatic cysts in children.

Intracranial aneurysms

These are rarely found in pediatric patients.

Cardiac abnormalities

The incidence of mitral valve prolapse is 12% in children. ADPKD children have a 5% incidence of congenital heart defects compared to 1% in unaffected family members.

Investigations

In PKD1 families, 60% of affected children under 10 years will have cysts rising to 80% at age 18 years. In PKD2 families the reliability of diagnosis with USS is reduced with a 50% detection rate at age <15 years.

Prenatal USS may show large hyperechoic kidneys but is not specific for ADPKD. In infancy kidneys can be normal or cystic. Cysts are scattered throughout the medulla and cortex. Asymmetrical or single kidney involvement has been reported.

The most crucial investigation in distinguishing early-onset ADPKD from ARPKD is for both parents to have a renal USS. If both parents (aged >30 years) have a normal renal USS the probability of ADPKD then reduces to that of a spontaneous mutation.

Genetic linkage studies and mutational analysis can be used but are not routine. The presence of unstable mutations and genetic imprinting have been discounted as underlying causes for early-onset presentations.

Treatment

Hypertension

This is a common feature occurring in 33–47% of patients. Activation of the renin angiotensin-aldosterone system has been documented and increased left ventricular mass has been documented in children. ACEIs and angiotensin receptor blockers (ARBs) are recommended.

Follow-up

The frequency of follow-up will depend on the degree of renal impairment but should occur in specialist pediatric and adult renal units.

Prognosis

Prognosis is good if onset is in childhood, but poor if onset is within the first year of life.

Future prospects

Potential drug treatments, including vasopressin type 2 (V2) receptor antagonists, sirolimus and everolimus, are currently being tested in adult patients.

Glomerulocystic kidney disease

Glomerulocystic kidney disease (GCKD) is characterised by bilateral cortical cysts from dilatation of Bowman's capsule and the proximal convoluted tubule. Glomerulocystic kidneys can be divided into three major categories:

1. GCKD comprising both sporadic and nonsyndromal inherited forms.
2. Glomerulocystic kidneys as a feature of malformation syndromes (e.g. orofacial–digital syndrome type 1): cysts are variably expressed.
3. Glomerular cysts in dysplastic kidneys: dysplastic features predominate.

A rare familial form of GCKD associated with hypoplastic kidneys has been documented. This autosomal dominant form is associated with maturity onset diabetes of the young (MODY) and is caused by mutations in hepatocyte nuclear factor (HNF)-1β.

Dilatation of glomeruli is also seen in ADPKD and other multisystem diseases, e.g. tuberous sclerosis and Von Hippel–Lindau disease.

Glomerular cysts tend to be small and are located predominantly in the subcapsular region although the entire cortex can be involved. High resolution USS, CT or MRI is needed for the diagnosis.

The clinical course is variable and the natural history is not well documented. Infants and children present with bilaterally enlarged kidneys with variable renal function. Adult patients may be asymptomatic or present with progressive renal failure. Early progression to renal failure with need for renal replacement therapy may occur.

Further reading

Bingham C, Bulman MP, Ellard S, et al. Mutations in the hepatocyte nuclear factor-1β gene are associated with familial hypoplastic glomerulocystic kidney disease. Am J Hum Genet 2001; **68**: 219–224.

Fick-Brosnahan GM, Tran ZV, Johnson AM, et al. Progression of autosomal dominant polycystic kidney disease in children. Kidney Int 2001; **59**: 1654–1662.

Guay-Woodford LM, Desmond RA. Autosomal recessive polycystic kidney disease: the clinical experience of North America. Pediatrics 2003; **111**: 1072–1080.

Lonergan GJ, Rice RR, Suarez ES. Autosomal recessive polycystic kidney disease: radiologic–pathologic correlation. RadioGraphics 2000; **20**: 837–855.

Peral B, Ong ACM, San Millan JL, et al. A stable nonsense mutation associated with a case of infantile autosomal dominant polycystic kidney disease. Hum Mol Genet 1996; **5**: 539–542.

Sweeney WE, Avner ED. Molecular and cellular pathophysiology of autosomal recessive polycystic kidney disease (ARPKD). Cell Tissue Res 2006; **326**: 671–685.

Zerres K, Rudnik-Schöneborn S, Deger F. Childhood onset autosomal dominant polycystic kidney disease in sibs: clinical picture and recurrence risk. J Med Genet 1993; **30**: 583–588.

Zerres K, Rudnik-Schöneborn S, Steinkamm C, et al. Autosomal recessive polycystic kidney disease. J Mol Med 1998; **76**: 303–309.

Internet resources

The Polycystic Kidney Disease Charity:

http://www.pkdcharity.co.uk/

National Kidney Federation:

http://www.kidney.org.uk/medical-info/kidney-disease/pckd.html

NIH (NIDDK) Information Clearing House:

http://kidney.niddk.nih.gov/kudiseases/pubs/polycystic/

Polycystic Kidney Disease Foundation:

http://www.pkdcure.org

See also

Autosomal dominant polycystic kidney disease, p. 590

Nephronophthisis, p. 600

Tuberose sclerosis and von Hippel–Lindau disease, p. 598

Rare syndromes with renal involvement, p. 640

Medullary sponge kidney, p. XXX

Chronic kidney disease in children, p. 462

Autosomal dominant polycystic kidney disease

Introduction

Autosomal dominant polycystic kidney disease (ADPKD) is the most common genetic cause of renal failure and accounts for 10% of patients on dialysis. Unlike other causes of chronic kidney disease, ADPKD is characterized by progressive kidney enlargement. It is also a systemic disorder characterized by cyst formation in other organs such as the liver and the pancreas as well as noncystic complications such as arterial aneurysm formation.

Epidemiology

ADPKD has a prevalence of 1:400 to 1:1000 live births.

The disease is usually evident by the 3rd and 4th decades of life but can present at any age.

Genetics

The inheritance pattern is autosomal dominant with 100% disease penetrance. Each offspring has therefore a 50% chance of inheriting the disease. There is a high rate of new mutation. Mutations in either of two genes can lead to ADPKD:

- *PKD1* (chromosome 16p13.3) accounts for 85–90% of cases. *PKD1* encodes for the polycystin-1 protein;
- *PKD2* (chromosome 4q21) accounts for 10–15% of cases. *PKD2* encodes for the polycystin-2 protein.

A small number of families unlinked to either gene could signify the potential existence of a third gene ('*PKD3*').

Polycystin-1 and polycystin-2 are integral membrane proteins.

Polycystin-1 is likely to act as a receptor and is found in primary cilium, focal adhesions, desmosomes, and adherens junctions.

Polycystin-2 is a nonselective cation channel which is highly permeable to calcium ions and is found in the endoplasmic reticulum, centrosome and primary cilium.

Both proteins are widely expressed in multiple tissues and cell types including epithelial cells, vascular smooth muscle cells and cardiac myocytes. They are thought to form a functional complex regulating key aspects of cellular behavior including proliferation, apoptosis, cell adhesion, morphogenesis and net transepithelial fluid secretion via multiple signal transduction pathways.

Cysts form in <1% of nephrons although all cells carry the germline mutation. This observation has led to the two-hit model of cystogenesis which proposes that a second mutation (second hit or somatic mutation) is required for cyst formation.

Environmental factors and modifying genes may influence the rate of second hits (Fig. 15.3.1).

A different mechanism underlying cystogenesis is the haploinsufficiency model where reduced expression of the normal allele below a threshold level may predispose cells to genetic/environmental triggers for cyst formation.

Genotype/phenotype correlations

PKD1 and *PKD2* gene mutations result in a similar clinical phenotype but PKD2 patients have a more favorable course and slower progression to ESRD (mean age of onset 54.3 years PKD1; 74 years in PKD2).

Female PKD2 patients have delayed ESRD compared to males.

There is considerable intrafamilial phenotypic variability indicating the major modifying effects of nonallelic and environmental factors on the phenotype compared to allelic factors.

True genetic anticipation does not occur.

Clinical features

As most patients are asymptomatic, the commonest modes of presentation are with asymptomatic hypertension, incidental USS findings or a positive family history.

Features at presentation

Flank, back and/or abdominal pain (60%).

Urinary tract infection.

Renal stones (20–30%).

Hematuria (gross 30–50%, microscopic 25%).

Hypertension (60%).

Intracerebral aneurysm or bleed (6–16%).

Symptoms of renal failure (usually in the 4th–6th decade of life):

- lethargy;
- poor appetite;
- fluid overload.

Family history of:

- ADPKD;
- cerebrovascular accident/intracranial bleed.

Cardiovascular (important for risk management).

Examination

Proteinuria >300 mg/day (18%).

Nephrotic range proteinuria is uncommon.

Palpable, bilateral flank masses from enlarged kidneys.

Nodular hepatomegaly.

Enlarged pancreas from pancreatic cysts.

Cardiac valve defects: aortic regurgitation, mitral valve prolapse, tricuspid regurgitation.

Hernia—inguinal and umbilical.

Differential diagnosis of renal cysts

Renal cysts are not unique to ADPKD. Other potential causes of renal cysts are listed in Table 15.3.1. The diagnosis of ADPKD can usually be made based on family history, extrarenal manifestations and radiological appearances.

Simple cysts

These become more common with age:

- 1.7% of 30–49-year-olds;
- 22.1% of >70-year-olds.

They are usually unilocular and are located in the cortex.

The kidneys are not normally enlarged and extrarenal manifestations should be absent.

Medullary sponge kidney

This involves cystic dilatation of the medullary collecting ducts resulting in cysts confined to the medulla with a typical appearance on excretory urogram.

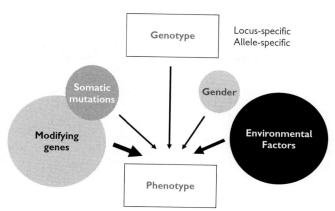

Fig. 15.3.1 Factors that could determine the severity of the cystic phenotype in an individual inheriting a germline *PKD1* or *PKD2* mutation.

Table 15.3.1 Renal cystic diseases

Genetic

Autosomal-dominant
- Autosomal-dominant polycystic kidney disease
- Tuberous sclerosis
- Von Hippel–Lindau disease
- Medullary cystic disease

Autosomal recessive
- Autosomal-recessive polycystic kidney disease
- Juvenile-onset nephronophthisis
- Other rare syndromes associated with multiple malformations

X-linked
- Orofaciodigital syndrome type 1

Chromosomal disorders
- Trisomy 21
- Trisomy 13
- Trisomy 18
- Trisomy C

Nongenetic

Acquired
- Simple cysts
- Acquired renal cystic disease
- Hypokalemia-related cysts

Developmental
- Medullary sponge kidney
- Multicystic dysplastic kidneys
- Pyelocalyceal cysts

Multicystic dysplastic kidneys or congenital multicystic kidneys
This is a unilateral and cystic kidney that has no excretory function.

Tuberous sclerosis complex
This should be suspected if cysts and solid masses (angiomyolipomas) coexist on renal scans. They also have skin lesions in the form of facial and periungual fibromas and CNS involvement.

Von Hippel–Lindau disease
This is characterized by multiple tumors in the cerebellum, spinal cord, retina, adrenal glands (pheochromocytoma), pancreas and kidney. There is a high risk of renal cell carcinoma.

Acquired cystic disease
Patients with a long duration of renal impairment or dialysis can develop acquired renal cysts. They tend to have shrunken kidneys and a negative family history.

Autosomal recessive polycystic kidney disease
ARPKD can be distinguished from ADPKD by the inheritance pattern, earlier age of onset (infancy or childhood) and the obligate presence of liver disease (congenital hepatic fibrosis or Caroli's disease).

Investigations
The diagnosis is based on family history and imaging. Renal USS is the most commonly used modality. Where the family history is unknown or negative, the diagnosis is supported by the presence of bilaterally enlarged cystic kidneys, hepatic cysts, and the absence of extrarenal manifestations that suggest a different renal cystic disease.

Laboratory studies
Serum chemistry profile, calcium and phosphate: for staging of renal function and CKD management.

Full blood count: patients tend to have preserved hemoglobin levels due to preserved erythropoietin secretion.

Urinalysis and culture. Microscopic hematuria is present in 25%, and overt proteinuria in 18%. Nephrotic range proteinuria is rare and should prompt further investigation for concomitant glomerulonephritis. Sterile pyuria is common.

Genetic testing
This can be performed by DNA linkage studies and sequence analysis.

Linkage studies require at least two affected and one unaffected relative for a diagnosis to be made.

Mutation analysis can be done by denaturing high performance liquid chromatography (DHPLC) or direct sequencing.

However, the pathogenicity of unclassified variants (missense mutations vs neutral polymorphisms), which can be seen in up to 40% of cases for *PKD1*, can be difficult to prove in the absence of a valid functional assay.

Imaging studies

Ultrasound

This is the most widely used diagnostic technique for ADPKD. Ultrasound is also useful for detecting liver or pancreatic cysts (Fig. 15.3.2).

Diagnostic criteria:
- at least two cysts in one kidney or one cyst in each kidney in at-risk patients aged <30 years;
- at least two cysts in each kidney in at-risk patients aged 30–59 years;
- at least four cysts in each kidney for at-risk patients aged ≥60 years.

This criterion has a sensitivity of 97–100% in PKD1 patients ≥30 years old but may have a higher false negative rate in younger PKD2 patients. In patients under 30 years of age, false-negative rates are quoted as 23% in PKD2 and 5% in PKD1.

CT and MRI

These are not routinely used for diagnostic purposes but can be helpful in identifying cyst hemorrhage, differentiating renal cell carcinoma from simple cysts, and investigating renal stones (Fig. 15.3.3).

MRI is able to detect renal volume changes with greater sensitivity and accuracy than USS.

Change in kidney volume by sequential MRI has been found to correlate inversely with GFR in the Consortium of Radiologic Imaging Studies of Polycystic Kidney Disease (CRISP) study of ADPKD. MRI can provide a growth rate 'signature' for individual patients and is likely to become widely adopted as the gold standard for estimating disease progression.

Magnetic resonance angiography

This is the preferred imaging technique for diagnosing intracerebral aneurysms (ICA). Screening is recommended where there is family history of ICA, if symptoms of ICA are described, when the patient has a high risk job, or when the patient has had a previous ICA. Presymptomatic screening of ADPKD patients is not otherwise recommended.

Other imaging

Barium enema for the investigation of symptoms suggestive of colonic diverticular disease.

Echocardiography only if valvular abnormalities are suspected on clinical grounds.

Treatment

There is no cure for ADPKD.

Treatment is aimed at:
- slowing the progression of renal failure;
- managing disease complications;
- managing the consequences of CKD.

Pain

This is a common symptom and has several possible causes:

Renal

Acute pain can be due to:
- infection;
- stones;

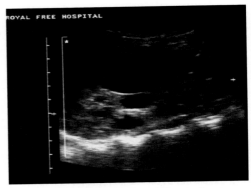

ROYAL FREE HOSPITAL

Fig. 15.3.2 Ultrasound scan showing multiple cysts of varying sizes within a kidney.

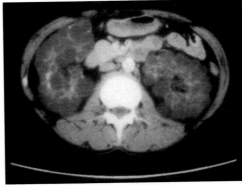

Fig. 15.3.3 CT scan showing bilateral enlarged polycystic kidneys.

- intracystic hemorrhage;
- urinary tract obstruction from stone or blood clot.

Chronic pain can be due to pressure, stretching of the renal capsule or structural distortion.

Nonrenal

This may be due to diverticulitis, liver and pancreatic enlargement, or infection.

Treatment of the underlying cause and simple analgesia is necessary.

NSAIDs should be avoided due to their potential impact on renal function.

Support, reassurance and counseling are important in the management of pain.

Lifestyle modification and avoidance of aggravating activities can be useful.

Patients may require specialist pain clinic involvement, and surgical management (cyst decompression, renal denervation or nephrectomy) may be necessary.

Hypertension

This is a very common early symptom (60% of patients with normal renal function) and is important in the context of cardiovascular risk.

Activation of the renin–angiotensin–aldosterone and sympathetic nervous systems, and endothelin and vasopressin release have been described.

The aim is to achieve a blood pressure of <130/80 mmHg.

Cardiovascular risk factor reduction, e.g. smoking cessation and hyperlipidemia, is important.

There is no specific evidence that any particular antihypertensive drug is more effective in ADPKD. A trial currently in progress (HALT-PKD) is investigating whether the use of ACEIs or ARBs in CKD stage 1–3 confers additional benefit.

Infection

The most common cause of pyrexia is urinary tract infection which can originate from any part of the urinary tract.

Urine cultures may be consistently negative in cyst infection.

Ureteric obstruction from stone or clot with associated infection should be excluded.

Infection can also be extrarenal in origin, i.e. diverticulitis, pancreatic or liver cyst infection.

Patients will require prompt antibiotic treatment that is adjusted according to renal function and culture results.

Cyst infection requires treatment with antibiotics that penetrate the cyst. The most commonly used are ciprofloxacin, trimethoprim and clindamycin. A prolonged course of antibiotics may be required.

Surgical intervention is rarely required. Patients may occasionally require drainage of a perinephric abscess or large infected cyst. Nephrectomy is only required in severe uncontrolled infections.

If there is evidence of recurrent infection, it would be prudent to start long-term prophylactic antibiotics.

If urinary tract instrumentation is ever required, antibiotic prophylaxis should be given.

Cyst hemorrhage and hematuria

Gross hematuria occurs in 30–50% of patients.

The incidence increases as kidney size increases.

It usually occurs spontaneously but may be related to:
- physical activity;
- trauma;
- stones;
- infection;
- tumor formation.

Conservative management with bed rest, hydration and analgesia is the mainstay of therapy as it is normally self-limiting and resolves within days.

Further investigation to exclude malignancy may be considered if episodes are frequent or prolonged, occur in older patients (aged >50 years), or are associated with other systemic symptoms.

Rarely, hemodynamically significant bleeding requiring hospital admission, transfusion and CT ± angiography can occur.

Persistent hemorrhage may require segmental arterial embolization or nephrectomy.

Nephrolithiasis

This occurs in 20–30% of patients.

Stones are commonly composed of calcium oxalate and uric acid.

Stone disease should be considered if acute pain, an acute deterioration in renal function, and hematuria are present.

The higher frequency of stone formation in ADPKD could relate to abnormalities in citrate and magnesium excretion or to prolonged urinary stasis.

Diagnosis by USS is often difficult due to the presence of large cysts; therefore, an IV pyelogram or CT scan is preferred.

Renal stones normally resolve with conservative measures including hydration, treatment of infection, and analgesia.

More complicated cases should be referred for extracorporeal shock wave lithotripsy and/or percutaneous nephrostolithotomy.

Massive polycystic kidneys and large renal cysts

Massive cysts can cause abdominal discomfort or pain.

Cyst reduction can be achieved using:
- alcohol sclerosis;
- percutaneous drainage;
- laparoscopic deroofing.

Laparoscopic renal denervation can be considered in rare cases of uncontrolled pain.

Infected cysts resistant to conventional antibiotic therapy may require surgical drainage under USS guidance.

Nephrectomy is indicated for massive kidneys as a prelude to transplantation (occupying surgical space), and for severe resistant recurrent infection, severe pain or malignancy.

Cancer

There is no evidence for an increased risk of renal cell carcinoma in the ADPKD population. However, if renal cancer is present it is more likely to be bilateral, multicentric and sarcomatous.

Hematuria and flank pain with anorexia and weight loss should prompt further investigation.

CT and MRI are required but can prove difficult to interpret due to the highly altered kidney architecture. Comparison with previous scans (if available) may prove useful.

Liver cysts

Hepatic cysts are the commonest extrarenal manifestation.

Their prevalence increases with age:
- 20% in the 3rd decade;
- 75% in the 7th decade

Hepatomegaly can be massive.

They occur more frequently and are more severe in females, correlating with estrogen exposure (e.g. pregnancy, contraceptive pill).

Liver cysts originate from bile ductules or peribiliary glands.

They are usually asymptomatic and do not lead to hepatic failure.

Pain from compression, feelings of satiety, cystic hemorrhage and infection are the commonest symptoms. Rarely, massive polycystic liver disease can result in portal hypertension (i.e. ascites, esophageal varices).

Cyst infection will require treatment with antibiotics that have good cyst penetration and are tailored to renal function and microbiological sensitivities. A prolonged course of antibiotics is often required. If the infection does not settle, patients may require cyst drainage or, in rare cases, hepatectomy.

If the patient develops problems with satiety that impact on their nutritional status, or has severe discomfort, a surgical debulking procedure can be considered.

The options include:
- cyst deroofing or fenestration;
- cyst drainage and sclerosis;
- transcatheter hepatic arterial embolization (TAE);
- partial hepatectomy.

A massive polycystic liver can rarely cause hepatic venous outflow obstruction resulting in ascites and portal hypertension. If portal hypertension is severe or the polycystic liver is very large with nonresectable areas, liver transplantation may be necessary.

Intracerebral aneurysms

Intracerebral aneurysms (ICAs) occur in:
- 6% of ADPKD patients with no family history of ICA;
- 16% of ADPKD patients with a family history of ICA.

There is a combined 35–55% risk of severe morbidity and mortality following aneurysm rupture.

The median age of ICA rupture among ADPKD patients is less than that in the general population (39 vs 51 years).

Kidney function and blood pressure are usually normal in most patients.

Acute rupture results in subarachnoid hemorrhage (SAH) that is characterized by sudden intense occipital headache.

20–50% of patients have symptoms of headache for up to a week before the acute bleed.

Other features include:
- focal neurological deficit;
- nausea and vomiting;
- photophobia;
- seizures;
- an altered conscious level.

However, the most common neurological event in ADPKD is hypertensive hemorrhage or ischemic stroke.

CT scanning (± lumbar puncture) should be performed if there is clinical suspicion.

Patients with a confirmed bleed need to be referred urgently for neurosurgical assessment.

The International Subarachnoid Aneurysm Trial (ISAT) of ruptured aneurysms showed that in aneurysms suitable for coiling or clipping, endovascular coiling reduced the absolute risk of death and dependency at 1 year by 7.4% compared to clipping. Successful obliteration by endovascular repair is quoted as 66% compared to 82% for open surgery.

The International Study of Unruptured Intracranial Aneurysms (ISUIA) showed that the likelihood of rupture of an aneurysm of <7 mm in diameter is 0.1% per year in patients with no history of SAH.

The decision to treat will have to be balanced against the likely complications of surgery.

Total mortality and morbidity rates for open surgical repair are 12.6% in patients with no history of SAH and 10.1% in patients with previous SAH.

Risk factors for a poor outcome following intervention are:
- age >50 years;
- large aneurysm;
- posterior circulation location;
- previous history of ischemic cerebrovascular disease;
- aneurysmal symptoms.

Conservative management is recommended for aneurysms <7 mm in size in the anterior circulation.

Larger aneurysms are treated by coil embolization or surgical clipping.

If an aneurysm <7 mm is detected, follow-up surveillance scans will be required at 6–12-monthly intervals with increasing duration between scans should the aneurysm be stable.

Control of hypertension and hyperlipidemia and cessation of smoking are advised.

The risk of a new aneurysm developing after an initial negative study is ~2.6% at 10 years in patients with a positive family history of ICA. Therefore a repeat scan may be deferred for 3–5 years unless there are other clinical indications.

Chronic kidney disease and renal replacement therapy

Patients with renal failure will require more frequent monitoring.

Management of CKD and its complications (e.g. bone mineral metabolism, fluid balance, acid–base balance, electrolyte abnormalities) should be started.

By the age of 60 years, ~50% of patients will require renal replacement therapy.

Both peritoneal dialysis and hemodialysis can be used in ADPKD patients.

If massive organomegaly is present, peritoneal dialysis may not be feasible without prior nephrectomy.

Transplantation is the treatment of choice.

There is no difference in patient or graft survival in ADPKD patients compared with other ESRD populations.

Pretransplant nephrectomy may be considered if there are space limitations.

Other extrarenal manifestations

Pancreatic cysts
These occur in 9% of patients aged >20 years.

This is not related to pancreatic dysfunction and no treatment is required.

Cardiac
Valvular abnormalities do not generally require valve replacement but, if present, antibiotic prophylaxis should be instituted for invasive procedures.

Diverticulitis
This has been found mainly in ADPKD patients on dialysis.

It tends to be asymptomatic and its clinical significance is unclear.

Other cystic phenomena
Isolated cysts have been reported in the thyroid, spleen, arachnoid membranes and seminal vesicles of ADPKD patients. These changes are usually asymptomatic and do not require specific treatment.

Follow-up

Patients are best followed up through a specialist renal or genetics clinic.

Genetic counseling should be made available to all at-risk family members.

The management of CKD and its complications should be undertaken according to accepted guidelines for CKD.

In future, the development of effective early treatment could validate mutation testing in presymptomatic individuals.

Prognosis

Patients are usually asymptomatic until the middle decades but 2–5% of patients present in childhood with significant morbidity.

By the age of 60 years, ~50% of patients with ADPKD will require renal replacement therapy.

Commonly, renal function remains normal for decades despite progressive enlargement of kidneys.

End-stage renal disease is not inevitable for all patients.

Poor prognostic indicators for renal survival are:
- male gender;
- Black race;
- hematuria before age 30 years;
- multiple pregnancies;
- hypertension before age 35 years;
- proteinuria;
- *PKD1* mutation.

ADPKD patients do not have a higher risk of mortality compared with other patients with ESRD.

The main cause of mortality is cardiovascular disease (in 36% of cases).

Family screening

Patients should be advised to inform all at-risk blood relatives of the diagnosis and the need for screening.

The autosomal dominant inheritance pattern should be explained with advice on methods of presymptomatic diagnosis including the possibility of prenatal diagnosis.

Each at-risk individual should be informed of the consequences of diagnostic screening.

The benefits and risks of establishing the diagnosis, including the possibility of false-negative USS tests in younger patients, should be discussed.

Pros for diagnosis

Allows early management of complications, particularly hypertension.

Allows for family planning.

Absence of ADPKD reassures the patient.

Cons for diagnosis

Psychological consequences as no specific treatment or cure is available at present.

Insurance and employment issues.

If a family member opts not to have screening, they should be advised to have yearly checks of:
- renal function;
- blood pressure;
- urinalysis.

They will need to inform their general practitioner of their risk of having ADPKD and developing CKD.

Pregnancy

Preconception counseling and referral to a specialist renal/obstetric service should be undertaken.

Prenatal diagnosis by chorionic villous sampling (CVS) can be done at the 9th week of pregnancy. This is not performed routinely due to the high intrafamilial phenotypic variability.

Prenatal screening may be considered in families with one severely affected child (early-onset PKD) who have a 45% recurrence risk for subsequent pregnancies.

The risk of renal function deterioration and ADPKD-related complications in pregnancy is higher with:
- moderate–severe renal impairment;
- proteinuria;
- hypertension.

Hypertensive complications including new and worsening hypertension have been reported in 25% of patients.

Pre-eclampsia occurs in 11% of patients.

Pregnant ADPKD patients require close monitoring for infection and hypertension to enable treatment to be started promptly.

Liver cysts are likely to enlarge in the context of increased estrogen exposure.

Future prospects

As our understanding of ADPKD pathophysiology grows, promising candidate drugs are being developed to treat this disease. Several of these are undergoing clinical trials:

Vasopressin type 2 (V2) receptor antagonists have been found to inhibit cyst development in animal models. A phase III clinical trial on such a compound (tolvaptan) started in 2007.

Octreotide, a somatostatin analogue, has been shown to retard the progression of hepatic and renal cyst growth in rat models. It has also been shown to inhibit renal growth in a few patients.

Sirolimus slows progression of cyst expansion in rodent models. Phase II clinical trials of sirolimus and everolimus have commenced.

Inhibitors of the protein kinases Erb-B1, MEK and CDK also have potential value in treating ADPKD.

Further reading

Grantham JJ, Torres VE, Chapman AB, et al. Volume progression in polycystic kidney disease. N Engl J Med 2006; **354**: 2122–2130.

Molyneux AJ, Kerr RSC, Yu LM, et al. International subarachnoid aneurysm trial (ISAT) of neurosurgical clipping versus endovascular coiling in 2143 patients with ruptured intracranial aneurysms: a randomised comparison of effects on survival, dependency, seizures, rebleeding, subgroups, and aneurysm occlusion. Lancet 2005; **366**: 809–817.

Ong ACM, Harris PC. Molecular pathogenesis of ADPKD: the polycystin complex gets complex. Kidney Int 2004; **67**: 1234–1247.

Ravine D, Gibson RN, Walker RG, et al. Evaluatation of ultrasonographic diagnostic criteria for autosomal dominant polycystic kidney disease 1. Lancet 1994; **343**: 824–827.

Rossetti S, Harris PC. Genotype–phenotype correlations in autosomal dominant and autosomal recessive polycystic kidney disease. J Am Soc Nephrol 2007; **18**: 1374–1380.

Schrier RW, Belz MM, Johnson AM, et al. Repeat imaging of intracranial aneurysms in patients with autosomal dominant polycystic kidney disease with initially negative studies: a prospective ten year follow up. *J Am Soc Nephrol* 2004; **15**: 1023–1028.

Takei R, Ubara Y, Hoshino J, et al. Percutaneous transcatheter hepatic artery embolization for liver cysts in autosomal dominant polycystic kidney disease. *Am J Kidney Dis* 2007; **49**: 744–752.

Torres VE, Harris PC. Mechanisms of disease: autosomal dominant and recessive polycystic kidney diseases. *Nature Nat Clin Prac Nephrol* 2006; **2**: 40–54.

Walz G. Therapeutic approaches in autosomal dominant polycystic kidney disease (ADPKD): is there light at the end of the tunnel? *Nephrol Dial Transplant* 2006; **21**: 1752–1757.

Wiebers DO, Whisnant JP, Huston J 3rd, et al. Unruptured intracranial aneurysms: natural history, clinical outcome, and risks of surgical and endovascular treatment. *Lancet* 2003; **362**: 103–110.

Internet resources

The Polycystic Kidney Disease Charity:

http://www.pkdcharity.co.uk/

National Kidney Federation:

http://www.kidney.org.uk/medical-info/kidney-disease/pckd.html

NIH (NIDDK) Information Clearing House:

http://kidney.niddk.nih.gov/kudiseases/pubs/polycystic/

Polycystic Kidney Disease Foundation:

http://www.pkdcure.org

See also

Polycystic kidney disease in children, p. 586

Tuberose sclerosis and von Hippel–Lindau disease, p. 598

Medullary sponge kidney, p. 664

Nephronophthisis, p. 600

Tuberous sclerosis

Introduction
Tuberous sclerosis complex (TSC) is a multisystem disease associated with the growth of hamartomatous lesions in multiple organs.

A definitive clinical diagnosis requires the presence of two major criteria or one major and two minor criteria:

Major criteria
- Cardiac rhabdomyoma.
- Cerebral cortical tuber.
- Hypomelanotic macule.
- Retinal hamartoma.
- Facial angiofibroma.
- Shagreen patch.
- Subependymal nodule.
- Subependymal giant-cell tumor.
- Renal angiomyolipoma.
- Ungual fibroma.
- Lymphangiomyomatosis.

Minor criteria
- Multiple renal cysts.
- Multiple pits in dental enamel.
- Hamartomatous rectal polyps.
- Bone cysts.
- Cerebral white-matter radial migration lines.
- Gingival fibromas.
- Retinal achromic patch.
- 'Confetti' skin lesions.

Epidemiology
Incidence: 1 in 6000 to 10 000 live births.

Prevalence: 1 in 23 000 from 15 to 45 years

1 in 97 000 age >45 years.

Genetics
Autosomal dominant disorder resulting from inactivating mutations in two genes:
- TSC1 : chromosome 9q34, encoding hamartin;
- TSC2 : chromosome 16p13, encoding tuberin.

More than 200 mutations have been identified.
- 26% of patients have mutations in TSC1;
- 55% of patients have mutations in TSC2;
- 20% of patients have no identified mutation.

A germline (inherited) mutation inactivates one allele and a somatic mutation or loss of heterozygosity inactivates the remaining allele. New mutations (sporadic cases) account for 65% of patients.

TSC1 and TSC2 proteins function as tumor suppressors; they form heterodimers that integrate growth factors, nutrients and the cell cycle via the mammalian target of rapamycin (mTOR). Mutations lead to increased activity of mTOR which has a central role in the control of cell growth and proliferation.

Clinical features
Most patients are identified due to central nervous system (CNS) disease (epilepsy or learning difficulties) and skin lesions. Renal manifestations are often identified during screening.

Renal involvement
Renal involvement occurs in 60% of patients:
- renal angiomyolipoma (AML)(70–80%);
- renal cysts (30–45%);
- renal cell carcinoma (4%).

There is a clear genotype/phenotype correlation with TSC2 mutations having a more severe renal phenotype:
- TSC2 60% AML vs TSC1 22% AML;
- TSC2 31% renal cysts vs TSC1 15% renal cysts.

With more numerous and bilateral lesions of both types with TSC2 mutations.

Angiomyolipoma
These are benign tumors composed of abnormal blood vessels, immature smooth muscle cells and fat cells.

They commonly appear by 7 years of age.

They may present with frank hematuria (uncommon occurring in 4–9%). Life-threatening hemorrhage may occur.

Like sporadic cases, AML in TSC are more common and more numerous in females.

The presence of multiple AML is a reliable indicator of TSC.

They are more likely than not to grow in size.

They become more vascular as they increase in size.

AML >4 cm are at increased risk of hemorrhage, ~50% will bleed vs 5% <4 cm.

AML are unlikely to develop in an individual who has not developed them by early adulthood.

It is unlikely that TSC-related AML progress to carcinoma.

Renal cysts
Cysts commonly appear by age 9 years.

They are often single or small and multiple. A contiguous deletion of TSC2 and autosomal dominant polycystic kidney disease (PKD1) on chromosome 16 leads to early-onset polycystic kidney disease. These cysts are numerous and large.

Cysts are more often associated with hypertension and renal impairment than AML but the majority are asymptomatic.

TSC should always be included in the differential diagnosis of cystic kidney disease.

Renal cell carcinoma
The mean age of occurrence is 28 years compared with 53 years in the general population.

There are variable histological subtypes; clear cell, papillary, chromophobe and oncocytomas are reported.

Chronic kidney disease
Renal impairment is an uncommon initial presentation of TSC (<1%).

CKD may occur as a consequence of renal compression by AML, treatment of AML or glomerulosclerosis but most commonly due to the polycystic phenotype.

Overall 1% of patients will develop ESRD with a mean age of onset of 36 years.

The TSC2 polycystic phenotype is more likely to be symptomatic and lead to CKD.

Investigations

Renal angiomyolipoma

AML need to be 0.4–0.5 cm in diameter to be reliably detected on USS. They are seen as hyperechoic lesions, equal to renal sinus fat.

Fat is an important identifying feature of AML. On CT scan there should be attenuation equal to that of subcutaneous fat and no enhancement with contrast. MRI scans show high signal on T1-weighted images.

Diagnostic difficulty can arise due to fat-poor AML that resemble carcinoma on imaging.

In cases of diagnostic doubt, surgical exploration should be considered, not percutaneous biopsy. There is a significant risk of bleeding from vascular AML and seeding of malignant tumors.

Indeterminate AML on imaging studies often have indeterminate pathology and may be mistakenly diagnosed as malignant lesions.

In female patients aged >16 years AML are associated with pulmonary lymphangiomyomatosis. Due to the significant morbidity, lung function and chest imaging should be undertaken.

Renal cysts

Cysts are sharply circumscribed smooth-walled anechoic structures on USS with water attenuation or fluid signals on CT/MRI. Complex lesions are not commonly seen in TSC and suggest carcinoma.

Genetic testing

In view of the genotype/phenotype correlation, blood for genetic mutation analysis should be taken.

Treatment

A multidisciplinary team approach is required to effectively manage patients with TSC. CNS symptoms often predominate; epilepsy is frequently the most prevalent and challenging clinical manifestation, occurring in 70–80% of patients.

Young patients and those with learning disability are likely to require general anesthetic for investigation and treatment.

Angiomyolipoma

Nephron-sparing strategies are required since renal involvement is typically bilateral.

Treatment should be considered for:
- AML >4 cm in diameter;
- symptomatic AML of any size;
- rapidly growing asymptomatic AML.

Selective arterial embolization is the treatment of choice. In experienced hands this allows almost complete preservation of surrounding normal parenchyma. Embolization can be performed on large AML, >20 cm.

Pharmacological therapy is currently under investigation. Sirolimus, an inhibitor of mTOR, is being trialled in a multicenter phase II study of AML in TSC patients.

Renal cysts

Cysts rarely require treatment and may be managed as simple renal cysts.

Renal transplantation

There is no significant increased risk of malignancy.

In the limited number of reported patients followed long term, no malignancy occurred.

The native kidneys do not need to be removed before transplant.

There is no evidence that neurological features worsen after renal transplantation.

Follow-up

Baseline renal USS should be performed in all patients before 5 years.

If normal it should be repeated every 2–3 years.

If abnormal it should be repeated every 12 months.

If suspicious of carcinoma, MRI or CT is required and this should be repeated after 6 months.

Prognosis

Overall life expectancy is normal. Renal manifestations are the second most common cause of death after complications of CNS disease.

Progression of AML and cysts is difficult to predict but lesions become more numerous with age.

Renal lesions may develop in adulthood after normal imaging in childhood (3% of cases with renal involvement).

Morbidity from renal involvement is low, <10% require intervention.

Future prospects

Detailed understanding of TSC1 and TSC2 interactions with multiple cellular pathways may identify potential antitumoral targets.

The consequences of mTOR inhibition (sirolimus) require further study.

Further reading

Crino PB, Nathanson KL, Henske EP. The tuberous sclerosis complex. *N Engl J Med* 2006;**355**:1345–1356.

Rakowski SK, Winterkorn EB, Paul E, *et al*. Renal manifestations of tuberous sclerosis complex: incidence, prognosis, and predictive factors. *Kidney Int* 2006;**70**:1777–1782.

Internet resources

UK Tuberous Sclerosis Association:

www.tuberous-sclerosis.org

TS Alliance (North America):

www.tsalliance.org

See also

von Hippel–Lindau disease

Introduction
von Hippel–Lindau disease (VHL) is a familial, autosomal dominant, multisystem cancer syndrome. Patients develop multiple benign and malignant tumors in many organs. The CNS, kidneys, adrenal glands and pancreas are most commonly affected.

A clinical diagnosis generally requires one major manifestation in a patient with a positive family history or two major manifestations (including one retinal or CNS) in isolated cases.

Major manifestations
- Retinal hemangioblastoma.
- CNS hemangioblastoma.
- Renal cell carcinoma.
- Pheochromocytoma.
- Pancreatic tumor.

Other manifestations
- Renal cysts.
- Pancreatic cysts.
- Endolymphsac tumor.
- Epididymal cystadenoma.

Epidemiology
Incidence: 1 in 36 000 live births.

90% penetrance by 65 years.

Genetics
The *VHL* gene, on chromosome 3p25-26, encodes a tumor suppressor protein.

Most patients (80%) inherit a germline mutation from an affected parent and normal wild type allele from an unaffected parent. Tumors develop after inactivation of the wild type allele in susceptible organs. The same gene is inactivated in sporadic renal cell carcinoma (RCC) and CNS hemangioblastoma.

The *VHL* gene product, pVHL, is pivotal in angiogenesis via an oxygen-sensing pathway involving hypoxia-inducible factor (HIF). Defective pVHL leads to increased activation of HIF and overproduction of vascular growth factors.

pVHL has multiple other functions with site-specific tumor risks dependent on the degree of expression.

Clinical features
Renal involvement occurs in up to 60% of patients and is found in the majority of patients as a result of screening:
- renal cysts (50–70%);
- renal cell carcinoma (25–45%);
- end-stage renal disease (20–25%).

Renal cysts
Cysts are usually few in number.

They are typically asymptomatic and rarely become infected or lead to hypertension and renal impairment.

VHL should be included in the differential diagnosis of cystic kidney disease.

The presence of numerous pancreatic cysts helps to identify VHL.

Cysts grow slowly (0.5 cm in diameter per year) and some may involute.

Foci of cancer are found in cyst walls but transition to solid RCC is rare.

Cysts generally precede the development of RCC by 5 years.

Renal cell carcinoma
This is uncommon before 18 years.

It occurs at a younger age and is more frequently bilateral or multicentric than sporadic cases.

It often remains asymptomatic for long periods of time.

Large tumors present with hematuria, flank pain or abdominal mass.

Neoplastic lesions uniformly enlarge (1.6 cm in diameter per year).

Histologically all are clear cell subtype.

Multiple (up to 600) microscopic tumors are present throughout both kidneys.

Small carcinomas, <3 cm, tend to be low grade and rarely, if ever, metastasize.

RCC is the leading cause of mortality for VHL patients.

Most will develop recurrence possibly requiring the removal of all renal tissue.

End-stage renal disease
One quarter (23%) of patients develop ESRD as a result of treatment of RCC.

Investigations
Renal ultrasound should be used to screen for renal involvement.

Cysts are thin-walled and have no solid component.

Complex cystic and solid lesions suggest RCC and require CT or MRI.

Lesions suspicious for RCC have attenuation greater than water and enhance with contrast.

Pheochromocytoma should be excluded, by 24 h urine collection for catecholamines and metanephrines, prior to surgery or pregnancy.

DNA should be sent for *VHL* gene mutation analysis.

Treatment
A multidisciplinary team approach is required. The management of progressive, multiple tumors in various organs must be co-ordinated with treatment of the renal involvement.

Renal cell carcinoma
Nephron-sparing surgical techniques should be employed; the goal is to remove lesions that could metastasize.

Treatment should be considered for RCC >3 cm in diameter.

Smaller lesions should be followed until >3 cm.

Arterial embolization, radiofrequency ablation, partial nephrectomy and tumor enucleation have been successfully employed.

Pharmacological agents blocking downstream targets of HIF have shown promise in early phase I studies.

Renal transplantation

Graft and patient survival is similar to that of matched controls. (Note: overall survival is better with surveillance and nephron-sparing surgery.)

A waiting period of 2 years to exclude recurrence of RCC should be considered. This may not be required in patients with low grade asymptomatic tumors found during screening.

Excluding VHL mutations in family members, by genetic screening, will allow living related donor transplantation.

Follow-up

Annual blood pressure from 5 years.

Renal imaging:
- renal USS from 8 years and annually thereafter;
- abdominal CT with contrast from 16 years;
- MRI as clinically indicated.

Annual 24 h urine for catecholamines and metanephrines from 11 years.

Prognosis

Any renal involvement is usually apparent between 18 and 30 years.

An initial onset after 60 years is very rare.

ESRD develops due to repeated surgical removal of renal tissue for the treatment of recurrent and multiple RCC.

Future prospects

Antiangiogenic therapies and specific inhibitors of HIF may be used for the treatment of VHL-related RCC and sporadic cases.

Further reading

Lonser RR, Glenn GM, Walther M, *et al.* von Hippel–Lindau disease. *Lancet* 2003; **361**: 2059–2067.

Shuin T, Yamasaki I, Tamura K, *et al.* Von Hippel–Lindau disease: molecular pathological basis, clinical criteria, genetic testing, clinical features of turmors and treatment. *Jpn J Clin Oncol* 2006; **36**: 37–43.

Internet resources

von Hippel–Lindau Family Alliance:

`www.vhl.org`

Cancerbackup:

`http://www.cancerbackup.org.uk/home`

See also

Polycystic kidney disease in children, p. 586

Autosomal dominant polycystic kidney disease, p. 590

Tumors of the kidney, p. 668

Nephronophthisis

Introduction

Nephronophthisis (NPHP), historically termed 'familial juvenile nephronophthisis', is a chronic tubulointerstial nephritis and frequent cause of CKD in children and adolescents. Inheritance is autosomal recessive, and constitutes the most frequent genetic cause for ESRD in the first three decades of life.

Epidemiology

NPHP is the commonest cause of genetic ESRD in children and is commonly associated with nonrenal abnormalities. NPHP1 is the commonest form, with an incidence of 1:5000, and constitutes ~25% of NPHP cases.

NPHP1 and medullary cystic kidney disease (MCKD) account for 10–20% of children with CKD and for 1–5% of all children undergoing dialysis or transplantation.

Genetics

Positional cloning has revealed seven monogenic recessive genes to date (NPHP1-6 and AHI1), suggesting that mutations in each of these genes is sufficient to cause NPHP, and mammalian data suggest that the encoded proteins function together.

NPHP1

Mutations in NPHP1 were identified as causing juvenile NPHP type 1. NPHP1 encodes nephrocystin-1, a protein that interacts with components of cell–cell and cell–matrix signaling. It also interacts with the products of other NPHP genes, such as nephrocystin-2/inversin, nephrocystin-3, and nephrocystin-4.

Polymerase chain reaction testing for the gene deletion causing type 1 disease is available.

NPHP2

The renal cystic changes of infantile NPHP (NPHP type 2) combine clinical features of NPHP and of polycystic kidney disease (PKD). Mutations in human inversin (INVS, the protein product of NPHP2) cause infantile NPHP (type 2) with and without situs inversus. Inversin interacts with nephrocystin-1 and with β-tubulin, which constitutes the microtubule axoneme of primary cilia (see below). In particular, inversin/NPHP2 function has been implicated in signaling mechanisms of planar cell polarity.

NPHP3

By positional cloning in a large Venezuelan kindred, mutations in NPHP3 have been shown to be responsible for adolescent NPHP. The protein product is termed nephrocystin-3.

NPHP4

Mutations in NPHP4 were identified by homozygosity mapping and total genome search for linkage. The encoded protein, nephrocystin-4/nephroretinin, is in a complex with other proteins that are involved in cell adhesion and actin cytoskeleton organization, such as nephrocystin-1, p130Cas, Pyk2, tensin, filamin, and β-tubulin. In polarized epithelial cells, nephrocystin-4 localizes to primary cilia, basal bodies, and the cortical actin cytoskeleton, whereas in dividing cells, it localizes to centrosomes.

NPHP5, 6 and AHI1 – see below

Clinical features (overview)

Three clinical forms of NPHP have been distinguished by onset of ESRD: infantile, juvenile, and adolescent NPHP,
which manifest with ESRD at the median ages of 1, 13 and 19 years, respectively.

Symptoms

Initial symptoms are relatively mild (except in infantile NPHP type 2). Typically it presents after 6 years of age through adolescence, but may become apparent in early childhood. At an average age of 9 years, a slightly raised serum Cr is noted. The clinical presentation is insidious, and the early symptoms of polyuria and polydipsia are often overlooked in the presence of a relatively normal urinalysis and in the absence of proteinuria, uremia, and hypertension.

Other typical symptoms to look out for include secondary enuresis and anemia. Thus most patients are not diagnosed until after the onset of renal failure.

If a patient presents with mild renal impairment, ESRD invariably develops within a few years. These children are excellent candidates for transplantation.

Disease recurrence has never been reported in kidneys that were transplanted to patients with NPHP.

Syndromic associations

NPHP is associated with several extrarenal features, often coming under eponymous names according to the systems involved. These syndromes include:

Senior–Løken syndrome (SLSN)
Retinal dystrophy, retinitis pigmentosa.

Joubert syndrome (JBTS)
Retinal degeneration, cerebellar vermis aplasia, diffuse hypotonia and mental retardation.

Cogan syndrome
Ocular motor apraxia.

Mainzer–Saldino syndrome
Retinal pigmentary dystrophy, cerebellar ataxia and skeletal dysplasia (cone-shaped epiphyses of the hands).

Leber's congenital amaurosis
Retinal dystrophy.

Jeune syndrome
Asphyxiating thoracic dysplasia.

Ellis–van Creveld syndrome
Chondroectodermal dysplasia.

RHYNS syndrome
Retinitis pigmentosa, hypopituitarism, NPHP, and skeletal dysplasia.

Alström syndrome
Retinitis pigmentosa, deafness, obesity, and diabetes without mental defect, polydactyly, or hypogonadism.

Meckel–Gruber syndrome

Additional NPHP-associated disorders are Sensenbrenner syndrome (cranioectodermal dysplasia) and Arima syndrome (cerebro-oculo-hepato-renal syndrome). NPHP has also been described in association with ulcerative colitis.

As can be seen in this chapter, the delineation of the genes responsible for these disorders is clarifying the phenotyping and classification of the disease. In some instances, there seems to be a genotype/phenotype correlation.

For instance, there is involvement of the retina in all known cases with mutations of NPHP5 or NPHP6. In other instances, such as NPHP1 mutations, the eyes are involved in <10% of patients. The molecular basis of eye involvement is unknown.

Extrarenal features

NPHP is variably associated with conditions affecting extrarenal organs, such as retinitis pigmentosa (SLSN) and ocular motor apraxia (Cogan syndrome).

Eyes

The renal–retinal involvement in SLSN can be explained by the fact that the primary cilium of renal epithelial cells is a structural equivalent of the connecting cilium of photoreceptor cells in the retina. SLSN has been associated with NPHP1, 3, 4 and 5, and it has been suggested to use the nomenclature SLSN1, SLSN2, SLSN4 and SLSN5 to correspond to the associated NPHS gene mutation. Similarly, patients with NPHP1 mutations as well as those with NPHP4 mutations have been described with Cogan syndrome, highlighting a possible pleiotropic effect of NPHP mutations.

The heterogeneity of the renal–retinal syndrome is indicated by the variable age of onset of the retinal abnormality. In some families it is congenital, whereas in others it behaves like isolated recessive retinitis pigmentosa. In children with recessive mutations in the NPHP1, 2, 3, and 4 genes, retinitis pigmentosa occurs in ~10% of all affected families, without any obvious genotype/phenotype correlation.

Three different terms have been used in the literature to describe the retinal findings of SLSN: retinitis pigmentosa, tapetoretinal degeneration, and retinal–renal dysplasia. This most likely reflects a spectrum within the pathogenesis that includes developmental defects (dysplasia) as well as defects of tissue maintenance (degeneration).

In the retinal dysplasia of NPHP, pale optic nerve head and attenuated blood vessels are seen, as in other forms of chorioretinal degeneration. Fundoscopic alterations are present in all patients with late-onset SLSN by the age of 10–years. The late-onset form manifests first with night blindness, followed by development of blindness during school age.

Retinal degeneration is characterized by a constant and complete extinction of the electroretinogram, which precedes the development of visual and fundoscopic signs of retinitis pigmentosa. The kidney involvement in SLSN is identical clinically to what is known from patients with NPHP without ocular involvement regarding age of onset, symptoms, and histology of renal disease.

Leber's congenital amaurosis is characterized by moderate to severe visual impairment identified at or within a few months of birth, infantile nystagmus, sluggish pupillary responses (and occasionally a paradoxical pupil response), and absent or poorly recordable electroretinographic responses early in life. Additional features include symmetric midfacial hypoplasia with enophthalmos and hypermetropic refractive errors.

Congenital oculomotor apraxia (in Cogan syndrome), is a condition characterized by (1) defective or absent horizontal voluntary eye movements, and (2) defective or absent horizontal ocular attraction movements.

Liver

Both NPHP and Bardet–Biedl syndrome can be associated with liver fibrosis. Autosomal recessive PKD is also associated with bile duct ectasia. Bile duct involvement in these cystic kidney diseases may be explained by the ciliary theory, because the epithelial cells lining bile ducts (cholangiocytes) possess primary cilia.

Patients develop hepatomegaly and moderate portal fibrosis with mild bile duct proliferation. This pattern differs from that of classical congenital hepatic fibrosis, whereby biliary dysgenesis is prominent. A recessive mutation in the NPHP3 gene has been described in a patient with NPHP and liver fibrosis. Hepatic involvement in NPHP type 2 (infantile NPHP) seems to involve only transient elevation of transaminases.

Central nervous system

Recent findings suggest that oculomotor apraxia type Cogan (associated with NPHP1 and NPHP4 mutations), cerebellar vermis hypoplasia (in JBTS), and mental retardation (in NPHP type 6) may be due to defects in microtubule-associated functions during neurite outgrowth and axonal guidance.

Cardiac

The phenotypic combination of NPHP2, situs inversus, and cardiac septal defect (one patient with a VSD has been reported) on the basis of inversin mutations is observed in humans, mice, and zebrafish.

Clinical features according to genotype

NPHP1 (juvenile form)

In the various reports, anemia, polyuria, polydipsia, and death in uremia have been features.

Hypertension and proteinuria are conspicuous by their absence. Excessive urinary loss of sodium accounts for the rarity of hypertension.

It has also been reported that decreased urine-concentrating ability might be a manifestation of heterozygotes.

Histologically the kidneys show morphologic changes affecting tubular basement membranes of all segments of the nephron, with or without cysts. These included extreme thinning and attenuation, layering, and thickening. Also reported are interstitial lymphohistiocytic cell infiltration, and development of cysts at the corticomedullary border of the kidneys.

NPHP2 (infantile form)

The specific clinical features of this disease are its early onset and rapid progression to ESRD. It presents within the first months of life with severe renal failure and acidosis, associated with hypertension and polyuria in the majority. In addition, some patients display severe cholestatic liver disease though others may have hepatomegaly without histological disease.

Renal ultrasound will confirm lack of distinct cysts, and some kindreds have been reported with enlarged and echogenic kidneys that lack corticomedullary differentiation.

Renal biopsy is characterized by a diffuse chronic tubulointerstitial nephritis and particularly by the presence of microcystic dilatation of proximal tubules and Bowman space. Pathologically, it differs from later-onset NPHP by the absence of medullary cysts and thickened tubular basement membranes and by the presence of cortical microcysts.

NPHP3 (adolescent form)

The history is similar to juvenile NPHP. Most patients suffer from anemia when they first come to medical attention.

In adolescent NPHP, onset of ESRD occurs significantly later (median age 19 years; quartile borders, 16.0 and 25.0 years) than in juvenile NPHP (median age 13.1 years; quartile borders, 11.3 and 17.3 years).

Histologic findings in adolescent NPHP are generally not distinguishable from those of juvenile NPHP. Renal pathology is thus characterized by alterations of tubular basement membranes, tubular atrophy and dilatation, sclerosing tubulointerstitial nephropathy, and renal cyst development predominantly at the corticomedullary junction.

NPHP4

This gene locus was discovered in patients without NPHP1–3, with clinical and biopsy features of NPHP and ESRD commencing within a wide age range, 11–34 years. This was additionally found to be a new locus for SLSN, an NPHP variant associated with retinitis pigmentosa.

NPHP5

Overall, one in 10 individuals with NPHP has retinitis pigmentosa, constituting SLSN. However, all individuals with NPHP5 mutations have retinitis pigmentosa, suggesting that mutation in NPHP5 is the most frequent cause of SLSN. Eight different mutations in the NPHP5 gene have been identified in patients with SLSN and NPHP mapping to chromosome 3q21.1 (SLSN5).

All patients have early-onset retinitis pigmentosa with no signs of cerebellar vermis aplasia or oculomotor apraxia (Cogan syndrome, associated with NPHP1 and 4).

NPHP6

Recently, recessive truncating mutations in a novel gene NPHP6/CEP290, which encodes a centrosomal protein, were identified as the cause of NPHP type 6 and Joubert syndrome type 5.

The clinical features of NPHP type 6 include renal cysts, retinitis pigmentosa, and cerebellar vermis aplasia.

AHI1

Mutations in AHI1, encoding jouberin, have been detected in patients with Joubert syndrome with and without renal involvement.

Patients reported with renal involvement develop ESRD in their 20s.

Other renal syndromes associated with NPHP

Bardet–Biedl syndrome (BBS)

BBS exhibits renal histology that is similar to NPHP. Positional cloning of recessive genes that are mutated in BBS has revealed that the molecular relation between NPHP and BBS may lie in coexpression of the respective gene products in primary cilia, basal bodies, and centrosomes of renal epithelial cells.

Distinction from MCKD

NPHP has previously been grouped together with the clinical entity of medullary cystic kidney disease (MCKD) because of similarities of clinical and pathologic features.

Both have normal or slightly small kidneys with corticomedullary cysts. However, MCKD follows autosomal dominant inheritance, and is due to mutations in MCKD1 and MCKD2 genes.

In MCKD ESRD occurs in the 4th decade and later.

In MCKD there is no extrarenal involvement other than hyperuricemia and gout.

Genetics of MCKD

There are now known to be 2 types of MCKD, 1 and 2, distinguished by chromosomal localization, with one form of medullary cystic kidney disease (MCKD2) known to be caused by mutation in the gene encoding uromodulin (UMOD), which is also the site of mutations causing juvenile hyperuricemic nephropathy.

Pathology: the ciliopathies

The cilium is a hair-like structure that extends from the cell surface into the extracellular space.

The interaction and colocalization to cilia of nephrocystin-1, inversin, and β-tubulin provide a functional link between the pathogenesis of NPHP, the pathogenesis of PKD (polycystic kidney disease), primary cilia function, and left–right axis determination.

The functional relationship between ciliary expression of these so-called 'cystoproteins' (proteins mutated in cystic kidney disease) and the renal cystic phenotype, however, is still somewhat unclear. One of the first concepts for this relationship proposes that cilia may act as mechanosensors to sense fluid movement in the kidney tubule, where polycystin-1 (the protein product of PKD1) transmits the signal to polycystin-2, which is a TRP type calcium channel. This would produce sufficient calcium influx to induce calcium release from intracellular storage, which then regulates numerous intracellular signaling activities that are linked to the regulation of cell cycle and planar cell polarity.

Taken together, these findings indicate that the nephrocystin proteins are involved in functions of sensory cilia, cell polarity, and cell division.

Treatment

No specific prophylaxis or treatment is available for NPHP currently. The only therapeutic options are supportive treatment once CKD has developed and dialysis and transplantation for ESRD.

Follow-up

Genetic counseling is important for this group of diseases. Genetic mutation analyses are increasingly being offered by genetics departments in major centers.

Prognosis

In both nephronophthisis (NPHP) and medullary cystic kidney disease (MCKD) patients typically progress to ESRD within 5–10 years of presentation.

Retinal involvement is very variable, and long-term information on outcome is not available.

Liver function at the time of renal failure is usually normal despite histological changes, though longer-term liver outcome may become a more significant feature as these patients survive longer.

Future prospects

The delineation of the biology underlying this group of conditions in recent years will lead to exciting potential advances in treatment. For example the renal cystic phenotype of pcy mice, which is the equivalent of human NPHP type 3, can be strongly mitigated or even reversed by treatment with the vasopressin V2 receptor antagonist OPC31260.

Table 15.6.1 Principal features of the different types of nephronophthisis

Nomenclature		Gene	Protein	Renal manifestations	Extrarenal manifestations
Juvenile NPHP	Type 1	NPHP 1	Nephrocystin-1	Presents at 4–6 years with ESRD at 13 years	Renal–retinal syndrome (retinitis pigmentosa, tapetoretinal degeneration). Joubert syndrome (uncommon)
Infantile NPHP	Type 2	NPHP 2	Inversin	Presents at 1–2 months with ESRD at 1 year	Retinitis pigmentosa. Hepatomegaly. Cholestatic liver disease. Situs inversus.
Adolescent NPHP	Type 3	NPHP3	Nephrocystin-3	Presents at 4–6 years ESRD at 19 years	Tapetoretinal degeneration and hepatic fibrosis, cerebellar ataxia, cone-shaped epiphyses, congenital oculomotor apraxia.
	Type 4	NPHP4	Nephrocystin-4 or nephroretinin	Wide range of ESRD onset, 11–34 years	Tapetoretinal degeneration; retinitis pigmentosa.
	Type 5	NPHP5 also known as IQCB1	Nephrocystin-5	Renal involvement in all. ESRD by second decade of life.	Retinitis pigmentosa in all patients
	Type 6	NPHP6	Nephrocystin-6	Either severe or absent	Retinitis pigmentosa; cerebellar vermis aplasia; Leber's congenital amaurosis.
Joubert syndrome		AHI1	Jouberin	ESRD in the 3rd decade of life, if renal involvement	Joubert syndrome: aplasia of the cerebellar vermis, ataxia, abnormal eye movements, an abnormal breathing pattern in the neonatal period and psychomotor mental retardation.

Further reading

Chang B, Khanna H, Hawes N, *et al.* In-frame deletion in a novel centrosomal/ciliary protein CEP290/NPHP6 perturbs its interaction with RPGR and results in early-onset retinal degeneration in the rd16 mouse. *Hum Mol Genet* 2006; **15**: 1847–1857.

Hildebrandt F, Zhou W. Nephronophthisis-associated ciliopathies. *J Am Soc Nephrol* 2007; **18**: 1855–1871.

Hildebrandt F, Otto E, Rensing C, *et al.* A novel gene encoding an SH3 domain protein is mutated in nephronophthisis type 1. *Nat Genet* 1997; **17**: 149–153.

Mangos JA, Opitz JM, Lobeck CC, *et al.* Familial juvenile nephronophthisis. An unrecognized renal disease in the United States. *Pediatrics* 1964; **34**: 337–345.

Olbrich H, Fliegauf M, Hoefele J, *et al.* Mutations in a novel gene, NPHP3, cause adolescent nephronophthisis, tapeto-retinal degeneration and hepatic fibrosis. *Nat Genet* 2003; **34**: 455–459.

Otto E, Hoefele J, Ruf R, *et al.* A gene mutated in nephronophthisis and retinitis pigmentosa encodes a novel protein, nephroretinin, conserved in evolution. *Am J Hum Genet* 2002; **71**: 1161–1167.

Otto EA, Schermer B, Obara T, *et al.* Mutations in INVS encoding inversin cause nephronophthisis type 2, linking renal cystic disease to the function of primary cilia and left–right axis determination. *Nat Genet* 2003; **34**: 413–420.

Otto EA, Loeys B, Khanna H, *et al.* Nephrocystin-5, a ciliary IQ domain protein, is mutated in Senior–Løken syndrome and interacts with RPGR and calmodulin. *Nat Genet* 2005; **37**: 282–288.

Parisi MA, Doherty D, Eckert ML, *et al.* AHI1 mutations cause both retinal dystrophy and renal cystic disease in Joubert syndrome. *J Med Genet* 2006; **43**: 334–339.

Sayer JA, Otto EA, O'Toole JF, *et al.* The centrosomal protein nephrocystin-6 is mutated in Joubert syndrome and activates transcription factor ATF4. *Nat Genet* 2006; **38** 674–681.

Yang H, Wu C, Zhao S, *et al.* Identification and characterization of D8C, a novel domain present in liver-specific LZP, uromodulin and glycoprotein 2, mutated in familial juvenile hyperuricaemic nephropathy. *FEBS Lett* 2004; **578**: 236–238.

Internet resources

Joubert Syndrome Foundation:

http://www.jsfrcd.org/

Genetic & Rare Diseases Information Centre:

http://rarediseases.info.nih.gov

See also

Rare syndromes with renal involvement, p. 640

Polycystic kidney disease in children, p. 586

CKD in children, p. 462

Thin membrane nephropathy

Thin membrane nephropathy (TMN) is a common autosomal dominant inherited glomerular disorder that results in persistent microscopic hematuria.

TMN is characterized by glomerular basement membranes (GBMs) which are thin but otherwise morphologically normal.

The term 'benign familial hematuria' was previously used in an era before the GBM abnormality had been identified.

Genetics

The similarity between the basement membrane changes seen in early Alport's syndrome and those seen in TMN suggested the presence of a similar underlying genetic defect.

40% of families with TMN have hematuria that segregates with the COL4A3/COL4A4 locus, and identical mutations have been described in both TMN and autosomal recessive Alport's syndrome.

TMN patients with such mutations can be considered as carriers of autosomal recessive Alport's syndrome.

Approximately 20 COL4A3 and COL4A4 mutations have been identified in families with TMN. The majority are single nucleotide substitutions that are different in each family.

Recently the association of TMN, focal segmental glomerulosclerosis and progressive CKD has been described in a cohort of patients with mutations in both COL4A3 and COL4A4 genes.

In some families linkage with the COL4A3 and COL4A4 genes has not been found. Whereas some of these cases may be explained by de novo mutations or incomplete penetrance, it is probable that the remainder are due to the presence of further TMN loci.

Clinical features

TMN is the underlying diagnosis in 20–25% of patients presenting to a nephrologist with isolated microscopic hematuria.

Autopsy and kidney transplant donor studies suggest that 5–9% of the population has TMN.

It is an autosomal dominant condition but may also be sporadic.

Persistent microscopic hematuria is typical and usually lifelong.

Episodic macroscopic hematuria may also occur in up to 1/5 of patients.

Up to 30% of patients experience flank pain. In a small number of cases TMN has been described in patients with loin-pain hematuria syndrome.

Hypertension may be more common than in the general population although this is not confirmed in all studies.

Proteinuria is uncommon and patients with nephrotic range proteinuria usually have a second, superadded diagnosis.

Progressive renal impairment is rare but has been described in a number of families.

Deafness and other extrarenal manifestations seen in Alport's syndrome are absent.

There is no specific treatment.

Pathology

The pathological findings in TMN are limited to diffuse thinning of the GBM which is otherwise morphologically normal (Fig. 15.7.1).

This contrasts with Alport's syndrome in which the GBM is thickened and lamellated and the normal lamina densa of the GBM is disrupted.

The normal range for GBM thickness must be determined in each laboratory because of the influence of techniques used for fixing the biopsy, but typically normal GBM thickness is 350–450 nm and a reduction to <250 nm involving >50% of the GBM is diagnostic of TMN.

An accurate assessment of GBM thickness can only be made on glutaraldehyde-fixed renal tissue. Reprocessing of formalin-fixed tissue for electron microscopy (for example when the glutaraldehyde-fixed sample contains no glomeruli) results in artifactual thinning of the GBM which precludes the accurate diagnosis of TMN.

Differential diagnosis

The two principal differential diagnoses are:
- IgA nephropathy;
- Alport's syndrome.

TMN can only be distinguished from IgAN by renal biopsy.

TMN and IgAN may coexist; whether this is a true association or simply due to the coincidence of two common glomerular disorders is unclear.

TMN must be distinguished from Alport's syndrome (hereditary nephritis with deafness), of which the commonest form is X-linked.

If there is a clear autosomal dominant pattern of hematuria without renal insufficiency or extrarenal problems a clinical diagnosis of TMN may be established with reasonable confidence, but a renal biopsy in at least one family member is still preferable.

Once the diagnosis is established in a kindred, biopsy is not required unless there are unexpected clinical changes.

Differentiation from the less common autosomal forms of Alport's syndrome may be less straightforward.

Subclinical deafness should be excluded by audiography if necessary.

The renal biopsy also requires careful assessment. In TMN there is uniform thinning; early in the course of Alport's syndrome, even if the typical structural disruption of the GBM has not yet developed, marked variability in GBM width is typical.

Staining of GBM for the α chains of type IV collagen is highly informative: in X-linked Alport's the α3, α4 and α5 are absent (mosaic expression in female carriers); in autosomal recessive Alport's the α3, α4 chains are absent; whereas in TMN normal α chain distribution is preserved.

Genetic testing for COL4A3 or COL4A4 mutations to diagnose TMN is clinically not practical because of the huge size of these genes, their frequent polymorphisms, and the likelihood of the existence of further gene loci.

Prognosis and follow-up

The prognosis is excellent in the great majority of families with TMN, though there is a small but definite risk of

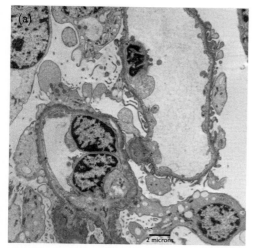

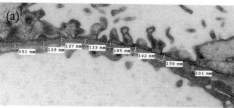

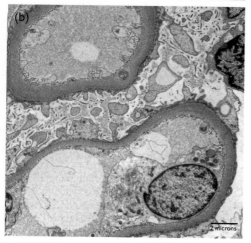

developing CKD, heralded by the onset of proteinuria and hypertension.

Long-term follow-up of patients with TMN is therefore mandatory with urinalysis, blood pressure measurement and renal function testing recommended every 1–2 years.

Further reading

Dische FE, et al. Incidence of thin membrane nephropathy: morphometric investigation of a population sample. *J Clin Pathol* 1990; **43**: 457–460.

Nieuwhof CM, deHeer F, de Leeuw P, van Brieda Vriesman PJ. Thin glomerular basement nephropathy. Premature glomerular obsolescence is associated with hypertension and late onset renal failure. *Kidney Int* 1997; **515**: 1596–1601.

Tiebosch AT, et al. Thin basement membrane nephropathy in adults with persistent hematuria. *New Engl J Med* 1989; **320**: 14–18.

Tryggvason K, Patrakka J. Thin basement membrane nephropathy. *J Am Soc Nephrol* 2006; **17**: 813–822.

Internet resources

Background information on Alport's and TMN:

http://www.genetests.org/query?dz=alport

See also

Urinalysis and microscopy, p. 8

Renal biopsy, p. 32

Alport's syndrome, p. 606

IgA nephropathy and Henoch–Schönlein purpura, p. 100

Fig. 15.7.1 Thin membrane nephropathy. (a) Electron micrograph of two capillary loops with abnormally thin basement membranes. The GBM is otherwise structurally normal. (a)¹ Measurement of the GBM shows that it is uniformly thinned. (b) Electron micrograph of two capillary loops with normal GBM for comparison. (Electron micrographs courtesy of Dr Nick Mayer, Consultant Histopathologist, University Hospitals of Leicester, UK.)

Alport's syndrome

Introduction
Alport's syndrome (also known as hereditary nephritis or Davidson's nephritis) is an inherited syndrome of hematuria and progressive renal impairment due to defects in synthesis of type IV collagen. Type IV collagen is a hexamer (Fig. 15.8.1) and a major component of basement membranes, predominantly found in the glomerular basement membrane (GBM), tubular basement membranes, Bowman's capsule and skin. In addition to the renal involvement there may be associated sensorineural deafness, anterior lentoconus and other ocular abnormalities.

Epidemiology
Alport's syndrome is rare, affecting 1 in 5000 live births.

There is no difference in inheritance by:
- gender;
- geography;
- ethnicity.

Males are more severely affected than females.

Severity of disease is consistent within kindreds but there is marked variability between families.

Novel mutations account for 20% of cases.

Patients with Alport's syndrome account for 2–3% of patients with ESRD.

Genetics
The constitutive proteins are coded on six genes found on three different chromosomes (Fig. 15.8.1).

Genes are located on chromosomes 2, 13 and X.

Theoretically these gene products could polymerize in 46 656 combinations but in fact only three are found.

Alport's syndrome can be inherited in three ways (Table 15.8.1):
- X-linked (80% of cases);
- autosomal recessive (15% of cases);
- autosomal dominant (5% of cases).

More than 200 distinct disease-causing mutations have been identified resulting in defects in type IV collagen (Fig. 15.8.2).

X-linked Alport's syndrome is most prevalent.

Mutations in COL4A2 have thus far not been identified in Alport's syndrome.

Mutations in COL4A1 have recently been implicated in a novel syndrome of hematuria, cystic kidney disease, intracranial aneurysms and muscle cramps.

Clinical features
Hematuria
Persistent microscopic hematuria can be seen from infancy.

Upper respiratory tract infections may be associated with paroxysmal macroscopic hematuria.

Male children without microscopic hematuria by the age of 10 years are unlikely to have Alport's syndrome.

Affected female patients (X-linked heterozygous) and autosomal dominant (AD) Alport's syndrome may have intermittent hematuria.

Proteinuria
Autosomal recessive (AR) Alport's syndrome and males with X-linked Alport's syndrome develop proteinuria in early adulthood.

Nephrotic syndrome occurs in 40%.

X-linked heterozygous females and AD Alport's syndrome rarely develop proteinuria but when present it is associated with worse prognosis.

Excretory renal dysfunction
Cases of AR Alport's syndrome and males with X-linked disease progress to ESRD.

Most patients reach ESRD in their third decade.

Some kindreds progress more slowly, reaching ESRD in their 5th decade.

X-linked disease in females and AD Alport's syndrome is generally benign.

Proteinuria or diffuse GBM thickening on electron microscopy is associated with progressive renal failure.

Hypertension
With progressive proteinuria and renal dysfunction hypertension is common.

Sensorineural deafness
Alport's syndrome is associated with deafness in most males with X-linked disease and patients with AR Alport's syndrome.

Hearing loss is progressive and usually clinically significant by the second decade.

In females with X-linked disease and AD Alport's syndrome hearing loss is less severe and develops later in life.

Ocular defects
Anterior lenticonus is associated with established progression to ESRD and occurs in 15% of males with X-linked disease.

Asymptomatic perimacular granulations can be observed in up to 30% of patients.

Related syndromes
Defects in type IV collagen are found in other conditions bearing some similarities to Alport's syndrome.

Benign familial hematuria is etiologically identical to AD Alport's syndrome and probably represents the most benign end of the spectrum of disease.

Nail–patella syndrome results from mutation of the LMX1B transcription factor altering expression of COL4A3 and COL4A4.

Differential diagnoses
- Thin membrane disease.
- IgA nephropathy.
- Familial membranous nephropathy.
- Focal segmental glomerulosclerosis (FSGS).
- Epstein and Fechner's syndromes.
- Urogenital neoplasia.
- Urinary calculi.

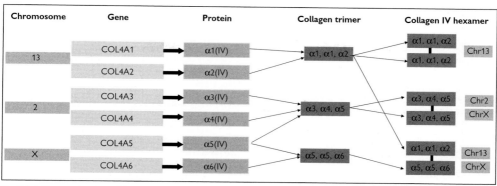

Fig. 15.8.1 The genetics of type IV collagen.

Table 15.8.1 Patterns of inheritance of Alport's syndrome

Inheritance	Family history	Prevalence	Genetic defect	Clinical features
X-linked males	Yes	40%	COL4A5 (Chr Xq22)	Hematuria from first decade
				Proteinuria and progression to ESRD in 3rd decade
				Associated with leiomyomas if defect extends to COL4A6 gene
X-linked females	Yes	40%	COL4A5 (Chr Xq22)	More benign
				Isolated microscopic hematuria may be the only manifestation
				Progression to ESRD occurs in 12% by 5th decade
Autosomal recessive	No	15%	COL4A3 (Chr 2q35-q37) COL4A4 (Chr 2q35-q37) De novo mutation in COL4A5 (Chr Xq22)	Similar to males with X-linked disease
Autosomal dominant	Yes	5%	COL4A3 (Chr 2q35-q37) COL4A4 (Chr 2q35-q37)	Marked heterogeneity
				Spectrum of disease from isolated microscopic hematuria to ESRD

Investigations

Alport's syndrome should be suspected in a patient with:

- hematuria;
- deafness;
- family history of kidney disease.

Biochemistry

Biochemical investigations are not diagnostic of Alport's syndrome.

They do help identify and monitor degree of renal impairment:

- urea, creatinine and electrolytes;
- urine protein excretion: spot PCR or 24 h collection.

Imaging

Imaging of the renal tract in Alport's will be normal.

Ultrasound examination of the urogenital tract is important to exclude alternative diagnoses for example structural abnormalities and neoplasia.

Plain abdominal X-ray may identify calculi within the urogenital system.

Genetic testing

Genetic screening by linkage analysis or gene sequencing is possible. However, this is time-consuming and often unreliable due to the large number of disease-causing mutations.

It may be useful for prenatal diagnosis in previously characterized kindreds.

Renal biopsy

Diagnosis is confirmed by renal biopsy.

Light microscopy

There are no pathognomonic lesions of Alport's syndrome on light microscopy but this can exclude other potential diagnoses including FSGS, membranous nephropathy and IgA nephropathy.

GBM thickening, glomerular sclerosis and tubulointerstitial fibrosis may be seen with progessive disease.

Immunofluorescence

Direct immunofluorescence is unhelpful in diagnosing Alport's syndrome but can exclude IgA nephropathy.

Immunostaining for components of type IV collagen can be diagnostic. Commercially available antibodies against $\alpha3(IV)$, $\alpha4(IV)$ and $\alpha5(IV)$ are available (Table 15.8.2).

Some female patients with X-linked disease have a mosaic pattern of immunostaining for type IV collagen.

Electron microscopy

Lamellation of the GBM is strongly suggestive of Alport's syndrome (Fig. 15.8.3).

Other abnormalities include variability in thickness of the GBM with both abnormally thick and thin areas.

Skin biopsy

Skin biopsy has been advocated by some as a less invasive alternative to renal biopsy.

An absence of $\alpha5(IV)$ collagen in skin biopsies is diagnostic of X-linked Alport's syndrome in patients with hematuria and a positive family history.

Treatment

Slowing progression of renal failure

There is no specific treatment for Alport's syndrome.

There are no randomized controlled trials of therapies to slow progression of CKD in Alport's syndrome.

Ciclosporin and ACEIs/ARBs

There is a single report of treatment with ciclosporin preserving renal function for more than a decade in eight children.

Data from a proteinuric animal model of Alport's syndrome suggests that ACEIs may reduce proteinuria and slow decline in renal excretory dysfunction.

It is likely that treatment of high blood pressure with an ACEI and/or ARB will reduce proteinuria and delay progression of renal decline in common with other progressive renal diseases.

Observational trials are in progress to assess the efficacy of this approach.

Renal transplantation

Renal transplantation is an effective treatment of ESRD in Alport's syndrome.

Post-transplant renal outcomes are comparable to other populations with reported 1 year and 5 year graft survival of 87% and 66% respectively.

Care must be taken when assessing potential living related donors.

Post-transplantation anti-GBM disease

Patients with Alport's syndrome are immunologically naive to subunits of type IV collagen. Following transplantation, exposure to these previously absent type IV collagen subunits in the renal allograft may trigger a significant immune response.

Post-transplantation anti-GBM disease is encountered in patients with Alport's syndrome, although it is less common than one might expect.

Antibodies against components of type IV collagen can be identified in up to 20% of renal allograft recipients.

Overt anti-GBM disease occurs in only 1.5–2.5%.

Post-transplantation anti-GBM disease differs from traditional Goodpasture's disease:

- the disease is always renal-limited;
- in traditional disease, antibodies usually form against the $\alpha3(IV)$ subunit of collagen but in patients with Alport's syndrome they may be against $\alpha3(IV)$, $\alpha4(IV)$, $\alpha5(IV)$ or $\alpha6(IV)$ depending on the genotype;
- laboratory testing for 'anti-GBM' antibodies is normally limited to $\alpha3(IV)$ collagen, so false-negative results may arise.

Diagnosis is confirmed by renal transplant biopsy showing linear IgG staining, crescentic glomerulonephritis, segmental necrosis and neutrophilic infiltrates.

There are no randomized controlled trials for the treatment of post-transplantation anti-GBM disease.

Graft outcomes are poor.

A trial of immunosuppressive therapy and plasma exchange may be considered.

Retransplantation of affected individuals is rarely successful and often associated with more rapid acute vascular rejection.

Follow-up

Patients with AR Alport's syndrome or males with X-linked disease will progress to ESRD.

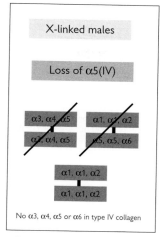

X-linked males

Loss of α5(IV)

α3, α4, α5   α1, α3, α2

α3, α4, α5   α5, α5, α6

α1, α1, α2

α1, α1, α2

No α3, α4, α5 or α6 in type IV collagen

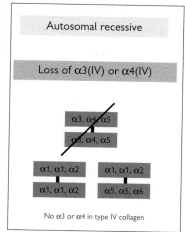

Autosomal recessive

Loss of α3(IV) or α4(IV)

α3, α4, α5

α3, α4, α5

α1, α1, α2   α1, α1, α2

α1, α1, α2   α5, α5, α6

No α3 or α4 in type IV collagen

Fig. 15.8.2 Phenotype of type IV collagen in Alport's syndrome.

Table 15.8.2 Type IV collagen immunostaining patterns in Alport's syndrome

	α3(IV)	α4(IV)	α5(IV)
Normal	✓	✓	✓
X-linked males	✗	✗	✗
X-linked females		Mosaic pattern	
Autosomal recessive	✗	✗	✗
Autosomal dominant	Reduced or absent	✓	✓

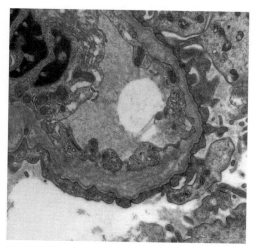

Fig. 15.8.3 Electron micrograph showing lamellation, thickening and thinning of the glomerular basement membrane in Alport's syndrome. (Courtesy of Nick Dr Mayer, Consultant Histopathologist, University Hospitals of Leicester, UK.)

Timely treatment of complications of CKD (hypertension, anemia, renal bone disease) and planning for renal replacement therapy improves morbidity and mortality as with other kidney diseases.

Pre-emptive renal transplantation is effective for patients with Alport's syndrome. Relatives offering kidneys for transplantation should be carefully assessed to exclude covert disease.

Patients should be offered genetic counseling if planning to start a family.

Ophthalmology and audiology input is often indicated.

Prognosis

Males with X-linked disease
ESRD develops in 90% of patients by the 5th decade.

Patients with deafness and ocular changes tend to progress more rapidly.

Increasing proteinuria and hypertension are associated with more rapid progression to ESRD.

Life expectancy is shortened due to complications of transplantation and dialysis.

Females with X-linked disease
This is usually a benign disorder of microscopic hematuria.

Progression to ESRD occurs in 12% by the 5th decade.

Associated deafness, ocular disorders, proteinuria and hypertension are associated with worse prognosis.

Autosomal recessive disease
Outcomes are similar to males with X-linked disease.

Absence of a family history and relative increase in severity in females may delay diagnosis.

Autosomal dominant disease
There is marked heterogeneity in clinical manifestations dependent on genotype.

Outcomes range from isolated microscopic hematuria to ESRD.

Future prospects
Bone marrow transplantation has been shown to ameliorate renal disease in a murine model of Alport's syndrome although we remain a long way from offering this or other forms of gene therapy for the treatment of Alport's syndrome.

Increased use of ACEIs, ARBs with stringent BP control may slow progression of excretory dysfunction and delay the onset of ESRD but this still needs to be confirmed.

Further reading
Hudson BG, Tryggvason K, Sundaramoorthy M, Neilson EG. Alport's syndrome, Goodpasture's syndrome and type IV collagen. N Engl J Med 2003; 348: 2543–2556.

Plasier E, Gribouval O, Alamowitch S, et al. COL4A1 mutations and hereditary angiopathy, nephropathy, aneurysms and muscle cramps. N Engl J Med 2007; 357; 2687–2695.

Saito A, Yamazaki H, Nakagawa Y, Arakawa M. Molecular genetics of renal diseases. Intern Med 1993; 36: 81–86.

Internet resources
The Alport Syndrome Foundation:

http://alportsyndrome.org/index.html

National Kidney Federation: Alport's syndrome:

http://www.kidney.org.uk/medical-info/alports/

See also
Antiglomerular basement membrane disease, p. 124

Selection and preparation of recipients, p. 544

Recurrent disease and de novo disease post renal transplantation, p. 566

Nail–patella syndrome, p. 608

Nail–patella syndrome

Introduction

Nail–patella syndrome (NPS) is an autosomal dominant disease characterized by dystrophic nails, hypoplastic or absent patellae, dysplasia of the elbows and iliac horns, and renal disease in some patients.

Epidemiology

Estimated incidence of NPS is 22 pmp.

NPS is described in populations throughout the world.

Equal gender distribution.

Genetics

NPS is caused by mutation of the *LMX1B* gene found on the long arm of chromosome 9 (9q34).

LMX1B is a LIM homeodomain-type transcription factor that regulates the transcription of genes critical for glomerular basement membrane formation (GBM) and podocyte function.

These are:

- type IV and probably type III collagen;
- podocin;
- CD2AP.

Loss of regulated expression of these glomerular components leads to abnormal GBM production and podocyte dysfunction, leading to the renal phenotype described below.

Clinical presentation

Renal manifestations

Renal disease is clinically apparent in less than one-half of patients with NPS.

Approximately 10% of NPS patients with nephropathy will develop ESRD.

NPS-related nephropathy usually becomes apparent in late adolescence or young adulthood.

The features of nephropathy are variable and typically include microscopic hematuria and low grade proteinuria, but may progress to nephrotic syndrome in association with hypertension. Urine concentrating ability may also be affected.

The frequency and severity of renal involvement varies between families and also in affected individuals within families.

Extrarenal manifestations

Skeletal defects

60% of patients have absent or hypoplastic patellae that results in lateral slippage of the patella on knee flexion. Joint effusions and osteoarthritis leading to knee pain may result.

Up to 80% of patients have iliac horns that are pathognomonic of NPS. These are symmetrical osseous processes arising from the iliac wings. They are asymptomatic but may be detected on clinical examination.

Elbow abnormalities are also common. These include hypoplasia of the radial heads leading to elbow subluxation, hypoplasia of the distal humerus, and formation of posterior processes from the distal humerus leading to limitations of extension, pronation and supination of the forearm.

Nail defects

80–90% of patients will have nail abnormalities.

These are present at birth and tend to be bilateral and symmetrical.

The fingernails are more commonly affected than toenails with the thumb and index finger particularly affected.

The nails may be absent but are more often hypoplastic or dysplastic with discoloration, koilonychia, longitudinal ridges, or triangular lunulae.

Other defects

Bony abnormalities of the feet and ankles, and scoliosis have been described.

In addition, symptoms of irritable bowel syndrome and vasomotor dysfunction are occasionally observed.

Renal pathology

Light microscopy

Essentially normal in those with normal renal function.

Heavy proteinuria and/or impaired renal function is manifested by basement membrane thickening and nonspecific focal and segmental glomerulosclerosis.

Immunofluorescence microscopy

Usually negative apart from nonspecific IgM and C3 reactivity in sclerotic areas.

Electron microscopy

Demonstrates irregular and lucent rarefactions of the lamina densa of the basement membrane.

These areas contain crossbanded collagen fibrils that are best demonstrated by staining with uranyl acetate and phosphotungstic acid.

These lesions are pathognomonic for NPS.

They may involve the whole or just segments of the GBM, may be seen in the mesangium, but are never seen in the tubular basement membrane.

These fibrils have been shown to be comprised of type III collagen (Fig. 15.9.1).

Note that these features can also be seen in NPS patients without clinical evidence of renal involvement and the severity of histological abnormality correlates poorly with clinical renal dysfunction in those with nephropathy.

Natural history

End-stage renal disease develops in ~10% of NPS patients with nephropathy.

Mean age when ESRD develops is 33 ± 18 years.

The clinical course can be highly variable suggesting that nongenetic factors influence outcome.

Other glomerular diseases have been described in patients with NPS-related nephropathy including:

- IgA nephropathy;
- membranous nephropathy;
- anti-GBM disease;
- pauci-immune vasculitis.

Whether these diseases occur in NPS with increased frequency is unknown.

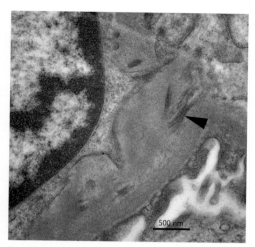

Fig. 15.9.1 Nail–patella syndrome. Electron micrograph showing the characteristic crossbanded collagen fibrils in the glomerular basement membrane (arrowhead).

Treatment

There is no specific treatment available.

A generic treatment approach with blood pressure control, the use of ACEIs and/or ARBs, and cardiovascular risk management is appropriate.

Renal transplantation is not associated with recurrent disease and is not complicated by anti-GBM disease (in contrast to Alport's syndrome).

Further reading

Bennett WM, Musgrave JE, Campbell RA, et al. The nephropathy of the nail–patella syndrome. Clinicopathologic analysis of 11 kindred. Am J Med 1973; **54**: 304.

Bongers EM, Gubler MC, Knoers NV. Nail–patella syndrome. Overview on clinical and molecular findings. Pediatr Nephrol 2002; **17**: 7037–7012.

Dunston JA, Hamlington JD, Zaveri J, et al. The human LMX1B gene: transcription unit, promoter, and pathogenic mutations. Genomics 2004; **84**: 565.

Sweeney E, Fryer A, Mountford R, Green A, McIntosh I. Nail patella syndrome: a review of the phenotype aided by developmental biology. J Med Genet 2003; **40**: 153–162.

Internet resources

Nail Patella Syndrome UK:

`http://www.npsuk.org/`

Nail Patella Syndrome Worldwide:

`http://www.nailpatella.org/`

See also

Proteinuria and/or hematuria, p. 76

Alport's syndrome, p. 606

Thin membrane nephropathy, p. 602

Congenital and infantile nephrotic syndrome

Introduction

Congenital nephrotic syndrome by definition develops within the first 3 months of life. The onset of nephrotic syndrome between 3 and 12 months of age is called infantile nephrotic syndrome.

Genetic abnormalities underlie the majority of cases of nephrotic syndrome that develop in the first year of life.

The renal outcome is generally poor.

Genetics

More than 85% of cases of congenital nephrotic syndrome are due to mutations of the following genes (Table 15.10.1):

NPHS1

Encodes the slit diaphragm component nephrin; mutations result in congenital nephrotic syndrome of Finnish type.

NPHS2

Encodes podocin; mutations result in familial FSGS.

WT1

Encodes the Wilms' tumor suppressor gene; mutations result in the Denys–Drash and Frasier syndromes.

LAMB2

Encodes β2-laminin; mutations result in the Pierson syndrome.

PLCE1

Encodes phospholipase Cε; mutations result in early-onset diffuse mesangial sclerosis.

NPHS1 and NPHS2 mutations account for >90% of cases of congenital nephrotic syndrome.

Congenital nephrotic syndrome may also result from non-genetic causes and these are listed in Table 15.10.1.

Congenital nephrotic syndrome of the Finnish type (CNF)

This is most frequent in Finland.

The incidence is between 0.9 and 1.2 per 10 000 live births but is now falling due to the availability of prenatal screening.

CNF has also been described in a variety of ethnic groups throughout the world.

Pathogenesis

CNF results from abnormalities of the NPHS1 gene.

This gene encodes for nephrin which is a component of the podocyte slit diaphragm.

The absence of nephrin from the slit diaphragm is thought to result in the breakdown of glomerular permselective function and the free movement of plasma proteins into the urine.

A wide variety of nephrin mutations has been described. However, ~90% of Finnish CNF patients have either the Fin-major (nt121delCT) or Fin-minor (R1109X) mutations.

In non-Finnish CNF patients >30 mutations have been identified. In addition, a small number of patients with features of classical CNF have no identifiable NPHS1 mutations, suggesting that the disease can be induced by promoter or intronic mutations or mutations of proteins that interact with nephrin.

Clinical features

Prematurity (35–38 weeks) is usual.

Babies are small for gestational age.

Cranial sutures are widely separated, the nose is small and ears are low-set. Flexion deformities of hips, knees and elbows are common.

The placenta is enlarged.

Edema present by the end of the 1st week of life in 50%.

Severe nephrosis with ascites is invariably present by 3 months.

Profound hypoalbuminemia and hypogammaglobulinemia develops.

Growth is poor.

Bacterial infections (peritonitis, respiratory infections) and thromboembolism may occur.

Hypothyroidism is common (urinary loss of thyroxine-binding proteins).

End-stage renal failure develops at 3–8 years of age.

Prolonged survival is possible with supportive treatment including dialysis and transplantation.

Pathology

Early changes are confined to mild mesangial hypercellularity with increased mesangial matrix expansion.

Later with further mesangial matrix deposition progressive glomerulosclerosis develops.

Immune deposits are absent.

On electron microscopy podocytes have profound foot process effacement and slit-diaphragms are absent.

Tubulointerstitial changes are prominent, with microcystic dilatation of tubules, progressive interstitial fibrosis and tubular atrophy developing later in the course of disease.

Treatment

Glucocorticoids and immunosuppressive agents are ineffective.

Management includes:
- daily or alternate day albumin infusions;
- gammaglobulin replacement;
- high-protein, low-salt diet (tube feeding/parenterally);
- vitamin and thyroxine supplementation;
- infection and thromboembolism prophylaxis.

Bilateral surgical nephrectomy may be required since even maximal supportive therapy may not avoid growth retardation and intercurrent complications of nephrosis.

The administration of indomethacin and ACEIs to reduce intraglomerular pressure is an alternative approach to surgery. In a small number of cases this has led to substantial reduction in proteinuria and subsequently an improvement in nutritional status and growth.

Renal transplantation can be undertaken once the child reaches a weight of 8–9 kg.

Recurrence of nephrotic syndrome can occur in ~20–25% of transplants. This is more common in Fin-major recipients (nephrin is absent in native kidneys) and has been shown to be due to the presence of circulating anti-nephrin

Table 15.10.1 Causes of congenital nephrotic syndrome

Genetic causes
Congenital nephrotic syndrome of the Finnish type
Diffuse mesangial sclerosis (idiopathic)
Diffuse mesangial sclerosis with Denys–Drash syndrome
Diffuse mesangial sclerosis with Frasier syndrome
Pierson syndrome
Galloway syndrome
Nail–patella syndrome

Nongenetic causes
Idiopathic nephrotic syndrome
Infection:
• congenital syphilis
• congenital toxoplasmosis
• cytomegalovirus
• rubella virus
• human immunodeficiency virus
• hepatitis B
Mercury exposure
Membranous nephropathy due to maternal neutral endopeptidase mutations

antibodies in the majority (analogous to the development of anti-GBM antibodies following the transplantation of patients with Alport's syndrome).

Recurrence of disease is associated with graft loss but graft survival may be improved by plasmapheresis and methylprednisolone.

Antenatal diagnosis

Amniotic and maternal plasma α-fetoprotein (AFP) levels are increased by 15–16 weeks gestation due to increased urinary loss of AFP by the fetus. This finding is not specific but in high risk families may be sufficient evidence to consider termination of pregnancy.

Heterozygous carrier fetuses also have increased amniotic AFP levels, but are not at risk of developing CNF. Therefore unnecessary terminations can be undertaken on the basis of AFP testing alone.

Prenatal genetic screening is now available using genetic linkage and haplotype analysis (the four major haplotypes accounting for 90% of CNF alleles in Finland have been identified). Haplotype testing is ~95% accurate.

NPHS2 mutations

A small number of patients with features typical of CNS have been found to have homozygous *NPHS2* mutations.

NPHS2 encodes podocin which is a podocyte-specific protein that interacts with nephrin and appears to be critical for normal slit-diaphragm function.

Combined *NPHS1* and *NPHS2* mutations have also been identified demonstrating the genetic heterogeneity of CNS.

The clinical manifestations and outcome are similar to that seen with *NPHS1* mutations.

Immunosuppressive treatment is ineffective.

Diffuse mesangial sclerosis

Pathogenesis

Mutations of the *PLCE1* gene appear to be the cause of isolated diffuse mesangial sclerosis. Diffuse mesangial

sclerosis may also be seen as part of Denys–Drash syndrome resulting from a mutation in the *WT1* gene.

PLCE1 encodes phospholipase Cε which is an enzyme that catalyzes the hydrolysis of phosphoinositides and results in the generation of signaling molecules.

The mechanism through which aberrant phospholipase Cε activity leads to podocyte dysfunction is unclear but a causal role is supported by the observation that targeted deletion of *PLCE1* gene in zebrafish leads to glomerular dysfunction.

Clinical features

Babies with diffuse mesangial sclerosis appear normal at birth, with normal size and no placental abnormalities.

Nephrotic syndrome may be present at birth but more usually develops during the first 2 years of life.

Various extrarenal manifestations have been reported including muscular dystrophy, myopia, microcephaly, mental retardation, cataract, and nystagmus.

End-stage renal failure is invariable and usually occurs before the age of 3 years.

Pathology

Early glomerular changes include mesangial matrix expansion without hypercellularity.

Capillary walls become thickened due to hypertrophy of podocytes.

Progression leads to massive mesangial matrix expansion, GBM thickening and reduction of capillary lumens.

Mesangial sclerosis eventually contracts resulting in a sclerotic mass within a dilated Bowman's space.

Immunohistochemistry demonstrates mesangial deposition of IgM, C3 and C1q probably as the result of nonspecific deposition in injured glomeruli.

Electron microscopy demonstrates hypertrophic mesangial cells, hypertrophic podocytes containing numerous vacuoles and irregular effacement of podocyte foot processes.

The same renal pathological appearances can be seen in the Denys–Drash syndrome, for which screening should therefore be instituted.

Treatment

Diffuse mesangial sclerosis is thought to be resistant to steroid and immunosuppressive treatment.

However, a small number of instances of remission of proteinuria with steroids or ciclosporin have been reported.

Nephrotic syndrome is less severe than that seen with CNF, therefore the intensive supportive treatment described for CNF is generally not required for patients with diffuse mesangial sclerosis.

Supportive treatment includes:
• maintenance of adequate nutrition;
• infection prophylaxis;
• management of renal dysfunction.

Renal transplantation is not complicated by disease recurrence.

Bilateral nephrectomy is considered at the time of transplantation given the potential risk of developing Wilms' tumor in those with *WT1* mutations. There is no consensus about this approach, however.

Denys–Drash syndrome (DDS)

This is the combination of:

- progressive renal disease (diffuse mesangial sclerosis);
- male pseudohermaphroditism;
- Wilms' tumor.

Most cases are sporadic.

It is caused by mutations of the *WT1* gene (chromosome 11) which encodes the Wilms' tumor suppressor gene (a zinc finger protein transcription factor).

In DDS most mutations are missense mutations affecting exons 8 and 9.

DDS patients are heterozygous for WT1 mutations with the abnormal WT1 protein acting in a dominant negative manner.

Loss of WT1 function predisposes to the development of Wilms' tumors (embryonic kidney tumors arising from aberrant mesenchymal stem cell differentiation).

Wilms' tumors develop when both alleles become abnormal (ie acquisition of a 2nd WT1 mutation).

Clinical features

Diffuse mesangial sclerosis is invariably seen in DDS and it follows the same clinical course as described previously.

Wilms' tumor may be the first manifestation of the syndrome, may be unilateral or bilateral, and may be associated with nephroblastomatosis.

Male pseudohermaphroditism (ambiguous genitalia or female phenotype, and dysgenetic testes or streak gonads) is seen in all 46XY patients. 46XX children in contrast have a normal female phenotype.

A normal male phenotype effectively excludes a diagnosis of DDS.

Progressive renal dysfunction is invariable with ESRD occurring <3 years of age.

Almost all patients will develop Wilm's tumor if they retain their native kidneys. Bilateral nephrectomy is performed prior to transplantation to avoid this complication.

Frasier syndrome

This also results from WT1 mutations (point mutations in the donor splice site in intron 9).

It consists of nephrotic syndrome, complete XY gonadal dysgenesis, and increased susceptibility to gonadal tumors, usually gonadoblastomas.

Classically, it has been described in 46XY patients with under-masculinized external genitalia that may range from ambiguous in appearance to normal-looking female genitalia.

Recently 46XX patients have been described with a normal female phenotype (and gonads) in association with nephropathy and Wilms' tumor.

The renal abnormalities may be either diffuse mesangial sclerosis or focal segmental glomerulosclerosis.

Renal dysfunction is progressive with ESRD occurring by late childhood.

Idiopathic nephrotic syndrome (INS)

This is rarely seen at birth but can develop during the first year of life.

Histological appearances of minimal change disease, FSGS and diffuse mesangial proliferation can be seen.

A response to steroids heralds a favorable prognosis; however, most children who present with INS <1 year of age are treatment resistant and tend to have progressive renal dysfunction.

Mutations of *NPHS2* can be seen in such patients.

Mutations in the α-actinin-4 gene can be identified in some patients. The protein is involved in maintenance of the podocyte cytoskeleton and abnormalities have been identified in some families with autosomal recessive FSGS.

Pierson syndrome

This is also known as microcoria-congenital nephrosis syndrome.

It is an autosomal recessive syndrome resulting from mutations in the *LAMB2* gene.

LAMB2 encodes laminin β2 which is a component of the glomerular basement membrane.

Mice with a targeted deletion of LAMB2 develop congenital nephrotic syndrome, retinal abnormalities, and neuromuscular junction defects.

In children the features are:

- congenital nephrotic syndrome with diffuse mesangial sclerosis on renal biopsy;
- microcoria (small unreactive pupils);
- abnormal lens (posterior lenticonus) with cataracts;
- retinal abnormalities.

Galloway syndrome

This is the constellation of:

- microcephaly;
- mental retardation;
- hiatus hernia;
- nephrotic syndrome.

Probable autosomal recessive inheritance.

Underlying cause is unknown.

The nephrosis develops at ~3 months of age, is treatment resistant, usually severe, and progresses to ESRD.

The histological appearances resemble either minimal change disease, FSGS, mesangioproliferative GN, or diffuse mesangial sclerosis.

Infection

Table 15.10.1 lists potential infectious causes of congenital nephrotic syndrome.

Congenital syphilis and cytomegalovirus are the most important clinically.

Renal biopsy reveals either membranous nephropathy or diffuse proliferative GN. Immune complexes containing microbial antigen can often be identified and probably mediate the onset of glomerular disease.

Successful treatment of the infection usually leads to resolution of the glomerular disease.

Other causes

- Membranous nephropathy secondary to maternal neutral endopeptidase mutations;
- Nail–patella syndrome;
- Mercury exposure.

Several cases of congenital membranous nephropathy have been described in which podocyte injury is induced in the fetus by the materno-fetal transfer of antibodies directed against the podocyte protein neutral endopeptidase. Antibodies are generated in mothers who lack this antigen and are then sensitized by the fetus.

Further reading

Habib R. Nephrotic syndrome in the first year of life. *Pediatr Nephrol* 1993; **7**: 347.

Heaton PA, Smales O, Won W. Congenital nephrotic syndrome responsive to captopril and indometacin. *Arch Dis Child* 1999; **81**: 174.

Kestilä M, Järvelä I. Prenatal diagnosis of congenital nephrotic syndrome (CNF, NPHS1). *Prenat Diagn* 2003; **23**: 323–324.

Little M, Wells C. A clinical overview of WT1 mutations. *Hum Mutat* 1997; **9**: 209.

Niaudet P. Genetic forms of nephrotic syndrome. *Pediatr Nephrol* 2004; **19**: 1313–1318.

Niaudet P, Gubler MC. WT1 and glomerular diseases. *Pediatr Nephrol* 2006; **21**: 1653–1660.

Patrakka J, Martin P, Salonen R, *et al*. Proteinuria and prenatal diagnosis of congenital nephrosis in fetal carriers of nephrin gene mutations. *Lancet* 2002; **359**: 1575.

VanDeVoorde R, Witte D, Kogan J, Goebel J. Pierson syndrome: a novel cause of congenital nephrotic syndrome. *Pediatrics* 2006; **118**: e501.

Internet resources

Congenital nephrotic syndrome: Family Factsheet:

http://www.gosh.nhs.uk/factsheets/families/F990283/index.html

Orpha.net: a database of rare diseases and orphan drugs:

http://www.orpha.net/

See also

Nail–patella syndrome, p. 608

Nephrotoxic metals, p. 236

Rare syndromes with renal involvement, p. 640

Nephronophthisis, p. 600

Fabry disease

Introduction

Fabry (or Fabry–Anderson) disease is a rare lysosomal storage disease that results from deficiency of the lysosomal enzyme α-galactosidase A (α-Gal A) and the inability to catabolize glycosphingolipids with terminal α-galactosyl residues. Glycosphingolipids are normal constituents of the plasma membrane and intracellular organelles and often circulate in association with apolipoproteins. In the absence of sufficient α-Gal A, these lipids, particularly globotriaosylceramide (GL-3; also known as Gb3, and ceramide trihexoside, CTH), accumulate progressively in the lysosomes of many cell types, particularly endothelial cells.

Epidemiology

Fabry disease is the second most prevalent lysosomal storage disorder after Gaucher's disease.

Population estimates range from 1 in 80 000 to 1 in 120 000 live births.

There is a slight preponderance of males with an increased incidence of 1 in ~50 000.

Genetics

The gene for α-Gal A is found on the long arm of the X chromosome (Xq21.33-q.22.1).

More than 100 mutations have been identified in the α-Gal A gene.

Most of the mutations described are associated with the classic Fabry phenotype, in which there is multisystem involvement.

Mutations that decrease but do not eliminate the enzyme's activity usually cause the milder, late-onset forms of Fabry disease that affect only the heart or kidneys.

Unlike other X-linked disorders, Fabry disease causes significant medical problems in many females, but the signs and symptoms usually begin later in life and are milder than those seen in their affected male relatives.

Some females who carry a mutation in one copy of the α-Gal A gene never have any of the signs and symptoms of Fabry disease.

Clinical features

Fabry disease may be classified into either a classic form or a cardiac variant.

Classic Fabry disease is a multisystem disorder involving the:
- skin;
- eyes;
- kidneys;
- heart;
- neurological system.

The variant form is characterized by cardiac abnormalities, most typically, conduction defects and cardiomyopathy.

Renal involvement

There is progressive glomerular damage resulting in proteinuria and microscopic hematuria.

Renal function slowly declines over years with secondary hypertension and ESRD usually developing by the 4th or 5th decades of life.

Heterozygote women may have abnormal urinary sediment, but ESRD is rare.

Cardiac involvement

Glycosphingolipid accumulation within the heart and coronary vessels leads to:
- progressive coronary occlusive disease;
- ischemic cardiomyopathy;
- conduction abnormalities;
- valvular heart disease;
- left ventricular hypertrophy.

Neurological involvement

Peripheral nervous system:
- autonomic dysfunction;
- hypohydrosis;
- painful extremities (acroparesthesia, occurs early).

Central nervous system:

Glycosphingolipid accumulation tends to occur in the vertebrobasilar circulation resulting in strokes characterized by:
- hemiparesis;
- ataxia;
- memory loss.

Skin involvement

Angiokeratomas are small dilated veins of the upper dermis that become covered by hyperkeratotic epidermis (Fig. 15.11.1).

They usually present early in the disease and tend to cluster on the lower trunk and extremities and appear as clusters of small, dark red spots.

Ocular involvement

Corneal opacities develop in the form of whitish curls that radiate from the centre (corneal verticillata).

Vascular lesions of the conjunctiva and retina may be identified with slit-light examination.

Pulmonary involvement

Deposition of glycosphingolipid in the bronchial tree causes airway narrowing leading to:
- cough;
- shortness of breath;
- a fixed deficit with airflow limitation on spirometry.

Investigations

Clinical examination including slit-lamp examination is often sufficient to secure the diagnosis.

The serum level of globotriaosylceramide (Gb3 with GL-3) may be elevated.

The urine may contain glycosphingolipid-laden epithelial cell aggregates containing oval fat bodies.

Confirmation of the diagnosis requires the demonstration of reduced or absent α-Gal A activity in serum, leukocytes, skin or other tissue.

Indeterminate results may be obtained from atypical variants or heterozygous females, in which case further evaluation is required.

This may include:
- urinary ceramide digalactoside and trihexoside;
- molecular diagnosis.

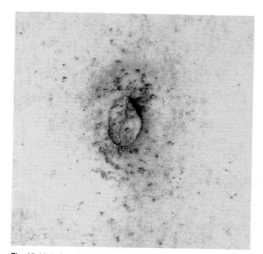

Fig. 15.11.1 Angiokeratoma corporis diffusum.

Renal biopsy

Light microscopy

This will show characteristic glomerular changes with secondary tubular and vascular abnormalities (Fig. 15.11.2).

Podocytes are enlarged and packed with small, clear vacuoles, which represent ceramide-lipid deposits.

Progressive disease leads to capillary loop collapse and segmental or global glomerulosclerosis.

Vacuoles may also be observed in endothelial and smooth muscle cells of arterioles and arteries.

Endothelial cell enlargement leading to occlusion of the vascular lumen of arterioles and tissue ischemia is common.

Electron microscopy

This reveals numerous inclusions contained in lysosomes, especially within podocytes (Fig. 15.11.2). These have a characteristic lamellated appearance and are known as myelin (myeloid) or zebra bodies.

Treatment

Recombinant human α-Gal A

The introduction of enzyme replacement therapy using recombinant human α-Gal A (agalsidase α and β) has transformed the treatment of Fabry disease.

Randomized clinical trials have reported that treatment with enzyme replacement for ≥6 months results in:

- reduced plasma and urine glycosphingolipid levels;
- less neuropathic pain;
- reduced organ deposition;
- improved cerebral blood flow;
- better quality-of-life scores.

Deteriorating renal function is also stabilized in most patients with mild–moderate CKD on treatment.

Adjunctive treatments

Gabapentin, carbamazepine, and opioids may be tried for neuropathic pain.

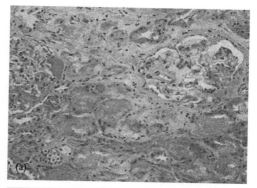

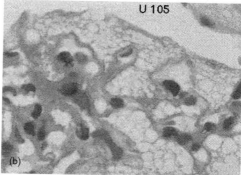

U 105

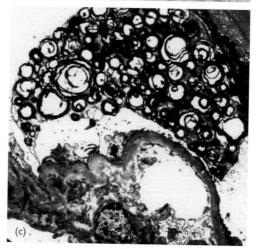

Fig. 15.11.2 Renal biopsy appearances of Fabry disease. (a) Normocellular glomeruli with prominent 'swollen' podocytes (H&E stain). (b) At higher power the podocyte cytoplasm is voluminous and clear and has a 'bubbly' appearance. Similar changes can also be observed in endothelial cells and smooth muscle cells of blood vessels (H&E stain). (c) At the ultrastructural level the podocyte cytoplasm is packed with characteristic concentric lysosomal inclusions known as myelin bodies. (Courtesy of Prof. Peter Furness and Dr Nick Mayer, Consultant Histopathologists, University Hospitals of Leicester, UK.)

Antihypertensive and antiplatelet therapies are useful in reducing overall cardiovascular risk.

Renal replacement therapy

In those on maintenance hemodialysis, α-Gal A may be safely given and there is minimal clearance during a dialysis session.

Renal transplantation is an effective treatment for advanced kidney disease but will not ameliorate the extrarenal manifestations.

α-Gal A treatment should be continued in allograft recipients.

Follow-up

Genetic counseling is necessary for affected individuals.

A careful pedigree should be obtained to identify all affected family members.

In X-linked recessive disease, all daughters of affected males are carriers, and sons of affected males will not carry the gene for Fabry disease.

It is usual for mothers of affected individuals to be considered carriers, and their siblings to be at risk.

Prognosis

In time, experience with the use of enzyme replacement therapy will determine its effectiveness in the prevention, reversal or stabilization of renal disease, which is the main determinant of morbidity in this disorder.

Both renal replacement therapy and transplantation are now recognized treatments for Fabry disease.

Future prospects

Future research will investigate the use of gene therapy strategies for Fabry disease.

Another area for future development is the use of small molecules ('pharmacologic chaperones') that rescue and enhance the activity of mutant α-Gal A enzymes with residual activity.

Further reading

Eng CM, Guffon N, Wilcox WR. Safety and efficacy of recombinant human alpha-galactosidase A replacement therapy in Fabry's disease. *N Engl J Med* 2001; **345**: 9–16.

Eng CM, Germain DP, Banikazemi M, *et al.* Fabry disease: guidelines for the evaluation and management of multi-organ system involvement. *Genet Med* 2006; **8**: 539–548.

Schiffmann R. Enzyme replacement in Fabry disease: the essence is in the kidney. *Ann Intern Med* 2007; **146**: 142–144.

Schiffmann R, Kopp JB, Austin HA, *et al.* Enzyme replacement therapy in Fabry disease: a randomized controlled trial. *J Am Med Assoc* 2001; **285**: 2743–1749.

Internet resources

Fabry Support & Information Group:

http://www.fabry.org

The Fabry Community:

www.fabrycommunity.com

National Institute of Neurological Disorders and Stroke:

http://www.ninds.nih.gov/disorders/fabrys/fabrys.htm

Fabrazyme website:

http://www.fabrazyme.com

GeneTests website detailing centres offering genetic testing for Fabry disease:

http://www.genetests.org/query?testid=2775

See also

Chronic kidney disease in children, p. 462

Other metabolic storage disorders with renal involvement, p. 624

Investigation of inherited renal disease, p. 582

Other metabolic storage disorders with renal involvement

Glycogen storage disease type I (Von Gierke's disease) (Glucose 6-phosphatase deficiency)

The glycogen storage disorders primarily affect the liver, heart, and muscle.

Patients are able to synthesize and store glycogen but are unable to break glycogen down to release stored glucose. The principle manifestations are therefore glycogen accumulation in the liver and repeated episodes of hypoglycemia.

More than ten distinct metabolic lesions contribute to this group of diseases but primary renal involvement only occurs in glycogen storage disease type 1 (GSD1). GSD1 is the commonest type of glycogen storage disease, accounting for ~25% of all cases.

GSD1 may be subdivided into two major forms:
- Type 1a: glucose-6-phosphatase (G6P) deficiency (~80% cases);
- Type 1b: glucose-6-phosphatase translocase deficiency (enzyme involved in intracellular trafficking of G6P).

Epidemiology
The incidence of GSD1 is 1 per 100 000 live births.

The incidence is higher in North Africa where it may be as high as 1 per 5000 live births.

Genetics
GSD1 is an autosomal recessive disorder and therefore affects males and females equally.

The gene for G6P lies at 17q21 and the gene for G6P translocase at 11q23.

Pathology
Glycogen and glucose-6-phosphate accumulate in the:
- liver;
- heart;
- kidneys;
- muscles.

Hyperlipidemia occurs as a result of increased hepatic lipogenesis.

Hepatic adenomas may develop. These are benign tumors usually first noted around the time of puberty. They typically do not cause symptoms and are identified by routine imaging studies of the liver. In rare instances they can undergo malignant transformation.

Renal involvement in GSD1
Deficiency of glucose 6-phosphatase in proximal and distal convoluted tubules results in glycogen accumulation and progressive renal enlargement.

Clinically this may be obscured by gross hepatosplenomegaly.

Tubular cell vacuolation leads to tubular dysfunction manifest by a Fanconi syndrome characterized by:
- aminoaciduria;
- glycosuria;
- phosphaturia.

Tubular damage leading to declining renal function is not usually a major problem.

Early hyperfiltration ultimately leads to secondary focal and segmental glomerulosclerosis and progressive CKD.

Clinical features
Presentation is usually with hypoglycemia.

Abdominal pain is a common feature and may be due to:
- hepatosplenomegaly;
- uric acid nephrolithiasis;
- pancreatitis.

Large and small joint involvement may also occur.

A protruding abdomen and short stature are the most common physical signs.

Hepatomegaly is common as the number and size of adenomas increase with time.

There may also be signs of hyperlipidemia (tendon xanthomata) and hyperuricemia (tophi).

Most patients by the time they are 20 years old will have some degree of:
- proteinuria;
- hypertension;
- nephrolithiasis;
- renal impairment.

The risk of developing ESRD is variable but the likelihood is increased with increasing proteinuria.

Diagnosis
Genetic testing is possible but the gold standard for establishing the diagnosis remains a liver biopsy and comparison of glycogen content to glucose 6-phosphatase levels.

Treatment
There is no cure.

Treatment focuses on correcting the associated metabolic changes and promoting growth and development.

Effectively this is managed through regular feeding to avoid hypoglycemia and avoidance/restriction of sucrose, fructose, lactose and galactose to prevent excessive glycogen accumulation.

Hyperlipidemia
Hyperlipidemia should initially be treated with dietary modification where possible.

There is no long-term effective therapy although fibrates and niacin may be useful.

Statins are contraindicated as they exacerbate triglyceride levels.

Hepatic adenomas
These require ongoing surveillance.

If they are complicated by pain, hemorrhage or necrosis they may need to be removed.

Renal involvement
There is no evidence for any specific intervention to retard progression of renal disease although the use of ACEIs and/or ARBs appears to be an attractive option in view of the associated hyperfiltration and proteinuria early in the disease.

Follow-up

The importance of monitoring, detecting, and correcting hypoglycemia in order to minimize the risk of long-term brain injury from hypoglycemic episodes should be reiterated at each visit.

Patients with multiple hepatic adenomas should be entered into a surveillance programme.

Prognosis

In the past, many patients with GSD1 did not survive beyond infancy and childhood.

Prompt recognition of this condition in the perinatal period allows effective therapy to be instituted early to improve the metabolic abnormalities and reverse the severe growth failure characteristic of untreated patients.

It is still unclear whether long-term complications can be prevented by dietary therapy alone.

With earlier diagnosis, appropriate diet, and better metabolic control, many individuals with GSD1 survive into adulthood.

Glycogen storage disease type V (McArdle disease) (Myophosphorylase deficiency)

In 1951 McArdle first described the clinical manifestations of GSD5 in a 30-year-old man who experienced pain, weakness and stiffness after exercise. Later work identified the cause of GSD5 to be deficiency of the enzyme myophosphorylase. More than half of patients with GSD5 experience acute muscle necrosis and myoglobinuria following vigorous exercise, which can in some individuals result in AKI.

Epidemiology

Estimated incidence is 1 per 100 000 population, but it may be more common.

The disorder is probably underdiagnosed because the symptoms are mild in many patients.

Genetics

There are two autosomal recessive forms of GSD5, a childhood-onset form and an adult-onset form.

There is also a rarer autosomal dominant form.

The gene for myophosphorylase has been mapped to chromosome 11q13.

Pathology

Myophosphorylase (α-1,4-glucan orthophosphate glycosyl transferase) normally initiates glycogen breakdown in skeletal muscle by removing 1,4-glucosyl groups from glycogen and releasing glucose-1-phosphate as an energy source.

Most sufferers have undetectable myophosphorylase activity and are therefore unable to release glucose from the glycogen stored in muscle.

Affected individuals have difficulty performing exercise, particularly anaerobic exercise, as they are unable to metabolize muscle glycogen, the main energy source in anaerobic exercise.

The lack of access to glycogen stores results in muscle breakdown in an attempt to release usable energy stores.

With time, bloodborne energy substrates such as glucose and free fatty acids enter skeletal muscle and are utilized. This may account for the 'second wind' phenomenon experienced by most individuals.

Clinical features

Typical features include:
- exercise intolerance with myalgia;
- early tiredness;
- muscle stiffness;
- cramps.

All of which resolve on rest.

Following a short period of rest, most patients experience a 'second wind' phenomenon which allows for a return to activity without much difficulty.

Exercise may be associated with myoglobinuria in ~1/3 of patients.

This may be associated with development of AKI.

Patients are of normal height and do not suffer episodes of hypoglycemia.

Diagnosis

Elevated serum creatinine kinase levels at rest are common.

Lactic acid production after exercise is absent.

50% of patients may have nonspecific myopathic changes on EMG.

Muscle biopsy shows accumulation of glycogen between myofibrils giving the fibers a vacuolar appearance. The glycogen is periodic acid–Schiff (PAS) positive. Electron microscopy demonstrates extensive accumulation of normal-appearing glycogen under the sarcolemma and between the myofilaments.

Treatment

There is no specific treatment.

Branched-chain amino acids represent an alternative fuel source for exercising muscle. A high protein diet may therefore be useful.

Strenuous and isometric exercise, which is most likely to cause symptoms and induce rhabdomyolysis, should be avoided.

Follow-up

In light of the genetic basis of GSD5 it is important to offer genetic counseling for future pregnancies.

Prognosis

It has a relatively benign course if not complicated by severe rhabdomyolysis and AKI.

Some patients have developed severe myopathies in later life.

The development of CKD and ESRD has not been described.

Further reading

Baker L, Dahlem S, Goldfarb S, et al. Hyperfiltration and renal disease in glycogen storage disease, type I. *Kidney Int* 1989; **35**: 1345–1350.

Chen YT, Coleman RA, Scheinman JI, et al. Renal disease in type I glycogen storage disease. *N Engl J Med* 1988; **318**: 7–11.

Internet resources

The Children's Fund for Glycogen Storage Disease Research:

http://www.curegsd.org/

Association for Glycogen Storage Diseases UK:

http://www.agsdus.org.uk

Association for Glycogen Storage Diseases US:

http://www.agsdus.org

See also

CKD in children, p. 462

Fabry disease, p. 620

Investigation of inherited renal disease, p. 582

Fanconi syndrome, p. 204

Pigment-induced acute kidney injury, p. 362

Cystinosis

Introduction

Cystinosis is an inherited disorder of systemic cystine accumulation resulting from defective lysosomal transport of the amino acid cystine. Lysosomes are intracellular organelles that accumulate breakdown products from the intracellular degradation of macromolecules. Lysosome cell membranes contain a variety of distinct transporters one of which is cystinosin. Cystinosin acts as the lysosomal cystine/H⁺ symporter, mediating saturable cystine transport out of the lysosome, and defects in this transporter result in lysosomal accumulation of cystine and cystinosis.

Cystinosis is a multisystem disorder with widespread cystine accumulation. It is not known why the kidneys and eyes are particularly sensitive, although there is a very high lysosomal density in the cornea and proximal renal tubule.

Cystinosis typically presents with features of the renal Fanconi syndrome of generalized proximal tubular dysfunction. Most cases (95% in UK Cystinosis Registry) present in early childhood but a very few patients present in adolescence or adult life. Such 'late-onset' cases present with manifestations of CKD usually without features of Fanconi syndrome. Some individuals with milder mutations can develop corneal cystine accumulation but no renal manifestations.

Epidemiology

This is a very rare disorder; about five children are diagnosed each year (UK Cystinosis Registry) and there are ~180 patients in the UK.

Cystinosis occurs in all ethnic groups and has a higher prevalence in communities with a higher rate of consanguinity.

Genetics

Cystinosis is inherited as an autosomal recessive trait. Mutations in *CTNS* (the gene encoding the protein cystinosin, chromosome 17p13) either cause no production of cystinosin or defective action leading to lysosomal cystine accumulation. The commonest mutation in cystinosis is a 57 kb deletion, found in 76% of patients of Northern European origin. This deletion can be readily detected in a PCR-based rapid diagnostic test for the disorder. Other mutations, mainly causing premature termination of cystinosin, are found in the severe, infantile-onset form of cystinosis.

Clinical features

These often appear towards first birthday.

Nonspecific symptoms

- poor feeding;
- vomiting;
- poor weight gain or weight loss;
- dehydration;
- gross salt and water craving;
- slow gross motor development (walking).

Signs

- poor growth;
- rickets (e.g. rickettic rosary);
- can occur in any ethnic group but often Caucasians, blond with fair complexion;
- corneal crystals on slit-lamp examination (specialized technique).

Rarely patients present later (adolescence/early adulthood) with proteinuria, CKD.

Long-term manifestations

Whilst kidney dysfunction (initially tubular and later glomerular) predominates in the first decade, systemic cystine accumulation causes multiple organ dysfunction. However, many of these chronic complications have been observed in patients who have not had long-term or adequate cysteamine therapy.

The frequency of complications, from a variety of published sources, has been defined below as very common if >50% affected, common if 25–50%, rare if <25%, very rare if <10%.

These frequencies are certainly affected by the extent and adequacy of cysteamine therapy.

Endocrine

Poor growth (very common): multifactorial, growth hormone secretion usually normal.

Hypothyroidism (very common).

Hypergonadotrophic hypogonadism (very common) with delayed puberty (affects males more severely than females and several pregnancies have been reported).

Impaired glucose tolerance (very common); diabetes mellitus (common).

Neurological

Swallowing problems (very common, even from young age).

Distal vacuolar myopathy (common, affects hands).

Respiratory insufficiency (late complication, severity related to myopathy).

Subtle psychometric defects (visuospatial and visuomotor problems), e.g. difficulty with writing, mathematics; although normal intelligence and speech (very common, apparent in childhood).

Memory loss, seizures (rare).

Stroke-like episodes (very rare).

Cerebral degeneration (very rare).

Ophthalmological

Progressive corneal crystal deposition and clouding (very common).

Retinopathy and visual impairment (rare).

Narrow angle glaucoma (rare).

Others

Pancreatic exocrine insufficiency (extremely rare).

Pancytopenia (rare but sometimes resistance to erythropoetin treatment).

Portal hypertension associated with nodular regenerating hyperplasia (rare).

Vascular calcification with relatively low calcium-phosphate product (compared with other ESRD patients) (common).

Investigations

Diagnostic confirmation

Leukocyte cystine concentration

This test requires specialist laboratory expertise.

Usually patients have >2 nmol cystine per mg protein (normal <0.2).

Demonstration of cystine crystals
These are usually found in the cornea by slit-lamp examination but may be hard to see especially in very young, or in a biopsy material (not usually necessary).

Molecular diagnosis of CTNS deletion
Use of rapid PCR assay for common deletion.

Other mutations more difficult to diagnose.

Serum biochemistry

- Hyperchloremic metabolic acidosis.
- Hypokalemia.
- Hypophosphatemia.

Very rarely with profound dehydration features of secondary hyperaldosteronism predominate with hypokalemic alkalosis ('pseudo-Bartter syndrome').

Urine biochemistry

- Excess phosphaturia (low TmP/GFR).
- Aminoaciduria.
- Glycosuria (not always evident).
- Low molecular weight proteinuria and enzymuria.

Pathology

Renal biopsy is not routinely undertaken in cystinosis as the diagnosis is better confirmed on clinical and biochemical evidence.

Histological sections show variation in size and shape of proximal tubules and irregularity of the brush border. There is also variation in the appearances of podocytes, sometimes forming a multinucleate giant cell.

Cystine crystals may be identified in the interstitium.

Chronic damage is associated with progressive tubulointerstitial, glomerular and vascular changes.

Treatment

General management

Rehydration
Rehydrate with 0.9% saline with added potassium (avoid glucose solutions which may exacerbate hypokalemia).

Correct acidosis
Slowly correct acidosis with sodium bicarbonate supplements (IV or oral) or combined sodium and potassium citrate solutions (tricitrates/polycitra). Rapid correction may precipitate 'hungry bone disorder' with acute hypocalcemia.

Fluid intake and nutrition
Provide high fluid intake (free access to water) and high calorie intake (many children need enteral feeding support).

Supplementation
Add supplements of potassium, phosphate and sometimes calcium and magnesium.

Add 1-alfacalcidol to correct the rickets.

Carnitine supplements may be used to restore the low plasma and muscle levels, although the clinical relevance is uncertain.

Growth hormone
Recombinant growth hormone may be necessary in children with sustained poor growth after optimal general management and adequate (e.g. 1 year at maintenance doses) cysteamine therapy – see below.

Psychosocial and other specialized support
Involvement of the multidisciplinary team is essential for both the long-term care of patients with cystinosis (e.g. feeding programs) and their relatives.

Specific cystine-depleting therapy with cysteamine (mercaptamine)

This reacts with intralysosomal cystine to form mixed-disulfide cysteamine–cysteine which can then leave the lysosome using the lysine transporter.

For children or patients aged <12 years or 50 kg, the recommended maintenance dose is 1.3 g/m²/day divided into four doses, as equally spaced as possible but starting at low dose and building up gradually over 4–6 weeks (see 'Adverse effects' below).

Doses >1.9 gm/m²/day are not recommended.

For patients aged >12 years or >50 kg, the maximal dose is 500 g four times a day.

Monitoring
The effect should be monitored (leukocyte cystine concentration taken 5–6 h after dose if given 4 times per day) approximately monthly for the first 3 months and thereafter 3-monthly, aiming for level of <1 nmol cystine per mg protein.

Adverse effects of cysteamine (mercaptamine) therapy
Nausea and breath smell (very common).

Vomiting (common, tolerance develops at each dose level).

Increased acid and gastrin production (consider proton pump inhibitor).

Rash, fever, lethargy (very rare and only at high doses).

Circumscribed bruising over elbows/knees and striae.

Bone lesions (very rare, associated with high doses: biopsy shows angioendotheliomatosis).

One death reported.

No interference with immunosuppression.

Benefits of cysteamine therapy
Treatment results in:

- Improvement of GFR in first 3 years life.
- Retardation of progression of CKD.
- Improvement in growth.
- Reduced frequency of nonrenal complications.

Follow-up

Initial correction of electrolyte imbalances requires very close monitoring (often as an inpatient) because rapid correction of acidosis can precipitate hypocalcemic cramps or seizures.

Thereafter it is important to gradually increase cysteamine therapy and monitor cystine levels (e.g. monthly in first 4–6 months, 3-monthly when stable).

Effective cysteamine therapy has reduced the frequency of clinical assessment to 3 or 4 times per year.

Adults with cystinosis usually require standard management of their renal replacement therapy and more specialist assessment of the treatment and mulitsystem problems of cystinosis every 3–4 months.

Prognosis

Untreated children risk life-threatening dehydration and electrolyte imbalance and progress to ESRD by 10 years.

Rickets, poor nutrition and systemic disorder contribute to poor growth.

Kidney transplantation (deceased or live donor) are both feasible and successful; although cystine may be seen in graft biopsies, the disorder does not recur within the kidney.

Systemic cystine accumulation causes progressive multisystem damage and dysfunction.

Future prospects

Effective cysteamine treatment has changed the outlook for cystinosis, from inevitable renal replacement therapy within the first decade to a disorder requiring intense medication but with prospects of reasonable growth and kidney survival through childhood. There is also encouraging evidence that cysteamine ameliorates the longer-term complications.

A better understanding of the pathogenetic mechanisms whereby cystine, accumulated within the lysosome, affects cell dysfunction should open new avenues of therapy.

Further reading

Bockenhauer D, van't Hoff W. Fanconi syndrome. In: Geary DF, Schaeffer F (eds), *Clinical pediatric nephrology*. Philadelphia: Mosby. Chap. 28. In press.

Gahl W, Thoene J, *et al.* Cystinosis: a disorder of lysosomal membrane transport. In: Scriver C, Beaudet A, Valle D, Sly W (eds), *The metabolic and molecular basis of inherited disease*. New York: McGraw-Hill; 2001. pp. 5085–5108.

Kleta R, *et al.* First NIH/Office of Rare Diseases Conference on Cystinosis: past, present, and future. *Pediatr Nephrol* 2005; **20**: 452–454.

Van't Hoff W. Cystinosis. In: *Evidence-based nephrology*. In press.

Internet resources

The Cystinosis Foundation:

http://www.cystinosisfoundation.org/

Cystinosis Research Foundation:

http://www.natalieswish.org/page.cfm

Cystinosis Foundation UK:

http://www.cystinosis.org.uk/index.php

See also

CKD in children, p. 462

Fanconi syndrome, p. 204

Investigation of inherited renal disease, p. 582

Conflict of interest

The author has a contract (nonpersonal) as a medical consultant to Orphan Europe, a distributor of Cystagon (mercaptamine).

Primary hyperoxalurias

Introduction

Primary hyperoxalurias are autosomal recessive disorders of hepatic enzymes leading to increased production of oxalate. More than 90% of the body's oxalate is excreted by the kidney with a small amount of excretion from the large intestines. Oxalate is poorly soluble and when present in excess can lead to calcium oxalate deposition in various tissues, primarily the kidney with formation of oxalate stones.

Two forms are recognized (Fig. 15.14.1):

PH type 1: defect in alanine-glycoxylate transferase (AGXT).

PH type 2: defect in glycoxylate reductase/hydroxypyruvate reductase (GR/HPR).

Epidemiology

PH1 occurs in ~1 in 100 000 live births.

PH2 is very rare, but may be underreported.

Genetics

More than 50 different disease-causing mutations have been identified in AGXT. The most common mutation leads to an amino acid replacement G170R. Interestingly, this mutation is only pathogenic if occurring on the same allele together with the polymorphism P11L, which in Caucasians has an allelic frequency of ~20%. On liver biopsy, these patients have demonstrable AGXT immuno- and enzyme activity (albeit reduced), but the enzyme is mistargeted to mitochondria, instead of peroxisomes. Thus, the presence of AGXT in liver biopsy does not rule out the diagnosis of PH1. There is enormous variability in genotype–phenotype correlation, even between individuals within a family with identical genotype, making genetic counseling difficult.

Clinical features

Age at presentation and severity of symptoms is highly variable even within families with identical genotype.

PH type 1

Most commonly presents in childhood with:
- recurrent nephrolithiasis or nephrocalcinosis;
- associated symptoms (polyuria, dysuria, hematuria).

Rarely, is diagnosed in late adulthood based on occasional stone passage.

In the most severe form, PH1 presents in infancy with rapidly progressive kidney failure and strikingly echobright kidneys (on USS), and extrarenal oxalosis, especially in bones, leading to pain and erythropoietin-resistant anemia. Other organs may be affected including:
- heart: arrhythmias, heart block;
- nerves: neuropathy;
- retina: flecked retinopathy.

PH type 2

Typically presents during adolescence with recurrent oxalate stones. Progressive CKD occurs in ~10% of patients.

Differential diagnosis

Secondary hyperoxaluria
Normal levels of glycolate and L-glycerate

Enteric
Fat malabsorption: fatty acids compete with oxalate to complex calcium in the gut, leaving more oxalate available for absorption.

Ascorbic acid intoxication
Metabolized to oxalate.

Deficiency in intestinal Oxalobacter formigenes
Normally degrades enteric oxalate, preventing absorption.

Investigations

Diagnostic confirmation

Stone analysis and urinary oxalate excretion
The presence of oxalate stones, especially recurrent ones, should always lead to the consideration of PH. The diagnosis is established by determination of oxalate and metabolites in an acidified urine sample (Table 15.14.1).

Genetic testing
If elevated levels of metabolites in the urine are detected, the diagnosis can be confirmed by genetic testing. If no mutation is identified or genetic testing is not feasible, a liver biopsy needs to be considered for determination of enzyme activity.

Monitoring

Plasma oxalate levels
With progressive CKD, renal excretion of oxalate decreases and plasma levels increase. If levels exceed ~40 µmol/L, saturation is reached and systemic oxalosis can occur.

Imaging
Calcium oxalate stones are radio-dense and thus easily imaged. Ultrasound is usually the preferred initial imaging modality. Routine imaging in the asymptomatic patient is unlikely to change management, but may be helpful in those patients with small parenchymal stones to assess the risk for dislodgement and thus obstructive urolithiasis.

Pathology

Both AGXT and GR/HPR are hepatic enzymes involved in the metabolism of glycoxylate to glycine (Fig. 15.14.1). Glycoxylate can be converted to glycine (AGXT), glycolate (GR/HPR) or oxalate (lactate dehydrogenase, LDH). Decreased function of one pathway leads to overproduction of the alternative metabolites, explaining the different patterns found in the urine of patients with either PH1 or 2 (Table 15.14.1). AGXT is a peroxisomal enzyme that requires pyridoxine as cofactor, whereas GR/HPR is a cytoplasmic enzyme.

Treatment

Treatment depends on the severity of symptoms.

Nephrolithiasis and normal GFR

High fluid intake (>1.5 L/m^2/day) is recommended.

Citrate can be used to inhibit crystal formation (0.5–1 mmol ~0.1–0.2 g/kg/day).

Dietary modification is less helpful, as the oxalate is derived from internal metabolism.

Pyridoxine, the cofactor of AGXT, in supraphysiologic doses (2–5 mg/kg starting dose, can be increased up to 20 mg/kg) should be tried early in patients with PH1.

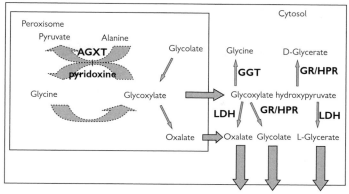

Fig. 15.14.1. Simplified diagram of a hepatic cell with metabolic pathways pertinent for the different types of primary hyperoxaluria. Decreased metabolism of glycoxylate by either AGXT or GR/HPR leads to increased conversion to oxalate. AGXT, alanine-glycoxylate aminotransferase (PH1); GR/HPR, glycoxylate/hydroxypyruvate reductase (PH2); LDH, lactate dehydrogenase; GGT: γ-glutamyl transpeptidase.

Approximately one-third of patients experience reduction of oxalate levels with pyridoxine, sometimes back to the normal range. Typically, these are patients with the G170R mutation, but there is no complete genotype–phenotype concordance (see above). Pyridoxine can rarely induce neuropathy and should be promptly discontinued in pyridoxine nonresponsive patients. PH2 patients do not benefit from pyridoxine.

Oxalobacter formigenes has been shown to decrease oxalate load in some patients, but treatment effects have been limited by loss of intestinal colonization with *Oxalobacter* over time.

Progressive chronic kidney disease

Liver transplantation

In more severe cases with progressive CKD not halted by medical interventions, liver transplantation should be considered, as it corrects the metabolic defect and thus prevents further excessive oxalate production.

Renal replacement therapy

If liver transplantation is not feasible, renal replacement therapy should be started early (GFR 30–40 mL/min/ 1.73 m^2), before systemic oxalosis occurs (see above).

Plasma oxalate levels need to be monitored and should be kept below the saturation level of ~40 μmol/l.

Unfortunately, oxalate is cleared poorly by dialysis. Hemodialysis with high flux membranes has the highest oxalate clearance, but even with daily sessions is often not sufficient to maintain plasma oxalate levels in the desired range. Occasionally, a combination of hemo- and peritoneal dialysis has been used.

Isolated renal transplantation improves oxalate clearance, but carries the high risk of graft failure due to recurrent oxalosis. Thus, combined liver and kidney transplantation is the preferred option in patients with advanced renal failure.

Follow-up

Follow-up depends on the severity of symptoms. It is important to recognize that patients after liver-kidney transplantation can still have elevated oxalate excretion for many months after transplantation, reflecting the systemic oxalosis that accumulated during renal failure. A large fluid intake and citrate supplementation should thus be continued until urinary levels normalize.

Prognosis

Prognosis depends on the severity of symptoms. Because of poor genotype–phenotype correlation, genetic analysis is not particularly helpful in determining prognosis, except that patients with PH2 seem to fare better than those with PH1, where roughly half progress to ESRD before the age of 25 years. Obviously, the earlier the presentation, the more severe the disease and the more likely progression will occur.

Future prospects

PH1 is an inherited disease and gene therapy would thus be the ideal cure, but is unlikely to become available in the foreseeable future. However, identification of mitochondrial mistargeting as the pathophysiologic basis of the most common mutation *G170R* has opened new possibilities. Already, proper targeting can be rescued *in vitro*. The determination of the crystal structure of AGXT is helping to identify the effect of other missense mutations and will aid the design of novel drugs.

Further reading

Cochat P. Primary hyperoxaluria type 1. *Kidney Int* 1999; **55**: 2533–2547.

Danpure CJ. Molecular etiology of primary hyperoxaluria type 1: new directions for treatment. *Am J Nephrol* 2005; **25**: 303–310.

Hoppe B, Beck B, Gatter N, *et al.* Oxalobacter formigenes: a potential tool for the treatment of primary hyperoxaluria type 1. *Kidney Int* 2006; **70**: 1305–1311.

Leumann E, Hoppe B. The primary hyperoxalurias. *J Am Soc Nephrol* 2001; **12**: 1986–1993.

Internet resources

Oxalosis and Hyperoxaluria Foundation:

http://www.ohf.org/about_disease.html

Genetics Home Reference (useful site for carers)

`http://ghr.nlm.nih.gov/condition+primaryhypero xaluria`

See also

Medical management of stone disease, p. 270

Surgical management of stone disease, p. 274

Renal and urinary tract stone disease in children, p. 282

Investigation of inherited renal disease, p. 582

Table 15.14.1 Age-appropriate reference values for oxalate and glycolate

Body fluid		<1 year	1–4 year	5–12 year	Adult
Urine	Oxalate/day (mmol/1.73 m²)	<0.46			<0.4
	Oxalate/creatinine (mmol/mmol)	<0.15	<0.13	<0.07	<0.08
	Glycolate/day (mmol/1.73 m²)		<0.55		<0.26
	Glycolate/creatinine (mmol/mmol)	<0.07	<0.09	<0.05	<0.04
	L-Glycerate/ creatinine (mmol/ mmol)			<0.03	
Plasma	Oxalate (mmol/l)		<7.4		<5.4
	Oxalate/creatinine (mmol/mmol)		<0.19		<0.06

Adapted from: Cochat (1999).

Table 15.14.2 Diagnostic pattern of urine metabolites in PH1 and 2

	Urine oxalate	Urine glycolate	Urine L-glycerate
PH1	High	High	Normal
PH2	High	Normal	High

Inherited disorders of purine metabolism and transport

Introduction

Inherited defects of purine metbolism may lead to the overproduction of uric acid or other purine end-products. Nephrotoxicity derives from the insolubility of uric acid and its analogues, and the ability of any crystals formed to initiate stone formation within the urinary tract, to generate inflammation leading to permanent renal damage within renal tissue, or sometimes both.

Insoluble purines include in order of decreasing solubility:
• uric acid > xanthine > 2,8-dihydroxyadenine.

Defects of purine metabolism (Fig. 15.15.1) are often overlooked as none are common (Table 15.15.1).

Hypoxanthine-guanine phosphoribosyltransferase (HPRT) deficiency Lesch–Nyhan and Kelly–Seegmiller syndromes

HPRT catalyzes salvage transfer of the phosphoribosyl moiety of PP-ribose-P to hypoxanthine and guanine to form IMP and GMP respectively (Fig. 15.15.1), thus saving most of the energy required to synthesize new purine bases. This process is a major downregulator of *de novo* purine synthesis. The presence of inactive mutant HPRT protein results in gross oversynthesis of purine nucleotides and uric acid. A number of mutations have been reported which can lead to a broad spectrum of presentations.

Lesch–Nyhan syndrome (LNS)

One of the highest concentrations of HPRT is in the brain. In addition to urate problems, severe neurological difficulties can develop, usually involving spasticity, developmental retardation, choreo-athetosis and self-mutilation (LNS). The biochemical origin of this neuropathology remains unclear.

Kelley–Seegmiller syndrome (KLS)

Partial enzyme defects may be associated only with uric acid overproduction and its consequences may present (usually with gout) in adolescence or early adulthood; this is sometimes known as the Kelley–Seegmiller syndrome.

Presentation

All degrees of HPRT deficiency may present in the first weeks of life with crystalluria, gout and AKI, sometimes leading to ESRD or death in infancy.

Diagnosis

The diagnosis can be advanced by measurement of plasma urate, remembering that the fractional excretion of filtered urate (FE_{urate}) is much higher in infants and children, and the plasma urate correspondingly lower than in adults. Renal failure leads to a rise in plasma urate concentration. A better guide to diagnosis is the excretion fo urate whilst taking a low-purine diet, to demonstrate over-production. Finally, diagnosis can be confirmed by using an enzyme assay on red cell lysates. Carrier detection is unsatisfactory with a low yield, but preimplantation diagnosis and chorionic villous sampling are possible.

Treatment

The elevated uric acid concentrations in either complete or partial deficiencies may be controlled by a high fluid intake, together with alkali and allopurinol.

Allopurinol should be used with care, however, since urinary oxypurine excretion in all HPRT-deficient patients is exquisitely sensitive to allopurinol, resulting in a rapid increase in concentrations of the extremely insoluble xanthine, with the possible appearance of xanthine nephropathy and stones. The allopurinol metabolite oxipurinol is itself also relatively insoluble, and both xanthine and oxipurinol calculi have been reported in patients with LNS on long-term allopurinol therapy.

As in all patients with renal impairment, the allopurinol dose must be carefully monitored, and reduced if necessary to no more than 5 mg/kg/24 h in children, or 100 mg/24 h in adults.

Some patients have progressed to ESRD and transplantation, but immunouppression using azathioprine will be ineffective, and mycophenolate mofetil could have catastrophic consequences (Fig. 15.15.1); ciclosporin alone has proved successful.

In children with the full LNS, management is dominated by the neurological problems, especially the distressing self-mutilation, often by biting, which may lead to requirement for prophylactic dental extractions. The long-term prognosis is good in children and adolescents with a partial defect, but patients with the full LNS rarely survive beyond adolescence. Death is usually due to aspiration pneumonia or ESRD. No successful treatment is yet available for the severe neurological complications.

Phosphoribosyl pyrophosphate synthetase (PRPS) superactivity

This much rarer condition has some clinical similarities to HPRT deficiency, as it is again sex-linked, leads to urate overproduction, and there may be a neurological component to the disease. The enzyme PRPS catalyzes the transfer of the pyrophosphate group of ATP to ribose 5-phosphate to form PP-ribose-P in the *de novo* pathway leading to purine synthesis (Fig. 15.15.1). The mutation leads to PRPS overactivity and overproduction of urate.

Presentation

In addition to crystalluria, gout and renal impairment, affected children may present with dysmorphic features, sometimes inherited nerve deafness, a family history of repeated attacks of bronchopneumonia and death in early infancy as well as developmental retardation. A much milder phenotype presents later in adolescence with kidney stones or severe gout.

Diagnosis

Although this defect is X-linked, it should be suspected in any child, female, or young adult of either sex with marked hyperuricemia and/or hyperuricosuria, but with normal HPRT activity in lysed red cells. The heterozygote females can be severely affected also, particularly mothers of male children with neurological deficits or urate overproduction who themselves have gout. These female carriers may also have sensorineural deafness.

Treatment

Allopurinol, again used with care to avoid xanthine nephropathy, will control plasma uric acid in patients with normal renal function and gout or kidney stones. A high fluid intake and alkalinization of the urine may help, and in CKD

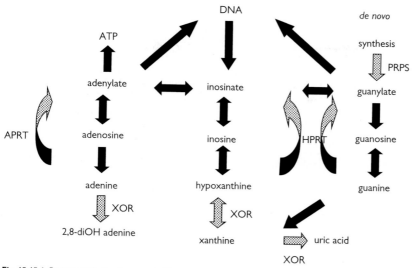

Fig. 15.15.1 Purine metabolism in summary. The reactions catalyzed by the enzymes HPRT, PRPS, APRT, and XOR are indicated by stippled arrows. XOR, xanthine oxidoreductase; PRPS, phosphoribosyl pyrophosphate synthetase; HPRT, hypoxanthine-guanine phosphoribosyltransferase; APRT, adenine phosphoribosyltransferase; DNA, deoxyribonucleic acid; ATP, adenosine triphosphate.

Table 15.15.1 Common defects of purine metabolism

Enzyme defect	Abbreviation	Gene location and mode of inheritance	Homo-/hemizygote frequency	Insoluble purine in crystals/stones	Associated features
Hypoxanthine-guanine ribosyltransferase **deficiency**	HPRT	Xq Sex-linked	1:380 000 (1/3 new mutations)	Uric acid[a]	Choreoathetosis Self-mutilation Developmental arrest
Phosphoribosyl pyrophosphate synthetase **overactivity**	PRPS	Xq.21ptr (*PRS1*) Xp.22.3 (*PRS2*) Sex-linked	?	Uric acid[a]	Dysmorphia Developmental arrest Deafness
Adenine phosphoribosy ltransferase **deficiency**	APRT	16q24 Autosomal recessive	1:33 000 to 1:250 000	2,8-Dihydroxyadenosine	None
Xanthine oxidoreductase **deficiency**	XOR	2p22 Autosomal recessive	1:45 000	Xanthine	None

[a] Also contain xanthine and/or oxypurinol in those treated with allopurinol.

the allopurinol dose must be reduced even further as indicated above.

To date, no successful therapy for the associated neurological complications in severe cases has been devised, and unfortunately death in childhood is frequent. Prognosis for patients presenting in adolescence is good.

Adenine phosphoribosyltransferase (APRT) deficiency

APRT is the companion salvage enzyme of HPRT which catalyses the conversion of adenine to AMP using PP-ribose-P (Fig. 15.15.1). Its prime function is the removal of adenine arising as a metabolic waste product from the polyamine pathway. In the congenital absence of APRT, adenine accumulates in quantity and is oxidized by xanthine dehydrogenase to 8-hydroxyadenine and then the very insoluble 2,8-dihydroxyadenine.

2,8-Dihydroxyadenine is extremely insoluble at any pH, and has a high renal clearance: 2,8-dihydroxyadenine is protein-bound but is actively secreted by the human kidney. The stones, unlike the hard, compact, yellowish urate stones, are bluish or putty-colored and crumbly, but often have been misidentified as uric acid because of their identical chemical behavior, giving positive tests in both the colorimetric and murexide reactions for urate.

Type I APRT deficiency
Subjects are predominantly Caucasian and have no detectable APRT activity in lysed erythrocytes. Various substitutions, insertions, and deletions have been identified in non-Japanese patients.

Type II APRT deficiency
Subjects have an erythrocyte lysate APRT activity up to 25% of normal, found almost exclusively in Japan, where APRT deficiency is common. A single mutation accounts for ~70% of Japanese patients.

Differentiation of these two types of defect requires intact cell studies.

Presentation
At least 15% of cases are without symptoms, which occur only when 2,8-dihydroxyadenine stones or crystals are formed. The picture may vary from benign to life-threatening. The age of onset of symptoms for both defects has varied from birth to the 7th decade. Crystalluria and renal damage may be worsened by a diet high in adenine. Both AKI from stones, and CKD may occur, and in some patients the diagnosis is only made following transplantation, sometimes with loss of the allograft.

Diagnosis
Renal USS may provide the first clue to the underlying crystal nephropathy in patients with AKI but in others it has taken more than 50 years before the nature of the kidney stones was recognized.

Subjects with complete APRT deficiency generally have normal amounts of uric acid in plasma and urine, in contrast to HPRT deficiency and PRPS superactivity.

Treatment
Treatment with allopurinol is highly effective, immediately and in the long term, with the usual proviso relating to allopurinol dose reduction in CKD. Unlike uric acid, alkali will not increase the solubility of 2,8-dihydroxyadenine. If ESRD occurs because of late diagnosis, renal transplantation can be successful. The allograft remains at risk, and

recipients will continue to need treatment with allopurinol; therefore, azathioprine should be avoided. If used, the dose of both drugs should be reduced (up to 200 mg for allopurinol and 25% of the daily dose for azathioprine).

Hereditary xanthinuria

Deficiency of xanthine oxidoreductase (XOR) results in an inability to oxidize hypoxanthine and xanthine to uric acid (Fig. 15.15.1). This leads to accumulation of xanthine (and to a lesser extent hypoxanthine) in place of uric acid. Xanthine concentrations in plasma and especially urine are increased. The nephrotoxicity of this purine, like that of 2,8-dihydroxyadenine, is due to its insolubility, which unlike uric acid can barely be increased by alkalinizing the urine. By contrast, hypoxanthine is very soluble and poses no problem. Xanthine lithiasis, like uric acid lithiasis, is climate dependent, being much more prevalent and associated with more severe renal complications in countries which fringe the Mediterranean.

Type 1 xanthinuria
Typically nonsense, missense, or frame-shift mutations are found in the XOR gene in patients with 'classical' type 1 xanthinuria. In most homozygotes uric acid is virtually undetectable in plasma and urine on a purine-free diet, and is replaced in the urine by xanthine and, to a lesser extent, hypoxanthine (which is extensively salvaged) in a ratio of 3–4:1. The potential toxicity of xanthine in xanthinuric subjects relates to its high renal clearance by filtration with little or no tubular reabsorption. In XOR-deficient homozygotes with normal renal function, plasma and urinary xanthine concentrations are generally well in excess of the solubility of xanthine in urine (0.9 mmol/L), even at pH 7.0. Therefore the potential for precipitation in the kidney or urinary tract is high. The condition predominates in males.

Type 2 xanthinuria (associated lack of aldehyde oxidase; MoCo deficiency)
Xanthinuria, as well as resulting from an isolated deficiency of XOR (type 1), may also arise from a dual deficiency of XOR and the related enzyme aldehyde oxidase (type 2). Aldehyde oxidase (AO), like XOR, contains molybdenum and a defect in the synthesis of the sulphide ligand of the molybdenum cofactor (MoCo) common to both enzymes deletes the activity of both – but leaves the activity of associated sulfite oxidase intact. This dual enzyme deficiency may account for up to 50 per cent of cases with supposed 'classical' xanthinuria. These subjects are at special risk for drugs that are normally metabolized by aldehyde oxidase, which include allopurinol, azathioprine, cyclophosphamide, methotrexate, and quinine.

A few infants have a deficiency of all three enzymes (XOR, AO and sulfite oxidase), due to the absence of MoCo from several genetic defects, with severe clinical features of sulfite oxidase deficiency (severe neonatal fitting, microcephaly, and other specific neurological deficits) which overshadow those of classical xanthinuria, although multiple renal calculi have been observed by ultrasonography.

Presentation
Although the age of onset of nephrotoxicity has varied from the first year of life to the 8th decade, nearly half of the cases presenting with urolithiasis have been children aged ≤10 years. Symptoms present from birth have included persistent vomiting, poor weight gain and urinary tract infection; irritability, sleeplessness, and gross hematuria have also been noted. Despite the insolubility of xanthine,

it is likely that up to half of XOR-deficient homozygotes never present with symptoms, and are picked up incidentally or not at all. Nevertheless, renal damage can be severe, leading in some to ESRD, nephrectomy and even death. Adults with the more serious renal complications frequently have a history of recurrent urolithiasis dating back to early childhood.

Inherited disorders of renal urate handling

Several inherited conditions arising from defects in the bidirectional transport of urate in the renal tubule lead to decreased or increased excretion of urate, with concomitant alterations in plasma urate concentrations.

Hypouricemia of renal tubular origin

Urate, being an anion, is handled mainly if not exclusively in the proximal nephron by a number of channels and transporters of varying specificities. Thus, among those patients noted to have hypouricemia (usually on screening, ~0.5% of the population) are some who have inherited disorders of these transport systems.

Some of these patients are found to have full Fanconi syndrome, with hypouricemia representing only one aspect of the generalized proximal tubular dysfunction present, e. g. cystinosis or Lowe's syndrome.

Mutations in URAT-1

URAT-1 is a relatively specific reabsorptive proximal tubular transporter of urate, mutations of which lead to a recessively inherited hyperuricosuria and hypouricemia. These individuals are usually without symptoms, but may suffer urate crystalluria, stones or exercise-associated AKI. This disorder is particularly common in Japan, where a single point mutation is usually (80%) responsible. The cause of the AKI episodes remains obscure – urate crystals have been found in the kidney only occasionally. The FE_{urate} usually varies from 35 to 80%, but in some instances may exceed the GFR.

Some other forms of renal hypouricemia may relate to mutations in others of the many transport systems which handle urate, none have yet been proven to be implicated in non-URAT-1 cases.

Familial hyperuricemia and gout

A group of related, dominantly inherited, disorders has been described including hyperuricemia and gout in a proportion of family members. These disorders include the symptom complexes of familial juvenile hyperuricemic nephropathy (FJHN) and medullary cystic kidney disease type 2 (MCKD2). They have been shown to be the result of mutations either of the gene for the major urinary protein uromodulin on chromosme 16p11-12 (*UMOD*), present in some 30–40% of families; or presumptively of some other gene(s) which is/are concerned with uromodulin assembly, traffic or excretion, since these other families generally show, as in those with a UMOD mutation, a low urinary excretion of uromodulin and abnormal patterns of uromodulin staining in their renal tubules. Loci have been identified tentatively on chromosomes 1 and 7, the latter as part of the syndrome of hepatocyte nuclear factor-1β, which can include medullary cystic kidney disease.

Patients, especially those with FJHN, show hyperuricemia and in some families gout. A low FE_{urate} ($\leq$3%) is present throughout the course of the condition until renal failure supervenes, and presents before any other signs of the condition are found in children; but the relationship between this and the uromodulin abnormalities remains obscure, since all major urate handing mechanisms so far defined seem to be present only in the proximal tubule, whereas uromodulin is found only in the thick ascending limb of the loop of Henle. There is some evidence also that treatment with allopurinol, if begun early, may be renoprotective, but this is disputed by others. If so, this would suggest some major role for urate in the pathogenesis of the condition. Otherwise, it may merely be a side-effect of secondary polyuria and volume contraction – features not particularly evident in the majority of patients, and urate deposits are in general absent from the kidneys. Moreover, inherited nephrogenic DI is not associated with renal failure, although gout may occur.

Otherwise onset or presentation may be from childhood to middle age, and females are equally affected as males, as one would expect of a dominantly inherited condition. Hypertension is usually absent, unless and until renal failure supervenes.

Further reading

Becker MA. Hyperuricemia and gout. In: Scriver CR, Beaudet AL, Sly WS, Valle D (eds), *The metabolic and molecular basis of inherited disease*, 8th edn. New York: McGraw-Hill; 2001. pp. 2513–2535.

Cameron JS, Moro F, Simmonds HA. Inherited disorders of purine metabolism and transport. In: Davison AM, Cameron JS, Grünfeld JP, et al. (eds), *Oxford textbook of clinical nephrology*, 3rd edn, Oxford: Oxford University Press; 2005. pp. 2381–2395.

Raivio KO, Saksela M, Lapatto R. Xanthine oxidoreductase – role in human pathophysiology and in hereditary xanthinuria. In: Scriver CR, Beaudet AL, Sly WS, Valle D (eds), *The metabolic and molecular basis of inherited disease*, 8th edn. New York: McGraw-Hill; 2001. pp. 2639–2652.

Sahota AS, et al. Adenine phosphoribosyltransferase deficiency and 2,8-dihydroxyadenine lithiasis. In: Scriver CR, Beaudet AL, Sly WS, Valle D (eds), *The metabolic and molecular basis of inherited disease*, 8th edn. New York: McGraw-Hill; 2001. pp. 2571–2584.

Scriver CR, Beaudet AL, Sly WS, Valle D (eds), *The metabolic and molecular basis of inherited disease*, 8th edn. New York: McGraw-Hill; 2001.

Internet resources

Purine Research Society:

http://www.purineresearchsociety.org/

Lesch–Nyhan Disease International Study Group:

http://www.lesch-nyhan.org/

See also

Medical management of stone disease, p. 270

Isolated defects of tubular function, p. 200

Rare syndromes with renal involvement

There are between 250 and 300 syndromes with recognized renal anomalies. Each of these syndromes may be individually rare, but collectively patients with syndromic conditions are seen relatively commonly in pediatric practice.

The disorders in this chapter have been selected for their broad relevance. With improved survival, it is likely that some of these conditions will be encountered by nephrologists in adult practice more frequently.

Alagille syndrome

Synonym: arteriohepatic dysplasia.

Genetic basis: mutation of *JAG1* gene (20p12), which encodes a ligand in the Notch signalling pathway involved in early determination of cellular fate during development.

Inheritance pattern: autosomal dominant (AD).

General features: characteristic facies (broad forehead, long nose, prominent chin in adults); ocular abnormalities (posterior embryotoxon); vertebral anomalies (butterfly vertebrae); right-sided congenital cardiac defects (peripheral pulmonary artery stenosis, tetralogy of Fallot); intrahepatic bile duct hypoplasia and chronic cholestasis (frequently presenting as prolonged neonatal jaundice); abdominal aortic coarctation has been documented in some cases.

Nephrourological features: variable—unilateral renal agenesis; renal dysplasia; renal artery stenosis; renal abnormalities are thought to occur in ~10% of affected individuals.

Bardet–Biedl syndrome

Genetic basis: genetically heterogeneous disorder, involving at least 12 loci (*BBS1–12*). Experimental studies suggest that the *BBS* genes may be involved in ciliary function. Other genes are thought to have a role in modifying expression of the BBS phenotype.

Inheritance pattern: generally regarded as autosomal recessive (AR). In some cases, clinical manifestation of the BBS phenotype may require two abnormal alleles of one *BBS* gene and a third mutation in another *BBS* gene (triallelic inheritance).

General features: incidence <1 in 100 000 in UK, but higher in some ethnic groups; short stature; obesity; postaxial polydactyly; ocular abnormalities (pigmentary retinopathy causing progressive visual impairment, Fig. 15.16.1); hypogonadism; developmental delay/learning difficulties.

Nephrourological features: >95% of affected individuals have demonstrable renal abnormalities, which may include: persistent fetal lobulation; abnormal calyces; renal dysplasia; renal scarring; pelviureteric duplication; vesicoureteric reflux (VUR); urinary concentrating deficit; renal tubular acidosis; progressive CKD, leading to ESRD in a minority of patients (~4%).

Additional notes: heterozygous relatives are thought to have a higher frequency of congenital renal malformations and an increased incidence of renal cell carcinoma, compared with the general population.

Beckwith–Wiedemann syndrome

Genetic basis: related to abnormalities of imprinted growth-regulation genes clustered on 11p15, including uniparental disomy and abnormalities of DNA methylation.

Inheritance pattern: 85% sporadic; 15% AD.

General features: affects ~1 in 13 700 individuals; macrosomia (birth weight and length typically ~97th centile, adult height 50–97th centiles); macroglossia (particularly notable in infancy); unusual skin creases on ear lobe and indentations on outer rim of ear pinna; omphalocele/umbilical hernia; visceromegaly, including pancreatic hyperplasia (associated with hyperinsulinemia and neonatal hypoglycemia); hemihypertrophy; increased risk of embryonal tumors (e.g. hepatoblastoma).

Nephrourological features: nephronomegaly with renal medullary dysplasia; Wilms' tumor predisposition (occurs in ~7% of cases); hypercalciuria is an occasional feature.

Additional notes: in view of risk of Wilms' tumor and other embryonal tumors, USS screening recommended at 3–4 month intervals until age 7–8 years.

Branchio-oto-renal (BOR) syndrome

Synonym: Melnick–Fraser syndrome.

Genetic basis: mutations of the EYA1 gene (8q13) account for ≥50% of cases (type 1); cases of BOR syndrome type 2 are due to mutation of the SIX5 gene (19q13).

Inheritance pattern: AD.

General features: BOR syndrome affects ~1 in 40 000 people; hearing loss (90% of cases may be sensorineural, conductive or mixed pattern); abnormal ear pinna (may be cup-shaped, flattened or hypoplastic); structural defects of middle ear, vestibular system and cochlea may be demonstrable on CT scan; pre-auricular pits (80%) or, less commonly, skin tags; branchial fistulae or cysts (50%); see Fig. 15.16.2.

Nephrourological features: spectrum of abnormalities includes unilateral or bilateral renal agenesis; renal hypoplasia or dysplasia (~65% of cases); cysts; pelviureteric duplication; VUR.

Additional notes: branchio-otic syndrome type1 and otofacio-cervical syndrome result from different mutations of the EYA1 gene; these disorders have phenotypic overlap with branchio-oto-renal syndrome, but do not include renal abnormalities.

CHARGE syndrome

Genetic basis: most affected individuals have mutations of the *chromodomain helicase binding protein 7* (*CHD7*) gene on 8q12; the phenotype may also be caused by mutations of the *semaphorin-3E* gene (*SEMA3E*) on 7q21.

Inheritance pattern: generally sporadic.

General features: affects ~1 in 12 000 individuals; CHARGE is an acronym representing the principal features; **C**oloboma; **H**eart defects; **A**tresia choanae; **R**etardation of growth and development; **G**enital anomalies and hypogonadism; **E**ar abnormalities ± deafness.

Nephrourological features: include renal agenesis; ectopic kidney; renal hypoplasia/dysplasia; lower urinary tract abnormalities (e.g. VUR).

Denys–Drash syndrome

Genetic basis: mutations of the *WT1* gene (11p13), usually located in exons 7–10, which encode the DNA-binding domains of a transcription factor expressed in renal and genitourinary tract tissues; a different type of WT1 mutation gives rise to Frasier syndrome.

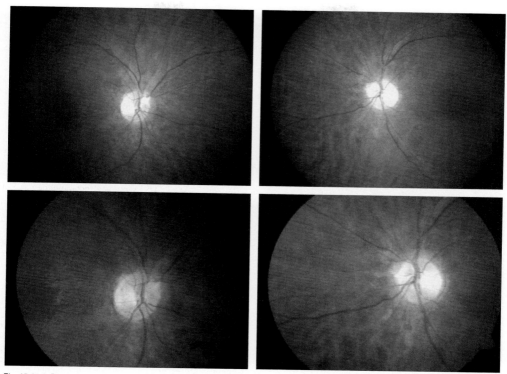

Fig. 15.16.1 Pigmentary retinopathy is associated with renal abnormalities in a number of conditions, including Bardet–Biedl syndrome and Senior–Løken syndrome (Retinal photograph courtesy of Dr Alan Fryer, Consultant in Clinical Genetics, Cheshire and Merseyside Clinical Genetics Service, Liverpool, UK).

Inheritance pattern: usually due to new mutation (nonpenetrance in carrier parent has been reported in some cases).

Nephrourological features: the classic triad consists of:

1. External genital abnormalities (variable severity; hypospadias and cryptorchidism may result in the appearance of pseudohermaphroditism in males).
2. Wilms' tumor predisposition.
3. Proteinuric nephropathy with progressive renal impairment (diffuse mesangial sclerosis histology on renal biopsy).

Additional notes:

- Karyotype should be checked in phenotypic females presenting with proteinuric nephropathy and diffuse mesangial sclerosis histology, to exclude male pseudohermaphroditism.
- In view of the Wilms' tumor predisposition, bilateral nephrectomy is advocated in Denys–Drash syndrome.
- The proteinuric nephropathy does not appear to recur after renal transplantation.

Down syndrome

Genetic basis: chromosomal (trisomy 21 in 95%; remainder due to mosaicism, translocation or complex chromosomal rearrangements).

General features: incidence ~1 in 800 live births; short stature; characteristic facial appearance; developmental delay/learning difficulties; congenital cardiac defects in 40–50% of affected individuals (notably septal defects); hypothyroidism in 20–40%; epilepsy in 8%; increased incidence of duodenal atresia, Hirschsprung's disease and several other congenital anomalies; also increased risk of leukemia (affects 1–2%); ligamentous laxity, associated with risk of atlanto-axial subluxation (often asymptomatic, may rarely cause spinal cord compression with alteration of bladder/bowel function or motor deficits; usually occurs prior to age 10 years).

Nephrourological features: may occur in ~20% of affected individuals and include: renal hypoplasia/dysplasia; pelviureteric junction obstruction; vesicoureteric junction obstruction; VUR; posterior urethral valves.

Additional notes: in the absence of significant comorbidity, Down syndrome is not considered to be a contraindication to successful management of ESRD.

Frasier syndrome

Genetic basis: mutation of the *WT1* gene (11p13), which encodes a transcription factor expressed in renal and genitourinary tract tissues; alternative splicing of mRNA transcripts leads to the production of four isoforms of the transcription factor; in Frasier syndrome, a mutation in intron 9 causes a splice site change, altering the ratio of

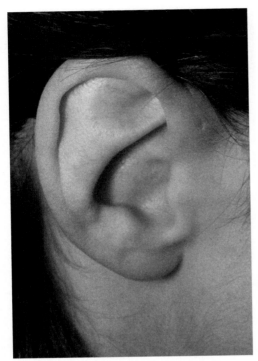

Fig. 15.16.2 Careful examination may be required to detect subtle features of branchio-oto-renal syndrome: note the pre-auricular pit. (Photograph courtesy of Dr Alan Fryer, Consultant in Clinical Genetics, Cheshire and Merseyside Clinical Genetics Service, Liverpool, UK.)

these isoforms (in contrast, exon mutations of *WT1* result in structurally abnormal transcription factor in Denys–Drash syndrome).

Inheritance pattern: new mutation.

Nephrourological features: male pseudohermaphroditism (normal female external genitalia with 46XY karyotype); childhood-onset proteinuric glomerulopathy with nephrotic syndrome (focal segmental glomerulosclerosis histology on renal biopsy), progressing to ESRD in adolescence or early adulthood; streak gonads with predisposition to gonadoblastoma (hence gonadectomy is usually advocated); relatively small increased risk of Wilms' tumor.

Additional notes: the proteinuric nephropathy does not appear to recur after renal transplantation.

Jeune syndrome

Synonym: Asphyxiating thoracic dystrophy.

Genetic basis: not fully elucidated; linkage to 15q13.

Inheritance pattern: AR.

General features: normal facial appearance; short stature; long narrow thorax with short ribs, associated with lung hypoplasia (may be fatal in infancy, due to respiratory insufficiency, particularly during viral respiratory tract infections; for those who survive, there is a gradual improvement in the relative growth of the thorax); postaxial polydactyly

in 50%; rhizomelic limb shortening; pelvic skeletal abnormalities; biliary dysgenesis with periportal hepatic fibrosis; pancreatic cysts and fibrosis in a minority of cases; retinal degeneration.

Nephrourological features: cystic renal dysplasia; progressive chronic renal impairment may manifest in early childhood; renal transplantation has been performed successfully in affected individuals.

MURCS Association

Genetic basis: unknown.

Inheritance pattern: usually sporadic, but familial cases have been reported in siblings.

General features: MURCS is an acronym representing the principal features: **MU**llerian duct anomalies (absent/hypoplastic uterus and absent upper 2/3 of vagina–known as the Rokitansky defect); **R**enal anomalies; **C**ervicothoracic **S**omite dysplasia (Klippel–Feil anomaly); many patients are diagnosed following investigation of primary amenorrhea (normal female secondary sexual characteristics develop, as the ovaries are present).

Nephrourological features: unilateral renal agenesis, renal dysplasia or ectopia are found in ~88% of cases.

Neurofibromatosis type 1

Synonym: von Recklinghausen disease.

Genetic basis: mutation in the *NF1* gene (17q11), which encodes neurofibromin, a GTPase-activating protein involved in cell cycle regulation.

Inheritance pattern: AD, but 50% of cases are due to new mutations.

General features: birth incidence ~1 in 2500 and prevalence ~1 in 4000; common features: café-au-lait spots (six or more; ≥0.5 cm before puberty or ≥1.5 cm after puberty); axillary/groin freckling; neurofibromas (skin, spinal, visceral); Lisch nodules (benign hamartomas of iris); distinctive dysplastic lesions of sphenoid or long bones; learning difficulties affect ~33%; less common features include scoliosis, epilepsy and tumor predisposition (optic gliomas in early childhood; CNS tumors, malignant peripheral nerve sheath tumors and rhabdomyosarcomas in adulthood); endocrine tumors occur in ~3% (e.g. pheochromocytomas).

Nephrourological features: neurofibromas may occur in the kidneys or bladder; renal artery stenosis occurs in ~2% of affected individuals.

Additional notes: regular blood pressure checks are recommended in all age groups; when hypertension is detected, it is important to investigate appropriately for renal artery stenosis and pheochromocytoma.

Noonan syndrome

Genetic basis: genetically heterogeneous; ~50% of cases are due to mutation of the *PTPN11* gene (12q24), which encodes a tyrosine phosphatase involved in multiple cellular cascades.

Inheritance pattern: AD.

General features: affects ~1 in 2500 people; short stature; characteristic facial appearance (hypertelorism, epicanthic folds, low-set ears, low posterior hair-line with short or webbed neck); cardiac defects in 50–80% (notably pulmonary valve stenosis, septal defects); thrombocytopenia or coagulation defects occur in up to 50% of cases; cryptorchidism is common in males; lymphatic abnormalities are associated with dorsal edema of the hands and feet.

Nephrourological features: renal dysplasia and ureteric abnormalities (duplication, VUR) are recognized in some cases.

Prune belly syndrome

Synonyms: Eagle–Barrett syndrome; early urethral obstruction sequence; (triad of megacystis-megaureter, cryptorchidism, deficient anterior abdominal wall musculature).

Genetic basis: unknown; occurrence in one member of a monozygotic twin pair suggests that nongenetic factors may be relevant.

Inheritance pattern: generally considered sporadic.

General features: incidence ~1 in 30 000; male predominance (>95%); oligohydramnios during pregnancy may lead to pulmonary hypoplasia and skeletal abnormalities (congenital talipes equinovarus and developmental dysplasia of the hip); cardiac anomalies are found in 10% of cases.

Nephrourological features: urethral narrowing/atresia may be present; bladder is typically large volume and low pressure with poor contractility; ureters typically dilated and tortuous with high grade VUR; in a minority of cases, there may be ureteric obstruction due to kinking or stenosis; renal dysplasia of variable severity; cryptorchidism and infertility in males; females may have vaginal atresia or uterine abnormalities; decompression of distended bladder and deficient abdominal wall musculature lead to the classical wrinkled 'prune belly' appearance in infants.

Additional notes: poor detrusor contractility and VUR contribute to incomplete bladder emptying and UTI risk; expert urological management is essential; the combination of renal dysplasia and acquired scarring may lead to progressive CKD; ESRD management may be successfully undertaken, but it is necessary to ensure adequacy of urinary drainage prior to renal transplantation.

Renal–Coloboma syndrome

Synonym: Papillorenal syndrome.

Genetic basis: mutation of paired box gene 2 (*PAX2*, 10q24).

Inheritance pattern: AD.

General features: wide range of ocular abnormalities, from mild optic disc dysplasia (difficult to recognize, no functional consequences) to colobomas of optic nerve and retina; high frequency sensorineural hearing loss in some affected individuals; Chiari malformation with hydrocephalus has been reported.

Nephrourological features: VUR; renal hypoplasia; CKD may progress to ESRD in childhood or adult life.

Senior–Løken syndrome

Synonym: juvenile nephronophthisis with Leber amaurosis; renal–retinal syndrome.

Genetic basis: genetically heterogeneous; Senior–Løken syndrome 1 is due to mutations in the nephrocystin gene (*NPHP1*, 2q13); mutations in *NPHP4* (1p36), *NPHP5* (3q21) and possibly *NPHP3* (3q22) are also associated with the Senior–Løken phenotype; other mutations in these genes may result in juvenile nephronophthisis without ocular abnormalities.

Inheritance pattern: AR.

General features: pigmentary retinopathy; in the early stages, impaired function of the rod photoreceptors manifests as reduced vision in dim illumination ('night blindness'); this is followed by restriction of peripheral visual fields and progressive visual loss; fundal examination shows pigmentary changes in the midperipheral retina (Fig. 15.16.1).

Nephrourological features: nephronophthisis; the earliest detectable clinical feature may be impaired urinary concentrating ability, manifesting as polyuria and polydipsia; followed by progressive CKD in childhood/adolescence.

Townes–Brock syndrome

Genetic basis: mutation of *SALL1* gene (16q12), which encodes a zinc finger transcription factor.

Inheritance pattern: AD; high proportion of cases are due to new mutations.

General features: ear anomalies (dysplastic ears, pre-auricular tags) with sensorineural hearing loss; various hand malformations (notably triphalangeal thumb or hypoplastic thumb; preaxial polydactyly); imperforate anus.

Nephrourological features: renal malformations (variable – may include: renal agenesis; unilateral or bilateral dysplastic/hypoplastic kidneys); lower urinary tract abnormalities (VUR; posterior urethral valves; urethral meatal stenosis; hypospadias; bifid scrotum); CKD occurs in some cases; life-long monitoring of renal function is recommended.

Turner syndrome

Genetic basis: chromosomal (karyotype 45X in ~50% of cases; remaining cases involve various combinations of mosaicism).

General features: affects 1 in 2500 live female births; phenotype is highly variable and features may be very subtle in some individuals; significant short stature (may be treated with growth hormone therapy); neck may be broad and webbed, with low posterior hair-line; cardiovascular abnormalities are present in 15–50% (notably aortic coarctation and ventricular septal defects; adults have an increased risk of aortic root dilatation and aortic dissection – regular surveillance is advised); lymphatic abnormalities are associated with edema of hands and feet, seen most commonly in newborn period but may be present at any age; gonadal dysgenesis leads to absent or limited spontaneous pubertal development and infertility in the majority of cases (estrogen treatment required from adolescence); other problems in adulthood include risk of osteoporosis and susceptibility to autoimmune diseases (hypothyroidism, diabetes mellitus, inflammatory bowel disease, chronic liver disease); mosaic 45X/46XY individuals have an increased risk of gonadoblastoma.

Nephrourological features: congenital renal anomalies are found in ~1/3 of cases (notably horseshoe kidney; unilateral renal agenesis; renal dysplasia/hypoplasia; pelviureteric duplication; VUR); hypertension may be more common than in the general adult population.

VATER/VACTERL association

Genetic basis: unknown; more frequent in offspring of diabetic mothers.

Inheritance pattern: sporadic.

General features: incidence ~1.6 in 10 000; VATER/ VACTERL are acronyms representing the principal features: **V**ertebral defects (typically hemivertebrae or fused vertebrae in thoracic or lumbar regions); **A**nal atresia; **C**ardiac abnormalities (80% of cases, various types); **T**racheo-esophageal fistula with **E**sophageal atresia; **R**enal anomalies; radial upper **L**imb defects; a secure diagnosis requires at least one defect each in limbs, thorax and lower abdomen/pelvis (probable diagnosis may be based upon two anomalies in each of two of these regions).

Nephrourological features occur in 80% of cases and may include: unilateral renal agenesis; renal dysplasia/hypoplasia; pelviureteric duplication; VUR; urethral atresia/stenosis; external genital defects (e.g. hypospadias, bifid scrotum).

Additional notes: extensive surgical treatment may be required over many years (neonatal repair of tracheo-esophageal fistula and esophageal atresia, colostomy, urological procedures), but most affected individuals achieve normal cognitive development; dialysis and renal transplantation are established treatments for those patients who progress to ESRD.

WAGR syndrome

Genetic basis: microdeletion of chromosome 11p13, encompassing the Wilms' tumor suppressor gene *WT1* and the adjacent aniridia gene *PAX6*.

Inheritance pattern: usually new deletion, but familial occurrence has been reported.

General features: WAGR is an acronym representing the principal features: **W**ilms' tumor predisposition; **A**niridia; **G**enitourinary abnormalities (hypospadias, cryptorchidism); mental **R**etardation.

Nephrourological features: Wilms' tumor occurs in up to 60% of cases; ≥20% develop CKD in later life.

Williams syndrome

Genetic basis: microdeletion of chromosome 7q11, encompassing ~17 genes, including the elastin gene (ELN); hemizygosity of the elastin gene is thought to be responsible for the vascular anomalies in this syndrome, while hemizygosity of other genes in this region may account for other features.

Inheritance pattern: usually sporadic, but AD inheritance has been reported.

General features: short stature; characteristic facial appearance (periorbital fullness, wide nasal tip, long philtrum, wide mouth with full lips, small widely spaced teeth; adults tend to develop a gaunt appearance); moderate–severe learning difficulties, but relatively good language skills and talkative personality; hypersensitivity to noise; congenital heart disease in 80% of cases (typically supravalvular aortic stenosis or supravalvular pulmonary stenosis; other arteries may also be affected by vascular stenosis – see below); ~15% of infants develop hypercalcemia of unknown cause (may require reduced dietary calcium intake; tends to improve during childhood).

Nephrourological features: several structural anomalies are recognized (including asymmetry of renal lengths; uni-lateral renal agenesis; pelvic kidney; VUR; bladder diverticulae; urethral stenosis); hypercalciuria may be present even in the absence of hypercalcemia and may lead to nephrocalcinosis; renal artery stenosis affects 40%; nonrenovascular hypertension is also recognized; ESRD has been successfully managed by renal transplantation.

22q11 deletion syndrome

Synonyms: velocardiofacial syndrome; DiGeorge syndrome.

Genetic basis: ~96% of patients have hemizygous 1.5–3 Mb deletions of 22q11, including 24–30 genes; other patients have specific deletions, translocations or point mutations of the *TBX1* gene, which lies within this chromosomal region.

Inheritance pattern: ~94% of cases are due to new deletions; 6% inherited in AD pattern (although there is intrafamilial variability in phenotypic expression).

General features: growth retardation/short stature; characteristic facial appearance (prominent wide nasal bridge and root, small mouth, round ears); velopharyngeal insufficiency ± cleft palate; congenital heart disease in 75% of cases (notably tetralogy of Fallot and other malformations of the cardiac outflow tract); variable defect in cell-mediated immunity (usually mild and improving in first 2 years of life; a minority have a persistent profound T-cell dysfunction); 60% are hypocalcemic at some stage (notably during neonatal period, but also during later childhood or pregnancy); several of these features (velopharyngeal defects; thymic and parathyroid abnormalities; cardiac outflow tract malformations) are attributed to abnormal development of the derivatives of the third and fourth branchial arches.

Nephrourological features: structural renal tract anomalies are found in 36% of cases (renal agenesis; multicystic dysplastic kidney; hydronephrosis; VUR).

Further reading

Firth HV, Hurst JA, Hall JG. *Oxford desk reference: clinical genetics.* Oxford: Oxford University Press; 2005.

Jones KL. *Smith's recognizable patterns of human malformation*, 6th edn. Philadelphia: Elsevier/Saunders; 2006.

Internet resources

Online Mendelian Inheritance in Man (OMIM).

www.ncbi.nlm.nih.gov

See also

Renal dysplasia, p. 646

Congenital abnormalities of the urinary tract, p. 658

Nephronophthisis, p. 600

Congenital and infantile nephrotic syndrome, p. 616

Wilms' tumor, p. 672

Structural and congenital abnormalities

Chapter contents

Renal dysplasia

Introduction
The term renal dysplasia is used to describe a specific type of parenchymal development due to abnormal metanephric development and is a histological diagnosis.

Dysplastic kidneys contain microscopic abnormalities that have been attributed to the persistence of mesonephric tissue, developmental arrests and faulty differentiation leading to persistence of primitive or fetal structures.

Hypoplastic kidneys are considered to have a significant reduction in nephron number.

A histological diagnosis is rarely made in clinical practice, rather the presence of kidneys with lack of normal coticomedullary differentiation (sometimes containing cysts) is often assumed clinically to denote renal dysplasia (Fig. 16.1.1).

Often, but not always, the kidneys are small.

Some authors prefer to group renal dysplasia and hypoplasia together as renal hypodysplasia.

Classification
Renal dysplasia is considered to be a common form of CAKUT (congenital abnormalities of the kidney and urinary tract).

Renal dysplasia can occur in isolation or together with other congenital abnormalities of the urinary tract.

CAKUT are an important cause of ESRD in childhood (accounting for almost half of patients with ESRD in childhood).

Renal dysplasia may occur less commonly as part of a complex syndrome with malformations of other organ systems or external features.

Epidemiology
Overall dysplastic kidneys are common malformations affecting ~1 in 1000 of the general population.

Severe forms of renal dysplasia account for ~20% of pediatric ESRD cases.

Genetics
Usually renal dysplasia occurs sporadically.

There are also >100 syndromes which include renal dysplasia and therefore clinical genetics advice should be consulted in cases with dysmorphic features or family history.

For example there may be a chromosomal abnormality or mutations in a single gene that may be helpful.

It is possible that a genetic diagnosis may be possible in some cases in association with syndromes:
- SALL1 mutations (Townes–Brock);
- PAX2 (renal coloboma syndrome);
- EYA1 or SIX1 mutations.

Currently the prevalence of mutations in developmental genes in children with renal hypodysplasia is ~16%.

Clinical features
Clinical examination of patients with suspected renal dysplasia should include looking for dysmorphic features, for example:
- fundoscopy examination to look for optic nerve colobomas even in the absence of visual impairment (PAX2 renal coloboma syndrome);
- external ear malformations, pre-auricular pits, branchial cysts and hearing loss (branchio-oto-renal syndrome);
- imperforate anus, thumb abnormalities, hearing defects, hypospadias (Townes–Brock syndrome);
- diabetes and uterus malformations (RCAD syndrome).

Management
Management of renal dysplasia depends on the level of renal function which may be variably impaired.

Isolated renal dysplasia may be difficult to detect on antenatal screening.

In children born with significantly impaired renal function the glomerular filtration rate may improve over the first year of life and sometimes up to 3 years of age.

Puberty is typically a time when renal insufficiency may need closer monitoring as renal function may decrease associated with growth.

Milder cases of renal dysplasia may not be detected in childhood and present later in life with established renal impairment.

Clinically when associated with other malformations including VUR it may be difficult to differentiate from scarring associated with ascending infections.

Clinical follow-up is required to assess renal function, renal growth as assessed by USS and monitoring for development of hypertension.

Multicystic dysplastic kidney (MCDK)
This is a developmental abnormality of the kidney in which the renal parenchyma is non-functioning and replaced by many large cysts of differing sizes which appear to be non-communicating.

It is nearly always associated with proximal ureteral atresia.

Epidemiology
The incidence is considered to be between 1 in 2000 and 1 in 4500.

MCDK occurs twice as often in males as in females.

Genetics
MCDK is usually sporadic although there are reported families with many affected individuals with MCDK in the literature.

Unusually, MCDK may occur in association with a number of rare syndromes:
- Meckel–Gruber;
- Jeune thoracic dystrophy;
- Zellweger cerebro-hepato-renal syndrome.

Hence an assessment for external dysmorphic features should be undertaken.

Clinical features
The presenting sign of a multicystic kidney is usually a unilateral mass.

They are unilateral in 90% of cases.

Abnormalities of the contralateral kidney may be present in up to 30% of cases, including vesicoureteric reflux, renal agenesis and pelviureteric junction obstruction.

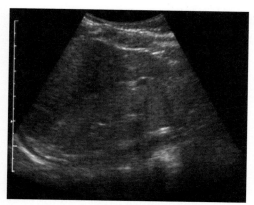

Fig. 16.1.1 Featureless renal ultrasound of renal dysplasia.

Investigations

MCDK are usually diagnosed on antenatal USS and confirmed by postnatal USS (Fig. 16.1.2) although historically they used to present as an abdominal mass.

DMSA isotope renogram postnatally will demonstrate absence of function in the multicystic dysplastic kidney (Fig. 16.1.3).

The micturating cystourethrogram (if performed) may show a blind-ending ureter and vesicoureteric reflux in the contralateral kidney.

Management

The management of MCDK is controversial.

The outcome in children with unilateral MCDK and a normal contralateral kidney is excellent as the normal contralateral kidney develops compensatory hypertrophy.

Surgical removal of the unilateral mass has been advocated for many years because of an anticipated risk of hypertension and malignancy.

Currently, if the renal diagnosis of MCDK is clear, conservative management with sequential renal USS is usually advocated unless symptoms develop.

Patients should be followed up regularly with measurement of BP and urinalysis and annual renal USS to ensure

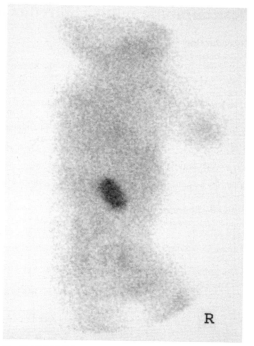

Fig. 16.1.3 DMSA isotope renogram in the same 3-month-old infant with left MCDK and no function on left side.

that the MCDK has regressed. This usually occurs at age ≤5 years.

Indications for surgery would include obstruction/gross abdominal distension or hypertension.

A few centers still advocate nephrectomy even if cysts have regressed because of a small chance of late complications.

Further reading

Firth HV, Hurst JA, Hall JG. *Clinical genetics*. Oxford: Oxford University Press; 2005.

Jones KL. *Smith's recognizable patterns of human malformation*, 6th edn. Philadelphia: Elsevier/Saunders; 2006.

Postlethwaite RJ, Webb N. *Clinical paediatric nephrology*, 3rd edn. Oxford: Oxford University Press; 2003.

Internet resources

Online mendelian inheritance in man:

http://www.ncbi.nlm.nih.gov/omim

Genetic & Rare Diseases Information Centre:

http://rarediseases.info.nih.gov

See also

Vesicoureteric reflux and reflux nephropathy, p. 648

Investigation of inherited renal disease, p. 582

Polycystic kidney disease in children, p. 586

Rare syndromes with renal involvement, p. 640

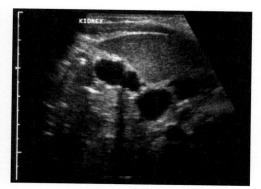

Fig. 16.1.2 Renal ultrasound of a 3-month-old infant with left MCDK.

Vesicoureteric reflux and reflux nephropathy

Introduction

Vesicoureteric reflux (VUR)

This is the retrograde passage of urine from the bladder towards the kidneys as demonstrated on radiological imaging.

Overall VUR is heterogeneous but can be defined as:

Primary:

- generally considered to be due to abnormal/more lateral insertion of the ureter into the bladder wall.

Secondary:

- to obstruction or bladder dysfunction.

VUR may be considered to be one feature of a malformed urinary tract.

Reflux nephropathy

Reflux nephropathy is defined as the renal disease resulting from VUR.

At least three different renal patterns of reflux nephropathy are seen:

- congenital dysplasia;
- focal defects associated with pyelonephritis;
- glomerular sclerosis associated with proteinuria and hypertension.

It is important to appreciate that the small shrunken kidney associated with urinary tract infections (UTIs) is not necessarily scarred due to infection and VUR and could equally represent renal dysplasia.

VUR is known to regress with age.

Classification

According to the International Reflux Study Committee (1981), VUR is classified according to severity (Fig. 16.2.1 and Table 16.2.1).

VUR can be classified as active (occurring during micturition) and passive (without micturition).

Epidemiology

The incidence of VUR is estimated to be 1–2%.

Reflux nephropathy accounts for ~15% of ESRD in teenagers and adults.

VUR is less common in Afro-Caribbean children compared with Caucasian children.

In older children VUR is reported in greater frequency in females but, in children who present with UTI, VUR is found in similar frequencies in both males and females.

The prenatal diagnosis of VUR is more common in males than females and this is usually in the context of a congenitally abnormal renal tract.

Genetics

Screening studies of relatives of children with VUR using micturating cystograms suggest that VUR occurs more frequently in first-degree relatives of individuals compared with the general population.

Overall the aetiology of VUR is multifactorial and the genetic component likely to be polygenic (due to many different genes) although in some families a single gene may play a major role.

A family history of VUR or recurrent UTI should be sought.

Most centers would not advocate routine screening of siblings with micturating cystograms to look for VUR but would focus on:

- awareness of urine infection symptoms;
- prompt diagnosis and treatment of infections;
- renal USS to look for dilating degrees of VUR/major renal tract abnormality.

Since VUR can occur in association with a malformed urinary tract in a genetic syndrome, careful examination of the patient for features of a syndrome is important (e.g. ear abnormalities, optic disc abnormalities).

There is no genetic diagnosis available unless VUR occurs as part of a syndrome in which the genetic defect is already known.

Clinical features

The two main presenting features of VUR are:

- antenatal diagnosis: hydronephrosis on fetal USS;
- urinary tract infection in childhood.

Febrile urinary tract infections are particularly important as they are more likely to be associated with VUR.

Other more unusual presentations include:

- loin pain;
- hypertension;
- proteinuria;
- enuresis.

Clinical examination of the spine and nervous system is important if there is inadequate bladder emptying due to a neuropathic bladder.

In bladder outflow obstruction, especially in boys, posterior urethral valves should be excluded.

Investigations

VUR is a radiological diagnosis.

Renal ultrasound scan

In the context of UTI, renal USS is a useful initial investigation to look for renal size, presence of hydronephrosis and hydroureter, bladder wall thickness and extent of bladder emptying.

Cystogram

The gold standard for diagnosis of VUR is a cystogram.

Micturating cystourethrogram (MCUG)

This is the method of choice for infants who are unable to void to command and those in whom it is important to delineate anatomy (Fig. 16.2.2).

A catheter is inserted into the bladder, filled with contrast and then withdrawn.

In male infants with VUR it is important to obtain a view of the urethra to exclude obstruction due to posterior urethral valves.

It is important to cover this investigation with antibiotic prophylaxis.

The timing of the MCUG with respect to UTI is not crucial in terms of false-positive VUR findings.

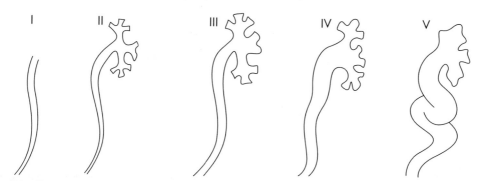

Fig. 16.2.1 Classification of grades of vesicoureteric reflux used by the International Reflux Study Committee.

Table 16.2.1 Classification of vesicoureteric reflux (International Reflux Study Committee, 1981)

Grade I	Reflux into ureter only with no dilatation.
Grade II	Reflux into ureter, pelvis and calyces with no dilatation.
Grade III	Mild or moderate dilatation of the pelvis.
	No or only slight blunting of the fornices.
Grade IV	Moderate dilatation and/or tortuosity of the ureter and moderate dilatation of the pelvis and calyces.
	Complete obliteration of the sharp angles of the fornices but maintenance of the papillary impressions of the majority of the calcyces.
Grade V	Gross dilatation and tortuosity of the ureter, pelvis and calyces.
	The papillary impressions are no longer seen in the majority of calyces.

Isotope cystogram

In older children (able to micturate when requested and in whom urethral catheter insertion is more traumatic) an indirect isotope cystogram using MAG3 radioisotope can be used instead although it is recognized that this investigation can be less sensitive (Fig. 16.2.3).

In this investigation, radioactive contrast is injected IV.

Uptake of the contrast occurs in the kidneys, excretion can be followed into the bladder and then on micturition, contrast can be seen to reflux back towards the kidneys if VUR is present.

Indirect cystography is not available in all centers.

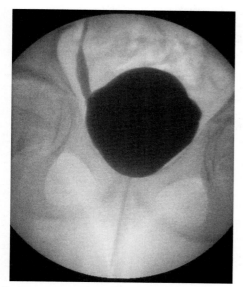

Fig. 16.2.2 MCUG showing grade IV/V vesicoureteric reflux on the right-hand side in an infant with recurrent febrile UTI.

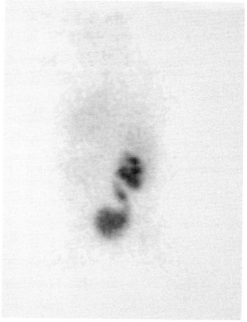

Fig. 16.2.3 MAG3 isotope renogram showing unilateral right-sided vesicoureteric reflux.

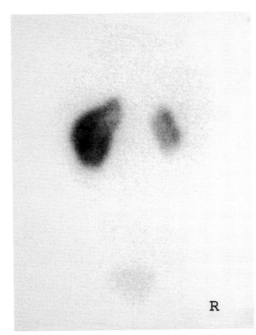

R

Fig. 16.2.4 DMSA isotope renogram showing bilateral focal defects and reduced function on the right-hand side (15% R, 85% L).

Further investigations if VUR confirmed

If VUR is demonstrated, some assessment of renal imaging needs to be made.

Renal USS is a useful initial assessment.

An isotope renogram using DMSA radioisotope is usually performed. This investigation gives an assessment of relative contribution to renal function of each kidney and whether or not there are focal defects due to scarring or dysplasia (Fig. 16.2.4).

The timing of DMSA isotope renogram with respect to urinary tract infection is important; at least 3–6 month delay after UTI is recommended so that acute changes have an opportunity to resolve.

An IV pyelogram is now not routinely used as an investigation for reflux nephropathy.

It is likely that new guidelines for the investigation of UTI will suggest less frequent use of MCUG in children with UTI.

Management

Secondary causes of VUR should be sought and managed as appropriate.

The rationale for management of VUR is aimed at two objectives:

- preventing further renal damage due to scarring with ascending urinary tract infection;
- improving symptoms of recurrent urine infection which can be debilitating for infants (e.g. may affect growth).

The most important aspect of management is to correctly diagnose and promptly treat UTI in children, especially if they are known to have VUR.

It is important to be aware that UTI in small children can present with a nonspecific range of symptoms including fever, failure to thrive, vomiting.

Simple measures

Advice regarding prevention of urine infections including:

- good fluid intake;
- regular voiding (including double voiding if VUR present);
- avoidance of constipation;
- perineal hygiene;
- advice to avoid perineal irritation (including avoidance of bubble baths and scented soaps).

Other options are:

- antibiotic prophylaxis;
- surgical management (reimplantation of ureters or endoscopic correction of VUR).

Antibiotic prophylaxis

Antibiotic prophylaxis is usually the first-line management.

Typically trimethoprim (1–2 mg/kg) once a day is used as first line although this may need to be changed if resistance to trimethoprim develops.

If no further infection occurs prophylaxis can eventually be discontinued. There is no clear guidance as to when this should be done and a reasonable time to do this is when the child comes out of nappies and urine collection becomes easier.

Prophylaxis may need to be stopped if there are evolving problems with antibiotic resistance.

There is controversy as to whether it is necessary to perform a cystogram before stopping antibiotic prophylaxis.

It would seem reasonable not to do this providing the child remains well.

Repeated DMSA isotope renograms may not be needed unless there are problems with ongoing urine infections.

Surgical management

Controversy exists as to the appropriate surgical management for VUR.

There is no clear evidence base that either reimplantation of the ureters or endoscopic correction of VUR provide a better outcome in terms of prevention of renal failure or symptoms (although some studies have suggested that surgery may be better for symptoms).

Usually invasive surgery (reimplantation of the ureters) is reserved for cases in which repeated symptomatic UTI occur despite antibiotic prophylaxis.

Newer methods such as noninvasive endoscopic correction may be used as an early alternative to antibiotic prophylaxis. Shared management with a pediatric nephrologist and urologist may be indicated.

Follow-up

The presence of persistent focal defects on DMSA isotope renograms indicates the possible need for indefinite follow-up of BP and urinalysis to look for proteinuria.

When bilateral focal defects on DMSA isotope renogram are present, continued follow-up and regular assessment of renal function is required.

Further reading

Cochrane Renal Group. Interventions for primary vesicoureteric reflux. Review.

Postlethwaite RJ, Webb N. *Clinical paediatric nephrology*, 3rd edn. Oxford: Oxford University Press; 2003.

Internet resources

Cochrane Renal Group:

http://www.cochrane-renal.org/

The Renal Registry:

http://www.renalreg.org

Great Ormond Street Hospital Family Factsheet on VUR:

http://www.ich.ucl.ac.uk/factsheets/families/F000277/index.html

UK Vesicoureteric reflux DNA collection:

http://www.vur.org.uk/

See also

Urinary tract infections in infancy and childhood, p. 252

Lower and upper urinary tract infection in the adult, p. 244

Renal dysplasia, p. 646

Congenital abnormalities of the urinary tract, p. 658

Urinary tract obstruction

Introduction

Obstruction of the urinary tract remains a major but preventable cause of chronic kidney disease (CKD) worldwide. Urinary tract obstruction can result from a number of different pathologies with the causes of obstruction varying according to the patient's age and sex. Immediately following acute obstruction, the changes within the kidney are mainly functional and potentially fully reversible. However, longstanding obstruction results in irreversible functional and structural damage. In order to avoid long-term structural and functional damage to the kidney, prompt investigation is required along with effective relief of the obstruction. Close collaboration between nephrologists, radiologists and urologists is essential for optimal investigation and management of the patient with urinary tract obstruction.

Definitions

Obstructive uropathy

The structural or functional changes in the urinary tract which impede normal urinary flow. It is classified according to the site, the degree, and the duration of the obstruction. It may be complete (high grade) or partial or incomplete (low grade).

Obstructive nephropathy

The renal disease resulting from impaired urine flow.

Hydronephrosis

Dilatation of the upper urinary tract. Obstruction is the commonest cause. It may also occur without obstruction (as in reflux nephropathy) and rarely can be absent in established obstruction.

Epidemiology

The frequency and etiology of obstruction varies with age and sex.

Antenatal USS commonly detects urinary tract dilatation in the fetus although the exact long-term significance of many such observations remains to be determined.

In children aged <10 years obstruction is commoner in males due to congenital anomalies of the urinary tract (urethral valves, PUJ obstruction). Congenital obstructive uropathy is a common cause of ESRD in this age group (up to 16%). With improved survival the impact of this disease can now be seen in adult life.

Between 10 and 20 years of age, the frequency of urinary tract obstruction is similar in males and females.

After 20 years of age, obstruction occurs more commonly in females, as a result of pregnancy and gynecologic malignancies.

>60 years of age obstruction is more common in males as a result of either benign or malignant prostatic disease.

80% of men >60 years of age have some symptoms of bladder outflow obstruction, and up to 10% have hydronephrosis.

The postmortem prevalence of hydronephrosis is 3.5–3.8%, with approximately equal distribution between males and females.

Etiology

It is useful to consider whether the obstruction is:
- congenital or acquired;
- due to disease intrinsic or extrinsic to the renal tract;
- unilateral (will not result in significant renal impairment as there is a functioning contralateral kidney) or bilateral (will result in renal impairment);
- affecting the lower or upper urinary tract (lower urinary tract obstruction always has the potential to result in significant renal impairment as it can inevitably affect the drainage of both kidneys).

The common sites and causes of obstruction are shown in Fig. 16.3.1.

Congenital urinary tract obstruction

This is commonest in males.

Causes include:
- posterior urethral valves;
- meatal strictures;
- ureteropelvic junction obstruction – this is bilateral in 20% of cases but, if low grade and unilateral, may not present until adulthood or as an incidental finding on abdominal USS.

Acquired urinary tract obstruction

Intrinsic causes of obstruction

Renal calculi: can be found anywhere along the renal tract but typically lodge at the ureteropelvic junction or vesicoureteric junction causing obstruction. Renal calculi affect 1–5% of the population and occur most commonly during the 2nd and 3rd decades of life. (male:female >3:1).

Sloughed papilla resulting from papillary necrosis which can occur in:
- diabetes mellitus;
- sickle cell trait or disease;
- analgesic nephropathy;
- renal amyloidosis;
- acute pyelonephritis.

Blood clots seen in:
- bleeding renal tumors;
- arteriovenous malformations;
- following renal trauma;
- patients with polycystic kidney disease.

Uroepithelial malignancy: may occur in the renal pelvis, ureter and bladder.

Ureteral strictures: secondary to radiotherapy or retroperitoneal surgery. Worldwide infection with *Schistosoma haematobium* is an important cause. Ova may lodge in the distal ureter and bladder causing ureteral strictures, and contraction of the bladder in up to 50% of chronically infected patients.

Urethral strictures: usually only in males secondary to urethral instrumentation or infection.

Neurological conditions: can result in either a contracted (spastic) or a flaccid (atonic) bladder (depending on whether the lesion affects upper or lower motor neurons) and cause impaired bladder emptying, e.g. multiple sclerosis, spinal cord trauma.

Extrinsic causes of obstruction

Females:
- carcinoma of the cervix: direct extension of the tumor to involve the urinary tract occurs in up to 30% of patients;

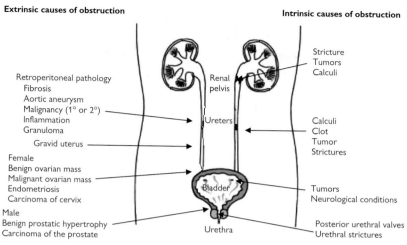

Extrinsic causes of obstruction

Intrinsic causes of obstruction

Retroperitoneal pathology
Fibrosis
Aortic aneurysm
Malignancy (1° or 2°)
Inflammation
Granuloma

Gravid uterus

Female
Benign ovarian mass
Malignant ovarian mass
Endometriosis
Carcinoma of cervix

Male
Benign prostatic hypertrophy
Carcinoma of the prostate

Renal
pelvis

Ureters

Bladder

Urethra

Stricture
Tumors
Calculi

Calculi
Clot
Tumor
Strictures

Tumors
Neurological conditions

Posterior urethral valves
Urethral strictures

Fig. 16.3.1 Diagrammatic representation of urinary tract showing the common sites and causes of obstruction.

- benign and malignant uterine and ovarian masses;
- pelvic pathology: abscesses, endometriosis, and pelvic inflammatory disease;
- inadvertent ligation of the ureter during surgical procedures;
- pressure from a gravid uterus on the pelvic rim: right ureter more commonly affected than the left. It is usually asymptomatic and the changes resolve rapidly following delivery (non-obstructed ureteral dilatation is also seen in pregnancy as a result of hormonal effects, especially progesterone on smooth muscle).

Males:
- benign prostatic hyperplasia: commonest cause;
- carcinoma of the prostate: either from direct extension of the tumor to the bladder outlet or ureters or from metastases to the ureter or lymph nodes.

Either sex:
- retroperitoneal malignancy: either primary (lymphoma and sarcoma) or metastases;
- retroperitoneal fibrosis: either idiopathic (rare) or secondary to inflammatory aortic aneurysms, drugs (methysergide, β-blockers bromocriptine), radiation, trauma or granulomatous disease (TB, Crohn's, sarcoid, Wegener's);
- vascular abnormalities: aneurysmal dilatation of the aorta or iliac vessels, aberrant vessels, or anatomic variations in the location of the ureter (retrocaval ureter).

Acquired urinary tract obstruction (mostly prostatic disease in men) accounts for 3–5% of the cases of ESRD in patients aged >65 years.

Pathophysiological changes within the kidney

Obstruction of the renal tract rapidly results in alteration in both glomerular and tubular function.

These changes depend on the duration of the obstruction, the patient's hydration state and whether there is a contralateral functioning kidney.

Ultimately irreversible structural damage leads to CKD.

Glomerular filtration

The glomerular effects of obstruction are complex.

Obstruction can alter all the determinants of glomerular filtration:
- mean hydraulic pressure gradient between the glomerular capillary lumen and Bowman's space;
- renal plasma flow;
- ultrafiltration coefficient of the glomerular capillary wall;
- mean oncotic pressure difference across the glomerular wall.

Early obstruction is typically characterized by:
- progressive intrarenal vasoconstriction;
- shunting of blood to nonfiltering areas;
- proportionately greater fall in GFR;
- fall in filtration fraction.

These changes are modulated by generation of vasoconstrictors such as thromboxane and angiotensin II, a decrease in the generation of vasodilatory prostaglandins and nitric oxide and an infiltrate of macrophages – the latter has also been implicated in the pathogenesis of the structural changes that occur following prolonged obstruction.

Whole kidney GFR will usually return to normal after short-term obstruction (days). However, even relatively short periods of obstruction may lead to a permanent loss of nephrons with whole kidney GFR recovering at the expense of hyperfiltration in the remaining functional nephrons.

Once extensive chronic structural changes have occurred within the kidney the patient will be left with a decreased GFR and CKD even after the effective relief of the obstruction.

Tubular function

Abnormalities in tubular function are common in urinary tract obstruction and may include:
- altered renal handling of electrolytes;
- changes in the regulation of water excretion;
- impairment of urinary concentrating ability;
- urinary acidification defects.

Recovery of tubular function following release of obstruction is slow and it may remain abnormal even after whole kidney GFR has returned to normal.

Clinical features

Symptoms

Symptoms depend on the patient's age and the site, duration, degree and cause of the obstruction.

Congenital obstruction may cause:

- oligohydramnios;
- distended bladder;
- failure to thrive;
- vomiting.

Acquired obstruction may cause:

- changes in urine output;
- flank pain;
- hematuria;
- lower urinary tract symptoms;
- urinary tract infections;
- no symptoms.

Changes in urine output: anuria occurs following complete bilateral obstruction or unilateral obstruction in patients with a single functioning kidney. In partial obstruction, urine output may be normal or increased (polyuria).

Flank pain and tenderness are typical of upper tract obstruction and may be severe and crescendo in nature radiating to the labia, the testicles, or the groin (renal colic) if the obstruction is acute.

Hematuria: trauma to the uroepithelium from calculi or a uroepithelial malignancy can result in either visible (macro) or invisible (microscopic) hematuria.

Lower urinary tract symptoms are typical of bladder outflow obstruction:

- poor urine stream;
- dribbling;
- hesitancy;
- nocturia.

Urgency, frequency, and urinary incontinence can also result from incomplete bladder emptying. 'Prostatism' is used to describe these symptoms in men as they are commonly (but not always) due to prostatic hypertrophy.

Urinary tract infections (UTIs): lower urinary tract obstruction predisposes to the development of UTIs because of urinary stasis. Further investigation to exclude obstruction should be undertaken following a single UTI in men or young children of either sex, recurrent infections in women or infections with an atypical organism.

Obstruction should be considered in any patient with CKD.

Signs

Physical examination may demonstrate:

- flank tenderness;
- a flank mass (enlarged hydronephrotic kidney);
- a distended bladder (bladder outflow obstruction);
- evidence of malignancy – rectal and pelvic examinations are important (enlarged prostate and gynecological malignancy);
- hypertension (sodium and water retention and abnormal release of renin);
- hypotension (polyuria and volume depletion);

Investigations

General investigations

Urinalysis

This is commonly negative but depending on the cause of obstruction can show:

- hematuria;
- bacteriuria;
- pyuria;
- crystalluria;
- low grade proteinuria.

Full blood count

Anemia may be found if obstruction has resulted in CKD, but polycythemia has been described in short-term obstruction from erythropoetin release.

Renal function tests

These may range form near normal (especially if the obstruction is unilateral or partial without damage to the upper renal tract) to advanced CKD.

Electrolytes

These may demonstrate a hyperchloremic hyperkalemic (type IV) metabolic acidosis and hypernatremia.

Imaging investigations

Imaging is key to diagnosing the site and cause of obstruction and may require complementary use of a number of different modalities.

No single investigation should be relied upon to rule out obstruction if the clinical suspicion is high.

The imaging techniques below have largely replaced the use of IVU in the evaluation of suspected renal tract obstruction.

Ultrasound (Fig. 16.3.2A)

Useful first-line investigation but operator dependent.

Avoids ionizing radiation.

Readily detects hydronephrosis but not its cause.

Can be used to assess bladder emptying in patients with lower urinary tract symptoms.

Should be combined with a KUB X-ray to look for areas of calcification in the line of the ureter (stones).

False positives (nonobstructed dilatation, as may be seen in reflux nephropathy) and false negatives (nondilated urinary tract obstruction) can occur.

CT scan (Fig. 16.3.2B)

Noncontrast helical CT is excellent at detecting stones and is therefore the imaging modality of choice for patients with acute flank pain.

It can provide good anatomical definition and define the nature and the site of the obstructing lesion, especially when this is extrinsic to the urinary tract.

IV contrast can improve the diagnostic potential but may be contraindicated in patients with renal impairment.

Exposure of the patient to ionizing radiation limits the ability to use it repetitively.

MR urography (Fig. 16.3.2C)

Can provide both functional and anatomic information without exposure to ionizing radiation (and may allow a diagnosis without using multiple investigations such as nuclear scans, voiding cystourethrography and USS).

Has similar accuracy to spiral CT (when used in conjunction with KUB).

The potential for gadolinium to cause nephrogenic sclerosing dermopathy limits the use of MR in patients with moderate–severe CKD.

Renography (Fig. 16.3.2D)
[⁹⁹ᵐTc]MAG-3 renography with IV furosemide at 20 min (diuresis renogram) can help determine whether a dilated collecting system is due to functional obstruction: persistence of the isotope suggests obstruction.

The test is unhelpful when renal function is poor.

It may overdiagnose obstruction in those aged <2 years (the renal pelvis normally expands during diuresis in this age group).

Retrograde/antegrade pyelography
Can be used to accurately localize and characterize obstructing lesions.

May be combined with therapeutic interventions (nephrostomy, ureteric stenting).

May be combined with functional tests of obstruction (Whitaker test, urodynamics).

Are invasive and have generally been replaced by USS, CT and MR.

Treatment

Close collaboration between nephrologists, radiologists and urologists is essential.

The treatment required is determined by the duration and location of the obstruction, the underlying cause, and the degree (if any) of renal impairment.

Goals of treatment must include:
• prompt relief of the obstruction to allow recovery of renal impairment and reduce the possibility of CKD in the long term;
• management of any metabolic and fluid and electrolyte disturbance;
• a long-term management plan to definitively deal with the pathology which caused the obstruction.

Dialysis should only be required in a minority, for example where life-threatening hyperkalemia or fluid overload has to be corrected to get the patient fit for the planned intervention.

Bladder outflow obstruction can usually be treated by a urethral catheter.

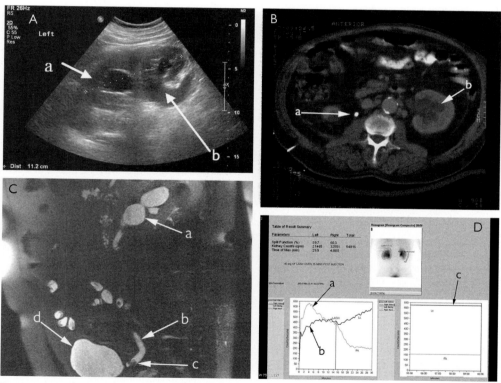

Fig. 16.3.2 (A) Longitudinal USS of an obstructed kidney showing well-preserved parenchyma (a) and a dilated pelvis (b). (B) Abdominal CT of a patient with bilateral renal stones. There is a calculus on the left (a) and a dilated renal pelvis on the right (b). (C) MR urogram showing a hydronephrotic kidney (a), a dilated lower ureter (b), a filling defect in the ureter (c) and bladder (d). (D) Diuresis renogram. The trace of the right kidney is normal (a), but the trace of the left obstructed kidney continues to rise after furosemide (b). On delayed images the left kidney has not emptied (c).

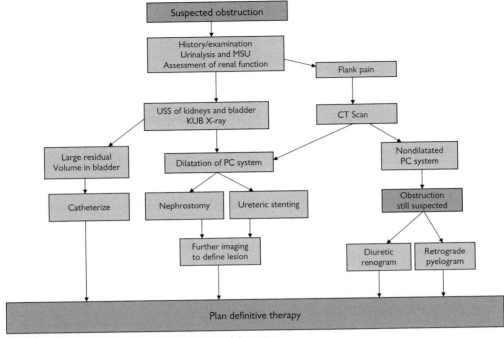

Fig. 16.3.3 Algorithm for the investigation and management of obstruction.

If a catheter cannot be passed per urethra a suprapubic catheter should be inserted.

Upper urinary tract obstruction can be rapidly relieved by placement of a nephrostomy under local anesthetic, and this is the treatment of choice in an emergency setting or where infection above the site of the obstruction is suspected.

When both kidneys are obstructed, the nephrostomy should be placed in the kidney with the best-preserved parenchyma.

A nephrostomy allows time for renal function to recover and to plan definitive therapy, although it may be used long term in patients who either have an incurable malignancy or who are unfit for surgery.

Antegrade stenting of the ureter may be possible following a nephrostomy to establish internal drainage of the kidney into the bladder.

Cystoscopy and retrograde stenting of the ureter(s) offers an alternative approach to relief of upper urinary tract obstruction.

Once the obstruction has been relieved and wherever possible, definitive treatment of the obstructing lesion should be undertaken. The therapy required depends on the site and nature of the obstructing lesion and a full discussion is beyond the scope of this chapter.

The general approach to the investigation and management of obstruction is shown in Fig. 16.3.3.

Postobstructive diuresis
This is typically seen following the release of bilateral obstruction or obstruction in a single functioning kidney.

It may result from both an appropriate excretion of retained salt and water and an inappropriate loss of salt and water due to tubular dysfunction following obstruction.

Without appropriate management volume depletion and electrolyte disturbances can occur with failure of the renal function to recover.

Management includes:
- regular assessment of the patient's fluid balance including hourly urine output and weighing daily;
- regular measurement of serum electrolytes: at least daily and more frequently if the diuresis is massive;
- appropriate fluid replacement: once the patient is euvolemic, replacement of urine losses plus an allowance for insensible losses is required. Intravenous therapy may be required and bicarbonate, potassium, calcium, phosphate, and magnesium replacement may be necessary.

Follow-up
Many patients will recover normal renal function following effective relief of the obstruction.

The follow-up of such patients relates to that required for the underlying condition which caused the obstruction or to the postoperative follow up required for any surgery that was undertaken to treat the obstruction.

However, if the kidney had sustained structural damage following prolonged obstruction, the patient may be left with a varying degree of CKD. Treatment is then the same as for any patient with CKD with attention paid to:

- control of blood pressure;
- use of ACEIs if there is ongoing significant proteinuria;
- aggressive management of cardiovascular risk factors.

Progression of CKD (even if severe) is likely to be slow if the obstruction has been effectively relieved and hypertension is controlled.

Further reading

Leyendecker JR, Barnes CE, Zagoria RJ. MR urography: techniques and clinical applications. *Radiographics* 2008; **28**: 23–46.

Proesmans W. The neurogenic bladder: introducing four contributions. *Pediatr Nephrol* 2008; **23**: 537–540.

Vaglio A, Palmisano A, Corradi D, Salvarani C, Buzio C. Retroperitoneal fibrosis: evolving concepts. *Rheum Dis Clin North Am* 2007; **33**: 803–817.

Internet resources

Retroperitoneal fibrosis patient and carer information:

`http://www.retroperitonealfibrosis.com/`

Schistosomiasis information:

`http://www.cdfound.to.it/html/gen1.htm#sh5`

See also

Imaging in renal disease, p. 20

Renal stone disease, p. 269

Congenital abnormalities of the urinary tract, p. 658

Malignancy of the kidney and urinary tract, p. 667

Congenital abnormalities of the urinary tract

Introduction

Antenatal USS screening has increased the prenatal detection and early postnatal management of a group of diseases of abnormal early renal development called congenital abnormalities of the kidney and urinary tract (CAKUT).

CAKUT comprise 1 in 500 fetal USS, up to 30% of all antenatally diagnosed fetal anomalies and are the most common cause of CKD and ESRD in infants and children.

Genetic studies have implicated mutations in various genes (including *HNF-1β*, *PAX2*, *EYA1*, *SIX1*, and *SALL1*) and are providing further evidence that there is a polygenic trait of inheritance with incomplete and variable penetrance.

Some of the diverse anatomical renal and ureteric anomalies are discussed in this and other chapters (Tables 16.4.1 and 16.4.2).

Commonly encountered CAKUT include:
- renal hypodysplasia;
- polycystic kidney disease;
- hydroureteronephrosis;
- vesicoureteric reflux (VUR);
- mega-ureter;
- ureteroceles;
- urinary tract obstruction (posterior urethral valves, pelviureteric and vesicoureteric junction obstruction).

Clinical evaluation of CAKUT

As in other birth defects, it is important to undertake a full evaluation with history, examination and appropriate investigations.

History

A detailed maternal history (including prescribed and recreational drug use) is important.

The history of the antenatal period is also important, including oligohydramnios or anhydramnios, results of antenatal USS (with degree of dilatation at various gestational ages).

A complete family history should be taken (diabetes mellitus, hearing and/or visual loss, congenital and urinary tract anomalies).

Examination

Any dysmorphic features should be identified including:
- pre-auricular tags or pits;
- branchial arch abnormalities;
- retinitis pigmentosa;
- coloboma;
- aniridia;
- abnormal number or shape of digits and/or toes;
- external genitalia.

Major and minor anomalies associated with syndromes including:
- VACTERL (**V**ertebral, **A**no-rectal **C**ardiac, **T**racheo-esophageal fistula, **E**sophageal atresia, **R**adial/renal, **L**imb) association;
- CHARGE (**C**oloboma (iris, choroids or retina), **H**eart defects, **A**tresia choanae, **R**etarded growth and development, **G**enital anomalies and **E**ar anomalies or deafness).

Investigations

Postnatal USS together with micturating cystourethrography and nuclear medicine imaging may noninvasively diagnose the specific CAKUT, although cystoscopy may be required (for example, when obstructive uropathy due to posterior urethral valves is suspected in a male infant).

Genetic testing may be appropriate if there are specific features of CAKUT-associated syndromes.

Multicystic dysplastic kidney

This is due to failure of union of the ureteric bud with renal mesenchyme resulting in a multiloculated mass with thin-walled cysts, atretic proximal ureter and no functional renal parenchyma (as seen on nuclear medicine scan). The renal parenchyma is replaced by multiple noncommunicating different-sized cysts.

Clinical features

90% of cases who survive are unilateral.

It is commoner in boys.

It is associated with contralateral renal anomalies including:
- contralateral renal agenesis (resulting in Potter's syndrome);
- pelviureteric junction obstruction;
- VUR.

Investigations

Renal ultrasound

This normally demonstrates hyperechoic scanty renal tissue among cysts in a nonreniform mass (Fig. 16.4.1).

If there is a normal contralateral kidney this will show compensatory hypertrophy although a normal bladder without ureteric dilatation should be identified.

DMSA scan

To assess the solitary functioning kidney.

Formal measurement of glomerular filtration rate

This should be considered in all infants at 12 months of age where there is no evidence of compensatory hypertrophy or concerns with renal dysfunction (such as elevated plasma creatinine).

Differential diagnosis

Renal dysplasia (or renal cystic dysplasia) where there is functioning tissue in the affected kidney(s), although some studies show different spectrums of disease with both renal dysplasia and multicystic dysplasia occurring within some families.

Prognosis

Multicystic dysplastic kidneys spontaneously involute (usually by 2 years of age when size is <5 cm), so that many solitary kidneys which were labeled as contralateral renal agenesis may now be detected on antenatal USS screening as multicystic dysplastic kidneys.

Recent evidence suggests that the risks of developing hypertension and/or malignancy are negligible and routine nephrectomy is not advised.

Hypertension and/or malignancy are more likely to occur when size is >7 cm (spontaneous involution is unlikely).

Table 16.4.1 Different patterns of renal anomalies

Agenesis	Unilateral or bilateral (without any functioning renal tissue resulting in Potter's syndrome).
Crossed renal ectopia	Fusion of upper to lower pole.
Duplication	Patients mostly asymptomatic.
Ectopia	Secondary to error in ascent. Pelvic location most common.
Fusion	Complete fusion of the kidneys is rare with lower pole fusion commoner (horseshoe kidney).
Multicystic dysplastic kidneys	Mostly congenital with no functioning renal parenchymal tissue and associated with vesicoureteric reflux (although hypothetical risks of hypertension and malignancy).
Polycystic kidneys	Autosomal recessive or dominant polycystic kidney disease with bilaterally enlarged echogenic kidneys and cysts.

Table 16.4.2 Other CAKUT conditions

Mega-ureter	Primary mega-ureter without infravesical obstruction and secondary mega-ureter with high intravesical pressure (obstruction, neuropathy).
Obstructive uropathy	Most commonly posterior urethral valves which affects male children only, although anterior urethral valves have been described in females. Accompanied by bilateral (can be unilateral) hydroureteronephrosis with or without VUR, renal dysplasia and CKD.
Pelviureteric junction obstruction	Functional obstruction of the junction between renal pelvis and ureter.
Ureterocele	Cystic dilatation of the terminal ureter which can be: • intravesical (less obstructive, often asymptomatic) or • extravesical (located at bladder neck, often associated with renal duplication).
Vesicoureteric junction obstruction	Functional obstruction of the junction between bladder and ureter.

Nephrectomy may be indicated if there are severe and recurrent infections as surgical intervention carries a low complication rate and obviates the need for long-term follow-up if the contralateral kidney and bladder are normal.

Follow-up
Long-term follow-up is required if there is evidence of CKD (usually due to solitary contralateral dysplastic kidney).

Duplication
Renal duplications of the upper urinary tract result in a duplex kidney and collecting system caused by the development of an accessory ureteric bud and are associated with chromosomal defects:
• Turner syndrome (45XO);
• trisomy 13 and 18.

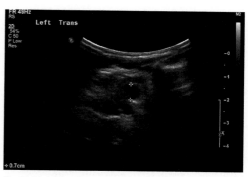

Fig. 16.4.1 A left multicystic dysplastic kidney with the largest cyst shown on USS image measuring 7 mm. There was no normal renal parenchyma tissue but only a few small cysts seen in the left flank (overall the collection of cysts measured 1.7 × 1 cm).

Bilateral duplication is relatively rare accounting for 15% of all duplication cases.

Duplication has been detected frequently in postmortem studies of asymptomatic individuals.

Clinical features
Kidneys are larger than normal.

Common occurrence (1% of population).

Usually familial.

Often asymptomatic (usually females).

Complete duplication
There are two moieties. Either both ureters enter the bladder with the upper pole ureter opening inferomedially or one ureter is ectopic, draining into the vagina or posterior urethra.

This carries an increased risk of complications including:
• obstruction of the upper moiety (ureterocele or VUJ obstruction);
• VUR of the lower moiety ureter due to its short intramural tunnel as it traverses the bladder wall.

Duplication is often associated with:
• ectopic ureters;
• ureteroceles;
• VUR;
• pelviureteric junction obstruction;
• dysplastic moiety;
• family history or as part of a syndrome.

Partial duplication
A functionally single, uncomplicated system with a divided pelvis or the ureters joining along their length (commonly over sacroiliac joint).

Investigations
Renal ultrasound
Ultrasound imaging can delineate the collecting systems and confirm the presence of dilatation and/or ureteroceles (Fig. 16.4.2).

No further imaging is required if the duplication is uncomplicated (for example no dilatation) and/or if the patient is asymptomatic where clinical detection was via abdominal USS for another cause.

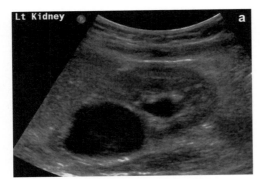

Fig. 16.4.2 An obstructed duplex in the upper pole of the left kidney on USS.

Intravenous pyelography
This is rarely performed in pediatric practice but can delineate a bladder ureterocele (which can also be seen on micturating cystourethrogram) and a dilated upper pole moiety compressing a dilated lower pole moiety due to VUR.

Nuclear medicine imaging
This is helpful in providing information on the differential function between the kidneys as well as of the respective moieties of the duplex kidney and delineating if there is an obstructive element.

Renal agenesis
This is caused by failure of the ureteric bud to communicate with the metanephric blastema during the first trimester of pregnancy.

It is associated with other malformations including:
- pelviureteric and vesicoureteric junction obstruction;
- VUR;
- genital abnormalities;
- genetic conditions;
- syndromes and nonsyndromic conditions.

Bilateral renal agenesis

This is rare and results in Potter's syndrome:
- facial appearance of flat face and nasal bridge;
- micrognathia, low-set malrotated ears;
- anhydramnios;
- foetal anuria;
- pulmonary hypoplasia.

Fetal or neonatal death results.

Unilateral renal agenesis
This may be as a result of spontaneous involution of a multicystic dysplastic kidney (which may have been detected on antenatal USS screening as above) or failure of the metanephros to develop.

Familial cases are common.

Parents can be reassured when the contralateral kidney and bladder are normal and when follow-up reveals normal renal function and contralateral compensatory hypertrophy.

Investigations
Abdominal and pelvic USS as well as nuclear medicine scanning with DMSA scan should be undertaken to exclude ectopic renal tissue (Fig. 16.4.3).

A MAG3 scan should be carried out where there is clinical suspicion of pelviureteric and/or vesicoureteric junction obstruction and micturating cystourethrogram if there is or has been ureteric dilatation.

Formal measurement of glomerular filtration rate should be considered in all infants at 12 months of age where there is no evidence of compensatory hypertrophy or concerns with renal dysfunction (such as elevated plasma creatinine).

Follow-up
Long-term follow-up is required if evidence of CKD (usually due to solitary contralateral dysplastic kidney).

There is no evidence base for any dietary or physical activity restrictions, although general advice regarding healthy lifestyle in patients with solitary kidneys should be given.

Renal ectopia
This is a developmental anomaly of abnormally shaped and (usually) functioning kidneys where there is a failure of ascent during embryogenesis usually resulting in pelvic placement (although rare cases can be found in the thorax and abdomen).

Ectopic kidneys are usually:
- unilateral (90%);
- pelvic (60%);
- hypoplastic;
- left-sided.

Renal ectopia can be associated with:
- ureteric abnormalities (including retrocaval and ectopic ureter);
- VUR;
- pelviureteric junction obstruction;
- genital abnormalities (including vaginal agenesis, and bicornuate uterus).

Antenatal USS screening may detect some cases, although some children present with pelvic masses incidentally where constipation and tumors remain the most likely differential diagnoses.

Crossed renal ectopia
This is an abnormally rotated kidney crossing the midline inferomedially to the normally sited kidney with its upper pole usually fused to the normal kidney's lower pole and the ureter from the ectopic kidney usually inserted to its normal position.

Crossed renal ectopia can occur with (85%) or without renal fusion and can be solitary or bilateral, often associated with ureteric, lower tract, cloacal and anorectal anomalies.

Crossed renal ectopia usually occurs in males with crossing occurring from left to right and can be associated with VACTERL and agenesis of the corpus callosum.

Fusion
Renal fusion is commonly associated with syndromes and other urological, neurological, skeletal, cardiovascular and gastrointestinal anomalies and is rarely complete resulting in a single renal mass.

Fusion commonly occurs at the poles with horseshoe kidney being the most common (95%) entity where embryological fusion of the lower poles of metanephric tissue interferes with the normal process of renal ascent, vascularization and rotation.

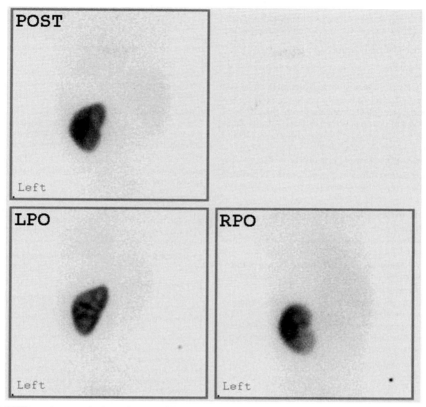

Fig. 16.4.3 DMSA scan in a case of right renal agenesis delineating a normal left kidney without evidence of a right or ectopic kidney.

Horseshoe kidney
This describes the configuration with fusion of the lower poles of the kidneys by a narrow isthmus, which usually comprises functioning tissue, but may be composed of dysplastic or fibrous tissue (Fig 16.4.4).

The isthmus can lie:
- beneath the origin of the inferior mesenteric artery at the level of L4 (40%);
- at the level of the lower poles of normally placed kidneys (40%);
- in the pelvis (20%).

Horseshoe kidneys are usually asymptomatic and undetected as they do not cause clinical problems. They lie more caudally than normal with the lower poles adjacent to the spine.

Horseshoe kidneys are commoner in males, although they are frequently associated with Turner syndrome (45XO) in females and with trisomy 13, 18 and 21.

Clinical presentation may be with:
- hematuria;
- abdominal pain;
- abdominal mass;
- urinary tract infection.

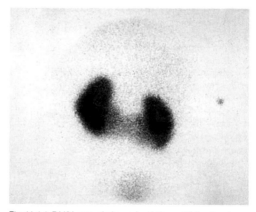

Fig. 16.4.4 DMSA scan of a horseshoe kidney with functional renal parenchyma in the isthmus.

Complications include:
- hypertension;
- VUR;
- pelviureteric junction obstruction;
- nephrolithiasis;
- malignancy;
- trauma to the isthmus due to its close relationship with the spine.

Obstruction occurs due to compression of the pelviureteric junction and proximal ureter by the aberrant vessels commonly found at the renal hilum or due to distortion of the proximal ureter as it loops over the renal isthmus.

The continuity of both lower poles may be missed on USS.

Intravenous pyelography is rarely performed in pediatric practice and confirmation of diagnosis by CT or MRI scanning is very infrequently required.

Lower and other urinary tract defects

Prune belly syndrome
Absent abdominal wall musculature, Eagle–Barrett or triad syndrome.

It is caused by failure of mesenchymal development predominantly in males (otherwise pseudo prune belly syndrome).

Clinical features include:
- deficiency or absence of anterior abdominal wall musculature with wrinkled, lax appearance;
- bilateral cryptorchidism with empty hypoplastic scrotum;
- ureter, bladder and urethral abnormalities (usually megacystis, mega-ureter due to dysplasia).

It is associated with:
- renal dysplasia;
- VUR;
- urinary stasis;
- narrowed urethra;
- obstruction of ureteric, pelviureteric and vesicoureteric junctions;
- poorly contractile, thick-walled (nontrabeculated) bladder with large diverticulae;
- urachal cyst or patent urachus;
- postmicturition residual volumes;
- malrotation;
- gastroschisis;
- imperforate anus;
- constipation;
- congenital heart disease;
- talipes equinovarus;
- developmental dysplasia of the hips.

Long-term follow-up is required if there is evidence of CKD. A formal measurement of GFR should be performed at 12 months of age when it is associated with renal dysplasia and/or there are concerns about renal dysfunction (such as elevated plasma creatinine).

Bladder extrophy
There is exposure of the posterior wall of the bladder.

It occurs due to a breakdown of the cloacal membrane caused by the infra-umbilical mesenchyme failing to separate the cloaca component that develops into the bladder from the overlying ectoderm.

It is commoner in boys with lower abdominal wall defects, symphisis pubis diastasis, pelvic, bladder, urethral and genital abnormalities, including inguinal herniae, epispadias, hemi-clitoris and anterior anus.

Neonatal bladder closure is required with pelvic bone osteotomies and latter reconstructive surgery to normalize the urogenital tract and ensure continence.

Infants with cloacal extrophy have the defects of bladder exstrophy with exomphalos, imperforate anus and lumbosacral spinal defects.

Cloacal anomaly
There is a urethra, vagina and colon single channel and opening in girls due to failure of the urorectal septum to develop. This may result in stenosis and obstruction of urinary tract, uterine cavity and gastrointestinal tract.

Surgical relief of obstruction and later reconstructive surgery may be required.

Urogenital sinus
There is a urethra and vaginal single channel and opening in girls due to failure of the urethrovaginal septum to develop. This may result in stenosis and obstruction of the urinary tract and/or uterine cavity (resulting in hydrocolpos).

Urological surgery is required to separate the urethra and vagina.

Further reading

Hiraoka M. Medical management of congenital anomalies of the kidney and urinary tract. *Pediatr Int* 2003; **45**: 624–633.

Limwongse C, Cassidy SB. Syndromes and malformations of the urinary tract. In: Avner ED, Harmon WE, Niaudet P (eds), *Pediatric nephrology*, 5th edn. Philadelphia: Lippincott Williams & Wilkins; 2004.

Miyazaki Y, Ichikawa I. Ontogeny of congenital anomalies of the kidney and urinary tract, CAKUT. *Pediatr Int* 2003; **45**: 598–604.

Nakai H, Asanuma H, Shishido S, Kitahara S, Yasuda K. Changing concepts in urological management of the congenital anomalies of kidney and urinary tract, CAKUT. *Pediatr Int* 2003; **45**: 634–641.

Nakanishi K, Yoshikawa N. Genetic disorders of human congenital anomalies of the kidney and urinary tract (CAKUT). *Pediatr Int* 2003; **45**: 610–616.

Schedl A. Renal abnormalities and their developmental origin. *Nat Rev Genet* 2007; **8**: 791–802.

Internet resources

Evaluation of congenital anomalies of the kidney and urinary tract (UpToDate):

http://patients.uptodate.com/topic.asp?file=pedineph/17792

Human Renal Tract Malformations: Unravelling The Genes – summary of lecture by Prof. A. Woolf at the XLIII ERA-EDTA Congress:

http://www.ndt-educational.org/woolfslide2006txt.asp

National Congenital Anomaly System:

http://www.statistics.gov.uk/downloads/theme_health/National_Congenital_Anomaly_System/CA_text_v2.pdf

NHS Perinatal Institute:

http://www.perinatal.nhs.uk/car/anomaly/renal/renal.htm

See also

Renal dysplasia, p. 646

Vesicoureteric reflux and reflux nephropathy, p. 648

Rare syndromes with renal involvement, p. 640

Medullary sponge kidney

Introduction
Medullary sponge kidney (MSK) is also called renal tubular ectasia or Cacchi–Ricci disease. It is a congenital renal developmental abnormality and part of a group of renal cystic disorders but rarely encountered even in pediatric nephrological practice. Its name is derived from the sponge appearance of the renal medulla which can occur focally in one or both kidneys (usually both kidneys) due to collecting duct ectasia and cyst formation in one or more renal pyramids.

MSK is believed to arise from hyperplasia or obstruction of fetal collecting tubules and hypercalciuria with increased urinary pH causing the associated nephrolithiaisis and structural changes.

Epidemiology
MSK is commoner in males than females (although more females are affected with hypercalciuria).

It affects children (from 2 years of age) and adults, although commoner in adolescents and young adults with progressive degeneration of the collecting tubules occurring later in life.

The prevalence is 1 in 5000–20 000 individuals but this is an underestimate as many patients are asymptomatic.

MSK is detected in 0.5–1% of patients undergoing intravenous pyelography.

Genetics
Most cases are sporadic.

Familial clustering (including autosomal dominant inheritance) has been described.

Clinical features
Presentation
Incidental finding in asymptomatic patient.

Failure to thrive (with growth failure due to distal renal tubular acidosis).

Loin pain

Microscopic (>90% of patients) and macroscopic (<20% of patients) hematuria.

Urinary tract infection (30% of symptomatic patients) with possible recurrent acute and chronic pyelonephritis due to urinary stasis and nephrolithiasis.

Associated renal features
Distal renal tubular acidosis.

Proximal renal tubular dysfunction.

Mild urinary concentration impairment and acidification defects.

Nephrocalcinosis and nephrolithiaisis (calcium oxalate and apatite calculi or struvite calculi from bacteria).

Risk of chronic kidney disease
Few cases progress with renal dysfunction.

Proteinuria and hypertension are rare, although pregnancy-induced hypertension has been reported.

Clinical associations
Autosomal dominant polycystic kidney disease (ADPKD).

Horseshoe kidney.

Renal duplication or malrotation.

Caroli's disease.

Congenital heart disease.

Pyloric stenosis.

Parathyroid adenoma.

Hemihypertrophy.

Beckwith–Wiedemann syndrome (with associated increased malignancy rates).

Marfan and Ehlers–Danlos syndrome.

Differential diagnosis
Polycystic kidney disease, especially ADPKD.

Renal papillary necrosis or tuberculosis.

Calyceal diverticulum.

Nephrolithiasis.

Investigations
Abdominal X-ray
Linear/rounded clusters of medullary nephrocalcinosis.

Nephrolithiasis within renal pelvis, ureter or bladder.

Renal ultrasound
Normal-sized kidneys or renal hypertrophy (especially if associated with ADPKD) with echogenic medullary pyramids with calcification.

Intravenous pyelography
Findings include:

Discrete linear papillary striations due to dilated collecting tubules of renal medulla (Fig. 16.5.1).

Nephrolithiasis arranged in groups around a calyx (bunch of grapes pattern).

Hypertrophy of renal pyramids.

Distorted calyces, which are broad and shallow (Fig. 16.5.2).

CT
Medullary nephrocalcinosis and tubular ectasia.

Contrast-enhanced scans may demonstrate papillary architecture (Fig. 16.5.3).

Interstitial nephritis and renal abscess formation.

MRI
This is not sensitive for calcification (CT preferred).

It has a limited role, especially in patients with known allergies to contrast media.

DMSA renogram
Photopenic areas of renal parenchymal scarring may be found and differential renal function can be assessed.

Pathology
MSK is a developmental defect with ectasia and cyst formation (of 1–8 mm size representing dilated terminal collecting tubules) with hyperplasia affecting the intrapyramidal or intrapapillary segments of renal medullary collecting tubules.

Noncommunicating, and more commonly communicating, cysts (proximally with collecting tubules and distally with papillary ducts or calyx) are occasionally associated with calculus formation.

Treatment and prognosis

Urinary tract infection, nephrocalcinosis and nephrolithiasis require standard treatment including antibiotics, increased fluid intake and thiazide diuretics.

A few cases are associated with CKD.

There is no associated increased mortality rate.

Further reading

Forster JA, Taylor J, Browning AJ, Biyani CS. A review of the natural progression of medullary sponge kidney and a novel grading system based on intravenous urography findings. *Urol Int* 2007; **78**: 264–269.

Gambaro G, Feltrin GP, Lupo A, Bonfante L, D'Angelo A, Antonello A. Medullary sponge kidney (Lenarduzzi–Cacchi–Ricci disease): a Padua Medical School discovery in the 1930s. *Kidney Int* 2006; **69**: 663–670.

Kasap B, Soylu A, Oren O, Türkmen M, Kavukçu S. Medullary sponge kidney associated with distal renal tubular acidosis in a 5-year-old girl. *Eur J Pediatr* 2006; **165**: 648–651.

Maw AM, Megibow AJ, Grasso M, Goldfarb DS. Diagnosis of medullary sponge kidney by computed tomographic urography. *Am J Kidney Dis* 2007; **50**: 146–150.

Internet resources

National Organisation for Rare Disorders:

http://www.rarediseases.org/

Medullary Sponge Kidney Support Group:

http://groups.msn.com/medullaryspongekidney

National Kidney Federation patient information:

http://www.kidney.org.uk/Medical-Info/kidney-disease/cysts.html

See also

Lower and upper urinary tract infection in the adult, p. 244

Nephrocalcinosis, p. 278

Medical management of stone disease, p. 270

Surgical management of stone disease, p. 274

Congenital abnormalities of the urinary tract, p. 658

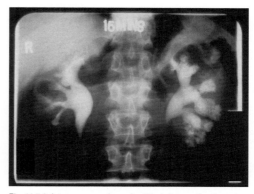

Fig. 16.5.2 Intravenous pyelography: 15 min image of patient who presented with hematuria and had renal calculi on control film with irregularity of calyces (dilated without cupping).

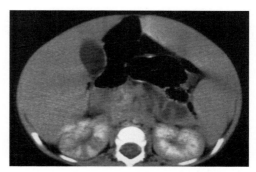

Fig. 16.5.3 CT scan performed for congenital hepatic fibrosis in a child with contrast nephrogram demonstrating medullary cysts.

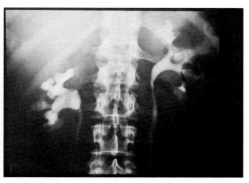

Fig. 16.5.1 Renal tubular ectasia without nephrolithiasis on intravenous pyelography.

Malignancy of the kidney and urinary tract

Chapter contents

Tumors of the kidney

Introduction
Renal cell carcinoma (RCC) is the most frequently occurring solid lesion within the kidney. It comprises different tumor subtypes with specific genetic characteristics. The study of the hereditary types of kidney cancer syndromes has helped to elucidate the genetic basis of sporadic renal tumor formation, and provided the background for developing molecular-targeted agents in the treatment of RCC. Levels of evidence are indicated as used by the US Department of Health and Human Services.

Definition
By far the most common renal tumor is renal cell carcinoma, followed by Wilms' tumor, which is found in children, and finally urothelial tumors of the calyces and renal pelvis. Because of their gross yellow color and resemblance of the tumor cells to clear cells of the adrenal cortex, it was once thought that they arose from adrenal tissue, accounting for the term hypernephroma. It is now clear that these tumors arise from tubular epithelium and are therefore renal adenocarcinomas.

Epidemiology
Kidney tumors account for 2–3% of all cancers.

Male predominance over female (1.5:1).

Within the European Union:
- ~30 000 patients were diagnosed with RCC in 1998;
- ~15 000 patients died of RCC in 1998.

The highest incidence is in developed countries.

The peak incidence is between 60 and 70 years of age.

Worldwide annual increase in incidence is ~2%.

Predisposing factors
Cigarette smoking (evidence: 2a).

Obesity (evidence: 2a).

Prolonged intake of antihypertensives (evidence: 2a).

Genetics
A number of genetic mutations have been found in association with sporadic and hereditary renal cell tumors (Table 17.1.1).

Of sporadic clear cell RCC, ~75% show loss of von Hippel–Lindau (VHL) activity and 13% of sporadic papillary type 1 tumors have activating mutations in the MET proto-oncogene.

VHL protein functions as a tumor suppressor and inhibits hypoxia-inducible genes.

These genes encode several proteins involved in:
- angiogenesis: vascular endothelial growth factor (VEGF);
- cell growth: transforming growth factor-α;
- glucose uptake: the GLUT-1 glucose transporter;
- acid–base balance: carbonic anhydrase IX.

When VHL protein is lost, these proteins are overexpressed, creating conditions favoring epithelial proliferation.

Clinical features
Symptoms
Asymptomatic: incidental detection of RCC using noninvasive imaging (> 50%).

The classic triad of flank pain, abdominal mass and gross hematuria (6–10%).

Presentation may alternatively be with symptoms associated with, but not directly caused by, metastatic disease (30%).

Paraneoplastic syndromes can occur in ~30% of patients with symptomatic RCC:
- hypertension;
- hypercalcemia;
- erythrocytosis;
- Stauffer's syndrome (paraneoplastic cholestatic jaundice).

Physical examination
- Abdominal mass.
- Cervical lymphadenopathy.
- Nonreducing varicocele.
- Bilateral lower limb edema.

All of these signs should initiate imaging.

Renal cell tumors and syndromes
A number of rare syndromes can be associated with the development of RCC (Table 17.1.1).

von Hippel–Lindau (VHL) disease
The commonest syndrome associated with RCC

Autosomal dominant.

1 in 35 000 individuals.

There is a spectrum of germline mutations of VHL in 99% of VHL families.

The three major manifestations are:
- clear cell RCC;
- CNS hemangioblastoma;
- pheochromocytoma.

Affected families may not have all three conditions.

The kidneys of affected patients often contain multiple, bilateral solid tumors and cysts. Nephron-sparing surgery is recommended when solid renal lesions reach 3 cm.

Investigations
Abdominal ultrasound
The detection of a solid renal mass with ultrasound always requires further investigation.

CT scan of the abdomen and chest with contrast
To determine the extent of any spread within the abdomen and to detect pulmonary metastases.

MRI of abdomen and chest
This is reserved for those with renal insufficiency or an allergy to intravenous contrast.

Percutaneous biopsy
This is usually only considered in selected cases (e.g. when there is suspicion that the renal mass is a secondary), although there is now a move towards biopsy of small lesions.

Other investigations
- Estimate of renal fuction (serum creatinine and eGFR);
- Full blood count.
- Bone profile and liver function tests if the disease is metastatic.

Table 17.1.1 Sporadic and hereditary renal cell tumors and genetic alterations

Sporadic renal cell tumors			Renal cell tumors in an inherited syndrome		
Histological appearance	Incidence	Gene alteration and freqency	Syndrome	Gene alteration	Chromosome affected
Clear cell	75%	VHL, 60%	VHL disease	VHL	3p
			FCRC		3p
			Hereditary paraganglioma	SDHB	1q
Papillary type 1	5%	MET, 13%	HPRC	MET	7q
Papillary type 2	10%	TFE3, <1%	HLRCC	FH	1q
Chromophobe	5%		Birt–Hogg–Dubé	BHD	17p
Oncocytoma	5%		Birt–Hogg–Dubé	BHD	17p
Collecting duct	Rare (<1%)	–	–	–	–
Medullary carcinoma	Rare	–	–	–	–

VHL, von Hippel–Lindau; FCRC, familial clear cell cancer; HPRC, hereditary papillary renal carcinoma; HLRCC, hereditary leiomyomatosis and renal cell cancer; SDHB, succinate dehydrogenase B; FH, fumarate hydratase.

- DMSA renogram if there is concern about the relative function of the contralateral kidney.

Pathology

Histological grading

Fuhrman nuclear grade (1–4) is the most widely accepted histological grading system in RCC.

Sporadic renal cell tumor subtypes

The current World Health Organization (2004) classification is based on the Heidelberg classification system (Table 17.1.1).

The trend for better prognosis in pT1–T2 RCC is:
- chromophobe > papillary > clear cell RCC.

Collecting-duct carcinoma is frequently metastatic at diagnosis. Renal medullary carcinoma has some morphological overlap, occurs in younger patients and is associated with sickle cell disease.

Papillary type 1 tumors are indolent compared with the more aggressive type 2 tumors.

Renal oncocytomas are almost invariably benign, but rare hybrid tumors with chromophobe RCC exist.

Pathology and natural history of small enhancing renal tumors (<4 cm) on CT

Approximately two-thirds are malignant.

The mean growth rate of these tumors managed by surveillance is slow (<3 mm per year) and the metastasis rate is 1%.

If RCC is proven, the growth rate is 4 mm per year and the metastasis rate is 2.8%.

Staging

The 2002 UICC TNM stage classification system is recommended (Table 17.1.2). The pT1 substratification, introduced in 2002, has been validated by a number of studies.

Table 17.1.2 TNM stage classification system for renal cell cancer

T	Primary tumor	
	T1a	Tumor ≤4 cm in greatest dimension, limited to the kidney
	T1b	Tumor >4 cm but ≤7 cm in greatest dimension
	T2	Tumor >7 cm in greatest dimension, limited to the kidney
	T3a	Tumor directly invades adrenal gland or perinephric tissues but not beyond
	T3b	Tumor grossly extends into renal vein(s) or its segmental branches, or the vena cava below the diaphragm
	T3c	Tumor grossly extends into vena cava or its wall above diaphragm
	T4	Tumor directly invades beyond Gerota's fascia
N	Regional nodes	
	N0	No regional lymph node metastasis
	N1	Metastasis in a single regional lymph node
	N2	Metastasis in more than one regional lymph node
M	Distant metastasis	
	M0	No distant metastasis
	M1	Distant metastasis

aUICC (International Union Against Cancer, 2002).

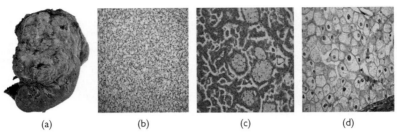

(a)   (b)   (c)   (d)

Fig. 17.1.1. Renal cell carcinoma (RCC). (a) Gross appearance of a large upper pole clear cell RCC. The adrenal gland is also included on the superior aspect of the specimen. (b) Typical morphology of clear cell RCC, solid pattern. (c) Papillary RCC (Type I), papillae lined by a single layer of small cuboidal cells. Also note prominent foamy macrophages. (d) Chromophobe RCC; characterized by large polygonal cells with prominent cell membranes and perinuclear halos.

Treatment

Treatment of localized RCC

Radical nephrectomy

Radical nephrectomy is the gold standard curative therapy for patients with localized RCC. The adrenal gland can be spared in the majority of patients.

Laparoscopic nephrectomy is a standard of care for patients with T1–2 RCCs.

Radical nephrectomy and thrombectomy can be performed for T3b and T3c tumors.

Lymph node dissection is not routinely performed.

Nephron-sparing surgery

Indications

- Absolute: anatomical or functional solitary kidney or bilateral RCC.
- Relative: a functioning opposite kidney that is affected by a condition that might impair renal function, and hereditary forms of RCC.

Open partial nephrectomy (OPN)

- OPN currently remains the standard of care for nephron-sparing surgery.
- It is used for T1a tumors in the presence of a normal contralateral kidney.
- It has gained popularity because OPN for patients with T1a tumors has long-term survival rates similar to those of radical nephrectomy (evidence: 2b).

Local recurrence rates after OPN for presumed RCC with 3–6 years of follow-up are low (0–4%).

Laparoscopic partial nephrectomy (LPN)

- This is feasible if time-sensitive intracorporeal suturing can be performed.
- LPN is associated with more complications than OPN.

Energy ablative techniques

These are used to destroy tissue *in situ*.

They are developmental (evidence: 2b).

Most published series have used cryotherapy or radiofrequency probes placed either laparoscopically or percutaneously depending on tumor position.

The 5 year local recurrence rate following renal cryoablation (RCA) is 6–10%; 5 year data for radiofrequency ablation are not available.

Treatment of metastatic RCC (mRCC)

Cytokines

Tumor nephrectomy in combination with interferon-α (INF-α) improves the survival of patients with mRCC and good performance status (evidence: 1b).

Those with a clear cell subtype derive clinical benefit from INF-α or interleukin-2 (IL-2) (evidence: 1b).

Angiogenesis inhibitor drugs

Sorafenib (an oral multikinase inhibitor of Raf-1, B-Raf, VEGFR-2, PDGFR, FLT-3, KIT) delays progression in cytokine-refractory patients (evidence: 1b).

Sunitinib (an oral multikinase inhibitor of PDGFR, VEGFR, KIT, FLT-3) improves progression-free survival compared with interferon in cytokine-naive, good and intermediate prognosis tumors (evidence: 1b).

Temsirolimus (an intravenous inhibitor of the kinase mTOR (mammalian target of rapamycin)) monotherapy in poor prognosis patients is more effective than INF-α or temsirolimus plus INF-α (evidence: 1b).

Follow-up

There is no evidence-based standard for the follow-up of patients with nonmetastatic RCC. Consequently, the European Association of Urology Guidelines (2006) makes no recommendations.

A number of scoring systems have divided patients with clear cell RCC into low, intermediate and high risk for developing metastases. This allows the urologist to be selective in the use of imaging and outpatient follow-up. An internationally validated algorithm which is increasingly used was created by Leibovich et al. from the Mayo Clinic. (see Further Reading)

Prognosis

The following contribute important prognostic information (evidence: 2):

- TNM stage.
- Fuhrman nuclear grade.
- RCC subtype.

Histological features carrying a poor prognosis:

- coagulative necrosis in clear cell RCC.
- microvascular invasion may be important.

Future prospects

A serum biomarker for RCC.

Percutaneous biopsy of small renal masses is likely to become more routine when fears concerning safety and diagnostic accuracy are allayed.

Ablative therapies for small nonmetastatic renal tumors may develop from being minimally invasive to noninvasive.

Molecular biological advances are likely to lead to the development of further targeted therapies.

Further reading

Chawla SN, Crispen PL, Hanlon AL, Greenberg RE, Chen DY, Uzzo RG. The natural history of observed enhancing renal masses: meta-analysis and review of the world literature. *J Urol* 2006; **175**: 425–431.

Cohen HT, McGovern FJ. Renal-cell carcinoma. *N Engl J Med* 2005; **353**: 2477–2490.

Escudier B, Eisen T, Stadler WM, *et al.* TARGET Study group. Sorafenib in advanced clear-cell renal-cell carcinoma. *N Engl J Med* 2007; **356**: 15–34.

Lane BR, Novick AC. Nephron-sparing surgery. *BJU Int* 2007; **99**: 1245–1250

Leibovich BC, Blute ML, Cheville JC, *et al.* Prediction of progression after radical nephrectomy for patients with clear cell renal cell carcinoma: a stratification tool for prospective clinical trials. *Cancer* 2003; **97**: 1663–1671.

McDougal WS. Radiofrequency ablation of renal cell carcinoma. *BJU Int* 2007; **99**: 1271–1272.

Motzer RJ, Hutson TE, Tomczak P, *et al.* Sunitinib versus interferon-alpha in metastatic renal-cell carcinoma. *N Engl J Med* 2007; **356**: 115–114.

Stein RJ, Kaouk JH. Renal cryotherapy: a detailed review including a 5-year follow-up. *BJU Int* 2007; **99**: 1265–1270.

Internet resources

European Association of Urology Guidelines:

`http://www.uroweb.org`

Cancerbackup:

`http://www.cancerbackup.org.uk/home`

See also

Wilms' tumor , p. 672

Tumors of the renal pelvis and ureter, p. 676

Tuberous sclerosis and von Hippel–Lindau disease, p. 578

Wilms' tumor

Introduction

Wilms' tumor is the most common renal malignancy in childhood. It was first described in 1899 by Max Wilms, when he noted what is now recognized as classic, triphasic histology. Multinational trials over the last 20 years have led to a significant improvement in outcome for patients with Wilms' tumor so that the majority are cured, usually with little or no long-term morbidity.

Definition

Wilms' tumor is an embryonal neoplasm arising in the kidney. Classical, 'triphasic' Wilms' tumor consists of stromal, blastemal and epithelial elements. Other renal tumors occurring in children are often included under the Wilms' tumor heading, but only anaplasia is a true variant. The bone-metastasizing renal tumor (clear cell sarcoma) and malignant rhabdoid tumor are pathologically and genetically distinct entities, and have distinct clinical courses. Renal cell carcinoma and peripheral neuroectodermal tumors may also occur.

Epidemiology

Wilms' tumors account for ~8% of all childhood neoplasia.

It ranks fifth in incidence among the solid tumors of childhood.

The annual incidence is ~8 per million children <15 years.

Racial and regional variation in incidence exist.

The peak ages for diagnosis are the 3rd and 4th years of life.

The frequency in males and females is equal.

It is very rare in the neonatal period and after the age of 10 years. Careful review of cases of 'Wilms' tumor' seen in adults will usually determine that the histology is in fact that of a peripheral neuroectodermal tumor or a renal cell carcinoma.

Predisposing factors

There are a number of conditions known to predispose to the development of Wilms' tumor, but this group of patients represents only a small proportion of the total number seen.

- Genitourinary abnormalities with or without aniridia (the WAGR syndrome).
- Aniridia.
- Hemihypertrophy.
- Beckwith–Wiedemann syndrome.
- Denys–Drash syndrome.
- Perlmann syndrome.
- Simpson–Golabi–Behmel syndrome.

There is no clear evidence that screening examinations and investigations leads to significant improvement in stage distribution or outcome. However, in patients with aniridia, Beckwith–Wiedemann syndrome and hemihypertrophy screening is recommended.

The incidence of familial Wilms' tumor is extremely low.

Genetics

Wilms' tumor was initially thought to represent a simple model for studying the genetics of the etiology of cancer. This belief is now known to be incorrect.

WT1 gene was the first Wilms' tumor gene to be identified at the 11p locus. The precise role of the protein product of the WT1 is unclear although it is known to be a transcription factor.

In WAGR there is a deletion of one copy each of the WT1 gene and the associated PAX6 gene on chromosome 11p13. Germline mutations in the WT1 gene are also found in Denys–Drash syndrome.

A second gene, WT2, has been identified on the basis of loss of heterozygosity at the 11p15 locus.

Genetic abnormalities have been consistently found in chromosomes 16q, 1p and 7p.

p53 mutations, β-catenin mutations, and deletions in the X chromosome have also been reported.

Clinical features

74% of patients present with an abdominal mass arising in the loin often detected by a parent. The mass may be rounded or lobulated, usually ballotable and does not move with respiration.

44% of patients present with abdominal pain.

Additional features may include:

- hematuria;
- fever;
- hypertension;
- pulmonary metastases.

Hypertension may arise from vascular compression of the tumor, excessive renin production or pre-existing renal disease. Blood pressure should be measured. Angiotensin-converting enzyme inhibitors, β-blockers, and calcium channel antagonists have been used to control BP in these patients.

Pulmonary metastases present at diagnosis are only rarely detected by clinical examination.

Physical examination should include a search for the signs of the various predisposing conditions such as Beckwith–Wiedemann syndrome, aniridia and hemihypertrophy.

Essential investigations

The major differential diagnosis of abdominal neuroblastoma must be excluded, not only to make a correct diagnosis, but because immediate surgery may then not be appropriate and catecholamine-secreting tumors pose anesthetic problems. The minimum set of investigations must include:

Abdominal ultrasound

- Confirm organ of origin.
- Determine extent of any spread within the abdomen.
- Confirm patency of the inferior vena cava.

Chest X-ray (PA and lateral)

- Detect pulmonary metastases.

Urinary catecholamines

- Exclude intrarenal neuroblastoma.
- Aid interpretation of imaging investigations which can occasionally be erroneous.

CT scan of the abdomen and chest

- Common practice, although role in detection of pulmonary metastases is not yet established and additional information gained about the anatomy of the tumor and surrounding organs is of less importance in patients who receive preoperative chemotherapy.

Other investigations

- FBC to detect anemia resulting from hemorrhage into the tumor
- PT and aPTT as some patients may have an acquired form of von Willebrand disease.
- Urea, creatinine and urinalysis to detect any gross abnormalities of renal function.
- It is important to know that the contralateral kidney is functioning adequately before surgery. IVU, DMSA scan or excretion of contrast at the end of CT scan of chest/abdomen are all useful for this.

Pathology

Two broad groups of tumors may be recognized by their histological appearances.

Favorable histology – by far the larger group

Classical triphasic histology: epithelial, blastemal, and stromal elements are all present.

An additional feature that may be seen in triphasic tumors is rhabdomyoblastic differentiation, such that the cells resemble fetal rhabdomyoblasts. This should not be confused with the malignant rhabdoid tumor of the kidney, which has a poor prognosis.

Monomorphic epithelial variant. This variant consists of entirely primitive tubules and is usually found in children aged <1 year. It has a favorable prognosis and patients are often treated by nephrectomy alone.

Unfavorable histology

Anaplasia: an unfavorable feature occasionally observed in triphasic tumors. It is often patchy. Histological characteristics include large hyperchromatic nuclei, an increased nuclear:cytoplasmic ratio, and abnormal mitoses.

The other major unfavorable histological types are distinct tumors, rather than true variants of Wilms' tumor:

Bone-metastasizing renal tumor of childhood (clear cell sarcoma)

This tumor has a propensity for skeletal metastasis and an aggressive clinical course. In NWTS3 (US National Wilms' Tumor Study Group) the tumor represented nearly 6% of cases making it the most frequent form of 'unfavorable' histology. In the second UKCCSG (United Kingdom Children's Cancer Study Group) Wilms' tumor study 5% of cases were bone-metastasizing renal tumor of childhood and patients had a 4 year overall survival of 82%, comparable with that of patients with favorable histology.

Malignant rhabdoid tumor

It is the least common of the unfavorable histological types and represented only 2% of cases entered in the American national studies. Malignant rhabdoid tumor is associated with various primary tumors arising in the midline of the posterior intracranial fossa. Genetic analysis of malignant rhabdoid tumors shows that they contain mutations of the hSNF5/INI1 gene that controls the shape of the DNA–histone complex. Hypercalcemia has been reported in a number of cases.

Staging

Most staging systems currently in use rely heavily on the system devised for the Third National Wilms' Tumor Study, which itself was a derivation of the systems used in NWTS

1 and 2 (Table 17.2.1). This staging system is based on tumor location at the time of surgery, before any adjuvant therapy has been given. By contrast the European staging system used by the SIOP (International Society of Pediatric Oncology) group is based on radiological, biopsy, and surgical findings after preoperative chemotherapy. The differences mean that trial data from the two groups cannot be easily compared. In the European model preoperative chemotherapy downstages the tumor and reduces the risks at the time of nephrectomy. However, it is argued by the North American group that by giving preoperative chemotherapy the virgin stage and histology of the tumor will be unknown and there is a risk of giving unneeded chemotherapy to benign tumors.

Treatment

There is overwhelming evidence that Wilms' tumor ought to be treated in recognized pediatric oncology centers and that there is no place for the casual therapist. Surgeons, radiotherapists, pediatricians, or nephrologists not working in a center with pediatric oncological expertise who find they are unexpectedly dealing with a child with Wilms' tumor should make an urgent referral to an appropriate unit. It has been shown that patients not treated in a recognized trial or at a recognized pediatric oncology center are overtreated compared to current recommendations and are more likely to receive radiotherapy.

Surgery

Surgical extirpation is, and almost certainly will remain, fundamental treatment for Wilms' tumor. There is debate about the timing of surgical intervention, the place of percutaneous needle biopsy, and the use of preoperative chemotherapy.

North American practice remains steadfastly in favor of immediate surgery followed by adjuvant therapy dictated by the surgical stage. In contrast, the SIOP group in Europe has conducted a series of trials based on the use of preoperative therapy. By downstaging the tumor fewer patients would be subjected the morbidities of abdominal radiation and anthracycline therapy. Between 1991 and 2001 the UKCCSG conducted a prospective randomized trial comparing immediate surgery with 6 weeks of chemotherapy and delayed surgery. The trial showed there was a significant improvement in stage distribution for patients with Wilms' histologies receiving preoperative chemotherapy compared to those having immediate nephrectomy, while maintaining excellent event-free and overall survival in children with nonmetastatic Wilms' tumor. Current SIOP trials aim to reduce the use of anthracyclines in stage II and III disease further. The debate as to the role of preoperative chemotherapy versus immediate nephrectomy continues but it is notable that the overall survival rates between North American and European groups are very similar.

Surgery for Wilms' tumor should start with a transverse abdominal incision that allows a thorough examination of the abdominal cavity and contralateral kidney. It will also ease tumor removal, which should be done en bloc with any associated tissue. Para-aortic lymph nodes are then biopsied, especially if they are enlarged.

Contraindications to surgery are bilateral disease, a large fixed tumor, hepatic invasion and extension of the tumor into the inferior vena cava.

Biopsy

In Europe the majority of patients with suspected Wilms' tumor will have preoperative chemotherapy for ~6 weeks with deferred surgery. Current UK practice is to biopsy the tumor using a Trucut needle. In the UKW3 trial, an analysis of biopsy results demonstrated that 10% of patients either had unfavorable histology or other diagnoses. However, many pediatric oncologists and surgeons feel that biopsy is unnecessary and there is a risk of providing an unrepresentative sample or causing local tumor spillage along the biopsy track.

Chemotherapy

The use of chemotherapy as an adjuvant to surgery is now an essential part of Wilms' tumor treatment. The major advances in treatment have come as a result of the multicenter co-operative trials run by the NWTS, the SIOP and the UKCCSG. Consecutive studies have confirmed the role of vincristine, actinomycin D and doxorubicin as adjuvant agents in the treatment of Wilms' tumor.

An integral part of all therapy protocols is the 'stage' of the tumor and progress has been made in optimizing treatments according to the stage and therefore the risk of relapse. The second UKCCSG Wilms' tumor study demonstrated that stage 1 favorable histology tumors treated with minimal therapy (nephrectomy and only 10 weekly doses of vincristine) had an excellent 4 year overall survival of 94%. This is a significant reduction in treatment compared to the NWTS3 study in which stage I favorable histology patients received a nephrectomy and 6 months of vincristine and actinomycin D with a similar 4 year overall survival of 97.4%. The neurotoxic effects of vincristine as well as the myelosuppressive and hepatotoxic effects of actinomycin D are therefore significantly decreased.

By contrast the treatment for stage IV Wilms' tumors is more intensive with delayed surgery, triple chemotherapy (vincristine, actinomycin, and doxorubicin), and abdominal radiotherapy. Pulmonary radiotherapy may also be required if pulmonary metastases are present.

Trials continue with the aim of reducing the amount of treatment, and hence the morbidity, for all stages of Wilms' tumor. It may be possible, even in those with stage IV tumors, to reduce the need for pulmonary radiotherapy and doxorubicin while maintaining overall survival rates.

The main outcome findings of the European trial SIOP study (SIOP 9) are summarized in Table 17.2.2. All patients were randomized to receive either 4 or 8 weeks preoperative actinomycin D and vincristine, followed by the postoperative chemotherapy listed.

Radiotherapy

The use of radiotherapy has decreased due to the long-term morbidity it imposes on growing tissues. Radiotherapy doses have been decreased as a consequence of the results of several trials. More effective and rational use of chemotherapy may allow it to supplant radiotherapy in some instances. The NWTS3 trial showed that survival was not significantly different in stage II patients who received 2000 cGy of radiotherapy compared with those who had chemotherapy alone. Furthermore in stage III patients 2000 cGy of irradiation did not improve overall survival or the risk of relapse compared to 1000 cGy. The result is that fewer patients will be exposed to the deleterious effect of poor muscle growth caused by radiotherapy. In SIOP 9 radiotherapy was reserved for those patients with stage II N1 and III favorable histology tumors and all unfavorable histology tumors greater than stage I. This was a total of 21% of patients. The total dose delivered to the midplane was 15 Gy, increased to 30 Gy in unfavorable histology.

Boosts were given for areas of residual disease or if lymph nodes were positive. As with chemotherapy, differences occur between patients treated in the American trials and the SIOP trials.

Follow-up

Pulmonary relapse is more common than local relapse. PA and lateral CXR should be obtained regularly during and after treatment.

Typically patients should have a CXR every 9 weeks during treatment, every 2 months for the first year and every 3 months for the 2nd and 3rd years after completing treatment.

Stage IV patients should continue to have CXR for a further year.

It is sufficient to screen for local relapse with an abdominal USS at the end of treatment and then 6-monthly for the next 2 years.

Evaluation of renal function in the remaining kidney shows some evidence of dysfunction in a third of cases with only about a half of patients undergoing significant compensatory renal hypertrophy.

Blood pressure measurement and assessment of proteinuria must be carried out at intervals.

Prognosis

The great majority of patients with Wilms' tumor will be cured as indicated in Table 17.2.2 (SIOP 9 results).

Long-term evaluation of cardiac function in those patients treated with anthracyclines must be carried out.

Patients who received radiotherapy will have a disturbance of growth, often asymmetrical.

Future prospects

To further refine therapy in patients with a good prognosis in order to minimize treatment-related morbidity.

To improve therapy for those few patients with an identifiable poor prognosis or who relapse.

To understand further the genetic basis for Wilms' tumor and its variants and to analyse the role these genetic markers may have in stratifying the therapy required.

Further reading

Barr RD, Chalmers D, De Pauw S, et al. Health-related quality of life in survivors of Wilms' tumor and advanced neuroblastoma: a cross-sectional study. J Clin Oncol 2000; **18**: 3280–3287.

Dome JS, Cotton CA, Perlman EJ, et al. Treatment of anaplastic histology Wilms' tumor: results from the fifth National Wilms' Tumor Study. J Clin Oncol 2006; **24**: 2352–2358.

Huang CC, Cutcliffe C, Coffin C, et al. Renal Tumor Committee of the Children's Oncology Group. Classification of malignant pediatric renal tumors by gene expression. Pediatr Blood Cancer 2006; **46**: 728–738.

Mitchell C, Pritchard-Jones K, Shannon R, et al. For the United Kingdom Cancer Study Group. Immediate nephrectomy versus preoperative chemotherapy in the management of non-metastatic Wilms' tumour: results of a randomised trial (UKW3) by the UK Children's Cancer Study Group. Eur J Cancer 2006; **42**: 2554–2562.

Reinhard H, Semler O, Bürger D, et al. Results of the SIOP 93-01/ GPOH trial and study for the treatment of patients with unilateral nonmetastatic Wilms tumor. Klin Padiatr 2004; **216**: 132–140.

Weirich A, Ludwig R, Graf N, et al. Survival in nephroblastoma treated according to the trial and study SIOP-9/GPOH with respect to relapse and morbidity. Ann Oncol 2004; **15**: 808–820.

Table 17.2.1 Wilms' tumor staging based on the Third National Wilms' Tumor Study

Stage	
Stage I	Tumor completely within renal capsule, completely resected.
Stage II	Extension of tumor outside renal capsule, but still completely resected. Includes vessel infiltration, tumor biopsy, or tumor spillage confined to the flank
Stage III	Residual nonhematogenous tumor, confined to the abdomen. Extension outside the renal capsule, with incomplete excision. Lymph node involved. Diffuse peritoneal contamination following tumor spillage either microscopically or macroscopically.
Stage IV	Hematogenous metastases to lung, liver, or brain.
Stage V	Bilateral renal tumors.

Internet resources

International Society of Pediatric Oncology:

http://www.siop.nl/

US National Wilms' Tumor Study Group:

http://www.nwtsg.org/

Children's Cancer and Leukaemia Group (formerly UKCCSG):

http://www.ukccsg.org/

Cancerbackup:

http://www.cancerbackup.org.uk/home

See also

Tumors of the kidney, p. 668
Rare syndromes with renal involvement, p. 640

Table 17.2.2 Percentage outcomes for patients in SIOP 9

Stage and histology	2 year event-free survival	5 year overall survival	Postoperative treatment
Stage I Favorable histology	100	100	None
Stage I Anaplasia/ standard histology	88	93	Acintomycin D and vincristine × 3 courses
Stage II N0 Standard histology	84	88	Actinomycin D and vincristine and anthracycline × 5 courses ± RT
Stage II N1/III Standard histology	71	85	Actinomycin D and vincristine and anthracycline × 5 courses
Stage II/III Anaplasia	71	71	Actinomycin D, vincristine, anthracycline and ifosphamide × 5 courses ± RT

SIOP, International Society of Pediatric Oncology RT, radiotherapy.

Tumors of the renal pelvis and ureter

Definition
Benign or malignant lesions arising from the lining of the upper renal tract anywhere between the renal calyces and the vesicoureteric junction.

Epidemiology
Upper tract transitional cell carcinoma (UTTCC) is rare, with ureteric tumors being less common than renal pelvic tumors. 70% of ureteric tumors occur in the distal ureter, 25% within the mid-ureter and 5% in the upper ureter. Bilateral tumors are very rare (1.5% of UTTCC). UTTCC represents 5% of all diagnosed transitional cell carcinomas (TCC). Tumor incidence increases with age and UTTCC is twice as common in men.

Predisposing factors
Smoking (dose-dependent effect, RR = 2.6–7.2).

Occupational exposure (aniline dyes, β-naphthylamine, benzidine, RR = 4.0–5.5).

Drug exposure:
- analgesic (phenacetin) abuse (RR = 3.3–3.6);
- cyclophosphamide exposure.

Chronic urinary infection/presence of urinary stones (typically cause squamous cell carcinoma, SCC).

Balkan nephropathy (degenerative interstitial nephropathy occurring in patients from Balkan countries) is typically associated with low grade, bilateral tumors (RR = 57.0–61.0).

Coffee consumption (RR = 1.3).

Hereditary syndromes, e.g. Lynch II syndrome (hereditary nonpolyposis colonic cancer, endometrial, ovarian and pancreatic adenocarcinoma and UTTCC).

Genetics
The chromosomal abnormalities underlying UTTCC mirror those of bladder TCC (deletions of chromosomes 9, 13 and 17). 5% of patients with bladder TCC will develop UTTCC, whereas 30–40% of patients with UTTCC will subsequently develop bladder TCC. Presence of synchronous/metachronous lesions correlates strongly with tumor stage. Metachronous tumors occurring after high grade UTTCC frequently share common specific genetic mutations supporting the theory of downstream tumor seeding.

Clinical features
Frank hematuria (60–100%).

Flank pain (30%).

Clot colic.

Symptoms of metastatic disease in 20% (abdominal mass, anorexia, loss of weight, and bone pain).

15% of patients are asymptomatic.

Investigations
IVU/CT urogram/retrograde studies
These studies will demonstrate a filling defect (Fig. 17.3.1).

They allow assessment of the contralateral kidney.

Cystoscopy
This is mandatory to assess for synchronous bladder TCC

Rigid/flexible ureteroscopy with or without biopsy (Fig. 17.3.2)
There is good concordance between biopsy and surgical specimen grade, but not stage.

It allows accurate assessment of tumor grade, permitting subsequent endoscopic/percutaneous management if appropriate.

The time delay performing ureteroscopy and biopsy does not negatively impact on survival, if radical surgery is required.

Selective upper tract saline washings for cytology
Only of value for high grade lesions.

Other investigations
Contrast CT of abdomen/chest and pelvis required for staging.

Bone scan is reserved for symptomatic patients.

Concern regarding contralateral renal function mandates that a DMSA renogram is performed to accurately assess differential function.

Pathology
Benign lesions are very rare and include:
- fibroepithelial polyps;
- neurofibromas;
- inverted papillomas.

Malignant lesions predominate:
- 98% TCC;
- 2% SCC, adeno-, sarcomatoid or small cell carcinomas.

Staging
Staging is described by the TNM system (Table 17.3.1). 40% of UTTCC are invasive at presentation (cf. 20% bladder TCC), which is thought to relate to the relative paucity of ureteric musculature. Tumor spread is epithelial (downstream seeding or field change), lymphatic (para-aortic, para-caval, ipsilateral common iliac and pelvic lymph nodes) or hematogenous (liver, lung and bone).

Treatment
Endoscopic/percutaneous strategies
Indications:
- solitary kidney;
- bilateral disease;
- impaired renal function;
- significant comorbidity precluding major surgical intervention;
- low grade/stage disease with normal contralateral kidney.

Choice of procedure
Ureteroscopy and laser ablation:
- rigid ureteroscope for distal/mid-ureteric tumors;
- flexible ureteroscope for more proximal/small renal pelvic tumors.

Percutaneous antegrade resection:
- suitable for larger renal pelvic lesions;
- minute risk of percutaneous tumor seeding.

Both procedures can be combined with retrograde and antegrade instillation of topical chemo- or immunotherapy.

Table 17.3.1 TNM classification of upper tract transitional cell carcinoma (UTTCC)

Stage	Description
TX	Primary tumor cannot be assessed
T0	No evidence of primary tumor
Ta	Papillary noninvasive carcinoma
Tis	Carcinoma *in situ*
T1	Tumor invades subepithelial connective tissue
T2	Tumor invades muscularis
T3	Tumor invades periureteric/peripelvic fat or into renal parenchyma
T4	Tumor invades adjacent organs or through kidney into perinephric fat
NX	Regional lymph nodes cannot be assessed
N0	No regional lymph node metastasis
N1	Single lymph node metastasis <2 cm
N2	Single lymph node metastasis 2–5 cm or multiple lymph nodes <5 cm
N3	Lymph node metastasis >5 cm
MX	Distant metastasis cannot be assessed
M0	No evidence of distant metastasis
M1	Distant metastasis present

Table 17.3.2 Five year UTTCC survival rates

Stage	5 year survival (%)
Ta/1/is	60–90
T2	43–75
T3	16–33
T4	0–5

Such treatments are technically feasible but no outcome data exists regarding efficacy.

Outcome

Endoscopic/percutaneous treatment regimens are associated with a 30–40% tumor recurrence rate (directly related to tumor grade). Several series report the efficacy of these strategies in low grade/stage tumors although it is common to require repeat treatments. Results for multifocal and/or high grade/stage tumors are less favorable. Such treatment strategies require intense patient and surgeon commitment to 3–6-monthly ureteroscopic surveillance.

Nephron-sparing techniques

• Segmental renal pelvis resection (rarely used).
• Segmental ureteric resection ± uretero-ureterostomy/ureteric reimplantation (suitable for large mid/distal ureteric tumors).

Any retained ureter requires careful inspection for concomitant lesions.

Nephroureterectomy

This is the gold standard procedure for management of UTTCC and can be performed:

• open;
• laparoscopically;
• combined open/laparoscopically.

Open procedures carry a higher morbidity (dual loin and lower abdominal incisions). Laparoscopic procedures permit more rapid recovery and recent series confirm the oncological safety of this approach.

Successful nephroureterectomy requires removal of the entire ureter in continuity, preventing spillage of tumor cells (Figs 17.3.3 and 17.3.4). Tumor recurrence occurs in 30% of retained ureteric stumps.

Ureterectomy

This can be achieved by:

• open distal ureterectomy
• endoscopic or laparoscopic transvesical ureteric detachment;
• distal ureteric stapling;
• ureteric intussusception ('stripping').

No evidence exists confirming the superiority of any of the above techniques.

Lymphadenectomy

This confers no survival benefit although it does permit more accurate tumor staging.

Adjuvant therapy

As high grade/stage disease is associated with poor outcome, effective adjuvant therapy should be beneficial. There is no evidence to support use of adjuvant radiotherapy. There are also no RCTs determining the efficacy of chemotherapy in this setting. Current regimens are based on (neo-)adjuvant bladder TCC regimens, i.e. methotrexate, vinblastine, adriamycin and cisplatin or gemcitabine and cisplatin.

Follow-up

This should aim to detect:

• local recurrence;
• metastatic spread;
• metachronous upper and/or lower tract TCC.

Follow-up depends on original tumor histology and the type of surgical intervention undertaken.

Typically the following are required:

Regular clinical, cystoscopic and, if ureter retained, ureteroscopic evaluation (initially 3-monthly, then 6-monthly and annually thereafter)

Regular evaluation of the contralateral upper tract using IVU/retrograde studies (3-yearly for low grade/stage disease and annually for all others).

Regular evaluation for metastatic disease using blood parameters and CT scanning.

Prognosis

Several factors have independent prognostic significance with respect to survival in UTTCC:

• stage (most important, Table 17.3.2);
• grade (low vs high grade);
• age;
• location (renal pelvis better prognosis);
• carcinoma *in situ*.

An extensive literature exists regarding numerous potential molecular makers associated with impaired survival (p53 status, lymphovascular invasion, microsatellite instability, tumor ploidy and p27). None reproducibly aid survival prognostication using multivariate analysis.

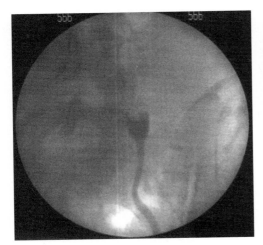

Fig. 17.3.1 Filling defect in the left mid-ureter seen on retrograde ureterogram.

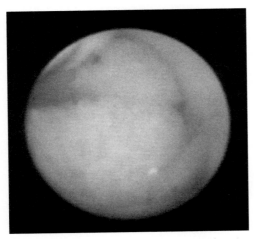

Fig. 17.3.2 Endoscopic view of same ureteric tumor as shown in Fig. 17.3.1.

Future prospects

The identification of reliable urine biomarkers may aid future follow-up of the bladder and contralateral upper tract in UTTCC. More clinical trials are needed to confirm that our current understanding of the behavior of bladder cancer can be extrapolated to UTTCC.

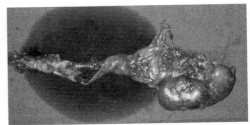

Fig. 17.3.3 *En bloc* kidney and ureter following nephroureterectomy.

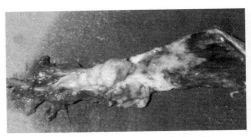

Fig. 17.3.4 Opened ureter demonstrating a distal papillary ureteric tumor. Reddened ureteric mucosa represents areas of carcinoma *in situ*.

Further reading

Flanigan RC. Urothelial tumours of the upper urinary tract. In: Wein AJ (ed.), *Campbell–Walsh Urology*, 9th edn. Philadelphia: WB Saunders; 2007. Vol. 2, pp. 1630–1652.

Sagalowsky AI, Jarrett TW. Management of urothelial tumours of the renal pelvis and ureter. In: Wein AJ (ed.), *Campbell–Walsh Urology*, 9th edn. Philadelphia: WB Saunders; 2007. Vol. 2, pp. 1653–1685.

Internet resources

European Association of Urology:

http://www.uroweb.org/

Cancerbackup:

http://www.cancerbackup.org.uk/home

See also

Tumors of the kidney, p. 668

Tumors of the bladder, p. 680

Tumors of the bladder

Introduction

Bladder cancer is the second commonest cancer of the genitourinary tract, with transitional cell carcinoma due to cigarette smoking being the predominant type. Accurate histopathological staging is crucial to ensure appropriate management which ranges from endoscopic surveillance only to radical combination therapy. It is hoped that urinary biomarkers will in due course reduce the need for repeat cystoscopies in patients who are being followed for bladder cancer. Radical surgery for bladder cancer has begun to be performed laparoscopically/robotically in increasing numbers of centers.

Epidemiology

Bladder cancer is the fifth commonest cancer in the UK but its incidence has been falling.

Incidence rises sharply after 55 years of age with the median age at diagnosis being 70 years.

It is 2.5-fold more common in men than women.

It is more common in the Caucasian compared with Afro-Caribbean population.

Survival by stage is more favorable in Caucasians.

Predisposing factors

Cigarette smoking is associated with a four-fold increased incidence. Known urothelial carcinogens in cigarette smoke include β-naphthylamine and 4-aminobiphenyl.

Occupational exposure to aromatic amines and polyaromatic hydrocarbons.

Exposure of the bladder to ionizing radiation such as following treatment for cervical or prostate cancer.

Cyclophosphamide and phenacetin.

Prolonged immunosuppression, e.g. in organ transplant recipients.

Chronic cystitis, bladder calculi, indwelling catheters and *Schistosoma hematobium* cystitis (bilharzia) predispose to squamous cell carcinomas.

Genetics

p73 (chromosome 1p36) and cyclin D1 (chromosome 11) are frequently amplified.

Losses from chromosome 9, especially 9q, are found frequently, even in early bladder cancer, but it is not known through which genes this alteration has its effect.

Altered expression of tumor suppressor genes *Rb* (chromosome 13q14) and *p53* (chromosome 17p13) are both commonly found in muscle invasive bladder cancer.

Clinical features

Hematuria is the cardinal feature, either frank or microscopic.

Any patient aged >40 years with persistent or intermittent microscopic hematuria (two or more dipsticks 1+ or more in the absence of signs of urinary tract infection or known glomerular disease) needs a full urological evaluation.

Irritative symptoms may occur such as frequency, urgency, nocturia and dysuria.

Irritative symptoms predominate with carcinoma *in situ* (CIS).

Loin pain may indicate ureteric obstruction due to bladder carcinoma.

Pelvic mass, weight loss and hepatomegaly are late signs.

Investigations

Urine cytology

The sensitivity of urinary cytology varies widely between centers. The sensitivity is higher for high grade disease including CIS.

Urine proteomics

Many tests for urinary molecules correlated with transitional cell carcinoma (TCC) have been proposed to reduce the need for cystoscopy, but they have not been widely adopted. Those urinary molecules with US Food and Drug Administration approval include:

- human complement factor H-related protein (BTA TRAK/BTA Stat);
- nuclear matrix protein 22 (NMP22 BladderChek);
- mucin glycoprotein and carcinoembryonic antigen combination (ImmunoCyt/uCyt+);
- aneuploidy of chromosomes 3, 7 and 17 with deletion of chromosome 9p21 (UroVysion).

Bimanual examination under anesthetic

To assess presence and mobility of a mass.

Cystoscopy

To assess size, number, position, morphology of tumors.

The sensitivity of cystoscopy can be increased by use of photodynamic diagnosis. The bladder is instilled with a solution containing aminolevulinic acid 2 h before cystoscopy. This accumulates in carcinoma tissue and fluoresces red under blue light.

Tumor resection/biopsy

Transuretheral resection should include muscularis propria in the specimen to enable accurate histological staging.

Bladder biopsies should be taken from any area showing abnormal urothelium or hyperemia. However, random biopsies to detect CIS should be reserved for cases with positive cytology.

Repeat transurethral resection should be performed after all high grade, Ta or T1 diagnoses to avoid understaging.

IVU/CT scan with contrast

All confirmed cases of bladder carcinoma should have assessment of the upper tracts by either IVU (Fig. 17.4.1) or contrast CT scan.

Other investigations

FBC, U&Es, alkaline phosphatase (ALP), urinalysis and urine culture.

Evaluation of muscle invasive disease also includes a CXR; a radionuclide bone scan in the case of bone pain or raised ALP; and MRI (Fig. 17.4.2) to assess the extent of extravesical extension and nodal involvement.

Pathology

More than 90% of bladder cancers are TCCs that arise from the urothelium.

TCCs of the bladder are often multifocal; 30–40% of cases have synchronous tumors at initial presentation.

Other possible bladder malignancies include:
- squamous carcinomas (5%);
- adenocarcinomas (2%);
- sarcomas (2%);
- secondary metastatic deposits and small cell carcinomas.

TCC is morphologically classified as:
- papillary;
- sessile;
- carcinoma *in situ*.

Grading of nonmuscle-invasive TCC is of more prognostic importance than in cases of muscle-invasive TCC.

The 1973 WHO grading system of TCC (papilloma, G1, G2 or G3) is still widely used but there are concerns about high rates of interobserver variability.

In 2004, the WHO grading system was updated (papillary neoplasm of low malignant potential (PNLMP), low and high grade papillary carcinoma).

Accurate identification of PNLMP allows the identification of patients requiring less intensive follow-up.

CIS, by definition, is composed of cytologically high grade tumor cells confined to the urothelium.

Staging

Bladder TCC is staged using the 2002 TNM system (Table 17.4.1).

About 70% of bladder carcinomas present as nonmuscle-invasive disease (Ta/T1), 25% as muscle-invasive disease (T2+) and 5% as CIS.

Treatment

Accurate staging is a prerequisite to the correct management of bladder TCC, as the management of nonmuscle-invasive versus muscle-invasive tumors differs significantly. Management of all but the lowest risk bladder transitional cell carcinomas should be discussed within multidisciplinary teams.

Nonmuscle-invasive TCC

Initial management is by transurethral resection (TURBT). Small tumors can often be resected in one chip which includes detrusor muscle; larger tumors may require more extensive resection followed by a separate deep muscle biopsy. For large tumors, the tumor edge should be resected separately to allow thorough pathological examination for CIS.

Bladder biopsies should also be taken of any abnormal areas within the bladder, or random biopsies taken from throughout an otherwise normal bladder if cytology is positive. If tumor is found at the bladder neck, or CIS is suspected, the prostatic urethra should also be biopsied in males.

Within 24 h of the initial TURBT, a single dose of an intravesical chemotherapy agent (commonly mitomycin-C, but epirubicin and doxorubicin are also used) should be given to reduce the risk of recurrence.

Subsequent management depends on a variety of factors related to the initial tumor and is based on the likelihood of the tumor either recurring or progressing.

Re-resection should be performed, usually within 6 weeks, if residual tumor is known to have been left, if no detrusor muscle is present in the TURBT specimen, or if high grade disease is reported. Re-resection decreases the risk of understaging and reduces recurrence; recurrence within three months is itself an important prognostic marker.

Low risk tumors
G1pTa.

Require continued surveillance (see 'Follow-up').

Intermediate risk tumors
Single G2pT1, multifocal G2pTa or G1pT1.

May be offered subsequent intravesical treatment to reduce recurrence (occurring in ~50% of these patients) and/or progression (~2%).

Intravesical therapy in these patients takes the form of either chemotherapy (mitomycin-C, epirubicin or doxorubicin) which reduces recurrence and is relatively well-tolerated, or immunotherapy (bacillus Calmette–Guérin, BCG) which reduces both recurrence and progression but is less well-tolerated and has greater risk of systemic complications (fever, arthralgia, hepatitis and pneumonitis).

High risk tumors
Any CIS, any G3 tumor(s) or multiple G2pT1 tumors.

These have an ~15% risk of progressing to muscle invasion. Clear evidence suggests that a maintenance course of intravesical BCG reduces the risk of progression by ~25%.

A response to intravesical BCG should occur within 6 months, therefore in patients who show treatment failure (development of higher stage or grade tumor, or CIS (new or refractory) during treatment, or recurrence of even the same stage/grade tumor at 3 and 6 months), radical treatment should be offered (as for muscle-invasive disease).

Muscle-invasive TCC

Patients found to have muscle-invasive disease (T2–T4a, N0–Nx, M0) or those with high risk nonmuscle-invasive disease in whom conservative treatment fails may be candidates for radical treatment in the form of either radical cystectomy or radical external beam radiotherapy.

Radical cystectomy with urinary diversion
This is currently regarded as the gold standard treatment. It also includes bilateral lymph node dissection, the limits of which are currently debated with recent evidence suggesting that a more radical lymph node dissection leads to a better outcome.

Three main options exist for the urinary diversion:
- ileal conduit using a segment of exteriorized ileum to form a stoma;
- orthotopic neobladder using a pouch formed from detubularized bowel segments anastomosed to the urethra;
- continent cutaneous pouches, similar to neobladders, but which are connected to the skin via the appendix or a bowel segment to allow catheterization for drainage.

Urethrectomy should be performed when tumor has been identified in the prostatic urethra in males or the bladder neck in females. This then precludes the creation of an orthotopic neobladder.

Radical cystectomy has an operative mortality rate of ~3%. Perioperative morbidity is between 20% and 56% and long-term morbidity is between 28% and 94%, mainly being due to the method of urinary diversion. Five year survival rates are 40–60%.

Radical external beam radiotherapy
Radiotherapy traditionally has been reserved for patients who are less fit or have poorer outlooks. A dose of 60–66

Gy with a subsequent boost can be given within a 6–7 week course, to give a 5 year survival rate of 40–60%. Patients who relapse or fail to respond to radiotherapy can be considered for salvage cystectomy.

Neoadjuvant chemotherapy

Chemotherapy has a role in managing muscle-invasive tumors. Good quality evidence supports the use of neoadjuvant rather than adjuvant chemotherapy, using regimes such as MVAC (methotrexate, vinblastine, doxorubicin and cisplatin) or newer ones such as GC (gemcitabine and cisplatin), along with radical cystectomy and radiotherapy to improve survival.

Metastatic disease

MVAC and GC chemotherapy regimes can prolong life, although outcome with metastatic disease is invariably poor.

External beam radiotherapy can also be used in the palliative setting to manage symptoms such as recurrent hematuria, urinary urgency and pain.

Squamous cell carcinoma

Both pure squamous cell carcinoma and bilharzial squamous cell carcinoma have poor long-term outcomes. The treatment of choice is radical cystectomy, although there is limited evidence for neoadjuvant chemotherapy and radiotherapy in bilharzial squamous cell carcinoma.

Adenocarcinoma

The treatment of choice for primary adenocarcinoma is radical cystectomy. Patients with urachal adenocarcinoma should be treated with *en bloc* resection of the urachus and umbilicus combined with partial cystectomy, or radical cystectomy for larger tumors.

Follow-up

Nonmuscle-invasive TCC – low risk tumors

Patients with low risk tumors (G1pTa) should have check flexible cystoscopies at 3, 12, 24, 36, 48 and 60 months, or until they develop a recurrence. Recurrences may be dealt with by repeat TURBT or cystodiathermy (electrocautery or laser) depending on size and equipment availability.

Non muscle-invasive TCC – intermediate risk tumors

The follow-up cystoscopy protocol for these patients is often intermediate to that of low and high risk patients and allows for patient factors and local availability.

Non muscle-invasive TCC – high risk tumors

Cystoscopic follow-up for these patients is 3-monthly for two years, then 4-monthly for 1 year, 6-monthly until 5 years and then yearly after, or until recurrence or progression intervenes.

Muscle-invasive TCC

In muscle-invasive disease, follow-up of patients after cystectomy or bladder preservation is recommended to detect local recurrence or distant metastasis as early as possible. Following cystectomy regular outpatient review is necessary. Early assessment of upper tract drainage with IVU or USS is necessary and annual urethroscopy when the urethra is left. In cases of node-positive disease, additional regular CT scans and bone scans are necessary. Patients treated with radiotherapy should undergo an early CT scan of the pelvis and regular cystoscopic examination.

Prognosis

60–70% of nonmuscle-invasive bladder cancers recur, 10–20% progress in stage or grade.

Risk factors that correlate with recurrence and progression of superficial disease are:

- lamina propria invasion (T1);
- grade;
- presence of CIS;
- >3 tumors;
- tumor >3 cm;
- previous recurrence.

Approximately half of patients with muscle-invasive bladder carcinoma have occult metastases at presentation, which become overt within 5 years.

Future prospects

For nonmuscle-invasive disease, urinary biomarkers have the potential to reduce the need for follow-up cystoscopy and newer methods of administering intravesical agents (e.g. hyperthermia, electromotive drug administration) and photodynamic therapy are gaining in popularity. For invasive tumors, laparoscopic and robotic cystectomy are being performed increasingly and new chemotherapeutic agents are being tested in clinical trials for this type of aggressive cancer.

Further reading

Jakse G, Algaba F, Fossa S, Stenzl A, Sternberg C. Guidelines on Bladder Cancer (Muscle-invasive and Metastatic). European Association of Urology Guidelines; 2006.

Oosterlinck W, van der Meijden A, Sylvester R, *et al.* Guidelines on TaT1 (Non-muscle-invasive) Bladder Cancer. European Association of Urology Guidelines; 2006.

Parekh DJ, Bochner BH, Dalbagni G. Superficial and muscle-invasive bladder cancer: principles of management for outcomes assessments. *J Clin Oncol* 2006; **24**: 5519–5527.

Table 17.4.1 TNM classification of transitional cell carcinoma

Stage	Description
Ta	Papillary tumor confined to the urothelium
T1	Invasion into the lamina propria
T2a	Invasion into the inner half of the muscularis propria
T2b	Invasion into the deeper half of the muscularis propria
T3a	Microscopic invasion into the perivesical fat
T3b	Macroscopic invasion into the perivesical fat
T4a	Invasion into prostate, uterus or vagina
T4b	Invasion into pelvic or abdominal wall
NX	Regional lymph nodes cannot be assessed
N0	No regional lymph node metastasis
N1	Single lymph node metastasis <2 cm
N2	Single lymph node metastasis 2–5 cm or multiple lymph nodes <5 cm
N3	Lymph node metastasis >5 cm
M0	No evidence of distant metastasis
M1	Distant metastasis present

Internet resources

A useful online calculator for recurrence and progression probabilities:

http://www.eortc.be/tools/bladdercalculator/

Hematuria referral guidelines:

http://www.emrn.org.uk/documents/HaematuriaGuidelines_25_4.pdf

European Association of Urology:

http://www.uroweb.org/

Cancerbackup:

http://www.cancerbackup.org.uk/home

See also

Tumors of the renal pelvis and ureter, p. 676

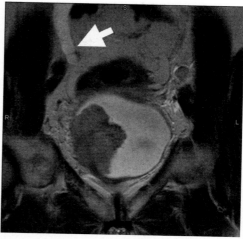

Figure 17.4.2 MRI demonstrating large right-sided invasive bladder cancer with right hydronephrosis (arrow).

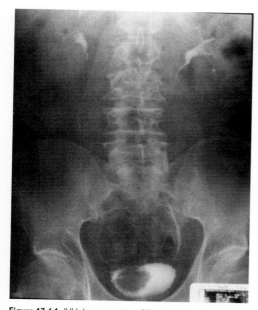

Figure 17.4.1 IVU demonstrating a filling defect consistent with a bladder tumor.

Tumors of the prostate

Introduction

Prostate cancer is the commonest solid organ malignancy diagnosed in men in Europe and the USA and is the second most frequent cause of cancer-related death in men. The age-adjusted incidence has increased from 21 per 100 000 in 1980 to 98 per 100 000 in 2004 in the UK, an almost four-fold increase. This is partly due to the increasing use of transurethral surgery leading to diagnosis, but mainly due to increasing levels of awareness caused by prostate-specific antigen (PSA) testing. In many patients the disease has an indolent course, hence surveillance is commonly recommended in localized disease.

Definition

Prostate cancer is most commonly an adenocarcinoma arising in the peripheral zone of the prostate, classically in a posterior location, making it readily palpable on digital rectal examination. Prostate cancer usually develops in a multifocal pattern; however, by the time symptoms develop, one or more focus will have grown to substantially replace the prostate.

It is difficult to define 'clinically relevant' prostate cancer. Histological (microscopic) prostate cancer is common in the asymptomatic population. Furthermore, advanced disease may not cause symptoms and as prostate cancer is a disease of old age, when there are many competing causes of morbidity and mortality, it is difficult to establish the true impact of histological prostate cancer.

Epidemiology

Since the introduction of PSA testing in 1990 the incidence of prostate cancer has been rising due to detection of asymptomatic disease. In parallel there has been a similar increase in the rates of prostate surgery.

Incidental disease

Postmortem studies reveal that 30% of men aged >50 years have microscopic prostate cancer. Only a small number of these will become clinically relevant.

Healthy men in the prostate cancer prevention trial had a prostate biopsy at the end of the study. In the placebo arm 15% of men with a normal PSA were found to have prostate cancer.

Prostate cancer

In 2004 there were 34 986 new cases of prostate cancer reported in the UK.

In 2005 there were 10 000 deaths from prostate cancer in the UK.

~70% of patients with metastases die from prostate cancer.

Screening for prostate cancer

Screening presents a dilemma.

Localized disease has a good prognosis and PSA is effective in its detection.

Screening detects many cases which may not progress and may miss cases destined to progress.

No adequate study has shown a benefit from screening.

Predisposing factors

The main predisposing factor is age.

Prostate cancer is very rare at ages <50 years and becomes the commonest malignancy in older men.

Ethnic origin is important as the incidence worldwide is highly variable.

Asian men have the lowest incidence whereas the Afro-Carribean population in the UK and African-American men have a high incidence.

The low incidence seen in the Japanese is increased if they move to Hawaii and rises to near that of the US population if they move to California, suggesting an environmental cause.

There is mounting evidence that exposure to sunlight and consumption of vegetables is protective.

Conversely red meat and animal fat consumption may contribute to its development.

Genetics

A family history is a strong predisposing factor.

If one first-degree relative has prostate cancer then the risk is doubled, but rises to 5–10-fold if two first-degree relatives have the disease.

A small proportion (9%) of patients are thought to have genetically linked prostate cancer.

For the majority of these the predisposing genetic abnormalities are unknown.

This is the subject of the 'UK genetic prostate cancer study' which is recruiting young patients and those with a family history, aiming to discover a shared germline mutation.

In a small proportion of these men, with a history of breast cancer in the female line, genetic linkage of the disease is established and linked to the BCRA-2 gene.

Clinical features

Symptoms

Localized disease
- Asymptomatic.
- Lower urinary tract symptoms.

Locally advanced disease
- Hematuria.
- Erectile dysfunction.
- Perineal or suprapubic pain.
- Uremic symptoms (from obstructive renal failure).
- Rectal obstruction.

Metastatic disease
- Bone pain.
- Paraplegia due to spinal cord compression.
- Cachexia.

Physical examination
- Abnormal rectal examination (Table 17.5.1).
- Palpable bladder.
- Lymphadenopathy which may cause lower limb. Edema due to venous or lymphatic obstruction.

Investigations
- PSA.
- Transrectal ultrasound (TRUS) and biopsy.

Prostate-specific antigen (PSA)

Is a serine protease.

Is prostate specific, not prostate cancer specific.

Rises with age and increasing prostate volume.

May be raised in:

- prostate cancer;
- benign prostatic hyperplasia;
- urinary tract infection;
- prostatitis;
- following instrumentation.

Around 30% of patients with a raised PSA will have prostate cancer.

15% of men with a normal PSA will have prostate cancer on biopsy.

The rate of rise is a strong predictor of tumor progression.

Is a valuable marker in follow-up where clinical relapse is usually preceded by a rise in PSA.

There are age-related reference ranges (Table 17.5.2).

TRUS and biopsy

The commonest definitive diagnostic test.

Local anesthetic procedure.

Other investigations

In patients with localized or locally advanced disease, staging investigations may include a bone scan and prostate MRI.

For those with advanced disease, alkaline phosphatase may indicate bone metastases.

Hypercalcemia is surprisingly rare despite bone metastases.

Renal failure and anemia, particularly a leukoerythroblastic anemia, are commonly seen in symptomatic advanced disease.

Pathology

The vast majority of prostate cancers are adenocarcinomas which may be multifocal in origin but at symptomatic presentation have usually coalesced. Rarer types include transitional cell carcinoma of the prostate ducts, epidermoid carcinoma and adenoid cystic carcinoma.

Tumor differentiation (grade) is measured by the Gleason score which ranges from 2 (well-differentiated) to 10 (poorly differentiated). The score is based on the degree of glandular differentiation and growth pattern of the tumor in relation to the stroma. The Gleason score correlates closely with the staging and prognosis.

Staging

The TNM stage classification system is recommended (Table 17.5.3).

T staging is most commonly decided using rectal examination (Table 17.5.1).

A small proportion of patients undergo cross-sectional imaging, which can determine T and N stage with reasonable accuracy.

Treatment

Localized disease

Watchful waiting

Defined as monitoring and subsequent treatment with hormone therapy on disease progression. This is a particularly suitable treatment for the elderly and those with comorbidity. It is inferior to surgery and so is little used in young fit men.

Active monitoring

Defined as monitoring with subsequent radical treatment on disease progression. This may be an effective means of selecting patients for radical treatment. The results of the ProtecT study (**P**rostate **te**sting for **c**ancer and **T**reatment) will confirm if this approach is comparable to surgery or radiotherapy.

Radical prostatectomy

This produces very good results in terms of cancer survival but at the expense of significant treatment-related morbidity including erectile dysfunction and incontinence. It has been shown to be superior to watchful waiting although the survival difference is relatively small currently. The real challenge is in defining which patients will benefit, since some will not be cured while many others will be overtreated.

Radical radiotherapy

The dilemma of who to treat is very similar to that with surgery. There is no proof that this is a better treatment than monitoring. Treatment-related morbidity includes lower urinary tract and rectal symptoms and erectile dysfunction.

Brachytherapy

The insertion of radioactive seeds into the prostate.

15 year survival data shows this to be effective but there is no randomized controlled trial evidence. It can be delivered in a single day-case procedure. Treatment-related morbidity mainly involves the lower urinary tract.

Locally advanced disease

Radical radiotherapy

This is a commonly offered treatment for patients with a long life expectancy. We know that survival is improved by the addition of hormone therapy. It remains unclear whether this treatment is more effective than hormone therapy alone.

Hormone therapy

This provides effective palliation and delays progression. There is mounting but incomplete evidence that it improves survival.

Radical prostatectomy

This may have a role in fit young patients with limited disease. A significant proportion of selected patients will have a pathologically complete excision. It is not known if surgery improves survival in this group.

Table 17.5.1 Prostate cancer staging by digital rectal examination

Digital rectal examination staging	Rectal examination findings
T1	Tumor clinically inapparent/not palpable. Normal texture prostate. Symmetrical.
T2	Tumor confined to prostate. No distortion of capsule.
T3	Tumor extends through capsule. Tumour mobile. Distortion of capsule.
T4	Tumor invades other organs locally. Immobile as other structures are involved.

Table 17.5.2 Age-related reference ranges for PSA

Age (years)	PSA (ng/mL)
40–49	≤2.5
50–59	≤3.5
60–69	≤4.5
>70	≤6.5

Metastatic disease

Hormone therapy

Early hormone therapy is superior to delayed therapy in terms of complications and mortality.

However, the differences are small and need to be balanced against long-term cardiovascular and bone demineralization risks.

Hormone therapy

Hormone therapy decreases androgenic stimulation of the prostate cancer which in turn leads to tumor regression and delayed progression in most patients.

Side-effects of hormone therapy include hot flushes, gynecomastia and loss of male characteristics.

Includes the following equivalent therapies:

Surgical orchidectomy
• Effective but unfashionable.

Medical orchidectomy
• Luteinizing hormone-releasing hormone (LHRH) agonists.

Antiandrogens.

Estrogens.

LHRH agonists are used with antiandrogens to prevent tumor flare.

Antiandrogens are oral drugs occasionally used alone for primary treatment.

Estrogen is commonly used second line or in combination therapy. It is effective but is used second line due to the risk of cardiovascular complications.

Palliative care

Common problems in those with progressive disease include:

Bladder outflow obstruction
Often managed by TURP.

Pelvic and bone pain
Treated with radiotherapy, chemotherapy (docetaxel) or bisphosphonates.

Renal failure
Prostate cancer causes renal failure by two mechanisms:
• Bladder outflow obstruction: usually high pressure chronic retention caused by locally advanced disease.
• Ureteric obstruction: caused by locally advanced disease or pelvic/retroperitoneal lymphadenopathy.

Renal failure has a poor prognosis but can occur in two settings:
• Hormone-naive patients in whom aggressive therapy for renal failure including nephrostomy is justified.
• Hormone-relapsed disease: patients are reaching the end of their lives. Patients and carers need to be involved in the decision-making process. It may be justified to

Table 17.5.3 TNM staging classification for prostate cancer

Stage	Description
TX	Primary tumor cannot be assessed
T0	No evidence of primary tumor
T1	Clinically inapparent tumor not palpable or visible by imaging
T1a	Tumor incidental histological finding in ≤5% of tissue resected
T1b	Tumor incidental histological finding in >5% of tissue resected
T1c	Tumor identified by needle biopsy (e.g. because of elevated PSA)
T2	Palpable tumor confined within prostate
T2a	Tumor involves half of a lobe or less
T2b	Tumor involves more than half of a lobe, but not both lobes
T2c	Tumor involves both lobes
T3	Tumor extends through the prostatic capsule
T3a	Extracapsular extention (unilateral or bilateral)
T3b	Tumor invades seminal vesicle(s)
T4	Tumor is fixed or invades adjacent structures other than seminal vesicles (bladder neck, external sphincter, rectum, levator muscles or pelvic wall)
NX	Regional lymph nodes cannot be assessed
N0	No regional lymph node metastasis
N1	Regional lymph node metastasis
MX	Distant metastasis cannot be assessed
M0	No evidence of distant metastasis
M1	Distant metastasis present
M1a	Nonregional lymph nodes
M1b	Bone metastasis present
M1c	Other metastasis present

offer nephrostomy in those well enough to receive chemotherapy.

Follow-up

Follow-up is heavily reliant on PSA as a tumor marker.

Following radical surgery any rise in PSA is indicative of recurrent disease, while following radical radiotherapy a rise of 2 ng/mL above the nadir defines treatment failure.

A rising PSA over time suggests disease progression; the rate of rise has important prognostic value.

However, disease progression can take place without a PSA rise, particularly in poorly differentiated disease.

Follow-up intervals are determined by the risk of progression, generally 3–6-monthly.

The forthcoming NICE guideline is likely to recommend that the majority of follow-up takes place in primary care.

Prognosis

Localized disease
~90% 10 year survival.

Tumor differentiation, clinical stage and PSA level are the important factors.

It is rare to diagnose prostate cancer with a Gleason score of ≤5 on needle biopsy and so in modern practice Gleason score 6 has a good prognosis, scores 8–10 a poor prognosis and score 7 an intermediate prognosis.

Metastatic disease

2–3 years median survival.

Hormone-relapsed metastatic disease

~6 months median survival if symptomatic.

Future prospects

New diagnostic tests, including the PCA3 urine test, may be more specific than those currently available. There is clearly a need to develop a test which identifies disease likely to progress and not indolent disease. Genomic studies may lead to such a development.

The ProtecT study, randomizing patients with localized disease between surgery, radiotherapy and active monitoring, should determine which of these is most effective, but will require 10–15 years of follow-up.

New technology is being used to manage prostate cancer in the form of cryotherapy, high-intensity-focused ultrasound (HIFU), laparoscopic surgery and intensity-modulated radiotherapy. These may replace current therapy as they promise treatment with low levels of morbidity.

Future developments in advanced disease will include combinations of treatments including chemotherapy and hormones. Vaccines and manipulation of androgen signaling appear promising for advanced disease.

Further reading

Bhatnagtar V, Kaplan RM. Treatment options for prostate cancer: Evaluating the evidence. *Am Fam Physician* 2005; **15**: 1915–1922.

Downes MR, Byrne JC, Pennington SR, Dunn MJ, Fitzpatrick JM, Watson RW. Urinary markers for prostate cancer. *BJU Int* 2007; **99**: 263–268.

Hamdy FC, Basler JW, Neal DE, Catalona WJ. *Management of urological malignancy*. Edinburgh: Churchill Livingstone; 2002.

Kirby RS, Brawer MK. *Fast facts – prostate cancer*. Health Press; 2004.

Internet resources

Age-standardized incidence and mortality rates for prostate cancer: Great Britain 1971 – 2004. Available at Cancer Research UK:

http://info.cancerresearchuk.org/cancerstats/

European Association of Urology:

www.uroweb.org

National Cancer Institute – Prostate cancer:

http://www.cancer.gov/cancertopics/types/prostate

ProtecT Study:

http://www.epi.tris.ac.uk/protect

See also

Tumors of the bladder, p. 680

Urinary tract obstruction, p. 652

Pharmacology and drug use in kidney disease

Chapter Contents

Handling of drugs in kidney disease

Introduction

The handling of drugs in the body (pharmacokinetics) is significantly altered in renal disease and also by the reduction in renal function with advancing age. Many drugs, and some active metabolites, are eliminated by the kidney, either by glomerular filtration or tubular secretion. Patients with kidney disease, and especially those who require dialysis, are often on multiple drugs.

There is the potential for the accumulation of many drugs even with modest decreases in renal function. In these circumstances, patients may be much more sensitive to their adverse effects.

In everyday clinical practice, the number of drugs for which changes in dose or interval are required is small and limited to those with a narrow therapeutic index or those that are associated with serious adverse effects.

Important factors that may reduce the risk of serious medication adverse effects in patients with kidney disease are:
- awareness of the presence or possibility of renal impairment;
- recognition that some medicines may be reliant on renal clearance;
- ability to monitor the therapeutic and adverse effects.

The main factor that determines the need for and the extent of the dose reduction is the glomerular filtration rate (GFR) and its impact on drug clearance. In practice, GFR is usually estimated from serum creatinine concentration and may be unreliable in patients with AKI. In some cases the GFR does not correlate well with the change in renal elimination.

As a general guide, alteration of drug dosage is only necessary if renal clearance exceeds 25% of total body clearance.

Pharmacokinetic alterations in kidney disease

The main effect of renal disease is to alter the rate of drug excretion but all phases of pharmacokinetics may be affected:
- absorption;
- distribution;
- metabolism;
- elimination.

In addition to its effects on pharmacokinetic handling, renal impairment may alter the sensitivity of target tissues to the therapeutic and adverse effects of drugs (pharmacodynamics).

For example, antiplatelet drugs may have an exaggerated effect in uremic patients (who already have impaired platelet aggregation), and there is a significantly increased risk of statin-induced myopathy. Some specific examples of pharmacokinetic variations are given in Table 18.1.1.

Absorption

Increased ammonia production in the stomach from urea hydrolysis buffers hydrochloric acid and raises pH. This may reduce absorption of ferrous sulphate and folic acid.

Aluminium hydroxide is occasionally used as a phosphate binding agent and may bind several drugs including aspirin, ferrous sulphate and ciprofloxacin.

Distribution

The build-up of acidic compounds in renal failure creates competition with various drugs for binding sites on albumin and other proteins.

Serum albumin levels are significantly reduced in the nephrotic syndrome. This means that, for a given amount of drug, the ratio of free to bound drug is increased and the fluctuation of free drug after each dose may be greater.

Importantly, the drug concentration reported by most assays includes both bound and free drug and these may not reflect increased tissue exposure.

Drugs where reduction in protein binding may be important include:
- warfarin;
- diazepam;
- phenytoin.

Increases in doses of drugs such as phenytoin should be small.

Fluid retention may lead to an expansion of both the intravascular and extracellular fluid compartments, which results in an increased volume of distribution (Vd) for many drugs. This decreases the plasma drug concentration resulting from a given dose of drug that is mainly distributed within those compartments.

Conversely, the tissue binding of some drugs (notably digoxin) is reduced and hence Vd decreases. This increases the plasma drug concentration resulting from a given dose.

Renal impairment is also associated with changes in body composition such as a reduction in the proportion of fat and reduced muscle mass. The former, in particular, may reduce the Vd of nonpolar (lipid-soluble) drugs.

Metabolism

Most drugs are excreted unchanged or as more polar (water-soluble) compounds produced after metabolism in the liver. Plasma drug assays must be interpreted with caution, not only because of the increase in free fraction noted above, but because some may pick up active or inactive metabolites making interpretation difficult.

The kidney itself is a site of metabolism of some drugs. The most notable example is the conversion of 25-(OH) vitamin D3 to its active form 1,25-$(OH)_2$ vitamin D3 which is reduced in renal impairment. The synthetic analogue 1α-(OH) vitamin D3 is converted to the active form and is used therapeutically.

Elimination

The rate of renal excretion of drugs depends on:
- glomerular filtration;
- active tubular secretion;
- active tubular reabsorption;
- passive diffusion.

This can be expressed mathematically by the equation:
- Clearance = $(F_{unbnd} \times GFR)$ + Secretion − Reabsorption

where F_{unbnd} is the fraction of drug unbound in the plasma. Clearance < $(F_{unbnd} \times GFR)$ means that active reabsorption is taking place.

Compounds with a molecular mass of <60 000 Da are filtered to an extent dependent on molecular size unless they are protein-bound when only the nonbound portion is filtered.

Table 18.1.1 Mechanisms of altered pharmacokinetics in renal disease

Pharmacokinetic phase	Pharmacokinetic change	Examples
Absorption	Raised stomach pH can reduce absorption of some drugs.	ferrous sulphate, folic acid
	Phosphate-binding agents such as aluminium hydroxide may interfere with the absorption of other drug.	aspirin, ferrous sulphate, ciprofloxacin
	Other factors influencing absorption: • reduced activity of intestinal drug transporters • prolonged gastric emptying • gut edema • nausea.	
Distribution	Protein concentration or protein binding reduced (more unbound (active) drug).	warfarin, diazepam, phenytoin
	Fluid volume expansion (increased volume of distribution of water-soluble drugs).	atenolol
	Tissue binding reduced (decreased volume of distribution).	digoxin
	Reduced proportion of body fat (decreased volume of distribution of fat-soluble drugs).	
Metabolism	Reduced liver metabolism for many drugs due to: • impaired transport into hepatocytes • impaired liver metabolic pathways.	aciclovir, cimetidine, metoclopramide, codeine, imipenem
	Reduced renal metabolism.	insulin
Renal excretion	Reduced GFR leading to the retention of: • unaltered drug • active metabolites.	digoxin, gentamicin, morphine-6-glucuronide

All aspects of renal elimination including glomerular filtration, reabsorption and secretion are altered in renal failure.

Nonpolar drugs easily diffuse across membranes while polar ones do not.

As the urine is progressively concentrated during its passage through the renal tubule, nonpolar drugs tend to be reabsorbed passively down their concentration gradient while polar drugs or the polar derivatives of nonpolar drugs produced in the liver are not.

Some polar drugs are actively excreted by the same mechanisms as organic acids and bases:
• organic acids (e.g. penicillins, cephalosporins, salicylates, furosemide and thiazides);
• organic bases (e.g. amiloride, procainamide and quinidine).

Some drugs interfere with the excretion of others:
• probenecid with penicillins;
• cephalosporins and furosemide;
• aspirin and paracetamol reduce the excretion of methotrexate.

A low protein diet reduces the acidity of the urine which may alter the ionization of drugs.

There is some evidence that filtration and secretion of drugs may fall in parallel and in proportion to the GFR. Some drugs are eliminated unchanged by the kidneys and are particularly vulnerable to accumulation in renal disorders. More commonly drugs are cleared by transformation into more water-soluble metabolites that can be eliminated in the urine. For most drugs the development of renal failure has a modest impact but, in some cases, the metabolite retains much of the activity of the parent drug and has the potential to cause adverse effects.

Renal blood flow

Renal blood flow can become an important independent influence on drug excretion when GFR has declined significantly.

In these circumstances, drug clearance may be adversely affected by hypovolemia or other drugs that impact on perfusion, e.g. NSAIDs (impair cortical blood flow by interfering with prostaglandin synthesis).

Assessing renal function before prescribing

The most important measure of renal function that might influence prescribing is the GFR.

Serum creatinine has been a widely used surrogate of renal function but is dependent not only on GFR but also on creatinine production and may significantly overestimate GFR in some groups (e.g. the elderly, those with low body mass).

Estimation of GFR from single creatinine measurements can be made by adjustment for body weight, age and gender using mathematical formulae (e.g. the Cockcroft–Gault formula). The modified MDRD formula is now commonly used to calculate 'eGFR'. The advantage is that it requires only the serum creatinine, age and gender (not height or weight). However, when using eGFR to make assessments of renal function that may influence decisions about therapeutic dose, there are important caveats:
• the eGFR is increasingly unreliable at the extremes of body weight and might lead to overdosing of small patients and underdosing of large patients;
• rises in serum creatinine (and hence reductions in eGFR) may lag behind the actual deterioration of GFR in AKI which is especially important in the intensive care setting;
• it is not valid in pregnant women or in children.

Concentration–time relationship

Most drugs eliminated by the kidneys exhibit first-order kinetics, i.e. the rate of removal is proportionate to the drug concentration. Under these circumstances a plot of concentration (C) versus time (t) displays an exponential decline (Fig. 18.1.1a) described by the equation

$$C(t) = C_0\, e^{-kt}$$

where C_0 is the concentration at time zero and k is the elimination rate constant.

Drugs that exhibit such kinetics can be described by their half-life ($t\frac{1}{2}$), the time taken for the concentration to halve (after absorption and distribution are complete). This has a major influence on the best dosing interval, the time required to achieve 'steady state' and the persistence of the drug effect after treatment is stopped (all are proportional to $t\frac{1}{2}$).

Most drugs are given repeatedly at regular intervals and their concentration increases to reach a steady state (after ~5 × $t\frac{1}{2}$) when the rate of intake matches the rate of excretion (Fig. 18.1.1b). Increases in the dose or frequency will result in a new, higher, steady state concentration profile producing the required elimination rate.

If renal function is impaired the clearance rate is reduced at any given concentration and the drug $t\frac{1}{2}$ is increased. If the dose and frequency remain the same, a higher steady state concentration (and hence drug exposure) will be required to produce the necessary elimination (Fig. 18.1.1b).

The increased steady state plasma concentration and drug exposure can be avoided by either a reduction in the drug dose or frequency (dose interval). It should be noted that these two strategies are not equivalent.

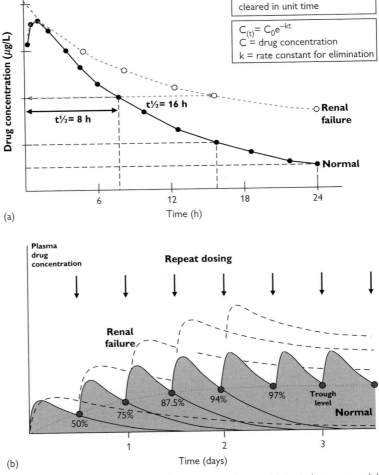

Fig. 18.1.1 Dose–response curves following (a) single dose administration or (b) repeated dosing in the presence and absence of renal impairment. Note the effect of reduced renal clearance on the half-life, time to steady state, and the steady state plasma concentration.

Dose reductions result in lower peak concentrations but maintained trough levels, which is ideal if a constant exposure is required.

Increased dose intervals preserve peak concentrations but allow lower trough levels to be reached.

The former strategy may be more suited to antihypertensive drugs while the latter is more suitable for aminoglycoside antibiotics where high peak concentration is required for bactericidal activity with low troughs to help avoid toxicity.

Single or 'loading' doses do not usually need to be altered in renal failure, even if the drug has a narrow therapeutic index. This is because, although drug exposure time may be increased, accumulation to high concentration will not occur.

Clearance of drugs in hemodialysis and peritoneal dialysis

Patients on dialysis will normally have a creatinine clearance/GFR of <10 mL/min.

Some drugs are actively removed from the circulation during dialysis, and this needs to be considered when deciding on the timing of administration as well as the dosage.

No form of dialysis is as effective as the normal kidney and the doses required will never be larger than those recommended in normal renal function.

Clearance by hemodialysis (HD) and hemofiltration (HF) follows first order kinetics.

Factors influencing clearance include:
- properties of the drug (e.g. molecular weight, protein binding and volume of distribution);
- delivery of drug to the filter (dependent on the blood flow through the filter);
- filter properties (e.g. pore size, surface area and duration of use).

HD drug clearance is based on diffusion down a concentration gradient from plasma to dialysate while hemofiltration clearance relies on convection only.

In the case of low molecular weight drugs, HD provides more efficient clearance.

With a pore size of only 0.001 μm, HD membranes will only clear molecules smaller than 500 Da.

Hemofilters have pore sizes of 0.01 μm and may clear molecules up to 5000 Da.

Peritoneal dialysis clears drugs much less efficiently than either HD or HF.

Although most antimicrobials are effectively cleared by HD, some important molecules such as vancomycin (1800 Da), amphotericin (960 Da) and erythromycin (734 Da) are retained.

Heavily protein-bound drugs such as propranolol (259 Da) are not successfully filtered even though they have a low molecular mass.

Water-soluble drugs pass through filters more readily than those that are lipid soluble.

Drugs with large volumes of distribution tend to have low plasma concentrations and so are less readily available for filtration (e.g. digoxin and antidepressants).

HD is normally performed for short periods every two or three days. Drugs that are cleared by HD are usually given after the session to avoid early postdose clearance.

The dose should take into account the diminished intrinsic renal function.

Therapeutic drug monitoring

Therapeutic drug monitoring describes the process of monitoring drug concentration or drug effect to tailor the drug regimen for individual patients (rather than relying on dosing considered appropriate for the average patient).

Monitoring is particularly important for drugs with a narrow therapeutic window (where there is a high risk of adverse effects) or in circumstances where pharmacokinetics are disturbed (notably renal impairment).

Drug concentrations are only helpful if there is an established relationship between concentration and adverse or beneficial effects.

Plasma concentration should normally be interpreted once steady state has been reached (e.g. digoxin). However, peak and trough levels after the first dose are important for some drugs (e.g. aminoglycosides). The timing of the peak is uncertain after oral dosing but measurement should be made 30 min after an IV dose.

Notes on specific drugs

When a drug with significant renal excretion is prescribed in renal impairment the dosing regimen can be adjusted in three ways:
- dose reduction;
- extending the dose interval;
- a combination of both.

For drugs with a narrow therapeutic index or serious adverse effects, monitoring plasma drug concentrations will be an important guide.

It should be noted that steady state concentration will only be reached after $5 \times t\frac{1}{2}$ and these may be longer in the presence of renal impairment.

Dose adjustment is normally only required when the creatinine clearance is <60 mL/min.

People who have been taking a drug for many years may need a dose adjustment as they age.

Some basic guiding principles are set out in Table 18.1.2.

Antimicrobials

Many antimicrobial drugs depend on renal excretion. Most have a wide therapeutic index and dose reductions are only required when GFR is <20 mL/min but gentamicin and vancomycin are notable exceptions.

Cephalosporins require dose reductions in more severe renal impairment. Cefotaxime, cephalexin and cephradrin can be used in normal doses until GFR is <10 mL/min but ceftazidime requires earlier dose reductions. Cephalosporins should be used cautiously when combined with loop diuretics.

Penicillins (e.g. amoxycillin, benzylpenicillin, co-amoxiclav), cefotaxime, ceftazidime, ciprofloxacin, clarithromycin, meropenem, metronidazole and trimethoprim are cleared by HD and should be given after the session.

β-Lactam accumulation significantly increases the risk of seizures when high doses are used in patients with renal impairment.

Aminoglycosides have the potential to cause severe nephrotoxocity and irreversible ototoxicity if they accumulate. Dose adjustment is required, even in mild renal failure.

Table 18.1.2 Issues for prescribers to consider in relation to renal impairment

Clinical issue	Comment
Age	Renal excretion of drugs is age dependent.
Weight	Drug dose may be calculated in mg/kg.
Renal function	May be assessed by measured creatinine clearance or estimated, e.g. eGFR.
Acute or chronic renal impairment	Estimated renal function may be misleading if there are rapid changes.
Is the patient being dialysed? If so, how?	Timing of drug clearance by dialysis needs to be taken into account
	Clearance varies with mode of dialysis.
Indication for the drug	Is the drug justified in the face of increased hazards?
	Always consider the risk–benefit balance.
	Some drugs cause serious adverse effects in patients with renal failure, e.g. sedation with morphine, lactic acidosis with metformin.
	Others rarely cause harm even with dose accumulation.
	Use nephrotoxic drugs with caution in lowest possible doses.
Comorbidities	These may also influence selection and dose, e.g. hepatic failure.
Other drugs	The drug effects may be additive, e.g. the patient may be taking several nephrotoxic or sedative drugs.
Active metabolites	Are there known metabolites that may have adverse effects?
Restrictions on fluid or sodium intake	These may influence drug selection.
How much data is available?	In many instances there may not be firm evidence to guide drug or dose selection and prescribing should be based on understanding of the principles involved.

Several factors increase the risk, including:
- prolonged treatment;
- dehydration;
- combination with diuretics;
- hypokalemia;
- hypomagnesemia;
- obstructive jaundice.

Dose adjustment is aimed at continuing to achieve bactericidal plasma levels but allowing subsequent clearance to reach a low trough level. This is monitored by measuring the peak plasma concentration (1 h post injection) and the trough (immediately before subsequent dose).

For gentamicin an adequate loading dose (1–1.5 mg/kg) is essential and the peak should be 8–12 mg/L while the trough should be <2 mg/L. Gentamicin is now commonly administered as a single daily dose of 5 mg/kg followed by a trough level at 24 h that can be used to predict the subsequent doses. Continued monitoring is necessary.

Vancomycin is widely used for staphylococcal infections including PD peritonitis and line sepsis. The peak (measured at 2 h) should be 20–30 mg/L while the trough should be <10 mg/L.

Neither gentamicin or vancomycin is effectively cleared by dialysis and doses are often days apart. Teicoplanin is a glycopeptide related to vancomycin but with an increased half-life.

Antimicrobials that do not require dose adjustment include macrolides, metronidazole, cloxacillin and clindamycin.

Antivirals
Many antivirals, including those used for treating herpes simplex, herpes zoster and cytomegalovirus infections (e.g. aciclovir, famciclovir, valganciclovir and ganciclovir), depend on renal clearance and tend to accumulate.

Even normal doses may precipitate neurological signs such as dizziness, confusion, hallucinations, somnolence and convulsions, as well as (more rarely) tremor, ataxia, dysarthria, seizures and encephalopathy.

These effects are dose-related and reversible, and more elderly patients and those taking other neurotoxic drugs are most at risk.

Lower doses are necessary when the GFR is <50 mL/min.

The dose of lamivudine should be reduced in mild renal impairment.

Analgesics
NSAIDs should generally be avoided in significant renal impairment, though in mild/moderate CKD they can be used after discussion and with monitoring if alternatives are much less effective.

Avoidance is not essential for dialysis patients although the risk of upper GI bleeding is increased.

The effects of opioid analgesics are often prolonged in renal failure because of the tendency of the parent drug and some active metabolites to accumulate.

Morphine and diamorphine are metabolized to morphine-3-glucuronide (M-3-G), morphine-6-glucuronide (M-6-G) and normorphine.

M-6-G is a potent analgesic and CNS depressant and, like morphine, accumulates in renal impairment.

Fentanyl is metabolized to inactive and nontoxic metabolites and may be a safer alternative.

All strong opioids should be used cautiously, with dose reduction and increased dosing interval.

Gastrointestinal system
Aluminium or bismuth-containing compounds should be avoided in renal impairment because of the potential for accumulation and neurotoxicity.

Cimetidine should be avoided in favor of ranitidine or other H2-blockers.

Proton pump inhibitors do not require dose reductions.

Anticoagulants
Patients with renal impairment already exhibit some degree of bleeding tendency and the decision to use anticoagulants should take this into account.

Low molecular weight heparins are renally excreted and their action is unpredictably prolonged, which may be hazardous when combined with a uremic bleeding tendency. They should not be used above prophylactic doses and the use of unfractionated heparin is still recommended for full anticoagulation.

A bolus of IV heparin (5000 U) is typically followed by an IV infusion at 1250 U/h. Anticoagulation should be regularly checked by aPTT ratio, the normal therapeutic range being 1.5–2.5.

Warfarin is metabolized in the liver and the anticoagulant effect depends only to a minor extent on renal function. No dose adjustment is necessary for patients with renal failure.

Cardiovascular drugs

ACEIs and ARBs reduce proteinuria and improve outcome in many patients with renal disease but need to be used with care because of the risks of hyperkalemia and renal function decline.

Those at greatest risk are:
- the elderly;
- those taking other high risk drugs (NSAIDs, spironolactone, loop diuretics);
- patients with diabetes (increased risk of renal artery stenosis).

A check of renal function is required after 3–4 days and again 7–10 days following introduction, dose titration or introduction of another interacting drug.

A small rise in creatinine is normal but a rise in creatinine of 20–30% should be regarded as significant.

Calcium channel blockers, nitrates, amiodarone and α-blockers do not normally require dose adjustments.

Statins and fibric acid derivatives are more likely to cause myopathy in patients with renal failure and their doses should be reduced.

Diuretics

Potassium-sparing diuretics such as spironolactone, amiloride and triamterene or potassium supplements are more likely to cause significant hyperkalemia in patients with renal failure and should be avoided unless there is continuing hypokalemia.

Further factors that may contribute to the risk of hyperkalemia in patients with renal impairment are age, higher doses, diabetes mellitus, and concomitant use of NSAIDs.

Frequent monitoring of serum potassium, creatinine and urea is essential, especially when starting spironolactone for heart failure.

Most diuretics are organic acids and have to compete with retained metabolites to reach their active site in the tubular lumen. Consequently higher doses are normally required.

Thiazide diuretics are ineffective in advanced renal impairment when higher doses of loop diuretics are required.

Diuretics should be carefully monitored since excessive volume contraction might further reduce GFR.

Digoxin

Digoxin is excreted by the kidneys and accumulates even in mild degrees of renal impairment necessitating reduced dose.

Digitoxin has been proposed as an alternative cardiac glycoside because it is cleared by the liver but its longer half-life increases the risk of toxicity.

Monitoring of digoxin levels helps to guide maintenance treatment.

Anticonvulsants

Phenytoin protein binding is reduced and its volume of distribution is significantly increased in renal failure.

The proportion of the reported total plasma concentration that is unbound, and therefore active, is likely to be increased.

For this reason a low plasma level may not necessarily be subtherapeutic.

Allopurinol

Allopurinol and its active principal metabolite, oxypurinol, are mainly excreted in the urine.

The dose should be reduced in patients with poor renal function to avoid accumulation.

Treatment is normally initiated at a dose of 100 mg/day and increased only if the serum or urinary urate is not satisfactorily controlled.

The frequency of hypersensitivity reactions (fever, chills, leukopenia, eosinophilia, arthralgia, and rash) is probably increased in patients with renal impairment, and in those who are concomitantly taking allopurinol and a thiazide diuretic. Caution is advised when using this combination in renal impairment.

The dose of colchicine should be halved for patients with GFR <10 mL/min.

Hypoglycemic drugs

Metformin is occasionally associated with fatal lactic acidosis when it accumulates and the risk is increased when clearance is reduced by renal impairment. Nausea is a common dose-related adverse effect that is more frequent in renal impairment.

Metformin should ideally be avoided in patients with a creatinine clearance of <30 mL/min and should be used with caution, at a reduced maximum daily dose of 1 g, in patients with a creatinine clearance of 30–60 mL/min. For those patients with a creatinine clearance of 60–90 mL/min, the recommended maximum daily dose is 2 g.

Metformin should also be withdrawn in patients undergoing surgery, suffering from dehydration, trauma or serious infections, or undergoing procedures likely to affect renal function (for example, contrast studies).

Sulfonylureas with more prolonged effects (e.g. glibenclamide and glimepiride) are known to increase the risk of hypoglycemia and this risk is even greater in patients with renal impairment. Gliclazide or glipizide have a shorter action and are a safer choice but should be introduced cautiously.

Insulin depends on renal clearance for up to half of its elimination. Dose requirements are often reduced and may reduce further if renal failure progresses. Diabetic nephropathy is often accompanied by unrecognized gastroparesis which delays food absorption, increasing the likelihood of insulin-induced hypoglycemia.

Psychoactive drugs

Benzodiazepines are metabolized in the liver but a number of active polar metabolites depend on renal clearance and have the potential to cause prolonged sedation. Chronic use should be avoided.

Lithium carbonate is excreted by the kidney and careful dose reduction and monitoring of plasma levels are required.

Antipsychotic drugs should be introduced cautiously at low dose. Tricyclic antidepressants are more likely to produce sedation and anticholinergic effects. The doses of selective-serotonin reuptake inhibitors should also be reduced.

Other drugs

The following drugs require dose reductions even in mild renal impairment (creatinine clearance 20–50 mL/min):

- atenolol
- buspirone
- carboplatin
- cimetidine
- disopyramide
- flecainide
- fludarabine
- imatinib
- methotrexate
- penicillamine
- procainamide
- rizatriptan
- tretinoin.
- baclofen
- capecitabine
- chloroquine
- duanorubicin
- ethambutol
- fluconazole
- gabapentin
- levetiracetam
- moxonidine
- pentamidine
- proguanil
- terbinafine

The following drugs are best avoided:

- acamprosate
- acetazolamide
- acitretin
- alendronate
- amphotericin
- cisplatin.

Further reading

Ashley C, Currie A (eds), The Renal Drug Handbook, 2nd edn. Oxford: Radcliffe Medical Press; 2004.

Bakris GL, Talbert R. Drug dosing in patients with renal insufficiency. Postgrad Med 1993; 94: 153–164.

Brier ME, Aronoff GR (eds), Drug prescribing in renal failure: dosing guidelines for adults and children, 5th edn. Philadelphia: American College of Physicians; 2007.

Davies JG, Kingswood JC, Sharpstone P, Street MK. Drug removal in continuous haemofiltration and haemodialysis. Br J Hosp Med1995; 54: 524–528.

DeBellis RJ, Smith BS, Cawley PA, Burniske GM. Drug dosing in critically ill patients with renal failure: a pharmacokinetic approach. J Intensive Care Med 2000; 15: 273–313.

Elliott R (ed.), Critical care therapeutics. London: Pharmaceutical Press; 1999.

Faull R. Prescribing in renal disease. Aust Prescriber 2007; 30: 17–20.

Kappel J, Calissi P. Safe drug prescribing for patients with renal insufficiency. Can Med Assoc J 2002; 166: 474–477.

Lam FYW, Banerji S, Hatfield C, Talbert RL. Principles of drug administration in renal insufficiency. Clin Pharmacokinet 1997; 32: 30–57.

Matzke GR, Frye RF. Drug administration in patients with renal insufficiency: minimizing renal and extrarenal toxicity. Drug Safety 1997; 16: 205–231.

Stevens LA, Coresh J, Greene T, Levey AS. Assessing kidney function – measured and estimated glomerular filtration rate. N Engl J Med 2006; 354: 2473–2483.

Internet resources

Nephrology Pharmacy Associates:

http://www.nephrologypharmacy.com/index.html

GlobalRPh.com. Guidelines for prescribing drugs in adults with impaired renal function:

http://www.globalrph.com/renaldosing2.htm

Joint Formulary Committee. British national formulary. 53rd ed. London: British Medical Association and Royal Pharmaceutical Society of Great Britain, 2007:

http://www.bnf.org/bnf/

UK Medicines Information. Specialist Services. Drugs in renal failure:

http://www.ukmi.nhs.uk/activities/specialistServices/default.asp?pageRef=5

South West Medicines Information Centre (UK). Drugs in renal failure:

http://www.swmit.nhs.uk/renal.htm

University of Pennsylvania Medical Center Guidelines for Antibiotic Use:

http://www.uphs.upenn.edu/bugdrug/antibiotic_manual/renal.htm

Royal Infirmary of Edinburgh Renal Unit:

http://renux.dmed.ed.ac.uk/edren/index.html

See also

Drug-induced nephropathies, p. 698

Clinical use of diuretics, p. 703

Drug-induced nephropathies

Introduction

The kidneys are particularly vulnerable to drug-related toxicity:

They are the principal organ of excretion for many drugs or their water-soluble metabolites.

High renal blood flow (25% of cardiac output) results in a high rate of drug delivery to the kidneys.

Some drugs are present in the tubular fluid at very high concentration (1000 times the plasma concentration).

Drug concentrations in the medullary interstitium are several times higher than in other tissues.

The thick ascending limb of Henle is highly sensitive to oxygen deprivation and/or decreased renal blood flow due to the local low partial pressure of oxygen.

Drug-induced renal syndromes

A variety of renal syndromes may be attributable to drug administration (Table 18.2.1). Given the diversity of drug-related renal syndromes clinicians should always conduct a comprehensive inquiry into all drugs taken by the patient, used or misused, prescribed or obtained over-the-counter, regular or alternative.

'False' renal failure

Seen with drugs inhibiting tubular Cr secretion such as cimetidine and trimethoprim.

Nephrotic syndrome

Nonsteroidal anti-inflammatory drugs (NSAIDs) can cause minimal change disease, focal glomerulosclerosis, membranous nephropathy. Gold therapy or penicillamine for rheumatoid arthritis can cause membranous nephropathy.

Tubulopathies

A variety of drugs may be associated with the development of tubular injury (Table 18.2.2).

Acute kidney injury

Drugs are an important etiologic factor for hospital-acquired AKI.

AKI may be due to prerenal reduction in renal blood supply, to direct acute tubular toxicity and tubular necrosis as well as to immunoallergic acute interstitial nephritis.

18–33% of in-hospital AKI may be attributed to drugs. The most frequently involved drugs are antibiotics, analgesics, NSAIDs, angiotensin-converting enzyme inhibitors (ACEIs) and contrast media.

Risk factors for drug-related AKI include congestive heart failure, severe liver disease, pre-existing renal failure, elderly population and dehydration.

In ~20% of AKI, some degree of renal impairment persists, especially in cases of NSAID-induced acute interstitial nephritis.

Acute interstitial nephritis (AIN)

All drugs can cause AIN. The mechanism is immune-mediated. AIN occurs in only a small percentage of individuals receiving the drug and is independent of the dosage. Drugs commonly associated with AIN are listed in Table 18.2.3.

Clinical presentation

- Renal failure (100%).
- Dialysis-dependent renal failure (40%).
- Hematuria (50%), proteinuria (60%).
- General symptoms (40%): fever, cutaneous rash, arthralgia.
- Eosinophilia (40%).

The sensitivity and specificity of noninvasive procedures (eosinophiluria and gallium scanning) is poor, so the diagnosis can only be confirmed by renal biopsy.

Typical renal biopsy findings are interstitial edema and infiltration by T-cells, monocytes–macrophages, plasma cells and eosinophils. Sometimes, infiltrating cells form non-necrotic granulomas with few giant cells (granulomatous interstitial nephritis).

Normal renal function is not always restored after AIN: CKD can be observed in 40% of these patients.

Treatment of drug-related AIN remains a matter of debate. The most important measure is the removal of the culprit drug. There is no evidence for the use of prolonged treatment with steroids. However, if there is no spontaneous recovery after 15 days, a brief course of pulse methylprednisolone (60 mg/day for 3 days) seems to quicken recovery.

Chronic kidney disease

CKD occurs secondary to chronic interstitial nephritis and may be a consequence of prolonged use of some drugs (calcineurin inhibitors, lithium) or of the misuse of others (analgesics, herbal medicine containing aristolochic acids).

Urinary tract syndromes

These include urinary retention (atropine), papillary necrosis (analgesics), stones formed by the drug itself (ephedrine, methotrexate, indinavir) or by the uricosuric properties of the drug (some NSAIDs), oxalate (vitamin C, cranberry juice) or xanthine (allopurinol).

Renal tract tumors

Some drugs are carcinogenic and may be responsible for urothelial carcinoma (analgesics, herbal medicine containing aristolochic acids).

Angiotensin-converting enzyme inhibitors (ACEIs) and angiotensin receptor blockers (ARBs)

Functional acute kidney injury

An intact renin–angiotensin system (RAS) is required for maintenance of GFR when renal perfusion pressure decreases. An acute and pronounced fall in GFR may be seen after blocking the RAS with ACEI or ARB, specifically in patients with:

- bilateral renal artery stenosis;
- renal artery stenosis in a solitary kidney (e.g. renal allograft);
- congestive heart failure;
- advanced CKD.

In any of these settings a fall in GFR is made more likely with volume depletion (e.g. diuretic therapy).

Prophylactic measures

For patients at risk, different measures are required:

- use of a short-acting drug;
- adaptation of dose to the renal function;
- start drug at a low dose with gradual titration;
- correction of volume depletion;
- temporary withdrawal of diuretics.

Combination with NSAIDs should be avoided (risk of severe hyperkalemia).

Table 18.2.1 Drug-induced renal syndromes

Renal syndrome	Mechanism/presentation	Drugs
'False' renal failure	Interference with creatinine tubular secretion	Creatine, fibrates, IV immunoglobulins, trimethoprim, cimetidine
Glomerular syndromes	Nephrotic syndrome	NSAIDs, gold, penicillamine, INF-α
	Nephritic syndrome (microangiopathy)	Ciclosporin, oral contraceptives, mitomycin C, quinine
Tubular syndromes	Fanconi syndrome	Old tetracyclines, streptozotocin, cisplatin, ifosfamide, adefovir, cidofovir, valproate, 6-mercaptopurine, herbal medicines
	Proximal tubular acidosis	Acetazolamide
	Hypokalemia (urinary wasting)	Amphotericin B, herbal medicines
	Hyperkalemia (hyporeninemia/ hypoaldosteronism syndromes)	β-Blockers, NSAIDs, ACEIs, ARBs
	Hypomagnesemia (urinary wasting)	Amphotericin B, cisplatin
	Distal renal tubular acidosis	Amphotericin B
	Diabetes insipidus	Lithium, demeclocycline, amphotericin B, cidofovir, didanoside, foscarnet
Acute kidney injury	Prerenal (reduced renal perfusion)	NSAIDs, ACEIs, ARBs, diuretics, contrast media, cyclosporin, interleukins
	Acute tubular toxicity	See Table 18.2.2
	Acute interstitial nephritis (including granulomatous nephritis)	See Table 18.2.3
Chronic kidney disease	Chronic interstitial nephritis	Analgesics, NSAIDs, herbal medicine (Table 18.2.4), indinavir, lithium, ciclosporin, tacrolimus, aminosalicylic acid
Urinary tract syndromes	Urinary retention	Atropine and related
	Papillary necrosis	Analgesics, NSAIDs
	Stones	
	Drug itself	Sulfonamides, glafenine, ephedrine (including herbal medicines) indinavir, methotrexate, aciclovir, ganciclovir
	Metabolite	Allopurinol (xanthine)
	Uric acid	Suprofene, phenylbutazone
	Oxalate	Vitamin C, herbal medicine (Table 18.2.4)
	Urinary tract carcinoma	Analgesics, herbal medicine (Table 18.2.4)

Membranous glomerulopathy
This has been reported in patients with pre-existing renal disease treated with high doses of captopril (a sulfhydryl-containing ACEIs).

Acute interstitial nephritis
This has been seen during treatment with captopril in a few cases.

Table 18.2.2 Drug-induced acute tubular toxicity

Class of drug	Typical examples
Antibiotics	Aminoglycosides, cephaloridine, cephalothin, amphotericin B, rifampicin, vancomycin, pentamidine
NSAIDs and analgesics	Diclofenac, indomethacin, glafenine, acetaminophen
Iodinated contrast media agents	Diatrizoate, iothalamate, metrizoate
Calcineurin inhibitors	Ciclosporin, tacrolimus
Antineoplastic drugs	Cisplatin
Antiviral drugs	IFN-α, foscarnet
Immunomodulators	IFN-α, IV immunoglobulins
Statins	Atorvastatin, simvastatin

Aminoglycosides
Aminoglycosides (AmGs) are filtered by the glomerulus and reabsorbed by the S1/S2 proximal convoluted tubules via megalin-mediated endocytosis. AmGs can accumulate in lysosomes and induce tubular apoptosis and necrosis.

Incidence of nephrotoxicity (generally manifesting as nono-liguric AKI) ranges from 5 to 25%.

Risk factors for nephrotoxicity
- Older age.
- Pre-existing renal disease.
- Female gender.
- Low intravascular volume.
- Hypokalemia and hypomagnesemia.
- Liver disease.
- Sepsis.
- Coadministration of other nephrotoxic drugs.

Prophylactic measures
- Use least toxic AmG (amikacin < gentamicin).
- Limit duration of treatment.
- Adapt dose to renal function.

Trough serum levels do not predict the risk of nephrotoxicity.

Table 18.2.3 Drug-induced acute interstitial nephritis

Antimicrobial agents	NSAIDs including salicylates	Diuretics
Acyclovir	Aclofenac	Chlorthalidone
Ampicillin	Azapropazone	Ethacrynic acid
Amoxicillin	Aspirin	Furosemide
Aztreonam	Benoxaprofen	Hydrochlorothiazide
Carbenicillin	Diclofenac	Indapamide
Cefaclor	Diflunisal	Tienilic acid
Cefamandole	Fenclofenac	Triamterene
Cefazolin	Fenoprofen	
Cephalexin	Flurbiprofen	**Others**
Cephaloridine	Ibuprofen	Allopurinol
Cephalothin	Indomethacin	α-Methyldopa
Cephapirin	Ketoprofen	Azathioprine
Cephradine	Mefenamic acid	Bethanidine
Cefixitin	Meloxicam	Bismuth salts
Cefotetan	Mesalazine (5-ASA)	Captopril
Cefotaxime	Naproxen	Carbimazole
Ciprofloxacin	Niflumic acid	Chlorpropamide
Cloxacillin	Phenazone	Cyclosporine
Colistin	Phenylbutazone	Cimetidine
Cotrimoxazole	Piroxicam	Clofibrate
Erythromycin	Pirprofen	Clozapine
Ethambutol	Sulfasalazine	Cyamethazine
Foscarnet	Sulindac	D-Penicillamine
Gentamicin	Suprofen	Fenofibrate
Indinavir	Tolementin	Griseofulvin
Interferon	Zomepirac	Interferon
Isoniazid		Interleukin-2
Gold salts	**Analgesics**	Omeprazole
Lincomycin	Aminopyrine	Phenindione
Methicillin	Antipyrine	Phenothiazine
Mezlocillin	Antrafenin	Phenylpropanolamine
Minocycline	Clometacin	Probenecid
Nafcillin	Floctafenin	Propranolol
Nitrofurantoin	Glafenin	Propylthiouracil
Norfloxacin	Metamizol	Ranitidine
Oxacillin	Noramidopyrine	Streptokinase
Penicillin G		Sulphinpyrazone
Piperacillin	**Anticonvulsants**	Warfarin
Piromidic acid	Carbamazepine	
Polymyxin acid	Diazepam	
Quinine	Phenobarbital	
Rifampicin	Phenytoin	
Spiramycine	Valproate sodium	
Sulfonamides		
Teicoplanin		
Tetracycline		
Vancomycin		

From: Rossert (2001).

Amphotericins

Amphotericin B (AmB) is a polyene macrolide, largely used in critically ill and immunocompromised patients for severe fungal infections.

AmB is associated with frequent and severe acute and chronic toxicity. Nephrotoxicity is its most restrictive adverse effect. Tubular (distal convoluted tubule and ascending limb of the loop) and glomerular damage has been reported resulting in:

Acute kidney injury
Generally limited to the duration of treatment, rarely causes CKD. Incidence varies between 50 and 90%. Risk factors are cumulative dose, rate of infusion (continuous infusion is less toxic), pre-existing renal disease, older age, and diuretic use (leading to electrolyte imbalance).

Distal renal tubular acidosis
Secondary to increased passive permeability of the luminal membrane to H^+ and impaired secretion of titratable acids. Occurs after a cumulative dose >500 mg of AmB. Reversible after therapy discontinuation.

Loss of concentrating ability of the kidney
Occurs early (1–2 weeks) from direct tubular toxicity (ADH hyporesponsiveness in the medullary collecting tubule).

Renal wasting of potassium and magnesium
Pathogenic mechanisms are unclear. Partial role of distal RTA (see above).

Hypokalemia occurs in ~75% of patients and may require up to 300 mmol of KCl supplementation per day (close monitoring necessary).

Hypomagnesemia generally develops after a cumulative dose of ~500 mg of AmB and is fully reversible.

Prophylactic measures
- Use of a 24 h infusion of AmB.
- Sufficient hydration.
- Supplementation with sodium (150 mmol/day above the normal intake), potassium and magnesium.

Frequent evaluation of serum electrolytes, serum Cr and hydration status are mandatory.

The lower nephrotoxicity of liposomal formulations remains unproven (for equally therapeutic doses to conventional AmB) and their use is often limited to patients with renal impairment, contraindications to sodium supplementation or to children.

Analgesics

Analgesics are widely used self-medicated compounds (5.3% of the US population).

Analgesic nephropathy is characterized by slowly progressive CKD and results from the daily use over many years of analgesic mixtures containing phenacetin (in the past) or paracetamol (now) with salicylates and addictive substances such as caffeine or codeine or both.

Pathological changes in analgesic nephropathy include interstitial renal fibrosis, predominantly in the medulla, with papillary necrosis and subendothelial capillary sclerosis.

In typical cases renal CT scan shows small kidneys, with irregular contours and papillary calcification.

The risk of developing ESRD secondary to analgesic abuse (daily consumption for years) has been calculated at ~1.7 per 1000 per year.

Analgesic nephrotoxicity remains a matter for debate. In the past, there was little doubt that analgesic mixtures involving phenacetin were responsible for chronic interstitial nephritis and urothelial carcinoma. Since phenacetin withdrawal, controversy persists about the relationship between nonphenacetin-containing analgesics and nephropathy. Some studies indicate that prolonged use of analgesics, even acetaminophen alone, leads to CKD.

Other studies fail to provide evidence for an increased risk of CKD in healthy subjects with chronic use (up to 14 years) of aspirin, acetaminophen and other NSAIDs.

Despite the controversy, it is reasonable to discourage the prolonged used of analgesic mixtures, especially those containing caffeine and/or codeine, as these drugs seem to favor addiction. Moreover, as exposure to analgesics (such as NSAIDs) may accelerate the progression of CKD, prolonged use of analgesics should be avoided in cases of pre-existing renal disease.

Antiviral therapy
Aciclovir

This may crystallize in renal tubules, mainly when administrated as a rapid IV bolus and in the setting of intravascular volume depletion. AKI often develops within 24–48 h, and may be severe enough to warrant temporary dialysis. Often asymptomatic, abdominal pain may be observed. Urinalysis reveals hematuria, pyuria, and birefringent needle-shaped crystals with polarizing microscopy. Most cases recover to baseline renal function after drug discontinuation and fluid infusion. Prophylactic measures include slow infusion, induction of high urine output and dosage adaptation to renal function.

Adefovir dipivoxil

This analogue of adenosine triphosphate induces mild–moderate proximal tubular toxicity (22–50% of patients) at a dose >60 mg/day. Renal injury may not resolve completely in ~15% of cases

Cidofovir

This nucleotide analogue has a dose-dependent nephrotoxicity leading to proteinuria (50% of cases), elevated serum Cr (12%), Fanconi syndrome (1%), rarely chronic interstitial nephritis and nephrogenic DI. Renal function generally returns to baseline levels after dosing adjustment or drug discontinuation.

Didanosine

Exceptionally this is associated with AKI and nephrogenic DI.

Foscarnet

This pyrophosphate analogue frequently causes AKI which can be effectively prevented by IV hydration. Nephrogenic DI has also been observed.

Ganciclovir

Like aciclovir, this may precipitate into the tubular lumen and cause AKI.

Indinavir

This is poorly soluble at urinary pH 5.5–7.0, and causes crystalluria and intrarenal tubular obstruction. Symptoms are classic renal colic, dysuria, back/flank pain or macroscopic hematuria. Stone formation (radiolucent) may occur. Renal impairment is often moderate and reversible. However, severe AKI and CKD have also been reported. Hydration (at least 2–3 L of fluid) is the main prophylactic measure; urinary acidification is generally not recommended. Nephrogenic DI has also been reported.

Interferon-α (INF-α)

See below 'IV immunoglobulins, recombinant cytokines, interferon-α'.

Ritonavir

This can induce AKI, particularly in patients with pre-existing renal insufficiency. Renal impairment is reversible after drug withdrawal.

Tenofovir disoproxil fumarate

A reverse-transcriptase inhibitor, rarely associated with proximal tubulopathy. Nephrogenic DI has been seen in patients concomitantly treated with tenofovir and ritonavir or lopinavir.

Calcineurin inhibitors

Ciclosporin A (CsA) and tacrolimus (FK 506) are immunosuppressive drugs inhibiting calcineurin, a key enzyme involved in T-cell activation. Both are effective in primary immunosuppressive regimens for solid organ and bone marrow transplantation (BMT) and in the treatment of nonimmune diseases (uveitis, psoriasis, rheumatoid arthritis). CsA is also used in steroid-resistant or relapsing nephrotic syndrome and in some forms of GN. An improved bioavailability has been obtained with the development of self-emulsifying formulations.

Two distinct forms of renal injury may be attributed to calcineurin inhibitors (CNIs):

Acute nephrotoxicity

This is hemodynamically mediated and characterized by the absence of permanent structural changes and by reversibility on dose reduction or CNI discontinuation.

Chronic nephrotoxicity

Characterized by the insidious development of irreversible and progressive renal interstitial fibrosis, leading to a significant decrease in renal function and possible ESRD.

General prophylactic measures

In all clinical situations, careful attention should be paid to concomitant administration of nephrotoxic drugs.

CNIs are metabolized by the cytochrome P450 liver microsomal enzyme system; many drugs interfering with this pathway can cause significant changes in CNI blood levels.

Compounds inhibiting P450 enzymes increase CNI blood concentration:

- e.g. ketoconazole, erythromycin, and diltiazem.
  Compounds inducing these enzymes can lower CNI levels and impair immunosuppression:
- e.g. phenobarbital, carbamazepine and rifampicin.

Acute CsA nephrotoxicity

There are four common presentations:

Asymptomatic increase in serum creatinine

The most frequent and dose-related presentation, even when CsA whole-blood trough levels are within the therapeutic range.

Distinction from kidney rejection may be difficult in kidney transplant recipients or from primary renal disease progression in the case of GN treated with CsA.

Renal histology is usually normal or shows nonspecific tubular changes (vacuolization, giant mitochondria).

Improvement in serum Cr is the rule after 1 week of drug discontinuation or dose reduction.

Acute kidney injury

This may be observed in 10–50% of patients in the postoperative period of heart, liver or BMT.

It is usually multifactorial: impaired pretransplant renal function is frequent in cardiac transplant recipients; liver transplant patients frequently present with intravascular volume depletion, hypotension, coagulopathy and have a high risk of sepsis; after BMT graft-versus-host disease, veno-occlusive liver disease, infection and hemodynamic instability are not uncommon.

Delayed graft function
This can be seen after renal transplantation when high CsA doses are combined with prolonged ischemic times.

Recurrent or de novo hemolytic uremic syndrome
This is a rare, but severe cause of AKI due to endothelial cell injury. Most often it is seen in BMT and kidney transplantation (where it can mimic acute vascular rejection). Prognosis of the renal graft is very poor. Biological parameters and renal biopsy abnormalities classically found in thrombotic microangiopathy may be highly variable in severity.

Chronic CsA nephrotoxicity
This clinicopathologic entity associates some degree of renal dysfunction with tubulointerstitial fibrosis in a striped pattern from the medulla to the medullary rays of the cortex, and degenerative hyaline changes in the afferent arteriole. This arteriolar lesion, classically absent in acute renal graft rejection, is actually reversible after CsA discontinuation, whereas tubulointerstitial changes never regress.

The contribution of chronic CsA nephrotoxicity to renal allograft survival is hard to delineate, as many combined factors may contribute to progressive structural and functional impairment. Therefore an improvement of renal function after CsA reduction or withdrawal occurs in only a small proportion of patients with biopsy-proven chronic CsA nephropathy.

In nonrenal solid organ transplantation, long-term use of CsA is associated with development of CKD. The frequency of ESRD after heart transplantation varies between 1 and 8%, with a mean time period to initiation of dialysis of 6–7 years.

Proposed risk factors for end-stage renal failure:
- individual susceptibility to CsA-induced injury;
- early decrease in GFR;
- CsA dose and length of exposure to CsA therapy;
- previous renal dysfunction;
- older age;
- hepatorenal syndrome in liver-transplanted patients;
- BMT.

Bone marrow transplantation
High doses of CsA (10–12 mg/kg) are used for prevention of graft-versus-host disease for limited time periods (ranging from 6 to 18 months). This may partially explain the high prevalence of chronic CsA nephrotoxicity. Other risk factors identified are: long duration of CsA therapy; more severe renal dysfunction in the first trimester post transplant; and the use of total body irradiation.

CsA use in autoimmune diseases
Chronic CsA nephrotoxicity may be detected even with low CsA doses (initial 5 mg/kg, tapered to 1–2 mg/kg). Histological lesions mainly consist of interstitial fibrosis and tubular atrophy, arteriolopathy is rarely demonstrated. Onset of chronic injury and its severity appear to depend on individual susceptibility to CsA. No correlation has been found between structural injury, cumulative CsA dose, and duration of treatment or decrease in GFR. The best predictors for the presence of fibrosis are the duration of renal dysfunction and the lack of reversibility of functional impairment after CsA discontinuation.

Clinical management of chronic CsA nephrotoxicity
This remains a matter for debate. Some potential diagnostic markers need to be validated (e.g. urinary enzymes or microproteins reflecting structural vs functional defects of the proximal tubule). Preventive measures or treatment are speculative. In many cases, decreasing dosages or CsA withdrawal result in renal function improvement but comparative renal biopsies to confirm this improvement structurally are often lacking.

Acute and chronic tacrolimus (FK 506) nephrotoxicity
Like CsA, tacrolimus induces acute and reversible functional changes in renal function, chronic renal lesions, electrolyte disturbances, RTA and HUS. However, tacrolimus induces less hypertension but more glucose metabolic impairment than CsA.

Tacrolimus trough levels correlate strongly with drug exposure and high trough levels are associated with episodes of nephrotoxicity. Dose should be adjusted to obtain efficient immunosuppression with minimal nephrotoxicity (usually blood levels of 10–15 ng/mL).

Chemotherapy in cancer (cisplatin and others)
Chemotherapeutic agents may induce nephrotoxicity as a result of two principal processes:
- a direct toxic cellular effect related to the pharmacological properties of the anticancer drug, usually seen with drugs which have a narrow therapeutic index and prescribed at high dose;
- a disturbed pharmacokinetic profile as a result of pre-existing CKD, which requires an adaptation of the dosage.

The frequency of renal disease in cancer patients is not well-defined despite the evaluation of renal function being mandatory before initiation of many chemotherapeutic treatments.

Clinical syndromes include AKI and CKD, tubular disorders and thrombotic microangiopathy.

Predisposing factors
- Underlying renal disease (e.g. diabetic nephropathy).
- Prerenal failure (common due to poor intake, diarrhea, sepsis).
- Coadministration of nephrotoxic drugs.

Cisplatin (and to a lesser extent carboplatin)
This alkylating agent has a direct toxic effect on tubular cells. Renal manifestations are more frequent when treatment is prolonged and repeated, and often irreversible.

Tubular toxicity
There may be severe hypomagnesemia (urinary waste of magnesium), which may be associated with hypocalcemia and tetany. About 50% of patients receiving 70 mg/m^2 cisplatin every 3 weeks may present with hypomagnesemia, which is more pronounced when other nephrotoxic agents are coadministered (e.g. aminoglycosides).

Proteinuria
This reflects defects in reabsorptive capacity of the tubular epithelium towards low molecular weight proteins such as β2-microglobulin.

Acute or progressive renal failure
CKD is related to the total cumulative dose and the frequency of administration. Irreversible tubulointerstitial lesions are commonly seen and may be worse in patients who have also received radiotherapy.

Thrombotic microangiopathy syndrome
This has been described but is uncommon.

Prophylactic measures
- Hydration and vigorous diuresis with saline.
- Use daily doses for 5 days instead of single infusion.
- Aim for cumulative dose <120 mg/m^2.

Cyclophosphamide and ifosfamide
Oxazophosporines are known to induce hemorrhagic cystitis, which may be prevented by aggressive hydration and Mesna®. Both agents are tubulotoxic and Fanconi syndrome may be observed. Reversible tubular lesions are reflected by transient increase in proximal tubule enzymuria. Although severe toxicity of ifosfamide is uncommon, tubular lesions may be irreversible, resulting in progressive CKD. Dose fractionation is recommended to minimize complications.

Streptozotocin
This belongs to the nitrosourea group of drugs and may cause Fanconi syndrome (severe hypophosphatemia) and glomerular toxicity. Long-term treatment with carmustine or >6 courses with the conventional dose of 200 mg/m^2 are associated with a high risk of developing renal failure.

Methotrexate
This antimetabolite has been associated with ATN and non-oliguric AKI, attributed to intrarenal obstructive uropathy (precipitation of intact methotrexate or metabolites in distal tubules if dose >50 mg/m^2). Enhanced toxicity has been reported when there has been previous treatment with cisplatin or NSAIDs. If dose >1 g/m^2, a rapid and dose-related fall in GFR is seen. Prevention of methotrexate nephrotoxicity is by urinary alkalinization and hydration. In cases of severe renal toxicity, charcoal hemoperfusion and sequential hemodialysis (high flux) has been shown to be effective.

Mitomycin
This antitumor antibiotic may induce HUS when high doses are used (>60 mg/m^2). Estimated risk ranges from 2 to 10%. Onset is late, occurring after 3–4 cycles. No predictive marker known. In order to prevent HUS the cumulative dose should not exceed 40 mg/m^2.

Mithramycin
A daily dose of 5–50 μg/kg may result in ATN and tubular atrophy in 40% of cases.

Gemcitabine
Thrombotic microangiopathy is a rare but serious complication (incidence 0.015–1.4%); risk increases with a cumulative dose ~20 000 mg/m^2. Discontinuation of the drug is recommended in association with antihypertensive therapy where necessary. In severe cases, plasma exchange or hemoperfusion should be considered.

Radiocontrast-induced nephropathy (RCIN)
RCIN is usually defined as otherwise unexplained AKI 48–72 h after iodinated contrast agent administration (increase in serum Cr of ≥25% or 0.5 mg/dL, or a reduction in GFR of >25% from the baseline value).

RCIN is the third commonest cause of hospital-acquired renal failure (incidence is variable, depending on the patient population studied and the definition used for RCIN), and is associated with significant patient morbidity and mortality.

In general, RCIN is attributed to a combination of direct tubular toxicity and sustained vasoconstriction at the corticomedullary junction. Histologic findings are mainly vacuolar changes in the proximal convoluted tubular cells.

Risk factors for RCIN are numerous and their effect additive (presence of multiple risk factors in the same patient can create a high risk ~50% for RCIN).

Risk factors for RCIN
- Pre-existing CKD (eGFR <60 mL/min/1.73 m^2).
- Diabetes.
- Periprocedural hemodynamic instability.
- Volume depletion.
- Congestive heart failure.
- Older age (>75 years).
- Nephrotoxic drug use (NSAIDs).
- Anemia.
- Hypoalbuminemia.
- High volume and high osmolar contrast media.

Strategies to prevent RCIN
All patients should be evaluated for their risk of RCIN (when serum Cr is not available, medical history of the patient can identify those who require further assessment of renal function).

Low osmolar contrast medium is recommended and the administered volume should be the minimum amount required for an interpretable study.

Optimal volume status: outpatients are encouraged to drink water liberally in the 12 h before contrast exposure. Inpatients 'at risk' require IV volume expansion adapted to the patient characteristics (time available prior to contrast exposure, cardiac status). Isotonic crystalloid (1.0–1.5 mL/kg/h) ≥6 h before the procedure and continued at least 6 h afterward is generally recommended. IV sodium bicarbonate infusion is not recommended unless efficacy confirmed by further trials.

The risk/benefit of discontinuing drugs with nephrotoxic potential (ACEIs, ARBs diuretics) prior to contrast exposure should be evaluated. In stable patients with chronic therapy, these agents do not need to be withheld.

Conflicting data regarding the efficacy of N-acetylcysteine (NAC) prevents a strong recommendation for the use of this drug for the prevention of RCIN. When given at the discretion of the physician, the recommended dose is 600–1200 mg orally given twice on day before and day of procedure. When time available before procedure is short, NAC may be given IV (150 mg/kg in 500 mL 0.9% saline before and 50 mg/kg in 500 mL 0.9% saline after procedure).

Other prophylactic agents are ineffective (e.g. dopamine, fenoldopam, calcium channel blockers) or deleterious (e.g. furosemide, mannitol, endothelin receptor antagonist). Any potential benefit of theophylline/aminophylline needs to be confirmed in further clinical trials.

Hemodialysis is not useful in lowering the risk for RCIN. Further trials are required before recommending hemofiltration as a prophylactic measure for patients at high risk for RCIN.

A follow-up serum Cr is necessary in all patients at high risk for RCIN.

Fibrates and statins
Fibric acid derivatives (fibrates) and HMG-CoA reductase inhibitors (statins) are lipid-lowering drugs associated

with myotoxicity, which ranges in severity from myalgia to rhabdomyolysis resulting in AKI and death.

Fibrates
These are generally well-tolerated and are not generally associated with an increased risk of renal failure but may be associated with:

- reversible increase in serum Cr (most likely due to an effect mediated by peroxisome proliferator-activated receptor-α).
- higher risk of rhabdomyolysis-associated AKI when used in combination with statins.

Gemfibrozil should be avoided and fenofibrate is preferred (it is not associated with inhibition of statin metabolism).

Ezetimide alone or with a statin may cause myopathy.

Serum Cr should be measured before fibrate initiation and the dose adjusted according to renal function. Routine monitoring of serum Cr is not required but could be useful in situations of possible drug interactions and/or in patients with advanced CKD.

Statins
There is limited information available on the potential benefit of statins in CKD in terms of reduction of cardiovascular morbidity and mortality. A beneficial effect on albuminuria has been proposed but is still controversial.

Statins are safe and usually well-tolerated even in advanced CKD and ESRD. However, the following adverse events have been reported:

Muscle pain or weakness
Seen in fewer than 1 in 10 000 patients on standard doses. Risk varies with statin, and increases with higher doses and interacting drugs. Drug discontinuation reverses these side-effects.

Potentiation of myotoxicity may be observed when atorvastatin is used with colchicine or quinine because of modifications of the pharmacokinetic profile of atorvastatin (colchicine is a P-glycoprotein inhibitor and quinine inhibits cytochrome P450 isoenzyme 3A4).

Acute hepatic injury and AKI secondary to rhabdomyolysis
This has been reported in patients receiving gemfibrozil and fluvastatin. Cerivastatin was banned after similar fatal cases.

Rhabdomyolysis with cardiac involvement and AKI
This has been reported with rosuvastatin combined with fenofibrate.

Tubular proteinuria
Rosuvastatin ($\geq$40 mg/day) may cause a mild form of tubular proteinuria without an increased risk of renal failure.

Thus it is recommended that statins are used carefully in CKD.

Herbal medicine
Herbal medicines are used by 75% of the world's population, mostly in the developing countries. Herbal medicine is also popular in the West with 15% of the population consulting a herbal medicine provider each year.

Herbal products may contain nephrotoxic compounds and, therefore, may be responsible for various renal syndromes (Table 18.2.4).

Herbal nephrotoxicity falls into four main categories

1. Herbal plants may be properly identified but may have unknown or underestimated toxicity. This is often the case for ATN secondary to some traditional African medicines, the mineralocorticoid activity of licorice used in many herbal prescriptions and the adrenergic effect of ephedra-containing herbal preparations.

2. Herbal medicines may contain undisclosed drugs and heavy metals (up to 35%). Contamination by cadmium may result in Fanconi syndrome. Adulteration by NSAIDs has led to a chronic 'analgesic'nephropathy.

3. Herbal plants may be incorrectly identified, resulting in patients being given toxic compounds (or compounds with an underestimated toxicity) under the false assumption that they are harmless natural herbal remedies. Chronic interstitial fibrosis (and urothelial carcinoma) secondary to the intake of medicinal herbs containing aristolochic acids is discussed in Chapter 6.6.

4. Herbal plants may interact with conventional drugs. *Hypericum perforatum* (St John's wort) activates the hepatic cytochrome system and thus can decrease plasma levels of a wide range of prescribed drugs, with clinical consequences such as a renal allograft rejection in patients treated by CsA or tacrolimus.

For patients with ESRD, it must also be stressed that some herbal compounds contain significant amounts of potassium and may induce hyperkalemia: alfala (*Medicago sativa*), dandelion (*Taraxacum officinale*), noni juice (*Morinda officinalis*).

Intravenous immunoglobulin, recombinant cytokines, interferon-α
High dose intravenous immunoglobulin (IVIG)
IVIG is generally well-tolerated. However, cases of AKI have been reported secondary to the tubular toxic effects of sucrose, maltose, glucose, or glycine contained in IVIG formulations. Advanced age, diabetes mellitus and pre-existing renal failure are risk factors. Slow rate of infusion and nonsucrose formulations may prevent renal complications. IVIG can also inhibit tubular secretion of Cr and, thus, may cause a 'false' renal failure.

Interferon-α (INF-α)
This is frequently used as an antiviral agent, immunomodulator and anticancer therapy. Administration may lead to mild–moderate proteinuria (25%) and an increase in serum Cr (10%), mostly in patients with hematological malignancies or hepatitis. Renal biopsies reveal minimal change disease, focal segmental hyalinosis or crescentic glomerulonephritis. Thrombotic microangiopathy has also been observed with INF-α.

Interleukin-2 (IL-2)
IL-2 is used in certain forms of renal carcinoma. The administration of IL-2 may result in a capillary leak syndrome with proteinuria and prerenal AKI secondary to an ineffective circulating blood volume.

Lithium
In Western countries ~1 in 1000 individuals is given lithium for the treatment of uni- or bipolar affective disorders. Lithium is eliminated by the kidney (glomerular filtration and proximal tubular reabsorption) and may accumulate in distal tubular cells. After long-term exposure, tubular cysts as well as tubular atrophy and interstitial fibrosis and sometimes glomerular sclerosis may develop.

Renal side-effects of lithium include:
- AKI (prerenal type);
- CKD (secondary to interstitial renal fibrosis);
- nephrogenic DI (most frequently);
- incomplete distal RTA (rare, no clinical consequence);
- nephrotic syndrome (rare, due to FSGS).

Lithium may also induce hypothyroidism and hyperparathyroidism. The latter is responsible for hypercalcemia (in 35% of the patients) which can aggravate renal lesions.

Nephrogenic diabetes insipidus
Lithium induces resistance to ADH: 50% of patients will have impaired urine concentration ability and 20% develop polyuria and polydypsia. In view of the efficacy of lithium therapy polyuria is commonly accepted as a side-effect. Treatment with amiloride (10–20 mg/day) can significantly reduce daily urine output.

Lithium-induced chronic kidney disease
Evidence exists that lithium is responsible for chronic interstitial nephritis sometimes leading to ESRD:
- Development and progression of CKD are related to the average serum lithium level and the cumulative lithium dose. Therefore, it is recommended to maintain a lithium serum concentration at the lowest level (if possible between 0.4 and 0.8 mmol/l) to adequately control affective symptoms.
- Once CKD is present, withdrawal of lithium after long-term use does not guarantee the stabilization of renal function and progressive evolution to ESRD is still the rule.

NSAIDs (including selective cyclo-oxygenase 2 inhibitors)
NSAIDs are inhibitors of cyclo-oxygenases (COX), which catalyze the production of prostaglandins (PG). Two COX isoforms have been isolated: COX-1 and COX-2. Selective COX-2 inhibitors are associated with fewer gastrointestinal adverse effects than nonselective NSAIDs.

Many of the renal effects of NSAIDs appear to be mediated by COX-2 inhibition rather than COX-1 inhibition.

COX-2 inhibition decreases urinary PG excretion and may result in decreased GFR and sodium retention.

This is particularly the case when renal PG secretion is required for the preservation of renal hemodynamics:
- volume depletion;
- reduced renal blood flow (cardiac failure);
- ineffective circulating blood volume (sepsis, cirrhosis, nephrotic syndrome);
- toxic injury (CsA, tacrolimus);
- advanced age;
- pre-existing renal failure.

In normal conditions, temporary use of NSAIDs produces negligible effects on renal hemodynamics. In the conditions mentioned above, NSAIDs may induce prerenal AKI or ATN.

Observational studies have shown that NSAIDs were responsible for 36% of in-hospital AKI.

All NSAIDs, including selective COX-2 inhibitors, may also induce AKI secondary to AIN. Most cases of NSAID-related AIN are associated with nephrotic syndrome (minimal change disease, rarely FSGS, membranous nephropathy).

Various fluid and electrolyte disorders (hyponatremia, hyperkalemia, acidosis, fluid retention) as well as hypertension and resistance to diuretics have been related to the use of NSAIDs.

The long-term (>2 years) daily use of NSAIDs has been associated with an increased risk for developing CKD secondary to chronic interstitial nephritis. Episodes of papillary necrosis have been reported with ibuprofen, indomethacin, phenylbutazone, fenoprofen and mefenamic acid.

Suprofen may give rise to AKI with unilateral or bilateral flank pain ('suprofen nephropathy'). This syndrome is probably due to the uricosuric properties of NSAIDs leading to an acute uric acid nephropathy.

Among all NSAIDs, aspirin is the only one that is clearly associated with a low risk of renal side-effects (with the exception of lupus nephropathy). Claims regarding the renal-sparing properties of particular NSAIDs (sulindac, nabumetone) lack convincing evidence. Thus caution must be applied when using NSAIDs (including selective COX-2 inhibitors) chronically or in situations associated with renal hemodynamic stress.

Sulphasalazines (5-amino salicylic acid, 5-ASA)
Sulphazalazine is effective in the treatment of patients with inflammatory bowel disease (IBD). Second generation sulphasalazines (mesalazine, olsazazine, balsalazine) free of sulphapyridine were developed in order to avoid the hematological side-effects of sulphazalazine.

5-ASA therapy in chronic IBD has been associated with renal impairment in 1.3 to 3.3 per 1000 patients.

Treatment with mesalazine and olsalazine has been reported to induce biopsy-proven AIN. In several cases, recovery of renal function did not occur.

Current recommendations are to monitor renal function in patients on 5-ASA derivatives every 3 months. If there is renal failure, a renal biopsy is required to confirm the diagnosis as patients with chronic IBD are at risk of diverse nephropathies (immune glomerulopathies, amyloidosis, oxalate stones).

Oral sodium phosphate solution (acute phosphate nephropathy)
Oral sodium phosphate solution (OSPS; Fleet® Phospho soda), widely used for bowel cleansing, may lead to acute phosphate nephropathy and AKI with a high risk of CKD.

While the incidence is low this entity is probably under-recognized.

Histologic findings are characterized by the presence of abundant calcium phosphate crystals in renal tubules.

Factors predisposing patients to acute phosphate nephropathy after OSPS are:
- volume depletion;
- older age;
- gender (female);
- hypertension;
- concurrent therapy with diuretics, NSAIDs, ACEIs or ARBs.

OSPS is contraindicated in CKD and should be used with caution in elderly patients and in patients with electrolyte disturbances.

Further reading
de Mattos A, Olyaei A, Bennett W. Nephrotoxicity of immunosuppressive drugs: long-term consequences and challenges for the future. *Am J Kidney Dis* 2000; **35**: 333–346.

Domenica D, Gehr T. 3-Hydroxy-3-methylglutaryl coenzyme A reductase inhibitors and rhabdomyolysis: considerations in the renal failure patient. *Curr Opin Nephrol Hypertens* 2002; **11**: 123–133.

Isnard Bagnis C, Deray G, et al. Herbs and the kidney. *Am J Kidney Dis* 2004; **44**: 1–11.

Izzedine H, Launay-Vacher V, Deray G. Antiviral drug-induced nephrotoxicity. *Am J Kidney Dis* 2005; **45**: 804–817.

Kintzel P. Anti-cancer drug-induced kidney disorders. *Drug Safety* 2001; **24**: 19–38.

Rossert J. Drug-induced acute interstitial nephritis. *Kidney Int* 2001; **60**: 804–817.

Stacul F, Adam A, et al. Strategies to reduce the risk of contrast-induced nephropathy. *Am J Cardiol* 2006; **98**: 59K–77K.

Wali R, Henrich W. Recent developments in toxic nephropathy. *Curr Opin Nephrol Hypertens* 2002; **11**: 155–163.

Internet resources

Epocrates® ONLINE provides continually updated information on brand and generic drugs (dosing, drug–drug interactions, adverse reactions and mode of action:

http://www.epocrates.com

A patient-friendly US-based site with drug information:

http://drugs.com

See also

Analgesic nephropathy, p. 226

NSAIDs and the kidney, p. 228

Aristolochic acid nephropathy ('Chinese herb nephropathy') and other rare causes of interstitial nephropathy), p. 240

Systemic Cancer therapies and the kidney, p. 714

Table 18.2.4 Renal syndromes related to herbal medicine

Hypertension	*Glycyrrhiza* spp. (Chinese herbal teas, gancao, Boui-ougi-tou)
	Ephedra spp. (ma huang)
Acute tubular necrosis	Traditional African medicine: toxic plants (*Securida longe pedunculata, Euphoria matabelensis, Callilepsis laureola, Cape aloes*) or adulteration by dichromate.
	Chinese medicine: *Taxus celebica*
	Marocco: *Takaout roumia* (para-phenylenediamine)
Acute interstitial nephritis	Peruvian medicine (*Uno degatta*)
	Tung Shueh pills (adulterated by mefenamic acid)
Fanconi syndrome	Chinese herbs containing AA (*Akebia* spp., *Boui, Mokutsu*)
	Chinese herbs adulterated by cadmium
Papillary necrosis	Chinese herbs adulterated by phenylbutazone
Chronic interstitial renal fibrosis	Chinese herbs or Kampo containing AA (*Aristolochia* spp., *Akebia* spp., *Mu-tong, Boui, Mokutsu*)
Urinary retention	*Datura* spp., *Rhododendron molle* (atropine, scopolamine)
Kidney stones	*Ma huang* (ephedrine)
	Cranberry juice (oxalate)
Urothelial carcinoma	Chinese herbs containing AA

AA, aristolochic acids.
From: Isnard Bagnis et al. (2004).

Clinical use of diuretics

Introduction

Diuretics are commonly used pharmacological agents. Alone, or in combination, they are used in the management of hypertension. They are especially useful in those pathophysiological conditions in which sodium retention is a central problem (renal failure, cardiac failure, hepatic failure, nephrotic syndrome).

Diuretics act by inhibiting sodium reabsorption in different segments along the nephron. The objective of therapy is to initiate and sustain an increased natriuresis until the patient has returned to euvolemia, at which new steady state it is easier to maintain homeostasis, particularly if dietary salt intake is restricted.

Clinical goals may not always be achieved easily and adverse effects are common. This relates, in part, to pathophysiologically determined variation in the pharmacokinetics of individual agents (a phenomenon often referred to as diuretic resistance) and, in part, to rapid changes in the pharmacodynamic response of the nephron (a phenomenon often referred to as diuretic blunting).

Although diuretic agents have been used for many decades, much prescribing still occurs in an *ad hoc* fashion. Basic and clinical research has expanded our knowledge of the mechanisms of action of these agents. Application of the pharmacokinetic and pharmacodynamic principles derived from these studies should improve the achievement of clinical objectives.

Classification of diuretic agents

Site of action in different nephron segments classifies the commonly used agents.

Although the bulk (60–70%) of filtered sodium is reabsorbed in the proximal tubule, agents acting at this site (e.g. acetazolamide) are of relatively little clinical utility in edematous states, as increased sodium loss here is offset by increased reabsorption further down the nephron, particularly in the thick ascending loop of Henle.

Diuretics may also have actions at other sites (e.g. many interfere with urate absorption and secretion in the proximal tubule).

Loop diuretics

Loop diuretics:

- furosemide;
- bumetanide;
- torasemide.

These are organic anions and are secreted into the lumen of the proximal tubule by the organic anion transporter-1 (OAT-1).

They then act upon the luminal aspect of the thick ascending loop of Henle.

Here, they exhibit high affinity for the chloride-binding site of the sodium-potassium-2 chloride transporter (NKCC2). This transporter is an integral membrane protein from Solute Carrier Family 12, and is encoded by the *SLC12A1* gene on chromosome 15.

Binding of diuretic directly inhibits sodium and chloride reabsorption.

This minimizes the usual luminal positive charge indirectly leading to decreased reabsorption of calcium and magnesium, and interferes with urinary concentrating and diluting mechanisms.

Up to 20% of filtered sodium can be excreted using these agents.

Individual agents differ in terms of bioavailability, duration of action and modes of excretion.

All can be administered orally or parenterally.

In general terms they achieve very similar clinical outcomes.

Ethacrynic acid is an uncommonly used loop diuretic indicated in patients known to have had hypersensitivity reactions to sulphonamides and related agents.

Thiazide and thiazide-like diuretics

Thiazide and related diuretics:

- bendroflumethiazide
- hydrochlorothiazide
- chlorthalidone
- indapamide
- metolazone
- mefruside.

Are also organic anions secreted by OAT-1.

These act upon the luminal aspect of the distal convoluted tubule and the connecting segment.

These agents have a high affinity for the chloride-binding site of another member of Solute Carrier Family 12 – the Sodium-Chloride Co-transporter (NCC), encoded by the *SLC12A3* gene on chromosome 16.

In this segment, diuretics directly inhibit sodium and chloride reabsorption. Calcium reabsorption is indirectly increased because of this.

The maximum natriuresis achieved is less than that with loop diuretics, but the combination of these classes can be especially potent.

Individual agents differ in terms of bioavailability, duration of action and modes of excretion.

All can be administered orally.

In general terms they achieve very similar clinical outcomes.

Potassium-sparing diuretics

Potassium-sparing diuretics:

- amiloride
- triamterene
- spironolactone
- eplerenone.

The first two of these are organic cations, secreted into the proximal tubule and subsequently blocking the luminal Epithelial Sodium Channel (ENaC) of the principal cells in the cortical collecting duct. ENaC, also referred to as Sodium Channel Nonvoltage-gated channel-1 (SCNN1), has three subunits encoded by different genes (*SCNN1A* on chromosome 12; *SCNN1B* and *SCNN1G* on chromosome 16).

Spironolactone and eplerenone, on the other hand, enter the principal cells from the blood and act intracellularly to inhibit the effect of aldosterone on the intracellular aldosterone receptor in these cells. This reduces the cellular drive to reabsorb sodium and decreases the expression of luminal ENaC channels.

Interference with sodium reabsorption affects potassium secretion by these cells – the greater the sodium reabsorption, the greater the potassium secretion. Thus, increased delivery of sodium to the cortical collecting duct consequent upon successful inhibition of reabsorption in the thick ascending loop of Henle and distal convoluted segment (as would happen with the combined use of a loop and thiazide diuretic) will lead to increased distal sodium reabsorption and an associated kalliuresis.

This can be inhibited by potassium-sparing diuretics which also (on the same principle) minimize the magnesuric effect of the sodium-magnesium antiporter also found in distal nephron segments.

Individual agents differ in terms of bioavailability, duration of action and modes of excretion.

All can be administered orally.

In general terms they achieve very similar clinical outcomes.

Other diuretics
Osmotic diuretics
Substances which are filtered at the glomerulus but not completely reabsorbed will act as osmotic diuretics. Examples are mannitol, glycerol, glucose (when glucose has exceeded its maximum reabsorption capacity) and urea (after relief of urinary tract obstruction).

Due to the risk of rapid expansion of intravascular volume and pulmonary edema in patients with impaired glomerular filtration rate, these drugs are rarely used in patients with AKI and CKD, and are reserved for patients with traumatic brain injury and acute angle-closure glaucoma.

Nesiritide
This is a recombinant form of the B-type natriuretic peptide and is licensed in the USA for treatment of acute decompensated heart failure.

Nesiritide binds to the natriuretic peptide receptor A and increases intracellular cyclic GMP.

It has to be given IV and is reported to induce vasodilation (reducing preload), natriuresis and diuresis.

Achieving clinical objectives
To achieve a decrease in total body salt and water requires that excretion exceeds intake.

Dietary sodium intake is frequently >100 mmol/day (~6 g salt/day).

Renal avidity for sodium is increased in the edematous clinical conditions.

To lose, for example, 5 kg of excess extracellular fluid (ECF) volume requires a net sodium loss of 700 mmol, over and above that needed to balance daily intake.

Thus, the diuretic regimen employed must initiate and sustain a sufficient increment in natriuresis to achieve this cumulative excretion within a reasonable period of time.

It is irrational not to concurrently prescribe a reduction in dietary salt intake in those taking diuretics; it may, however, be difficult to achieve.

Many patients find diets containing <80 mmol/day unpalatable and most salt intake is nondiscretionary because of addition during food processing.

Unexpected failure to lose weight/ECF volume in a patient on a seemingly appropriate dose of diuretic should prompt a systematic enquiry into salt intake.

Measurement of 24 h urinary sodium excretion may help.

If a patient is passing ≥150 mmol sodium per day but not losing weight it is likely that excess salt intake is the problem.

If a patient is passing ≤100 mmol sodium per day it will be difficult to lose weight/ECF volume as this does not greatly exceed the likely minimum dietary restriction. A change in strategy to increase natriuresis will be needed.

Pharmacokinetic and pharmacodynamic considerations are the main reasons why patients fail to achieve and sustain an adequate natriuretic response. Pharmacokinetics are important in the initiation of natriuresis; pharmacodynamics in sustaining it.

Pharmacokinetic considerations
The natriuretic response is proportional to the rate at which diuretic is excreted in the tubular fluid, and there is a threshold level of excretion required before it initiates. To overcome pharmacokinetic problems in initiating natriuresis it is most important to progressively increase the initial dose (or otherwise modify the regimen) until the natriuretic threshold has been exceeded.

Giving an ineffective dose more frequently (as is often observed in clinical practice) will not help. In difficult cases, measurement of 24 h sodium excretion may guide dosing.

The barriers between administering an apparently adequate dose and achieving an adequate amount excreted in the urine need to be identified. Exceeding the natriuretic threshold may be difficult because of:

Decreased bioavailability
Furosemide has an oral bioavailability of ~60%.

This may be decreased with an edematous GI tract.

Increasing the oral dose, switching to IV or using an equivalent oral dose of bumetanide (which has a higher bioavailability) may be chosen to help overcome this.

Increased volume of distribution
Diuretics are highly protein-bound.

Secretion into the nephron is predominantly of bound drug.

In patients with hypoalbuminemia, free diuretic passes out of the vascular space leading to a decreased amount available for secretion into the tubule.

Increasing dose or taking the steps above may help.

Low glomerular filtration rate
In heart failure and renal failure the delivery of diuretic to the kidney will be decreased (as will the initial filtered sodium load).

Increasing dose, taking the steps above or enhancing cardiac output by other means (e.g. ACEIs) may help.

Competition for secretion in the proximal tubule
Many organic ions accumulate in liver and renal failure: these compete for secretion via OAT-1, decreasing the amount of diuretic reaching the tubular lumen.

Certain medications (e.g. cimetidine) also have this effect.

Avoiding such agents and taking the steps above may help.

It was formerly speculated that loop diuretic excretion was increased if the drug was administered with albumin. Similarly it was felt that proteinuria might decrease the effective tubular concentration, by binding free drug within the tubule. Recent studies do not support these views.

Pharmacodynamic considerations
In a very short time (days) after the initiation of natriuresis more distal parts of the tubule will increase reabsorption of sodium, thereby blunting the natriuretic effect.

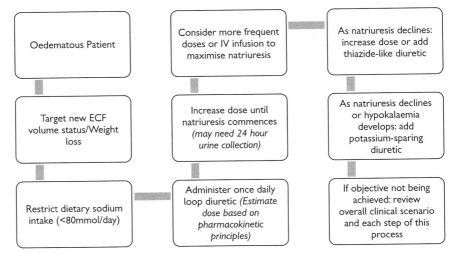

Fig. 18.3.1 Simplified schema illustrating basic steps in achieving clinical objectives. In individual patients each step may be simple/easily achieved or quite difficult. Potential problems are detailed in the text.

This is principally a local response to an increased delivery of tubular sodium to these segments, particularly following administration of loop and thiazide diuretics where downstream ENaC channel abundance increases.

There is now evidence that allelelic variations in the *SLC12A3* and the *SCNN1B* genes influence the intensity of this adaptation.

Furthermore, chronic administration of both loop and thiazide diuretics seems to increase the abundance of their respective target transporters.

Strategies should anticipate the inevitable occurrence of these pharmacodynamic adaptations and may include:

More frequent dosage
Furosemide acts for ~6 h and no enhanced natriuresis will occur for the rest of the day.

Once the initial natriuretic threshold has been exceeded, twice- or thrice-daily dosing allows for a higher cumulative daily loss of sodium until blunting of the response begins.

Studies indicate that continuous drug infusion may achieve a greater cumulative sodium loss than repeated boluses.

Sequential nephron blockade
As the initial response to loop diuretics declines, a structured inhibition of the distal nephron sites is indicated.

Initially, thiazide diuretics should be administered and subsequently potassium-sparing agents.

The latter may, in fact, be required quickly – combination therapy with the other classes markedly increases potassium loss and this may be an additional limiting factor.

Sequential strategies have been shown to be successful even in patients with advanced renal failure and cardiac failure.

In crossover studies there appears to be little difference in the response to equipotent doses of different thiazides used in this fashion – personal choice may be the best guide.

Careful application of these principles should achieve the objectives of therapy – in difficult cases therapy adjustment and clinical evaluation may be time-consuming and therapy prolonged.

Other uses or indications for specific diuretic agents
The hypocalciuric effects of thiazides may be employed in reducing the frequency of stone events in some hypercalciuric patients. However, other measures to achieve this should also be used; not all patients benefit, and therapy usually needs to continue for at least 2–3 years.

In some clinical circumstances, choice of agent may be informed by other outcomes.

Patients with heart failure, particularly with more marked left ventricular impairment and low/normal serum potassium concentrations, may have an excess mortality if potassium-sparing diuretics are not used.

Similarly the survival benefit of treating hypertension with nonpotassium-sparing diuretics may be attenuated as a consequence of an increase in cardiac deaths.

In addition, spironolactone may have specific beneficial effects in some patients with severe heart failure.

Diuretics do not alter outcomes in AKI. Previously they were used in protocols attempting to diminish anticipated nephrotoxicity but they have now been shown to be more likely to increase nephrotoxicity.

Adverse events
These are common and include:

ECF volume depletion
This is particularly common in patients who develop other ECF-depleting problems such as diarrhea and vomiting while continuing on diuretics.

Coadministration of loop and thiazide diuretics can also rapidly deplete the ECF volume.

This adverse event is often associated with raised blood urea concentrations because of renal hypoperfusion. In many patients, glomerular filtration rate (GFR) is relatively preserved due to autoregulation, but impaired renal blood flow causes enhanced tubular urea reabsorption.

Decreased GFR
This can occur as a consequence of ECF depletion and is more commonly seen in older patients, those with pre-existing CKD, chronic heart failure and low mean arterial pressure.

Electrolyte disturbances
Including:

- hyponatremia (commoner with thiazides);
- hypomagnesemia (commoner with thiazides);
- hypokalemia (most common when combinations of loop and thiazide diuretics are used).

Avoiding a high water intake (>1.5 L/day) may reduce the incidence of hyponatremia, which is more common in the elderly.

Hypokalemia is usually manifest within 5–7 days of establishing therapy; 'routine screening' is not indicated in the absence of changes in clinical circumstances, dose or other medications.

Potassium-sparing diuretics may cause hyperkalemia, especially in the presence of renal impairment.

Hypercalcemia, dyslipidemia, and glucose intolerance (especially with associated hypokalemia) are common side-effects of thiazide diuretics.

Metabolic alkalosis
This results from chloride loss and ECF volume contraction.

Potassium-sparing diuretics may, alternatively, cause acidosis.

Hyperuricemia and gout
Tubular handling of uric acid is complex, with both reabsorption and secretion occurring in the proximal tubule.

Diuretics (particularly thiazides) can interfere with either of these processes with the usual consequence being hyperuricemia.

This effect is usually dose dependent and frequently asymptomatic.

Combination therapy with ACEIs or ARBs may blunt the effect.

Clinical gout is more likely if the patient is also ECF volume-depleted.

Thiamine depletion
This may follow prolonged diuretic use (is a water-soluble vitamin), potentially leading to impaired cardiac function.

Chronic hypercalciuria and magnesiuria
This is induced by long-term use of loop diuretics.

It may lead to osteopenia, subclinical hyperparathyroidism and alteration in intracellular cations leading to a potentially proinflammatory vascular phenotype.

Activation of the renin–angiotensin–aldosterone system
Use of loop diuretics as the sole therapy for cardiac failure may lead to chronic activation of the renin–angiotensin–aldosterone system and other harmful neuroendocrine alterations.

Hypersensitivity reactions
These include skin rashes and interstitial nephritis.

Muscle cramps
Ototoxicity
This is a major but uncommon potential side-effect.

It has been reported with high dose (>2 g/day) infusion therapy in patients with renal failure.

The mechanism is believed to be mediated via the NKCC1 transporter in the inner ear, which is structurally similar to the NKCC2 transporter in the kidney.

Pregnancy
Diuretics should be avoided in pregnancy.

They can cross the placenta and may cause fetal electrolyte disturbances.

Placental perfusion may be compromised.

Diuretics enter breast milk.

Further reading

Agarwal R, Gorski JC, Sundblad K, Brater DC. Urinary protein binding does not affect response to furosemide in patients with nephrotic syndrome. J Am Soc Nephrol 2000; **11**: 1100–1105.

Brater DC. Pharmacology of diuretics. Am J Med Sci 2000;**319**:38–50.

Brater DC. Diuretic therapy. New Eng J Med 1998; **339**: 387–395.

Channer KS, McLean KA, Lawson-Matthew P, Richardson M. Combination diuretic treatment in severe heart failure: a randomised controlled trial. Br Heart J 1994; **71**: 146–150.

Cooper HA, Dries DL, Davis CE, Shen YL, Domanski MJ. Diuretics and risk of arrhythmic death in patients with left ventricular dysfunction. Circulation 1999; **100**: 1311–1315.

Delpire E, Lu J, England R, Dull C, Thorne T. Deafness and imbalance associated with inactivation of the secretory Na-K-2Cl co-transporter. Nature Genet 1999; **22**: 192–195.

Ellison DH. Diuretic drugs and the treatment of edema: from clinic to bench and back again. Am J Kidney Dis 1994; **23**: 623–643.

Fliser D, Schroter M, Neubeck M, Ritz E. Coadministration of thiazide diuretics increases the efficacy of loop diuretics even in patients with advanced renal failure. Kidney Int 1994; **46**: 482–488.

Fliser D, Zurbruggen I, Mutschler E, et al. Coadministration of albumin and furosemide in patients with the nephrotic syndrome. Kidney Int 1999; **55**: 629–634.

Gupta S, Neyses L. Diuretic usage in heart failure: a continuing conundrum in 2005. Eur Heart J 2005; **26**: 644–649.

Ho KM, Sheridan DJ. Meta-analysis of frusemide to prevent or treat acute renal failure. Br Med J 2006; **333**: 406–407.

Hoes AW, Grobbee DE, Lubsen J, Man in 't Veld, AJ, van der Does E, Hofman, A. Diuretics, beta-blockers, and the risk of sudden cardiac death in hypertensive patients. Ann Intern Med 1995; **123**: 481–487.

Kim JH. Long-term adaptation of renal ion transporters to chronic diuretic treatment. Am J Nephrol 2004; **24**: 595–605.

Meisler MH, Barrow LL, Canessa CM, Rossier BC. SCNN1, an epithelial cell sodium channel gene in the conserved linkage group on mouse chromosome 6 and human chromosome 12. Genomics 1994; **24**: 185–186.

Pitt B, Zannad F, Remme WJ, et al. The effect of spironolactone on morbidity and mortality in patients with severe heart failure. N Engl J Med 1999; **341**: 709–717.

Rudy DW, Voelker JR, Greene PK, Esparza FA, Brater DC. Loop diuretics for chronic renal insufficiency: a continuous infusion is more efficacious than bolus therapy. Ann Intern Med 1991; **115**: 360–366.

Salvador DRK, Rey NR, Ramos GC, Punzalan FER. Continuous infusion versus bolus injection of loop diuretics in congestive heart failure. Cochrane Database Syst Rev 2004; (1): CD003178. pub3.

Simon DB, Nelson-Williams C, Bia MJ, et al. Gitelman's variant of Bartter's syndrome, inherited hypokalaemic alkalosis, is caused by mutations in the thiazide-sensitive Na-Cl cotransporter. Nature Genet 1996; **12**: 24–30.

Simon DB, Karet FE, Hamdan JM, Di Pietro A, Sanjad SA, Lifton, RP. Bartter's syndrome, hypokalaemic alkalosis with hypercalciuria, is caused by mutations in the Na-K-2Cl transporter NKCC2. *Nature Genet* 1996; **13**: 183–188.

Sun WY, Reiser IW, Chou S-Y. Risk factors for acute renal insufficiency induced by diuretics in patients with congestive heart failure. *Am J Kidney Dis* 2006; **47**: 798–808.

Voilley N, Bassilana F, Mignon C, *et al.* Cloning, chromosomal localization, and physical linkage of the beta and gamma subunits (SCNN1B and SCNN1G) of the human epithelial amiloride-sensitive sodium channel. *Genomics* 1995; **28**: 560–565.

Vormfelde SV, Sehrt D, Toliat MR, *et al.* Genetic variation in the renal sodium transporters NKCC2, NCC, and ENaC in relation to the effects of loop diuretic drugs. *Clin Pharmacol Ther* 2007; **82**: 300–309.

Weber KT. Furosemide in the long-term management of heart failure: the good, the bad and the uncertain. *J Am Coll Cardiol* 2004; **44**: 1308–1310.

Internet resources

NICE guidelines for treatment of hypertension and heart failure:

http://www.nice.org.uk

National Prescribing Centre:

http://www.npc.co.uk/

See also

Systemic cancer therapies and the kidney

Introduction

Many chemotherapeutic agents are filtered by the kidneys with some also undergoing tubular secretion. The kidneys are therefore vulnerable to the toxic effects of cytotoxic drugs with nephrotoxicity often the dose-limiting side-effect in chemotherapeutic regimens.

Drug pharmacokinetics may be altered in patients with renal impairment if renal excretion plays a significant role in drug elimination. Dose adjustment tailored to patients' renal function is necessary to avoid exposure to excessive drug levels and subsequent toxicity.

Assessment of renal function

Renal function is assessed prior to chemotherapy dosing.

Methods include:

- EDTA-GFR (gold standard: radioisotope to measure GFR);
- timed urine collection to calculate creatinine clearance:

$$CrCl \ (mL/min) = \frac{(Urine \ Cr \times Urine \ Vol)}{(Plasma \ Cr \times Time \ (min))};$$

- formulae to estimate GFR.

Formulae developed to estimate creatinine clearance are based on point sampling of serum creatinine and incorporate patient-related factors including age, weight and gender.

Formulae include:

- Cockcroft and Gault (see below);
- Jeliffe;
- Wright;
- Chatelut;
- Modification of Diet in Renal Disease (MDRD) study formula. (most commonly employed, see Appendix)

Formulae require stable creatinine and are influenced by muscle mass and fluid balance.

Cockcroft and Gault formula

$$CrCl \ (mL/min) = \frac{(140 - age) \times Weight \ (kg) \times 'Y'}{Serum \ Cr \ (mg/dL)}$$

Y = 1.23 in men and 1.04 in women.

Chemotherapy

The aim of treatment in patients with cancer needs to be clearly defined. Potential side-effect profiles should be considered in the context of whether treatment is curative or palliative.

Drugs causing significant nephrotoxicity such as methotrexate and cisplatin should be avoided in patients with renal insufficiency.

Renal impairment and pharmacokinetics

Anticancer drugs can be eliminated from the body through metabolism, excretion in the urine, bile or feces, or through the respiratory tract.

Patients with renal dysfunction receiving chemotherapy which is primarily eliminated via the kidneys have decreased clearance in the urine. This results in increased systemic exposure as indicated by increased area under the curve (AUC) of plasma concentration vs time (Table 18.4.1).

Hemodialysis and chemotherapy

There is limited data on the clearance of chemotherapeutic agents by dialysis.

Clearance of the drug by hemodialysis can lead to decreased drug exposure and therapeutic efficacy.

Dialysable drugs

- cisplatin
- carboplatin
- cyclophosphamide
- ifosfamide
- methotrexate.

Nephrotoxicity of chemotherapy agents

Chemotherapy agents can affect the microvasculature, glomeruli and tubules.

Clinical manifestations (examples given below) depend on the site of nephron most adversely affected and include:

- tubulointerstitial injury causing asymptomatic decrease in GFR;
- hemolytic microangiopathy resembling hemolytic uremic syndrome (HUS);
- tubular dysfunction with electrolyte imbalance;
- AKI necessitating dialysis.

Agents causing tubulointerstitial damage

Cisplatin

Heavy metal alkylating-like agent.

Widely used in many treatment sites including:

- testicular;
- gynecological;
- urological;
- head and neck cancers.

Cisplatin rapidly becomes protein-bound but concentrates in the kidneys by undetermined mechanisms.

15–75% cleared in the urine as unchanged drug.

Nephrotoxicity is major dose-limiting side-effect.

Cisplatin should be avoided if GFR <30 mL/min.

Cisplatin nephrotoxicity manifestations:

- subclinical reduction in GFR with each cycle;
- AKI;
- salt-wasting nephropathy;
- magnesium-wasting nephropathy.

Prevention of nephrotoxicity:

- vigorous prehydration;
- 0.9% saline infusion; aim for urine output >150 mL/h;
- magnesium replacement as cisplatin-induced hypomagnesemia potentiates nephrotoxicity;
- consider mannitol.

Carboplatin

A second generation platinum agent.

Nephrotoxicity is rarely clinically significant.

Carboplatin dosing is safe in patients with renal impairment.

Renal clearance is closely correlated with GFR.

The dose is calculated using the Calvert formula (see below), which considers the GFR and desired AUC (normally 4–7 mg/mL/min).

Carboplatin = target AUC × (EDTA-GFR + 25) dose (mg)

Table 18.4.1 Chemotherapy dosing in patients with renal impairment

Drugs requiring dose adjustment	Bleomycin	Etoposide	Melphalan
	Capecitabine	Epirubicin	Methotrexate
	Cisplatin	Fludarabine	Nitrosoureas
	Carboplatin	Ifosfamide	Raltitrexed
	Dacarbazine	Irinotecan	
Drugs not generally requiring dose adjustment	Docetaxel		
	Fluorouracil		
	Gemcitabine		
	Oxaliplatin		

Methotrexate (MTX)
An antifolate drug which depletes cellular tetrahydrofolate.

High dose MTX (1–12 g/m^2) is used in the treatment of CNS lymphoma and osteosarcomas.

It is exclusively eliminated via the kidneys.

Parent drug and metabolite are highly insoluble in acid and urine.

Toxicity is related to level and duration of elevated MTX levels.

  AKI can occur due to precipitation of drug within tubules and potentially a direct nephrotoxic effect.

  Normally it is self-limiting with recovery over 12 ± 7 days. Prevention of nephrotoxicity:
* adequte hydration;
* IV bicarbonate (alkalinize urine);
* leukovorin rescue (tetrahydrofolic acid derivative) commencing 24–36 h post MTX.

Ifosfamide
An alkylating drug similar to cyclophosphamide.

Indications include sarcomas and hematological cancers.

Side-effects: nephrotoxicity, neurotoxicity and myelosuppression.

Ifosfamide and cyclophosphamide can also cause hemorrhagic cisitis.

Ifosfamide can cause tubular injury presenting with Fanconi's anemia:
* hyperchloremic metabolic acidosis;
* hypophosphatemia;
* hypokalemia;
* renal glycosuria;
* aminoaciduria.

Agents causing hemolytic uremic syndrome
Mitomycin C (MMC)
An alkylating antibiotic used in the treatment of breast, gastrointestinal, pancreatic and lung cancers.

MMC nephrotoxicity normally presents with HUS 6–20 months after initiation of chemotherapy.

There is a classical triad of:
* microangiopathic hemolytic anemia;
* thrombocytopenia;
* AKI.

It is dose dependent, usually occurring after a cumulative dose >60 mg/m^2.

Mortality ~50%.

Gemcitabine
A nucleoside analogue which interferes with DNA synthesis.

It is used in breast, bladder, lung, gastrointestinal, gynecological and germ cell tumors.

Mild proteinuria and microscopic hematuria occur in up to 50% of patients and elevated creatinine in 8%.

It rarely develops into profound HUS with no clear relationship between dose or time interval post therapy.

Agents causing urinary tract obstruction
Ifosfomide and cyclophosphamide

Both drugs can cause obstruction secondary to hemorrhagic cystitis.

This complication is caused by metabolites including acrolein excreted in the urine.

Prevention:
* vigorous hydration and frequent bladder emptying;
* IV Mesna® (binds acrolein to produce nontoxic compound).

Biological and targeted therapies
There has been a marked increase in the use of biological therapies in cancer management over recent years.

The side-effect profiles of most of these therapies are favorable compared to conventional cytotoxic chemotherapy.

Monoclonal antibodies
Humanized monoclonal antibodies are directed against a variety of proteins including:
* growth factor receptors;
* angiogenesis-promoting factors;
* tumor cell surface antigens.

Nephrotoxicity is rare and not usually of clinical significance with these agents.

Bevacizumab
A monoclonal antibody to vascular endothelial growth factor (VEGF).

Hypertension, proteinuria and rarely nephritic syndrome have been reported.

Renal biopsy demonstrates an immune-complex-mediated glomerulonephritis.

Tyrosine kinase inhibitors
Tyrosine kinase inhibitors are metabolized in the liver with excretion predominantly in the feces.

Dose reduction not usually required but multiple new agents are in development and each must be assessed individually.

Immune response modifiers
Interferon
An antiviral and antineoplastic agent which modifies the host response to cancer (e.g. renal cell carcinoma and melanoma).

It has a spectrum of renal toxicity from mild elevation of creatinine and proteinuria to nephrotic syndrome and AKI (rare).

Other drugs

Bisphosphonates

These are potent inhibitors of osteoclast-mediated bone resorption.

They are used in the treatment and prevention of bone metastasis in breast and prostate cancer and also in the treatment of hypercalcemia of malignancy.

Dose-dependent renal tubular injury occasionally develops after several months of treatment and is recognized by an asymptomatic elevation in serum creatinine.

NSAIDs

These analgesics are used widely in cancer pain management.

Adverse renal effects include AKI, nephrotic syndrome, hyperkalemia and papillary necrosis.

Further reading

Cohen EP. *Cancer and the kidney*. Oxford: Oxford University Press; 2005.

COIN Guidelines. Renal function and chemotherapy. *Clin Oncol* 2001; **13**: S222.

Fischer DS, et al. *The cancer chemotherapy handbook*, 6th edn. St Louis: Mosby; 2003.

Kintzel PE. Anticancer drug-induced kidney disorders. *Drug Safety* 2001; **24**: 19–38.

Souhami RL, Tannock I, Hohenberger P, Horiot J-C. *Oxford textbook of oncology*. Oxford: Oxford University Press; 2002.

Internet resources

Clinical Oncology Information Network (COIN):

`http://www.rcr.ac.uk/index.asp?pageid=148`

Cancerbackup:

`http://www.cancerbackup.org.uk/home`

Epocrates® ONLINE provides continually updated information on brand and generic drugs (dosing, drug–drug interactions, adverse reactions and mode of action:

`http://www.epocrates.com`

See also

Drug-induced nephropathies, p. 698

Cancer and the kidney, p. 196

Clinical approach to acute kidney injury, p. 318

Appendix

Anatomy of the kidney and nephron

Gross anatomy of the kidney

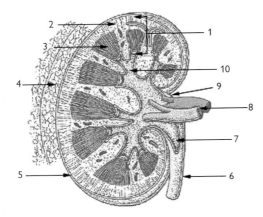

1	Parenchyma	6	Ureter
2	Cortex	7	Pelvis of the kidney
3	Medulla	8	Renal vessels
4	Perirenal fat	9	Hilum
5	Capsule	10	Calyx

Anatomical divisions of the nephron

The drawing (not to scale) depicts a short-looped (superficial) and a long-looped (juxtamedullary) nephron. Within the cortex, a dashed line delineates a medullary ray.

1   Renal corpuscle, including glomerulus and Bowman's capsule
2   Proximal convoluted tubule
3   Proximal straight tubule (pars recta)
4   Thin descending limb
5   Thin ascending limb
6   Thick ascending limb
7   Macula densa
8   Distal convoluted tubule
9   Connecting tubule
9* Connecting tubule of juxtamedullary nephron that forms an arcade
10 Cortical collecting tubule
11 Outer medullary collecting duct
12 Inner medullary collecting duct

Reproduced with permission from Davison AMA, Cameron JS, Grunfeld J-P et al. (eds) (2005) *Oxford Textbook of Nephrology*, 3rd edn. Oxford: Oxford University Press.

Microanatomy of the glomerulus

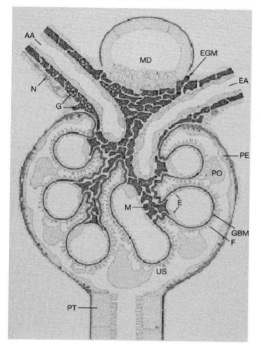

Electron micrograph of a glomerular lobule

The capillary (C) is outlined by a flat fenestrated endothelium (E).

The podocyte layer (PO) and the glomerular basement membrane (GBM) do not encircle the capillary completely, they form a common surface cover around the entire lobule.

In the peripheral portion of the capillary the filtration barrier is formed (see below).

Two subdomains of the GBM are delineated from each other by mesangial angles (arrows): the pericapillary GBM (cGBM) faced by the podocyte and endothelial layer, and the perimesangial GBM (mGBM) bordered by the podocyte layer and the mesangium.

Within the mesangium two types of mesangial cells are shown: contractile mesangial cells proper (M) and a cell (*) that is probably a macrophage that has invaded the mesangium.

US, urinary space.

The renal corpuscle and juxtaglomerular apparatus

The capillary tuft consists of a network of specialized capillaries, which are outlined by a fenestrated endothelium (E). At the vascular pole an afferent arteriole (AA) enters and an efferent arteriole (EA) leaves the tuft. The capillary network is surrounded by Bowman's capsule, comprising two different epithelia: the visceral and the parietal epithelium. The visceral epithelium consists of highly branched podocytes (PO) and directly follows, together with the glomerular basement membrane (GBM), the surface of the capillaries and the mesangium (M). At the vascular pole, the visceral epithelium and the GBM are reflected into the parietal epithelium (PE) of Bowman's capsule (and its basement membrane), which passes over into the epithelium of the proximal tubule (PT) at the urinary pole. Mesangial cells (M) are situated in the axes of glomerular lobules. At the vascular pole the glomerular mesangium is continuous with the extraglomerular mesangium (EGM), consisting of cells and matrix.

The EGM, together with the terminal portion of the afferent arteriole containing the granular cells (G), the efferent arteriole, and the macula densa (MD), establish the juxtaglomerular apparatus.

F, foot processes; N, sympathetic nerve terminals; US, urinary space.

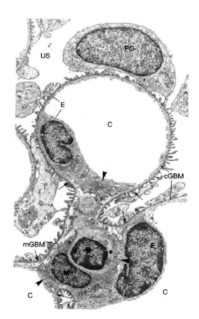

Electron micrograph of the filtration barrier

The peripheral part of the glomerular capillary wall comprises the fenestrated endothelial layer (E), the GBM, and the interdigitating foot processes (F). The filtration slits between the foot processes are bridged by thin diaphragms (long arrows). Arrowheads point to the endothelial pores. The GBM shows a lamina densa (2) bounded by the lamina rara interna (1) and the lamina rara externa (3). C, capillary lumen.

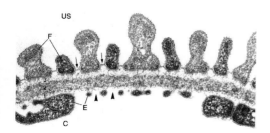

Calculations for acid–base balance and extracellular fluid volume

Renal and respiratory compensation for primary acid–base disturbances

Disorder	Primary change	Compensatory response
Metabolic acidosis	$\downarrow [HCO_3^-]$	0.16 kPa (1.2 mmHg) decrease in PCO_2 per 1 mmol/L decrease in $[HCO_3^-]$
Metabolic alkalosis	$\uparrow [HCO_3^-]$	0.093 kPa (0.7 mmHg) increase in PCO_2 per 1 mmol/L increase in $[HCO_3^-]$
Respiratory acidosis	$\uparrow PCO_2$	
Acute		1 mmol/L increase in $[HCO_3^-]$ per 1.33 kPa (10 mmHg) increase in PCO_2
Chronic		3.5 mmol/L increase in $[HCO_3^-]$ per 1.33 kPa (10 mmHg) increase in PCO_2
Respiratory alkalosis	$\downarrow PCO_2$	
Acute		2 mmol/L decrease in $[HCO_3^-]$ per 1.33 kPa (10 mmHg) decrease in PCO_2
Chronic		4 mmol/L decrease in $[HCO_3^-]$ per 1.33 kPa (10 mmHg) decrease in PCO_2

Metabolic acidosis
Serum anion gap (AG)

$[Na^+] - [HCO_3^-] - [Cl^-]$ (normal range 12 ± 2)

or

$[Na^+] + [K^+] - [HCO_3^-] - [Cl^-]$ (normal range 16 ± 2)

Normal AG metabolic acidosis	Increased AG metabolic acidosis

• Renal tubular acidosis (types 1, 2, and 4)
• Diarrhea and other intestinal losses (e.g. biliary or pancreatic drainage)
• Carbonic anhydrase inhibitors
• Ureteral diversion (e.g. ileal conduit)
• Toluene ingestion
	• Lactic acidosis
	• Ketoacidosis
	  • diabetic
	  • alcohol-associated
	  • starvation
	• Ingestions
	  • methanol
	  • ethylene glycol
	  • aspirin
	• Renal failure

Serum osmolal gap (OG)

Measured − calculated osmolality ($2[Na^+]$ + [glucose] + [urea]). Normal OG <10 mosm/L.

In the presence of metabolic acidosis, an OG >10 mosm/L suggests the presence of methanol or ethylene glycol.

Urine anion gap (to differentiate causes of normal gap metabolic acidosis)
Urine $[Na^+] + [K^+] - [Cl^-]$
• Positive value = lack of ammonium in urine = Type 1 RTA, Type 4 RTA
• Negative value = presence of ammonium in urine = All other causes

Calculations for the evaluation of disorders of water balance
To calculate the sodium requirement (in mmol) for a patient with hyponatremia

TBW × (desired serum $[Na^+]$ − actual serum $[Na^+]$)

To calculate the water excess (in liters) in a patient with hyponatremia

$$TBW \times \left(\frac{1 - \text{actual serm } [Na^+]}{\text{desired serum } [Na^+]} \right)$$

To calculate the change in serum $[Na^+]$ after 1 liter of IV fluid is infused

$$\left(\frac{[Na^+] \text{ concentration in IV fluid} - \text{actual serum } [Na^+]}{TBW + 1} \right)$$

To calculate the water deficit (in liters) in a patient with hypernatremia

$$\text{TBW} \times \left\{ \left(\frac{\text{actual serum [Na}^+]}{\text{desired serum [Na}^+]} \right) - 1 \right\}$$

Total body water (in liters) is estimated as body weight multiplied by 0.6 in men and by 0.5 in women.

Calculations of the glomerular filtration rate

Creatinine clearance

$$CrCl = \frac{(U_{creat} \times V)}{(P_{creat} \times f)}$$

Creatinine clearance in mL/min.

Where
- U_{creat} is the urinary creatinine concentration (mmol/L)
- V is the volume of collected urine (mL)
- P_{creat} is the plasma creatinine concentration (μmol/L)
- t is the collection time (min)

Estimates of GFR (eGFR)

The Cockcroft–Gault formula

$$eGFR = \frac{(140 - age) \times \text{lean body weight}}{(P_{creat}/88.4) \times 72}$$

eGFR in mL/min

where
- Lean body weight is in kg
- P_{crea} is the plasma creatinine concentration (μmol/L)

The MDRD (Modification of Diet in Renal Disease) Study formulae

Four-variable (most widely used)

eGFR = $186 \times (P_{creat}/88.4)^{-1.154} \times (age)^{-0.203} \times (0.742$ if female$) \times (1.21$ if Black$)$

eGFR in mL/min/1.73 m^2

where
- P_{creat} is the plasma creatinine concentration (μmol/L)
- Age is in years

Six-variable (original formula)

eGFR = $170 \times (P_{creat}/88.4)^{-0.999} \times (age)^{-0.176} \times (P_{urea}/0.166)^{-0.170} \times (P_{alb})^{+0.318} \times (0.762$ if female$) \times (1.18$ if Black$)$

eGFR in mL/min/1.73 m^2

where
- P_{creat} is the plasma creatinine concentration (μmol/L)
- P_{urea} is the plasma urea concentration (mmol/L)
- P_{alb} is the plasma albumin concentration (g/dL)
- Age is in years.

Relationship of glomerular filtration rate with age

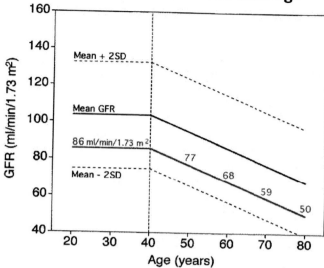

GFR is constant up to the age of 40 years and then declines at the rate of 9 mL/min/1.73 m^2 per decade.
- Mean GFR (solid black line).
- Outer dashed lines show the +2 population standard deviation limits.
- The grey line shows the safety limit for living donation of 86 mL/min/1.73 m^2 for young adults declining to 50 mL/min/1.73 m^2 at age 80 years.

The reference plot is based on an analysis of data for 428 live renal transplant donors who had [^{51}Cr]ETDA GFR measurements performed according to the method described in the British Nuclear Medicine Society GFR guidelines.

Reproduced with permission from: United Kingdom Guidelines for Living Donor Kidney Transplantation (http://www.bts.org.uk).

Calculations of dialysis adequacy

Hemodialysis

Formulae for quantifying urea removal on hemodialysis and hemodiafiltration.

Urea reduction ratio

The urea reduction rate (URR) is measured as follows:

$$URR = (1 - R) \times 100\%$$

where
- R is the ratio of $Urea_{post}/Urea_{pre}$
- $Urea_{post}$ is postdialysis blood urea concentration
- $Urea_{pre}$ is the predialysis blood urea concentration.

Single pool Kt/V

spKt/V urea may be estimated by the second generation equation described and validated by Daugirdas:

$$spKt/V \text{ urea} = -Ln(R - 0.008 \times t) + (4 - 3.5 \times R) \times UF/W$$

where
- Ln is the natural logarithm
- R is the ratio of $Urea_{post}/Urea_{pre}$
- t is the dialysis session length in hours
- UF is the ultrafiltration volume in liters
- W is the postdialysis weight in kilograms.

Direct measurement of equilibrated Kt/V urea (eKt/V)

The single pool model equation does not allow for tissue rebound of blood urea and can be used with a 30 min post-dialysis blood urea concentration to calculate equilibrated Kt/V urea (eKt/V):

$$eKt/V = -Ln(R30 \text{ min} - 0.008 \times t) + (4 - 3.5 \times R30 \text{ min}) \times UF/W$$

where
- Ln is the natural logarithm
- R30 min is the ratio of 30 min $Urea_{post}/Urea_{pre}$
- t is the dialysis session length in hours
- UF is the ultrafiltration volume in liters
- W is the postdialysis weight in kilograms.

Estimation of equilibrated Kt/V (eKt/V)

Most HD patients do not wish to wait 30 min after the end of HD to have a blood sample taken and so formulae have been developed to predict the 30 min blood urea concentration.

Formulae for estimating eKt/V have been derived for the stop dialyzate flow and slow flow methods of postdialysis blood sampling.

Both methods were derived and validated in HD patients by direct comparison with the gold standard of using a measured 30 min postdialysis blood urea concentration to calculate eKt/V.

For the stop dialyzate flow method of blood sampling

$$eKt/V = -Ln(R30 \text{ min} - 0.008 \times t) + (4 - 3.5 \times R30 \text{ min}) \times UF/W$$

where
- R30 min is estimated from the 5 min postdialysis blood urea concentration obtained by the stop dialyzate flow method
- R30 min is the ratio of estimated 30 min (e30 min) $Urea_{post}/Urea_{pre}$
- e30 min $Urea_{post} = 1.06 \times (5 \text{ min } Urea_{post}) + 0.22$.

For the slow flow method of blood sampling

$$eKt/V = Kt/V - (0.6(Kt/V)/t) + 0.03$$

where
- Kt/V is as in formula for spKt/V
- t is time on dialysis in hours.

Urea kinetic modeling (Formal UKM)

This requires multiple data inputs to a computer to calculate Kt/V by iteration, which makes this method less practical in busy renal units.

It requires the following data:
- measurement of pre- and postdialysis blood urea concentrations;
- record of blood and dialyzate flow rates and the dialyser used;
- measurement of weight loss during dialysis;
- measurement of urea removal in the interdialytic urine collection;
- measurement of predialysis blood urea concentration from the subsequent dialysis session.

Further reading

Daugirdas JT, Schneditz D. Overestimation of hemodialysis dose depends on dialysis efficiency by regional blood flow but not by conventional two pool kinetic analysis. *ASAIO J* 1995; **41**: M719–M724.

Daugirdas JT. Second generation logarithmic estimates of single-pool variable volume Kt/V; an analysis of error. *J Am Soc Nephrol* 199; **4**: 1205–1213.

Geddes CC, Traynor J P, Walbaum D, et al. A new method of post-dialysis blood urea sampling: the "stop dialysate flow" method. *Nephrol Dial Transplant* 2000; **15**: 517–523.

Gotch FA, Sargent JA. A mechanistic analysis of the National Cooperative Dialysis Study (NCDS). *Kidney Int* 1985; **28**: 526–534.

Owen WF, Lew NL, Lowrie EG, et al. The urea reduction ratio and serum albumin concentration as predictors of mortality in patients undergoing haemodialysis. *N Eng J Med* 1993; **329**: 1001–1006.

Priester-Coary A, Daugirdas JT. A recommended technique for obtaining the post dialysis BUN. *Semin Dial* 1997; **10**: 23–25.

Traynor JP, Geddes CC, Ferguson C, Mactier RA. Predicting 30-minute post-dialysis blood urea concentration using the stop dialysate flow method. *Am J Kidney Dis* 2002; **39**: 308–314.

Online adequacy calculators

http://www.kt-v.net/

http://www.hdcn.com/calcf/dzer.htm

Peritoneal dialysis

Weekly dialysis creatinine clearance

$$CrCl = \frac{(D_{creat} \times D \text{ vol})}{P_{creat}} \times (1.73/BSA) \times 7$$

Creatinine clearance in L/1.73 m²/week

where
- D_{creat} is the dialyzate creatinine concentration (corrected for glucose)
- P_{creat} is the plasma creatinine concentration
- BSA is body surface area
- D vol is the dialyzate volume in liters.

Weekly residual renal creatinine clearance

$$CrCl = \frac{\left[\frac{(U_{urea} \times Uv)}{P_{urea}} + \frac{(U_{creat} \times Uv)}{P_{creat}}\right]}{} \times (1.73/BSA) \times (7/2)$$

Creatinine clearance in L/1.73 m²/week

where

- U_{urea} is the urine urea concentration
- Uv is the urine volume
- P_{urea} is the plasma urea concentration
- U_{creat} is the urine creatinine concentration
- P_{creat} is the plasma creatinine concentration.

Total weekly creatinine clearance

Weekly dialysis + Weekly residual renal
    CrCl   CrCl

Creatinine clearance in L/1.73 m²/week.

Weekly dialysis Kt/V_urea

$Kt/V = (D_{urea} \times \text{Dialyzate volume}/P_{urea}) \times (7/V)$

where

- D_{urea} is dialyzate urea concentration
- P_{urea} is the plasma urea concentration
- V is the patient's total body water (see below).

Weekly residual renal Kt/V_urea

$Kt/V = (U_{urea} \times \text{Urine volume}/P_{urea}) \times (7/V)$

where

- U_{urea} is the urine urea concentration
- P_{urea} is the plasma urea concentration
- V is the patient's total body water (see below).

Total weekly Kt/V_urea

Weekly dialysis + Weekly residual renal
   Kt/V_urea   Kt/V_urea

Body surface area

Dubois method:

$BSA = 0.007184 \times (\text{height} \times 0.725) \times (\text{weight} \times 0.425)$

where

- weight is in kg
- height is in cm.

Total body water

V as estimated by the Watson equation:

Males

$V = 2.447 - (0.09516 \times \text{age}) + (0.1074 \times \text{height}) + (0.3362 \times \text{weight})$

Females

$V = 2.097 + (0.1069 \times \text{height}) + (0.2466 \times \text{weight})$

where

- weight is in kg
- height is in cm
- age is in years.

Normalized protein equivalent of total nitrogen appearance

nPNA as estimated by the Randerson equation:

$nPNA = [10.76 \, (UNA/1.44 + 1.46)]/\text{body weight}$

where

- UNA is the urea appearance in dialyzate and urine in g/day.

Alternatively the nPNA can be calculated using:

$nPNA = 5.02 \times [(UGR \times 60.06) + 3.12]/\text{body weight}$

where

- UGR is the urea generation rate in mmol/min.

Further reading

Lysaght MJ, Farrell PC. Membrane phenomena and mass transfer kinetics in peritoneal dialysis. *J Membr Sci* 1989; **44**: 5–33.

Lysaght MJ, Pollock CA, Hallet MD, Ibels LS, Farrell PC. The relevance of urea kinetic modeling to CAPD. *ASAIO Trans* 1989; **35**: 784–790.

Online adequacy calculators

http://www.kt-v.net/

http://www.hdcn.com/calcf/dzer.htm

Classification of chronic kidney disease

Classification of CKD based on the NKF K/DOQI recommendations

CKD stage	Description	GFR (mL/min/1.73 m^2)
1	Kidney damage with a normal or increased GFR There must be other evidence of kidney damage: • persistent microalbuminuria • persistent proteinuria • persistent hematuria • structural abnormalities of the kidneys demonstrated • on USS or other radiological tests • biopsy-proven chronic glomerulonephritis	>90
2	Kidney damage with mild reduction in GFR There must be other evidence of kidney damage (as above)	60–89
3	Moderate reduction in GFR	30–59
4	Severe reduction in GFR	15–29
5	Kidney failure	<15 (or dialysis)

This classification is based on the NKF K/DOQI recommendations.
http://www.kidney.org/professionals/kdoqi/index.cfm

Proposed changes according to the draft NICE National Clinical Guideline for the Management of Adults with Chronic Kidney Disease

It has been proposed that the suffix P should be used to denote the presence of proteinuria when staging CKD:

For this purpose proteinuria is defined as:
• urinary albumin to creatinine ratio ≥30 mg/mmol
• urinary protein excretion ≥0.5 g/24 h

Stage 3 should be split into two subcategories defined by:
• GFR 45–59 mL/min/1.73 m^2 CKD stage 3A
• GFR 30–44 mL/min/1.73 m^2 CKD stage 3B

http://www.nice.org/guidance/index.jsp?action=download&o=39959

Internet resources

Journals

Advances in Chronic Kidney Disease
An official Journal of the National Kidney Federation:
http://journals.elsevierhealth.com/periodicals/xackd

American Journal of Kidney Diseases
Journal of the National Kidney Federation:
http://www.ajkd.org/

American Journal of Nephrology
http://content.karger.com/ProdukteDB/produkte.asp?Aktion=JournalHome&ProduktNr=223979

American Journal of Physiology – Renal Physiology
Journal of the American Physiological Society:
http://ajprenal.physiology.org/

American Journal of Transplantation
Journal of the American Society of Transplant Surgeons and the American Society of Transplantation:
http://www.blackwellpublishing.com/journal.asp?ref=1600-6135

British Journal of Renal Medicine
http://www.bjrm.co.uk/bjrm/

Clinical and Experimental Nephrology
Journal of the Japanese Society of Nephrology:
http://www.springerlink.com/content/103835/

Clinical Journal of the American Society of Nephrology
An official Journal of the American Society of Nephrology:
http://cjasn.asnjournals.org/

Clinical Nephrology
http://www.clinnephrol.com

Clinical Transplantation
http://www.blackwellpublishing.com/journal.asp?ref=0902-0063

Current Opinion in Nephrology and Hypertension
http://www.co-nephrologyandhypertension.com

Experimental and Clinical Transplantation
http://www.ectrx.org/

Hypertension, Dialysis and Clinical Nephrology
An official educational program of the Renal Physicians Association and American Society of Nephrology:
http://www.hdcn.com/

Journal of Nephrology
Journal of the Italian Society of Nephrology:
http://www.jnephrol.com/index.asp?a= current

Journal of the American Society of Nephrology
http://jasn.asnjournals.org/

Kidney and Blood Pressure Research
http://content.karger.com/ProdukteDB/produkte.asp?Aktion=JournalHome&ProduktNr=224258

Kidney International
Journal of the International Society of Nephrology:
http://www.nature.com/ki/index.html

Nature Clinical Practice Nephrology
http://www.nature.com/ncpneph/index.html

Nephrology
Journal of the Asian Pacific Society of Nephrology:
http://www.blackwellpublishing.com/journal.asp?ref=1320-5358&site=1

Nephrology Dialysis and Transplantation
Journal of the European Renal Association – European Dialysis and Transplant Association:
http://ndt.oxfordjournals.org/

Nephron Journals
Incorporating:
- *Nephron Clinical Practice*
- *Nephron Experimental Nephrology*
- *Nephron Physiology*

http://content.karger.com/ProdukteDB/produkte.asp?Aktion=JournalHome&ProduktNr=223854

Pediatric Nephrology
Journal of the International Pediatric Nephrology Association:
http://link.springer-ny.com/link/service/journals/00467/ index.htm

Pediatric Transplantation
Journal of the International Pediatric Transplant Association:
http://www.blackwellpublishing.com/journal.asp?ref=1397-3142&site=1

Peritoneal Dialysis International
Journal of the International Society for Peritoneal Dialysis:
http://www.pdiconnect.com/

Renal Failure
http://www.informaworld.com/smpp/title~db=all~content=t713597293~tab=issueslist

Seminars in Nephrology
http://www.seminarsinnephrology.org/

Seminars in Dialysis
http://www.blackwellpublishing.com/journal.asp?ref=0894-0959&site=1

Journal of Renovascular Disease
http://www.journalrenovasculardisease.com

Transplantation
Journal of the Transplantation Society:
http://www.transplantjournal.com/

Professional societies

American Society for Artificial Organs
http://www.asaio.com/

American Society of Diagnostic and Interventional Nephrology
http://www.asdin.org/

American Society of Nephrology
http://www.asn-online.org/

American Society of Pediatric Nephrology
http://www.aspneph.com/

American Society of Transplantation
http://www.a-s-t.org/

Asian Pacific Society of Nephrology
http://www.apsneph.org/

Association of Renal Technologists (UK)
http://www.artery.org.uk/site/ART/home

Australia and New Zealand Society of Nephrlology
http://www.nephrology.edu.au/

British Association for Paediatric Nephrology
http://www.bapn.org/

British Renal Society
http://www.britishrenal.org/

British Society for Histocompatibility and Immunogenetics
http://www.bshi.org.uk/

British Transplantation Society
http://www.bts.org.uk/

Canadian Society of Nephrology
http://www.csnscn.ca/

Commission for the Global Advancement of Nephrology
http://www.nature.com/isn/society/outreach/index.html

European Renal Association – European Dialysis and Transplant Association
http://www.era-edta.org/

European Kidney Health Alliance
http://www.ekha.eu/

European Society for Organ Transplantation
http://www.esot.org/

International Pediatric Transplant Association
http://www.iptaonline.org/

International Society for Hemodialysis
http://www.ishd.net/

International Society of Blood Purification
http://www.isbp.org

International Society of Nephrology
http://www.nature.com/isn/index.html

International Society of Peritoneal Dialysis
http://www.ispd.org/

International Society of Renal Nutrition and Metabolism
http://www.renalnutrition.com/

National Kidney Foundation (US)
http://www.kidney.org/

Renal Association, UK
http://www.renal.org/pages/

Renal Pathology Society
http://www.renalpathsoc.org/

Renal Physicians Association (US)
http://www.renalmd.org/

The Transplantation Society
http://www.transplantation-soc.org/

UK Transplant
http://www.uktransplant.org.uk/

Vascular Access Society (UK)
http://www.vascularaccesssociety.com/

Clinical practice guidelines and renal registries

ANZDATA Australia and New Zealand Dialysis and Transplant Registry
http://www.anzdata.org.au/ANZOD

Australian and New Zealand Organ Donation Registry
http://www.anzdata.org.au/anzod/anzodwelcome.htm

British Transplantation Society Guidelines
http://www.bts.org.uk/standards.htm

CARI Guidelines (Australian)
http://www.cari.org.au/

Canadian Registry
http://secure.cihi.ca/cihiweb/splash.html

Canadian Society of Nephrology Guidelines
http://www.csnscn.ca/english/professional%20practice/programmes/default.asp?s=1

Collaborative Transplant Study
http://www.ctstransplant.org/

Dialysis Outcomes and Practice Patterns Study D.O.P.P.S Study
http://www.dopps.org/

European Renal Registry
http://www.era-edta-reg.org/index.jsp

Eurotransplant
http://www.transplant.org/

Guidelines of the European Best Practice Group of the ERA–EDTA
http://www.ndt-educational.org/

International Federation of Renal Registries
http://www.ifrr.net/

Israel Penn Transplant Tumor Registry:
http://www.ipittr.uc.edu/Home.cfm

K/DOQI Guidelines (USA) Kidney Disease Outcomes Quality Initiative
http://www.kidney.org/professionals/kdoqi/index.cfm

Kidney Disease: Improving Global Outcomes (KDIGO)
http://www.kdigo.org/

Renal Association (UK) Clinical Practice Guidelines
http://www.renal.org/pages/pages/clinical-affairs/guidelines.php

Scottish Renal Registry
http://www.srr.scot.nhs.uk/

UK Renal Registry
http://www.renalreg.com/

United States Renal Data System
http://www.usrds.org/

United States Transplant Registry
http://www.ustransplant.org

Information resources for professionals

Atlas of Diseases of the Kidney
http://www.kidneyatlas.org/

Calculation tools for nephrologists
Dialysis adequacy tools
http://www.kt-v.net/
http://www.hdcn.com/calcf/dzer.htm

eGFR calculator
http://www.renal.org/eGFRcalc/GFR.pl

Renal SI Conversion Centre
http://nephron.com/cgi-bin/SI.cgi

Cochrane Renal Group
http://www.cochrane-renal.org/

CyberNephrology
http://www.kidney.org/professionals/cyber/index.cfm#

East Midlands Renal Network
http://www.eastmidlandsrenalnetwork.org.uk/

EdREN, the website of the Renal Unit at the Royal Infirmary of Edinburgh
www.edren.org

European Uraemic Toxin (EUTox) work group of the European Society of Artificial Organs
http://www.uremic-toxins.org/

Great Ormond Street Hospital
http://www.gosh.nhs.uk/clinical_information/

Kidney Disease Quality of Life Working Group
http://www.gim.med.ucla.edu/kdqol/

Kidney Health Australia
http://www.kidney.org.au/

Kidney & Urologic Disease Dictionary Index
http://kidney.niddk.nih.gov/kudiseases/a-z.asp

Kidney School
http://www.kidneyschool.org/

Family Practice Notebook
http://www.fpnotebook.com/REN.htm

Medmark
http://www.medmark.org/neph/nep2.html

National Institute for Health and Clinical Excellence
http://www.nice.org.uk

National Institute of Diabetes & Digestive & Kidney Diseases (US)
http://www.niddk.nih.gov/index.htm

NDT Educational
http://www.ndt-educational.org/Nephrology

Nephrology Rounds
http://www.nephrologyrounds.org

Nephron Information Center
http://nephron.com/

NephrOnline
http://www.nephronline.org/

PREVEND Study (Prevention of Renal and Vascular End-Stage Disease)
http://www.prevend.org/

RenalNet
http://www.renalnet.org/

Renal Resource Centre
http://www.renalresource.com/

RenalWEB
http://www.renalweb.com/

UKidney–Internet School of Nephrology
http://ukidney.com/

Information resources for patients and carers

Associations

American Association of Kidney Patients
http://www.aakp.org/

British Organ Donor Society
http://body.orpheusweb.co.uk/index.html

Diabetes UK
http://www.diabetes.org.uk/

European Kidney Health Alliance
http://www.ekha.eu/

European Kidney Patients Federation
http://www.ceapir.org/HP/

European Transplant and Dialysis Sport Federation
http://www.etdsf.org/

International Federation of Kidney Foundations
http://www.ifkf.net/

National Kidney Federation (US)
http://www.kidney.org/patients/

Scottish Kidney Federation
http://scotskidneyfederation.org/

The British Kidney Patients Association
http://www.britishkidney-pa.co.uk/

The Kidney Alliance
http://www.kidneyalliance.org.uk/

UK National Kidney Federation
http://www.kidney.org.uk/

World Transplant Games Federation
http://www.wtgf.org/

Understanding kidney disease

How Your Kidneys Work
http://www.howstuffworks.com/kidney.htm

Kidney directions
http://www.kidneydirections.com

Kidney disease community
http://www.ikidney.com/

Kidney diseases in childhood
http://www.kidshealth.com/parent/medical/kidney/kidney_diseases_childhood.html

Nephcure
http://www.nephcure.org

RenalInfo
http://www.kidneydirections.com/

The Kidney Patient Guide
http://www.kidneypatientguide.org.uk/

The Kidney School
http://www.kidneyschool.org/

National Kidney Disease Education Program
http://www.nkdep.nih.gov/

Transplantation

Living Kidney Donors' Experiences
http://www.transweb.org/people/live_don.htm

Transplants in Mind
http://www.transplantsinmind.org.uk/

TransWeb
http://www.transweb.org/

The Transplant Support Network
http://www.transplantsupportnetwork.org.uk/

Travel and dialysis

Bulgarian holiday dialysis units
http://www.dialysisbulgaria.com/

Cyprus holiday dialysis unit
http://www.cyprodial.com.cy/

Dialysis at sea
http://www.dialysisatsea.com/

Eurodial
http://www.eurodial.org/index.html

Fresenius holiday dialysis
http://www.hditravel.com/hdi/index.html

Global holiday dialysis facilities
http://www.globaldialysis.com/

NKF (UK) holiday Pages
http://www.kidney.org.uk/holidays/index.html

Renal recipes

List of cookbooks for renal patients
http://www.kidney.org/professionals/CRN/cookbooks.cfm

Culinary Kidney Cooks
http://www.culinarykidneycooks.com

DaVita (US)
http://www.davita.com/recipes/

Patient counseling tools

Clinical presentations

Hematuria
http://www.emrn.org.uk/documents/Haematuria%20.pdf

http://www.bjrm.co.uk/ext/200831749395.pdf

http://renux.dmed.ed.ac.uk/EdREN/EdRenINFObits/HaematuriaLong.html

Proteinuria
http://renux.dmed.ed.ac.uk/EdREN/EdRenINFObits/ProteinuriaLong.html

Nephrotic syndrome
http://www.emrn.org.uk/documents/Nephrotic%20Syndrome.pdf

http://www.bjrm.co.uk/ext/200831749357.pdf

http://renux.dmed.ed.ac.uk/EdREN/EdRenINFObits/NephroticShort.html

High blood pressure
http://www.emrn.org.uk/documents/High%20Blood%20Pressure.pdf

http://www.bjrm.co.uk/ext/200831749651.pdf

http://renux.dmed.ed.ac.uk/EdREN/EdRenINFObits/BPshort.html

http://renux.dmed.ed.ac.uk/EdREN/EdRenINFObits/malighypert.html

Investigations

Blood and urine tests
http://www.bjrm.co.uk/ext/200831748650.pdf

http://renux.dmed.ed.ac.uk/EdREN/EdRenINFObits/kidneytests.html

Kidney biopsy
http://www.emrn.org.uk/documents/Kidney%20Biopsy.pdf

http://www.bjrm.co.uk/ext/200831749487.pdf

http://renux.dmed.ed.ac.uk/EdREN/EdRenINFObits/RenalBiopsyShort.html

http://www.kidney.org.uk/Medical-Info/kidney-disease/biopsy.html

Kidney transplant biopsy
http://www.kidney.org.uk/Medical-Info/kidney-disease/biopsy-transplant-kidney.html

Renal angiogram
http://www.emrn.org.uk/documents/Kidney%20Renal%20Angiogram.pdf

http://renux.dmed.ed.ac.uk/EdREN/EdRenINFObits/angioshort.html

Glomerular disease

Alport syndrome
http://renux.dmed.ed.ac.uk/EdREN/EdRenINFObits/AlportLong.html

Crescentic nephritis
http://renux.dmed.ed.ac.uk/EdREN/EdRenINFObits/CrescenticShort.html

Diabetic nephropathy
http://www.emrn.org.uk/documents/Diabetic%20Nephropathy.pdf

http://www.bjrm.co.uk/ext/200831749996.pdf

http://www.bjrm.co.uk/ext/200831750033.pdf

http://renux.dmed.ed.ac.uk/EdREN/EdRenINFObits/Diabetic_nephLong.html

Focal and segmental glomerulosclerosis
http://www.emrn.org.uk/documents/Glomerulosclerosis%20FSGS.pdf

http://renux.dmed.ed.ac.uk/EdREN/EdRenINFObits/FSGSLong2.html

Goodpasture's disease
http://renux.dmed.ed.ac.uk/EdREN/EdRenINFObits/GoodpastureShort.html

Hemolytic uremic syndrome
http://www.bjrm.co.uk/ext/200831749680.pdf

http://renux.dmed.ed.ac.uk/EdREN/EdRenINFObits/HUS.Long.html

IgA nephropathy
http://www.emrn.org.uk/documents/IgANephropathy.pdf

http://renux.dmed.ed.ac.uk/EdREN/EdRenINFObits/IgALong.html

Lupus and the kidney
http://renux.dmed.ed.ac.uk/EdREN/EdRenINFObits/LupusNonRen.html

http://renux.dmed.ed.ac.uk/EdREN/EdRenINFObits/LupusLong.html

Membranous nephropathy
http://www.bjrm.co.uk/ext/200831749420.pdf

http://renux.dmed.ed.ac.uk/EdREN/EdRenINFObits/Membranous.Long.html

Minimal change nephropathy
http://www.emrn.org.uk/documents/Minimal%20Change%20nephropathy.pdf

http://renux.dmed.ed.ac.uk/EdREN/EdRenINFObits/MinChangeShort.html

Scleroderma and the kidney
http://renux.dmed.ed.ac.uk/EdREN/EdRenINFObits/Scleroderma.html

Vasculitis
http://www.bjrm.co.uk/ext/200831748943.pdf

http://renux.dmed.ed.ac.uk/EdREN/EdRenINFObits/VasculitisLong.html

Other kidney diseases

Interstitial nephritis
http://www.bjrm.co.uk/ext/200831749588.pdf

http://renux.dmed.ed.ac.uk/EdREN/EdRenINFObits/Interstitial.html

Kidney stones
http://www.bjrm.co.uk/ext/200831749458.pdf

http://renux.dmed.ed.ac.uk/EdREN/EdRenINFObits/
KidStonesLong.html

Loin pain hematuria syndrome
http://renux.dmed.ed.ac.uk/EdREN/EdRenINFObits/
Loin_painLong.html

Polycystic kidney disease
http://www.bjrm.co.uk/ext/200831749214.pdf
http://renux.dmed.ed.ac.uk/EdREN/EdRenINFObits/
PCKDShort.html

Renal artery stenosis
http://www.emrn.org.uk/documents/Renal%20Arter
y%20Stenosis%20RAS.pdf
http://www.bjrm.co.uk/ext/200831749116.pdf
http://renux.dmed.ed.ac.uk/EdREN/EdRenINFObits/
RAS.html

Reflux nephropathy
http://www.bjrm.co.uk/ext/200831749155.pdf
http://renux.dmed.ed.ac.uk/EdREN/EdRenINFObits/
reflux.html

Renal tract obstruction
http://renux.dmed.ed.ac.uk/EdREN/EdRenINFObits/
Obstruction.html

Urinary tract infections
http://renux.dmed.ed.ac.uk/EdREN/EdRenINFObits/
urineinfs.html

Drugs in renal disease
Immunosuppressive drugs in renal disease
http://renux.dmed.ed.ac.uk/EdREN/EdRenINFObits/
ISdrugs.html

Over-the-counter medications
http://www.bjrm.co.uk/ext/200831749328.pdf

Chronic kidney disease, its complications and treatment
General
http://www.emrn.org.uk/documents/Patient%20
information%20Chronic%20Kidney%20Disease.pdf
http://www.emrn.org.uk/documents/RCP%20CKD%20
patient%20info%20Leaflet.pdf
http://www.emrn.org.uk/documents/Kidney%20Care
%20modernisation%20initiative.pdf
http://www.emrn.org.uk/documents/Kidney%20
Disease%20Leaflet%201006.pdf
http://www.bjrm.co.uk/ext/200831749901.pdf
http://renux.dmed.ed.ac.uk/EdREN/EdRenINFObits/
CRFLong.html

Intravenous iron
http://www.bjrm.co.uk/ext/200831749561.pdf

Kidney disease and pregnancy
http://www.emrn.org.uk/documents/Kidney%20Dise
ase%20&%20Pregnancy.pdf
http://www.bjrm.co.uk/ext/200831749183.pdf
http://renux.dmed.ed.ac.uk/EdREN/EdRenINFObits/
PregnancyLong.htmf

Renal anemia
http://www.emrn.org.uk/documents/Renal%20
Anaemia.pdf

Renal diets
http://www.bjrm.co.uk/ext/200831749262.pdf
http://renux.dmed.ed.ac.uk/EdREN/EdRenINFObits/
Diet_CRF.html

Sex and renal failure
http://www.bjrm.co.uk/ext/200831749088.pdf

Procedures
Dialysis line insertion
http://www.bjrm.co.uk/ext/200831749713.pdf
http://www.kidney.org.uk/Medical-Info/
haemodialysis/dialysis-line-insertion.html

Formation of a fistula
http://www.bjrm.co.uk/ext/200831749811.pdf
Inde

Peritoneal catheter insertion
http://www.kidney.org.uk/Medical-Info/pd/
pdcatheter.html

Dialysis
General
http://renux.dmed.ed.ac.uk/EdREN/
EdRenINFObits/Dialysis_ESRFLong.html

Hemodialysis
http://www.bjrm.co.uk/ext/200831749776.pdf
http://renux.dmed.ed.ac.uk/EdREN/EdRenINFObits/
HDShort.html

Home hemodialysis
http://www.bjrm.co.uk/ext/200831749739.pdf

Infections and hemodialysis
http://www.bjrm.co.uk/ext/200831749620.pdf

Peritoneal dialysis
http://www.bjrm.co.uk/ext/200831749963.pdf
http://renux.dmed.ed.ac.uk/EdREN/EdRenINFObits/
PDShort.htm

Transplantation
General
http://www.bjrm.co.uk/ext/200831749056.pdf
http://renux.dmed.ed.ac.uk/EdREN/EdRenINFObits/
TransplantShort.html
http://www.kidney.org.uk/Medical-Info/trans-
plant.html

Living kidney donation
http://www.bjrm.co.uk/ext/200831749838.pdf
http://www.bjrm.co.uk/ext/200831749870.pdf

Pancreas transplantation
http://www.bjrm.co.uk/ext/200831749292.pdf

Conservative management of kidney failure
http://www.bjrm.co.uk/ext/200831749932.pdf
http://renux.dmed.ed.ac.uk/EdREN/EdRenINFObits/
NoRRTshort.html

Pediatric nephrology
Acute kidney injury
http://www.ich.ucl.ac.uk/factsheets/families/
F060416/

Chronic kidney disease
http://www.kidney.org.uk/kids/crf/index.html

http://www.ich.ucl.ac.uk/factsheets/families/F060426/

Dialysis access
http://www.gosh.nhs.uk/factsheets/families/F060406/index.html

http://www.gosh.nhs.uk/factsheets/families/F000297/index.html

http://www.gosh.nhs.uk/factsheets/families/F060405/index.html

Hemodialysis in children
http://www.bjrm.co.uk/ext/200831748699.pdf

http://www.gosh.nhs.uk/factsheets/families/F040280/index.html

Hemolytic uremic syndrome
http://www.kidney.org.uk/kids/hus/

http://www.gosh.nhs.uk/factsheets/families/F060408/index.html

http://www.gosh.nhs.uk/factsheets/families/F060409/index.html

HSP and IgA nephropathy
http://www.gosh.nhs.uk/factsheets/families/F050244/index.html

http://www.gosh.nhs.uk/factsheets/families/F060415/index.html

Medications
http://www.kidney.org.uk/kids/medication/

Nephritis
http://www.kidney.org.uk/kids/nephritis/nephritis.html

Nephrotic syndrome
http://www.kidney.org.uk/kids/neph_syn/index.html

Multicystic dysplastic kidney
http://www.kidney.org.uk/kids/mcdk/

Renal tract problems detected antenatally
http://www.bjrm.co.uk/ext/200831749521.pdf

http://www.kidney.org.uk/kids/ultrasound/index.html

Renal transplants in children
http://www.bjrm.co.uk/ext/200831749024.pdf

http://www.kidney.org.uk/kids/transplant/

http://www.gosh.nhs.uk/factsheets/families/F070146/index.html

Urinary tract infections and reflux in children
http://www.bjrm.co.uk/ext/200831748977.pdf

http://www.kidney.org.uk/kids/uti/index.html

http://www.gosh.nhs.uk/factsheets/families/F050192/index.html

Investigations
General

http://www.kidney.org.uk/kids/crf_tests/page01.html

DMSA scan

http://www.kidney.org.uk/kids/dmsa_scan/page01.html

Ultrasound scan

http://www.kidney.org.uk/kids/us_scan/page01.html

http://www.gosh.nhs.uk/factsheets/families/F010093/index.html

Mag 3 scan

http://www.kidney.org.uk/kids/mag3_scan/page01.html

Micturating cystourethrogram

http://www.kidney.org.uk/kids/mict_cyst/mict_cyst.html

Renal biopsy

http://www.kidney.org.uk/kids/biopsy/

http://www.gosh.nhs.uk/factsheets/families/F990377/index.html

Vasculitis
http://www.ich.ucl.ac.uk/factsheets/families/F040127/

Other useful information sheets are also available at :

http://www.ich.ucl.ac.uk/gosh/clinicalservices/Nephrology/InformationforFamilies

Biochemistry conversion table

Parameter	SI to conventional unit conversion factor	
Bilirubin	µmol/l to mg/dl	÷ 17
Calcium	mmol/l to mg/dl	× 4
Carbon dioxide	kP to mmHg	× 7.5
Cholesterol	mmol/l to mg/dl	× 38.7
Creatinine	µmol/l to mg/dl	÷ 88
Glucose	mmol/l to mg/dl	× 18
Magnesium	mmol/l to mg/dl	× 2.4
Oxalate	µmol/l to mg/dl	÷ 11
Oxygen	kP to mmHg	× 7.5
Phosphate	mmol/l to mg/dl	× 3.1
Potassium	mmol/l to meq/l	× 1
Sodium	mmol/l to meq/l	× 1
Triglyceride	mmol/l to mg/dl	× 88.6
Urea / blood urea nitrogen	mmol/l to mg/dl	× 2.82
Uric acid	µmol/l to mg/dl	÷ 59.5

Index

Please note that page references to Figures or Tables are in *italic* print